Essentials of

Plastic Surgery

Q&A Companion

Essentials of
Plastic Surgery

Q&A Companion

Second Edition

ALEX P. JONES, FRCS (PLAST), MBCHB, BSc

Consultant Plastic Reconstructive and Aesthetic Surgeon
Department of Plastic and Reconstructive Surgery
James Cook University Hospital, Middlesbrough;
Nuffield Tees Hospital;
Norton and Tees Valley Hospital
Middlesbrough, UK

JEFFREY E. JANIS, MD, FACS

Professor
Department of Plastic and Reconstructive Surgery;
Chief of Plastic Surgery (University Hospital);
Adjunct Professor, Departments of Neurosurgery,
Neurology, and Surgery;
Co-Director, Center for Abdominal Core Health
The Ohio State University Wexner Medical Center;
Past President, American Society of Plastic Surgeons,
American Council of Academic Plastic Surgeons,
and Migraine Surgery Society;
President, American Hernia Society
Columbus, Ohio, USA

With the Assistance of Dr. Anna R. Barnard

With Illustrations by:

**Brenda L. Bunch, MA, MS; Amanda L. Tomasikiewicz, MA; Sarah J. Taylor, MS, BA;
Jennifer N. Gentry, MA, CMI; and Graeme Chambers, BA (Hons.)**

395 illustrations

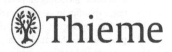

New York • Stuttgart • Delhi • Rio de Janeiro

Library of Congress Cataloging-in-Publication Data is available from the publisher.

Illustrators: Brenda L. Bunch, MA, MS; Amanda L. Tomasikiewicz, MA; Sarah J. Taylor, MS, BA; Jennifer N. Gentry, MA, CMI; and Graeme Chambers, BA (Hons.)

Thieme Medical Publishers, Inc.
333 Seventh Avenue, 18th Floor,
New York, NY 10001, USA
www.thieme.com
+1 800 782 3488, customerservice@thieme.com

Cover design: © Thieme
Cover image source: Picasso, Pablo (1881-1973)
© Artist Rights Society (ARS), NY. Girl Before a
Mirror. Boisgeloup, March 1932. Oil on canvas,
64″ × 51.″ Gift of Mrs. Simon Guggenheim. (2.1938).
The Museum of Modern Art, New York, NY, USA.
Digital Image © The Museum of Modern Art/
Licensed by SCALA/Art Resource, NY. © 2006 Estate
of Pablo Picasso/ARS, New York.

Typesetting by Thomson Digital, India

Printed in Canada by Marquis
Book Printing Inc.   5 4 3 2 1

ISBN 978-1-68420-090-0

Also available as an e-book:
eISBN (PDF): 978-1-68420-091-7
eISBN (epub): 978-1-63853-657-4

Important note: Medicine is an ever-changing science undergoing continual development. Research and clinical experience are continually expanding our knowledge, in particular our knowledge of proper treatment and drug therapy. Insofar as this book mentions any dosage or application, readers may rest assured that the authors, editors, and publishers have made every effort to ensure that such references are in accordance with **the state of knowledge at the time of production of the book**.

Nevertheless, this does not involve, imply, or express any guarantee or responsibility on the part of the publishers in respect to any dosage instructions and forms of applications stated in the book. **Every user is requested to examine carefully** the manufacturers' leaflets accompanying each drug and to check, if necessary in consultation with a physician or specialist, whether the dosage schedules mentioned therein or the contraindications stated by the manufacturers differ from the statements made in the present book. Such examination is particularly important with drugs that are either rarely used or have been newly released on the market. Every dosage schedule or every form of application used is entirely at the user's own risk and responsibility. The authors and publishers request every user to report to the publishers any discrepancies or inaccuracies noticed. If errors in this work are found after publication, errata will be posted at www.thieme.com on the product description page.

Some of the product names, patents, and registered designs referred to in this book are in fact registered trademarks or proprietary names even though specific reference to this fact is not always made in the text. Therefore, the appearance of a name without designation as proprietary is not to be construed as a representation by the publisher that it is in the public domain.

Thieme addresses people of all gender identities equally. We encourage our authors to use gender-neutral or gender-equal expressions wherever the context allows.

To my family and friends for their love and support,
to my mentors for sharing their skills and knowledge,
and to my patients for making the art of plastic surgery so worthwhile.

Alex P. Jones, FRCS (Plast), MBChB, BSc

To my parents and sisters for their unwavering support and love.
To my friends and colleagues for their encouragement and influence.
To my teachers and mentors for their guidance and wisdom.
To my former, current, and future residents for their inspiration.
And most of all to my wife, partner, and best friend, Emily, and our three
absolutely incredible children, Jackson, Brinkley, and Holden—for everything.

Jeffrey E. Janis, MD, FACS

Contents

Foreword

When considering textbooks on plastic, reconstructive, and aesthetic surgery, there are a myriad of choices. The majority of textbooks are beautifully written, nicely illustrated, and take a deep dive into the various aspects of plastic surgery with the goal of facilitating one's ability to learn and retain complex information. Despite the beautiful construction of these books, it is difficult to assess how effective they are when it comes to knowledge assessment and information retention. The best way to demonstrate learning is via the testing and examination process that is usually in a verbal or written question format. The question then becomes, wouldn't it behoove us to learn in a question-and-answer format rather than the traditional lecture or textbook format?

In this textbook, *Essentials of Plastic Surgery: Q&A Companion*, Second Edition, Alex P. Jones and Jeffrey E. Janis have carefully organized and compiled more than 1,600 questions into 127 different chapters focused on the various aspects of plastic, reconstructive, and aesthetic surgery that mirror the content that is contained in the (newly released and long-awaited) parent book, *Essentials of Plastic Surgery*, Third Edition. These are slated for simultaneous "release," making them a perfect match for the delivery and testing of the content.

The chapters are arranged into seven sections focused on the different categories that comprise our specialty. These include: Fundamentals and Basics; Skin and Soft Tissue; Head and Neck; Breast; Trunk and Lower Extremity; Hand, Wrist, and Upper Extremity; and Aesthetic Surgery. The ability to prepare such a book requires not only an exceptional grasp of the material at hand, but also a tremendous understanding of what is relevant and important, and to be able to assimilate that information in such a way that the reader is immersed and completely interested in learning the material. Anyone who has prepared questions and answers for examination purposes understands that this is not an easy task. It takes tremendous thought and knowledge to be able to tease out what is important and what is not and to properly format the questions. All of us can attest to the fact that examination questions are effective to assess not only how much we know, but also where we are deficient. The question-and-answer format is a valuable tool for education and learning, especially when the questions are organized into a clinically relevant format. The process of answering the question requires problem solving as we think about the potential possibilities and solutions. Reading *Essentials of Plastic Surgery: Q&A Companion*, Second Edition is a unique experience because it facilitates the learning process by making it fun, enjoyable, sustainable, and, most importantly, effective.

Determining the ideal format for textbook-based learning is not an easy task, with many theories about what constitutes the most effective method to optimize retention. The unfortunate reality is that most textbooks on plastic surgery do not force us to think and problem solve in the same manner as taking an examination. Test taking is an exceptionally effective learning tool because when posed with a question, we are forced to think critically and explore possibilities. In addition, we process information differently when posed with a question compared to when we are spoon-fed information or when we read an exhaustive amount of material. Learning in a problem-solving format via questions and answers is an active process, whereas traditional didactic learning is passive. Individuals tend to learn more effectively when posed with questions that they have to think about to formulate an answer. When our answers are correct, we can assume that we have a good understanding of the specific topic and the explanation will reinforce it. If our answers are incorrect, then having the ability to immediately review the explanations will facilitate our ability to better comprehend and understand it.

The art of preparing questions that are conducive to the learning process cannot be overemphasized. The best questions are those in which the important principles and concepts are embedded and also where the readers can place themselves in the clinical situation being described. This is essentially how board examination and in-service examination questions are created, and also how the *Essentials of Plastic Surgery: Q&A Companion*, Second Edition is created. The clinical situation usually piques our interest; we think about the possibilities and review the choices. This is in contrast to traditional textbook learning in which the material is presented in a structured format that sometimes lacks clinical relevance.

In conclusion, *Essentials of Plastic Surgery: Q&A Companion*, Second Edition is an excellent textbook for students, residents, and practicing clinicians and should be included in the armamentarium of plastic surgeons on our shelves and computers. It is organized so that it covers each section from the basics to the nuances and provides a strong foundation for focused learning, and at the same time preparatory learning with the goal being to obtain a superb understanding of the essential educational aspects of our specialty. This textbook is an effective means to assess one's knowledge, to acquire new knowledge, and for exam preparation focused on plastic, reconstructive, and aesthetic surgery.

Maurice Y. Nahabedian, MD FACS
Professor of Plastic Surgery
VCU College of Medicine - Inova Branch
National Center for Plastic Surgery
McLean, Virginia, USA

Foreword

Most of us love a quiz, whether to test our knowledge privately or to compete as a team. The satisfaction of knowing an answer is balanced by dismay at failing on a question while not understanding why. This volume is comprehensive not only in its scope but in the excellent explanations of the answers, each of which is clearly delineated and referenced.

By this method, the pleasure of quizzing is combined with the joy of learning, and any candidate for any higher exam in the specialty who can master these questions need not fear their future inquisitors. The scope goes beyond the essentials of our specialty to test and provide a breadth of knowledge and insight which I believe surpasses that of most practicing surgeons. I doubt many will resist the impulse to follow up some of the references that appear at the end of each answer and so take their learning further. Moreover the subject matters also serve as an excellent portal to new advances in our specialty for more senior surgeons to refresh their knowledge. A book this enjoyable and instructive deserves a place in every surgeon's library.

Simon Kay, OBE, FRCS
Professor of Hand Surgery
University of Leeds, UK
Consultant Plastic Surgeon
Leeds Teaching Hospitals NHS Trust
Leeds, UK

Preface

Almost a decade has passed since we first discussed producing a Q&A companion to the second edition of the popular *Essentials of Plastic Surgery*. We felt there was a paucity of texts available for self-assessment and that the market could benefit from a comprehensive, clinically oriented Q&A book to help readers cement the core principles covered within the *Essentials* text.

The third edition of *Essentials* has grown considerably over time, going from 88 to 102 to 127 chapters, paralleling the increased scope, breadth, and depth of plastic surgery.

The second edition of the Q&A companion has also grown, mirroring the equivalent chapters from *Essentials*, third edition, with the same style and format and pertinent illustrations reproduced as well as some additional images created for this text.

The new edition of the Q&A companion book contains more than 1,600 questions, all of which are now formatted as multiple-choice questions (MCQ) to match the style used in most international, professional examinations.

The questions are specifically designed to test the reader on the content of each source *Essentials* chapter, with key emphasis on clinical application of the knowledge.

This learning resource is accompanied by an electronic version (e-book), which means that it can be readily accessed on smartphones and tablets.

For those who prefer traditional books, the format is both compact and portable and presented with high-quality production.

We hope that readers find this second edition to be an even more useful and clinically relevant adjunct to the third edition of *Essentials* on which it is based, and that it can be used to assess one's knowledge base of the spectrum of plastic surgery as presented in the parent book. We hope it will prove useful through your training and revalidation and in developing career as a plastic surgeon.

Alex P. Jones, FRCS (Plast), MBChB, BSc
Jeffrey E. Janis, MD, FACS

Acknowledgments

The creation of this book has required teamwork by a significant number of talented people, and I would like to express my gratitude for each person's part in its development.

First, my appreciation to Dr. Jeff Janis for providing us with the superb *Essentials of Plastic Surgery*, now in its third edition, as the source text and inspiration for this *Q&A Companion*. I would like to thank him for his great teamwork, insightful collaboration, commitment, dedication, and enthusiasm throughout the development of both editions of the *Q&A Companion* book. It has been a real pleasure working with him. I would also like to thank all of the original contributors to the source text for providing such a wealth of information on which to base questions.

A particular thank you is also due to Karen Berger and her team, who first expressed their belief in and support for the first edition.

Anna Barnard has been a significant contributor to both editions, providing feedback and editing advice throughout and for this am I truly grateful. Furthermore, she provided specific expert inputs in the upper limb sections, for which she created and updated the majority of questions alongside juggling our baby twins, clinical work, and our 4-year-old daughter. Our excellent colleague Donald Dewar also provided insightful feedback for some of the early chapters. With infinite patience and tenacity, developmental editor Judith Tomat spent endless hours keeping us on track, while shaping the book into a cohesive whole. Most impressively, she achieved this while simultaneously doing the same for the parent book to ensure close alignment in content and completion time between the two. The size of this task is not to be underestimated. Praise must also be given to Brenda Bunch and her team for providing such high-quality illustrations. A special thank you to the illustrators including Sarah Taylor, Amanda Tomasikiewicz, and Graeme Chambers. My thanks also go to the many members of the Thieme editing and production team, fully supported by Sue Hodgson and Karen Edmonson.

Our goal was to produce a valuable resource for the plastic surgeons of today and tomorrow as they expand and refine their knowledge of our ever-growing field. The nature of plastic surgery demands innovators, and it is our hope that through *Essentials of Plastic Surgery* and this *Q&A Companion*, readers will reinforce their mastery of the fundamentals, which may prove necessary for the very next patient they see.

Alex P. Jones, FRCS (Plast), MBChB, BSc

Acknowledgments

A tremendous debt of gratitude is owed to a great number of people who put an incredible amount of time, energy, and effort into the creation, editing, and production of this second edition of the *Q&A Companion* to the third edition of *Essentials of Plastic Surgery*.

It goes without saying that there could not be a companion book without a parent book, and to that end, I would like to thank the authors of the original chapters on whose work these questions were crafted and founded.

I also acknowledge with sincere appreciation Alex Jones, who once again poured his heart and soul into this new edition, just as he did in the first. As you will see from the quality of the book, these questions and answers were not written overnight, but rather were painstakingly written over a long period of time with many meticulous revisions and modifications. Alex's dedication, time, sweat, and passion come through in the final result, and it has been a distinct pleasure to work closely with him. His European perspective gives international flavor and relevance to the book and the types of questions it contains to make it applicable to plastic surgeons worldwide. Credit clearly is also due to Anna Barnard, who helped Alex on many of the chapters and whose work and effort absolutely need to be recognized.

I would also like to recognize Judith Tomat, the Developmental Editor for both this book and its parent book, *Essentials of Plastic Surgery*. Through her experience, expertise, and indefatigable work ethic, she simultaneously worked on both titles to make them fully and seamlessly integrated—a true companion volume! Massive credit is also due to Brenda Bunch, who managed all artwork associated with both titles. With the incredible number of tables and figures, this was no small task! And finally, I would also like to recognize Sue Hodgson and Karen Edmonson from Thieme Publishing, whose leadership and oversight, and most importantly support, were invaluable. Without each of these individuals, this project simply could not have come to fruition. Their skill and expertise are clearly represented in every page.

Most of all, I would like to deeply and sincerely thank my wife, Emily, and our beautiful children, Jackson, Brinkley, and Holden. Their love, support, patience, and understanding is unequaled and unparalleled and is the only reason a book like this is possible in the first place. I owe them more than I could ever hope to repay, and I take nothing for granted.

Jeffrey E. Janis, MD, FACS

PART I

Fundamentals and Basics

1. Wound Healing

See *Essentials of Plastic Surgery,* third edition, pp. 3-11

PHASES OF WOUND HEALING

1. **Which one of the following statements is true of the process of wound healing?**
   A. It is comprised of five key phases.
   B. Vasodilatation is the initial response after injury.
   C. Each of the key phases are distinct entities.
   D. Each of the phases are of similar duration.
   E. The wound healing process differs in fetal tissue.

CELLS IN WOUND HEALING

2. **In the first 24 hours after a soft tissue injury, which one of the following represents the dominant cell type?**
   A. The neutrophil
   B. The macrophage
   C. The lymphocyte
   D. The fibroblast
   E. The myofibroblast

COLLAGEN SUBTYPES

3. **Which one of the following collagen subtypes is most commonly found in the skin?**
   A. Type I
   B. Type II
   C. Type III
   D. Type IV
   E. Type V

WOUND HEALING

4. **Which one of the following is true in a 6-week-old healing wound?**
   A. Net collagen production is positive.
   B. Net glycosaminoglycan production is positive.
   C. Net vasculogenesis is positive.
   D. Net glycosaminoglycan production is static.
   E. Net collagen production is static.

COLLAGEN SUBTYPES

5. **Which one of the following collagen subtypes predominates in a 3-week-old healing wound?**
   A. Type I
   B. Type III
   C. Type V
   D. Type VII
   E. Type IX

WOUND HEALING STRENGTH

6. **After 10 weeks of direct closure of a wound to the forearm, what proportion of preinjury tensile strength can be expected across the scar?**
   A. 20%
   B. 40%
   C. 60%
   D. 80%
   E. 100%

GROWTH FACTORS IN WOUND HEALING

7. A patient sustains a wound to the right arm following trauma. After wash-out in the emergency department, the wound is left to heal by secondary intention. *Which one of the following is correct regarding the effect of growth factors in this process?*
   A. Fibroblast growth factor (FGF) will decrease fibroblast proliferation.
   B. Transforming growth factor (TGF)-beta promotes fibroblast migration and proliferation.
   C. Vascular endothelial growth factor (VEGF) is produced by endothelial cells.
   D. Epidermal growth factor (EGF) promotes endothelial proliferation.
   E. Platelet-derived growth factor (PDGF) promotes keratinocyte proliferation.

CELL TYPES IN WOUND HEALING

8. *Which one of the following cell types is chiefly responsible for reducing the surface area of a granulating wound because of its contractile properties?*
   A. Fibroblast
   B. Keratinocyte
   C. Macrophage
   D. Lymphocyte
   E. Myofibroblast

CELLULAR PROCESS IN EPITHELIALIZATION

9. *Which one of the following is an important cellular process that facilitates mobilization of keratinocytes during healing of a split-thickness skin graft donor site?*
   A. Diapedesis
   B. Margination
   C. Loss of contact inhibition
   D. Differentiation
   E. Epithelialization

TYPES OF WOUND HEALING

10. *Which one of the following most accurately defines whether primary or secondary healing occurs within a cutaneous wound?*
    A. The mechanism of injury
    B. The amount of tissue damage
    C. The time healing takes to occur
    D. The method of wound closure
    E. How closely the wound edges are apposed

FACTORS AFFECTING WOUND HEALING

11. *In which one of the following conditions is normal wound healing expected after surgery?*
    A. Ehlers-Danlos
    B. Progeria
    C. Werner syndrome
    D. Cutis laxa
    E. Smokers

VITAMINS IN WOUND HEALING

12. *Which one of the following vitamins can be particularly useful to help wound healing in patients on long-term steroids?*
    A. Vitamin A
    B. Vitamin B
    C. Vitamin C
    D. Vitamin D
    E. Vitamin E

FAILURE OF WOUND HEALING

13. *What is the single most important cause of a wound to fail to heal?*
    A. Poor oxygen supply
    B. Denervation
    C. Dry wound base
    D. Radiation injury
    E. Poor nutrition

SMOKING CESSATION

14. A 35-year-old lady is planning to undergo augmentation mastopexy on the understanding that she will have to stop smoking preoperatively. *Which one of the following tests would be most useful to assess her compliance with smoking cessation?*
    A. Platelet count
    B. Blood nicotine
    C. Exhaled carbon dioxide
    D. Urine cotinine
    E. Blood hydrogen cyanide

EFFECTS OF NICOTINE ON WOUND HEALING

15. You see a patient who wishes to undergo a face lift. She has given up smoking after your advice and now uses only nicotine replacement medications. *Which one of the following represents a well-recognized effect of nicotine on tissues?*
    A. Reduced oxyhemoglobin concentrations
    B. Reduced platelet adhesion
    C. Reduced local inflammation
    D. Reduced local blood supply
    E. Toxic effects on keratinocytes

CHEMOTHERAPY AND WOUND HEALING

16. You have a patient with a large wound to the calf after a fall and have closed this directly. He is due to start chemotherapy very soon. *When can the chemotherapy be started without detrimental effects on healing of this wound?*
    A. Immediately
    B. In 3 days
    C. In 14 days
    D. In 1 month
    E. There is no evidence to guide this decision

BIOFILMS

17. *When considering the formation of a biofilm around a breast implant, which one of the following is true?*
    A. Its presence can be detected with routine blood or wound cultures.
    B. It would probably respond well to systemic antibiotic therapy.
    C. It is associated with an acute inflammatory reaction with release of histamine.
    D. It would be effective at evading a host immune response.
    E. It would be unlikely to reform following thorough debridement.

ABNORMAL SCARRING

18. *When examining a patient with an abnormally thickened scar, what is the key factor that will differentiate a keloid from a hypertrophic scar?*
    A. Elevation of the scar
    B. Erythema within the scar
    C. Growth beyond the original wound borders
    D. A biopsy of the scar tissue is the only way to differentiate
    E. The shape of the scar

TREATMENT FOR KELOID SCARS

19. A 23-year-old lady presents with a 1-cm keloid scar to the left pinna following ear piercing 12 months before. *Which one of the following approaches to treatment would be optimal for scar reduction with least risk of recurrence?*
    A. Silicone sheeting
    B. Steroid injection
    C. Radiation
    D. Combination therapy
    E. Surgical excision

Answers

1. Wound Healing

PHASES OF WOUND HEALING

1. *Which one of the following statements is true of the process of wound healing?*

   E. The wound healing process differs in fetal tissue.

Fetal wound healing during the first two trimesters differs from the normal wound healing process and is the subject of much research because of the perceived potential for scarless healing. The process is more of a regenerative process than a repair process often with the absence of an inflammatory phase.[1]

Wound healing after birth represents a highly evolved and complex defense mechanism that helps to limit infection and further injury. The normal wound healing process is comprised of three (not five) phases. These are the inflammatory, the fibroproliferative, and the remodeling phases. The phases are not distinct entities and have overlap both in terms of timing and function. Each phase has a different duration and it can be quite variable. The inflammatory phase typically lasts for 1 week, the fibroproliferative phase lasts for 2–3 weeks, and the remodeling phase lasts for up to 1 year. Vasoconstriction is the initial response to injury in order to limit blood loss and lasts for 5–10 minutes after injury. Vasodilatation and increased tissue permeability follow this as part of the inflammatory phase to promote cellular access to the injured area. Knowledge of the key processes in wound healing is often tested in examinations and a solid understanding of these principles is important for clinical practice with respect to the management of different wound types.[2–5]

REFERENCES

1. Hu MS, Maan ZN, Wu JC, et al. Tissue engineering and regenerative repair in wound healing. Ann Biomed Eng 2014;42(7):1494–1507
2. Broughton G, Rohrich RJ. Wounds and scars. Sel Read Plast Surg 2005;10(7):1–56
3. Glat P, Longaker M. Wound healing. In: Aston SJ, Beasley RW, Thorne CH, et al, eds. Grabb and Smith's Plastic Surgery. 5th ed. Philadelphia: Lippincott-Raven; 1997
4. Janis JE, Kwon RK, Lalonde DH. A practical guide to wound healing. Plast Reconstr Surg 2010;125(6):230e–244e
5. Janis JE, Harrison B. Wound healing: Part I. Basic science. Plast Reconstr Surg 2016;138(3, Suppl):9S–17S

CELLS IN WOUND HEALING

2. *In the first 24 hours after a soft tissue injury, which one of the following represents the dominant cell type?*

   A. The neutrophil

There are a number of key cell types involved in the wound healing process and they are generally specific to a particular phase of wound healing. For example, the neutrophil is the dominant cell type in the first 24 hours after injury. It serves to produce inflammatory mediators and undertake phagocytosis of damaged cells but is not actually critical to wound healing. After 48 hours the macrophage becomes the dominant cell type. In contrast to neutrophil, this is critical to wound healing because it orchestrates growth factors such as TGF-beta, which promotes collagen production, remodeling, epithelialization, and chemotaxis. Lymphocytes are involved in the inflammatory phase, although their role is poorly defined. They are typically present toward the end of the first week after injury. The fibroblast is key to wound healing and moves into the wound after 48 hours. By the end of the first week, it represents the dominant cell type. Along with the myofibroblast, it has a key role in the fibroproliferative phase with the production of collagen.[1]

REFERENCE

1. Janis JE, Harrison B. Wound healing: Part I. Basic science. Plast Reconstr Surg 2016;138(3, Suppl):9S–17S

COLLAGEN SUBTYPES

3. *Which one of the following collagen subtypes is most commonly found in the skin?*

   A. Type I

Collagen is a protein that forms the key building block for skin, bone, cartilage, and tendon. The basic structure consists of three left-handed polypeptide helices wound together to form a right-handed helix. It comprises two alpha-1 and one alpha-2 chains; each of these are formed by amino acid sequences: glycine-prolene-X and glycine-X-hydroxyprolene. There are more than 20 different collagen subtypes and type I is the most common in humans, representing 90% of all body collagen. It predominates in the skin, tendon, and bone. Type II is found in the cornea and articular cartilage. Type III is found in the vessel and bowel walls. Type IV is found in the basement membrane only.

WOUND HEALING

4. *Which one of the following is true in a 6-week-old healing wound?*

E. Net collagen production is static.

At 6 weeks, the healing wound should be in the remodeling phase of wound healing. During this phase, net collagen production is static because an equilibrium is reached between collagen breakdown and collagen synthesis. Although there is no change in quantity, collagen continues to undergo remodeling with increased organization and formation of stronger cross-links. The ratio of different collagen subtypes also changes. Glycosaminoglycan production and vasculogenesis decrease as does the water content and cellular population.[1,2]

REFERENCES

1. Glat P, Longaker M. Wound healing. In: Aston SJ, Beasley RW, Thorne CH, et al, eds. Grabb and Smith's Plastic Surgery, 5th ed. Philadelphia: Lippincott-Raven; 1997

2. Janis JE, Harrison B. Wound healing: Part I. Basic science. Plast Reconstr Surg 2016;138(3, Suppl):9S–17S

COLLAGEN SUBTYPES

5. *Which one of the following collagen subtypes predominates in a 3-week-old healing wound?*

B. Type III

There are more than 20 different types of collagen with type I representing 90% of all total body collagen. The normal adult ratio of type I to type III collagen within the skin is around 4:1. However, in the healing wound, type III collagen is made first and this subtype predominates in the proliferation and early remodeling phases until it is gradually replaced by type I collagen.

WOUND HEALING STRENGTH

6. *After 10 weeks of direct closure of a wound to the forearm, what proportion of preinjury tensile strength can be expected across the scar?*

D. 80%

In spite of the impressive ability of wounds to heal, tissues never regain 100% of their preinjury tensile strength. It is estimated that a completely healed wound will have, at best, around 80% of its preinjury tensile strength and this will be achieved between 60 days and 1 year after the injury, typically around 90 days. The evidence for this stems from a 1965 study by Levenson et al[1] where healing in rat skin wounds was assessed at various time intervals. Knowledge of skin strength at various time points following repair is clinically useful when considering suture selection, such that the suture is able to satisfactorily support the wound until adequate strength has been regained. For example, placement of buried dermal sutures in the face allows for external skin sutures to be removed at 5 days although the repair will still be weak at this stage. It also helps guide the clinician and patient with regard to resumption of normal activities following surgery.[1]

REFERENCE

1. Levenson SM, Geever EF, Crowley LV, Oates JF III, Berard CW, Rosen H. The healing of rat skin wounds. Ann Surg 1965;161:293–308

GROWTH FACTORS IN WOUND HEALING

7. A patient sustains a wound to the right arm following trauma. After wash-out in the emergency department, the wound is left to heal by secondary intention. *Which one of the following is correct regarding the effect of growth factors in this process?*

B. TGF-beta promotes fibroblast migration and proliferation.

Many growth factors are involved in the wound healing process and most of these positively influence cell proliferation and migration. Similarly, TGF-beta will promote fibroblast migration and proliferation. FGF will increase both fibroblast and keratinocyte proliferation. It also affects fibroblast chemotaxis. VEGF will promote endothelial cell proliferation and is produced by many different cell types in response to hypoxia or injury. EGF promotes keratinocyte and fibroblast division rather than endothelial cell proliferation. PDGF promotes fibroblast, endothelial cell, and smooth muscle proliferation rather than keratinocyte proliferation.

CELL TYPES IN WOUND HEALING

8. *Which one of the following cell types is chiefly responsible for reducing the surface area of a granulating wound because of its contractile properties?*

   E. Myofibroblast

   Fibroblasts are the key cells responsible for forming extracellular matrix and collagen. They are present in both the early and late stages of wound healing and have a permanent presence in the dermis. Myofibroblasts are specialized fibroblasts that have contractile cytoplasmic microfilaments and distinct cellular adhesion structures. They are present in the early stages of wound healing and serve to collectively decrease the size of a wound. They usually remain within the wound for the first few weeks following injury. Keratinocytes are the major cells of the epidermis and are involved in wound healing and normal skin cell turnover. Macrophages and lymphocytes are both inflammatory cells that are involved in the orchestration of wound healing.

CELLULAR PROCESS IN EPITHELIALIZATION

9. *Which one of the following is an important cellular process that facilitates mobilization of keratinocytes during healing of a split-thickness skin graft donor site?*

   C. Loss of contact inhibition

   The process of healing a split-thickness skin graft donor site is termed reepithelialization. This involves a series of cellular processes that enable keratinocytes from the wound edges to proliferate and move toward the center of the wound. Cells are usually held at the wound edge by contact inhibition and this must be lost to enable cells to mobilize. Following a loss of contact inhibition, cells move across the wound until they meet cells from the other side and contact inhibition is reestablished. While cells at the wound edge are migrating, basal cells further back from the wound edge proliferate to support the cell numbers required to bridge the wound. Differentiation of keratinocytes subsequently occurs to reestablish normal epithelial layers from basal layer to stratum corneum. Margination refers to the process of leukocytes moving from the axial zone (central higher flow zone) to the plasmatic zone (peripheral lower flow zone) within blood vessels and adhering to the vessel walls in order to exit the blood stream. Diapedesis refers to the process of cells passing through vessel walls once margination has taken place during the inflammatory phase of wound healing.

TYPES OF WOUND HEALING

10. *Which one of the following most accurately defines whether primary or secondary healing occurs within a cutaneous wound?*

    E. How closely the wound edges are apposed

    Healing is defined as primary, secondary, or tertiary (delayed primary). The key factor that differentiates whether primary or secondary healing occurs is how closely the wound edges are apposed. When the wound edges are reapproximated, such as when an incised wound is sutured, primary healing can occur. This results in the least amount of scar tissue production. In contrast, where there is a gap between the wound edges, such as when a finger pulp injury with tissue loss is left open, secondary wound healing will occur in order to fill in the missing tissue. More scar tissue is formed and the process involves a combination of contraction and epithelialization. Neither the mechanism of injury, the amount of tissue damage, nor the method of wound closure, per se, define whether healing by primary or secondary intention occur, only the reapproximation of the wound edges. Even when tissue loss has occurred, primary healing is possible providing that the wound edges are debrided and well apposed. Complete healing is normally achieved most quickly in wounds that are closed primarily, but this is not a defining factor. Wound closure can be satisfactorily achieved with sutures, staples, or glue, and each of these techniques allows primary healing to take place. Tertiary healing and delayed primary healing are the same thing. They refer to wounds that are initially left open and then closed after debridement at a later stage. This is an approach commonly employed in infected wounds where closure is delayed until the infection has been satisfactorily treated.

FACTORS AFFECTING WOUND HEALING

11. *In which one of the following conditions is normal wound healing expected after surgery?*

    D. Cutis laxa

    Cutis laxa is a condition where there is a mutation in elastin fibers and this results in loose wrinkled skin and hypermobile joints. Some patients can benefit from resection of excess skin and this is safe as wound healing is normal.

    The other conditions are all associated with abnormal wound healing. Ehlers-Danlos syndrome is also known as cutis hyperelastica and is a genetic connective tissue disorder with abnormal collagen cross-linking. The condition is associated with thin friable skin, poor wound healing, hypertrophic scarring, and hypermobile joints. Progeria is also known as Hutchinson-Gilford syndrome and is also a genetic condition observed in children. Patients have premature aging with skin laxity and poor wound healing. Werner syndrome is adult progeria with similar features to Hutchinson-Gilford syndrome. In each of these conditions, surgery is best avoided where possible.

It is well accepted that there is an association between smoking and delayed wound healing, although the precise mechanism is not well understood. The constituents implicated within tobacco smoke include nicotine, carbon monoxide, and hydrogen cyanide. Sørensen undertook a systematic review in 2012[1] to consider the effects of smoking on wound healing and found that smoking temporarily decreases tissue oxygenation and aerobic metabolism, while it also attenuates both the inflammatory and proliferation phases of wound healing, thereby decreasing collagen production. Cessation of smoking for 4 weeks before surgery appears to reverse some, but not all, of the processes described.

REFERENCE

1. Sørensen LT. Wound healing and infection in surgery: the pathophysiological impact of smoking, smoking cessation, and nicotine replacement therapy: a systematic review. Ann Surg 2012;255(6):1069–1079

VITAMINS IN WOUND HEALING

12. Which one of the following vitamins can be particularly useful to help wound healing in patients on long-term steroids?

A. Vitamin A

Vitamins are vital to normal wound healing processes, but supplements typically help wound healing only when there is a deficiency present. Vitamin A is also known as retinol and has important functions in immunity, vision, and wound healing. It can help reverse delayed wound healing due to steroids and increase epithelialization in healing wounds. It is well accepted that steroids delay wound healing and animal and human studies have shown these negative effects to be reversed when vitamin A is used either topically or systemically. The mechanism is not well understood, and the benefit of using vitamin A is absent when steroids are not being given. Given this evidence, it may be particularly useful to prescribe vitamin A during the perioperative period in patients on long-term steroids such as for rheumatoid arthritis or ulcerative colitis.[1]

There are a number of different B vitamins including thiamine, folic acid, pyridoxine, and cobalamin which have important roles in metabolism and oxygen transport. Deficiencies of the B vitamins can therefore result in a broad range of conditions. Vitamin C is vital for hydroxylation reactions in collagen synthesis and a deficiency leads to scurvy, with immature fibroblasts, deficient collagen synthesis, capillary hemorrhage, and decreased tissue strength. Vitamin D is important for calcium regulation and a deficiency can lead to rickets in children or osteomalacia in adults. Vitamin E is an antioxidant that stabilizes membranes. Large doses inhibit healing and may cause dermatitis.

REFERENCE

1. Hunt TK, Ehrlich HP, Garcia JA, Dunphy JE. Effect of vitamin A on reversing the inhibitory effect of cortisone on healing of open wounds in animals and man. Ann Surg 1969;170(4):633–641

FAILURE OF WOUND HEALING

13. What is the single most important cause of a wound to fail to heal?

A. Poor oxygen supply

The single most common reason for a wound not to heal is tissue hypoxia. This can occur secondary to a number of causes such as poor vascularity, smoking, previous injury, or radiation therapy. The presence of infection with microorganisms greater than 10^5 per gram of tissue will decrease oxygen tension, lower the pH, and increase collagenase activity. Denervation of a wound will make it more susceptible to pressure damage and is a major factor in the development of sacral sores in paraplegic patients and foot ulcers in diabetic patients. A moist wound is thought to be beneficial to healing so wounds are often kept moist until reepithelialization is complete, but a dry wound is not the most significant factor in failure of a wound to heal. Radiation injury is a significant factor in wound healing and results from damage to blood vessels, which in turn causes poor oxygen supply to local tissues.

Nutritional status is a key component in wound healing and needs to be considered pre- and postoperatively, with dietician support requested in more complex cases.

SMOKING CESSATION

14. A 35-year-old lady is planning to undergo augmentation mastopexy on the understanding that she will have to stop smoking preoperatively. Which one of the following tests would be most useful to assess her compliance with smoking cessation?

D. Urine cotinine

Cotinine is the body's key metabolite of nicotine and is considered the gold standard biomarker for smoking assessment. It has a half-life of up to 20 hours in contrast to nicotine which has a half-life of up to 2 hours. Measurement of nicotine itself is therefore less useful than cotinine because it is more rapidly metabolized from the body, so would only be measurable very shortly after a recent cigarette. In contrast, cotinine levels would remain elevated some weeks following a patient's last cigarette if he or she is a regular smoker. Cotinine levels can be measured in the urine, blood, saliva, or hair follicles. Urine testing is generally preferred because blood testing of cotinine can be affected by diet due to the presence of thiocyanate, which is found in green vegetables such as broccoli and cabbage. Hair or saliva testing of cotinine is less commonly used. One advantage of the hair sampling over saliva is that longer exposure estimates may be obtained.[1]

Exhaled carbon monoxide (not carbon dioxide) is another useful measurement for assessing smoking. It is recorded in parts per million (ppm). It is generally accepted that a level of 7 ppm is the upper limit to show evidence of recent smoking. Measurement of exhaled carbon monoxide has some drawbacks including the fact it is not specific to tobacco intake as it is influenced by atmospheric carbon monoxide, passive smoking, occupational exposure, or smoke from biomass or coal burning. It too has a short half-life so tends to provide an assessment of smoking behavior primarily over a 6–8 hours period.[2]

Smoking can lead to increased platelet adhesiveness due to nicotine itself; however, the platelet count would not be expected to be measurably altered. Some other blood parameters can be affected by smoking and these include hemoglobin, white cell count, and mean corpuscular volume.[3] Hydrogen cyanide inhibits oxygen transport and is increased in smokers. However, it is not routinely measured in relation to smoking cessation.

REFERENCES

1. Miron R, Trofor L, Bucur D, Man M, Cernat R, Trofor A. Biomarkers of tobacco exposure-relevant diagnostic implications in daily practice. Romanian Journal of Oral Rehabilitation 2014;6(1)
2. Cope GF, Wu HHT, O'Donovan GV, Milburn HJ. A new point of care cotinine test for saliva to identify and monitor smoking habit. Eur Respir J 2012;40(2):496–497
3. Malenica M, Prnjavorac B, Bego T, et al. Effect of cigarette smoking on haematological parameters in healthy population. Med Arh 2017;71(2):132–136

EFFECTS OF NICOTINE ON WOUND HEALING

15. You see a patient who wishes to undergo a face lift. She has given up smoking after your advice and now uses only nicotine replacement medications. *Which one of the following represents a well-recognized effect of nicotine on tissues?*

   D. Reduced local blood supply

   Nicotine is a vasoconstrictor that reduces nutritional blood flow to the skin, resulting in tissue ischemia and the potential for impaired healing of injured tissues. Nicotine also increases platelet adhesiveness (not decreases it), raising the risk of thrombotic microvascular occlusion and further tissue ischemia. In addition, it can reduce red blood cells, fibroblast, and macrophage proliferation. Nicotine is therefore one of the components within cigarette smoke that may be responsible for the increased risk of wound complications associated with tobacco smoking.

   There have been a number of studies to explore the precise role of nicotine in wound healing, both as a single agent and as part of cigarette smoking. However, the mechanisms involved are complex and remain incompletely understood. At present, in spite of the effects of nicotine on wound healing, there is no clinical evidence to show that nicotine replacement therapy in patients abstaining from smoking will significantly affect their wound healing. In high-risk procedures such as face lifting, it is still probably best to avoid both smoking and nicotine replacement therapy in order to minimize risk of wound complications. Other products in cigarette smoke such as carbon monoxide and hydrogen cyanide are responsible for reduced oxyhemoglobin concentrations, altered inflammation, and toxic cellular effects.[1–3]

REFERENCES

1. Sørensen LT. Wound healing and infection in surgery: the pathophysiological impact of smoking, smoking cessation, and nicotine replacement therapy: a systematic review. Ann Surg 2012;255(6):1069–1079
2. Silverstein P. Smoking and wound healing. Am J Med 1992;93(1A):22S–24S
3. Warner DO. Perioperative abstinence from cigarettes: physiologic and clinical consequences. Anesthesiology 2006;104(2):356–367

CHEMOTHERAPY AND WOUND HEALING

16. You have a patient with a large wound to the calf after a fall and have closed this directly. He is due to start chemotherapy very soon. *When can the chemotherapy be started without detrimental effects on healing of this wound?*

   C. In 14 days

   It is well accepted that antineoplastic agents affect wound healing. This evidence is based on both lab-based animal studies and clinical studies in humans. However, there is unlikely to be any significant effect on wound healing, providing that chemotherapy treatment is delayed for 10–14 days after the wound has been closed. This makes sense given the anticipated healing time for a typical soft tissue wound.[1,2]

REFERENCES

1. Falcone RE, Nappi JF. Chemotherapy and wound healing. Surg Clin North Am 1984;64(4):779–794
2. Shamberger RC, Devereux DF, Brennan MF. The effect of chemotherapeutic agents on wound healing. Int Adv Surg Oncol 1981;4:15–58

BIOFILMS

17. *When considering the formation of a biofilm around a breast implant, which one of the following is true?*

   D. **It would be effective at evading a host immune response.**

   Biofilms have a significant role in plastic surgery, particularly where implants are used. They can be a major saboteur to wound healing and the reconstructive process. In addition, there has been much debate as to their importance in formation of capsular contracture in breast augmentation, where their presence has been implicated as a key causal factor.[1]

   One of the most challenging factors in managing biofilms is their effectiveness at evading the host's immune system. Biofilms are fundamentally different from free floating bacteria (termed the planktonic state). They require a surface for growth, which can be either a prosthetic implant or one occurring within the body's own soft tissues. They are difficult to detect and treat. Routine culture is not effective at detection of biofilms and they are recalcitrant to treatment with systemic antimicrobials. Even following debridement, they have a tendency to recur.

REFERENCE

1. Barker JC, Khansa I, Gordillo GM. A formidable foe is sabotaging your results: what you should know about biofilms and wound healing. Plast Reconstr Surg 2017;139(5):1184e–1194e

ABNORMAL SCARRING

18. *When examining a patient with an abnormally thickened scar, what is the key factor that will differentiate a keloid from a hypertrophic scar?*

   C. **Growth beyond the original wound borders**

   Keloid and hypertrophic scars each represent abnormal scarring processes and are differentiated clinically. The key defining feature of a keloid scar is that it grows beyond the original scar border, whereas a hypertrophic scar does not. Both keloid and hypertrophic scars are typically elevated and erythematous. The histological appearances are similar with high concentrations of type III collagen in each. Keloid scars are only seen in humans, and typically observed in younger patients, i.e., 10–30 years of age. They can occur spontaneously or secondary to injury or infection. They tend to affect patients with darker skin tones most commonly. Females are more commonly affected than males. They commonly occur on the ear or anterior chest and rarely regress spontaneously. Hypertrophic scars have an equal sex ratio, are typically seen in younger age groups (less than 20 years of age), and appear soon after injury such as in children who have sustained a burn. All skin tones can be affected (**Fig. 1.1**).[1,2]

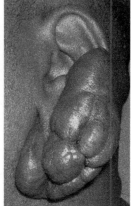

Fig. 1.1   Keloid scar.

REFERENCES

1. Sidle DM, Kim H. Keloids: prevention and management. Facial Plast Surg Clin North Am 2011;19(3):505–515
2. Chike-Obi CJ, Cole PD, Brissett AE. Keloids: pathogenesis, clinical features, and management. Semin Plast Surg 2009;23(3):178–184

TREATMENT FOR KELOID SCARS

19. A 23-year-old lady presents with a 1-cm keloid scar to the left pinna following ear piercing 12 months before. *Which one of the following approaches to treatment would be optimal for scar reduction with least risk of recurrence?*

   D. **Combination therapy**

   Keloid scars can develop following body piercings, as in this case, following tattoos, acne, insect bites, vaccinations, trauma, or surgery. Effective management of them can be challenging. There are a number of potential options for treatment including silicone sheeting, corticosteroids, interferon, radiation, surgical excision, and cryotherapy.

Recurrence rates tend to be high in many cases, so multimodality or combination therapy is generally accepted as the best practice approach for their treatment.[1,2]

In this case, initial treatment with steroid injection followed by surgical excision or debulking may be effective. Additional scar management therapies such as silicone sheeting or pressure may also be helpful. Alternatively, surgical excision combined with radiotherapy may provide the most effective solution if this treatment is available. Radiation treatment for keloids is typically commenced on the same day as surgery with dose ranges of 12–30 gray (Gy), delivered over 5–7 days.[3,4]

Silicone sheeting would be recommended for wounds as soon as epithelialization is complete so it would be too late for this duration of scar as primary treatment and would be unlikely to show any effect. Steroid injections can reduce collagen synthesis and inflammatory mediators to soften keloid scars. Radiation inhibits angiogenesis and fibroblasts and can be associated with lower rates of recurrence than some treatments.

REFERENCES

1. Sidle DM, Kim H. Keloids: prevention and management. Facial Plast Surg Clin North Am 2011;19(3):505–515
2. Chike-Obi CJ, Cole PD, Brissett AE. Keloids: pathogenesis, clinical features, and management. Semin Plast Surg 2009;23(3):178–184
3. Zainib M, Amin NP. Radiation Therapy in the Treatment of Keloids. StatPearls; 2019
4. Mankowski P, Kanevsky J, Tomlinson J, Dyachenko A, Luc M. Optimizing radiotherapy for keloids: a meta-analysis systematic review comparing recurrence rates between different radiation modalities. Ann Plast Surg 2017;78(4):403–411

2.   General Management of Complex Wounds

See Essentials of Plastic Surgery, third edition, pp. 12–20

BLOOD GLUCOSE CONTROL

1. A diabetic patient is scheduled to undergo abdominal wall reconstruction. Preoperative hemoglobin A_1C is 12% and random blood glucose (RBG) level is 200 mg/dL. *Which one of the following is correct?*
   A. A normal A_1C should be 8.5 when expressed as a percentage of glycosylated hemoglobin.
   B. The A_1C represents the patient's average glucose control over the previous 180 days.
   C. Postoperative infection risk is significantly increased for this patient because the blood glucose level is higher than 180 mg/dL.
   D. Tight blood glucose control (<70 mg/dL) during the perioperative period will reduce the postoperative mortality risk.
   E. An elevated A_1C level linearly correlates with an increased risk of surgical site infections.

PREOPERATIVE ASSESSMENT OF NUTRITION

2. *When assessing a patient's preoperative nutritional status before major surgery by monitoring blood albumin levels, which one of the following is correct?*
   A. The half-life of albumin is 3 days.
   B. A preoperative value of 4.3 g/dL is outside the normal range.
   C. Assessment is based on the "rule of fives."
   D. Severe malnutrition would be suggested by preoperative values less than 3.0 g/dL.
   E. A low preoperative level is a strong predictor for postoperative mortality risk.

IMAGING IN COMPLEX WOUNDS

3. A 67-year-old smoker has exposed hardware after a wound breakdown over his tibial fracture. The hardware has been removed, but his wound is not progressing. His dorsalis pedis pulse is not palpable, and the posterior tibial pulse is weak. *Which one of the following modalities is the most accurate and least harmful for imaging of this patient's peripheral arterial disease status and leg vessel anatomy?*
   A. Magnetic resonance angiography (MRA)
   B. Plain radiographs
   C. Computerized tomography angiography (CTA)
   D. Ultrasound
   E. Contrast angiography

VASCULAR ULCER MANAGEMENT

4. After assessing a patient who is malnourished and has a punched-out ulcer on the lower lateral leg, you decide to perform an ankle-brachial pressure test, which shows a value of 0.4. *What does this result suggest?*
   A. Normal lower limb vasculature.
   B. Imminent ischemic gangrene is likely.
   C. Critical stenosis is present that warrants further intervention.
   D. Vessels are significantly calcified.
   E. Predominantly venous disease.

TISSUE RECONSTRUCTION AND WOUND CLOSURE

5. *What was the main limitation of the original reconstructive ladder concept?*
   A. It did not include free tissue transfer.
   B. The concept could only be practiced by plastic surgeons.
   C. It did not include dermal matrices or negative pressure therapy.
   D. The reconstructive process was performed in a stepwise manner.
   E. Primary closure was the first rung on the ladder.

NEGATIVE PRESSURE WOUND THERAPY

6. You are planning to temporize an abdominal wound with a negative pressure dressing after debridement. *Which one of the following is correct regarding negative pressure wound therapy?*
   A. It increases local blood flow and granulation tissue production.
   B. It reduces fluid exudate.
   C. It is contraindicated in recently debrided wounds.
   D. It can be useful for treating fistulas.
   E. It reduces mitotic activity in the wound.

WOUND DEBRIDEMENT

7. A 47-year-old paraplegic patient presents with a grade 3 sacral pressure sore. Examination shows a 7 × 8 cm chronic wound with eschar, fibrinous exudate, and granulation in the wound bed. *In order to optimize accuracy at the time of surgical debridement, which one of the following adjuncts would be most useful intraoperatively?*
   A. Quantitative tissue cultures
   B. Frozen section biopsy
   C. Iodine brown solution
   D. Methylene blue dye
   E. Indocyanine green dye

COMPLICATIONS OF RADIOTHERAPY

8. A 68-year-old male has undergone postsurgical radiotherapy to the right side of the neck and mandible for management of an intraoral squamous cell carcinoma (SCC). He now presents with symptoms of pain and swelling over the mandible and has reduced mouth opening. Examination shows bone exposed through the skin surface (sequestrum). *Which one of the following would be the most useful for treatment of this clinical problem?*
   A. Hyperbaric oxygen
   B. Transcutaneous oxygen tension
   C. Stem cell therapy
   D. Platelet-rich plasma
   E. Tissue biopsy and cultures

SELECTION OF SKIN SUBSTITUTES

9. You are considering the use of a biologic skin substitute in a patient with a burn. Your patient is concerned about the use of tissues from animals and states that he would only consent to products that are purely synthetic or human derived. *Which one of the following products is acceptable for use in this patient?*
   A. Biobrane   D. SurgiMend
   B. Apligraf   E. AlloDerm
   C. Transcyte

BIOLOGIC SKIN SUBSTITUTES

10. *Which one of the following biologic dressings is a bilayer construct containing bovine collagen, human fibroblasts, and keratinocytes?*
    A. Matriderm
    B. ReCell
    C. Acelagraft
    D. Epicel
    E. Apligraf

Answers

BLOOD GLUCOSE CONTROL

1. A diabetic patient is scheduled to undergo abdominal wall reconstruction. Preoperative hemoglobin A_1C is 12% and random blood glucose (RBG) level is 200 mg/dL. *Which one of the following is correct?*

   C. Postoperative infection risk is significantly increased for this patient because the blood glucose level is higher than 180 mg/dL.

   In patients with or without diabetes, perioperative hyperglycemia (>180 mg/dL) carries a significantly increased risk of postoperative wound infection.[1]

   The hemoglobin A_1C is a blood test used to assess the long-term control of blood glucose. Because hemoglobin molecules remain in the blood for 3 months, it is possible to gauge glucose control over a 120-day period (not 180 days) by measuring glycosylated hemoglobin levels. A normal hemoglobin A_1C is around 6%. Tight blood glucose control with intensive insulin therapy and normoglycemia (<110 mg/dL) has shown a reduction in hospital deaths in some trials.[2] However, where glucose control is <7 mg/dL, there is an increased risk of death in critically ill patients.[3] Although postoperative hyperglycemia and undiagnosed diabetes increase the risk of surgical site infections, elevated hemoglobin A_1C does not linearly correlate.[4,5]

REFERENCES

1. Kwon S, Thompson R, Dellinger P, Yanez D, Farrohki E, Flum D. Importance of perioperative glycemic control in general surgery: a report from the Surgical Care and Outcomes Assessment Program. Ann Surg 2013;257(1):8–14
2. Vanhorebeek I, Langouche L, Van den Berghe G. Tight blood glucose control: what is the evidence? Crit Care Med 2007;35(9, Suppl):S496–S502
3. Finfer S, Liu B, Chittock DR, et al; NICE-SUGAR Study Investigators. Hypoglycemia and risk of death in critically ill patients. N Engl J Med 2012;367(12):1108–1118
4. King JT Jr, Goulet JL, Perkal MF, Rosenthal RA. Glycemic control and infections in patients with diabetes undergoing noncardiac surgery. Ann Surg 2011;253(1):158–165
5. Latham R, Lancaster AD, Covington JF, Pirolo JS, Thomas CS Jr. The association of diabetes and glucose control with surgical-site infections among cardiothoracic surgery patients. Infect Control Hosp Epidemiol 2001;22(10):607–612

PREOPERATIVE ASSESSMENT OF NUTRITION

2. *When assessing a patient's preoperative nutritional status before major surgery by monitoring blood albumin levels, which one of the following is correct?*

   E. A low preoperative level is a strong predictor for postoperative mortality risk.

   Albumin can provide a useful indication of nutrition. Its half-life is 20 days, and a normal value is 3.6–5.4 g/dL. A value of 2.8–3.5 g/dL suggests mild malnutrition, 2.1–2.7 g/dL suggests moderate malnutrition, and less than 2.1 g/dL indicates severe malnutrition. A large study published in 1999 involving more than 50,000 patients showed that as preoperative albumin levels decreased, early postoperative mortality and morbidity increased exponentially.[1] The authors concluded that albumin was a useful predictor of outcome in major surgical procedures.

   Prealbumin, rather than albumin, has a half-life of 3 days and can be assessed by the rule of fives. A normal value is greater than 15 mg/dL, mild deficiency is less than 15 mg/dL, moderate is less than 10 mg/dL, and severe is less than 5 mg/dL.

   Prealbumin, also known as transthyretin, is a transport protein for thyroxine and is actually unrelated to albumin. It earned its name because it runs faster than albumin on gel electrophoresis. Although prealbumin levels can be a useful marker of nutritional status, they are less reliable during infective or inflammatory processes as prealbumin is an acute phase protein.

REFERENCE

1. Gibbs J, Cull W, Henderson W, Daley J, Hur K, Khuri SF. Preoperative serum albumin level as a predictor of operative mortality and morbidity: results from the National VA Surgical Risk Study. Arch Surg 1999;134(1):36–42

IMAGING IN COMPLEX WOUNDS

3. A 67-year-old smoker has exposed hardware after a wound breakdown over his tibial fracture. The hardware has been removed, but his wound is not progressing. His dorsalis pedis pulse is not palpable, and the posterior tibial

pulse is weak. *Which one of the following modalities is the most accurate and least harmful for imaging of this patient's peripheral arterial disease status and leg vessel anatomy?*

A. Magnetic resonance angiography (MRA)

A systemic review of imaging in the lower limb confirmed that peripheral arterial disease is best imaged using magnetic resonance angiography (MRA) because this has an overall better diagnostic accuracy than computerized tomography angiography (CTA) or ultrasonography. It also showed patients' preference of MRA over standard contrast angiography.[1] MRA uses magnetic fields to evaluate blood vessels. It requires no radiation dose (in contrast to CTA) and can be performed with or without intravenous (IV) delivered contrast (normally gadolinium). This has a lower risk of contrast reaction in terms of anaphylaxis or renal injury compared with the iodine-based contrasts generally used for computed tomography (CT). MRI will visualize the surrounding soft tissues more effectively than CT, but is generally less useful for bony imaging. In the trauma setting, patients with long bone fractures such as this patient, with metal hardware (external fixation devices, internal plates, or intramedullary nails), may not be able to have MRI if the hardware is not MRI compatible. In such circumstances, CT or plain film angiography may be required as an alternative. Plain film radiography is more invasive than CT or MRA because it involves cannulation of the arterial tree, usually from the groin. Dye is then injected directly into the arterial system. Plain radiographic films can demonstrate calcification of vessels and may be useful for assessment of fractures, foreign bodies, and osteomyelitis, rather than vascular imaging.

In spite of the usefulness of imaging, clinical examination with palpation of distal pulses and the use of handheld Doppler machines can provide accurate assessment of limb vessels and are still preferred by many surgeons as the primary modality for assessment. Maintaining skills in this assessment is vital for plastic and reconstructive surgeons.

REFERENCE

1. Collins R, Cranny G, Burch J, et al. A systematic review of duplex ultrasound, magnetic resonance angiography and computed tomography angiography for the diagnosis and assessment of symptomatic, lower limb peripheral artery disease. Health Technol Assess 2007;11:iii–iv, xi–xiii, 1–184

VASCULAR ULCER MANAGEMENT

4. After assessing a patient who is malnourished and has a punched-out ulcer on the lower lateral leg, you decide to perform an ankle-brachial pressure test, which shows a value of 0.4. *What does this result suggest?*

C. Critical stenosis is present that warrants further intervention.

The ankle-brachial pressure index is a noninvasive test used to investigate the lower limb vasculature. It compares a patient's lower limb arterial pressure with that of the upper limb and expresses it as a ratio. A normal ankle-brachial pressure index is between 0.9 and 1.2. A value greater than 1.2 suggests calcification as vessels become noncompressible. A value of 0.5–0.9 is associated with mixed arteriovenous disease. A value of less than 0.5 suggests critical arterial stenosis, and a value of less than 0.2 indicates that ischemic gangrene is likely. The clinical picture is consistent with the appearance of an arterial ischemic ulcer, and referral for a vascular opinion is recommended.

TISSUE RECONSTRUCTION AND WOUND CLOSURE

5. *What was the main limitation of the original reconstructive ladder concept?*

D. The reconstructive process was performed in a stepwise manner.

The reconstructive ladder was a concept described by Mathes and Nahai[1] to categorize options for wound closure, progressing in a stepwise manner of complexity from healing by secondary intention to free tissue transfer, with the simplest option being preferentially used first. The major conceptual understanding of the original concept was that each rung was mandatory to climb before hitting the next rung. This was corrected by Gottlieb and Krieger[2] who coined the term "reconstructive elevator," which they described in the Editorial section of *Plastic Reconstructive Surgery* in 1994 to emphasize that reconstruction is flexible and does not have to proceed in a stepwise fashion. Reconstruction should immediately proceed to the best option in any given scenario, taking into consideration the patient, the wound, and the resources available. The original reconstructive ladder did not include negative pressure dressings or dermal matrices; however, this was not its major caveat. Janis et al[3] refined the reconstructive ladder to include dermal matrices and negative pressure wound therapy. Other models for reconstruction have included the reconstructive triangle[1] and the reconstructive matrix.[4] The reconstructive triangle includes tissue expansion, local flaps, and free tissue transfer. The reconstructive matrix contains three axes representing technological sophistication, surgical complexity, and patient's surgical risk (see Figs. 2.1 and 2.2, *Essentials of Plastic Surgery*, third edition).

REFERENCES

1. Mathes SJ, Nahai F. Reconstructive Surgery: Principles, Anatomy, & Technique. St Louis: Quality Medical Publishing; 1997
2. Gottlieb LJ, Krieger LM. From the reconstructive ladder to the reconstructive elevator. Plast Reconstr Surg 1994;93(7):1503–1504
3. Janis JE, Kwon RK, Attinger CE. The new reconstructive ladder: modifications to the traditional model. Plast Reconstr Surg 2011;127(Suppl 1):205S–212S
4. Erba P, Ogawa R, Vyas R, Orgill DP. The reconstructive matrix: a new paradigm in reconstructive plastic surgery. Plast Reconstr Surg 2010;126(2):492–498

NEGATIVE PRESSURE WOUND THERAPY

6. You are planning to temporize an abdominal wound with a negative pressure dressing after debridement. **Which one of the following is correct regarding negative pressure wound therapy?**

A. It increases local blood flow and granulation tissue production.

Negative pressure wound therapy is commonly used to accelerate wound healing either as a sole means of wound closure or to prepare a wound for skin grafting. Argenta and Morykwas[1] first described the term in 1997 after their clinical experience. It is believed to cause deformation of cells that leads to an increase in their mitotic activity. Fluid exudate is removed during negative pressure therapy, but the production of fluid per se is not affected. Production of granulation tissue is increased. Use of negative pressure therapy should be avoided in wounds with exposed vessels, fistulas, active infection, or malignancy. It can safely be used after wound debridement providing that hemostasis is adequate and the points described above are addressed with respect to the other contraindications.

REFERENCE

1. Argenta LC, Morykwas MJ. Vacuum-assisted closure: a new method for wound control and treatment: clinical experience. Ann Plast Surg 1997;38(6):563–576, discussion 577

WOUND DEBRIDEMENT

7. A 47-year-old paraplegic patient presents with a grade 3 sacral pressure sore. Examination shows a 7 × 8 cm chronic wound with eschar, fibrinous exudate, and granulation in the wound bed. **In order to optimize accuracy at the time of surgical debridement, which one of the following adjuncts would be most useful intraoperatively?**

D. Methylene blue dye

Traditional approaches to surgical debridement are based on clinical examination of the wound to assess for nonviable and viable tissues with the intention to surgically remove all nonviable tissues, while preserving all viable tissues. In general, sharp debridement is performed progressively with a scalpel, scissors, curette, or high-powered water jet stream (hydrosurgery) until bleeding healthy tissues are visualized in the wound bed. With clinical experience, this can be performed accurately and consistently to a high level. However, in order to help accuracy of debridement, a technique of using methylene blue dye has been described as a particularly useful adjunct. Using this approach, methylene blue dye is applied to the wound bed and the peripheral wound edges are also marked. The wound edges are sharply refreshed, and the wound base is debrided such that all of the blue stained tissues are removed. Once the blue stained tissues have been removed, there should remain only healthy tissues. Further assessment of this can be via a colorimetric approach where three colors will signify healthy tissue: Red (muscle), white (fascia and paratenon), and yellow (fat, bone). Other colors such as gray, green, purple, or black are not normally found in healthy wound beds and should be further debrided.[1]

Quantitative tissue cultures are considered by some to be an important adjunct to wound debridement, especially where there is or there has been a prosthesis or chronic wound. For example, in cases of orthopedic metalwork infection and associated osteomyelitis, multiple tissue samples of bone and soft tissue can be sent for culture before and after wound debridement to assess infection status and obtain microbiologic characterization. However, this will not provide on-table results to guide debridement. Most microbiological testing requires at least 36 hours to process. Furthermore, there may be difficulties in ensuring accuracy, which is affected by many factors.[2]

Frozen section biopsy is another useful assessment tool for characterizing tissue and is most commonly performed to assess for tumor presence. Key diagnostic indications are to prove or disprove malignancy and confirm a tissue diagnosis. Frozen section biopsy is also strongly indicated to assess for tumor clearance at the margin where larger, more complex tumors have been resected. In principle, it is possible to have frozen section to assess tissue normality and viability, but in reality, it is not used in this form.[3]

Iodine solution is commonly used as a skin preparation for its microbial effects and so is important in surgical wound preparation, but it is not specifically helpful to guide the surgical debridement process per se.

Indocyanine green (ICG) dye is generally indicated for use in plastic surgery to assess flap perfusion intraoperatively, for example, when planning and executing a perforator flap design. It forms part of an angiographic imaging modality. Intravenous ICG is delivered so that tissue perfusion can be assessed using dynamic laser fluorescence videography. It uses a digital video camera system and a near-infrared light. It has been used to help assess wounds following trauma and burns so it may have a role in cases such as that described in future practice. However, it may be best used to plan surgery prior to reaching the operating room and at present still remains more experimental than in mainstream use.[4]

REFERENCES

1. Anghel EL, DeFazio MV, Barker JC, Janis JE, Attinger CE. Current concepts in debridement: science and strategies. Plast Reconstr Surg 2016;138(3, Suppl):82S–93S
2. Kallstrom G. Are quantitative bacterial wound cultures useful? J Clin Microbiol 2014;52(8):2753–2756
3. Jaafar H. Intra-operative frozen section consultation: concepts, applications and limitations. Malays J Med Sci 2006;13(1):4–12
4. Kamolz LP, Andel H, Auer T, Meissl G, Frey M. Evaluation of skin perfusion by use of indocyanine green video angiography: rational design and planning of trauma surgery. J Trauma 2006;61(3):635–641

COMPLICATIONS OF RADIOTHERAPY

8. A 68-year-old male has undergone postsurgical radiotherapy to the right side of the neck and mandible for management of an intraoral squamous cell carcinoma (SCC). He now presents with symptoms of pain and swelling over the mandible and has reduced mouth opening. Examination shows bone exposed through the skin surface (sequestrum). *Which one of the following would be the most useful for treatment of this clinical problem?*

A. Hyperbaric oxygen

Osteoradionecrosis (ORN) is a condition where bone death occurs secondary to radiation and is most commonly seen in the mandible following treatment of head and neck cancers. Symptoms of ORN can be severe with significant impact on patients' quality of life. Key problems include chronic pain, nonhealing wounds, limited mouth opening, and mouth ulcers. It is related to high doses of radiation and occurs because of the damaging effects of radiation on tissue vascularity. The condition is difficult to treat and the main approaches include hyperbaric oxygen therapy and surgery to remove the affected bone.

Hyperbaric oxygen therapy involves breathing pure oxygen in a pressurized room. It is used for many conditions ranging from decompression sickness, carbon monoxide poisoning, infections, and wound healing problems. Patients are positioned in a chamber either individually or with other patients and the air pressure in the chamber is increased to three times the normal air pressure at sea level, providing supranormal levels of oxygen. There is a substantial research evidence base to support its use, but not all centers will have access to this treatment modality. For ORN, patients will need multiple episodes in the hyperbaric chamber.[1]

Transcutaneous oxygen tension (TcPO2) is a measure (not a treatment) of a response to oxygen administration as a surrogate marker for reversible ischemia. Normal levels are 400 mm Hg or greater. It has been used to provide a measure of lower limb peripheral vascular insufficiency.

Stem cell therapy has a number of potential uses in plastic and reconstructive surgery including the potential for regeneration of skin, cartilage, and bone. However, its use in general wound healing presently lacks high level evidence. There have been small studies evaluating the effects of stem cells in ORN as well as animal models in rats, which may, in future, provide some benefit for ORN patients.[2]

Platelet-rich plasma contains high concentrations of growth factors and is used in a number of situations including sports medicine, orthopedics, general surgery, dermatology, and plastic surgery. It is thought to help in wound healing and have beneficial effects on skin quality as a rejuvenation procedure. It may also help male pattern baldness. However, its use still lacks high level evidence in terms of precise usage and outcomes. One study assessed the benefits of platelet-rich plasma in prevention of ORN, but failed to show any significant benefit.[3]

A diagnosis of ORN is made on clinical grounds with the exposure of necrotic bone (sequestra) with ulceration of the skin and/or mucous membranes in the absence of evidence of tumor recurrence. In a patient with a clinical diagnosis of ORN, although tissue biopsies and cultures can be helpful to exclude tumor, to prove evidence of necrosis, and provide information on infection, they would not specifically help treat the condition.

REFERENCES

1. Fan H, Kim SM, Cho YJ, Eo MY, Lee SK, Woo KM. New approach for the treatment of osteoradionecrosis with pentoxifylline and tocopherol. Biomater Res 2014;18:13
2. Manimaran K, Sankaranarayanan S, Ravi VR, Elangovan S, Chandramohan M, Perumal SM. Treatment of osteoradionecrosis of mandible with bone marrow concentrate and with dental pulp stem cells. Ann Maxillofac Surg 2014;4(2):189–192

3. Batstone MD, Cosson J, Marquart L, Acton C. Platelet rich plasma for the prevention of osteoradionecrosis. A double blinded randomized cross over controlled trial. Int J Oral Maxillofac Surg 2012;41(1):2–4

SELECTION OF SKIN SUBSTITUTES

9. You are considering the use of a biologic skin substitute in a patient with a burn. Your patient is concerned about the use of tissues from animals and states that he would only consent to products that are purely synthetic or human derived. *Which one of the following products is acceptable for use in this patient?*

E. AlloDerm

A number of biologic skin substitutes are available. They can be classified according to composition: human derived, animal derived, synthetic, or a combination of these. All of the products listed contain animal derivatives, with the exception of AlloDerm (LifeCell, Branchburg, NJ). This is a regenerative tissue matrix derived from cadaveric human dermis. It has been used successfully in burn patients to reduce joint contracture.[1] It has also been used in breast and abdominal wall reconstruction. Biobrane (Smith and Nephew, London) is a biologic skin substitute comprising of silicone, nylon, and porcine collagen. It is used in the acute setting for management of partial-thickness burns, especially in children. It can accelerate healing, decrease pain, and reduce dressing changes. ACell line of products (Columbia, MD) are comprised of porcine urinary bladder matrix and are available in powder and sheet formations. They are intended for use in burn wounds, and pressure and venous ulcers. Integra is a bilayer of outer silicone combined with inner bovine collagen and glygosaminoglycans. It is used in burn surgery in both the acute and elective settings. SurgiMend (Integra LifeSciences, Plainsboro, NJ) is a bovine-derived acellular dermal matrix and is used in abdominal wall reconstruction. (See question 8 answer and Chapter 9, *Essentials of Plastic Surgery,* third edition.)

REFERENCE

1. Yim H, Cho YS, Seo CH, et al. The use of AlloDerm on major burn patients: AlloDerm prevents post-burn joint contracture. Burns 2010;36(3):322–328

BIOLOGIC SKIN SUBSTITUTES

10. *Which one of the following biologic dressings is a bilayer construct containing bovine collagen, human fibroblasts, and keratinocytes?*

E. Apligraf

Apligraf (Organogenesis Canton, MA) is a bioengineered skin substitute marketed for use in diabetic foot and venous leg ulcers. It has FDA approval for use in both of these conditions. It comprises a bilayer of bovine collagen and human foreskin-derived fibroblast matrix under human foreskin-derived keratinocytes. It therefore provides both cells and matrix for the nonhealing wound.[1]

Matriderm (Medskin Solutions, DR, Suwelack AG, Billerbeck, Germany) is a dermal matrix with bovine dermal collagen (Types I, III, and IV), elastin, and silicone sheeting. It is used beneath split skin grafts to provide a thicker soft tissue cover with the intention of providing superior cosmetic results than split skin graft alone.

ReCell (Avita Medical, Cambridge, UK) is an autologous noncultured cell therapy delivered as a cellular suspension. It is marketed for use in acute thermal burn injury and involves harvesting cells from the patient intraoperatively (as a very small split skin graft) which can then be sprayed as a suspension onto the burn injury following chemical and mechanical breakdown. The spray is then applied instead of using a split-thickness skin graft. A proposed benefit of ReCell is the very significantly reduced donor site, which in one trial was reduced by 40 times.[2]

Acelagraft (Celgene Cellular Therapeutics, Cedar Knolls, NJ) is a decellularized, dehydrated, frozen human amniotic membrane product that is marketed for use in wounds including the corneal and conjunctival surfaces of the globe. Epicel (Genzyme Biosurgery, Cambridge, MA) is a cultured epidermal autograft derived from the patients' own skin. It is intended for use in management of deep dermal or full-thickness burns and has FDA approval for this. Epicel grafts are made by harvesting skin cells from a patient and growing them in an incubator on mouse cells. The skin sample is typically the size of a postage stamp. The finished grafts are used to provide skin cover either with split skin grafts or instead of them. Epicel grafts can be grown in a relatively short time frame with 100% of total body surface area (TBSA) in less than 4 weeks.

REFERENCES

1. Zaulyanov L, Kirsner RS. A review of a bi-layered living cell treatment (Apligraf) in the treatment of venous leg ulcers and diabetic foot ulcers. Clin Interv Aging 2007;2(1):93–98
2. Holmes JH, Molnar JA, Carter JE, et al. A comparative study of the ReCell® device and autologous split-thickness meshed skin graft in the treatment of acute burn injuries. J Burn Care Res 2018;39(5):694–702

3.   Sutures and Needles

See Essentials of Plastic Surgery, third edition, pp. 21–31

SUTURE CHARACTERISTICS

1. *Following closure of an abdominoplasty with 2-0 Vicryl sutures, which one of the following is correct?*
   A. The sutures will lose half of their tensile strength within 1 week.
   B. The absorption process will occur through proteolysis.
   C. The rate of suture absorption will be unpredictable.
   D. The absorption process will be enzyme mediated.
   E. Inflammation will be less than if a natural suture was used.

NONABSORBABLE SUTURES

2. *Which one of the following statements is correct regarding nonabsorbable sutures?*
   A. Suture materials with greater memory form more secure knots.
   B. Monofilament sutures display superior knot security compared with braided sutures.
   C. *Elasticity* is the tendency of a suture to return to its original length after stretching.
   D. Sutures with more memory are also more pliable and easier to handle.
   E. *Capillarity* refers to the tendency of a suture to absorb fluid and swell.

SUTURE SPECIFICATION

3. *What does the #-0 value refer to in a 3-0 nylon suture?*
   A. The suture diameter in Imperial measurement.
   B. The suture diameter in Metric measurement.
   C. The suture diameter in French measurement.
   D. The suture USP breaking strength.
   E. The relative breaking strength compared to stainless steel.

NEEDLE CONFIGURATIONS

4. The configuration of a needle varies according to its intended use. *Which one of the following statements is correct regarding needle selection?*
   A. A conventional cutting needle is ideal for suturing skin under tension.
   B. Taper needles are occasionally used for tendon repairs.
   C. The reverse cutting needle is more likely to result in *cheese wiring* of the dermis.
   D. Blunt tip needles are reserved for ophthalmic surgery.
   E. The point of a standard cutting needle is on the inner curve of the needle.

CURVED NEEDLE CHARACTERISTICS

5. Curved suture needles are commonly used in plastic surgery. *Which one of the following statements is correct regarding their needle characteristics?*
   A. Needle length is usually the same as chord length.
   B. Chord length is unaffected by needle curvature.
   C. Chord length is the direct distance between the needle point and swage.
   D. Needle diameter is the same as chord length.
   E. Curve radius can vary with five-eighths circle being most popular for plastic surgery applications.

ABSORBABLE SUTURES

6. *Which one of the following absorbable sutures is unusual in that it is available in either monofilament or braided versions?*
   A. Vicryl
   B. Vicryl Rapide
   C. Caprosyn
   D. Monocryl
   E. Dexon

NONABSORBABLE SUTURES

7. *Which one of the following nonabsorbable sutures is a braided synthetic available in coated or uncoated variants with moderate reactivity and good memory and handling?*
   A. Polyester
   B. PDS
   C. Chromic gut
   D. Silk
   E. Nylon

WOUND CLOSURE

8. *Which one of the following statements is true regarding wound closure?*
   A. Braided sutures are popular for closure of animal bite wounds.
   B. Infection within a wound will slow the process of suture absorption and result in more suture granuloma problems.
   C. In the rat model, skin can be expected to regain 20% of its original strength after 1 week, and almost 95% by 6 weeks.
   D. Polydiaxone (PDS) is unlikely to adequately support a healing wound until 50% of original wound strength has been regained.
   E. Closure with stainless steel staples is rapid and causes a low amount of local tissue ischemia.

RAILROAD SCARS

9. *Why does the punctuate component of the railroad scar develop?*
   A. Localized pressure necrosis
   B. Over-tightening of sutures
   C. Localized wound infection
   D. Re-epithelialization around the suture
   E. Premature suture removal

MICROSURGICAL SUTURES

10. *When selecting appropriate sutures for microsurgical anastomoses, which one of the following statements is correct?*
    A. A 10-0 nylon suture is the best choice for repair of a 100% divided radial artery.
    B. Different microsuture materials have broadly similar handling characteristics.
    C. An 8-0 suture is the best choice for repair of an adult proper digital artery.
    D. Sutures used for microsurgery are commonly nylon, polypropylene, or polyglytone.
    E. Microsuture needle characteristics decrease uniformly as suture material diameter decreases.

WOUND CLOSURE ADJUNCTS

11. A patient is undergoing closure of the abdomen after a belt lipectomy and reinforcement of the lower anterior abdomen. *Which one of the following may be helpful to reduce both operating time and the suture material bulk within the wound?*
    A. Mesh suture
    B. Barbed suture
    C. Suture bridge device
    D. Embrace
    E. Pop off suture

WOUND CLOSURE ADJUNCTS

12. When closing the skin in a wound following a debridement of a facial bite injury, you advise your resident to use an antibacterial suture. *Which one of the following is the active component included in such an antibacterial suture design?*
    A. Flucloxacillin
    B. Augmentin
    C. Triclosan
    D. Chlorhexidine
    E. Bacitracin

Answers

SUTURE CHARACTERISTICS

1. *Following closure of an abdominoplasty with 2-0 Vicryl sutures, which one of the following is correct?*

E. Inflammation will be less than if a natural suture was used.

Absorption of suture material can be either hydrolytic (which is more common and results in less tissue inflammation) or proteolytic. There is variation in the rate of suture absorption depending on material type (see **Table 3.1**), but Vicryl sutures will take 2–3 weeks for their strength to decrease to 50%. Most absorbable sutures lose half their strength within the first 4 weeks and will eventually be completely absorbed. The rate of absorption is proportional to the degree of polymerization and is quite predictable for any given suture. Some sutures such as Vicryl Rapide and Caprosyn (Polyglytone 6211) should be avoided in areas that require longer support as they lose half their strength in the first week. Proteolytic absorption is enzyme mediated and is associated with natural sutures such as those derived from beef or sheep intestine, which are often referred to as cat gut. Synthetic sutures such as polydiaxone (PDS) and polyglactin (Vicryl) absorb by the process of hydrolysis where water from tissues is absorbed into the suture material resulting in disruption of cross-links within the polymeric structure.[1]

Table 3.1   *Qualities of Absorbable Sutures*

Composition (Proprietary Name)	Time to 50% Strength	Configuration	Reactivity	Memory
Gut	Unpredictable			
Fast	5-7 days	Monofilament	High	Low
Plain	7-10 days	Monofilament	High	Low
Chromic	10-14 days	Monofilament	High	Low
Polyglytone 6211 (Caprosyn*)	5-7 days	Monofilament	Low	Medium
Poliglecaprone 25 (Monocryl†)	7-10 days	Monofilament	Low	Medium
Glycomer 631 (Biosyn†)	2-3 weeks	Monofilament	Low	Medium
Glycolide/lactide copolymer Low molecular weight (Vicryl Rapide*)	5 days	Braided	Low	Low
Regular (Polysorb†, Vicryl*)	2-3 weeks	Braided	Low	Low
Polyglycolic acid (Dexon S†)	2-3 weeks	Monofilament or braided	Low	Low
Polyglyconate (Maxon†)	4 weeks	Monofilament	Low	High
Polydioxanone (PDS II*)	4 weeks	Monofilament	Low	High

*Ethicon
†Covidien

REFERENCE

1. Friedman J, Mosser SW. Closure material. In: Evans G, ed. Operative Plastic Surgery. New York: McGraw-Hill; 2000

NONABSORBABLE SUTURES

2. *Which one of the following statements is correct regarding nonabsorbable sutures?*

C. *Elasticity* is the tendency of a suture to return to its original length after stretching.

Elasticity is the tendency of a suture to return to its original length after stretching and can be helpful in wounds where postoperative swelling is anticipated by ensuring that the suture retains sufficiently tight closure after the swelling reduces. Memory refers to the tendency of a suture to return to its original shape and sutures with more memory are usually less pliable, more difficult to handle, and have less knot security. For example, PDS has greater memory than Monocryl or Dexon. Knot security refers to the force required to cause a knot to slip and will be increased with braided sutures such as Vicryl or Ethibond, compared with monofilament sutures such as Monocryl. Fluid absorption is the amount of fluid retained by a suture and capillarity refers to the movement of fluid along the suture. Sutures with greater capillarity (for example, braided subtypes) are more likely to become colonized with bacteria, potentially leading to wound infection. The braided nature of these sutures also provides a greater surface area and recesses for organisms to adhere. For these reasons, sutures such as nylon are less likely to harbor infection when compared with a braided alternative such as Vicryl.

SUTURE SPECIFICATION

3. *What does the #-0 value refer to in a 3-0 nylon suture?*

    D. The suture USP breaking strength.

It is a common misconception that the #-0 rating refers to the diameter of a suture. However, the rating for sutures refers to the United States Pharmacopeia (USP) breaking strength rating, rather than suture diameter.[1] Therefore, two different types of 3-0 suture can have different diameters but share the same breaking strength. As #-0 rating increases for any given suture, the diameter and breaking strength will both decrease.

REFERENCE

1. United States Pharmacopeia, Vol. 29. Rockville, MD: United States Pharmacopeia; 2006

NEEDLE CONFIGURATIONS

4. The configuration of a needle varies according to its intended use. *Which one of the following statements is correct regarding needle selection?*

    E. The point of a standard cutting needle is on the inner curve of the needle.

There are five main types of needles: conventional cutting, reverse cutting, side cutting, taper point, and blunt tip. Each has a particular use/indication (**Fig. 3.1**).

A standard cutting needle has its cutting surface or point on the inner curve and is at risk of tearing through the tissues causing cheese wiring when closing wounds under tension. In contrast, a reverse cutting needle has its

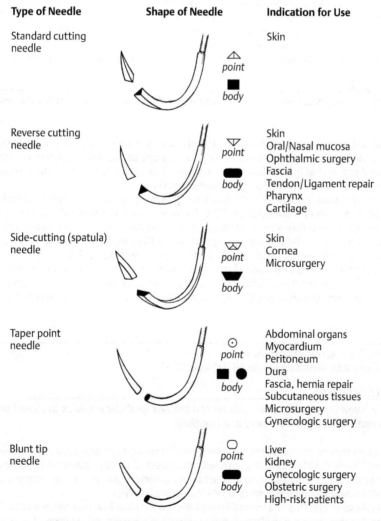

Type of Needle	Shape of Needle	Indication for Use
Standard cutting needle	point / body	Skin
Reverse cutting needle	point / body	Skin Oral/Nasal mucosa Ophthalmic surgery Fascia Tendon/Ligament repair Pharynx Cartilage
Side-cutting (spatula) needle	point / body	Skin Cornea Microsurgery
Taper point needle	point / body	Abdominal organs Myocardium Peritoneum Dura Fascia, hernia repair Subcutaneous tissues Microsurgery Gynecologic surgery
Blunt tip needle	point / body	Liver Kidney Gynecologic surgery Obstetric surgery High-risk patients

Fig. 3.1 Needle shapes and their indications in surgery.

cutting edge on the outer curve and is therefore less likely to cause cheese wiring. Side cutting needles have two cutting surfaces or points and can be used in skin closure to reduce cheese wiring. Taper point or round bodied needles do not have a cutting surface on the needle beyond the sharp tip and are the standard choice for tendon repair to prevent cutting through the tendon fibers and previously placed suture passes/knots. Blunt tip needles are used for intra-abdominal surgery and some high-risk patients.

CURVED NEEDLE CHARACTERISTICS

5. Curved suture needles are commonly used in plastic surgery. *Which one of the following statements is correct regarding their needle characteristics?*

   C. Chord length is the direct distance between the needle point and swage.

   Fig. 3.2 shows the key components of a curved needle. A needle has a point or tip at the leading edge and a swage at the other end where the thread is attached. Needle length is the distance from the swage to the needle point along the length of the needle body. Chord length is the direct or shortest distance between the swage and the needle point. It is therefore shorter than needle length in a curved needle. The curvature of a needle refers to the amount of a full circle involved and ranges from one-fourth to five-eighths, with three-eighths being most common in plastic surgery applications. Chord length will differ according to needle curvature and will be greatest with the half-circle needle. Needle diameter refers to the thickness of the needle itself and is determined by the balance between providing sufficient material strength yet maintaining the smallest diameter possible for the required size suture.

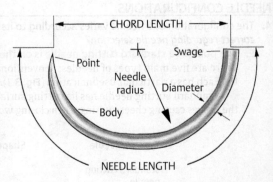

Fig. 3.2   Characteristics of a curved needle.

ABSORBABLE SUTURES

6. *Which one of the following absorbable sutures is unusual in that it is available in either monofilament or braided versions?*

   E. Dexon

   Dexon is an absorbable suture made from polyglycolic acid. It is unusual in that it is available in either braided or monofilament versions, where most sutures are generally one or the other. It shares similar characteristics, and hence uses, to Vicryl in that it has a low reactivity, with low memory, and loses 50% strength in 2–3 weeks. It is useful in skin closure for dermal and subcuticular situations.

   Vicryl is a braided suture made from Polyglactin 910 that is popular for use in the skin and closure of the oral lining, muscle, and tying off blood vessels. Vicryl Rapide is a similar braided suture to Vicryl but has a lower molecular weight and therefore loses its strength in just 5 days rather than 2–3 weeks. This suture is often used as an external skin suture in infants and younger children. Caprosyn is made from Polyglytone 6211 and shares some characteristics with Vicryl Rapide in that it has a rapid rate of absorption giving it a time to 50% strength for 5–7 days. It is a monofilament with low reactivity and medium memory. Monocryl is another monofilament and is made from poliglecaprone. It is a popular choice for buried skin closure in plastic surgery as it handles well and has a low reactivity. Biosyn (Glycomer 631) is similar to Monocryl but retains its strength for 1–2 weeks longer.[1,2]

REFERENCES

1. Covidien, 2012. Available at www.covldlen.com
2. Ethicon. Wound Closure Manual. Somerville, NJ: Ethicon; 2005

NONABSORBABLE SUTURES

7. *Which one of the following nonabsorbable sutures is a braided synthetic available in coated or uncoated variants with moderate reactivity and good memory and handling?*

   A. Polyester

   Polyester sutures may be uncoated such as Mersilene (Ethicon) or coated such as Ethibond (Ethicon), Surgidac (Covidien), and Ticron (Covidien). Coating involves the process of adding a lubricant to improve suture passage and handling. Polyester sutures may be used for tendon or ligament repair and some surgeons use them for securing the superficial musculoaponeurotic system (SMAS) during face lifts.

   PDS is polydiaxone and this is a monofilament suture that has low reactivity and maintains 50% strength until 4 weeks. For this reason, it is often useful in closure of deep wounds such as closing Scarpa's fascia during abdominoplasty. Gut is an absorbable suture available in different subtypes. Plain gut loses half its strength in 1 week and chromic gut loses half its strength in 2 weeks. Silk is a nonabsorbable braided suture that will still lose its strength over time and is often used for vessel ties and marker sutures (see **Tables 3.1 and 3.2**).

Nylon is a permanent suture, which is most often a monofilament (Ethilon) but is sometimes braided (Nurolon). It is commonly used for external wound closure in plastic surgery for the head and neck regions. It may also be used for deep permanent sutures as an alternative to polypropylene (Proline). It has a low reactivity and memory differs depending on whether it is a monofilament or braided product.

Table 3.1   *Qualities of Absorbable Sutures*

Composition (proprietary name)	Time to 50% Strength	Configuration	Reactivity	Memory
Gut	Unpredictable			
Fast	5-7 days	Monofilament	High	Low
Plain	7-10 days	Monofilament	High	Low
Chromic	10-14 days	Monofilament	High	Low
Polyglytone 6211 (Caprosyn*)	5-7 days	Monofilament	Low	Medium
Poliglecaprone 25 (Monocryl†)	7-10 days	Monofilament	Low	Medium
Glycomer 631 (Biosyn†)	2-3 weeks	Monofilament	Low	Medium
Glycolide/lactide copolymer Low molecular weight (Vicryl Rapide*)	5 days	Braided	Low	Low
Regular (Polysorb†, Vicryl*)	2-3 weeks	Braided	Low	Low
Polyglycolic acid (Dexon S†)	2-3 weeks	Monofilament or braided	Low	Low
Polyglyconate (Maxon†)	4 weeks	Monofilament	Low	High
Polydioxanone (PDS II*)	4 weeks	Monofilament	Low	High

*Ethicon
†U.S. Surgical Corporation

Table 3.2   *Qualities of Nonabsorbable Sutures*

Composition (Proprietary Name)	Tensile Strength	Configuration	Reactivity	Memory/ Handling
Silk	Lost in 1 year	Braided	High	–/Good
Nylon Monofilament (Ethilon*, Monosof-Dermalon†)	81% at 1 year, 72% at 2 years,	Monofilament	Low	+/Fair
Braided (Nurolon*, Surgilon†)	66% at 11 years	Braided	Low	–/Good
Polypropylene (Prolene*, Surgipro†)	Indefinite	Monofilament	Low	+ +/Poor
Polybutester Uncoated (Novafil†)	Indefinite	Monofilament	Low	+/Fair
Coated (Vascufil†)	Indefinite	Monofilament	Low	–/Good
Polyester Uncoated (Mersilene*)	Indefinite	Braided	Moderate	–/Good
Coated (Ethibond*, Surgidac†, Ticron†)	Indefinite	Braided	Moderate	–/Good
Surgical steel	Indefinite	Monofilament or braided	Low	+ +/Poor

*Ethicon
†Covidien

WOUND CLOSURE

8. Which one of the following statements is true regarding wound closure?
  E. Closure with stainless steel staples is rapid and causes a low amount of local tissue ischemia.
  Stainless steel clips have a number of advantages over sutures for wound closure. Closure is faster and they cause less local tissue ischemia. Some surgeons feel that there is little or no difference in the cosmetic outcome when comparing skin staples to sutures and they certainly can be useful in certain situations such as closure of scalp wounds where they also have a useful hemostatic effect. When using staples on the trunk or limbs, it is important to ensure that a deep layer of sutures is still present if the staples are to be removed sufficiently early (5–7 days) in order to avoid permanent staple marks.[1]

In general, monofilament sutures are a better choice than braided alternatives for closing wounds that have a high risk of developing postoperative infection (e.g., debrided bite wounds) because bacteria may be less adherent to them (as discussed in question 2). Infection in a wound will accelerate the process of suture absorption.

In the rat model, as described by Levenson et al,[2] skin strength can be expected to regain 5% of its original strength in 1 week, 50% by 4 weeks, and 80% by 6 weeks. In this model, wound strength at 1 year is thought to reach only 80% of original strength. PDS will have retained 50% of its original strength at 4 weeks and will remain in the wound for longer than 12 weeks. It will therefore support a wound until at least 60–70% of its original strength has been regained (see Fig. 3.4, *Essentials of Plastic Surgery*, third edition).

One downside to staples is that they are rigid and thus provide no ability to give or expand to accommodate postoperative soft tissue swelling. Hence, there may be an increased risk of pressure damage to the skin surface which is associated with development of the parallel row component of "railroad scars."

REFERENCES

1. Shuster M. Comparing skin staples to sutures. Can Fam Physician 1989;35:505–509
2. Levenson SM, Geever EF, Crowley LV, Oates JF III, Berard CW, Rosen H. The healing of rat skin wounds. Ann Surg 1965;161:293–308

RAILROAD SCARS

9. *Why does the punctuate component of the railroad scar develop?*
   D. Re-epithelialization around the suture
   A railroad scar has two main components: punctuate scars and parallel rows of scar between them. The punctuate component occurs because of re-epithelialization around the suture which causes a cylindrical cuff leading to a permanent suture tract. Early suture removal may help avoid this process. The parallel rows result from pressure necrosis on the skin and subcutaneous tissues and are exacerbated by over-tightening of sutures and delayed suture removal (**Fig. 3.3**).

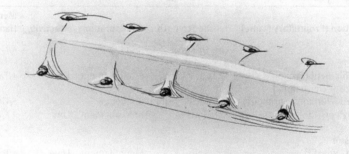

Fig. 3.3 Appearance of a railroad scar following delayed suture removal.

MICROSURGICAL SUTURES

10. *When selecting appropriate sutures for microsurgical anastomoses, which one of the following statements is correct?*
   B. Different microsuture materials have broadly similar handling characteristics.
   Handling characteristics are largely similar between different microsuture materials, although differences can occur between needles depending on their size, shape, and needle point. The choice of suture size depends on the vessel or structure size. For example, repair of the radial artery is satisfactorily achieved with an 8-0 nylon (Ethilon). A 10-0 is usually unnecessarily small and is more appropriate for repair of an adult digital vessel. Suture materials in microsurgery are monofilament permanent materials like nylon and polypropylene (Prolene and Surgipro). Polyglytone is an absorbable suture material used for wound closure (Caprosyn). It has a rapid absorption similar to Vicryl Rapide and would therefore not be well suited for use in microvascular anastomoses nor microsurgical nerve repair. Moving from a 9-0 to a 10-0 does not necessarily mean the needle will be smaller so needle size should always be confirmed before opening the suture material.

WOUND CLOSURE ADJUNCTS

11. A patient is undergoing closure of the abdomen after a belt lipectomy and reinforcement of the lower anterior abdomen. *Which one of the following may be helpful to reduce both operating time and the suture material bulk within the wound?*

B. Barbed suture

Barbed sutures have been designed with the intention of reducing the total internal suture volume and decreasing surgical operating time, by reducing the number of internal knots tied. They have one-way barbs along the length of the suture placed evenly and may help distribute and maintain tension across or along a wound. A caveat with this type of suture is that the surgeon is unable to backtrack and remove or revise suture placement and also the tightness of the suture pull through cannot be adjusted once tightened antegrade in a way that a traditional subcuticular monofilament suture can be. Most of the major suture manufacturers have a barbed suture in their range and their use for skin closure is driven by surgeon's preference.[1]

The use of a mesh suture has been described for high tension internal abdominal wall closures/repairs, as well as patients with an abdominal ventral wall hernia.[2] It also has intended uses within orthopedic surgery. The principle of using polypropylene mesh as a suture tie technique has been described by Lanier et al.[2] In this study, strips of polypropylene mesh were passed through the abdominal wall without an integrated swaged needle. The Duramesh suture is a device made from macroporous polypropylene with an integrated swaged needle.

Using this device reduces suture pull through by redistributing forces over a broader surface area. Once tied, the knots maintain porosity and should allow improved tissue incorporation. Souza et al[3] neatly illustrated use of this suture in an animal model displaying improved resistance to suture pull through compared with traditional polypropylene sutures. This device is intended for deep suture repair but not the skin.

Embrace (Neodyne Biosciences Inc, Menlo Park, Ca) is a silicone elastomeric dressing that is used following wound closure. It is applied to the incision site and is changed on a weekly basis for 60 days. The dressing is intended to contract and offload the skin's natural tension. In one multicenter randomized controlled trial (RCT), scar quality was improved when using this device.[4,5]

The suture bridge device is currently an experimental device used to lift sutures away from the skin in order to disperse pressure from the skin and ideally reduce both pressure effects and epidermal inflammation. In animal studies, it has been shown to increase tensile strength in the early days following tissue injury and repair.[6]

REFERENCES

1. Rubin JP, Hunstad JP, Polynice A, et al. A multicenter randomized controlled trial comparing absorbable barbed sutures versus conventional absorbable sutures for dermal closure in open surgical procedures. Aesthet Surg J 2014;34(2):272–283
2. Lanier ST, Dumanian GA, Jordan SW, Miller KR, Ali NA, Stock SR. Mesh Sutured Repairs of Abdominal Wall Defects. Plast Reconstr Surg Glob Open 2016;4(9):e1060
3. Souza JM, Dumanian ZP, Gurjala AN, Dumanian GA. In vivo evaluation of a novel mesh suture design for abdominal wall closure. Plast Reconstr Surg 2015;135(2):322e–330e
4. Lim AF, Weintraub J, Kaplan EN, et al. The embrace device significantly decreases scarring following scar revision surgery in a randomized controlled trial. Plast Reconstr Surg 2014;133(2):398–405
5. Longaker MT, Rohrich RJ, Greenberg L, et al. A randomized controlled trial of the embrace advanced scar therapy device to reduce incisional scar formation. Plast Reconstr Surg 2014;134(3):536–546
6. Townsend KL, Akeroyd J, Russell DS, Kruzic JJ, Robertson BL, Lear W. Comparing the Tolerability of a Novel Wound Closure Device Using a Porcine Wound Model. Adv Wound Care (New Rochelle) 2018;7(6):177–184

WOUND CLOSURE ADJUNCTS

12. When closing the skin in a wound following a debridement of a facial bite injury, you advise your resident to use an antibacterial suture. *Which one of the following is the active component included in such an antibacterial suture design?*

C. Triclosan

There are a number of manufacturers offering antibacterial sutures. Ethicon's range of Monocryl, Vicryl, and PDS are all available in antibacterial versions, each designated as "Plus." The antibacterial component is triclosan, which is an antibacterial and antifungal, that blocks fatty acid synthesis. There have been many studies assessing the benefits of using such sutures to reduce the risk of surgical site infections (SSIs), and in general it is thought that there is an advantage to using this type of sutures (level I evidence). However, the benefits will depend on factors such as the site and type of wounds being closed.[1,2] Flucloxacillin and Augmentin are both systemic antibiotics given either orally or intravenously. Each is potentially useful in reducing surgical site infections. Augmentin is generally the selected antibiotic of choice in human bite wounds such as in this case. Chlorhexidine is a useful skin preparation with antiseptic and disinfectant qualities rather than antibacterial qualities. Cleaning the wound with this can be a useful adjunct in management of a human bite injury prior to debridement and closure. Bacitracin is an antibacterial that can be used topically in preparations as a single agent or combined with polymyxin B in Polyfax ointment. This may be useful postoperatively in such cases. As appropriate debridement has already been performed, there is probably little real indication in this case for their use.

REFERENCES

1. Leaper D, Wilson P, Assadian O, et al. The role of antimicrobial sutures in preventing surgical site infection. Ann R Coll Surg Engl 2017;99(6):439–443
2. Konstantelias AA, Andriakopoulou CS, Mourgela S. Triclosan-coated sutures for the prevention of surgical-site infections: a meta-analysis. Acta Chir Belg 2017;117(3):137–148

4.   Basics of Flaps

See *Essentials of Plastic Surgery*, third edition, pp. 32–56

BLOOD SUPPLY TO FLAPS

1. **Which one of the following is correct regarding blood supply to flaps?**
   A. Fasciocutaneous flaps rely most heavily on the subfascial vascular plexus.
   B. Axial pattern flaps are based on the subdermal plexus and are limited by set width to length ratios.
   C. An *angiosome* is defined as an area of skin only supplied by a named source artery.
   D. The parasympathetic system is most important in regulating blood flow to the skin.
   E. Neurocutaneous flaps are based on perforating arteries accompanying a cutaneous nerve.

FLAP CLASSIFICATION

2. Flaps can be classified in a number of ways. **Which one of these is most clinically relevant?**
   A. Method of movement
   B. Tissue composition
   C. Vascular supply
   D. Size and depth
   E. Geometric configuration

PERFORATOR FLAPS

3. **Which one of the following is the key advantage of a perforator flap versus a muscle (myocutaneous) flap in free tissue transfer?**
   A. Ease and speed of harvest
   B. Preservation of donor site function
   C. Reduced fat necrosis and wound healing problems
   D. More consistent vessel anatomy
   E. Reduced anastomotic complications

VENOUS FLAPS

4. **Which one of the following is correct regarding venous flaps?**
   A. They tend to have very predictable survival outcomes.
   B. They are traditionally classified into five groups according to vascular anatomy.
   C. They are commonly sensate given the proximity of cutaneous nerves.
   D. The mechanism of flap perfusion is poorly understood.
   E. Donor site morbidity is typically increased compared to arterial flaps.

CLASSIFICATION OF MUSCLE FLAPS

5. Muscle flaps may be grouped according to their vascular anatomy. **Which one of the following is correct regarding the Mathes and Nahai classification of muscle flaps?**
   A. The tensor fascia lata (TFL) flap is a type III flap.
   B. Type IV flaps have one dominant pedicle with secondary segmental pedicles.
   C. The gluteus maximus represents a type II muscle flap.
   D. Flap types I, III, and V have the most reliable vascularity.
   E. The gracilis flap has two dominant pedicles but no secondary segmental pedicles.

FLAP SELECTION

6. **Which one of the following would be a potential advantage of a free muscle flap rather than a free fasciocutaneous flap for reconstruction following resection of osteomyelitis of the tibia?**
   A. It would be more pliable.
   B. It would avoid the need for a split skin graft.
   C. It would accelerate postsurgical rehabilitation.
   D. It would decrease wound bacterial concentration.
   E. It would create less donor site morbidity.

BONE FLAPS

7. *Which one of the following is true of a vascularized compared with a nonvascularized bone reconstruction?*
   A. It will undergo callous formation and secondary healing.
   B. It will withstand subsequent radiation treatment poorly.
   C. It cannot reliably be used as a composite flap with skin.
   D. It will decrease the surgical procedure time.
   E. It can be combined with integrated implants.

FLAP MANIPULATION

8. Prefabrication and prelamination refer to processes that may be applied to flaps used in tissue reconstruction. *What is the key principle involved in prefabrication that is not part of the prelamination process?*
   A. Insertion of a new blood supply prior to transfer
   B. Insertion of cartilage graft prior to transfer
   C. Insertion of skin graft prior to transfer
   D. Insertion of bone graft prior to transfer
   E. Insertion of nerve graft prior to transfer

LOCAL FLAP TECHNIQUES

9. *Which one of the following statements regarding local flaps is correct?*
   A. Advancement flaps are traditionally single-pedicle rectangular flaps.
   B. Rotation flaps can be facilitated by the use of Burow's triangles or back-cuts.
   C. Transposition flaps are usually rotated laterally about a pivot point into a distant defect.
   D. A Z-plasty is a variation of an advancement flap.
   E. Limberg and Dufourmentel flaps have identical angles.

Z-PLASTY DESIGN

10. You are selecting the internal angles for a Z-plasty procedure. *What angle should provide a theoretical 50% increase in central limb length?*
    A. 10 degrees
    B. 30 degrees
    C. 45 degrees
    D. 60 degrees
    E. 90 degrees

USE OF THE Z-PLASTY

11. *Which one of the following is correct regarding Z-plasty procedures?*
    A. A 75-degree Z-plasty provides the best compromise for central limb lengthening.
    B. Multiple Z-plasties in series are more effective for increasing skin length than a single, large Z-plasty.
    C. The double-opposing semicircular flap modification can effectively close circular defects.
    D. Actual gain in central limb length is very close to the theoretically predicted values.
    E. A Z-plasty with 90-degree internal angles provides the least tension on closure.

FLAP PHYSIOLOGY

12. *Which one of the following acts as a vasoconstrictor on flap microcirculation?*
    A. Thromboxane A_2
    B. Bradykinin
    C. Acidosis
    D. Prostaglandin E_1
    E. Hypercapnia

FLAP DELAY

13. You are planning to delay a flap for reconstruction of a large skin defect to the head and neck. *Which one of the following is correct regarding flap delay?*
    A. It will require two surgical procedures spaced 3–5 days apart.
    B. It will specifically improve long-term survival of the entire flap.
    C. Delay preconditions the flap to ischemia but often results in early tissue necrosis.
    D. Flap tip viability is improved as a result of increased blood flow coupled with a decreased oxygen requirement.
    E. Of the five proposed mechanisms of flap delay, sympathetic stimulation is probably most important.

PHARMACOLOGIC INFLUENCES ON FREE FLAP SURVIVAL

14. *Based on reliable evidence, which one of the following is recommended for use in free tissue transfer to improve anastomotic patency during the first week?*
    A. Dextran
    B. Unfractionated heparin
    C. Low-molecular-weight heparin
    D. Calcium channel blockers
    E. Aspirin

FLAP FAILURE

15. *What is the most common primary reason for a flap to fail in the early postoperative period?*
    A. Venous insufficiency
    B. Arterial insufficiency
    C. Intrinsic flap swelling
    D. Mechanical trauma
    E. Systemic patient factors

FLAP RECONSTRUCTION

16. *Which one of the following is true regarding flap reconstruction?*
    A. A tubed-pedicled groin flap can be used to reconstruct the neck in two stages.
    B. Functional muscle transfer will always require coaptation of a nerve.
    C. Skin and bone flaps are more tolerant of ischemia than muscle flaps.
    D. A transferred functional muscle should be inset tighter than its original tension.
    E. Ischemia-induced reperfusion injury is greatest in pedicled tissue transfer.

LEECH THERAPY

17. You are reviewing a congested skin flap on the ward 12 hours following surgery. Your resident suggests treatment with medicinal leeches. *Which one of the following is true regarding this type of treatment?*
    A. The risk of anaphylaxis is low unless patients have a nut allergy.
    B. A short course (1 week) of amoxicillin/clavulanate is recommended.
    C. The leeches will release substances which provide an anticoagulant effect.
    D. Secretion of hyaluronic acid by the leeches will result in tissue swelling.
    E. Bacterial infection with mycobacterium is commonly observed.

FREE FLAP MONITORING

18. You are asked to assess a patient 24 hours after breast reconstruction with a deep inferior epigastric perforator (DIEP) flap. *Which one of the following is the least helpful discriminator between arterial and venous occlusion in this flap?*
    A. Capillary refill time
    B. Flap tissue turgor
    C. Flap skin color
    D. Flap surface temperature
    E. Flap dermal bleeding

FREE FLAP MONITORING

19. *Which one of the following is considered to be the most effective method for monitoring free flaps postoperatively?*
    A. External Doppler ultrasound
    B. Transcutaneous oxygen tension
    C. Surface temperature
    D. Fluorescein injection
    E. Clinical observation

FREE FLAP SALVAGE

20. A 48-year-old female undergoes free tissue transfer for breast reconstruction. She returns to operating room for re-exploration of the flap 12 hours following the surgery as there are concerns about its viability. Intraoperative findings show thrombus within the flap pedicle beyond the anastomosis. *Which one of the following agents may be most useful to help salvage this flap?*
    A. Nitroglycerin
    B. Lidocaine
    C. Pentobarbitol
    D. Calcium channel blocker
    E. Tissue plasminogen activator

FLAP MONITORING

21. You are writing the postoperative instructions for monitoring of a free ALT flap following reconstruction of a mastoid defect. *What frequency of flap observations will you advise for the initial postsurgical period based on the principles of flap salvage?*
    A. Half hourly for the first 24 hours and hourly for the following 48 hours
    B. Half hourly for the first 24 hours and 2 hourly for the following 48 hours
    C. Hourly for the first 24 hours and 4 hourly for the following 48 hours
    D. 2 hourly for the first 24 hours and 3 hourly for the following 48 hours
    E. 4 hourly for the first 24 hours and 6 hourly for the following 48 hours

Answers

BLOOD SUPPLY TO FLAPS

1. *Which one of the following is correct regarding blood supply to flaps?*

    E. **Neurocutaneous flaps are based upon perforating arteries accompanying a cutaneous nerve.**

    Neurocutaneous flaps (such as the sural flap) receive their blood supply through the arteries accompanying the nerve.[1] Fasciocutaneous flaps are supplied by different levels of vascular plexus including the subfascial, intrafascial, and the intradermal layers, but the suprafascial and subdermal plexuses are considered to be the most important. *Axial pattern flaps* contain a specific direct cutaneous artery within the longitudinal axis of the flap. Examples include the pedicled groin and paramedian forehead flaps. This means they are not limited by specifically set width to length ratios. An angiosome refers to a composite unit of skin and the underlying deep tissue supplied by a source artery, not just the skin area alone. The sympathetic (not parasympathetic) system is most important in regulating blood flow to the skin. Flaps based on the subdermal plexus that are limited to particular width to length ratios are described as *random pattern flaps;* for example, a transverse rectangular advancement flap on the forehead.[2–4]

REFERENCES

1. Masquelet AC, Romana MC, Wolf G. Skin island flaps supplied by the vascular axis of the sensitive superficial nerves: anatomic study and clinical experience in the leg. Plast Reconstr Surg 1992;89(6):1115–1121
2. Nakajima H, Fujino T, Adachi S. A new concept of vascular supply to the skin and classification of skin flaps according to their vascularization. Ann Plast Surg 1986;16(1):1–19
3. Taylor GI, Caddy CM, Watterson PA, Crock JG. The venous territories (venosomes) of the human body: experimental study and clinical implications. Plast Reconstr Surg 1990;86(2):185–213
4. McGregor IA, Morgan G. Axial and random pattern flaps. Br J Plast Surg 1973;26(3):202–213

FLAP CLASSIFICATION

2. Flaps can be classified in a number of ways. *Which one of these is most clinically relevant?*

    C. **Vascular supply**

    A flap is a unit of tissue that has its own blood supply and may be transferred from one part of the body to another using this blood supply. There are a number of different ways to classify flaps including the vascularity, the method of movement, and the tissue composition. Having a thorough understanding of the classification categories and their subtypes is useful in understanding the principles of flaps. Furthermore, although there are merits in each of the different classifications used, the most clinically valid is the intrinsic vascularity, as it is the most critical determinant of a successful transfer.[1,2]

REFERENCES

1. Daniel RK, Kerrigan CL. Principles and physiology of skin flap surgery. In: McCarthy JG, ed. Plastic Surgery, Vol. 1. Philadelphia: Saunders; 1990
2. Taylor GI, Palmer JH. The vascular territories (angiosomes) of the body: experimental study and clinical applications. Br J Plast Surg 1987;40(2):113–141

PERFORATOR FLAPS

3. *Which one of the following is the key advantage of a perforator flap versus a muscle (myocutaneous) flap in free tissue transfer?*

    B. **Preservation of donor site function**

    Both perforator and muscle free flaps each have advantages and disadvantages (see **Boxes 4.1** and **4.2**).

Advantages	Disadvantages
Numerous potential donor sites	Tedious pedicle dissection
Often able to incorporate muscle, fat, and bone into flap design	Variation in perforator anatomy and size
Preserve muscle function	Increased risk of fat necrosis compared with myocutaneous flaps
Minimal donor site morbidity	
Reduced postoperative recovery time and pain medication requirements	
Versatility of size and thickness	

BOX 4.2   *ADVANTAGES AND DISADVANTAGES OF MUSCLE AND MYOCUTANEOUS FLAPS*

Advantages	Disadvantages
Potential to obliterate dead space with vascularized tissue	Donor site morbidity (functional deficit)
Increased resistance to infection	Flap bulk

Perforator flaps typically consist of skin and subcutaneous tissues supplied by a single isolated perforating vessel or multiple isolated perforating vessels joined to a main vascular pedicle. The key advantage to using a perforator flap compared with a muscle flap is that the underlying muscle function is preserved and donor site morbidity is reduced. For example, the skin and subcutaneous tissues of the lower anterior abdomen can be raised on one or more perforators of the deep inferior epigastric vessels (DIEP) without causing significant damage or loss of function to the rectus abdominis muscles or abdominal wall, through which the vessels pass. The same area of skin and soft tissue can also be harvested by sacrificing the rectus abdominis on one side by keeping attachment of the muscle, fascia, subcutaneous tissues, and skin en bloc (transverse rectus abdominis myocutaneous [TRAM] flap). The DIEP flap is the gold standard for autologous breast reconstruction, so it is very commonly used in plastic surgery.

Other advantages of perforator flaps include versatility of size and tissue thickness.

Incorporating muscle within a flap increases tissue bulk, so perforator flaps tend to be thinner and more pliable and also have less donor site morbidity in general. They are also associated with the potential for reduced postoperative pain and more rapid recovery.

The other options listed are all potential disadvantages to perforator flaps except option E. Perforator flaps are generally more technically challenging to raise and so it can often take longer to raise than a muscle-based flap. They tend to have higher rates of fat necrosis and hence may carry an increased risk of wound healing complications. The perforator vessel anatomy is not always consistent in terms of vessel size and location. For this reason, preoperative handheld Doppler assessment and sometimes computed tomography (CT) angiography are helpful. There should be no difference in terms of anastomotic complications between muscle and perforator flaps as the anastomoses are ultimately performed on the same vessels, e.g., TRAM versus DIEP (**Fig. 4.1**).[1-4]

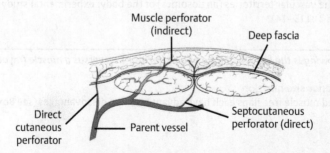

Fig. 4.1   Perforator flaps allow preservation of muscle and hence donor site function. There are different types of perforator. These include direct and indirect vessels. Direct perforators perforate deep fascia only, indirect muscle perforators travel through muscle before piercing the deep fascia, and indirect septal perforators travel through the intermuscular septum before piercing the deep fascia.

REFERENCES

1. Geddes CR, Morris SF, Neligan PC. Perforator flaps: evolution, classification, and applications. Ann Plast Surg 2003;50(1):90–99
2. Nahabedian MY, Momen B, Galdino G, Manson PN. Breast Reconstruction with the free TRAM or DIEP flap: patient selection, choice of flap, and outcome. Plast Reconstr Surg 2002;110(2):466–475, discussion 476–477
3. Celik N, Wei FC, Lin CH, et al. Technique and strategy in anterolateral thigh perforator flap surgery, based on an analysis of 15 complete and partial failures in 439 cases. Plast Reconstr Surg 2002;109(7):2211–2216, discussion 2217–2218
4. Chen HC, Tang YB. Anterolateral thigh flap: an ideal soft tissue flap. Clin Plast Surg 2003;30(3):383–401

VENOUS FLAPS

4. *Which one of the following is correct regarding venous flaps?*

D. The mechanism of flap perfusion is poorly understood.

The mechanism of flap perfusion is not well understood for venous flaps. Suggested mechanisms of venous flap perfusion include plasmatic imbibition, perfusion pressure, arteriovenous anastomoses, perivenous arterial networks, vein-to-vein interconnections, and circumvention of venous valves. Not only is their physiology poorly understood, survival can be unpredictable. Thatte and Thatte[1] have classified the following three types (not five) of venous flaps according to their vascular anatomy:

Type I is a unipedicled venous flap with a single cephalad vein as the only vessel.

Type II is a bipedicled flow-through venous flap.

Type III is an arterialized venous flap in which one end of the vein is anastomosed to a feeding artery.

Venocutaneous flaps are not usually sensate; it is neurocutaneous flaps such as the sural flaps that have this quality. Donor site morbidity is sometimes said to be reduced when compared to an arterial flap because no arterial sacrifice is required (see Fig. 4.2).

REFERENCE

1. Thatte MR, Thatte RL. Venous flaps. Plast Reconstr Surg 1993;91(4):747–751

CLASSIFICATION OF MUSCLE FLAPS

5. Muscle flaps may be grouped according to their vascular anatomy. *Which one of the following is correct regarding the Mathes and Nahai classification of muscle flaps?*

D. Flap types I, III, and V have the most reliable vascularity.

The Mathes and Nahai classification[1] of muscle flap supply is as follows:

Type I: One vascular pedicle (e.g., tensor fascia lata)

Type II: One dominant and one or more minor pedicles (e.g., gracilis)

Type III: Two dominant pedicles (e.g., gluteus maximus)

Type IV: Segmental vascular pedicle (e.g., sartorius)

Type V: One dominant pedicle with secondary segmental pedicles (e.g., latissimus dorsi)

Types I, III, and V have the most reliable blood supply for transfer as the entire muscle can be moved based on a single pedicle or segmental branches.

The TFL flap is a type I flap as it has one dominant pedicle arising from the lateral circumflex femoral artery. It may be harvested with an anterolateral thigh (ALT) flap: The gluteus maximus is a type III flap (not type II) as it has two dominant vascular pedicles, namely, the superior and inferior gluteals. This means that the entire muscle can be based on either vessel.

An example of a type IV flap is the sartorius. The challenge of using such a flap for reconstruction is that the segmental blood supply limits movement as a pedicled flap to ensure vascularity is maintained. It would not be useful as a free flap because only part of the muscle can be harvested on any given segmental supply. One scenario where the sartorius is used clinically is in a switch procedure during groin dissection for large vessel coverage. In this setting, the upper segmental supply is sacrificed to allow movement of the muscle. The latissimus dorsi muscle is a real workhorse muscle flap in plastic surgery and is classified as type V by the Mathes and Nahai classification. It can be moved as a pedicled flap on either the segmental supply or main pedicle to reconstruct the chest wall and back areas, or as a free flap based on the main pedicle (thoracodorsal artery) (**Fig. 4.2**).

REFERENCE

1. Mathes SJ, Nahai F. Classification of the vascular anatomy of muscles: experimental and clinical correlation. Plast Reconstr Surg 1981;67(2):177–187

Single-pedicled venous flap

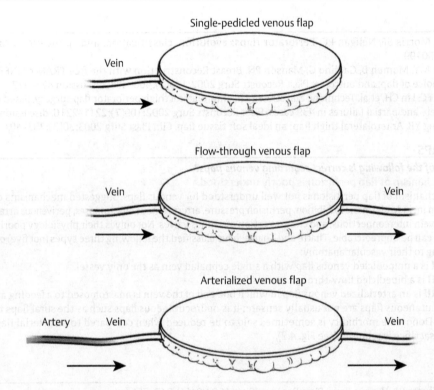

Fig. 4.2 Three types of venous flaps. (Adapted from Inoue G, Suzuki K. Arterialized venous flap for treating multiple skin defects of the hand. Plast Recontr Surg 91:299–302; discussion 303–306, 1993.)

FLAP SELECTION

6. **Which one of the following would be a potential advantage of a free muscle flap rather than a free fasciocutaneous flap for reconstruction following resection of osteomyelitis of the tibia?**

    D. **It would decrease wound bacterial concentration.**

    The use of myocutaneous flaps has been associated with a decrease in bacterial contamination within wounds compared with the use of fasciocutaneous flaps to reconstruct the same defect.[1,2] They are therefore generally accepted to be preferable in wounds associated with recent infection such as an osteomyelitis case or a delayed open fracture soft tissue cover. Muscle flaps are also well suited for coverage of irradiated and more general traumatic wounds. Other advantages include the ability to obliterate dead space, and relative ease for flap raising. The pliability of a muscle flap is generally less than the equivalent fasciocutaneous flap due to flap bulk, and muscle flaps require split skin grafting unless a skin paddle is included. Taking muscle is likely to slow the postoperative rehabilitation rather than accelerate it, and would also tend to increase the donor site morbidity.[3,4]

REFERENCES

1. Gosain A, Chang N, Mathes S, Hunt TK, Vasconez L. A study of the relationship between blood flow and bacterial inoculation in musculocutaneous and fasciocutaneous flaps. Plast Reconstr Surg 1990;86(6):1152–1162, discussion 1163
2. Calderon W, Chang N, Mathes SJ. Comparison of the effect of bacterial inoculation in musculocutaneous and fasciocutaneous flaps. Plast Reconstr Surg 1986;77(5):785–794
3. Mathes SJ. Clinical Applications for Muscle and Myocutaneous Flaps. St Louis: Mosby; 1981
4. Mathes SJ, Nahai F. Classification of the vascular anatomy of muscles: experimental and clinical correlation. Plast Reconstr Surg 1981;67(2):177–187

BONE FLAPS

7. Which one of the following is true of a vascularized compared with a nonvascularized bone reconstruction?

E. It can be combined with integrated implants.

There are a number of advantages of vascularized bone flaps over nonvascularized alternatives. One of the main advantages is the ability to insert osseointegrated implants into the vascularized flap at the time of transfer. This is particularly useful in mandibular and maxillary reconstruction to provide dentition. The other key advantages are that larger bone defects can be reconstructed, they tend to undergo primary bone healing, and they withstand irradiation well (particularly important if adjuvant radiotherapy is indicated following tumor resection and reconstruction). Furthermore, most bone flaps can be harvested with skin or muscle to provide lining for the defect. The downsides are that a different set of surgical skills are required and surgical time is increased. Donor site morbidity may also be increased, although the disability associated with bone flap harvest is relatively low (see **Box 4.3**).[1-3]

BOX 4.3   *ADVANTAGES AND DISADVANTAGES OF VASCULARIZED BONE FLAPS*

Advantages	Disadvantage
Can reconstruct large bony defects	Donor site morbidity
Undergo primary bony healing	
Withstand radiation and implantation	
Can be transferred as a composite with other tissue types (e.g., scapular flap and free toe transfers)	

REFERENCES

1. Frodel JL Jr, Funk GF, Capper DT, et al. Osseointegrated implants: a comparative study of bone thickness in four vascularized bone flaps. Plast Reconstr Surg 1993;92(3):449–455, discussion 456–458
2. Foster RD, Anthony JP, Sharma A, Pogrel MA. Vascularized bone flaps versus nonvascularized bone grafts for mandibular reconstruction: an outcome analysis of primary bony union and endosseous implant success. Head Neck 1999;21(1): 66–71
3. Klein L, Stevenson S, Shaffer JW, Davy D, Goldberg VM. Bone mass and comparative rates of bone resorption and formation of fibular autografts: comparison of vascular and nonvascular grafts in dogs. Bone 1991;12(5):323–329

FLAP MANIPULATION

8. Prefabrication and prelamination refer to processes that may be applied to flaps used in tissue reconstruction. What is the key principle involved in prefabrication that is not part of the prelamination process?

A. Insertion of a new blood supply prior to transfer

Prefabrication is a form of flap manipulation where a new dominant vascular pedicle is buried in the planned flap territory prior to transfer. Approximately 6 weeks later, the flap is then elevated based on the new pedicle and transferred. Prefabrication is not a commonly used technique, in contrast to prelamination, which also involves two stages. The principle of prelamination is to reconstruct the new body part with composite tissues **prior** to transfer. In this way bone, cartilage, or skin grafts may be added to the flap in its original position based on the native blood supply. Examples of this in clinical practice include nasal reconstruction with either the forehead or radial forearm flaps. In fact, this is an approach typically reserved for head and neck reconstruction.[1-3]

REFERENCES

1. Pribaz JJ, Fine N, Orgill DP. Flap prefabrication in the head and neck: a 10-year experience. Plast Reconstr Surg 1999;103(3):808–820
2. Pribaz JJ, Fine NA. Prefabricated and prelaminated flaps for head and neck reconstruction. Clin Plast Surg 2001;28(2):261–272, vii
3. Sinha M. "Prefabricated" and "prelaminated" flaps: two very different techniques. J Plast Reconstr Surg 2007;60(12):13701372

LOCAL FLAP TECHNIQUES

9. Which one of the following statements regarding local flaps is correct?

B. Rotation flaps may be facilitated by the use of Burow's triangles or back-cuts.

Local flaps can be subclassified as *rotation, advancement, transposition,* or *interpolation*.

Rotation flaps often have a semicircular design and rotate about a pivot point into an adjacent defect (**Fig. 4.3**). Direct closure of the donor site is usually possible. Use of a back-cut or Burow's triangle at the base will change the pivot point which can increase the reach of the flap tip.

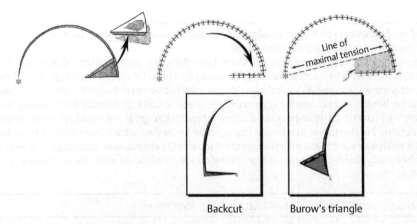

Fig. 4.3 Rotation flap. (*, Pivot point.)

Advancement flaps slide into an adjacent defect by stretching the skin or releasing subcutaneous tissues without rotation or lateral movement. They can be rectangular or V-Y shaped, and may be of single or double pedicle design. Incorporating small Burow's triangles at the base can increase advancement distance (**Figs. 4.4 and 4.5**). Transposition flaps have elements of rotation and lateral advancement, and they rotate around a pivot point into an adjacent defect. Common examples include rhomboid flaps and Z-plasty flaps (**Fig 4.6**).

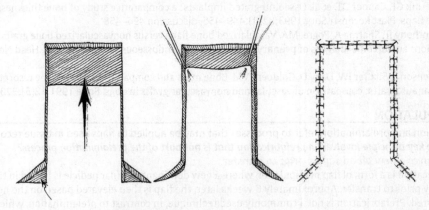

Fig. 4.4 Rectangular advancement flap. Burow's triangles allow increased advancement and eliminate dog-ears.

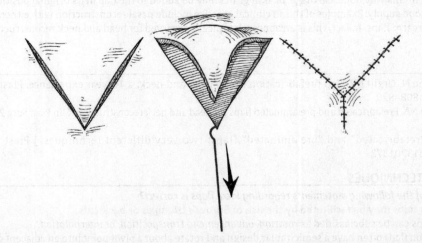

Fig. 4.5 V-Y advancement flap. The triangle of skin should have a length two to three times the diameter of the primary defect and a width equal to the greatest width of the primary defect.

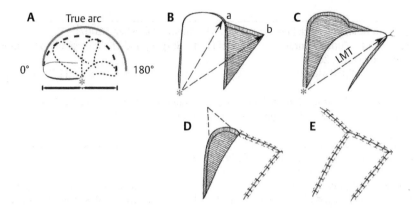

Fig. 4.6 *A*, The effective length of a flap becomes shorter the farther the flap is rotated. Therefore, it should be designed longer than the defect. *B–E*, Transposition flap. (*, Pivot point; *LMT*, line of maximal tension.)

Although Limberg and Dufourmentel flaps are both transposition flaps of a rhomboid design, they differ in the individual internal angles used. The Limberg flap is a rhomboid flap that uses two 60-degree angles and two 120-degree angles. The Dufourmentel flap is a narrower design with internal angles that are not fixed to specific numbers. The benefit of this flap is that it has a lesser arc of pivot and therefore reduces the likelihood of a dog-ear being created.[1]

REFERENCE

1. Jackson I. Local Flaps in Head and Neck Reconstruction. NY: Thieme Publishers; 2007

Z-PLASTY DESIGN

10. You are selecting the internal angles for a Z-plasty procedure. *What angle should provide a theoretical 50% increase in central limb length?*

   C. **45 degrees**

     A *Z-plasty* is a type of transposition flap with two adjacent triangular flaps that are reversed. Key factors in the design are that the three limbs should be of equal length, and the two internal angles should be equivalent (see Table 4.1, *Essentials of Plastic Surgery*, third edition). There is a consistent theoretical relationship between internal angle and percentage gain in central limb length. An angle of 30 degrees will allow an increase of 25%. Thereafter, for each increase in angle of 15 degrees, length increases by 25% (e.g., a 45-degree increase in angle gives a 50% increase in length, and a 60-degree increase in angle gives a 75% increase in length). In clinical practice actual gains in length may differ from the theoretical values because of skin laxity and adherence (**Fig. 4.7**).[1-5]

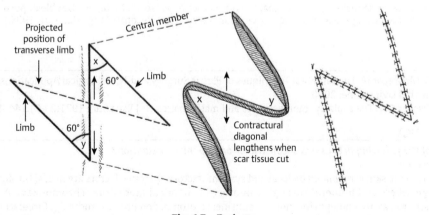

Fig. 4.7 Z-plasty.

REFERENCES

1. Jackson I. Local Flaps in Head and Neck Reconstruction. NY: Thieme Publishers; 2007
2. McGregor AD, McGregor IA. Fundamental Techniques of Plastic Surgery and Their Surgical Applications. 10th ed. Philadelphia: Churchill Livingstone; 2000
3. Rohrich RJ, Zbar RI. A simplified algorithm for the use of Z-plasty. Plast Reconstr Surg 1999;103(5):1513–1517, quiz 1518
4. Furnas DW, Fischer GW. The Z-plasty: biomechanics and mathematics. Br J Plast Surg 1971;24(2):144–160
5. Seyhan A. A V-shaped ruler to detect the largest transposable Z-plasty. Plast Reconstr Surg 1998;101(3):870–871

USE OF THE Z-PLASTY

11. Which one of the following is correct regarding Z-plasty procedures?

   C. The double-opposing semicircular flap modification can effectively close circular defects.

   The double-opposing Z-plasty technique involves a curvilinear modification of the Z-plasty principle and is used to close circular defects (**Fig. 4.8**). A 60-degree, rather than a 75-degree Z-plasty, provides the best compromise for achieving increased central limb length without significant lateral tension (see **Fig. 4.7**).

   Although combining multiple Z-plasties in series is a useful technique, more effective skin lengthening is achieved with a single, large Z-plasty. A number of techniques involve Z-plasties, such as the jumping-man flap and four-flap Z-plasty. Both of these can be useful for correction of first web space tightness (see Fig. 72.7, *Essentials of Plastic Surgery,* third edition). The jumping-man flap or double-opposing Z is created with a combination of Z-plasty flaps and a central V-Y advancement flap. The four-flap Z-plasty moves flaps from an initial ABCD orientation to CADB orientation following transfer. The actual gain in the central limb length following a standard Z-plasty differs from the theoretically predicted value. This can range from 55 to 84%. Use of the 90-degree Z-plasty provides a large theoretical gain in length but results in high tension across the wound closure.[1,2]

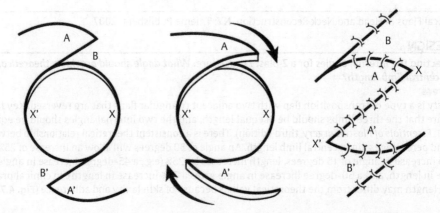

Fig. 4.8 Double-opposing semicircular flaps. (Adapted from Keser A, Sensoz O, Mengi AS. Double opposing semicircular flap: a modification of opposing Z-plasty for closing circular defects. Plast Reconstr Surg 102:1001, 1998.)

REFERENCES

1. McGregor AD, McGregor IA. Fundamental Techniques of Plastic Surgery and Their Surgical Applications. 10th ed. Philadelphia: Churchill Livingstone; 2000
2. Furnas DW, Fischer GW. The Z-plasty: biomechanics and mathematics. Br J Plast Surg 1971;24(2):144–160

FLAP PHYSIOLOGY

12. Which one of the following acts as a vasoconstrictor on flap microcirculation?

   A. Thromboxane A_2

   Blood flow to the skin is regulated by local and systemic factors. Systemic factors are neural through sympathetic adrenergic fibers and humeral through a number of chemical mediators. Thromboxane A_2 is a humoral vasoconstrictor, as are epinephrine, norepinephrine, serotonin, and prostaglandin F_{2a}. Circulating vasodilators include bradykinin, histamine, and prostaglandin-E_1. Local control is affected by metabolic factors including hypercapnia, hypoxia, and acidosis. Each of these acts primarily as a vasodilator.[1,2]

REFERENCES

1. Daniel RK, Kerrigan CL. Principles and physiology of skin flap surgery. In: McCarthy JG, ed. Plastic Surgery, Vol. 1. Philadelphia: Saunders; 1990
2. Peter FW, Franken RJ, Wang WZ, et al. Effect of low dose aspirin on thrombus formation at arterial and venous micro-anastomoses and on the tissue microcirculation. Plast Reconstr Surg 1997;99(4):1112–1121

FLAP DELAY

13. You are planning to delay a flap for reconstruction of a large skin defect to the head and neck. *Which one of the following is correct regarding flap delay?*

D. **Flap tip viability is improved as a result of increased blood flow coupled with a decreased oxygen requirement.**

Flap delay involves surgical interruption of a portion of the blood supply to a flap prior to transfer. It may be useful to improve the viable length of a given flap (i.e., improve tip viability) but it does not significantly affect more proximal areas such as the base which would have survived anyway. It requires two surgical procedures typically spaced 10–21 days apart. Although in animal models, flaps have been successfully divided at 3 days, this time interval is not normally advised in clinical cases. Flap delay should not result in tissue necrosis as vascularity should not be compromised to such an extent. The process should cause a milder degree of tissue ischemia.

There are two main theories regarding delay: that delay conditions tissues to ischemia allowing them to survive on less nutrient blood flow and that delay improves vascularity by opening up choke vessels between adjacent vascular territories. It is likely that a combination of these effects is responsible.

The five mechanisms believed to be involved in delay are sympathectomy, vascular reorganization, reactive hyperemia, acclimatization to hypoxia, and a nonspecific inflammatory reaction. Therefore, loss of sympathetic stimulation, as opposed to an increase in sympathetic stimulation, is proposed to be a factor in delay.[1,2]

REFERENCES

1. Chiu-Collins LL, Epstein JS, Chu EA. Delay of flap. In: Kountakis Stilianos E, ed. Encyclopedia of Otolaryngology, Head and Neck Surgery. ed. Springerlink; 2013
2. Hamilton K, Wolfswinkel EM, Weathers WM, et al. The delay phenomenon: a compilation of knowledge across specialties. Craniomaxillofac Trauma Reconstr 2014;7(2):112–118

PHARMACOLOGIC INFLUENCES ON FREE FLAP SURVIVAL

14. *Based on reliable evidence, which one of the following is recommended for use in free tissue transfer to improve anastomotic patency during the first week?*

C. **Low-molecular-weight heparin**

Of the medications listed, low-molecular-weight heparin has been shown to improve anastomotic patency while minimizing hemorrhage.[1] Dextran was originally used as a volume expander and can decrease platelet adhesiveness and procoagulant activity. It also increases bleeding time and has been shown to improve short-term microvascular patency. However, it is not routinely used because of its poor side effect profile including anaphylaxis, pulmonary edema, renal failure, and cardiac complications.[2–6]

Calcium channel blockers act on vascular smooth muscle and have been shown to improve flap survival in animal models, with no significant publications in human free flaps.[7] Aspirin acts on the cyclooxygenase pathway and decreases the synthesis of thromboxane A_2, a potent vasoconstrictor. Although some evidence suggests that anastomotic patency may be improved in the first 24 hours, beyond this time no further improvement is observed. There is currently no evidence to support the routine use of aspirin following free flap surgery.[8]

REFERENCES

1. Ritter EF, Cronan JC, Rudner AM, Serafin D, Klitzman B. Improved microsurgical anastomotic patency with low molecular weight heparin. J Reconstr Microsurg 1998;14(5): 331–336
2. Rothkopf DM, Chu B, Bern S, May JW Jr. The effect of dextran on microvascular thrombosis in an experimental rabbit model. Plast Reconstr Surg 1993;92(3):511–515
3. Zhang B, Wieslander JB. Improvement of patency in small veins following dextran and/or low-molecular-weight heparin treatment. Plast Reconstr Surg 1994;94(2):352–358
4. Salemark L, Knudsen F, Dougan P. The effect of dextran 40 on patency following severe trauma in small arteries and veins. Br J Plast Surg 1995;48(3):121–126
5. Hein KD, Wechsler ME, Schwartzstein RM, Morris DJ. The adult respiratory distress syndrome after dextran infusion as an antithrombotic agent in free TRAM flap breast reconstruction. Plast Reconstr Surg 1999;103(6):1706–1708

6. Brooks D, Okeefe P, Buncke HJ. Dextran-induced acute renal failure after microvascular muscle transplantation. Plast Reconstr Surg 2001;108(7):2057–2060
7. Huby M, Rem K, Moris V, Guillier D, Revol M, Cristofari S. Are prostaglandins or calcium channel blockers efficient for free flap salvage? A review of the literature. J Stomatol Oral Maxillofac Surg 2018;119(4):297–300
8. Peter FW, Franken RJ, Wang WZ, et al. Effect of low dose aspirin on thrombus formation at arterial and venous micro-anastomoses and on the tissue microcirculation. Plast Reconstr Surg 1997;99(4):1112–1121

FLAP FAILURE

15. What is the most common primary reason for a flap to fail in the early postoperative period?

   A. Venous insufficiency

   There are a number of potential reasons for flaps to fail including local factors such as a lack of arterial supply into the tissues, infection, bleeding, swelling, technical error, and trauma, as well as systemic factors such as poor nutrition, poor oxygenation, and poor compliance with postoperative care. However, the most common primary cause of flap failure across all flap types is venous insufficiency and this itself may occur secondary to some of the causes mentioned above.

   Venous insufficiency initially presents with signs of congestion including purple/blue discoloration and brisk capillary refill. Later, deepening of the purple color and fixed staining are key features. In free flaps, the venous insufficiency may be due to venous thrombus, or twisting or compression on the main vascular pedicle near to the anastomosis. Alternatively, there may be intrinsic venous failure within a flap as is seen in failing random pattern flaps and in the later stages of free or regional flaps where intravascular flap thrombi are features. It is important to recognize venous insufficiency early post surgery, as there may be steps taken to reduce or reverse this and avoid flap failure.[1–6]

REFERENCES

1. Smit JM, Zeebregts CJ, Acosta R, Werker PMN. Advancements in free flap monitoring in the last decade: a critical review. Plast Reconstr Surg 2010;125(1):177–185
2. Brown JS, Devine JC, Magennis P, Sillifant P, Rogers SN, Vaughan ED. Factors that influence the outcome of salvage in free tissue transfer. Br J Oral Maxillofac Surg 2003;41(1):16–20
3. Adams JF, Lassen LF. Leech therapy for venous congestion following myocutaneous pectoralis flap reconstruction. ORL Head Neck Nurs 1995;13(1):12–14
4. Novakovic D, Patel RS, Goldstein DP, Gullane PJ. Salvage of failed free flaps used in head and neck reconstruction. Head Neck Oncol 2009;1:33
5. Kroll SS, Schusterman MA, Reece GP, et al. Timing of pedicle thrombosis and flap loss after free-tissue transfer. Plast Reconstr Surg 1996;98(7):1230–1233
6. Hidalgo DA, Disa JJ, Cordeiro PG, Hu QY. A review of 716 consecutive free flaps for oncologic surgical defects: refinement in donor-site selection and technique. Plast Reconstr Surg 1998;102(3):722–732, discussion 733–734

FLAP RECONSTRUCTION

16. Which one of the following is true regarding flap reconstruction?

   C. Skin and bone flaps are more tolerant of ischemia than muscle flaps.

   Different tissues are able to tolerate periods of ischemia differently. This is clinically relevant in free flap transfer because the flap "off time" or ischemia time needs to be carefully limited. This is particularly true of flaps containing muscle or bowel, which tolerate prolonged ischemia poorly. It is generally accepted that the safe ischemia times for skin and bone are longer than those for other tissues (up to 3 hours).

   Tubed-pedicled reconstruction is an older method of reconstruction that has been largely superseded by free flap surgery. However, there may be situations where such an "old school" approach is warranted. One example is the tubed paramedian forehead flap for nasal reconstruction which is still in use. This type of procedure takes at least two stages in all cases, but to move a distance such as the groin to the neck would take additional stages.

   Functional muscle transfer is a useful way of replacing lost active joint function after nerve or muscle damage. The process can be performed with locoregional, pedicled transfer such as the latissimus dorsi for elbow flexion. Free flap functional muscle transfer includes the gracilis for facial reanimation. Any muscle transfer will require a blood and nerve supply, but coaptation is usually only required in free transfer as the usual nerve supply otherwise remains intact, e.g., latissimus dorsi transfer (thoracodorsal nerve). In free tissue transfer such as the gracilis to face, the nerve to gracilis (obturator nerve) may be coapted onto the hypoglossal nerve, nerve to masseter, or a cross face facial nerve graft. In terms of muscle tension for functional transfer, this should be set at the same tension as the transferring muscle was set for its original function, not tighter.

   Ischemia-induced reperfusion injury (IIRI) describes a process whereby direct cytotoxic injury occurs from accumulation of oxygen derived free radicals during flap ischemia. It is therefore a phenomenon of free tissue transfer rather than one of pedicled flaps.[1]

REFERENCE

1. Carroll WR, Esclamado RM. Ischemia/reperfusion injury in microvascular surgery. Head Neck 2000;22(7):700–713

LEECH THERAPY

17. You are reviewing a congested skin flap on the ward 12 hours following surgery. Your resident suggests treatment with medicinal leeches. *Which one of the following is true regarding this type of treatment?*

C. The leeches will release substances which provide an anticoagulant effect.

Medicinal leeches (*Hirudo medicinalis*) are used in patients where there is significant venous compromise in a flap and there are no surgical alternatives to improve venous outflow. They secrete a number of substances that affect coagulation. First, they inject hirudin (a naturally occurring anticoagulant that inhibits conversion of fibrin to fibrinogen) at the site of a bite. Second, they secrete hyalase which facilitates spread of hirudin through tissues, and third, they secrete a vasodilatory substance that also contributes to bleeding. They also have a mechanical effect of creating physical channels through which venous drainage can occur.

Use of medicinal leeches carries a risk of infection from the gram-negative rod (*Aeromonas hydrophila*) (not mycobacterium) and for this reason, antibiotics should be prescribed prophylactically. The antibiotic of choice would not be amoxicillin/clavulanate as there is resistance to this antibiotic by *Aeromonas hydrophila*. Instead, all patients having leech therapy should be prescribed fluroquinolones such as Ciprofloxacin.

The other risks of leech therapy include anaphylaxis, irrespective of nut allergy status, persistent bleeding, and excessive scarring. Furthermore, many patients will find them difficult to tolerate. That said, they can be beneficial in some cases.[1–3]

REFERENCES

1. Hackenberger PN, Janis JE. A comprehensive review of medicinal leeches in plastic and reconstructive surgery. Plast Reconstr Surg Glob Open 2019;7(12):e2555
2. Soucacos PN, Beris AE, Malizos KN, Kabani CT, Pakos S. The use of medicinal leeches, Hirudo medicinalis, to restore venous circulation in trauma and reconstructive microsurgery. Int Angiol 1994;13(3):251–258
3. Patel KM, Svestka M, Sinkin J, Ruff P IV. Ciprofloxacin-resistant Aeromonas hydrophila infection following leech therapy: a case report and review of the literature. J Plast Reconstr Aesthet Surg 2013;66(1):e20–e22

FREE FLAP MONITORING

18. You are asked to assess a patient 24 hours after breast reconstruction with a DIEP flap. *Which one of the following is the least helpful discriminator between arterial and venous occlusion in this flap?*

D. Flap surface temperature

Cutaneous free flap monitoring is predominantly based on clinical assessment, although a number of adjuncts are available.

Common clinical features assessed are tissue color, capillary return, tissue turgor, flap temperature, and dermal bleeding characteristics. Of these features, all can usually be used to discriminate between venous and arterial insufficiency with the exception of temperature, which is usually reduced in either case. A healthy flap should have a capillary refill time of 2–3 seconds. It should be a healthy pink color in pale skinned individuals. Tissue turgor should be normal. Low turgor indicates underfilling of the flap (i.e., arterial compromise) and increased turgor indicates venous congestion. Needle testing of the dermis can be helpful as a healthy flap should bleed bright red blood. No blood or serous fluid indicates there is no inflow and dark red blood suggests there is inadequate venous outflow (**Table 4.1**).[1]

Table 4.1 *Signs of Arterial Occlusion and Venous Congestion*

	Arterial Occlusion	Venous Congestion
Skin color	Pale, mottled, bluish, or white	Cyanotic, bluish, or dusky
Capillary refill	Sluggish	Brisker than normal
Tissue turgor	Prune like; turgor decreased	Tense, swollen; turgor increased
Dermal bleeding	Scant amount of dark blood or serum	Rapid bleeding of dark blood
Temperature	Cool	Cool

REFERENCE

1. Smit JM, Zeebregts CJ, Acosta R, Werker PMN. Advancements in free flap monitoring in the last decade: a critical review. Plast Reconstr Surg 2010;125(1):177–185

FREE FLAP MONITORING

19. *Which one of the following is considered to be the most effective method for monitoring free flaps postoperatively?*

E. Clinical observation

Despite a number of technologically advanced tools for monitoring free flaps, clinical observation remains the most widely used and consistent method for monitoring a free flap. Of the clinical assessment modalities, bleeding from a dermal wound is an accurate positive test, as the absence of bleeding indicates no arterial inflow, and dark red blood indicates venous outflow insufficiency. A failed flap will leak serous straw-colored fluid on dermal scratch testing. It is paramount to educate nursing and medical staff in accurate flap monitoring so that changes in flap appearance are identified and managed early. In buried flaps such as a bony fibula flap for reconstruction of the humerus, direct clinical observation of the flap is not possible so an internal Doppler placed on the artery or vein can be helpful. This involves securing a cuff around the vessel with ligaclips. The cuff is placed distal to the anastomosis and has a wire attached that connects to an external box providing audible confirmation of blood flow.[1]

REFERENCE

1. Smit JM, Zeebregts CJ, Acosta R, Werker PMN. Advancements in free flap monitoring in the last decade: a critical review. Plast Reconstr Surg 2010;125(1):177–185

FREE FLAP SALVAGE

20. A 48-year-old female undergoes free tissue transfer for breast reconstruction. She returns to operating room for re-exploration of the flap 12 hours following the surgery as there are concerns about its viability. Intraoperative findings show thrombus within the flap pedicle beyond the anastomosis. *Which one of the following agents may be most useful to help salvage this flap?*

E. Tissue plasminogen activator

Free flaps most commonly fail in the early postoperative period due to failure of the main flap anastomoses. When taken back to the operating room, a common finding is thrombus. A number of studies have shown successful flap salvage using intra-arterial injection of tissue plasminogen activator (TPA). Thrombolytic agents such as this stimulate the conversion of plasminogen to plasmin, which acts to cleave fibrin and breaks down thrombus. The first-generation agents included streptokinase and urokinase. Second-generation agents include tissue plasminogen activator (t-PA) and acylated plasminogen-streptokinase activator complex (APSAC). To use a product like t-PA successfully, it must be delivered directly into the flap vessels, so it is necessary to create an arteriotomy or open a small branch proximally in order to flush it through.[1-4]

Drugs that reduce vasospasm (i.e., vasodilators) are important in free flap surgery as dissection of vessels and general handling of them in preparation for the transfer tend to cause vasoconstriction. However, none of these are especially helpful in free flap salvage as in this case. Examples include lidocaine, calcium channel blockers such as verapamil, pentobarbitol, and papavarine. Nitroglycerin is also a topical vasodilator but its use in plastic surgery has been associated with improved survival of local skin flaps in animal models.[5] More recently, a large review compared the use of intraoperative use of nitroglycerin to prevent vasospasm as an alternative to papavarine and the results suggest this is an effective alternative for this purpose.[6]

REFERENCES

1. Serletti JM, Moran SL, Orlando GS, O'Connor T, Herrera HR. Urokinase protocol for free-flap salvage following prolonged venous thrombosis. Plast Reconstr Surg 1998;102(6): 1947–1953
2. Yii NW, Evans GR, Miller MJ, et al. Thrombolytic therapy: what is its role in free flap salvage? Ann Plast Surg 2001;46(6):601–604
3. Senchenkov A, Lemaine V, Tran NV. Management of perioperative microvascular thrombotic complications—the use of multiagent anticoagulation algorithm in 395 consecutive free flaps. J Plast Reconstr Aesthet Surg 2015;68(9):1293–1303
4. Casey WJ III, Craft RO, Rebecca AM, Smith AA, Yoon S. Intra-arterial tissue plasminogen activator: an effective adjunct following microsurgical venous thrombosis. Ann Plast Surg 2007;59(5):520–525
5. Rohrich RJ, Cherry GW, Spira M. Enhancement of skin-flap survival using nitroglycerin ointment. Plast Reconstr Surg 1984;73(6):943–948
6. Ricci JA, Singhal D, Fukudome EY, Tobias AM, Lin SJ, Lee BT. Topical nitroglycerin for the treatment of intraoperative microsurgical vasospasm. Microsurgery 2018;38(5):524–529

FLAP MONITORING

21. You are writing the postoperative instructions for monitoring of a free anterolateral thigh (ALT) flap following reconstruction of a mastoid defect. *What frequency of flap observations will you advise for the initial postsurgical period based on the principles of flap salvage?*

C. Hourly for the first 24 hours and 4 hourly for the following 48 hours

Postoperative free flap monitoring is very important in terms of the ability to salvage a flap if it changes in the early postoperative period and that change is identified early. Free flaps are most likely to stop flowing within the first 24 hours and then the risk of problems progressively decreases over the following days.

Given this, it is important to have very regular observations in the first 24-hour period following surgery. Therefore, most surgeons will request hourly observations of the flap itself and other key patient parameters such as blood pressure, pulse, fluid balance, oxygen saturations, and respiratory rate. Flap observations for skin flaps will normally include tissue turgor and capillary refill and may include either internal or external Doppler assessment and temperature assessment.

Hourly observations in this time frame provide a balance between overly arduous assessments, e.g., every 30 minutes, and yet a sufficiently early opportunity for the nursing and medical teams to act swiftly if a return to the operating room is required. Observations 2, 3, or 4 hourly in the first 24 hours would not provide this.

Recognition of a failing flap can enable the clinician to arrange a return to the operating room on an urgent basis. The cause of the failing flap can be identified and hopefully corrected. In a number of studies, it has been shown that salvage of failing free tissue transfers is most effective in the first 24 hours.[1]

In the second and third 24-hour periods, the risk of flap failure is less and therefore it is generally considered acceptable to reduce the intensity of the observations in this time period. There will be variations in the precise timing and factors specific to each case need to be considered. However, a sensible approach would be to drop down the observations to 4 hourly at this stage post surgery. This again provides a balance of reasonable monitoring. In general, the ability for successful flap salvage decreases as the time interval since surgery increases, while at the same time, the likelihood of the flap failing spontaneously also decreases. For this reason, the intensity within the first and second time periods will normally be different.

REFERENCE

1. Brown JS, Devine JC, Magennis P, Sillifant P, Rogers SN, Vaughan ED. Factors that influence the outcome of salvage in free tissue transfer. Br J Oral Maxillofac Surg 2003;41(1):16–20

5. Perforator Flaps

See *Essentials of Plastic Surgery*, third edition, pp. 57–68

ANATOMY OF PERFORATOR FLAPS

1. **Which one of the following statements is correct regarding perforator flaps?**
   A. An indirect perforator originates from the source artery and pierces the deep fascia without traversing any deeper structures.
   B. The terms *perforasome* and *angiosome* may be used interchangeably, given they are the same thing.
   C. A direct perforator passes directly through an intermediary structure before crossing the deep fascia en route to the skin.
   D. Vessels that are septocutaneous perforators are considered to be direct perforators.
   E. Any given perforasome is composed of multiple angiosomes arising from the same source vessel.

ANATOMY OF PERFORATOR FLAPS

2. **When attending a conference on recent flap reconstruction advances, there is discussion regarding "hot spots" in plastic surgery. *What does this term refer to?***
   A. A "hot spot" refers to any given flap's most reliable perforator
   B. Mapped areas of the body with high-density areas of perforators
   C. Cutaneous zones associated with elevated pain levels to avoid in flap design
   D. An invasive temperature-based method for intraoperative flap assessment
   E. Geographic areas of high intensity use of plastic surgical services

CLASSIFICATION OF PERFORATOR FLAPS

3. **Which one of the following is correct regarding the classification of perforator flaps?**
   A. The Gent consensus recommends the use of suffixes to indicate the muscles involved.
   B. The Canadian classification system considers the anatomic region and muscle name.
   C. The only difference between the Canadian and Gent classification systems is the use of the word *artery* within the flap title.
   D. No single universally accepted classification system exists for perforator flaps.
   E. The Gent consensus names flaps according to the nutrient source vessel only.

ANTEROLATERAL THIGH FLAP

4. **Which one of the following statements is correct regarding the anterolateral thigh flap?**
   A. It is a fasciocutaneous flap which obtains its dominant supply from the transverse branch of the lateral circumflex femoral artery.
   B. The correct Canadian nomenclature is anterior lateral thigh perforator (ALTAP) flap.
   C. The correct Gent consensus nomenclature is lateral circumflex femoral artery perforator (LCFAP).
   D. LCFAP-*s* indicates that an anterolateral thigh flap is based on a septocutaneous perforator.
   E. It is normally a type A fasciocutaneous flap using the Mathes and Nahai classification.

THE ANTEROLATERAL THIGH (ALT) FLAP

5. You are planning to reconstruct a 12 by 6 cm defect on the dorsal foot and ankle of a woman following leiomyosarcoma resection. She has a body mass index (BMI) of 38 and is hypertensive but is otherwise medically well. **Which one of the following is correct regarding the use of an ALT flap for this patient's reconstruction?**
   A. The standard ALT flap is ideal for reconstruction in this scenario.
   B. The ALT donor site will require skin grafting in this case.
   C. Preoperative donor site angiography is needed in this setting.
   D. A super thin perforator flap may be best for this woman's case.
   E. Pedicle length will be insufficient to reach to the posterior tibial vessels.

THE DEEP INFERIOR EPIGASTRIC ARTERY FLAP

6. **When considering the deep inferior epigastric artery flap, which one of the following represents a potential disadvantage to its use?**

A. Vascular pedicle length
B. Donor site morbidity
C. Lack of lifeboat options
D. Inflexibility to convert to a myocutaneous flap
E. Unpredictable perforator anatomy

TECHNIQUES FOR RAISING PERFORATOR FLAPS

7. While raising a deep inferior epigastric perforator (DIEP) flap for breast reconstruction, you are concerned regarding the size of the venae comitantes. The flap has been cut to size, preserving zones I through III. You have completed a satisfactory anastomosis and have inset the flap. The flap is running but capillary refill is very brisk and the flap is becoming blue. *Which one of the following is most likely to improve the flap viability?*
A. Further reduction of flap volume
B. Staged flap inset
C. Postoperative use of leech therapy
D. Anastomosis of the superficial inferior epigastric vein (SIEV)
E. Administration of systemic heparin

RAISING A PERFORATOR FLAP

8. You are planning to use a perforator flap to reconstruct a soft tissue defect and will be supervising your resident during the process. *Which one of the following should you tell them?*
A. The minimal perforator diameter should be 2.0 mm.
B. The inability to identify a visible perforator pulse does not matter.
C. The plane of dissection should be close to the perforator.
D. The perforator must be sited centrally in the skin flap.
E. Including two perforators is required for optimal flap viability.

DESIGNING A PERFORATOR FLAP

9. *When designing a freestyle perforator flap for reconstruction of a 9 cm diameter shoulder defect, which one of the following is the most useful preoperative investigation?*
A. Handheld Doppler
B. CT angiography
C. Laser Doppler flowmetry
D. Indocyanine green
E. Tissue oximetry

LATERAL CIRCUMFLEX FEMORAL ARTERY PERFORATOR FLAP

10. You are planning to use a pedicled lateral circumflex femoral artery perforator (LCFAP) flap to reconstruct an abdominal wall defect. *Which muscle often requires dissection when raising this flap?*
A. Vastus medialis
B. Gracilis
C. Gastrocnemius
D. Biceps femoris
E. Vastus lateralis

Answers

ANATOMY OF PERFORATOR FLAPS

1. **Which one of the following statements is correct regarding perforator flaps?**

   D. **Vessels that are septocutaneous perforators are considered to be direct perforators.**

   Perforator flaps are vascularized areas of skin and subcutaneous tissue receiving blood supply from one or more perforators originating from a named source vessel. The perforating vessels can pass directly from the source vessel without traversing any deep structures or indirectly through muscle. This has clinical relevance with regard to the ease and speed with which flaps can be raised. Flaps with an intramuscular perforator path are more challenging and time consuming to raise. Angiosomes and perforasomes are not identical. Taylor and Palmer[1] described the 40 angiosomes in 1987, and Taylor[2] subsequently related them to perforator flaps in 2003. Angiosomes represent a composite unit of skin and the underlying tissue supplied by a given source vessel. However, it was Saint-Cyr et al[3] who described the perforasome theory, representing a similar concept, but the composite tissue is based on a single perforator from a given source vessel. This means that multiple perforasomes form each angiosome and in consequence there are around 300 perforasomes described (**Fig. 5.1**).

REFERENCES

1. Taylor GI, Palmer JH. The vascular territories (angiosomes) of the body: experimental study and clinical applications. Br J Plast Surg 1987;40(2):113–141
2. Taylor GI. The angiosomes of the body and their supply to perforator flaps. Clin Plast Surg 2003;30(3):331–342, v
3. Saint-Cyr M, Wong C, Schaverien M, Mojallal A, Rohrich RJ. The perforasome theory: vascular anatomy and clinical implications. Plast Reconstr Surg 2009;124(5):1529–1544

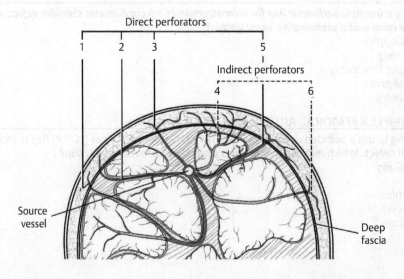

Fig. 5.1   The classic six distinct types of deep fascia perforators originally described by Nakajima.

ANATOMY OF PERFORATOR FLAPS

2. **When attending a conference on recent flap reconstruction advances, there is discussion regarding "hot spots" in plastic surgery. *What does this term refer to?***

   B. **Mapped areas of the body with high-density areas of perforators**

   "Hot spots" are described as cutaneous areas of the body which are known to have high perforator density. Accordingly, areas of lower density are described as "cold spots." The clinical relevance of this is that flap design incorporating a "hot spot" should ensure maximum inclusion of perforators and their required linking vessels, leading to more robust flap design and better chances of complete flap survival. The key hot spot areas are shown in **Fig. 5.2**.

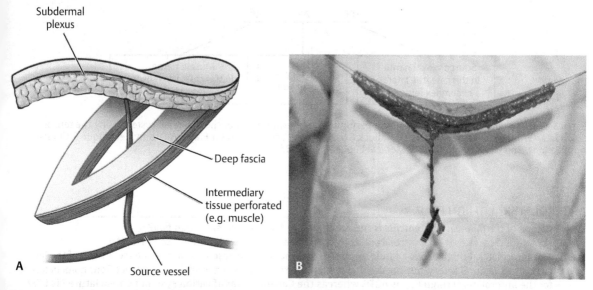

Fig. 5.2 A, Common perforator flap (myocutaneous type). **B,** Harvested perforator flap. Notice that the perforating vessel has been released from the source vessel and intermediary tissue (e.g., muscle).

The term is not related to high-density areas of nerve endings which would lead to increased pain levels associated with surgery. Although there are temperature-based modalities available which can be used for postoperative flap monitoring, such as surface temperature assessment and differential thermometry, they do not have an association with the "hot spot" terminology.

REFERENCE

1. Mohan AT, Sur YJ, Zhu L, et al. The concepts of propeller, perforator, keystone, and other local flaps and their role in the evolution of reconstruction. Plast Reconstr Surg 2016;138(4):710e–729e

CLASSIFICATION OF PERFORATOR FLAPS

3. *Which one of the following is correct regarding the classification of perforator flaps?*

D. No single universally accepted classification system exists for perforator flaps.

No single classification system for perforator flaps is universally accepted, but the two most commonly used are the Canadian classification system and the Gent consensus. In the Gent consensus, the flap is either named after the nutrient source vessel (e.g., deep inferior epigastric perforator [DIEP] flap) or the associated muscle or anatomic region in cases in which the source vessel supplies many other flaps (e.g., anterolateral thigh perforator [ALTP] or tensor fascia lata perforator [TFLP] flap).[1]

The Canadian classification system also names the flap according to the source vessel, with the addition of the word *artery* (e.g., deep inferior epigastric artery perforator [DIEAP] flap). In this system, when the source vessel supplies more than one flap, additional abbreviations are added. For example, a lateral circumflex femoral artery perforator flap involving the tensor fascia lata is named LCFAP-*tfl*[2] (**Fig. 5.3**).

REFERENCES

1. Blondeel PN, Van Landuyt KH, Monstrey SJ, et al. The "Gent" consensus on perforator flap terminology: preliminary definitions. Plast Reconstr Surg 2003;112(5):1378–1383, quiz 1383, 1516, discussion 1384–1387
2. Geddes CR, Morris SF, Neligan PC. Perforator flaps: evolution, classification, and applications. Ann Plast Surg 2003;50(1):90–99

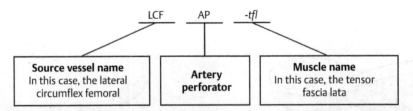

Fig. 5.3 An example of standardized muscle perforator nomenclature as per the Canadian system using the tensor fascia lata. (From Blondeel PN, Morris SF, Hallock GG, Neligan PC, eds. Perforator Flaps: Anatomy, Technique & Clinical Applications, 2nd ed. St Louis: Quality Medical Publishing, 2013.)

ANTEROLATERAL THIGH FLAP

4. *Which one of the following statements is correct regarding the anterolateral thigh flap?*

    D. LCFAP-*s* indicates that an anterolateral thigh flap is based on a septocutaneous perforator.

    The anterolateral thigh flap is a fasciocutaneous flap that may be based on the transverse branch of the lateral circumflex femoral artery, but the dominant supply is the descending branch. The correct Gent nomenclature[1] for the anterolateral thigh flap is ALTP, whereas the Canadian classification system nomenclature [2] is LCFAP. This becomes LCFAP-*vl* when the vastus lateralis is perforated (myocutaneous) and LCFAP-*s* when it is purely septocutaneous. The flap can be described using the Mathes and Nahai system according to the course of the perforator. This classification contains three subtypes: A, B, and C. Type A is a direct cutaneous flap, type B is a septocutaneous flap, and type C is a musculocutaneous or myocutaneous flap.[3]

    The ALT can be a septocutaneous flap (i.e., type B) and this is most easy to raise as no intramuscular dissection is required. Often there are perforators passing through the vastus lateralis and in this case it would be a type C flap. This dissection is more time consuming and risks damage to the perforating vessels.

REFERENCES

1. Blondeel PN, Van Landuyt KH, Monstrey SJ, et al. The "Gent" consensus on perforator flap terminology: preliminary definitions. Plast Reconstr Surg 2003;112(5):1378–1383, quiz 1383, 1516, discussion 1384–1387

2. Geddes CR, Morris SF, Neligan PC. Perforator flaps: evolution, classification, and applications. Ann Plast Surg 2003;50(1):90–99

3. Mathes SJ, Nahai F. Reconstructive Surgery: Principles, Anatomy, and Technique. St Louis: Quality Medical Publishing; 1997

THE ANTEROLATERAL THIGH (ALT) FLAP

5. You are planning to reconstruct a 12 by 6 cm defect on the dorsal foot and ankle of a woman following leiomyosarcoma resection. She has a body mass index (BMI) of 38 and is hypertensive but is otherwise medically well. *Which one of the following is correct regarding the use of an anterolateral thigh (ALT) flap for this patient's reconstruction?*

    D. A super thin perforator flap may be best for this woman's case.

    The ALT flap is a versatile flap that in many cases would be ideal for reconstructing the dorsum of the foot and ankle because it is often thin, pliable, and has a long pedicle enabling reach to the anterior or posterior tibial vessels. Furthermore, it can be raised as a chimeric flap with two separate skin paddles if there are separate defects involving medial and lateral malleoli, and it can limit surgery to a single limb.[1] However, in obese individuals such as in this patient, the ALT flap is often too thick and bulky for dissection for reconstruction of the dorsal foot. For this reason, flap thinning would be required to convert the flap to a "super thin" perforator flap. Alternatively, a thinner flap such as a radial forearm could be used instead as obese patients' radial forearm flap normally remains relatively thin.[2,3]

    ALT skin paddle dimensions may be as large as 25 by 35 cm in some cases and flaps less than 10 cm width, such as in this case, can usually be closed directly. Those wider than 10 cm are likely to require a skin graft to the donor site. However, this figure is still variable depending on individual patient's tissue characteristics. Preoperative angiography can be useful for evaluation of perforator flap vascularity but is not essential. It is more likely to be useful to confirm leg vascularity and availability of recipient vessels, particularly in cases following lower limb trauma or in patients with peripheral vascular disease.[4]

REFERENCES

1. Wei FC, Jain V, Celik N, Chen HC, Chuang DC, Lin CH. Have we found an ideal soft-tissue flap? An experience with 672 anterolateral thigh flaps. Plast Reconstr Surg 2002;109(7):2219–2226, discussion 2227–2230
2. Kimura N, Satoh K, Hosaka Y. Microdissected thin perforator flaps: 46 cases. Plast Reconstr Surg 2003;112(7):1875–1885
3. Ogawa R, Hyakusoku H. Flap thinning technique: the effect of primary flap defatting. Plast Reconstr Surg 2008;122(3):987–988
4. Zenn M, Jones G. Reconstructive Surgery: Anatomy, Technique, & Clinical Applications. St Louis: Quality Medical Publishing; 2012

THE DEEP INFERIOR EPIGASTRIC ARTERY FLAP

6. *When considering the deep inferior epigastric artery flap, which one of the following represents a potential disadvantage to its use?*
   E. Unpredictable perforator anatomy

   The deep inferior epigastric artery (DIEP) flap is a commonly used flap for both free tissue transfer in breast reconstruction, and locoregional transfer for reconstructing defects of the abdomen, genital region, and thighs. It has many advantages including a favorable donor site, a long vascular pedicle, low donor site morbidity, and the ability to convert to a traditional myocutaneous flap if the perforating vessels are poor.

   A disadvantage to this flap is that there is significant anatomic variation from patient to patient. Even within a single patient, there can be unpredictable side-to-side differences in perforator anatomy. This means it can be hard to anticipate the precise anatomical path and location of any given perforator. For this reason, preoperative imaging with computed tomography (CT) angiography is considered by many surgeons to be both useful and worthwhile in order to map the perforators and their relations to the skin and underlying muscle and fascia. Not only can perforator location present a challenge to the surgeon, perforators may also have a long intramuscular course and be closely located with the inscriptions of the rectus abdominis, thereby making their safe dissection more difficult. Intraoperative decision-making is probably the most challenging part of DIEP flap elevation as the wrong choice of perforator can result in partial or full flap loss.[1-3]

REFERENCES

1. Blondeel PN, Morris SF, Hallock GG, Neligan PC, eds. Perforator Flaps: Anatomy, Technique, & Clinical Application. 2nd ed. St Louis: Quality Medical Publishing; 2013
2. Baumann DP, Lin HY, Chevray PM. Perforator number predicts fat necrosis in a prospective analysis of breast reconstruction with free TRAM, DIEP, and SIEA flaps. Plast Reconstr Surg 2010;125(5):1335–1341
3. Hamdi M, Rebecca A. The deep inferior epigastric artery perforator flap (DIEAP) in breast reconstruction. Semin Plast Surg 2006;20(2):95–102

TECHNIQUES FOR RAISING PERFORATOR FLAPS

7. While raising a deep inferior epigastric perforator (DIEP) flap for breast reconstruction, you are concerned regarding the size of the venae comitantes. The flap has been cut to size, preserving zones I through III. You have completed a satisfactory anastomosis and have inset the flap. The flap is running but capillary refill is very brisk and the flap is becoming blue. *Which one of the following is most likely to improve the flap viability?*
   D. Anastomosis of the superficial inferior epigastric vein (SIEV)

   The flap as described is showing signs of venous compromise. This can occur in DIEP flaps where there is inadequate connection between the superficial and deep inferior epigastric vascular systems. In cases such as this, where the venae comitantes are small, it is likely that the superficial system is large. When raising a DIEP flap the SIEV should be identified and preserved at the inferior margin of the flap and where compromise occurs, it can be anastomosed to a suitable vein. This is the most appropriate step in this scenario.

   In general, venous compromise can be due to a number of factors which must be systematically addressed. First, the anastomotic patency must always be checked to ensure flow and that no external compression or twisting of the pedicle has occurred. In this case, the anastomoses are working satisfactorily. If one area of the flap (usually zone IV) is congested, this may be removed; but this has been done already. If the flap becomes brisk after inset, it may be that compression is the cause and release of inset and staged closure may be helpful. Systemic heparin is not likely to benefit in this situation given the venous compromise. Use of leeches can help small flaps such as those on the digits that have congested venous but would not be the first choice in this scenario.[1-4]

REFERENCES

1. Villafane O, Gahankari D, Webster M. Superficial inferior epigastric vein (SIEV): "lifeboat" for DIEP/TRAM flaps. Br J Plast Surg 1999;52(7):599

2. Wechselberger G, Schoeller T, Bauer T, Ninkovic M, Otto A, Ninkovic M. Venous superdrainage in deep inferior epigastric perforator flap breast reconstruction. Plast Reconstr Surg 2001;108(1):162–166

3. Boyd JB, Taylor GI, Corlett R. The vascular territories of the superior epigastric and the deep inferior epigastric systems. Plast Reconstr Surg 1984;73(1):1–16

4. Rozen WM, Ashton MW. The venous anatomy of the abdominal wall for deep inferior epigastric artery (DIEP) flaps in breast reconstruction. Gland Surg 2012;1(2):92–110

RAISING A PERFORATOR FLAP

8. You are planning to use a perforator flap to reconstruct a soft tissue defect and will be supervising your resident during the process. *Which one of the following should you tell them?*

   C. The plane of dissection should be close to the perforator.

   When raising perforator flaps, dissection around the perforator must be meticulous with limited vessel manipulation such as twisting, stretching, and grasping. Dissection should be close to the vessel within the loose areolar plane as this facilitates good visibility of the vessel and minimizes risk of inadvertent damage. The minimal perforator diameter is 0.5 mm rather than 2.0 mm and the presence of a visible or palpable pulse is a strong indicator of a good perforator. Having the perforator centrally within the skin paddle is not required and in some propeller freestyle flaps the perforator is deliberately offset (**Fig. 5.4**).

   The number of perforators that should be included in a flap is debated. DIEP flaps can be satisfactorily raised on single perforators, but some authors suggest that fat necrosis is reduced where more perforators are included.[1,2] Perforator quality is probably more important than perforator quantity for any given flap.[2]

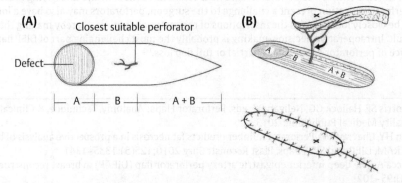

Fig. 5.4 *A,* Propeller flap concept. *B,* Propeller flap. (A and B Adapted from Zenn MR, Jones G, eds. Reconstructive Surgery: Anatomy, Technique, and Clinical Applications. St Louis: Quality Medical Publishing, 2012.)

REFERENCES

1. Baumann DP, Lin HY, Chevray PM. Perforator number predicts fat necrosis in a prospective analysis of breast reconstruction with free TRAM, DIEP, and SIEA flaps. Plast Reconstr Surg 2010;125(5):1335–1341

2. Lindsey JT. Perforator number does not predict fat necrosis. Plast Reconstr Surg 2011;127(3):1391–1392

DESIGNING A PERFORATOR FLAP

9. *When designing a freestyle perforator flap for reconstruction of a 9 cm diameter shoulder defect, which one of the following is the most useful preoperative investigation?*

   A. Handheld Doppler

   Preoperative methods for assessing perforator flaps include handheld Doppler, CT angiography duplex ultrasonography, and magnetic resonance angiography (MRA). Of these, the handheld Doppler will be ideal for most applications like this case where a freestyle flap is to be used because it is simple and reliable to help locate individual perforating vessels. CT angiography is more useful in flaps with variable anatomy such as the DIEP or superior gluteal artery perforator (SGAP) flap but is not essential when handheld methods can suffice. Indocyanine green is a useful *intraoperative* technique to help identify zones of adequate perfusion before committing to flap design. Laser Doppler flowmetry and tissue oximetry are methods used to monitor flaps postoperatively. They have high positive and negative predictive values but are expensive and not routinely used. Thermal smartphone imaging is a newly described and potentially useful tool for preoperative flap planning. It may also find a role in intraoperative assessment and postoperative monitoring. It utilizes infrared radiation that can detect dense areas of perforating vessels and tissue perfusion via temperature variations. It does not involve intravenous (IV) contrast or ionizing radiation exposure. In one study by Pereira et al in 2018,[1] this modality was compared with CT angiography in 20 patients undergoing ALT harvest for limb reconstruction. Within these patients, a total of 120 ALT flap perforators in 38 territories were identified. This study showed very high specificity and sensitivity (98 and 100% respectively) in detecting perforators identified by CT angiography.

REFERENCE

1. Pereira N, Valenzuela D, Mangelsdorff G, Kufeke M, Roa R. Detection of perforators for free flap planning using smartphone thermal imaging: a concordance study with computed tomographic angiography in 120 perforators. Plast Reconstr Surg 2018;141(3):787–792

LATERAL CIRCUMFLEX FEMORAL ARTERY PERFORATOR FLAP

10. You are planning to use a pedicled lateral circumflex femoral artery perforator (LCFAP) flap to reconstruct an abdominal wall defect. *Which muscle often requires dissection when raising this flap?*

  E. **Vastus lateralis**

As discussed in question 3, the LCFAP flap (also known as the ALT flap) is based on the lateral circumflex femoral artery and perforating vessels from this source vessel may pass through a portion of the vastus lateralis en route to the skin. In some cases, the perforators may be completely septal, and in this situation intramuscular dissection is not required.

Dissection of the gracilis muscle is required when raising an MCFAP flap which arises from the medial circumflex femoral vessels or the transverse upper gracilis (TUG) flap.[1,2] Intramuscular dissection of the medial head of gastrocnemius is required when raising a medial sural artery perforator (MSAP) flap.[3]

Perforator flaps have also been described based on the short head of biceps femoris and these may arise from either the popliteal or profunda femoris vessels.[4] In spite of a number of new perforator flaps having been described, the LCFAP and ALT remain the most popular workhorse flaps in reconstructive surgery.

REFERENCES

1. Hallock GG. The development of the medial circumflex femoral artery perforator flap. Semin Plast Surg 2006;20:121–126
2. Yousif NJ. The transverse gracilis musculocutaneous flap. Ann Plast Surg 1993;31(4):382
3. Cavadas PC, Sanz-Giménez-Rico JR, Gutierrez-de la Cámara A, Navarro-Monzonís A, Soler-Nomdedeu S, Martínez-Soriano F. The medial sural artery perforator free flap. Plast Reconstr Surg 2001;108(6):1609–1615, discussion 1616–1617
4. Cavadas PC, Sanz-Jiménez-Rico JR, Landin L, Correa J. Biceps femoris perforator free flap for upper extremity reconstruction: anatomical study and clinical series. Plast Reconstr Surg 2005;116(1):145–152

6.   Tissue Expansion

See *Essentials of Plastic Surgery*, third edition, pp. 69–81

VISCOELASTIC PROPERTIES OF SKIN

1. *Which one of the following statements is correct regarding biologic tissue creep?*
   A. It forms the basis of intraoperative expansion.
   B. It involves displacement of water from ground substance.
   C. The elastic fibers become microfragmented.
   D. Collagen fibers undergo realignment.
   E. Cellular ingrowth and tissue regeneration are initiated.

SOFT TISSUE CHANGES DURING TISSUE EXPANSION

2. You have placed a submuscular tissue expander for immediate breast reconstruction following skin-sparing mastectomy. *Which one of the following will occur in the soft tissues during tissue expansion?*
   A. The dermis will initially thicken but will normalize within 3 months.
   B. A capsule will form around the implant leading to improved skin flap viability.
   C. The pectoralis major muscles will stretch and increase in bulk.
   D. The number and size of blood vessels within the overlying skin will decrease.
   E. The subcutaneous fat layer will thicken, thereby helping to provide additional implant cover.

EXPANDER SUBTYPES

3. *Which one of the following is a consistent feature of all internal tissue expanders?*
   A. Permanence
   B. Shape
   C. Filling portal
   D. Silicone elastomer shell
   E. Inflation method

BREAST IMPLANT ASSOCIATED ANAPLASTIC LARGE CELL LYMPHOMA (BIA-ALCL)

4. *When considering the risk of developing BIA-ALCL during tissue expansion of the breast, which one of the following factors is believed to minimize the risk for patients?*
   A. Using an expander with an integrated port
   B. Placing the implant beneath the pectoralis major muscle
   C. Using a smooth surface expander device
   D. Providing a 1-week course of antibiotics following expander placement
   E. Limiting the expansion process to 3 months' duration

BREAST RECONSTRUCTION WITH TISSUE EXPANSION

5. *Which type of expansion device has the potential advantage of avoiding a second surgical stage for women undergoing breast reconstruction?*
   A. A self-inflating expander
   B. A dual chamber expander
   C. An expander with an integrated fill port
   D. An expander with an air fill port
   E. An expander with an integrated drainage port

TISSUE EXPANSION

6. *Which one of the following is correct regarding tissue expansion?*
   A. Expanders with remote ports require a magnet for accurate port location.
   B. Round expanders typically achieve 75% of their mathematically predicted tissue expansion.
   C. Expanders with differential expansion are useful in immediate breast reconstruction.
   D. Crescentic expanders achieve a greater percentage of their calculated expansion than any other implant shapes.
   E. Osmotic, self-inflating expanders are commonly used in clinical practice.

ADVANTAGES OF TISSUE EXPANSION

7. You are describing the risks and benefits of tissue expansion to a parent whose child requires excision of a giant cell nevus from the occipital scalp. *Which one of the following is the key advantage of tissue expansion for this child?*
   A. The number of general anesthetic procedures is minimized.
   B. The number of hospital clinic visits is reduced.
   C. The reconstruction can be completed more quickly.
   D. The defect is more likely to be closed directly using a hair-bearing skin flap.
   E. There is minimal functional and aesthetic impact during the expansion process.

TISSUE EXPANSION PLANNING

8. You are planning to expand tissue to resurface a scalp burn scar in an adult. *Which one of the following is correct regarding this tissue expansion?*
   A. The base diameter of the expander should be 5 times the defect diameter.
   B. The expander should not be inflated beyond the listed volume.
   C. Selection of a crescentic expander is a good choice in this scenario.
   D. The access incision is best placed parallel to the intended direction of expansion.
   E. The expander should be placed superficial to the galea.

THE EXPANSION PROCESS

9. You have placed an expander with an integrated port for delayed breast reconstruction. *Which one of the following is correct regarding the expansion process?*
   A. It should begin 6 weeks after implantation of the expander.
   B. It is best performed aseptically with a 14-gauge needle and sterile water.
   C. Expansion in the clinic should only be stopped once the patient feels discomfort.
   D. Skin blanching is a useful sign to guide expansion in a clinic setting.
   E. Risk of extrusion is reduced by early expansion.

ESTIMATION OF TISSUE AVAILABILITY AFTER EXPANSION

10. You are resurfacing a scalp defect using three expanders. *The amount of tissue available from each expander can be estimated by which of the following?*
    A. Base radius multiplied by circumference (dome length)
    B. Circumference (dome length) minus base radius
    C. Base radius divided by circumference (dome length)
    D. Circumference (dome length) minus base diameter
    E. Dome height minus base radius

CLINICAL APPLICATIONS OF EXPANSION

11. You see a 20-year-old girl in clinic with a large congenital nevus on the scalp measuring 10 by 10 cm. She would like it to be removed and you plan to use tissue expansion. *What is the maximum percentage of the scalp that can usually be reconstructed with tissue expansion without causing significant thinning of the remaining hair?*
    A. 15%   D. 65%
    B. 30%   E. 75%
    C. 50%

EXPANSION IN NOSE RECONSTRUCTION

12. *Why is tissue expansion not generally advocated for standard nasal reconstruction with a forehead flap?*
    A. Forehead skin does not expand well.
    B. The donor site is fully closed directly without expansion.
    C. The risk of implant extrusion is high.
    D. The donor site heals well by secondary intention.
    E. A general anesthetic can be avoided.

COMPLICATIONS OF TISSUE EXPANSION

13. *When considering the anatomic location for tissue expansion, which one of the following has the highest complication rates?*
    A. Neck   D. Arm
    B. Scalp   E. Leg
    C. Chest

EXPANSION IN BREAST RECONSTRUCTION

14. You see a patient following insertion of a submuscular breast expander for delayed breast reconstruction. She had 100 mL injected at the time of surgery and a small contour was created. She has had two further documented sessions of normal expansion with 80 mL on each occasion through the integrated port, but the chest wall now appears flat. *What is the most likely reason?*
    A. Insufficient volume injected at this stage
    B. Faulty valve on the integrated port
    C. Intraoperative damage to the implant
    D. Failure to inject the volumes directly into the expander
    E. Expander puncture during injection

Answers

VISCOELASTIC PROPERTIES OF SKIN

1. *Which one of the following statements is correct regarding biologic tissue creep?*
   E. **Cellular ingrowth and tissue regeneration are initiated.**

   Creep refers to a permanent elongation in tissues subjected to an external force. There are two types of creep: mechanical and biologic. Mechanical creep occurs where tissue is acutely stretched and results in collagen realignment, elastic fiber microfragmentation, water displacement, and recruitment of adjacent tissue. In contrast, biologic creep occurs where tissues are stretched for a prolonged period and cellular ingrowth is initiated. Changes include an increase in collagen production, angiogenesis, and epidermal proliferation.[1-5]

REFERENCES

1. Siegert R, Weerda H, Hoffmann S, Mohadjer C. Clinical and experimental evaluation of intermittent intraoperative short-term expansion. Plast Reconstr Surg 1993;92(2):248–254
2. Wilhelmi BJ, Blackwell SJ, Mancoll JS, Phillips LG. Creep vs. stretch: a review of the viscoelastic properties of skin. Ann Plast Surg 1998;41(2):215–219
3. Takei T, Mills I, Arai K, Sumpio BE. Molecular basis for tissue expansion: clinical implications for the surgeon. Plast Reconstr Surg 1998;102(1):247–258
4. Austad ED, Pasyk KA, McClatchey KD, Cherry GW. Histomorphologic evaluation of guinea pig skin and soft tissue after controlled tissue expansion. Plast Reconstr Surg 1982;70(6):704–710
5. Johnson TM, Lowe L, Brown MD, Sullivan MJ, Nelson BR. Histology and physiology of tissue expansion. J Dermatol Surg Oncol 1993;19(12):1074–1078

SOFT TISSUE CHANGES DURING TISSUE EXPANSION

2. You have placed a submuscular tissue expander for immediate breast reconstruction following skin-sparing mastectomy. *Which one of the following will occur in the soft tissues during tissue expansion?*
   B. **A capsule will form around the implant leading to improved skin flap viability.**

   There are a number of changes that occur in the skin and subcutaneous tissue during tissue expansion. A key factor is an increase in vascularity within expanded soft tissue because of an increased size and number of vessels secondary to angiogenesis. The highest vessel density is found at the junction of the capsule and host tissue, and this was demonstrated by Pasyk et al[1] who analyzed the capsule, identifying four distinct layers. The outermost layer had a high density of collagen and blood vessels. This has clinical relevance in that the capsule itself can increase skin flap viability and should be left in situ following expansion where possible.

   The dermis thins, not thickens, fibroblasts and myofibroblasts increase in number, and sweat glands and hair follicles become less dense. Thickness does not return to normal until approximately 2 years after expansion. The epidermis thickens secondary to hyperkeratosis and normalizes after 6 months. Muscle tends to decrease in thickness and mass due to either compression or stretch from the expander (depending on which level the expander is placed). In this scenario muscle function is not usually significantly reduced by the expansion process itself, although the medial release and muscle undermining may do so. Fat is extremely sensitive to mechanical force and aggressive expansion is likely to cause fat necrosis. In general, the subcutaneous layer thins and some permanent loss of fat occurs.[2]

REFERENCES

1. Pasyk KA, Argenta LC, Austad ED. Histopathology of human expanded tissue. Clin Plast Surg 1987;14(3):435–445
2. Johnson TM, Lowe L, Brown MD, Sullivan MJ, Nelson BR. Histology and physiology of tissue expansion. J Dermatol Surg Oncol 1993;19(12):1074–1078

EXPANDER SUBTYPES

3. *Which one of the following is a consistent feature of all internal tissue expanders?*
   D. **Silicone elastomer shell**

   Internal tissue expanders are formed with a silicone elastomer shell surrounding an internal reservoir. They may be classified by shape, permanence, inflation mechanism, or filling portal type. Shapes include round, crescentic, and rectangular. Implants are commonly temporary but may be permanent such as some breast prostheses with a second inner compartment filled with silicone. Inflation is usually manual but can be self-filling as a result of osmosis when hypertonic expanders are used. The filling portal can be integrated or placed externally.[1]

REFERENCE

1. Bauer B. Tissue expansion. In: Thorne CH, Beasley RW, Aston SJ, et al, eds. Grabb & Smith's Plastic Surgery. 6th ed. Philadelphia: Lippincott-Raven; 2007:84–90

BREAST IMPLANT ASSOCIATED ANAPLASTIC LARGE CELL LYMPHOMA (BIA-ALCL)

4. *When considering the risk of developing BIA-ALCL during tissue expansion of the breast, which one of the following factors is believed to minimize the risk for patients?*
    C. Using a smooth surface expander device

    Breast implant associated anaplastic large cell lymphoma (BIA-ALCL) is a rare type of non-Hodgkin's lymphoma, with more than 500 cases worldwide. In most reported cases, it has been identified within the breast capsule and seroma fluid surrounding the implant at a range of time points following primary implantation. It may also be found as a solid tumor mass within the breast parenchyma. This condition has been most often associated with specific brands of textured breast implants and at present there are no cases of BIA-ALCL identified with smooth surfaced implants worldwide. The FDA has recommended that certain textured implant types are no longer used, and a number of these have now been removed from the market. The use of an integrated port, placement beneath the pectoralis muscle, nor a rapid expansion process have been associated with a reduced risk of BIA-ALCL. There may well be a link between infection, biofilms, and development of capsular contracture, but there is currently no strong evidence to substantiate that BIA-ALCL is caused by infection. Nonetheless, meticulous care must be taken to minimize infection with any breast implants and a single dose of antibiotics (rather than a 1-week course) is accepted to represent best practice in most centers.

    Overall, the use of a tissue expander in the breast presents a low risk for patients for development of BIA-ALCL. However, the use of a smooth shelled device may be a factor in minimizing overall risk for the patient. The downside is that smooth devices are more likely to migrate in the early postoperative phase, and in the longer term, may be more likely to develop capsular contracture.[1,2]

REFERENCES

1. Fitzal F, Turner SD, Kenner L. Is breast implant-associated anaplastic large cell lymphoma a hazard of breast implant surgery? Open Biol 2019;9(4):190006
2. FDA.gov The FDA requests Allergan Voluntarily Recall Natrelle BIOCELL Textured breast implants and tissue expanders from the market to protect patients: FDA Safety Communication, 2019

BREAST RECONSTRUCTION WITH TISSUE EXPANSION

5. *Which type of expansion device has the potential advantage of avoiding a second surgical stage for women undergoing breast reconstruction?*
    B. A dual chamber expander

    Expanders are most commonly filled with saline, and this is injected via either an integrated or remote port. Methylene blue dye may be added to the saline to help confirm correct placement of the injection needle for subsequent expansion. The expansion process is commenced a few weeks after surgery by the clinician in the office setting. Where a normal expander is used, it has a single chamber which is filled purely with saline and when fully inflated to the required size, is then exchanged for a permanent silicone implant.

    The dual chamber device, known as a "Becker" implant after its inventor, has an inner compartment which is progressively filled via a remote port, and an outer compartment which is filled with silicone gel. It is therefore intended to be a permanent implant requiring only a single operating procedure.[1]

    The original device was round and has since been updated to be available in both round and anatomical variants. Mentor currently manufactures a Becker style implant in an anatomical shape, which has a 35% gel fill and a 65% saline fill potential. Although still popular with some surgeons and patients, a two-stage approach remains the most popular approach overall.[2]

    Self-expanding expanders are not really used in clinical practice. Of note, however, in 2016 the FDA approved the use of carbon dioxide within tissue expanders as an alternative to saline. The potential benefit for patients was that expansion with such devices could be controlled by the patient using a remote dosage controller. One study had shown that when patients were allowed control over their expansion in this manner, the number of office visits was reduced and the time to complete expansion and overall reconstruction was shortened.[3,4] Unfortunately, since then, the sole manufacturer of these devices has stopped trading, so at present no further progress is being made with this concept.

    While saline is most commonly used in expanders, air is another potential option, especially in the initial setting post mastectomy. Air is lighter than saline and so results in less tissue stress and tension, thereby reducing the risk of vascular compromise of mastectomy skin flaps. Once the mastectomy flaps' vascularity and swelling has stabilized, the air within the implant is often exchanged for saline at subsequent clinic visits, so this technique, although useful in helping wound healing, would not avoid a second surgical stage.

A recent interesting development in breast tissue expanders was the introduction of an expander with an integrated drainage port in addition to the traditional injection port. This facilitates drainage of fluid from the periprosthetic space through this integrated drainage port allowing for treatment of seroma and diagnostic fluid sampling from around the implant. In 2018, preliminary results using this device (Sientra AlloX2 breast tissue expander) were published and 40 patients were included in the study. They were all followed up for 6 months. In this group of patients, the most common complication was development of a seroma around the expander and in most cases, these were successfully managed with the use of a second port to drain them. The authors concluded that this expander device was successful in treating seromas and should be considered a tool for doing so. At present, further research is warranted to define the full indications, contraindications, safety efficacy, and outcomes.[5]

REFERENCES

1. Becker H. Breast reconstruction using an inflatable breast implant with detachable reservoir. Plast Reconstr Surg 1984;73(4):678–683
2. American Society of Plastic Surgeons. Reconstructive Breast Surgery Statistics 2012. Available online: https://www.plasticsurgery.org/documents/News/Statistics/2012/reconstructive-procedure-trends-2012.pdf
3. Morrison KA, Ascherman BM, Ascherman JA. Evolving approaches to tissue expander design and application. Plast Reconstr Surg 2017;140(5S Advances in Breast Reconstruction):23S–29S
4. Ascherman JA, Zeidler K, Morrison KA, et al. Carbon dioxide-based versus saline tissue expansion for breast reconstruction: results of the XPAND prospective, randomized clinical trial. Plast Reconstr Surg 2016;138(6):1161–1170
5. Zeidler KR, Capizzi PJ, Pittman TA. Sientra AlloX2 short-term case study, surgical pearls, and roundtable discussion. Plast Reconstr Surg 2018;141(4S Sientra Shaped and Round Cohesive Gel Implants):29S–39S

TISSUE EXPANSION

6. *Which one of the following is correct regarding tissue expansion?*

   C. Expanders with differential expansion are useful in immediate breast reconstruction.

   The use of permanent expanders is popular in breast reconstruction and they can be shaped with differential expansion of the upper/lower poles. This can help recreate a more natural breast contour with ptosis. They are comprised of a more highly projecting lower pole and a more modestly projecting upper pole. Expanders can have integrated or remote ports. Remote ports are either placed externally or subcutaneously and are palpable and therefore do not require a magnetic locator, which is reserved for integrated ports.[1]

   Expander geometry affects the amount of surface area gained. Expanders that are rectangular (not crescentic) achieve the greatest percentage of their calculated expansion at 38%. Crescentic expanders usually achieve values of approximately 32%, and round expanders typically achieve values of approximately 25%.

   Osmotic, self-inflating expanders contain hypertonic sodium chloride crystals and fill by osmosis. The rate of expansion cannot be altered after insertion. Although commercially available, they are not commonly used in clinical practice. They tend to be occasionally used in pediatric patients with scalp or periorbital defects and are otherwise largely experimental.[2]

REFERENCES

1. Spear SL, Pelletiere CV. Immediate breast reconstruction in two stages using textured, integrated-valve tissue expanders and breast implants. Plast Reconstr Surg 2004;113(7):2098–2103
2. van Rappard JH, Molenaar J, van Doorn K, Sonneveld GJ, Borghouts JM. Surface-area increase in tissue expansion. Plast Reconstr Surg 1988;82(5):833–839

ADVANTAGES OF TISSUE EXPANSION

7. You are describing the risks and benefits of tissue expansion to a parent whose child requires excision of a giant cell nevus from the occipital scalp. *Which one of the following is the key advantage of tissue expansion for this child?*

   D. The defect is more likely to be closed directly using a hair-bearing skin flap.

   Tissue expansion is useful because it can facilitate closure of defects that otherwise require importation of distant tissue, but it has several disadvantages. It is staged and requires at least two surgical procedures; multiple surgical outpatient appointments are needed for expansion; completion of reconstruction is delayed; and appearance and function may be unacceptable for the patient and/or family during the expansion process. Placement of an expander also carries a risk of infection. Should this occur, the expander would need to be removed.

   A further risk of tissue expansion is implant extrusion and this is a particular risk in high-risk areas of the body where skin blood supply is reduced and following other treatments such as radiation.[1-3]

REFERENCES

1. O'Reilly AG, Schmitt WR, Roenigk RK, Moore EJ, Price DL. Closure of scalp and forehead defects using external tissue expander. Arch Facial Plast Surg 2012;14(6):419–422
2. MacLennan SE, Corcoran JF, Neale HW. Tissue expansion in head and neck burn reconstruction. Clin Plast Surg 2000;27(1):121–132
3. Joss GS, Zoltie N, Chapman P. Tissue expansion technique and the transposition flap. Br J Plast Surg 1990;43(3):328–333

TISSUE EXPANSION PLANNING

8. You are planning to expand tissue to resurface a scalp burn scar in an adult. *Which one of the following is correct regarding this tissue expansion?*

   C. Selection of a crescentic expander is a good choice in this scenario.

   Shape selection of the expander depends on location and crescent shapes are often used in the scalp. These are normally placed subgaleally. Precise expander volume is not usually a concern because most can be safely overinflated beyond their recommended maximum volume. The base diameter of the expander should be 2 to 2.5 times the defect diameter (not 5 times).

   The access incision for initial expander placement should ideally be perpendicular to the main axis of expansion (long axis of the expander), not parallel, to reduce tension across the scar. It should be placed at the edge of the defect so that it can be removed at the time of reconstruction.[1–3]

REFERENCES

1. O'Reilly AG, Schmitt WR, Roenigk RK, Moore EJ, Price DL. Closure of scalp and forehead defects using external tissue expander. Arch Facial Plast Surg 2012;14(6):419–422
2. MacLennan SE, Corcoran JF, Neale HW. Tissue expansion in head and neck burn reconstruction. Clin Plast Surg 2000;27(1):121–132
3. Wagh MS, Dixit V. Tissue expansion: concepts, techniques and unfavourable results. Indian J Plast Surg 2013;46(2):333–348

THE EXPANSION PROCESS

9. You have placed an expander with an integrated port for delayed breast reconstruction. *Which one of the following is correct regarding the expansion process?*

   D. Skin blanching is a useful sign to guide expansion in a clinic setting.

   Expansion typically begins 2–3 weeks after surgery to allow time for the wound to heal sufficiently without tension. Expansion is best performed with a small needle (23 gauge or smaller). It is performed using sterile saline, which has a similar osmolarity to tissue fluids. Patient discomfort and blanching are both indicators that expansion for that appointment is complete. Tissue expansion is normally safely repeated weekly or every 2 weeks until final fill volume is achieved. Rapid expansion is associated with a greater risk of extrusion. Rapid or early expansion can lead to a greater risk of implant extrusion so a conservative approach to expansion is warranted.[1–3]

REFERENCES

1. Morrison KA, Ascherman BM, Ascherman JA. Evolving approaches to tissue expander design and application. Plast Reconstr Surg 2017;140(5S Advances in Breast Reconstruction):23S–29S
2. Manders EK, Schenden MJ, Furrey JA, Hetzler PT, Davis TS, Graham WP III. Soft-tissue expansion: concepts and complications. Plast Reconstr Surg 1984;74(4):493–507
3. Radovan C. Tissue expansion in soft-tissue reconstruction. Plast Reconstr Surg 1984;74(4):482–492

ESTIMATION OF TISSUE AVAILABILITY AFTER EXPANSION

10. You are resurfacing a scalp defect using three expanders. *The amount of tissue available from each expander can be estimated by which of the following?*

   D. Circumference (dome length) minus base diameter

   The amount of extra tissue available can be estimated by measuring the dome length and subtracting the base diameter (**Fig. 6.1**).

REFERENCES

1. van Rappard JH, Molenaar J, van Doorn K, Sonneveld GJ, Borghouts JM. Surface-area increase in tissue expansion. Plast Reconstr Surg 1988;82(5):833–839

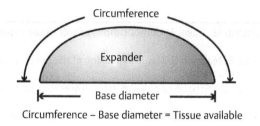

Fig. 6.1   Amount of tissue available equals circumference minus base diameter.

2. Wilhelmi BJ, Blackwell SJ, Mancoll JS, Phillips LG. Creep vs. stretch: a review of the viscoelastic properties of skin. Ann Plast Surg 1998;41(2):215–219
3. Manders EK, Schenden MJ, Furrey JA, Hetzler PT, Davis TS, Graham WP III. Soft-tissue expansion: concepts and complications. Plast Reconstr Surg 1984;74(4):493–507

CLINICAL APPLICATIONS OF EXPANSION

11. You see a 20-year-old girl in clinic with a large congenital nevus on the scalp measuring 10 by 10 cm. She would like it to be removed and you plan to use tissue expansion. *What is the maximum percentage of the scalp that can usually be reconstructed with tissue expansion without causing significant thinning of the remaining hair?*
    C. 50%
    The scalp is well suited to reconstruction using tissue expansion providing patients are motivated and willing to tolerate a prolonged period with a deformed appearance of the head. Applications include tumor excision as in this case, burn alopecia, and other traumatic defects (such as delayed procedures). Reconstruction outcomes will be specific to each individual patient and hair thinning will be dependent on both the site and size of the defect as well as the density of the patient's hair; however, 50% is considered to be the maximum defect size that can be reconstructed in postburn patients without causing significant hair thinning.[1]

REFERENCE

1. MacLennan SE, Corcoran JF, Neale HW. Tissue expansion in head and neck burn reconstruction. Clin Plast Surg 2000;27(1):121–132

EXPANSION IN NOSE RECONSTRUCTION

12. *Why is tissue expansion not generally advocated for standard nasal reconstruction with a forehead flap?*
    D. The donor site heals well by secondary intention.
    Forehead tissue expanders can be placed before raising a forehead flap with the intended benefit of facilitating direct closure of the donor defect. In practice this is not commonly performed because, in most cases, the caudal part of the donor site is closed directly and the residual defect on the scalp heals well by secondary intention. The forehead skin does expand well and has a relatively low rate of extrusion. A general anesthetic is standard practice for nasal reconstruction when using a forehead flap.[1]

REFERENCE

1. Burget GC. Axial paramedian forehead flap. In: Strauch B, ed. Grabb's Encyclopedia of Flaps. Philadelphia: Lippincott; 1998

COMPLICATIONS OF TISSUE EXPANSION

13. *When considering the anatomic location for tissue expansion, which one of the following has the highest complication rates?*
    E. Leg
    In general, extremity tissue is associated with the highest complication rate when using tissue expansion techniques. The main complications are poor wound healing, implant extrusion, and infection. Of the extremities, the lower limb has the highest complication rate, especially when used below the knee. This does not mean tissue expansion cannot be used successfully in these locations, rather that patients and clinicians must be aware of the increased risks and these are taken into account. Other contributory risk factors such as diabetes, peripheral vascular disease, previous burn surgery, and previous radiation therapy must also be factored into the decision-making process.[1–4]

REFERENCES

1. Antonyshyn O, Gruss JS, Mackinnon SE, Zuker R. Complications of soft tissue expansion. Br J Plast Surg 1988;41(3): 239–250
2. Casanova D, Bali D, Bardot J, Legre R, Magalon G. Tissue expansion of the lower limb: complications in a cohort of 103 cases. Br J Plast Surg 2001;54(4):310–316
3. Manders EK, Oaks TE, Au VK, et al. Soft-tissue expansion in the lower extremities. Plast Reconstr Surg 1988;81(2): 208–219
4. Pandya AN, Vadodaria S, Coleman DJ. Tissue expansion in the limbs: a comparative analysis of limb and non-limb sites. Br J Plast Surg 2002;55(4):302–306

EXPANSION IN BREAST RECONSTRUCTION

14. You see a patient following insertion of a submuscular breast expander for delayed breast reconstruction. She had 100 mL injected at the time of surgery and a small contour was created. She has had two further documented sessions of normal expansion with 80 mL on each occasion through the integrated port, but the chest wall now appears flat. *What is the most likely reason?*

   E. Expander puncture during injection

   The most likely reason for an expander not to retain volume following injection of fluid is damage to the outer shell, which allows fluid to leak out of the expander into the subcutaneous tissues. With modern implants, spontaneous volume loss is very unlikely to be due to faulty manufacture and is most likely due to the surgical team causing damage to the shell either during placement of the expander or during the expansion process itself.

   A risk of using an expander with an integrated port is that the shell can fold over on itself when underfilled, so that when the injecting needle is passed into the valve it also passes through the shell. This is most likely to have occurred in this scenario. The expander is also at risk of damage during wound closure as the suture needle may inadvertently be passed through the silicone shell. If implants or expanders are returned to the manufacturer to assess deflation, the manufacturer is able to identify whether needle damage has occurred. However, in most cases it is immediately obvious if the implant has been punctured, once it is removed.

   It is unlikely that the fluid has not been injected into the expander providing that the magnetic finder has been used and the backing plate palpated during expansion, but this could potentially occur.[1-3]

REFERENCES

1. Poppler LH, Mundschenk MB, Linkugel A, Zubovic E, Dolen UC, Myckatyn TM. Tissue expander complications do not preclude a second successful implant-based breast reconstruction. Plast Reconstr Surg 2019;143(1):24–34
2. Radovan C. Tissue expansion in soft-tissue reconstruction. Plast Reconstr Surg 1984;74(4):482–492
3. Antonyshyn O, Gruss JS, Mackinnon SE, Zuker R. Complications of soft tissue expansion. Br J Plast Surg 1988;41(3):239–250

7. Vascularized Composite Allografts and Transplant Immunology

See *Essentials of Plastic Surgery*, third edition, pp. 82–87

TRANSPLANT TISSUE TYPES

1. *Which transplant type best describes the transfer of tissues between unrelated members of the same species?*
   A. Autograft
   B. Xenograft
   C. Allograft
   D. Isograft
   E. Vascularized graft

MAJOR HISTOCOMPATIBILITY COMPLEX ANTIGENS

2. *Which one of the following is correct regarding major histocompatibility complex (MHC) antigens?*
   A. There are three classes of MHC molecules.
   B. MHC molecules encode proteins responsible for identifying foreign antigens.
   C. Class I molecules display peptides from outside the cell.
   D. Class II molecules are present on all nucleated cells.
   E. Human leukocyte antigen (HLA)-DP, HLA-DR, and HLA-DQ are all class I molecules.

ADAPTIVE (ACQUIRED) IMMUNE SYSTEM

3. *When considering the adaptive (acquired) immune system, which one of the following is true?*
   A. It plays no significant role in transplant immunology.
   B. The key cells involved are neutrophils and macrophages.
   C. The response is nonspecific in nature.
   D. It displays an enhanced secondary response (memory).
   E. The response typically occurs within 24 hours.

ALLOGRAFT REJECTION

4. *Which one of the following is correct regarding allograft rejection?*
   A. Acute rejection occurs within the first few hours and is mediated by donor-specific antibodies.
   B. The direct pathway of donor organ recognition predominates in chronic rejection.
   C. Chronic rejection occurs over weeks to months and may be satisfactorily treated with steroids.
   D. Acute rejection is difficult to treat, and at present no reliable treatment exists.
   E. Chronic rejection was initially thought to have little role in vascularized composite allograft (VCA) immunology.

VASCULARIZED COMPOSITE ALLOGRAFT TRANSPLANTATION

5. You are part of a team preparing a patient for a full-face transplant. Tissue components to be included are skin, muscle, nerve, vessels, mucosa, and bone. An immunosuppressive regimen needs to be selected. *Which one of the following is the most antigenic tissue?*
   A. Fat
   B. Muscle
   C. Nerve
   D. Bone
   E. Skin

BANFF GRADING FOR ACUTE REJECTION

6. A patient presents with diffuse erythema of the skin after facial transplantation and frank epidermal necrosis is confirmed histologically. *Which one of the following grades best describes the problem according to the Banff criteria?*
   A. Grade 0
   B. Grade I
   C. Grade II
   D. Grade III
   E. Grade IV

IMMUNOSUPPRESSION

7. *What drugs are usually prescribed for maintenance therapy following VCA?*
   A. Tacrolimus, mycophenolate mofetil, and corticosteroid
   B. Polyclonal antithymocyte globulin (ATG), daclizumab, and OKT3
   C. Clobetasol, sirolimus, and corticosteroid
   D. Corticosteroid, basiliximab, and sirolimus
   E. OKT3, corticosteroid, and mycophenoplate mofetil

TREATMENT WITH TACROLIMUS

8. *What is the main caveat of using tacrolimus in transplant antirejection medication?*
   A. It causes hypertension, hyperlipidemia, and hyperglycemia.
   B. It causes bone marrow suppression.
   C. It has a high association with lung toxicity.
   D. It is associated with cytokine release syndrome.
   E. It has a narrow therapeutic index.

IMMUNOSUPPRESSION THERAPY

9. A patient attends weekly review 3 months after hand transplant surgery. On examination, erythema and papules to the skin are found have developed. *Which one of the following represents part of the first-line management of this patient, assuming that the tacrolimus levels are therapeutic?*
   A. Add sirolimus
   B. Add monoclonal antibodies
   C. Add polyclonal antithymocyte globulin
   D. Increase prednisolone
   E. Increase mycophenolate mofetil

COMPLICATIONS OF IMMUNE SUPPRESSION

10. *Following VCA, what would be the most likely presentation of malignancy secondary to immunotherapy?*
   A. Hemoptysis
   B. Keratotic skin lesion
   C. Pathologic fracture
   D. Lymphadenopathy
   E. Change in bowel habit

Answers

TRANSPLANT TISSUE TYPES

1. *Which transplant type best describes the transfer of tissues between unrelated members of the same species?*

   C. Allograft

   An *allograft* is transplanted from an unrelated member of the same species (e.g., a cadaveric split-thickness skin graft or donor kidney transplant). An *isograft* is tissue that is transferred from one individual to another who is genetically identical. An *autograft* is tissue that is transplanted within the same individual (e.g., a split-thickness skin graft or free deep inferior epigastric artery perforator [DIEP] flap). A *xenograft* is tissue that is transplanted from one species to another, such as a porcine heart valve when implanted in a human. Grafts can be vascularized such as a hand transplant or nonvascularized such as a split-thickness graft and can be transferred between individuals or within the same individual depending on the graft in question.[1]

REFERENCE

1. Thorne CH, Bartlett SP, Beasley RW, et al, eds. Grabb and Smith's Plastic Surgery. 6th ed. Philadelphia: Lippincott Williams & Wilkins; 2007

MAJOR HISTOCOMPATIBILITY COMPLEX ANTIGENS

2. *Which one of the following is correct regarding major histocompatibility complex (MHC) antigens?*

   B. MHC molecules encode proteins responsible for identifying foreign antigens.

   The MHC antigens are part of the cell-mediated immune response and in humans they are referred to as *human leukocyte antigen* (HLA) *molecules*. They are relevant to allograft rejection and provide an immunological fingerprint. The HLA complex is a group of genes that encode proteins responsible for identifying foreign antigens to the immune system. They present antigen fragments to T-cells and bind T-cell receptors. There are two classes of molecules (not three) and they differ in a number of ways. Class I (HLA-A, HLA-B, and HLA-C) molecules are present on all nucleated cells, whereas class II (HLA-DP, HLA-DQ, and HLA-DR) are only found on antigen-presenting cells such as monocytes, macrophages, and B-cells. Class I molecules present target peptides generated from within the cell, whereas class II molecules target peptides acquired from outside the cell following processes such as phagocytosis.[1-3]

REFERENCES

1. Siemionow M, Klimczak A. Basics of immune responses in transplantation in preparation for application of composite tissue allografts in plastic and reconstructive surgery: part I. Plast Reconstr Surg 2008;121(1):4e–12e
2. Etra JW, Raimondi G, Brandacher G. Mechanisms of rejection in vascular composite allotransplantation. Curr Opin Organ Transplant 2018;23(1):28–33
3. Kaufman CL, Marvin MR, Chilton PM, et al. Immunobiology in VCA. Transpl Int 2016;29(6):644–654

ADAPTIVE (ACQUIRED) IMMUNE SYSTEM

3. *When considering the adaptive (acquired) immune system, which one of the following is true?*

   D. It displays an enhanced secondary response (memory).

   The adaptive or acquired immune system plays an important role in rejection of transplanted tissue. Activation of this pathway results in an antigen targeted immune response which is capable of memory. Furthermore, there is an enhanced secondary response that is more vigorous and has a faster onset. The primary cells involved in the adaptive response are the T- and B-cell lymphocytes with antigen-specific surface receptors. The T-cell activation requires three signals: (1) Foreign antigen recognition, (2) costimulatory signal, and (3) cytokine release. This process involves CD4 and CD8 cell types.

   In contrast, the innate immune system is a nonspecific, rapid-acting response (within minutes to hours) driven by neutrophils, macrophages, and monocytes. Its role within transplant rejection is less well defined and understood (see **Table 7.1**).[1,2]

Table 7.1 *Innate versus Adaptive (Acquired) Immunity*

	Innate	Adaptive
Components	Neutrophils, monocytes, macrophages, dendritic cells, natural killer cells, complement	Lymphocytes (T- and B-cells)
Characteristics	Occur rapidly (minutes to hours) Nonspecific	Develops over long periods Capable of memory (faster and more vigorous) Antigen-specific

REFERENCES

1. Siemionow M, Klimczak A. Basics of immune responses in transplantation in preparation for application of composite tissue allografts in plastic and reconstructive surgery: part I. Plast Reconstr Surg 2008;121(1):4e–12e
2. Etra JW, Raimondi G, Brandacher G. Mechanisms of rejection in vascular composite allotransplantation. Curr Opin Organ Transplant 2018;23(1):28–33

ALLOGRAFT REJECTION

4. *Which one of the following is correct regarding allograft rejection?*
   E. Chronic rejection was initially thought to have little role in vascularized composite allograft (VCA) immunology.

   Types of allograft rejection may be categorized as *hyperacute, accelerated, acute,* or *chronic.* Chronic rejection occurs over months to years via the indirect pathway of donor organ recognition. Treatment is very challenging, with no successful treatment available. Chronic rejection was initially thought to have no significant role in VCA transplants compared with solid organ transplants. However, as duration of ongoing VCA transplants has increased, longer term analysis has shown chronic rejection to occur in both hand and face transplants. Hyperacute rejection occurs within minutes to hours and is mediated by donor-specific antibodies that circulate before transplantation. These antibodies are acquired by prior exposure to an alloantigen after pregnancy, blood transfusion, or previous transplants. Accelerated rejection occurs within the first few days after a transplant. It represents a secondary immune response that is mediated by sensitized T-cells. Treatment involves steroids and lymphocyte-depleting agents. Acute rejection occurs in the weeks or months following a transplant and may be cell mediated (T-cell–mediated response) or humoral (B-cell/antibody–mediated response). However, the only type of acute rejection reported in VCAs is cell mediated. Treatment for cell-mediated acute rejection involves pulse steroids, optimization of maintenance therapy, and lymphocyte-depleting agents.[1,2]

REFERENCES

1. Siemionow M, Klimczak A. Basics of immune responses in transplantation in preparation for application of composite tissue allografts in plastic and reconstructive surgery: part I. Plast Reconstr Surg 2008;121(1):4e–12e
2. Etra JW, Raimondi G, Brandacher G. Mechanisms of rejection in vascular composite allotransplantation. Curr Opin Organ Transplant 2018;23(1):28–33

VASCULARIZED COMPOSITE ALLOGRAFT TRANSPLANTATION

5. You are part of a team preparing a patient for a full-face transplant. Tissue components to be included are skin, muscle, nerve, vessels, mucosa, and bone. An immunosuppressive regimen needs to be selected. *Which one of the following is the most antigenic tissue?*
   E. Skin

   Vascularized composite allografts (VCAs) contain numerous tissue types within a single graft such as skin, bone, muscle, and nerve. Of these tissue components, skin is the most antigenic, and as a result, direct inspection is important to identify acute rejection. This may manifest as erythematous macules, diffuse redness, or asymptomatic papules.[1–3]

REFERENCES

1. Etra JW, Raimondi G, Brandacher G. Mechanisms of rejection in vascular composite allotransplantation. Curr Opin Organ Transplant 2018;23(1):28–33
2. Kaufman CL, Marvin MR, Chilton PM, et al. Immunobiology in VCA. Transpl Int 2016;29(6):644–654
3. Issa F. Vascularized composite allograft-specific characteristics of immune responses. Transpl Int 2016;29(6):672–681

BANFF GRADING FOR ACUTE REJECTION

6. A patient presents with diffuse erythema of the skin after facial transplantation and frank epidermal necrosis is confirmed histologically. *Which one of the following grades best describes the problem according to the Banff criteria?*

   E. Grade IV

   The Banff 2007 grading system (**Box 7.1**) for acute rejection has five categories ranging from 0 to IV.[1] Grade 0 represents no rejection. Grade IV is the most severe rejection, and these patients present with frank necrosis of the epidermis or other skin structures. In face allografts, the transplanted mucosal surfaces may be similarly affected.

BOX 7.1   *BANFF 2007 GRADING SYSTEM FOR ACUTE REJECTION*[1]

Grade 0 (no rejection)
- No or rare inflammatory infiltrates

Grade I (mild rejection)
- Mild perivascular infiltration
- No involvement of the overlying epidermis

Grade II (moderate rejection)
- Moderate to severe perivascular inflammation with or without mild epidermal and/or adnexal involvement (limited to spongiosis and exocytosis)
- No epidermal dyskeratosis or apoptosis

Grade III (severe rejection)
- Dense inflammation and epidermal involvement, with epithelial apoptosis, dyskeratosis, and/or keratinolysis

Grade IV (necrotizing acute rejection)
- Frank necrosis of the epidermis or other skin structures

REFERENCE

1. Cendales LC, Kanitakis J, Schneeberger S, et al. The Banff 2007 working classification of skin-containing composite tissue allograft pathology. Am J Transplant 2008;8(7):1396–1400

IMMUNOSUPPRESSION

7. *What drugs are usually prescribed for maintenance therapy following VCA?*

   A. Tacrolimus, mycophenolate mofetil, and corticosteroid

   Following VCA transplant, a standard maintenance therapy involves three key drugs: A calcineurin inhibitor such as tacrolimus, an antimetabolite such as mycophenolate mofetil, and corticosteroids.

   In contrast, induction therapy, which is given at the time of transplantation, to prepare the recipient to receive foreign tissue, includes polyclonal antithymocyte globulin (ATGs), monoclonal anti-IL receptor antibodies (e.g., daclizub or basiliximab), and monoclonal anti-CD3 antibodies (OKT3) as in option B. Rescue therapy involves an increase in maintenance immunosuppression combined with steroid boluses, clobetasol, and sirolimus, as in option C.[1]

REFERENCE

1. Howsare M, Jones CM, Ramirez AM. Immunosuppression maintenance in vascularized composite allotransplantation: what is just right? Curr Opin Organ Transplant 2017;22(5):463–469

TREATMENT WITH TACROLIMUS

8. *What is the main caveat of using tacrolimus in transplant antirejection medication?*

   E. It has a narrow therapeutic index.

   Tacrolimus is a calcineurin inhibitor and is one of the key components in maintenance antirejection therapy following transplant surgery. It blocks intracellular signaling pathways that lead to IL-2 release and amplification of the immune response. The main problems with tacrolimus are twofold: It has a narrow therapeutic index and hence requires regular monitoring of drug levels, and it can cause nephrotoxicity. It has also been found to cause neurotoxicity at higher levels but has conversely been found to enhance nerve recovery after coaptation at lower doses, which may have additional benefits in VCA patients.[1]

   Corticosteroids are also important in transplant antirejection medications and can cause hypertension, hyperlipidemia, and hyperglycemia as well as weight gain and osteoporosis. Antiproliferative agents such as mycophenolate mofetil are also part of maintenance therapy and inhibit purine metabolism and DNA synthesis. They can cause bone marrow suppression. Cell cycle inhibitors such as sirolimus prevent T-cell proliferation and can cause lung toxicity. Biological agents such as OKT3, antithymocyte globulin (ATG), basiliximab, and daclizimab are monoclonal antibodies targeting CD3 or IL-2 receptors and are associated with cytokine release syndrome (see Table 7.4, *Essentials of Plastic Surgery*, third edition).[2]

REFERENCES

1. Konofaos P, Terzis JK. FK506 and nerve regeneration: past, present, and future. J Reconstr Microsurg 2013;29(3):141–148
2. Howsare M, Jones CM, Ramirez AM. Immunosuppression maintenance in vascularized composite allotransplantation: what is just right? Curr Opin Organ Transplant 2017;22(5):463–469

IMMUNOSUPPRESSION THERAPY

9. A patient attends weekly review 3 months after hand transplant surgery. On examination, erythema and papules to the skin are found have developed. *Which one of the following represents part of the first-line management of this patient, assuming that the tacrolimus levels are therapeutic?*

   D. Increase prednisolone

   This patient displays signs of acute rejection. This is managed with rescue therapy and involves systemic corticosteroids often alongside topical immunosuppressants such as clobetasol and protopic. It is important to confirm that calcineurin inhibitors such as tacrolimus are at therapeutic levels and if not, this must be addressed. Second-line agents include induction therapy agents, sirolimus and high-dose tacrolimus. Monoclonal antibodies and polyclonal antithymocyte globulin are part of a standard induction therapy regimen.[1,2]

REFERENCES

1. Howsare M, Jones CM, Ramirez AM. Immunosuppression maintenance in vascularized composite allotransplantation: what is just right? Curr Opin Organ Transplant 2017;22(5):463–469
2. Janis JE, MacKenzie KD, Wright SE, et al. Management of steroid-resistant late acute cellular rejection following face transplantation: a case report. Transplant Proc 2015;47(1):223–225

COMPLICATIONS OF IMMUNE SUPPRESSION

10. *Following VCA, what would be the most likely presentation of malignancy secondary to immunotherapy?*

    B. Keratotic skin lesion

    The most common malignancy after transplant surgery is skin cancer. The most likely subtype is squamous cell carcinoma (SCC) and this would first present as a keratotic skin lesion. The reason for the increased risk is immune suppression therapy. This is one of a number of reasons why close follow-up by a plastic surgery team is required.

    Hemoptysis is a sign of lung cancer, pathologic fractures are signs of bone metastases, and lymphadenopathy may represent metastatic spread of an SCC or other tumor. Alternatively, post-transplant lymphoproliferative disease may occur. This is a B-cell proliferation due to neutropenic immune suppression. Symptoms range from infectious mononucleosis-like lesions to frank lymphoma. Change in bowel habit is associated with benign and malignant processes in the gastrointestinal (GI) tract but not specifically to immune suppression therapy.[1]

REFERENCE

1. Chapman JR, Webster AC, Wong G. Cancer in the transplant recipient. Cold Spring Harb Perspect Med 2013;3(7):a015677

8. Basics of Microsurgery

See *Essentials of Plastic Surgery*, third edition, pp. 88–104

CONTRAINDICATIONS TO FREE TISSUE TRANSFER

1. You are giving a lecture to residents, which includes patient selection for free tissue transfer and microsurgery. *Which one of the following should you tell them to help guide their clinical practice?*
   A. Free tissue transfer is contraindicated in certain age groups.
   B. Free tissue transfer in smokers is associated with increased flap loss.
   C. Preoperative irradiation is a contraindication to free tissue transfer.
   D. Smoking after digital replantation significantly increases failure rates.
   E. Patients with a history of multiple venous thromboembolism (VTE) should not undergo free tissue transfer.

EQUIPMENT AND INSTRUMENTATION

2. *When performing a microvascular anastomosis for free tissue transfer, which one of the following is correct?*
   A. Heparinized saline is used in concentrations of 10,000 U/mL.
   B. Topical papaverine is a sodium channel blocker used to reduce vasospasm.
   C. Microvascular clamps should have a closing pressure of less than 30 g/mm^2.
   D. Operating loupes should not be routinely used for vascular anastomoses.
   E. Coupler devices should be reserved for end-to-end venous anastomoses.

TECHNICAL CONSIDERATIONS IN MICROVASCULAR SURGERY

3. *Which one of the following is correct regarding microvascular surgery?*
   A. Vessel inflow should be checked with the strip test before the anastomosis is performed.
   B. The adventitia should be trimmed flush to the vessel end.
   C. It is advisable to start with the simplest and most accessible anastomosis.
   D. Vessels are best manipulated by holding the adventitia.
   E. A set number of sutures will be required depending on vessel diameter.

INTRAOPERATIVE DECISION-MAKING

4. You have just completed a microsurgical anastomosis and released the clamps. Flow seems to be partially impaired, the vessel is not completely tubular, and there is a significant single-point leak in the anterior vessel wall. *What is the next step in the management of this situation?*
   A. Place an additional suture to close the leak.
   B. Clamp the vessels and cut out the anastomosis.
   C. Flush the anastomosis with heparinized saline.
   D. Apply lidocaine to reduce vessel spasm.
   E. Clamp the vessel and carefully inspect suture placement.

SIZE DISCREPANCY IN MICROVASCULAR ANASTOMOSES

5. During anastomosis of a lower-limb free flap, a size discrepancy of 2 mm between the donor artery and the recipient artery is found. *How will this challenge be best addressed?*
   A. Spatulation of the larger vessels
   B. Triangular wedge excision from the smaller vessels
   C. Use of a coupler device
   D. Perform an end-to-side technique
   E. Cut the larger vessels obliquely

END-TO-SIDE ANASTOMOSES

6. *When reconstructing an open Gustilo IIIB tibial fracture with a free latissimus dorsi (LD) muscle, what is the major advantage of using an end-to-side arterial anastomosis to the posterior tibial artery?*
   A. Operating time will be reduced.
   B. Anastomotic patency will be improved.
   C. Fewer sutures would be required.
   D. The anastomosis is technically easier.
   E. In-line flow to the foot can be maintained.

FREE FLAP MONITORING

7. You see a patient on the first evening after a free transverse rectus abdominis myocutaneous (TRAM) flap breast reconstruction. *Which one of the following is correct regarding monitoring of this flap?*
   A. Arterial insufficiency presents with a purple, swollen flap.
   B. Doppler monitoring is consistently reliable.
   C. Thermography is most reliable for intraoral flaps.
   D. Venous insufficiency presents with slow egress of bright red blood to pinprick.
   E. Transcutaneous tissue oximetry can detect vascular compromise before clinical signs alter.

FREE FLAP MONITORING

8. *Following circumferential reconstruction of a pharynx with a jejunal free flap, which one of the following represents the best modality for postoperative monitoring?*
   A. Clinical examination
   B. Implantable Doppler device
   C. Tissue oximetry
   D. Laser Doppler flowmetry
   E. Handheld Doppler device

FREE FLAP FAILURE

9. *Which one of the following is correct regarding failure of free flaps?*
   A. Success rates for free flaps are between 70 and 80% in experienced hands.
   B. The no-reflow phenomenon is the most common cause of flap failure.
   C. The no-reflow phenomenon is due to the absence of a patent anastomosis.
   D. Time from recognition of a failing flap to restoration of flow is most critical to successful salvage.
   E. The no-reflow phenomenon is usually reversible in the first 48 hours after surgery.

ANTICOAGULANTS IN MICROSURGERY

10. *Which one of the following is correct regarding heparin use in free flap surgery?*
    A. Heparin inhibits platelet aggregation via cyclooxygenase.
    B. Heparin binds to antithrombin and activates factor Xa.
    C. Heparin may be indicated when an anastomosis clots intraoperatively.
    D. Microvascular anastomotic patency is improved with systemic heparin.
    E. Systemic anticoagulation with heparin has minimal effect on hematoma rates.

MICRONEURAL REPAIR

11. After a laceration to the arm, a patient requires repair to the ulnar nerve. *Which one of the following is correct regarding repair of the transected nerve?*
    A. Direct repair under tension is preferable to interpositional grafting.
    B. Perineural repair is more difficult but has superior outcomes.
    C. Outcomes with sural nerve grafts are superior to those with vein grafts and synthetic tubes.
    D. Epineural repair with 10-0 sutures has the best overall outcomes.
    E. Accurate fascicular alignment with trimming where necessary will optimize outcomes.

HEALTH ECONOMICS

12. You are preparing a business case to the operating room management team to support routine use of a venous coupler in microsurgical cases. *Which one of the following is true and would best support your case?*
    A. Their use can reduce operative time compared with hand-sewn anastomoses.
    B. They avoid the need for a take back to the operating room due to venous thrombosis.
    C. Their use obviates the need for an operating microscope.
    D. They avoid the need for a surgical assistant in the operating room.
    E. As standard, they incorporate a postoperative monitoring Doppler device.

OCCUPATIONAL CONSIDERATIONS IN SURGERY

13. A recent survey of plastic surgeons has identified some health risks for microsurgeons. *Which one of the following microsurgeons have been shown to experience more than other surgeons?*
    A. Vertigo
    B. Migraine headaches
    C. Wrist and elbow pain
    D. Upper back and shoulder pain
    E. Visual disturbances

Answers

CONTRAINDICATIONS TO FREE TISSUE TRANSFER

1. **You are giving a lecture to residents, which includes patient selection for free tissue transfer and microsurgery.** *Which one of the following should you tell them to help guide their clinical practice?*

   D. **Smoking after digital replantation significantly increases failure rates.**

   Smoking can have significant detrimental effects on wound healing and success in digital replantation, but it does not appear to lead to an increase in free flap loss.[1,2] Free tissue transfer has been performed on young and old patients with good outcomes, and age, per se, is not a major concern. Rather, it is the overall general health of a patient that is important. A patient must be able to tolerate the potentially long general anesthetic and insult of major surgery and be compliant with postoperative therapy. A natural concern with regard to free tissue transfer in children is vessel size, but often the vessels are of good caliber and will also be free of atherosclerotic disease, making the procedure more straightforward. In elderly patients, vessels may be more friable or stiff and have atherosclerosis, which makes free tissue transfer more challenging. Preoperative radiation can also make vessel dissection and anastomosis more difficult, but it does not represent a contraindication to surgery. Many breast reconstructions are performed after radiation therapy, as are salvage cases in head and neck cancer. Additional care must, however, be taken with vessel handling as the vessels tend to be more fragile and are more prone to intimal damage.[3] If patients have a history of multiple venous thromboembolism (VTE) then a hypercoagulable disorder should be excluded; however, VTE, per se, is not a contraindication to free tissue transfer. Adequate prophylaxis with calf compression garments/hose/stocking and low-molecular-weight heparin will of course be required. Additional intraoperative heparin may be given. The risk of VTE can be assessed using the Caprini score.[4]

REFERENCES

1. Reus WF III, Colen LB, Straker DJ. Tobacco smoking and complications in elective microsurgery. Plast Reconstr Surg 1992;89(3):490–494
2. Chang LD, Buncke G, Slezak S, Buncke HJ. Cigarette smoking, plastic surgery, and microsurgery. J Reconstr Microsurg 1996;12(7):467–474
3. Bengtson BP, Schusterman MA, Baldwin BJ, et al. Influence of prior radiotherapy on the development of postoperative complications and success of free tissue transfers in head and neck cancer reconstruction. Am J Surg 1993;166(4):326–330
4. Pannucci CJ, Bailey SH, Dreszer G, et al. Validation of the Caprini risk assessment model in plastic and reconstructive surgery patients. J Am Coll Surg 2011;212(1):105–112

EQUIPMENT AND INSTRUMENTATION

2. *When performing a microvascular anastomosis for free tissue transfer, which one of the following is correct?*

   C. **Microvascular clamps should have a closing pressure of less than 30 g/mm².**

   It is important to use the correct microvascular equipment in order to avoid damage to vessels and anastomoses. Microvascular clamps are specifically designed to prevent trauma to the endothelium and should have a closing pressure of less than 30 g/mm². Heparinized saline is used in concentrations of 100 U/mL (not 10,000 U/mL). Topical papaverine works by blocking calcium (not sodium) channels and is useful to reduce vasospasm. Alternatively, 1–2% lidocaine or verapamil can be used. Ideally a microscope with at least 10× magnification should be used for vascular anastomoses; however, it is acceptable to use higher magnification loupes such as 3 to 4.5× for larger vessels.[1,2] The coupler device is ideally suited to venous anastomoses, and can be used in both end-to-end and end-to-side connections.[3] Although originally intended for venous anastomoses, it has been adopted by many surgeons for arterial anastomoses too. Spector et al[4] used them routinely in the artery for breast reconstruction in transverse rectus abdominis myocutaneous (TRAM) and deep inferior epigastric perforator (DIEP) flaps with good results when the thoracodorsal pedicle was the arterial source vessel.

REFERENCES

1. Acland RD. Instrumentation for microsurgery. Orthop Clin North Am 1977;8(2):281–294
2. Cox GW, Runnels S, Hsu HS, Das SK. A comparison of heparinised saline irrigation solutions in a model of microvascular thrombosis. Br J Plast Surg 1992;45(5):345–348
3. Jandali S, Wu LC, Vega SJ, Kovach SJ, Serletti JM. 1000 consecutive venous anastomoses using the microvascular anastomotic coupler in breast reconstruction. Plast Reconstr Surg 2010;125(3):792–798

4. Spector JA, Draper LB, Levine JP, Ahn CY. Routine use of microvascular coupling device for arterial anastomosis in breast reconstruction. Ann Plast Surg 2006;56(4):365–368

TECHNICAL CONSIDERATIONS IN MICROVASCULAR SURGERY

3. *Which one of the following is correct regarding microvascular surgery?*

D. Vessels are best manipulated by holding the adventitia.

During microvascular surgery, it is vital that vessel trauma, desiccation, and tension across the anastomosis are minimized. Carefully grasping the adventitia is preferred to stabilize the vessel during dissection. The strip test is sometimes called an *Acland test* and is performed *after* the anastomosis has been completed. It involves carefully grasping the vessel distal to the anastomosis with two forceps and then gently milking blood distally so the vessel is empty between the two forceps. On release of the proximal forceps, the vessel should fill if the anastomosis is working correctly. The *spurt test* is used to check inflow *before* anastomosis is performed. This involves releasing all clamps from the input vessel, flushing with heparinized saline solution, and testing blood flow. Most surgeons advocate trimming of the adventitia to preserve 2–5 mm of exposed vessel end. The most difficult anastomosis should be done first as should the most difficult sutures within a given anastomosis.

Although the size of vessel generally determines the number of stitches, there is no "set number" per vessel diameter. Essentially the aim should be to use "just enough" sutures to approximate and seal the vessel accurately. Insufficient sutures will leave potential openings for leakage and development of thrombus, while excessive sutures risk backwalling and causing vessel damage.[1,2]

REFERENCES

1. Acland RD. Instrumentation for microsurgery. Orthop Clin North Am 1977;8(2):281–294
2. Yap LH, Butler CE. Principles of microsurgery. In: Thorne CH, ed. Grabband Smith's Plastic Surgery. Philadelphia: Lippincott Williams & Wilkins; 2007

INTRAOPERATIVE DECISION-MAKING

4. You have just completed a microsurgical anastomosis and released the clamps. Flow seems to be partially impaired, the vessel is not completely tubular, and there is a significant single-point leak in the anterior vessel wall. *What is the next step in the management of this situation?*

E. Clamp the vessel and carefully inspect suture placement.

This scenario describes the appearance of having backwalled the anastomosis. This is evidenced by the reduced flow and misshapen vessel appearance with high pressure causing a leak at the anterior wall. In this situation, reapplication of the clamps is necessary and careful progressive suture removal is advocated so that the suture causing the backwalling can be identified and replaced. In some situations, it may be better to cut out the anastomosis and start again but in the first instance careful inspection is a better choice. Placing an additional suture would be appropriate if flow was good and no backwalling was suspected. Flushing the vessel may be helpful if the occlusion was secondary to a small amount of debris or thrombotic material. Application of lidocaine is useful to reduce spasm but not required in this case. The number of sutures required for an anastomosis will depend on the diameter of the vessel and the suture used. It is best to use the least number of sutures that will achieve a satisfactory seal.[1]

REFERENCE

1. Yap LH, Butler CE. Principles of microsurgery. In: Thorne CH, ed. Grabb and Smith's Plastic Surgery. Philadelphia: Lippincott Williams & Wilkins; 2007

SIZE DISCREPANCY IN MICROVASCULAR ANASTOMOSES

5. During anastomosis of a lower-limb free flap, a size discrepancy of 2 mm between the donor artery and the recipient artery is found. *How will this challenge be best addressed?*

D. Perform an end-to-side technique

A number of techniques are available to overcome size discrepancies between vessels. These include methods to increase the smaller vessel (spatulation) or to reduce the larger vessel (triangular wedge). Cutting the smaller vessel obliquely can also be helpful. In this case, an end-to-side anastomosis would be advisable, given the ratio of vessel mismatch is likely to be greater than 1.5:1 or even 2:1. Significant vessel mismatch results in alteration or disruption of flow mechanics and can promote vessel thrombosis so needs to be managed carefully. A further reason for using an end-to-side approach in this scenario is that distal limb blood flow through the anterior or posterior tibial vessels can be maintained. The use of an end-to-side anastomosis is often undertaken in head and neck cases where the flap vein is anastomosed into the internal jugular vein. Further options to address vessel mismatch include incorporation of a vein graft, but this introduces additional risk by doubling the number of anastomoses required and also adds a potential donor site harvest to the procedure.[1-4] Alternatively, a modified geometric Kunlin's technique can be used.[5] This adds an axial incision to further lengthen the aperture in spatulated vessels. The coupler device can be very useful for managing size discrepancy between donor and recipient veins and may also be useful in some arterial anastomoses. However, in the lower limb the vessels are likely to be too thick or stiff walled to work well with a coupler and it is not routinely used in this setting (**Figs. 8.1, 8.2, 8.3, and 8.4**).

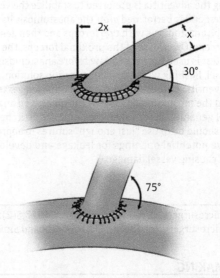

Fig. 8.1   Ideal characteristics of an end-to-side anastomosis.

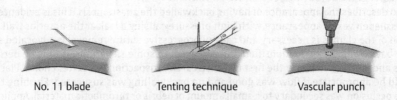

No. 11 blade   Tenting technique   Vascular punch

Fig. 8.2   Methods of performing an arteriotomy.

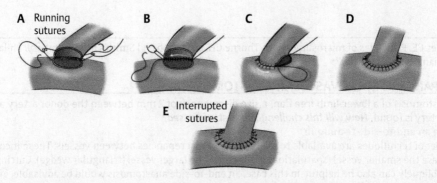

Fig. 8.3   End-to-side anastomosis. *A–D,* Running suture technique. *E,* Interrupted sutures.

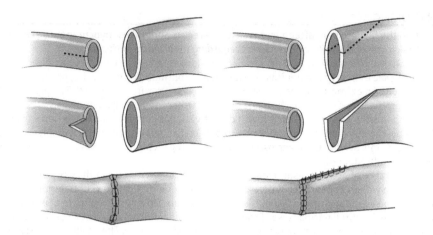

Fig. 8.4 Size discrepancies can be corrected by spatulation or longitudinal wedge resection.

REFERENCES

1. Alghoul MS, Gordon CR, Yetman R, et al. From simple interrupted to complex spiral: a systematic review of various suture techniques for microvascular anastomoses. Microsurgery 2011;31(1):72–80
2. Pederson WC. Principles of microsurgery. In: Green DP, Hotchkiss RN, Pederson WC, Wolfe SW, eds. Green's Operative Hand Surgery. 5th ed. Philadelphia: Elsevier Churchill Livingstone; 2005
3. Weiss DD, Pribaz JJ. Microsurgery. In: Achauer BM, ed. Plastic Surgery, Indications, Operations, and Outcomes. St Louis: Mosby-Year Book; 2000
4. Yap LH, Butler CE. Principles of microsurgery. In: Thorne CH, ed. Grabb and Smith's Plastic Surgery. Philadelphia: Lippincott Williams & Wilkins; 2007
5. Inbal A, Collier ZJ, Ho CL, Gottlieb LJ. Modified Kunlin's technique for microsurgical end-to-end anastomoses: a series of 100 flaps. J Reconstr Microsurg 2019;35(6):430–437

END-TO-SIDE ANASTOMOSES

6. ***When reconstructing an open Gustilo IIIB tibial fracture with a free latissimus dorsi (LD) muscle, what is the major advantage of using an end-to-side arterial anastomosis to the posterior tibial artery?***

  E. **In-line flow to the foot can be maintained.**

The main benefit of using an end-to-side anastomosis in this situation is the preservation of distal flow through the posterior tibial artery. This is particularly relevant given the history of trauma. An alternative is to use a flow-through flap (e.g., anterolateral thigh [ALT]) with two in-line anastomoses.[1,2] End-to-side and end-to-end anastomoses both have equivalent patency and generally require a similar amount of sutures and operating time. Surgeons often find end-to-end anastomoses easier to perform than end-to-side, but it will depend on personal preference.

When performing an end-to-side anastomosis, an arteriotomy is required in the source vessel. This is performed with either a beaver blade, scissors, or vascular punch. The angle of entry should be set between 30 and 70 degrees. The anastomosis is then performed with either interrupted or continuous sutures one side then the other (see **Figs. 8.1 and 8.3**).[3]

REFERENCES

1. Bullocks J, Naik B, Lee E, Hollier L Jr. Flow-through flaps: a review of current knowledge and a novel classification system. Microsurgery 2006;26(6):439–449
2. Aggarwal A, Singh H, Mahendru S, et al. A case series of flow-through free anterolateral thigh flap to augment the vascularity of ischaemic limbs with soft tissue defect. Indian J Plast Surg 2016;49(1):35–41
3. Alghoul MS, Gordon CR, Yetman R, et al. From simple interrupted to complex spiral: a systematic review of various suture techniques for microvascular anastomoses. Microsurgery 2011;31(1):72–80

FREE FLAP MONITORING

7. You see a patient on the first evening after a free transverse rectus abdominis myocutaneous (TRAM) flap breast reconstruction. *Which one of the following is correct regarding monitoring of this flap?*

   E. Transcutaneous tissue oximetry can detect vascular compromise before clinical signs alter.

   Transcutaneous tissue oximetry is a noninvasive method of continuously measuring perfusion quality of a free flap postoperatively. An oximetry probe measures tissue oxygen saturation (SpO2). The probe is placed on the skin flap intraoperatively to determine the baseline SpO2. Other than being a noninvasive technique, the main benefit of this monitoring approach is that it will detect vascular compromise of the flap earlier than clinical examination alone, thereby facilitating earlier re-exploration in operating theater if a problem arises. A study by Lin et al[1] has shown improved flap salvage using this monitoring technique. However, its use in routine practice has not been uniformly adopted.

   The usual appearance of arterial insufficiency is a pale, cool flap with no capillary return and no bleeding to pinprick. A purple, swollen appearance with egress of dark blood (not bright red) to pinprick is characteristic of a congested flap secondary to venous outflow obstruction. Doppler imaging is a useful adjunct to flap monitoring, but it can be unreliable because of transmission of signals from adjacent vessels. Another modality for postoperative flap monitoring is thermography. This measures skin surface. Thermography measures skin surface temperature using a thermocouple device. Both venous and arterial occlusion can cause flap surface temperature to drop. Khouri and Shaw[2] reported that a relative difference in flap surface temperature versus reference surface temperature of more than 1.8° C had a 98% sensitivity for vascular compromise and a 75% predictive value; however, accuracy was considered to be poor in intraoral flaps. Absolute flap temperature changes are less reliable without a reference nonflap temperature, because they are affected by changes in ambient or body temperature.

REFERENCES

1. Lin SJ, Nguyen MD, Chen C, et al. Tissue oximetry monitoring in microsurgical breast reconstruction decreases flap loss and improves rate of flap salvage. Plast Reconstr Surg 2011;127(3):1080–1085
2. Khouri RK, Shaw WW. Monitoring of free flaps with surface-temperature recordings: is it reliable? Plast Reconstr Surg 1992;89(3):495–499, discussion 500–502

FREE FLAP MONITORING

8. *Following circumferential reconstruction of a pharynx with a jejunal free flap, which one of the following represents the best modality for postoperative monitoring?*

   B. Implantable Doppler device

   In the situation of a buried free flap, the most reliable monitoring method is to use an implantable Doppler device. This can be placed directly on either the anastomosed artery or vein and secured with a small ligaclip. Rates of salvage are reported to be very high using this device but sometimes the signal can be lost when in fact the vessel is still running. Clinical examination is difficult with buried flaps other than systemic parameters such as blood pressure and urine output. A handheld Doppler can be useful for some buried flaps but transmission from other vessels can compromise reliability. Laser Doppler and tissue oximetry each require the presence of a skin paddle for monitoring. Some surgeons will incorporate a small monitoring skin paddle where possible in otherwise buried flaps and this can be helpful. The downside is that this may require further surgery to remove it for aesthetic reasons and it tends to be quite small, thereby making assessment of it more difficult.[1-4]

REFERENCES

1. Roehl KR, Mahabir RC. A practical guide to free tissue transfer. Plast Reconstr Surg 2013;132(1):147e–158e
2. Chang EI, Ibrahim A, Zhang H, et al. Deciphering the sensitivity and specificity of the implantable Doppler probe in free flap monitoring. Plast Reconstr Surg 2016;137(3):971–976
3. Chadwick SL, Khaw R, Duncan J, Wilson SW, Highton L, O'Ceallaigh S. The use of venous anastomotic flow couplers to monitor buried free DIEP flap reconstructions following nipple-sparing mastectomy. JPRAS Open 2019;23:50–54
4. Kempton SJ, Poore SO, Chen JT, Afifi AM. Free flap monitoring using an implantable anastomotic venous flow coupler: analysis of 119 consecutive abdominal-based free flaps for breast reconstruction. Microsurgery 2015;35(5):337–344

FREE FLAP FAILURE

9. *Which one of the following is correct regarding failure of free flaps?*

   D. Time from recognition of a failing flap to restoration of flow is most critical to successful salvage.

   Early recognition and surgical re-exploration of a failing flap are critical to optimization of outcomes in free flap surgery. Most flaps can be salvaged if surgery is performed within the first 2 hours following recognition of the problem. Accurate postoperative free flap monitoring is therefore key to free flap success. It is tailored to specific flaps but in general a combined approach of clinical examination to assess color, capillary refill, turgor, and temperature, along with Doppler assessment, is advised for free flap monitoring. The most common cause of flap failure is an anastomotic problem, leading to venous or arterial insufficiency. The no-reflow phenomenon is believed to be caused by endothelial swelling, platelet aggregation, and leaky capillaries in the presence of a patent anastomosis. It is less commonly seen as a cause of flap failure and although it may be reversible at approximately 4–8 hours, this is unlikely after 12 hours.[1,2] One retrospective study reviewed late salvage cases (i.e., beyond 1 week) and highlighted the futile nature of attempts at such late flap salvage. Surgeons need to be realistic about the chances of saving a failing flap at any stage and remain objective about when a second reconstruction would be a preferable option.[3]

REFERENCES

1. Chang EI, Chang EI, Soto-Miranda MA, et al. Comprehensive evaluation of risk factors and management of impending flap loss in 2138 breast free flaps. Ann Plast Surg 2016;77(1):67–71
2. Roehl KR, Mahabir RC. A practical guide to free tissue transfer. Plast Reconstr Surg 2013;132(1):147e–158e
3. Largo RD, Selber JC, Garvey PB, et al. Outcome analysis of free flap salvage in outpatients presenting with microvascular compromise. Plast Reconstr Surg 2018;141(1):20e–27e

ANTICOAGULANTS IN MICROSURGERY

10. *Which one of the following is correct regarding heparin use in free flap surgery?*
  C. **Heparin may be indicated when an anastomosis clots intraoperatively.**
  Some surgeons give a dose of intravenous heparin just before disconnecting or just after reconnecting the flap with the intention of reducing thrombosis at the anastomotic site. Others will reserve this for when the first anastomosis has clotted and the anastomosis must be redone. Aspirin inhibits platelet aggregation via cyclooxygenase. Heparin binds antithrombin III and results in inhibition of both antithrombin and factor Xa. No evidence suggests that systemic heparin will improve anastomotic patency, except perhaps in cases in which intraoperative clotting has occurred or the anastomosis requires revision. The use of systemic heparin increases the risk of postoperative bleeding, but its action is short-lived compared with low molecular heparin.[1–3]

REFERENCES

1. Pugh CM, Dennis RH II, Massac EA. Evaluation of intraoperative anticoagulants in microvascular free-flap surgery. J Natl Med Assoc 1996;88(10):655–657
2. Kroll SS, Miller MJ, Reece GP, et al. Anticoagulants and hematomas in free flap surgery. Plast Reconstr Surg 1995;96(3):643–647
3. Conrad MH, Adams WP Jr. Pharmacologic optimization of microsurgery in the new millennium. Plast Reconstr Surg 2001;108(7):2088–2096, quiz 2097

MICRONEURAL REPAIR

11. After a laceration to the arm, a patient requires repair to the ulnar nerve. *Which one of the following is correct regarding repair of the transected nerve?*
  E. **Accurate fascicular alignment with trimming where necessary will optimize outcomes.**
  Different techniques exist to repair transected nerves. They include epineural, perineural, or grouped fascicular. Outcomes are similar with all techniques, but perineural techniques may be technically more difficult. Grouped fascicular techniques can be helpful for larger nerves such as the ulnar nerve at the wrist, where specific branches can be identified. It is vital that neither excessive tension nor buckling of fascicles occurs at the repair site. For this reason, accurate trimming and use of interpositional grafts are advocated where necessary. The choice of graft in short defects in sensory nerves may be less important because vein grafts and polyglycolic acid tubes can have comparable outcomes to donor nerves such as the sural and antebrachial cutaneous nerves. Processed allograft conduits provide a further option, with results superior to those obtained with polyglycolic acid tubes. However, in larger defects autologous sural nerve grafts are the benchmark.[1–5]

REFERENCES

1. Walton RL, Brown RE, Matory WE Jr, Borah GL, Dolph JL. Autogenous vein graft repair of digital nerve defects in the finger: a retrospective clinical study. Plast Reconstr Surg 1989;84(6):944–949, discussion 950–952
2. Wang H, Lineaweaver WC. Nerve conduits for nerve reconstruction. Oper Tech Plast Reconstr Surg 2002;9(2):59–66
3. Chiu DT, Strauch B. A prospective clinical evaluation of autogenous vein grafts used as a nerve conduit for distal sensory nerve defects of 3 cm or less. Plast Reconstr Surg 1990;86(5):928–934
4. Mackinnon SE, Dellon AL. Clinical nerve reconstruction with a bioabsorbable polyglycolic acid tube. Plast Reconstr Surg 1990;85(3):419–424

5. Weber RA, Breidenbach WC, Brown RE, Jabaley ME, Mass DP. A randomized prospective study of polyglycolic acid con-duits for digital nerve reconstruction in humans. Plast Reconstr Surg 2000;106(5):1036–1045, discussion 1046–1048

HEALTH ECONOMICS

12. You are preparing a business case to the operating room management team to support routine use of a venous coupler in microsurgical cases. *Which one of the following is true and would best support your case?*

   A. Their use can reduce operative time compared with hand-sewn anastomoses.

   When considering a business case for new operating room (OR) equipment, management will be interested in cost effectiveness of a product or device. As surgeons we are aware of many clinical benefits of the coupler device and these include its rigid ring configuration which stents the anastomosis open, a low rate of venous thrombosis (<1%), a minimal operator learning curve, ease of use, and the ability to manage intraoperative vessel size mismatches effectively. From the perspective of the managers, factors which reduce OR time and increase OR efficiency will have highest importance on their radar. OR time is expensive and hence any factors which can safely and consistently reduce OR time requirement will be valuable. The use of the coupler device has been shown to be significantly quicker to perform than a hand-sewn anastomosis. It has been associated with a 16-minute decrease in time compared with a hand-sewn anastomosis in one recently published study.[1] With OR time expenses, the time saving would be likely to cover the costs of the device.

   A further potential cost benefit is the low thrombosis rate and hence need to return to OR. However, although this is lower than with hand-sewn anastomoses, couplers can still fail and need a return to the OR or indeed to be redone in the OR at the first sitting. Reasons for the coupler to fail include tearing of the vessel leaving a hole in the vessel wall, failure of the device to properly load or be detached from the applicator device, failure to remain closed (particularly if the vessel wall is thick and stiff), or residual thrombus or inadvertent injury to the intimal surface.

   Couplers do still need a microscope for their application and they don't necessarily obviate the need for a surgical assistant in the OR, in spite of it being possible to use one independently. As standard, they do not incorporate an implantable Doppler device for postoperative monitoring although there is one device available on the market which does so. Couplers are mainly used for venous anastomoses; however, they have been used successfully in some settings within the arterial anastomosis.[2-4]

REFERENCES

1. Head LK, McKay DR. Economic comparison of hand-sutured and coupler-assisted microvascular anastomoses. J Reconstr Microsurg 2018;34(1):71–76
2. Coroneos CJ, Voineskos SH, Heller AM, Avram R. Reduced venous thrombosis and re-exploration time with anastomotic coupling device: a cohort study. Microsurgery 2016;36(5):372–377
3. Kulkarni AR, Mehrara BJ, Pusic AL, et al. Venous thrombosis in handsewn versus coupled venous anastomoses in 857 consecutive breast free flaps. J Reconstr Microsurg 2016;32(3):178–182
4. Spector JA, Draper LB, Levine JP, Ahn CY. Routine use of microvascular coupling device for arterial anastomosis in breast reconstruction. Ann Plast Surg 2006;56(4):365–368

OCCUPATIONAL CONSIDERATIONS IN SURGERY

13. A recent survey of plastic surgeons has identified some health risks for microsurgeons. *Which one of the following microsurgeons have been shown to experience more than other surgeons?*

   D. Upper back and shoulder pain

   There is growing interest in surgical ergonomics and occupational health of surgeons. A recent study by Khansa et al[1] explored work-related musculoskeletal injuries in plastic surgeons. This study showed that microsurgery is more likely than any other subset of procedures to exacerbate symptoms of musculoskeletal problems and that microsurgeons are more likely to have upper back and shoulder problems than other surgeons (odds ratios were 1.64 and 1.47, respectively). Surgeons' posture and position are therefore essential to prevent fatigue, tremor, and avoid chronic musculoskeletal problems for surgeons.

   Recommendations for surgeons undertaking microsurgery, therefore, are to ensure a satisfactory position is maintained for both ease of microsurgery and hence effectiveness as well as surgeons' occupational health benefits. The surgeon should sit with their feet flat on the floor, hips, knees and elbows at right angles, and with their back and neck straight. The hands and forearms should be supported with stacks or towels to minimize tremor and ensure comfort. Avoiding standing or stooping over the microscope is important as is avoiding having the cervical spine flexed for extended periods.

REFERENCE

1. Khansa I, Khansa L, Westvik TS, Ahmad J, Lista F, Janis JE. Work-related musculoskeletal injuries in plastic surgeons in the United States, Canada, and Norway. Plast Reconstr Surg 2018;141(1):165e–175e

9.   Biomaterials

See *Essentials of Plastic Surgery*, third edition, pp. 105–120

GENERAL PRINCIPLES OF BIOMATERIALS

1. Biomaterials are commonly used in plastic surgery for a variety of different applications. *Which one of the following statements is correct regarding biomaterials?*
   A. Biomaterials are by definition synthetic materials.
   B. Biocompatibility describes the permanence of an implant.
   C. *Alloplasts* are implants derived from synthetic material.
   D. *Allografts* represent living tissue derived from the host.
   E. *Xenografts* are derived from the same species animal donor.

GRAFT SUBTYPES

2. *Which one of the following statements is correct regarding graft substitutes?*
   A. Allografts represent the benchmark for biomaterials.
   B. Autografts must be processed to reduce their antigenicity.
   C. The use of alloplastic materials prevents donor site morbidity and host reaction.
   D. The use of allogenic materials prevents the risk of disease transmission.
   E. Xenografts have more antigenic potential than homografts.

AUTOGRAFTS IN GENERAL

3. *Which one of the following is an advantage of using an autograft?*
   A. Reduced duration of surgery
   B. Natural function and incorporation
   C. Avoidance of a donor site
   D. Limitless tissue quantity
   E. Reduced early morbidity

FOREIGN BODY REACTION

4. *Which one of the following is true with regards to a foreign body reaction associated with implantation of a biomaterial?*
   A. It only affects a proportion of implanted biomaterials.
   B. It involves a two-stage process.
   C. It is a uniformly unhelpful process.
   D. It refers specifically to formation of granuloma.
   E. It includes incorporation of acellular matrices.

ACELLULAR DERMAL MATRIX

5. You see a patient 14 days after mastectomy and immediate implant reconstruction with an acellular dermal matrix (ADM) sling. A large patch of erythema has developed over the lower pole of the reconstruction. The patient remains systemically well and afebrile. *Which one of the following is correct?*
   A. This is unusual and the patient must be closely monitored.
   B. A course of oral antibiotics should be prescribed.
   C. This is unrelated to the surgical technique.
   D. The patient is likely to need surgery to remove the implant.
   E. The patient requires reassurance only at this stage.

SYNTHETICS IN ABDOMINAL WALL RECONSTRUCTION

6. You are considering the use of Permacol to augment an abdominal wall repair and read that it is a crosslinked porcine dermal matrix. *Which one of the following is the main advantage of cross-linking in an ADM?*
   A. Improved tissue incorporation
   B. Increased material strength and stiffness
   C. Reduced local tissue inflammation
   D. Fewer bowel wall adhesions
   E. Lesser chance of infection

ACELLULAR DERMAL MATRIX USAGE

7. You are discussing the merits of using an ADM in implant-based breast reconstruction with a patient. *Which one of the following may be decreased when using an ADM in this situation?*
   A. The total procedural costs
   B. The risk of seroma development
   C. The risk of capsular contracture formation
   D. The amount of soft tissue cover
   E. The amount of intraoperative expander fill

ALLOGRAFT MATERIALS

8. You see a patient who has undergone breast reconstruction with AlloDerm and an implant. *Which one of the following is true of this ADM?*
   A. It is manufactured from bovine dermis.
   B. It is classified by the Food and Drug Administration (FDA) as a medical device.
   C. Incorporation into the host tissue is rare.
   D. It contains no cellular elements.
   E. Resorption rates are very consistent.

INTEGRA USE FOR RECONSTRUCTION

9. A patient has a 10 by 10 cm defect over the posterior ankle, exposing the Achilles tendon. A 2 by 2 cm area of tendon lacks paratenon cover centrally. You are planning to use Integra. *Which one of the following is correct regarding Integra?*
   A. It has a trilaminar complex biologic structure.
   B. It compromises of two porcine components, collagen and glycosaminoglycans.
   C. Fraying of the superficial layer is a good indicator for grafting.
   D. A salmon pink color at 3 weeks indicates scaffold process failure.
   E. It is contraindicated in areas of exposed tendon.

BONE REPAIR

10. *Which one of the following best describes the process of surface mediated bone growth such as that which occurs at the margin of a bone graft?*
    A. Osteogenesis
    B. Osteoinduction
    C. Osteoconduction
    D. Osseointegration
    E. Osteofibrosis

SYNTHETIC BONE SUBSTITUTES

11. You are using polymethylmethacrylate (PMMA) to reconstruct the calvarium. *What is the main problem with using this biomaterial?*
    A. High cost
    B. Difficulty conforming
    C. Poor biocompatibility
    D. Lack of strength
    E. Risk of adjacent tissue damage

ALLOPLASTIC MATERIALS

12. You are considering the use of alloplastic facial implants in your aesthetic practice. *Which one of the following materials represents a nonresorbable alloplastic material made with high-density polyethylene?*
    A. Gore-Tex
    B. Medpor
    C. Marlex
    D. PEEK
    E. Phasix

THE FOREIGN BODY RESPONSE

13. *In two-stage flexor tendon reconstruction of the hand, how is the body's natural foreign body response specifically utilized to be advantageous to the reconstructive process?*
    A. It negates the need for tendon autograft.
    B. It accelerates the timing of rehabilitation.
    C. It facilitates smooth gliding of the tendon.
    D. It helps reduce bacterial load.
    E. It means the two stages can be performed 1 week apart.

BREAST IMPLANT ASSOCIATED ALCL (BIA-ALCL)

14. *Which one of the following is true with regards to BIA-ALCL?*
    A. Clinical presentation is most likely with an acute onset hot, red, painful breast.
    B. The mainstay of treatment is systemic oral tumor suppressing agents.
    C. The most likely cause is rupture of a smooth silicone breast implant.
    D. Diagnosis is made by sampling the capsule and fluid surrounding it.
    E. Prophylactic removal of implants older than 10 years is generally advocated.

FDA AND BREAST IMPLANTS

15. *Which one of the following is true regarding the FDA and the use of silicone gel-filled breast implants?*
    A. FDA approval is currently limited to reconstruction purposes only.
    B. FDA approval is currently permitted for all patients for either reconstruction or augmentation purposes.
    C. Regular imaging is advocated by the FDA following silicone breast implantation.
    D. The FDA has approved the use of textured implants manufactured using salt loss techniques.
    E. In 2019, the FDA advised the withdrawal of all textured breast implants from the market.

RECONSTRUCTION WITH COMPOSITE MESH

16. *What is the main clinical indication for using composite materials such as Proceed, Sepramesh, and TiMesh?*
    A. Breast reconstruction
    B. Scalp reconstruction
    C. Abdominal wall reconstruction
    D. Chest wall reconstruction
    E. Lower limb reconstruction

SILICONE AS A MEDICAL DEVICE MATERIAL

17. *Which one of the following is a consistent finding with silicone as a biomaterial?*
    A. Fibrous encapsulation
    B. Resorption
    C. Incorporation
    D. Rejection
    E. Degradation

Answers

GENERAL PRINCIPLES OF BIOMATERIALS

1. Biomaterials are commonly used in plastic surgery for a variety of different applications. *Which one of the following statements is correct regarding biomaterials?*

    C. *Alloplasts* are implants derived from synthetic material.

    Biomaterials can be either naturally occurring (autograft, allograft, or xenograft) or synthetic (alloplastic). Biocompatibility is the term used to describe desirable physicochemical and biologic properties of a material for its intended application rather than the permanence of the implant. There are a number of elements that contribute to biocompatibility including the absence of undesirable effects such as low toxicity, low host reaction, resistance to infection, and physical properties such as easy handling and manipulation. Permanence is an important clinical aspect of an implanted material and is achieved when harmony exists between host and implant. It refers to the long-term biocompatibility between host and implant. Allografts are either living or nonliving tissue derived from the same species donor (e.g., cadaveric skin grafts), whereas autografts are derived from the host (e.g., traditional skin grafts). Xenografts are derived from a different species donor (e.g., bovine/porcine) and include skin substitutes and acellular dermal matrices.

GRAFT SUBTYPES

2. *Which one of the following statements is correct regarding graft substitutes?*

    E. Xenografts have more antigenic potential than homografts.

    Xenografts are nonliving tissue derived from a different species, i.e., a nonhuman source, most commonly bovine or porcine. They will naturally cause a strong immunologic response with host tissue inflammatory reaction and strong antigenicity, and must be acellular to minimize this.

    Autografts, not allografts, represent the benchmark to which biomaterials are compared. They do not require processing to reduce their antigenicity because they originate from the host. Although donor site morbidity is not a problem with alloplastic materials, they cause a host reaction such as capsule formation around a breast implant. Allogenic materials include allografts and homografts. Each carries a risk of infectious disease transmission.

AUTOGRAFTS IN GENERAL

3. *Which one of the following is an advantage of using an autograft?*

    B. Natural function and incorporation

    Autografts are the benchmark for reconstruction because they are well tolerated by the host and become incorporated into adjacent tissue to provide lifelong reconstruction. However, the disadvantages include the need for a donor site, potential for donor site morbidity, increased surgical time for harvest, and a finite amount of available tissue.

    An example is the use of alveolar bone graft in cleft lip and palate patients. This can provide permanent bone stock in the alveolus at the expense of temporary donor site morbidity at the hip, which results in a prolonged surgical time and lengthened hospital stay. Hydroxyapatite synthetic material is an alternative substitute that could be used in this setting.

FOREIGN BODY REACTION

4. *Which one of the following is true with regards to a foreign body reaction associated with implantation of a biomaterial?*

    E. It includes incorporation of acellular matrices.

    The foreign body reaction is exhibited by all biomaterials and involves a multistaged process involving protein adsorption, fibrinogen deposition, formation of a provisional matrix, recruitment of inflammatory cells, and resolution or formation of a foreign body granuloma. The spectrum of responses includes rejection (e.g., xenograft), fibrous encapsulation (e.g., porous polyethylene or titanium plates), resorption (e.g., suture material breakdown), and incorporation (e.g., acellular matrices and grafts). Therefore, although unhelpful in some situations, the foreign body response is not uniformly so.[1,2]

REFERENCES

1. Anderson JM, Rodriguez A, Chang DT. Foreign body reaction to biomaterials. Semin Immunol 2008;20(2):86–100
2. Bellón JM, Buján J, Contreras L, Hernando A. Integration of biomaterials implanted into abdominal wall: process of scar formation and macrophage response. Biomaterials 1995;16(5):381–387

ACELLULAR DERMAL MATRIX

5. You see a patient 14 days after mastectomy and immediate implant reconstruction with an acellular dermal matrix (ADM) sling. A large patch of erythema has developed over the lower pole of the reconstruction. The patient remains systemically well and afebrile. *Which one of the following is correct?*

E. **The patient requires reassurance only at this stage.**

ADMs are immunologically inert, but they can mimic cellulitis when used in conjunction with implants or expanders in breast reconstruction. This is termed *red breast syndrome*.[1-3] It does not indicate active infection and therefore does not warrant antibiotic therapy. The manufacturers suggest thorough washing of the product before use because the chemicals and/or preservatives within the ADM are likely responsible for this phenomenon. It is unlikely the patient will need further treatment and will just require reassurance at this time. If she was febrile with a red, hot breast, this would be a different matter and would indicate the presence of an infectious process.

REFERENCES

1. Basu CB, Jeffers L. The role of acellular dermal matrices in capsular contracture: a review of the evidence. Plast Reconstr Surg 2012;130(5, Suppl 2):118S–124S
2. Danino MA, El Khatib AM, Doucet O, et al. Preliminary results supporting the bacterial hypothesis in red breast syndrome following postmastectomy acellular dermal matrix- and implant-based reconstructions. Plast Reconstr Surg 2019;144(6):988e–992e
3. Nahabedian MY. Prosthetic breast reconstruction and red breast syndrome: demystification and a review of the literature. Plast Reconstr Surg Glob Open 2019;7(5):e2108. Published online

SYNTHETICS IN ABDOMINAL WALL RECONSTRUCTION

6. You are considering the use of Permacol to augment an abdominal wall repair and read that it is a crosslinked porcine dermal matrix. *Which one of the following is the main advantage of cross-linking in an ADM?*

B. **Increased material strength and stiffness**

Acellular dermal matrices are nonliving dermal components from an allogenic or xenogenic donor comprised of collagen, elastin, laminin, and glycosaminoglycans. They have a broad range of uses in plastic surgery. A limited number of ADMs are cross-linked and this serves to strengthen the material, prolong its lifespan, and reduce antigenicity. However, this comes at the expense of delayed incorporation, prolonged inflammation, increased infection rate, and bowel adhesion formation. In essence cross-linking tends to make biologic material behave more like a synthetic material.[1]

REFERENCE

1. Janis JE, Nahabedian MY. Acellular dermal matrices in surgery. Plast Reconstr Surg 2012;130(5, Suppl 2)7S–8S

ACELLULAR DERMAL MATRIX USAGE

7. You are discussing the merits of using an ADM in implant-based breast reconstruction with a patient. *Which one of the following may be decreased when using an ADM in this situation?*

C. **The risk of capsular contracture formation**

The use of an ADM in implant-based breast reconstruction has become a popular option as it is believed to carry a number of potential advantages. First, it provides internal support to the reconstruction, and second, it provides additional thickness of implant coverage. When used with a subpectoral implant placement, it can essentially extend the muscle layer cover in the lower pole where otherwise the implant would only be covered by skin and subcutaneous tissues. When used pre-pectorally, the implant is fully wrapped in ADM and this provides additional cover subcutaneously in both upper and lower poles of the breast. Because the expander/implant is held in place more securely and potentially with less tension, it may enable the surgeon to increase the expander fill or go direct to implant with greater control. There is some evidence that ADM in this setting can reduce the capsular contracture rate. However, the disadvantages include a potential increase in seroma rate and increased total procedural costs.[1-3] There has been much debate about the overall benefits of using ADM in breast reconstruction, and an in-depth FDA review in 2019 considered evidence for and against their use. It is currently used off label for this purpose as use is mainly guided by surgeon and patient preference.[4,5]

REFERENCES

1. Jordan SW, Khavanin N, Fine NA, Kim JYS. An algorithmic approach for selective acellular dermal matrix use in immediate two-stage breast reconstruction: indications and outcomes. Plast Reconstr Surg 2014;134(2):178–188
2. Kim JYS, Davila AA, Persing S, et al. A meta-analysis of human acellular dermis and submuscular tissue expander breast reconstruction. Plast Reconstr Surg 2012;129(1):28–41

3. Krishnan NM, Chatterjee A, Rosenkranz KM, Powell SG, Nigriny JF, Vidal DC. The cost effectiveness of acellular dermal matrix in expander-implant immediate breast reconstruction. J Plast Reconstr Aesthet Surg 2014;67(4):468–476
4. United States of America, Department of Health and Human Services, Food and Drug Administration; Center for Devices and Radiological Health Medical Devices Advisory Committee. General and Plastic Surgery Devices Panel. March 26, 2019 Transcript. https://www.fda.gov/media/123746/download. Accessed June 28, 2019
5. American Society of Plastic Surgeons. ADM Update: The use of acellular dermal matrices (ADMs). https://www.plasticsurgery.org/for-medical-professionals/publications/psn-extra/news/adm-update-the-use-of-acellular-dermal-matrices

ALLOGRAFT MATERIALS

8. You see a patient who has undergone breast reconstruction with AlloDerm and an implant. *Which one of the following is true of this ADM?*

D. It contains no cellular elements.

AlloDerm is an acellular dermal matrix manufactured from human cadaveric tissue, not a bovine source. It has a minimal host response because it no longer contains antigenic cells. It is well incorporated into tissues, but it can have variable resorption rates. AlloDerm is the most extensively used ADM in the US for breast surgery and has the largest body of evidence in this setting.[1] However, it is not licensed for use in the European marketplace and a porcine alternative is offered instead (Strattice). It is also available for off-label use in the US for breast reconstruction according to the FDA.[2,3]

The FDA classifies human derived and animal derived products differently. This means that a human derived allograft, such as AlloDerm, is classified as a human cell and tissue-based product, while porcine or bovine derived ADMs are medical devices. This impacts the hops through which companies have to pass with product development, and usage differs quite significantly.

REFERENCES

1. Jansen LA, De Caigny P, Guay NA, Lineaweaver WC, Shokrollahi K. The evidence base for the acellular dermal matrix AlloDerm: a systematic review. Ann Plast Surg 2013;70(5):587–594
2. United States of America Department of Health and Human Services Food and Drug Administration; Center for Devices and Radiological Health Medical Devices Advisory Committee. General and Plastic Surgery Devices Panel March 26, 2019 Transcript. https://www.fda.gov/media/123746/download. Accessed June 28, 2019
3. American Society of Plastic Surgeons. ADM Update: The use of acellular dermal matrices (ADMs). https://www.plasticsurgery.org/for-medical-professionals/publications/psn-extra/news/adm-update-the-use-of-acellular-dermal-matrices

INTEGRA USE FOR RECONSTRUCTION

9. A patient has a 10 by 10 cm defect over the posterior ankle, exposing the Achilles tendon. A 2 by 2 cm area of tendon lacks paratenon cover centrally. You are planning to use Integra. *Which one of the following is correct regarding Integra?*

C. Fraying of the superficial layer is a good indicator for grafting.

Integra is a bilaminar dermal regeneration template used for skin replacement. It consists of a collagen and glycosaminoglycan base with a silicone upper layer that acts as a temporary epidermis. The silicone layer is removed after 3–4 weeks and is replaced with a skin graft. There are a number of ways to assess readiness for autograft when using Integra. One is that the silicone outer layer starts to fray at the edges away from the underlying neodermis. Also, granulation buds become visible at perforating staple or suture sites. In addition, the wound is ready for grafting when it appears a "salmon pink" color. Integra is useful for achieving soft tissue cover over exposed tendon where there is absence of paratenon, or bone without periosteum, as it helps convert a nongraftable wound bed to a graftable one. It is most often used in scar contracture release, venous leg ulcers, pressure ulcers, and burn surgery.[1-5]

REFERENCES

1. Yannas IV, Orgill DP, Burke JF. Template for skin regeneration. Plast Reconstr Surg 2011;127(Suppl 1):60S–70S
2. Snyder DL, Sullivan N, Schoelles KM. AHRQ technology assessments. In: Skin Substitutes for Treating Chronic Wounds. Rockville, MD: Agency for Healthcare Research and Quality (US); 2012
3. Moiemen NS, Staiano JJ, Ojeh NO, Thway Y, Frame JD. Reconstructive surgery with a dermal regeneration template: clinical and histologic study. Plast Reconstr Surg 2001;108(1):93–103
4. Komorowska-Timek E, Gabriel A, Bennett DC, et al. Artificial dermis as an alternative for coverage of complex scalp defects following excision of malignant tumors. Plast Reconstr Surg 2005;115(4):1010–1017

5. Valerio IL, Masters Z, Seavey JG, Balazs GC, Ipsen D, Tintle SM. Use of a dermal regeneration template wound dressing in the treatment of combat-related upper extremity soft tissue injuries. J Hand Surg Am 2016;41(12):e453–e460

BONE REPAIR

10. **Which one of the following best describes the process of surface mediated bone growth such as that which occurs at the margin of a bone graft?**
    C. Osteoconduction

    Osteoconduction is the process of surface mediated bone growth, such as from the margin of a graft. Osteoconductive materials are scaffolds (e.g., demineralized bone matrix). Osteogenesis is the overall term used to describe new bone formation. Osteoinduction is the process of recruiting and stimulating osteogenic precursor cells from surrounding tissue into osteoblasts for new bone formation (e.g., bone morphogenic protein). Osseointegration is the direct anchorage of an implant through the formation of a stable bone device (e.g., dental implant, ear prosthesis, or bone anchored hearing device). Currently only bone autografts are osteogenic, i.e., comprised of both cellular and scaffolding components.[1–3]

REFERENCES

1. Greenwald AS, Boden SD, Goldberg VM, Khan Y, Laurencin CT, Rosier RN; American Academy of Orthopaedic Surgeons. The Committee on Biological Implants. Bone-graft substitutes: facts, fictions, and applications. J Bone Joint Surg Am 2001;83-A(Suppl 2 Pt 2):98–103
2. Albrektsson T, Johansson C. Osteoinduction, osteoconduction and osseointegration. Eur Spine J 2001;10(Suppl 2): S96–S101
3. Pryor LS, Gage E, Langevin CJ, et al. Review of bone substitutes. Craniomaxillofac Trauma Reconstr 2009;2(3):151–160

SYNTHETIC BONE SUBSTITUTES

11. **You are using polymethylmethacrylate (PMMA) to reconstruct the calvarium. What is the main problem with using this biomaterial?**
    E. Risk of adjacent tissue damage

    Polymethylmethacrylate (PMMA) is a nonresorbable, high-density porous polymer used as a bone cement that also has clinical application in cranial reconstruction, forehead augmentation, and filling gaps in fractures. It is inexpensive, easily molded, inert, biocompatible, and has a high compression strength. However, it involves an exothermic reaction when mixed and can lead to local tissue damage unless adequate tissue cooling is achieved.[1,2]

REFERENCES

1. Pryor LS, Gage E, Langevin CJ, et al. Review of bone substitutes. Craniomaxillofac Trauma Reconstr 2009;2(3):151–160
2. Morselli C, Zaed I, Tropeano MP, et al. Comparison between the different types of heterologous materials used in cranioplasty: a systematic review of the literature. J Neurosurg Sci 2019;63(6):723–736

ALLOPLASTIC MATERIALS

12. **You are considering the use of alloplastic facial implants in your aesthetic practice. Which one of the following materials represents a nonresorbable alloplastic material made with high-density polyethylene?**
    B. Medpor

    Medpor is a high-density polyethylene material available as mesh and various implants, including chin, nasal, malar, and temporal prostheses. Gore-Tex is expanded polytetrafluoroethylene (ePTFE) that is available as mesh, tubes, and blocks. In mesh form it is used for chest and abdominal wall reconstruction; as a solid it is used for facial augmentation.[1–3] Marlex is a heavyweight polypropylene mesh that is used in chest and abdominal wall reconstruction.[4]

    Polyether ether ketone (PEEK) is polyether ketone and is a semi-crystalline polymer which has mechanical properties similar to cortical bone. It is resistant to heat and ionizing radiation and is nonferromagnetic which can be useful for postoperative monitoring. Patient-specific implants are becoming increasingly popular especially in craniofacial applications where computed tomography (CT) imaging combined with computer generated three-dimensional modeling can be used to create bespoke custom implants.[5]

    Phasix is an example of a newer absorbable (rather than nonresorbable) polymer used in abdominal wall surgery. It is made from poly-4-hydroxybutyrate (P4HB) and resorbs more slowly than more traditional alternatives such as polylactic acid (e.g., Vicryl, LactoSorb) or polydioxanone (PDS).[6]

REFERENCES

1. Patel K, Brandstetter K. Solid implants in facial plastic surgery: potential complications and how to prevent them. Facial Plast Surg 2016;32(5):520–531
2. Chim H, Gosain AK. Biomaterials in craniofacial surgery: experimental studies and clinical application. J Craniofac Surg 2009;20(1):29–33
3. Rubin JP, Yaremchuk MJ. Complications and toxicities of implantable biomaterials used in facial reconstructive and aesthetic surgery: a comprehensive review of the literature. Plast Reconstr Surg 1997;100(5):1336–1353
4. Usher FC, Hill JR, Ochsner JL. Hernia repair with Marlex mesh. A comparison of techniques. Surgery 1959;46:718–724
5. Honigmann P, Sharma N, Okolo B, Popp U, Msallem B, Thieringer FM. Patient-specific surgical implants made of 3D printed PEEK: material, technology, and scope of surgical application. BioMed Res Int 2018;2018:4520636
6. Scott JR, Deeken CR, Martindale RG, Rosen MJ. Evaluation of a fully absorbable poly-4-hydroxybutyrate/absorbable barrier composite mesh in a porcine model of ventral hernia repair. Surg Endosc 2016;30(9):3691–3701

THE FOREIGN BODY RESPONSE

13. In two-stage flexor tendon reconstruction of the hand, how is the body's natural foreign body response specifically utilized to be advantageous to the reconstructive process?

    C. It facilitates smooth gliding of the tendon.

Two-stage flexor tendon reconstruction in the hand involves first reconstructing the flexor sheath and then incorporating new tendon tissue to reconstruct the deficit. By placing a silicone rod (Hunter rod) within the tendon sheath and leaving it in place for a number of weeks, the natural foreign body response is used advantageously. During this time a response to the presence of the silicone rod occurs forming a smooth lined, longitudinal, circumferential capsule around the rod. Then in the second stage when tendon is brought into place, there is a smooth lined pseudo-sheath in place for it. The foreign body response does not negate the need for a tendon autograft, nor accelerate the process of rehabilitation directly. It has no impact on the bacterial load. There needs to be sufficient time between procedures for the pseudo-sheath to form and this is usually around 3 months.[1]

REFERENCE

1. Chattopadhyay A, McGoldrick R, Umansky E, Chang J. Principles of tendon reconstruction following complex trauma of the upper limb. Semin Plast Surg 2015;29(1):30–39

BREAST IMPLANT ASSOCIATED ALCL (BIA-ALCL)

14. Which one of the following is true with regards to BIA-ALCL?

    D. Diagnosis is made by sampling the capsule and fluid surrounding it.

Breast implant associated anaplastic large cell lymphoma (BIA-ALCL) is an uncommon condition which has been noted to occur in patients some years after having breast implants inserted. It is thought to be associated with specific types of textured implants (some of which have now been withdrawn from the market). It develops in the capsule around the implant and patients present with late-onset, peri-implant seromas, rather than an acute-onset red breast which would be more in keeping with infection. Diagnosis is made by sampling the fluid surrounding the implant or from tissue obtained from the capsule. Treatment involves first removing the capsule in its entirety as well as the implant (capsulectomy and explantation), and in most cases this is sufficient treatment. In some cases, further systemic treatment may be warranted. There is no evidence to support the prophylactic removal of implants at a specific time point following their placement. Instead, exchange or removal of implants is generally guided by other factors such as a changing in shape due to capsular contracture or evidence of rupture. Some patients will however elect to have implants changed at a certain time point in the absence of any visible concerns in aesthetics or altered function.[1,2]

REFERENCES

1. FDA Update on the Safety of Silicone Gel-Filled Breast Implants. Center for Devices and Radiological Health U.S. Food and Drug Administration, 2011
2. Clemens MW, Brody GS, Mahabir RC, Miranda RN. How to diagnose and treat breast implant-associated anaplastic large cell lymphoma. Plast Reconstr Surg 2018;141(4):586e–599e

FDA AND BREAST IMPLANTS

15. Which one of the following is true regarding the FDA and the use of silicone gel-filled breast implants?

    C. Regular imaging is advocated by the FDA following silicone breast implantation.

The FDA closely monitors and reports on the evidence in the use of silicone breast implants. Their current recommendation in terms of follow-up is to perform ultrasound for asymptomatic rupture 5–6 years after implantation and every 2–3 years thereafter and magnetic resonance imaging (MRI) for all symptomatic patients. This has changed from previous advice, which was to have regular MRI 3 years after implantation and every 2 years thereafter. FDA approval is present for breast augmentation in patients over 22 years of age and is unrestricted in patients requiring reconstruction. Breast implants may be textured using different techniques including salt loss or foam imprint stamping. Recently, a particular product by Allergan termed "Biocell," which uses a salt loss technique for texturing, was withdrawn from the market due to concerns over Breast implant associated anaplastic large cell lymphoma (BIA-ALCL). However, the FDA has not advised that all textured implants are withdrawn.[1,2]

REFERENCES

1. Breast Implants. https://www.fda.gov/medical-devices/implants-and-prosthetics/breast-implants
2. FDA Update on the Safety of Silicone Gel-Filled Breast Implants. Center for Devices and Radiological Health U.S. Food and Drug Administration; 2011. https://www.fda.gov/files/medical%20devices/published/Update-on-the-Safety-of-Silicone-Gel-Filled-Breast-Implants-%282011%29.pdf

RECONSTRUCTION WITH COMPOSITE MESH

16. What is the main clinical indication for using composite materials such as Proceed, Sepramesh, and TiMesh?

C. Abdominal wall reconstruction

The new breed of composite mesh materials includes Proceed, Sepramesh, Parietex, C-Qur, and TiMesh. These products are mostly used in ventral hernia repairs of the abdominal wall. They can be subdivided into two groups: (1) tissue separating meshes such as Proceed, Sepramesh, and Parietex; (2) coated meshes such as C-Qur and TiMesh.

The tissue separating meshes include a nonresorbable polymer on one surface and a biologic or resorbable material on the other side. The porous synthetic is placed against the abdominal wall to encourage host tissue incorporation, while the bioresorbable surface is placed against the viscera to limit bowel adhesions. The polymer is commonly polypropylene and the resorbable material commonly contains cellulose. Coated meshes comprise of a synthetic mesh such as polypropylene coated on both sides with a low inflammatory material such as titanium or omega fatty acids.[1–3]

REFERENCES

1. Judge TW, Parker DM, Dinsmore RC. Abdominal wall hernia repair: a comparison of Sepramesh and Parietex composite mesh in a rabbit hernia model. J Am Coll Surg 2007;204(2):276–281
2. Doctor HG. Evaluation of various prosthetic materials and newer meshes for hernia repairs. J Minim Access Surg 2006;2(3):110–116
3. Köckerling F, Schug-Pass C. What do we know about titanized polypropylene meshes? An evidence-based review of the literature. Hernia 2014;18(4):445–457

SILICONE AS A MEDICAL DEVICE MATERIAL

17. Which one of the following is a consistent finding with silicone as a biomaterial?

A. Fibrous encapsulation

Silicone is a nonresorbable polymer based on the element silicon. It has FDA approval as a solid and is most commonly used in breast implant prostheses. Fibrous encapsulation is a consistent finding with silicone implants and this is the basis of capsule formation and subsequent capsular contraction. Fibrous encapsulation can be a useful feature in the context of tissue expansion as the capsule develops a reliable blood supply that can be left in situ under local skin flaps.

Silicone is nonporous so it does not facilitate tissue ingrowth in the form of incorporation. However, it is inert so it is not rejected by tissues and is resistant to degradation, thereby having a long lifespan following implantation.[1,2]

REFERENCES

1. Rohrich RJ, Potter JK. Liquid injectable silicone: is there a role as a cosmetic soft-tissue filler? Plast Reconstr Surg 2004;113(4):1239–1241
2. Peters W, Fornasier V. Complications from injectable materials used for breast augmentation. Can J Plast Surg 2009;17(3):89–96

10. Negative Pressure Wound Therapy

See *Essentials of Plastic Surgery*, third edition, pp. 121–130

THEORIES OF NEGATIVE PRESSURE WOUND THERAPY

1. *Which one of the following represents a key part of the mechanism of action with negative pressure wound therapy (NPWT)?*
   A. The addition of interstitial fluid to aid oxygen delivery at a cellular level
   B. The generation of higher levels of matrix metalloproteases and acute phase proteins
   C. An increase in cellular proliferation due to altered mechanical stresses
   D. A reduction in both bacterial load and contraction at the wound edges
   E. An alteration of the collagen ratio in favor of type III to I production

MECHANICAL MECHANISMS IN NEGATIVE PRESSURE WOUND THERAPY

2. *Which one of the following is thought to be largely responsible for wound edges drawing closer together during negative pressure wound therapy (NPWT)?*
   A. Microstrain
   B. Macrostrain
   C. Nanostrain
   D. Equilibration of stresses
   E. Strain neutralization

CONTACT LAYERS IN NEGATIVE PRESSURE WOUND THERAPY

3. Different foam dressings can be used with negative pressure dressing systems. *What is the main theoretical clinical benefit of using foam with a larger pore size?*
   A. Reduced infection
   B. Increased tissue production
   C. Increased fluid removal
   D. Reduced pain
   E. Lower financial cost

CONTACT LAYERS IN NEGATIVE PRESSURE WOUND THERAPY

4. *Which one of the following base layers has the largest volume of evidence supporting its use in negative pressure wound therapy (NPWT)?*
   A. Polyvinyl foam
   B. Polypropylene foam
   C. Polyurethane foam
   D. Silver-coated sponge
   E. Honeycomb gauze

CONTACT LAYERS IN NEGATIVE PRESSURE WOUND THERAPY

5. A number of different base layers can be used in conjunction with negative pressure wound therapy (NPWT) and selection can affect outcome. *Which one of the following is correct regarding base layer selection?*
   A. Silver-coated sponge dressings are indicated in contaminated wounds.
   B. Polyvinyl alcohol (PVA) white foam should be used when rapid granulation is required.
   C. Use of gauze as a base layer tends to increase pain compared with foam dressings.
   D. Healing times are reduced when using foam rather than gauze.
   E. NPWT avoids the need for a nonadherent base layer on skin grafts.

PRESSURE SELECTION IN NEGATIVE PRESSURE WOUND THERAPY

6. You are choosing a setting for a negative pressure dressing. *Which one of the following represents the traditional industry standard for continuous pressure?*
   A. −25 mm Hg
   B. −50 mm Hg
   C. −75 mm Hg
   D. −100 mm Hg
   E. −125 mm Hg

FACTORS TO OPTIMIZE NEGATIVE PRESSURE WOUND THERAPY

7. *Which one of the following is most likely to accelerate granulation tissue production during negative pressure wound therapy (NPWT)?*
   A. Adjunctive fluid instillation
   B. A continuous pressure of −150 mm Hg
   C. Intermittent pressure mode
   D. A polyvinyl alcohol foam base layer
   E. Dressing changes every other day

CLINICAL USE OF NEGATIVE PRESSURE WOUND THERAPY

8. *In which one of the following scenarios can negative pressure wound therapy (NPWT) be indicated?*
   A. After sentinel node biopsy of the axilla
   B. Over a directly closed ankle wound
   C. On a cellulitic wound to the hand after a dog bite debridement
   D. Over a chronic wound to the elbow with eschar present
   E. Over a latissimus dorsi reconstruction of an open tibial fracture

MULTIDISCIPLINARY WORKING FOR WOUND CARE

9. You are setting up a new wound multidisciplinary team in your hospital and will be working alongside specialists from vascular, general, orthopedics, and cardiothoracic surgery to develop the use of negative pressure wound therapy (NPWT) across departments. *Which one of the following is correct and should be taken into account when planning the service?*
   A. There is no strong evidence to support the use of NPWT in diabetic foot disease.
   B. The incidence of limb amputation in diabetic foot disease is unaffected by NPWT.
   C. The evidence supporting NPWT as a primary treatment in venous ulcers is weak.
   D. NPWT on large abdominal or chest wall defects has no beneficial effect on respiratory function.
   E. NPWT with split-thickness skin grafts can improve their appearance but is not cost effective.

Answers

THEORIES OF NEGATIVE PRESSURE WOUND THERAPY

1. *Which one of the following represents a key part of the mechanism of action with negative pressure wound therapy (NPWT)?*

   C. An increase in cellular proliferation due to altered mechanical stresses

   The precise mechanism of action of negative pressure therapy is largely unknown, but three common theories prevail. The fluid-based theory proposes that interstitial fluid, which may otherwise compromise the microcirculation and oxygen delivery, and contain substances that negatively impact wound healing, is removed from the wound.[1] The second is a mechanically driven process in which cell proliferation is increased in response to mechanical tissue stress. This stimulates angiogenesis and cellular growth and helps to draw in the wound edges.[2] The third mechanism is a reduction in bacterial load.[3,4] It is not proven that negative pressure therapy will specifically alter collagen ratios.[5]

REFERENCES

1. Argenta LC, Morykwas MJ. Vacuum-assisted closure: a new method for wound control and treatment: clinical experience. Ann Plast Surg 1997;38(6):563–576, discussion 577
2. Lancerotto L, Bayer LR, Orgill DP. Mechanisms of action of microdeformational wound therapy. Semin Cell Dev Biol 2012;23(9):987–992
3. Urschel JD, Scott PG, Williams HTG. The effect of mechanical stress on soft and hard tissue repair; a review. Br J Plast Surg 1988;41(2):182–186
4. Plikaitis CM, Molnar JA. Subatmospheric pressure wound therapy and the vacuum-assisted closure device: basic science and current clinical successes. Expert Rev Med Devices 2006;3(2):175–184
5. Morykwas MJ, Argenta LC, Shelton-Brown EI, McGuirt W. Vacuum-assisted closure: a new method for wound control and treatment: animal studies and basic foundation. Ann Plast Surg 1997;38(6):553–562

MECHANICAL MECHANISMS IN NEGATIVE PRESSURE WOUND THERAPY

2. *Which one of the following is thought to be largely responsible for wound edges drawing closer together during negative pressure wound therapy (NPWT)?*

   B. Macrostrain

   Macrostrain refers to the process whereby negative pressure will cause the contact wound dressing to collapse. Negative pressure becomes equally distributed across the wound and force is transferred to the wound edges, bringing them closer together. *Microstrain* refers to the microdeformation that occurs across a foam dressing in a negative pressure system. This leads to induction of mechanical stress and stimulation of angiogenesis. There has been much research into the mechanical effects of negative pressure on the healing wound with trials of different pressure effects as part of this research. The other terms are not used to describe processes in NPWT.[1–3]

REFERENCES

1. Lancerotto L, Bayer LR, Orgill DP. Mechanisms of action of microdeformational wound therapy. Semin Cell Dev Biol 2012;23(9):987–992
2. Orgill DP, Bayer LR. Update on negative-pressure wound therapy. Plast Reconstr Surg 2011;127(Suppl 1):105S–115S
3. Agha R, Ogawa R, Pietramaggiori G, Orgill DP. A review of the role of mechanical forces in cutaneous wound healing. J Surg Res 2011;171(2):700–708

CONTACT LAYERS IN NEGATIVE PRESSURE WOUND THERAPY

3. Different foam dressings can be used with negative pressure dressing systems. *What is the main theoretical clinical benefit of using foam with a larger pore size?*

   B. Increased tissue production

   Black polyurethane foam is hydrophobic and has pore sizes of 400–600 µm compared with a pore size between 60 and 270 µm in polyvinyl alcohol white foam. The theoretical benefit is that tissue growth is maximized. However, there is no clear evidence to show that pore size makes a significant difference in the clinical setting.

   Clearly, reductions in infection rates, patient pain levels, wound exudate formation, and financial costs are all highly desirable with any given treatment. Indeed, negative pressure dressings have been shown to achieve these goals. However, there does not seem to be strong evidence to suggest that pore size will specifically alter any of these other parameters. Many studies have actually focused more on the comparison between foam and gauze in negative pressure therapy. Foam seems to be better suited for uniform contractible wounds, and gauze for shallow wounds and both remain popular. Reduced pain may be achieved by gauze in some settings.[1-6]

REFERENCES

1. Dorafshar AH, Franczyk M, Gottlieb LJ, Wroblewski KE, Lohman RF. A prospective randomized trial comparing subatmospheric wound therapy with a sealed gauze dressing and the standard vacuum-assisted closure device. Ann Plast Surg 2012;69(1):79–84

2. Malmsjö M, Ingemansson R, Martin R, Huddleston E. Negative-pressure wound therapy using gauze or open-cell polyurethane foam: similar early effects on pressure transduction and tissue contraction in an experimental porcine wound model. Wound Repair Regen 2009;17(2):200–205

3. Malmsjö M, Ingemansson R, Martin R, Huddleston E. Wound edge microvascular blood flow: effects of negative pressure wound therapy using gauze or polyurethane foam. Ann Plast Surg 2009;63(6):676–681

4. Borgquist O, Gustafsson L, Ingemansson R, Malmsjö M. Micro- and macromechanical effects on the wound bed of negative pressure wound therapy using gauze and foam. Ann Plast Surg 2010;64(6):789–793

5. Hu KX, Zhang HW, Zhou F, et al. [A comparative study of the clinical effects between two kinds of negative-pressure wound therapy]. Zhonghua Shao Shang Za Zhi 2009;25(4):253–257

6. Fraccalvieri M, Zingarelli E, Ruka E, et al. Negative pressure wound therapy using gauze and foam: histological, immunohistochemical and ultrasonography morphological analysis of the granulation tissue and scar tissue. Preliminary report of a clinical study. Int Wound J 2011;8(4):355–364

CONTACT LAYERS IN NEGATIVE PRESSURE WOUND THERAPY

4. *Which one of the following base layers has the largest volume of evidence supporting its use in negative pressure wound therapy (NPWT)?*

C. Polyurethane foam

Polyurethane foam was used as the original contact dressing for NPWT and most published evidence relates to this dressing. Polyurethane foam has a pore size designed to maximize tissue growth and is typically a black-colored synthetic with hydrophobic qualities. More recently, different foam types and gauze alternatives have become available as other manufacturers have entered into the market for NPWT devices. These include polyvinyl alcohol "white" foam which is hydrophilic and has a denser pore distribution (60–270 μm). Foam is considered better suited to uniform contractible wounds and gauze for shallow wounds. However, product availability, wound characteristics, patient factors, and surgeon's choice should be taken into consideration when selecting the base layer.[1-6]

REFERENCES

1. Dorafshar AH, Franczyk M, Gottlieb LJ, Wroblewski KE, Lohman RF. A prospective randomized trial comparing subatmospheric wound therapy with a sealed gauze dressing and the standard vacuum-assisted closure device. Ann Plast Surg 2012;69(1):79–84

2. Malmsjö M, Ingemansson R, Martin R, Huddleston E. Negative-pressure wound therapy using gauze or open-cell polyurethane foam: similar early effects on pressure transduction and tissue contraction in an experimental porcine wound model. Wound Repair Regen 2009;17(2):200–205

3. Malmsjö M, Ingemansson R, Martin R, Huddleston E. Wound edge microvascular blood flow: effects of negative pressure wound therapy using gauze or polyurethane foam. Ann Plast Surg 2009;63(6):676–681

4. Borgquist O, Gustafsson L, Ingemansson R, Malmsjö M. Micro- and macromechanical effects on the wound bed of negative pressure wound therapy using gauze and foam. Ann Plast Surg 2010;64(6):789–793

5. Hu KX, Zhang HW, Zhou F, et al. [A comparative study of the clinical effects between two kinds of negative-pressure wound therapy]. Zhonghua Shao Shang Za Zhi 2009;25(4):253–257

6. Fraccalvieri M, Zingarelli E, Ruka E, et al. Negative pressure wound therapy using gauze and foam: histological, immunohistochemical and ultrasonography morphological analysis of the granulation tissue and scar tissue. Preliminary report of a clinical study. Int Wound J 2011;8(4):355–364

CONTACT LAYERS IN NEGATIVE PRESSURE WOUND THERAPY

5. A number of different base layers can be used in conjunction with negative pressure wound therapy (NPWT) and selection can affect outcome. *Which one of the following is correct regarding base layer selection?*

A. Silver-coated sponge dressings are indicated in contaminated wounds.

Silver impregnated dressings can be used in conjunction with NPWT with foam or gauze contact dressings. Their use is indicated in contaminated wounds and can be helpful in reducing malodor. Silver likely achieves this by reducing bacterial cell counts.[1] PVA white foam should be used in areas where rapid rates of granulation are less desirable, not more. Gauze may actually decrease pain during dressing changes compared with foam but no differences have been observed between the two dressings in terms of decreasing wound size, healing time, or time to prepare for grafting. Gauze does tend to be more conformable and is therefore useful is unusual wound shapes and contours.[2-6] Using negative pressure in conjunction with skin grafting is a well-recognized technique. The dressing helps to minimize graft disruption with splintage, keep the wound sealed, manage fluid egress from the wound, and maintain appropriate pressure. It is especially useful in complex three-dimensional wounds and anatomic areas such as the perineum, axilla, neck, and lower extremity provided a good lasting seal can be achieved. Graft take is improved and hospital stay can subsequently be reduced in some cases. When using NPWT with skin grafts, it is recommended to use a nonadherent base layer underneath the foam or gauze dressing.[7]

REFERENCES

1. Gerry R, Kwei S, Bayer L, Breuing KH. Silver-impregnated vacuum-assisted closure in the treatment of recalcitrant venous stasis ulcers. Ann Plast Surg 2007;59(1):58–62
2. Dorafshar AH, Franczyk M, Gottlieb LJ, Wroblewski KE, Lohman RF. A prospective randomized trial comparing subatmospheric wound therapy with a sealed gauze dressing and the standard vacuum-assisted closure device. Ann Plast Surg 2012;69(1):79–84
3. Hu KX, Zhang HW, Zhou F, et al. [A comparative study of the clinical effects between two kinds of negative-pressure wound therapy]. Zhonghua Shao Shang Za Zhi 2009;25(4):253–257
4. Fraccalvieri M, Zingarelli E, Ruka E, et al. Negative pressure wound therapy using gauze and foam: histological, immunohistochemical and ultrasonography morphological analysis of the granulation tissue and scar tissue. Preliminary report of a clinical study. Int Wound J 2011;8(4):355–364
5. Malmsjö M, Ingemansson R, Martin R, Huddleston E. Negative-pressure wound therapy using gauze or open-cell polyurethane foam: similar early effects on pressure transduction and tissue contraction in an experimental porcine wound model. Wound Repair Regen 2009;17(2):200–205
6. Jeffery SL. Advanced wound therapies in the management of severe military lower limb trauma: a new perspective. Eplasty 2009;9:e28
7. Llanos S, Danilla S, Barraza C, et al. Effectiveness of negative pressure closure in the integration of split thickness skin grafts: a randomized, double-masked, controlled trial. Ann Surg 2006;244(5):700–705

PRESSURE SELECTION IN NEGATIVE PRESSURE WOUND THERAPY

6. You are choosing a setting for a negative pressure dressing. *Which one of the following represents the traditional industry standard for continuous pressure?*

   E. –125 mm Hg

   Subatmospheric pressure is used in NPWT. This may be continuous or intermittent. The pressures commonly used range from –50 to –125 mm Hg. The industry standard has traditionally been –125 mm Hg and much of the evidence on pressures has been assessing blood flow, microdeformation, and granulation tissue production in porcine models at varying pressures. For example, Morykwas et al found that –125 mm Hg was most effective at producing granulation tissue in a porcine model and for a long time this has been considered to be the optimal pressure.[1] However, in clinical practice, higher pressures can be less well tolerated by patients so reducing the pressure may be helpful. For this reason, studies have been conducted to assess parameters including blood flow at lower pressures, but remaining within the therapeutic range. For example, another animal study compared blood flow at a variety of pressures and found that pressures of –80 mm Hg gave comparable blood flow to –125 mm Hg. However, this paper did not assess granulation production or wound healing.[2] In general, a higher negative pressure is considered beneficial in highly exudative wounds, whereas lower pressures should be considered in poorly perfused wounds. An international consensus meeting published guidelines in 2011 having reviewed available evidence at the time. This report suggested that it is increasingly apparent that there may not be one single optimal level of pressure but an effective therapeutic range of negative pressure levels between –40 and –150 mm Hg. More research is still required in this area to clarify the optimal settings.[3,4]

REFERENCES

1. Morykwas MJ, Faler BJ, Pearce DJ, Argenta LC. Effects of varying levels of subatmospheric pressure on the rate of granulation tissue formation in experimental wounds in swine. Ann Plast Surg 2001;47(5):547–551
2. Borgquist O, Ingemansson R, Malmsjö M. Wound edge microvascular blood flow during negative-pressure wound therapy: examining the effects of pressures from –10 to –175 mmHg. Plast Reconstr Surg 2010;125(2):502–509
3. Ahearn C. Intermittent NPWT and lower negative pressures—exploring the disparity between science and current practice: a review. Ostomy Wound Manage 2009;55(6):22–28

4. Birke-Sorensen H, Malmsjö M, Rome P, et al; International Expert Panel on Negative Pressure Wound Therapy [NPWT-EP]. Evidence-based recommendations for negative pressure wound therapy: treatment variables (pressure levels, wound filler and contact layer)—steps towards an international consensus. J Plast Reconstr Aesthet Surg 2011;64(Suppl):S1–S16

FACTORS TO OPTIMIZE NEGATIVE PRESSURE WOUND THERAPY

7. Which one of the following is most likely to accelerate granulation tissue production during negative pressure wound therapy (NPWT)?

C. Intermittent pressure mode

The use of intermittent pressure (5 minutes on, 2 minutes off) has been shown to produce more rapid granulation tissue deposition in animal models.[1-3]

In spite of this there remains debate as to whether intermittent therapy is helpful in clinical practice as the results are not proven to be better and patients can find it painful to experience the transition between pressure "off and on." In addition, where there is a high level of exudate in the wound, fluid can tend to accumulate during the "off" period leading to loss of dressing contact with the skin and loss of the seal leading to fluid leakage. Because of these limitations, continuous settings remain most popular. Polyvinyl alcohol foam is less likely to produce rapid granulation compared with polyurethane foam. No evidence supports changing a dressing every other day to accelerate granulation and it is common to change NPWT dressings twice weekly providing the wound is clean. This may be increased to three times per week in highly exudative wounds and those with recent contamination. Fluid instillation can be used with either continuous or intermittent pressures. This technique involves instillation of isotonic solution containing saline, antibiotic, or antibacterial products and may contribute to improved infection control by virtue of its irrigating the wound and diluting the bacterial load.[4,5]

REFERENCES

1. Morykwas MJ, Argenta LC, Shelton-Brown EI, McGuirt W. Vacuum-assisted closure: a new method for wound control and treatment: animal studies and basic foundation. Ann Plast Surg 1997;38(6):553–562
2. Morykwas MJ, Faler BJ, Pearce DJ, Argenta LC. Effects of varying levels of subatmospheric pressure on the rate of granulation tissue formation in experimental wounds in swine. Ann Plast Surg 2001;47(5):547–551
3. Borgquist O, Ingemansson R, Malmsjö M. The effect of intermittent and variable negative pressure wound therapy on wound edge microvascular blood flow. Ostomy Wound Manage 2010;56(3):60–67
4. Birke-Sorensen H, Malmsjö M, Rome P, et al; International Expert Panel on Negative Pressure Wound Therapy [NPWT-EP]. Evidence-based recommendations for negative pressure wound therapy: treatment variables (pressure levels, wound filler and contact layer)—steps towards an international consensus. J Plast Reconstr Aesthet Surg 2011;64(Suppl):S1–S16
5. Kim PJ, Attinger CE, Steinberg JS, et al. Negative-pressure wound therapy with instillation: international consensus guidelines. Plast Reconstr Surg 2013;132(6):1569–1579

CLINICAL USE OF NEGATIVE PRESSURE WOUND THERAPY

8. In which one of the following scenarios can negative pressure wound therapy (NPWT) be indicated?

B. Over a directly closed ankle wound

Although it may seem counterintuitive to use negative pressure therapy on a directly closed wound, incisional NPWT has been universally adopted as a useful treatment modality for some specific wound care settings. Incisional NPWT may be indicated in certain clinical situations where either incision-related or patient-related factors place the wound at an increased risk of healing complications. Patient-related factors include diabetes mellitus, American Society of Anesthesiologists (ASA) ≥ 3, advanced age, obesity (body mass index [BMI] ≥ 30 kg/m²), tobacco use, hypoalbuminemia, and corticosteroid use. Incision-related factors include prolonged surgical time, reoperation or re-exploration, edema, extensive undermining, contamination, traumatized soft tissue, and high-tension closure.

Incisional NPWT is thought to provide splinting of incisions by reducing edema and tension across the wound while continuously evacuating excessive drainage, thereby avoiding skin irritation and bacterial colonization. It may have a positive effect on local wound blood supply and offloading of pressure. It has been used in a number of settings including internal fixation of lower limb fractures and complex abdominal wall reconstruction.[1-4] The technique involves placement of thin strips of adhesive dressing just lateral to the suture or staple line and placement of a nonadherent contact dressing over the incision. Sponge is then placed along the length of the incision over the nonadherent dressing, thereby avoiding contact with the skin. There are also "off the shelf" products designed for this purpose. Although these are neat and user friendly, they do not generally allow absorption of higher volumes of exudate compared with traditional negative pressure dressings and this must be taken into consideration when selecting the appropriate dressing.[1-5] NPWT should not be used in the following scenarios: exposed vessels and nerves, malignancy in the wound, untreated osteomyelitis, fresh anastomotic site, or in a site with necrotic tissue with eschar still present.[5]

REFERENCES

1. Willy C, Agarwal A, Andersen CA, et al. Closed incision negative pressure therapy: international multidisciplinary consensus recommendations. Int Wound J 2017;14(2):385–398

2. Condé-Green A, Chung TL, Holton LH III, et al. Incisional negative-pressure wound therapy versus conventional dressings following abdominal wall reconstruction: a comparative study. Ann Plast Surg 2013;71(4):394–397

3. Semsarzadeh NN, Tadisina KK, Maddox J, Chopra K, Singh DP. Closed incision negative-pressure therapy is associated with decreased surgical-site infections: a meta-analysis. Plast Reconstr Surg 2015;136(3):592–602

4. Chopra K, Gowda AU, Morrow C, Holton L III, Singh DP. The economic impact of closed-incision negative-pressure therapy in high-risk abdominal incisions: a cost-utility analysis. Plast Reconstr Surg 2016;137(4):1284–1289

5. Birke-Sorensen H, Malmsjö M, Rome P, et al; International Expert Panel on Negative Pressure Wound Therapy [NPWT-EP]. Evidence-based recommendations for negative pressure wound therapy: treatment variables (pressure levels, wound filler and contact layer)—steps towards an international consensus. J Plast Reconstr Aesthet Surg 2011;64 (Suppl):S1–S16

MULTIDISCIPLINARY WORKING FOR WOUND CARE

9. You are setting up a new wound multidisciplinary team in your hospital and will be working alongside specialists from vascular, general, orthopedics, and cardiothoracic surgery to develop the use of negative pressure wound therapy (NPWT) across departments. *Which one of the following is correct and should be taken into account when planning the service?*

   C. The evidence supporting NPWT as a primary treatment in venous ulcers is weak.

   Evidence is currently lacking for the use of NPWT as a primary treatment in venous ulcers, although its use as an adjunct to skin grafting in these cases is supported. In contrast there is Level I evidence to support the use of NPWT in the primary management of diabetic foot ulcers both in terms of time to wound closure and decreased incidence of limb amputation.[1-4] In large abdominal wall and chest defects, NPWT can be beneficial to respiratory function with decreased ventilator support requirement and shorter duration in high dependency care.[5-8] The use of NPWT on split-skin grafts has Level I evidence to support its use and is especially useful in areas such as the perineum and axilla. It not only improves graft appearance, but also improves graft take in some situations and has been shown to reduce subsequent hospital stay. Pressures may be reduced in this setting and continuous settings are preferred. This increased effectiveness would have a major impact on cost savings that would potentially outweigh the NPWT costs.[9]

REFERENCES

1. Körber A, Franckson T, Grabbe S, Dissemond J. Vacuum assisted closure device improves the take of mesh grafts in chronic leg ulcer patients. Dermatology 2008;216(3):250–256

2. Vuerstaek JD, Vainas T, Wuite J, Nelemans P, Neumann MH, Veraart JC. State-of-the-art treatment of chronic leg ulcers: a randomized controlled trial comparing vacuum-assisted closure (V.A.C.) with modern wound dressings. J Vasc Surg 2006;44(5):1029–1037, discussion 1038

3. Armstrong DG, Lavery LA; Diabetic Foot Study Consortium. Negative pressure wound therapy after partial diabetic foot amputation: a multicentre, randomised controlled trial. Lancet 2005;366(9498):1704–1710

4. Blume PA, Walters J, Payne W, Ayala J, Lantis J. Comparison of negative pressure wound therapy using vacuum-assisted closure with advanced moist wound therapy in the treatment of diabetic foot ulcers: a multicenter randomized controlled trial. Diabetes Care 2008;31(4):631–636

5. Boele van Hensbroek P, Wind J, Dijkgraaf MGW, Busch OR, Goslings JC. Temporary closure of the open abdomen: a systematic review on delayed primary fascial closure in patients with an open abdomen. World J Surg 2009;33(2):199–207

6. Zomerlei T, Janis JE. Negative pressure wound therapy. In: Novitsky YW, ed. Current Principles of Surgery of the Abdominal Wall. Springer Publishing; 2015:337–349

7. Singh D. The role of closed incision negative pressure therapy in abdominal wall reconstruction: a current review of the evidence. Plast Reconstr Surg 2018;142(3, Suppl):156S–162S

8. Agarwal JP, Ogilvie M, Wu LC, et al Vacuum-assisted closure for sternal wounds: a first-line therapeutic management approach. Plast Reconstr Surg 2005;116(4):1035–1040

9. Azzopardi EA, Boyce DE, Dickson WA, et al. Application of topical negative pressure (vacuum-assisted closure) to split-thickness skin grafts: a structured evidence-based review. Ann Plast Surg 2013;70(1):23–29

11. Lasers in Plastic Surgery

See *Essentials of Plastic Surgery*, third edition, pp. 131–142

LASER PHYSICS

1. *Which one of the following is true regarding laser physics?*
   A. The duration of laser energy delivery must be less than the thermal relaxation time.
   B. Wavelength and absorption length are inversely related.
   C. Laser light is typically noncoherent, polychromatic, and noncollimated.
   D. Fluence refers to the speed with which laser energy is transferred to tissues.
   E. Laser energy is most commonly delivered in a continuous fashion.

TARGET CHROMOPHORES

2. Laser therapy relies on the process of photothermolysis, which targets specific tissue chromophores according to laser characteristics. *What is the target chromophore when performing laser hair removal?*
   A. Oxyhemoglobin
   B. Melanin
   C. Collagen
   D. Keratin
   E. Water

WAVELENGTHS FOR COMMON LASERS

3. *Which one of the following lasers uses a wavelength of 1064 nm?*
   A. Potassium titanyl phosphate (KTP)
   B. Alexandrite
   C. Neodymium-doped yttrium aluminum garnet (Nd:YAG)
   D. CO_2
   E. Erbium-doped yttrium aluminum garnet (Er:YAG)

LASER SAFETY

4. *When using the CO_2 laser to treat an intraoral malignancy, which one of the following statements is correct?*
   A. The operating site must be free of wet towels and drapes as they represent a fire hazard.
   B. Only operating room staff directly involved in the delivery of the laser therapy will need to wear eye protection.
   C. An optical density of less than 2 is recommended for any protective goggles used.
   D. Laser specific warning signs must be placed at all entrances to the treatment room or operating room.
   E. A standard endotracheal tube must be used instead of a laryngeal mask in the anaesthetized patient.

TISSUE COOLING

5. *What is the main goal of cooling tissues during laser treatment?*
   A. To increase the speed of treatment
   B. To provide anesthesia to the patient
   C. To cool the target chromophore
   D. To protect the dermal–epidermal junction
   E. To allow higher powered lasers to be used

VASCULAR LESIONS

6. A 30-year-old woman is referred to clinic with a bright red spot on her cheek. It measures 2 mm in diameter with radiating telangiectasia. It disappears on digital pressure and rapidly reappears. *How can this be best treated with laser therapy?*
   A. KTP
   B. Green dye
   C. Er:YAG
   D. CO_2
   E. Fraxel

7. A patient is seen in clinic with rosacea and telangiectasia to the cheeks and central face. Your usual preferred KTP laser for this treatment is broken. *Which one of the following would still be a suitable treatment modality in this case while minimizing risk of purpura?*
   A. Yellow dye
   B. Green dye
   C. Ruby
   D. Er:YAG
   E. Nd:YAG

8. *Which one of the following vascular conditions is most likely to require multimodality treatment rather than isolated laser therapy?*
   A. Capillary venous malformations
   B. Early stage hemangiomas
   C. Venous and venolymphatic malformations
   D. Facial telangiectasia and rosacea
   E. Spider veins

9. A patient presents with a purple discolored patch to the left side of her face. It has been present since birth and has always grown in proportion to the patient's overall growth. It currently measures 6 cm by 8 cm. A plan is made for treatment with a pulsed dye laser. *When treating these lesions, when is treatment most likely to be effective?*
   A. In darker skinned individuals
   B. In adult patients
   C. When the lesion is in the trigeminal nerve V_2 distribution
   D. When the lesion is lightly pigmented
   E. When the lesion is on the hands or feet

HAIR REMOVAL

10. You see a young blonde patient in your office who wishes to have hair removal treatment. *Which one of the following laser modalities would be ineffective for this clinical indication?*
    A. Diode
    B. Alexandrite
    C. Nd:YAG
    D. Ruby
    E. Intense pulsed light (IPL)

TATTOO REMOVAL

11. You see a patient in your office following treatment to remove a multicolored tattoo. The initial treatment has been partly successful but there remains residual green pigment. *Which laser would be best to target these areas in subsequent treatment?*
    A. Q-switched Nd:YAG
    B. Q-switched alexandrite
    C. Nd:YAG
    D. Er:YAG
    E. Pulsed dye

12. You see a patient in clinic with a tattoo of a multicolored cartoon bear character. She wishes to have this removed with laser treatment. *Which color ink is most likely to be resistant to laser treatment?*
    A. Black
    B. Green
    C. Red
    D. Yellow
    E. Brown

LASERS IN BURN SCARS

13. You are asked to see a young girl in clinic following a 10% total body surface area (TBSA) superficial dermal burn that was treated conservatively 1 year ago. Most areas healed well but some areas remained thickened and were treated with steroids. The scars have now flattened but remain erythematous. *What laser treatment is most appropriate to reduce the residual hyperpigmentation of her scar?*
    A. Ruby
    B. Alexandrite
    C. Diode
    D. Pulsed dye
    E. Er:YAG

FACIAL REJUVENATION

14. You consult with a 70-year-old white female in clinic who has deep rhytids and has requested ablative skin resurfacing. *Which one of the following is best for this patient?*
    A. Er:YAG
    B. Alexandrite
    C. IPL
    D. Fraxel
    E. Nd:YAG

LASER RESURFACING

15. A patient is seen in clinic requesting laser skin resurfacing of the face. *Which one of the following medications should be discontinued prior to treatment to reduce the risk of scarring?*
    A. Acyclovir
    B. Hydroquinone
    C. Tretinoin
    D. Metronidazole
    E. Isotretinoin

LASER LIPOSUCTION

16. You see a patient in the office who requests liposuction and states a preference for laser liposuction over power assisted liposuction. *Which one of the following would be true about the use of laser liposuction in general?*
    A. There is a strong evidence base to support its use over standard liposuction.
    B. A major benefit would be a reduction in surgical procedure time.
    C. It should be avoided in the head and neck region.
    D. The risk of associated thermal injury is more than 10%.
    E. A 980-nm diode laser may be effective on areas with large amounts of fat.

Answers

LASER PHYSICS

1. **Which one of the following is true regarding laser physics?**

    A. **The duration of laser energy delivery must be less than the thermal relaxation time.**

    The energy delivery time or exposure time during laser treatment is termed the "pulse width" and achieving the correct pulse width is key to successful laser outcomes. The energy provided to the tissues by the laser must be introduced into the target faster than it can dissipate to adjacent tissues. The thermal relaxation time is defined as the time for the target tissue to dissipate 51% of the energy absorbed. The pulse width must be less than this and the ideal pulse time is usually half of the thermal relaxation time. If the process of heating to the required thermal temperature takes too long, then surrounding tissue temperature will build up causing unwanted damage and the target chromophore will not be adequately treated either.

    Laser light works at different wavelengths and the longer the wavelength, the longer the absorption length observed in the tissues, rather than the two properties being inversely proportional to one another. Each given wavelength will propagate to a specific tissue depth due to its own unique absorption characteristic.

    Laser light has a number of specific qualities including coherence (light is in phase), monochromaticity (light is one color only), and it is collimated (within a tight formation). In contrast, intense pulsed light (IPL) has the opposite features; it is noncoherent, polychromatic, and noncollimated.

    Fluence does not relate to the speed of energy transfer to the tissues, but instead refers to the energy density as measured in joules/cm^2. It is a product of the power and the spot size used.

    Laser energy delivery was previously continuous but is rarely so anymore because this is likely to cause scarring secondary to thermal damage. Instead, pulsed energy delivery is commonly used such that the timing can be matched between the size of the target and its thermal relaxation time.[1,2]

REFERENCES

1. Low DW, Thorne C. Lasers in plastic surgery. In: Thorne CH, Bartlett SP, Beasley RW, et al, eds. Grabb and Smith's Plastic Surgery. 6th ed. Philadelphia: Lippincott Williams & Wilkins; 2007
2. Farkas JP, Hoopman JE, Kenkel JM. Five parameters you must understand to master control of your laser/light-based devices. Aesthet Surg J 2013;33(7):1059

TARGET CHROMOPHORES

2. Laser therapy relies on the process of photothermolysis, which targets specific tissue chromophores according to laser characteristics. **What is the target chromophore when performing laser hair removal?**

    B. **Melanin**
    - Vascular lesions—hemoglobin and oxyhemoglobin
    - Pigmented skin lesions—melanin
    - Tattoo pigment—tattoo pigment
    - Ablative resurfacing—water
    - Laser liposuction—water and fat

    Hair removal works best on dark hairs given the chromophore target is melanin within the hair. Water is the chromophore for ablative lasers such as CO_2 and Er:YAG. The target chromophores for vascular lesions are hemoglobin and oxyhemoglobin.

    Skin constituents such as collagen or elastin are not chromophores, but may be affected by laser treatment. For example, use of a resurfacing laser, such as CO_2, will target water in the dermis and stimulate the regeneration of collagen and elastin which can tighten the skin.[1-3]

REFERENCES

1. Low DW, Thorne C. Lasers in plastic surgery. In: Thorne CH, Bartlett SP, Beasley RW, et al, eds. Grabb and Smith's Plastic Surgery. 6th ed. Philadelphia: Lippincott Williams & Wilkins; 2007
2. Farkas JP, Hoopman JE, Kenkel JM. Five parameters you must understand to master control of your laser/light-based devices. Aesthet Surg J 2013;33(7):1059–1064
3. Nahai F. The Art of Aesthetic Surgery: Principles & Techniques. 2nd ed. St Louis: Quality Medical Publishing; 2011

WAVELENGTHS FOR COMMON LASERS

3. *Which one of the following lasers uses a wavelength of 1064 nm?*

   C. Neodymium-doped yttrium aluminum garnet (Nd:YAG)

   The electromagnetic spectrum relevant to lasers in plastic surgery includes the ultraviolet (UV) (200–400 nm), visible (400–750 nm), near-infrared (750–1400 nm), and mid-infrared (1400–20,000 nm). Most vascular lasers are within the visible range (as this corresponds to the wavelength of hemoglobin), and most that target melanin are in the near-infrared spectrum. Those that target water are within the mid-infrared spectrum.

   Nd:YAG is in the near-infrared spectrum and can target both oxyhemoglobin and melanin as well as tattoo pigment. The wavelengths of common lasers are shown in **Box 11.1**.

   Wavelengths of commonly used lasers are often asked in written examinations.[1-4]

BOX 11.1 *WAVELENGTHS OF COMMON LASERS*

Vascular
KTP: 532 nm
Pulsed dye: 585 nm
Nd:YAG: 1064 nm
Ablative Resurfacing
CO_2: 10,600 nm
Er:YAG: 2940 nm
Melanin Target (hair removal, solar lentigines, or tattoo removal)
Alexandrite: 755 nm
Ruby: 694 nm
Diode: 810 nm

KTP, Potassium titanyl phosphate; Er:YAG, erbium-doped yttrium aluminum garnet; Nd:YAG, neodymium-doped yttrium aluminum garnet.

REFERENCES

1. Farkas JP, Hoopman JE, Kenkel JM. Five parameters you must understand to master control of your laser/light-based devices. Aesthet Surg J 2013;33(7):1059–1064
2. Nahai F. The Art of Aesthetic Surgery: Principles & Techniques. 2nd ed. St Louis: Quality Medical Publishing; 2011
3. Fankhauser F, Kwasniewska S. Applications of the neodymium:YAG laser in plastic surgery of the face and lacrimal surgery. Wound repair. A review. Ophthalmologica 2002;216(6):381–398
4. Stübinger S, Klämpfl F, Schmidt M, Zeilhofer HF. Lasers in Oral and Maxillofacial Surgery. SpringerLink; 2020

LASER SAFETY

4. *When using the CO_2 laser to treat an intraoral malignancy, which one of the following statements is correct?*

   D. Laser specific warning signs must be placed at all entrances to the treatment room or operating room.

   When using a laser for therapeutic interventions, it is vital that strict safety measures are in place. The responsibility of this falls on both the surgeon and **operating room (**OR) lead to ensure the safety measures are maintained. It is important to have formal training and accreditation in laser prior to using it in clinical practice.

   A key component to achieving adequate safety is ensuring that laser specific signs are placed at all entrances to the treatment room or operating room. These signs must indicate that a laser procedure is in progress and that eye protection is required. They must also show what wavelength and power of laser is being used. Furthermore, they should not be permanently posted, but instead should be removed when the laser treatment session is complete. The windows of the room must also have opaque coverings that correspond to the wavelengths of any laser being used.

   Eye protection with laser specific goggles/glasses is mandatory for all personnel in the treatment room or operating room. It is not limited to those actually giving the treatment. The optical density should be 5 or more (not less than 2) to adequately protect the eye. In addition to eye protection, masks should be worn, particularly in cases with malignancy or risk of viral transmission. Plume evacuation is required when using CO_2 or erbium lasers. Wet swabs should be placed around the operative site to reduce the chance of local burns and ignition risks when using the CO_2 laser. In this case a reinforced endotracheal tube must also be used with low FiO_2 flows (less than 30%) to reduce the risk of flash burn or inhalation.[1-3]

REFERENCES

1. Farkas JP, Hoopman JE, Kenkel JM. Five parameters you must understand to master control of your laser/light-based devices. Aesthet Surg J 2013;33(7):1059–1064
2. Rohrich RJ, Burns AJ. Lasers in office-based settings: establishing guidelines for proper usage. Plast Reconstr Surg 2002;109(3):1147–1148
3. Schmidt M, Zeilhofer HF. Lasers in Oral and Maxillofacial Surgery. SpringerLink; 2020

TISSUE COOLING

5. *What is the main goal of cooling tissues during laser treatment?*

   D. **To protect the dermal–epidermal junction**

   The main goal of cooling tissues during laser treatment is to protect them from unwanted damage, specifically the skin at the dermal–epidermal junction. Complications of damage to the dermal–epidermal junction are blistering and subsequent hypo- or hyperpigmentation. Cooling does have a secondary benefit for patients in that it can provide anesthesia, but this is not usually its primary purpose. Treatment speed is not affected by cooling and excessive cooling is not effective because the target chromophore will be less responsive to the treatment being given and therefore will itself require higher energy to achieve a result. There would be no benefit in using a higher-powered laser to account for overcooling of the tissues.[1,2]

REFERENCES

1. Rohrich RJ, Burns AJ. Lasers in office-based settings: establishing guidelines for proper usage. Plast Reconstr Surg 2002;109(3):1147–1148
2. Schmidt M, Zeilhofer HF. Lasers in Oral and Maxillofacial Surgery. SpringerLink; 2020

VASCULAR LESIONS

6. A 30-year-old woman is referred to clinic with a bright red spot on her cheek. It measures 2 mm in diameter with radiating telangiectasia. It disappears on digital pressure and rapidly reappears. *How can this be best treated with laser therapy?*

   A. **KTP**

   KTP is a popular choice for laser treatment of spider nevi. A spider nevus is an enlarged artery with radiating vessels supplied by it. This gives the appearance of a spider body with legs. On examination, pressure on the area makes the spot disappear and then on release it reappears as blood fills the empty vessel lumen. The cause is not known but they can be associated with liver or thyroid disease. Most commonly, they present as an isolated condition and can often resolve spontaneously. Laser therapy can be useful for the treatment of persistent spider nevi in a single visit. Other vascular lasers may also be considered such as yellow pulsed dye, ruby, alexandrite, and diode as they all target hemoglobin and cause local coagulation to the main source vessel.[1-4] Green dye is used for café au lait macules. Er:YAG, fraxel, and CO_2 are all used for resurfacing.[2]

REFERENCES

1. Erceg A, Greebe RJ, Bovenschen HJ, Seyger MM. A comparative study of pulsed 532-nm potassium titanyl phosphate laser and electrocoagulation in the treatment of spider nevi. Dermatol Surg 2010;36(5):630–635
2. Nahai F. The Art of Aesthetic Surgery: Principles & Techniques. 2nd ed. St Louis: Quality Medical Publishing; 2011
3. Hare McCoppin HH, Goldberg DJ. Laser treatment of facial telangiectases: an update. Dermatol Surg 2010;36(8):1221–1230
4. Hoopman JE. Lasers in Medicine. Dallas: University of Texas Southwestern Medical Center; 2000

---

7. A patient is seen in clinic with rosacea and telangiectasia to the cheeks and central face. Your usual preferred KTP laser for this treatment is broken. *Which one of the following would still be a suitable treatment modality in this case while minimizing risk of purpura?*

   E. **Nd:YAG**

   Nd:YAG is a very versatile laser choice because it can be used to target both oxyhemoglobin and melanin chromophores. Therefore, it can be effective in treating hemangiomas, telangiectasia, and spider veins, as well as pigmented skin lesions, tattoo pigment, hair removal, and scar management. Yellow dye is a good choice for vascular lesions including hemangiomas, port-wine stains, and telangiectasia. However, it is best for superficial lesions and is associated with a higher rate of post-treatment purpura.

   Green dye is useful for managing café au lait macules, rather than vascular lesions, given its chromophore is melanin. Ruby also targets melanin and is popular for tattoo removal. Er:YAG uses water as its target chromophore and is used for skin resurfacing, not vascular lesions.[1-3]

REFERENCES

1. Hare McCoppin HH, Goldberg DJ. Laser treatment of facial telangiectases: an update. Dermatol Surg 2010;36(8):1221–1230
2. Hoopman JE. Lasers in Medicine. Dallas: University of Texas Southwestern Medical Center; 2000
3. Juliandri J, Wang X, Liu Z, Zhang J, Xu Y, Yuan C. Global rosacea treatment guidelines and expert consensus points: The differences. J Cosmet Dermatol 2019;18(4):960–965

8. *Which one of the following vascular conditions is most likely to require multimodality treatment rather than isolated laser therapy?*

C. **Venous and venolymphatic malformations**

There are a number of vascular lesions which are effectively treated with isolated laser modalities. The target chromophores for such lesions are hemoglobin and oxyhemoglobin. Laser causes damage to the vessel intima, coagulation, and stasis. Most vascular lesions, particularly more superficial ones, will respond well to treatment, although multiple sessions are usually required. However, venous and mixed venous lymphatic malformations tend to respond less well to laser therapy alone, because they are often too large or too deep for isolated laser therapy to be effective. Their management is more commonly combined with other nonlaser techniques such as surgical debulking or intralesional sclerotherapy with agents such as bleomycin or OK451.[1,2]

Early stage, ulcerated, and regressed hemangiomas can be treated with laser monotherapy. However, its use is contraindicated when the hemangioma is in the proliferative phase as the treatment itself can induce ulceration and tissue necrosis. Nonlaser mainstays of treatment are now propranolol, which is taken orally, or intralesional injection with substances such as bleomycin or steroid.

Capillary venous malformations, facial telangiectasia, rosacea, and spider veins are generally all effectively treated with laser monotherapy. Common laser types for such treatments are KTP, Nd:YAG, or intense pulsed light (IPL).[3–6]

REFERENCES

1. Sainsbury DCG, Kessell G, Fall AJ, Hampton FJ, Guhan A, Muir T. Intralesional bleomycin injection treatment for vascular birthmarks: a 5-year experience at a single United Kingdom unit. Plast Reconstr Surg 2011;127(5):2031–2044
2. McMorrow L, Shaikh M, Kessell G, Muir T. Bleomycin electrosclerotherapy: new treatment to manage vascular malformations. Br J Oral Maxillofac Surg 2017;55(9):977–979
3. Seront E, Vikkula M, Boon LM. Venous malformations of the head and neck. Otolaryngol Clin North Am 2018;51(1):173–184
4. Love Z, Hsu DP. Low-flow vascular malformations of the head and neck: clinicopathology and image guided therapy. J Neurointerv Surg 2012;4(6):414–425
5. Richter GT, Braswell L. Management of venous malformations. Facial Plast Surg 2012;28(6):603–610
6. Fowell C, Verea Linares C, Jones R, Nishikawa H, Monaghan A. Venous malformations of the head and neck: current concepts in management. Br J Oral Maxillofac Surg 2017;55(1):3–9

9. A patient presents with a purple discolored patch to the left side of her face. It has been present since birth and has always grown in proportion to the patient's overall growth. It currently measures 6 cm by 8 cm. A plan is made for treatment with a pulsed dye laser. *When treating these lesions, when is treatment most likely to be effective?*

D. **When the lesion is lightly pigmented**

The patient described has a port-wine stain or capillary malformation. Port-wine stains represent a collection of abnormally formed capillaries within the skin, resulting in a red or purple colored mark. Most port-wine stains are present at birth, as in this case, but they can also be acquired. They are relatively common and occur in 1:300 infants with an equal sex distribution.

The pulsed dye laser is commonly used to improve the appearance of port-wine stains as it targets oxyhemoglobin within the abnormal vessels using a 585 nm wavelength. Cases generally require a series of treatments at regular intervals. These often require general anesthesia in children. Treatment outcomes can be quite successful although most lesions never fully disappear. In general, the outcome following treatment with pulsed dye laser is best in lighter colored lesions, in children, and in patients with lighter skin tones (Fitzpatrick I–III). Treatment can be started from the age of 6 months. Better responses are observed in the head and neck region with the exception of the trigeminal nerve V_2 distribution. The anatomic area associated with the poorest response is the extremities.[1–3] Long-term follow-up shows that these lesions darken again over time once treatment has finished. In most cases the port-wine stain at 10 years after treatment has an appearance midway between the before and after injury color. For this reason, patients must be informed of the risk of darkening over time.[4]

REFERENCES

1. Lee JW, Chung HY. Capillary malformations (portwine stains) of the head and neck: natural history, investigations, laser, and surgical management. Otolaryngol Clin North Am 2018;51(1):197–211
2. Maguiness SM, Liang MG. Management of capillary malformations. Clin Plast Surg 2011;38(1):65–73
3. Sadick M, Müller-Wille R, Wildgruber M, Wohlgemuth WA. Vascular anomalies (Part I): classification and diagnostics of vascular anomalies. Rofo 2018;190(9):825–835
4. Huikeshoven M, Koster PH, de Borgie CA, Beek JF, van Gemert MJ, van der Horst CM. Redarkening of port-wine stains 10 years after pulsed-dye-laser treatment. N Engl J Med 2007;356(12):1235–1240

HAIR REMOVAL

10. You see a young blonde patient in your office who wishes to have hair removal treatment. *Which one of the following laser modalities would be ineffective for this clinical indication?*

    D. Ruby

    There are a number of different laser types used in hair removal, each with its own advantages and disadvantages. These lasers include Diode, Alexandrite, and Nd:YAG. Ruby is not a hair removal laser choice and is indicated for tattoo removal and treating pigmented skin lesions. Alexandrite is commonly used for hair removal in patients with lighter skin tones. Nd:YAG is safest for darker skin tones to reduce the risk of hypopigmentation.[1,2]

    In general, laser hair removal is most effective in patients with fair skin and dark hairs because the target chromophore is melanin. Laser is therefore generally less effective in blonde patients although it does still work. Intense pulsed light (IPL) is an alternative option for hair removal and can be quite effective in fair-skinned, fair-haired individuals such as in this patient.[2,3]

REFERENCES

1. Haedersdal M, Beerwerth F, Nash JF. Laser and intense pulsed light hair removal technologies: from professional to home use. Br J Dermatol 2011;165(Suppl 3):31–36
2. Gan SD, Graber EM. Laser hair removal: a review. Dermatol Surg 2013;39(6):823–838
3. Nahai F. The Art of Aesthetic Surgery: Principles & Techniques. 2nd ed. St Louis: Quality Medical Publishing; 2011

TATTOO REMOVAL

11. You see a patient in your office following treatment to remove a multicolored tattoo. The initial treatment has been partly successful but there remains residual green pigment. *Which laser would be best to target these areas in subsequent treatment?*

    B. Q-switched alexandrite

    Green tattoo inks are best treated with a laser of wavelength 650 nm. Suitable choices include alexandrite (755 nm) and ruby (694 nm). Q-switched lasers are preferable over pulsed for tattoo removal. They use high bursts of energy in short time intervals and create acoustic waves that result in mechanical pigment disruption. The pigments that are fragmented can then be phagocytized by macrophages.[1,2]

REFERENCES

1. Kent KM, Graber EM. Laser tattoo removal: a review. Dermatol Surg 2012;38(1):1–13
2. Nahai F. The Art of Aesthetic Surgery: Principles & Techniques. 2nd ed. St Louis: Quality Medical Publishing; 2011

12. You see a patient in clinic with a tattoo of a multicolored cartoon bear character. She wishes to have this removed with laser treatment. *Which color ink is most likely to be resistant to laser treatment?*

    D. Yellow

    Multicolored tattoos are very difficult to treat and will require multiple therapies with different lasers. Of the colors listed, yellow will be most difficult to treat as this and orange are highly resistant to treatment. These colors best absorb light in the UV range which is absorbed by, and damages, melanocytes. This affects the ability of light to penetrate the dermis.[1–3]

REFERENCES

1. Kent KM, Graber EM. Laser tattoo removal: a review. Dermatol Surg 2012;38(1):1–13
2. Nahai F. The Art of Aesthetic Surgery: Principles & Techniques. 2nd ed. St Louis: Quality Medical Publishing; 2011
3. Naga LI, Alster TS. Laser tattoo removal: an update. Am J Clin Dermatol 2017;18(1):59–65

LASERS IN BURN SCARS

13. You are asked to see a young girl in clinic following a 10% total body surface area (TBSA) superficial dermal burn that was treated conservatively 1 year ago. Most areas healed well but some areas remained thickened and were treated with steroids. The scars have now flattened but remain erythematous. *What laser treatment is most appropriate to reduce the residual hyperpigmentation of her scar?*

    D. Pulsed dye

    Scars that remain erythematous due to increased vascularity may be treated with either pulsed dye, Nd:YAG, or KTP lasers. These cause coagulation necrosis and decrease the number and proliferation of fibroblasts as well as the deposition of type III collagen. Sometimes, ablative lasers such as Er:YAG or CO_2 are used for scars to reduce the texture and thickness, but their effects on decreasing the pink coloration within a scar are very limited.[1,2]

REFERENCES

1. Parrett BM, Donelan MB. Pulsed dye laser in burn scars: current concepts and future directions. Burns 2010;36(4):443–449
2. Nahai F. The Art of Aesthetic Surgery: Principles & Techniques. 2nd ed. St Louis: Quality Medical Publishing; 2011

FACIAL REJUVENATION

14. You consult with a 70-year-old white female in clinic who has deep rhytids and has requested ablative skin resurfacing. *Which one of the following is best for this patient?*

    A. Er:YAG

    Water is the target chromophore for ablative resurfacing and the two key traditional options for this are Er:YAG (2940 nm) and CO_2 (10,600 nm). Of the two, Er:YAG is generally preferred currently because energy absorption by water is far more efficient (by about 13 times) with ER:YAG compared with CO_2 lasers. It allows for a more controlled depth penetration without collateral thermal damage. It is also more suitable for areas of the face that have thinner skin and is associated with less erythema and an overall reduced downtime compared with CO_2. Nd:YAG is a nonablative resurfacing laser. Fraxel and intense pulsed light (IPL) are also nonablative techniques that may be used for less aggressive resurfacing.[1–3]

REFERENCES

1. Perrotti JA, Thorne C. Cutaneous resurfacing: chemical peeling, dermabrasion, and laser resurfacing. In: Thorne CH, ed. Grabb and Smith's Plastic Surgery. 6th ed. Philadelphia: Wolters Kluwer/Lippincott Williams & Wilkins; 2007
2. Chen KH, Tam KW, Chen IF, et al. A systematic review of comparative studies of CO_2 and erbium:YAG lasers in resurfacing facial rhytides (wrinkles). J Cosmet Laser Ther 2017;19(4):199–204
3. Nahai F. The Art of Aesthetic Surgery: Principles & Techniques. 2nd ed. St Louis: Quality Medical Publishing; 2011

LASER RESURFACING

15. A patient is seen in clinic requesting laser skin resurfacing of the face. *Which one of the following medications should be discontinued prior to treatment to reduce the risk of scarring?*

    E. Isotretinoin

    Isotretinoin is related to vitamin A and is taken orally to treat acne. The precise mechanism of action is not known but it works by suppressing activity in the sebaceous glands of the skin and by decreasing the amount of oil produced. It can make the skin fragile and cause delayed wound healing and scarring. This may be a direct result of damage to the epithelial cells of the adnexal structures which usually provide cells that repopulate the resurfaced skin wound. It can also increase the risk of wound infection and sensitivity to UV light. Therefore, isotretinoin should be stopped 6–12 months before resurfacing treatment to minimize the risk of scarring, poor wound healing, and hyperpigmentation. Using tretinoin and hydroquinone for 4–6 weeks pretreatment will stimulate rapid healing and help prevent post-treatment hyperpigmentation. Antivirals, such as Acyclovir, should be given 48 hours before and 7–10 days after ablative laser resurfacing. Use of sunblock before and after treatment is normally also advised. Metronidazole is used for treating acne and does not specifically need to be stopped for laser surgery. However, laser therapy should not be given during a bout of active acne as it will likely result in poor scarring.[1–3]

REFERENCES

1. Chen KH, Tam KW, Chen IF, et al. A systematic review of comparative studies of CO2 and erbium:YAG lasers in resurfacing facial rhytides (wrinkles). J Cosmet Laser Ther 2017;19(4):199–204

2. Perrotti JA, Thorne C. Cutaneous resurfacing: chemical peeling, dermabrasion, and laser resurfacing. In: Thorne CH, ed. Grabb and Smith's Plastic Surgery, 6th ed. Philadelphia: Wolters Kluwer/Lippincott Williams & Wilkins; 2007

3. Nahai F. The Art of Aesthetic Surgery: Principles & Techniques. 2nd ed. St Louis: Quality Medical Publishing; 2011

LASER LIPOSUCTION

16. You see a patient in the office who requests liposuction and states a preference for laser liposuction over power assisted liposuction. *Which one of the following would be true about the use of laser liposuction in general?*

E. A 980-nm diode laser may be effective on areas with large amounts of fat.

Laser liposuction can be performed with either Nd:YAG or Diode lasers. The Nd:YAG has the longest track record for use and can be useful for providing a skin tightening effect due to effects on collagen. Diode at 980 nm can be particularly effective on areas with large amounts of fat. However, although laser liposuction is purported to have benefits of causing adipocyte membrane rupture, coagulation of small blood vessels, and coagulation of dermal collagen, there is not enough evidence to show an increased efficacy compared with standard liposuction approaches. It can be associated with a steep learning curve for the operator and risks thermal injury, although this is only 1% rather than 10%. It can be used in the head and neck areas including the face, neck, and chin. In general, laser liposuction is associated with a longer, not shorter, operating time.[1-3]

REFERENCES

1. Fakhouri TM, El Tal AK, Abrou AE, Mehregan DA, Barone F. Laser-assisted lipolysis: a review. Dermatol Surg 2012;38(2):155–169

2. Collins PS, Moyer KE. Evidence-based practice in liposuction. Ann Plast Surg 2018;80(6S, Suppl 6):S403–S405

3. Pereira-Netto D, Montano-Pedroso JC, Aidar ALES, et al. Laser-assisted lipolysis: a review. Aesthetic Plast Surg 2018;42(2):376–383

12. Anesthesia

See *Essentials of Plastic Surgery*, third edition, pp. 143–158

AMERICAN SOCIETY OF ANESTHESIOLOGISTS CLASSIFICATION

1. You are planning surgery on a patient who will require a general anesthetic. The medical history includes well-controlled diabetes mellitus and hypertension. These conditions do not presently limit the patient's functional status. *According to the American Society of Anesthesiologists (ASA) classification, what is the ASA status of this patient?*
   A. ASA 1
   B. ASA 2
   C. ASA 3
   D. ASA 4
   E. ASA 5

INDUCTION OF GENERAL ANESTHESIA

2. A patient is to have breast reduction surgery under general anesthesia and has requested a gas induction due to fears of intravenous (IV) cannulation. *Which one of the following anesthetic induction agents would be best for this purpose?*
   A. Isoflurane
   B. Desflurane
   C. Nitrous oxide
   D. Sevoflurane
   E. Propofol

GENERAL ANESTHESIA

3. A patient is planned for elective reconstructive surgery and during the preoperative assessment it becomes evident the patient has a family history of malignant hyperthermia. *Which one of the following agents is most likely to cause this and must therefore be avoided in this case?*
   A. Vecuronium
   B. Rocuronium
   C. Succinylcholine
   D. Atracurium
   E. Cisatracurium

LOCAL ANESTHETIC ACTION

4. You have injected a local anesthetic agent as a digital ring block prior to digital nerve repair. *Which one of the following statements is true regarding how the anesthetic agent will take effect?*
   A. The first clinical effect will be a loss of proprioception.
   B. Nerve blockade will occur secondary to an effect on calcium channels.
   C. The agent needs to be in an ionized state to take effect.
   D. Propagation of action potentials is unaffected.
   E. The mechanism of action is the same for all agents.

LOCAL ANESTHETICS

5. *Which one of the following statements regarding lidocaine as an injectable local anesthetic agent is correct?*
   A. The maximum safe dose is 750 mg.
   B. Metabolism is predominantly renal.
   C. It is an amide local anesthetic compound.
   D. True allergies occur secondary to paraaminobenzoic acid (PABA) production.
   E. Onset of action usually takes 5–6 minutes.

SAFE DOSE SELECTION OF LOCAL ANESTHETICS

6. A woman weighing 55 kg (121 pounds) is having several basal cell carcinomas excised from her face. Lidocaine with epinephrine is given. *Based on a safe working dose of 7 mg/kg, what would be the maximum safe dose of local anesthetic agent she can receive?*
   A. 11 mL of 1% lidocaine with epinephrine
   B. 16 mL of 1% lidocaine with epinephrine
   C. 38 mL of 1% lidocaine with epinephrine
   D. 16 mL of 0.5% lidocaine with epinephrine
   E. 76 mL of 2% lidocaine with epinephrine

SAFE DOSE SELECTION OF LOCAL ANESTHETICS

7. A patient weighing 60 kg (132 pounds) is under general anesthesia and has a 25 cm by 15 cm split-thickness skin graft donor site on the thigh. Postoperative pain relief is needed. *Based on a maximum safe dose of 2 mg/kg, how much bupivacaine (Marcaine) can she receive?*
   A. 12 mL of 2%
   B. 16 mL of 0.5%
   C. 24 mL of 0.75%
   D. 48 mL of 0.25%
   E. 96 mL of 1%

LOCAL ANESTHETIC ADDITIVES

8. *What is the main effect of adding sodium bicarbonate to a local anesthetic solution?*
   A. It prolongs the duration of the anesthetic.
   B. It reduces localized bleeding.
   C. It allows a higher dose of anesthetic agent to be administered.
   D. It speeds the onset of anesthetic blockade.
   E. It helps stop precipitation of the anesthetic.

LOCAL ANESTHETICS CONTAINING EPINEPHRINE

9. You are planning an excisional biopsy and local flap reconstruction of a large basal cell carcinoma on the face. *Which one of the following is the main disadvantage of adding epinephrine to the anesthetic solution?*
   A. The effect on duration of anesthesia
   B. The effect on anesthetic absorption rate
   C. The effect on patient discomfort
   D. The effect on anesthetic dosage allowance
   E. The effect on localized bleeding

CONTRAINDICATIONS TO USING EPINEPHRINE IN LOCAL ANESTHETICS

10. *Which one of the following is only a relative contraindication to giving epinephrine with a local anesthetic?*
    A. Anesthesia of the penis
    B. A skin flap with limited perfusion
    C. Digital vessels compromised by infection or trauma
    D. Diabetic patients
    E. Dilutions of less than 1:60,000 to block a digit

CARDIOTOXICITY IN LOCAL ANESTHESIA

11. *Which one of the following is the most cardiotoxic local anesthetic agent?*
    A. Lidocaine
    B. Bupivacaine
    C. Lidocaine with epinephrine
    D. Cocaine
    E. Ropivacaine

TOXICITY WITH LOCAL ANESTHETIC AGENTS

12. You are operating on a patient and have just completed an injection of local anesthetic. The patient becomes unwell. *Which one of the following is most commonly the first sign of systemic toxicity?*
    A. Perioral numbness and a metallic taste in the mouth
    B. Cardiac or respiratory arrest

C. Muscle twitching or convulsion
D. Visual disturbances
E. Disorientation and hallucinations

LOCAL ANESTHETIC DELIVERY

13. *When administering local anesthetic prior to blepharoplasty, which one of the following is most likely to minimize patient discomfort?*
   A. Using a 21-gauge needle
   B. Administering rapidly
   C. Adding epinephrine
   D. Cooling the anesthetic agent first
   E. Adding sodium bicarbonate

LOCAL ANESTHETIC TOXICITY

14. *Which one of the following is true regarding local anesthetic toxicity?*
   A. When mixing local anesthetics, onset, duration, and potency become less predictable.
   B. Features of CNS toxicity are generally unrelated to dose of anesthetic agent.
   C. Methemoglobinemia is associated with the majority of anesthetic agents.
   D. The initial action following toxicity should be to administer 100% oxygen.
   E. Aspiration before injection can avoid its occurrence.

BIER BLOCK

15. *Which one of the following is true when performing a Bier block?*
   A. The block is usually performed using bupivacaine mixed with lidocaine.
   B. Care must be taken to avoid intravenous injection of anesthetic.
   C. Two separate tourniquets are inflated simultaneously at the start.
   D. The effect of the block normally lasts for between 16 and 24 hours.
   E. The minimum tourniquet time should be 40 minutes.

SPINAL AND EPIDURAL ANESTHESIA

16. *When comparing spinal and epidural anesthetic techniques, which one of the following is a key benefit of the epidural approach?*
   A. Lower volumes of anesthetic are required.
   B. The risk of hematoma is markedly reduced.
   C. The likelihood of developing a post-tap headache is avoided.
   D. There is flexibility to add more anesthetic later.
   E. The risk of developing urinary retention is removed.

CONSCIOUS SEDATION

17. A patient has requested conscious sedation for a mini facelift procedure. *Which one of the following is true regarding conscious sedation?*
   A. Preoperative fasting is not usually required.
   B. Surgical control of the airway is still required.
   C. It should be reserved for ASA 1 and 2 patients.
   D. Routine monitoring of carbon dioxide is not mandatory.
   E. It negates the need for local anesthetic agents.

TOPICAL LOCAL ANESTHETIC AGENTS

18. Topical local anesthetics are useful preoperatively, especially in the pediatric population. *Which one of the following is a topical anesthetic that contains lidocaine and prilocaine in equal concentrations?*
   A. EMLA
   B. LMX-4
   C. Betacaine
   D. Topicaine
   E. Tetracaine

GENERAL ANESTHETIC STARVATION TIMES

19. You are producing a patient information leaflet for general anesthetic guidance. *When considering the presurgical starvation times, which one of the following would normally be advised prior to the planned start time for anesthesia?*
    A. Avoidance of food and clear fluids for 6 hours
    B. Avoidance of food for 4 hours and clear fluids for 2 hours
    C. Avoidance of food for 2 hours and clear fluids for 1 hour
    D. Avoidance of food for 6 hours and clear fluids for 2 hours
    E. Avoidance of food for 8 hours and clear fluids for 3 hours

Answers

AMERICAN SOCIETY OF ANESTHESIOLOGISTS CLASSIFICATION

1. You are planning surgery on a patient who will require a general anesthetic. The medical history includes well-controlled diabetes mellitus and hypertension. These conditions do not presently limit the patient's functional status. *According to the American Society of Anesthesiologists (ASA) classification, what is the ASA status of this patient?*
   B. ASA 2

   The ASA physical status grade has six classes (1–6) ranging from a normal healthy patient (1) to one that is brain dead (6). The full categories are shown below:
   Class 1: A normal healthy patient
   Class 2: Mild systemic disease with no functional limitation
   Class 3: Severe systemic disease with functional limitation
   Class 4: Severe systemic disease that is a constant threat to life
   Class 5: Moribund and not expected to survive without surgery
   Class 6: Brain dead patient for organ retrieval

   This has clinical relevance for assessing the risk of surgery for individual patients and can help to guide which procedures can safely be offered and the appropriate level of care a patient will require (e.g., day case versus overnight admission and postoperative ward care versus high dependency). The ASA status also forms part of the World Health Organization (WHO) surgical checklist and facilitates communication between the surgeon and the anesthetist about a patient's general fitness for surgery. A patient's ASA status will also impact the billing costs for medical care in most medical systems as well as the clinical outcomes following surgery.[1,2]

REFERENCES

1. Dripps RD. New classification of physical status. Anesthesiol 1963;24:111
2. Hurwitz EE, Simon M, Vinta SR, et al. Adding examples to the ASA-physical status classification improves correct assignment to patients. Anesthesiology 2017;126(4):614–622

INDUCTION OF GENERAL ANESTHESIA

2. A patient is to have breast reduction surgery under general anesthesia and has requested a gas induction due to fears of intravenous (IV) cannulation. *Which one of the following anesthetic induction agents would be best for this purpose?*
   D. Sevoflurane

   Both induction and maintenance of anesthesia can be achieved with intravenous or inhalational agents. Of all the volatile inhalational agents, sevoflurane is the preferred choice for inhalational induction because it is well tolerated due to its having a low odor and being nonpungent. In contrast, other inhalational agents such as desflurane and isoflurane are extremely pungent and not suitable for induction of anesthesia; they would be likely to cause airway irritation and may cause laryngospasm or bronchospasm if used for that purpose.

   Nitrous oxide is a gas, which is used as an adjuvant to general anesthesia and as an analgesic during labor and other painful procedures. It can also be used in liquid form for cryotherapy for skin lesions. Entonox is the trade name for a 50:50 mix of oxygen and nitrous oxide which is typically used for analgesia, e.g., dressing changes, labor pains, and in the pre-hospital/emergency room setting.

   Intravenous induction can be achieved with a number of different substances of which propofol is a very commonly used example. Other agents include etomidate, thiopental, and ketamine.[1]

REFERENCE

1. Scarth E, Smith S. Drugs in Anaesthesia and Intensive Care. Oxford University Press; 2016

GENERAL ANESTHESIA

3. A patient is planned for elective reconstructive surgery and during the preoperative assessment it becomes evident the patient has a family history of malignant hyperthermia. *Which one of the following agents is most likely to cause this and must therefore be avoided in this case?*
   C. Succinylcholine

Malignant hyperthermia (MH) is a rare and potentially fatal genetic disorder that affects calcium regulation within skeletal muscle. It can be precipitated by a variety of drugs used in anesthesia including succinylcholine and inhalational volatile agents. Succinylcholine is a neuromuscular blocking agent used to induce rapid and profound paralysis, e.g., to facilitate endotracheal intubation and for modification of convulsions after electroconvulsive therapy (ECT). Historically, it was also used to maintain neuromuscular blockade during short procedures. Other potential triggers for malignant hyperthermia include volatile anesthetic agents such as desflurane, isoflurane, and sevoflurane. If given these drugs, people at risk for malignant hyperthermia may develop life-threatening multiorgan failure.

Early features of MH include an increase in end-tidal carbon dioxide (even with increasing minute ventilation), tachycardia, tachypnea, muscle rigidity, and hyperkalemia. Later features include fever, myoglobinuria, and multiple organ failure.

Patients often have no idea they are susceptible to MH unless they have a first-degree relative who has experienced problems or they themselves have experienced problems previously. There is a muscle biopsy test called the Caffeine Halothane Contracture Test, which can be performed at limited centers throughout the US. However, this is an expensive test to perform costing thousands of dollars. Any concerns raised with respect to MH during preassessment need to be escalated to the anesthetic team for further advice.[1-2]

REFERENCES

1. Ellinas H, Albrecht MA. Malignant hyperthermia update. Anesthesiol Clin 2020;38(1):165–181
2. Scarth E, Smith S. Drugs in Anaesthesia and Intensive Care. Oxford University Press; 2016

LOCAL ANESTHETIC ACTION

4. You have injected a local anesthetic agent as a digital ring block prior to digital nerve repair. *Which one of the following statements is true regarding how the anesthetic agent will take effect?*
   E. The mechanism of action is the same for all agents.
   Local anesthetic agents work in a broadly similar manner by interfering with sodium channels, thereby preventing an influx of sodium within the neuronal membrane. This does not affect the resting membrane potential but does impair propagation of the action potential. Penetration of the nerve membrane by the local anesthetic agent requires an unionized state (i.e., to be in base form). The pKa determines the ratio of ionized and nonionized local anesthetic and the closer the pKa is to the body pH, the faster the onset of action.[1-3]

   There is a differential sensitivity of nerve fibers that results in smaller fibers and those that are myelinated being blocked more quickly (**Fig. 12.1**). The clinical sequence is as follows:
   1. Vasodilatation
   2. Loss of pain and temperature
   3. Loss of proprioception
   4. Loss of pressure sensation
   5. Loss of motor function

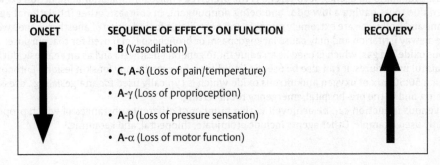

Fig. 12.1   Sequence of local anesthetic blockade.

REFERENCES

1. Becker DE, Reed KL. Local anesthetics: review of pharmacological considerations. Anesth Prog 2012;59(2):90–101, quiz 102–103
2. Butterworth J. Clinical pharmacology of local anesthetics. In: Hadzic A, ed. Textbook of Regional Anesthesia and Acute Pain Management. New York: McGraw-Hill; 2007
3. Moore PA, Hersh EV. Local anesthetics: pharmacology and toxicity. Dent Clin North Am 2010;54(4):587–599

LOCAL ANESTHETICS

5. *Which one of the following statements regarding lidocaine as an injectable local anesthetic agent is correct?*

C. It is an amide local anesthetic compound.

Local anesthetic agents are classified as either amides or esters depending on their chemical composition. Amides are more commonly used in clinical practice and may be identified by the presence of the letter *i* in their prefix. For example, lidocaine, bupivacaine, mepivacaine, and prilocaine. The maximum safe dose for lidocaine with epinephrine is 7 mg/kg, but without epinephrine it is only 3–5 mg/kg. Absolute maximum safe dose is 300 mg (not 750 mg). Lidocaine is metabolized in the liver (not the kidney) and its onset of action is rapid (usually within 2 minutes). The elimination half-life is 90–120 minutes and the duration of action is up to 1 hour without and 6 hours with epinephrine. True allergies are rare for amide anesthetic agents such as lidocaine. Paraaminobenzoic acid (PABA) is a by-product of metabolism of esters (such as procaine and tetracaine) not amides and is often responsible for hypersensitivity reactions following administration of these compounds. Methylparaben is a preservative found in some ester and amide local anesthetics that resembles PABA and may cause an allergic reaction.[1,2]

REFERENCES

1. Butterworth J. Clinical pharmacology of local anesthetics. In: Hadzic A, ed. Textbook of Regional Anesthesia and Acute Pain Management. New York: McGraw-Hill; 2007
2. Moore PA, Hersh EV. Local anesthetics: pharmacology and toxicity. Dent Clin North Am 2010;54(4):587–599

SAFE DOSE SELECTION OF LOCAL ANESTHETICS

6. A woman weighing 55 kg (121 pounds) is having several basal cell carcinomas excised from her face. Lidocaine with epinephrine is given. *Based on a safe working dose of 7 mg/kg, what would be the maximum safe dose of local anesthetic agent she can receive?*

C. 38 mL of 1% lidocaine with epinephrine

Lidocaine is a short-acting local anesthetic commonly used in plastic surgery. It is an amide that has a rapid onset of action and is often combined with epinephrine. The safe dose of lidocaine with epinephrine is 7 mg/kg. The safe dose without epinephrine is 3–5 mg/kg. This lady can therefore safely have 38 mL of 1% lidocaine with epinephrine.[1-3] The calculation is shown below:

7 mg × 55 kg = 384 mg
A 1% solution contains 10 mg in 1 mL
Therefore, she can have 384/10 = 38.4 mL

Option A is based on a calculation of 2 mg/kg which is a maximum safe dose for levobupivacaine. Option B is based on a calculation of 3 mg/kg which is a maximum safe dose for lidocaine with epinephrine. Option D refers to a safe maximum volume for 2% lidocaine with epinephrine, not 0.5%. Option E refers to a safe volume for 0.5% lidocaine with epinephrine, but would exceed the maximum safe dose for 2% lidocaine with epinephrine by four times. In the clinical setting it is vital to have a good understanding of safe dosing for commonly used local anesthetic agents.[1-4]

REFERENCES

1. British National Formulary. Available at www.bnf.org
2. Moore PA, Hersh EV. Local anesthetics: pharmacology and toxicity. Dent Clin North Am 2010;54(4):587–599
3. Burlacu CL, Buggy DJ. Update on local anesthetics: focus on levobupivacaine. Ther Clin Risk Manag 2008;4(2):381–392
4. Drasner K. Local anesthetic neurotoxicity: clinical injury and strategies that may minimize risk. Reg Anesth Pain Med 2002;27(6):576–580

SAFE DOSE SELECTION OF LOCAL ANESTHETICS

7. A patient weighing 60 kg (132 pounds) is under general anesthesia and has a 25 cm by 15 cm split-thickness skin graft donor site on the thigh. Postoperative pain relief is needed. *Based on a maximum safe dose of 2 mg/kg, how much bupivacaine (Marcaine) can she receive?*

D. 48 mL of 0.25%

The safe dose of bupivacaine is 2 mg to 2.5 mg per kg and is not significantly altered by the addition of epinephrine.[1] This patient can therefore safely have 48 mL of 0.25% bupivacaine or levobupivacaine. The calculation is shown below:

2 mg × 60 kg = 120 mg
A 0.25% solution contains 2.5 mg in 1 mL
Therefore, she can have 120/2.5 = 48 mL

Option A is the maximum safe volume of 1% not 2% bupivacaine. Option B is the maximum safe volume of 1% bupivacaine. Option C is the maximum safe volume of 0.5% bupivacaine. Option E is the maximum safe volume of 0.125% bupivacaine. Levobupivacaine and ropivacaine (Naropin) are both isomers of bupivacaine developed to reduce the cardiotoxicity of bupivacaine. They have become popular alternatives to bupivacaine as a result in many countries. Safe doses are 2–3 mg/kg for levobupivacaine and 3–4 mg/kg for ropivacaine, with maximum recommended doses of 150 and 200 mg, respectively. Use of local anesthetic in patients who have skin grafts taken under general anesthetic is very useful and should be routinely performed. This has the benefit of reducing intraoperative and postoperative pain. Often patients who have split-graft harvest state that the donor site is the most painful part of the procedure so anything that can be performed to minimize this is recommended.[1-6]

REFERENCES

1. British National Formulary. Available at www.bnf.org
2. Moore PA, Hersh EV. Local anesthetics: pharmacology and toxicity. Dent Clin North Am 2010;54(4):587–599
3. Drasner K. Local anesthetic neurotoxicity: clinical injury and strategies that may minimize risk. Reg Anesth Pain Med 2002;27(6):576–580
4. Burlacu CL, Buggy DJ. Update on local anesthetics: focus on levobupivacaine. Ther Clin Risk Manag 2008;4(2):381–392
5. Chahar P, Cummings KC III. Liposomal bupivacaine: a review of a new bupivacaine formulation. J Pain Res 2012;5:257–264
6. Candiotti K. Liposomal bupivacaine: an innovative nonopioid local analgesic for the management of postsurgical pain. Pharmacotherapy 2012;32(9, Suppl)19S–26S

LOCAL ANESTHETIC ADDITIVES

8. *What is the main effect of adding sodium bicarbonate to a local anesthetic solution?*

   D. It speeds the onset of anesthetic blockade.

   Sodium bicarbonate can be added to local anesthetic solutions to speed the onset of blockade. This works by reducing the acidity of the anesthetic and releasing unionized anesthetic agent. The dose should be 8.4% NaHCO$_3$ added in a ratio of 1:9 with lidocaine. Care should be taken with agents such as bupivacaine as bicarbonate can lead to precipitation. An additional benefit of using bicarbonate is that it can decrease pain during injection, presumably as a result of the decreased acidity and perhaps in part to a more rapid onset of anesthesia.[1,2]

REFERENCES

1. Mutalik S. How to make local anesthesia less painful. J Cutan Aesthet Surg 2008;1(1):37–38
2. Brandis K. Alkalinisation of local anaesthetic solutions. Aust Prescr 2011;34:173–175

LOCAL ANESTHETICS CONTAINING EPINEPHRINE

9. You are planning an excisional biopsy and local flap reconstruction of a large basal cell carcinoma on the face. *Which one of the following is the main disadvantage of adding epinephrine to the anesthetic solution?*

   C. The effect on patient discomfort

   Using epinephrine with a local anesthetic serves a number of useful purposes but it may increase pain on injection as it requires the solution to be more acidic. This is because epinephrine is unstable in solution at physiological pH.[1,2]

   Other potential disadvantages to utilizing epinephrine include increased myocardial irritability leading to tachycardia, hypertension, or arrhythmias. For this reason, particular caution should be exercised when using epinephrine in patients with cardiac disease.

   There are multiple beneficial effects of adding epinephrine to a local anesthetic solution. It causes local vasoconstriction and therefore maintains the anesthetic agent at the required site. It reduces bleeding and increases the duration of action. It also enables higher doses to be given safely. For example, lidocaine can be administered at doses of 3–5 mg/kg without epinephrine and up to 7 mg/kg when epinephrine is added. In addition, it will shorten the time to onset of anesthesia.

   Factors to reduce pain during injection of a local anesthetic include slow infiltration, the addition of bicarbonate, using hyaluronidase,[3] and ensuring the product is not cold (particularly relevant in products that are stored in the refrigerator).

REFERENCES

1. Mutalik S. How to make local anesthesia less painful. J Cutan Aesthet Surg 2008;1(1):37–38
2. Brandis K. Alkalinisation of local anaesthetic solutions. Aust Prescr 2011;34:173–175
3. Nevarre DR, Tzarnas CD. The effects of hyaluronidase on the efficacy and on the pain of administration of 1% lidocaine. Plast Reconstr Surg 1998;101(2):365–369

CONTRAINDICATIONS TO USING EPINEPHRINE IN LOCAL ANESTHETICS

10. *Which one of the following is only a relative contraindication to giving epinephrine with a local anesthetic?*

D. Diabetic patients

Contraindications to using epinephrine in local anesthetics can be classified as absolute or relative. Absolute contraindications include use in the penis, skin flaps with limited perfusion, and when the digital vessels are already compromised. The use of epinephrine in healthy digits is considered safe but dilutions greater than 1:200,000 are recommended. Most of the time a digital tourniquet can be used to reduce bleeding in a digit, negating the need for epinephrine. Relative contraindications for epinephrine use include hypertension, diabetes, cardiac disease, thyrotoxicosis, and certain drug interactions such as with the monoamine oxidase inhibitors (MAO). These can cause a hypertensive crisis when epinephrine is used, secondary to formation of a pool of available endogenous catecholamines.[1-4]

REFERENCES

1. Thornton PC, Grant SA, Breslin DS. Adjuncts to local anesthetics in peripheral nerve blockade. Int Anesthesiol Clin 2010;48(4):59–70
2. Becker DE, Reed KL. Local anesthetics: review of pharmacological considerations. Anesth Prog 2012;59(2):90–101, quiz 102–103
3. Butterworth J. Clinical pharmacology of local anesthetics. In: Hadzic A, ed. Textbook of Regional Anesthesia and Acute Pain Management. New York: McGraw-Hill; 2007
4. Moore PA, Hersh EV. Local anesthetics: pharmacology and toxicity. Dent Clin North Am 2010;54(4):587–599

CARDIOTOXICITY IN LOCAL ANESTHESIA

11. *Which one of the following is the most cardiotoxic local anesthetic agent?*

B. Bupivacaine

Bupivacaine is known to have the greatest cardiac toxicity, especially after inadvertent intravascular injection. Levobupivacaine is the L isomer of bupivacaine and was developed to help reduce these cardiotoxic effects. It is often marketed as Chirocaine. An advantage over lidocaine is the prolonged effects of pain relief which can be typically 6–8 hours after injection as a local anesthetic agent. However, the onset of action is delayed compared with lidocaine. Ropivacaine was also developed to provide a long duration of action with less cardiac toxicity and is a popular alternative. Symptoms of cardiovascular toxicity include hypotension, arrhythmias, and cardiovascular collapse. The use of epinephrine can also cause cardiac problems and should be carefully monitored.[1-3]

REFERENCES

1. Chahar P, Cummings KC III. Liposomal bupivacaine: a review of a new bupivacaine formulation. J Pain Res 2012;5:257–264
2. Candiotti K. Liposomal bupivacaine: an innovative nonopioid local analgesic for the management of postsurgical pain. Pharmacotherapy 2012; 32(9, Suppl):19S–26S
3. Moore PA, Hersh EV. Local anesthetics: pharmacology and toxicity. Dent Clin North Am 2010;54(4):587–599

TOXICITY WITH LOCAL ANESTHETIC AGENTS

12. You are operating on a patient and have just completed an injection of local anesthetic. The patient becomes unwell. *Which one of the following is most commonly the first sign of systemic toxicity?*

A. Perioral numbness and a metallic taste in the mouth

Toxicity due to local anesthetics can be unpredictable but generally parallels increasing plasma concentration and tongue numbness and a metallic taste are early signs (**Fig. 12.2**). Toxicity can be subclassified into central nervous system (CNS), cardiovascular, or idiosyncratic effects. CNS effects include dizziness, metallic taste in the mouth, perioral numbness, tinnitus, and seizures. Cardiovascular effects include hypotension and arrhythmias. Idiosyncratic effects include anaphylaxis in patients with hypersensitivity to esters, increased relative toxicity associated with liver disease and the effects of epinephrine.[1-4]

REFERENCES

1. Hadzic A, Vloka JD. Clinical pharmacology of local anesthetics. In: Hadzic A, ed. Hadzic's Peripheral Nerve Blocks and Anatomy for Ultrasound-Guided Regional Anesthesia. 2nd ed. New York: McGraw-Hill; 2012
2. Heavner JE. Pharmacology of local anesthetics. In: Longnecker DE, Brown DL, Newman MF, et al, eds. Anesthesiology. 2nd ed. New York: McGraw-Hill; 2012

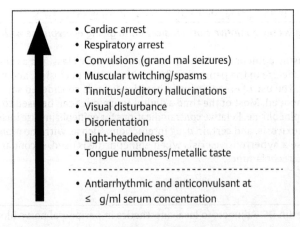

- Cardiac arrest
- Respiratory arrest
- Convulsions (grand mal seizures)
- Muscular twitching/spasms
- Tinnitus/auditory hallucinations
- Visual disturbance
- Disorientation
- Light-headedness
- Tongue numbness/metallic taste

- Antiarrhythmic and anticonvulsant at
  ≤ g/ml serum concentration

Fig. 12.2   Features of local anesthetic toxicity with increasing plasma concentration.

3. Hjelm M, Holmdahl MH. Biochemical effects of aromatic amines. II. Cyanosis, methaemoglobinaemia and heinz-body formation induced by a local anaesthetic agent (prilocaine). Acta Anaesthesiol Scand 1965;9:99–120
4. Neal JM, Bernards CM, Butterworth JF IV, et al. ASRA practice advisory on local anesthetic systemic toxicity. Reg Anesth Pain Med 2010;35(2):152–161

LOCAL ANESTHETIC DELIVERY

13. When administering local anesthetic prior to blepharoplasty, which one of the following is most likely to minimize patient discomfort?

E. Adding sodium bicarbonate

Ensuring patient comfort when administering local anesthetic agents is vital and there are a number of key steps that can be taken to minimize patient discomfort during this time. Adding sodium bicarbonate at a ratio of 1:9 parts lidocaine can be helpful in reducing patient discomfort, particularly when the solution contains epinephrine. However, sodium bicarbonate can cause some local anesthetics such as bupivacaine to precipitate, so may be best avoided or used in lower doses such as 0.1–10 mL bupivacaine. In addition, other factors include using a small needle such as 27 or 30 gauge, minimizing number of injection points, administering the agent slowly, using agents without epinephrine where possible (as epinephrine causes the agent to be more acidic), and warming the agent prior to injection. In addition, adding hyaluronidase can reduce pain on local anesthetic administration.[1]

REFERENCE

1. Nevarre DR, Tzarnas CD. The effects of hyaluronidase on the efficacy and on the pain of administration of 1% lidocaine. Plast Reconstr Surg 1998;101(2):365–369

LOCAL ANESTHETIC TOXICITY

14. Which one of the following is true regarding local anesthetic toxicity?

A. When mixing local anesthetics, onset, duration, and potency become less predictable.

Mixing of local anesthetics is generally encouraged as there are different benefits involved although the onset, duration, and potency may become less predictable. A mixture of lignocaine and bupivacaine, for example, will combine the benefits of a rapid onset and also a prolonged duration of action. Mixing amides and esters allows for different modes of elimination, which can be potentially helpful. Caution should be exercised when mixing local anesthetics of the same class, e.g., amides, as the documented maximum/toxic doses should be reduced in proportion to the mix. It is vital when doing this to ensure careful calculation of maximum doses by weight.

Features of CNS toxicity tend to be dose dependent. Local anesthetics readily cross the blood–brain barrier. Other factors such as acidosis, decreased protein binding, vasoconstriction, and hyperdynamic circulation affect CNS toxicity. Methemoglobinemia is primarily associated with prilocaine use rather than most anesthetics. Liver metabolism of prilocaine forms orthotoluidine which oxidates hemoglobin to methemoglobin.

When toxicity is suspected, the initial action should be to stop the injection immediately, then commence supportive/resuscitative care with basic and advanced cardiac life support. Key factors to consider are airway management with high-flow oxygen and management of blood pressure. IV lipid emulsion binds free local anesthetic and should be used in patients with suspected CNS or cardiovascular system (CVS) toxicity.

A number of steps can be taken to minimize toxicity, but will not necessarily avoid it. These include using frequent syringe aspirations to reduce intravascular anesthetic delivery, small test doses, and divided dose injection.[1-3]

REFERENCES

1. Hadzic A, Vloka JD. Clinical pharmacology of local anesthetics. In: Hadzic A, ed. Hadzic's Peripheral Nerve Blocks and Anatomy for Ultrasound-Guided Regional Anesthesia. 2nd ed. New York: McGraw-Hill; 2012
2. Heavner JE. Pharmacology of local anesthetics. In: Longnecker DE, Brown DL, Newman MF, et al, eds. Anesthesiology. 2nd ed. New York: McGraw-Hill; 2012
3. Neal JM, Bernards CM, Butterworth JF IV, et al. ASRA practice advisory on local anesthetic systemic toxicity. Reg Anesth Pain Med 2010;35(2):152–161

BIER BLOCK

15. Which one of the following is true when performing a Bier block?

E. The minimum tourniquet time should be 40 minutes.

A Bier block relies upon intravenous injection of a local anesthetic agent infiltrating the soft tissues of an exsanguinated limb. Due to the cardiac and central nervous system toxicity of local anesthetic agents, the limb must be isolated with a tourniquet and either lidocaine or prilocaine is the preferred agent to minimize risk in the event of unintended systemic spread. A double tourniquet is ideal, allowing greater patient comfort. The proximal tourniquet is inflated first while the block is established. Subsequently the more distal adjacent tourniquet is inflated, which is on tissue which is now insensate, and the proximal tourniquet can be deflated to reduce tourniquet discomfort. A tourniquet must remain inflated for at least 40 minutes to minimize the risk of releasing local anesthetic agent into the systemic circulation. Up to 2 hours of effective block can be achieved.[1-3]

REFERENCES

1. Burstein B, Bretholz A. A novel smartphone app to support learning and maintaining competency with Bier blocks for pediatric forearm fracture reductions: protocol for a mixed-methods study. JMIR Res Protoc 2018;7(12):e10363
2. Vaughn N, Rajan N, Darowish M. Intravenous regional anesthesia using a forearm tourniquet: a safe and effective technique for outpatient hand procedures. Hand (N Y) 2020;15(3):353–359
3. Dekoninck V, Hoydonckx Y, Van de Velde M, et al. The analgesic efficacy of intravenous regional anesthesia with a forearm versus conventional upper arm tourniquet: a systematic review. BMC Anesthesiol 2018;18(1):86

SPINAL AND EPIDURAL ANESTHESIA

16. When comparing spinal and epidural anesthetic techniques, which one of the following is a key benefit of the epidural approach?

D. There is flexibility to add more anesthetic later.

Spinal and epidural anesthesia have a key role to play in a variety of surgical procedures, particularly of the lower limb and pelvis. Although the two have some similarities, they are quite different procedures with different advantages and disadvantages.

Epidural anesthesia involves injection of local anesthetic via a temporary catheter placed in the epidural space. The advantage of this over a spinal injection is that the catheter allows titration of the block as well as later administration of further anesthetic for postoperative pain control.

In contrast, a spinal anesthetic involves direct injection of local anesthetic into the cerebrospinal fluid (CSF) at the level of the lumbar vertebrae. Smaller volumes of local anesthetic are required, but it is not possible to increase levels afterwards as no catheter is in situ. A spinal anesthetic typically has a more profound motor block than an epidural which, depending on the site, may have very little motor blockade of the lower limbs.

Both types of anesthesia carry risks including hypotension, urinary retention, and headaches. Epidural injections can also be associated with hematoma which, although rare, is important as it must be identified early and evacuated swiftly. Confirmation of diagnosis is usually with magnetic resonance imaging (MRI) scan.[1]

REFERENCE

1. Smith HM, Wedel DJ. Spinal and epidural anesthesia. Anesth Analg 2007;105(1):298 PubMed

CONSCIOUS SEDATION

17. A patient has requested conscious sedation for a mini facelift procedure. *Which one of the following is true regarding conscious sedation?*

  D. Routine monitoring of carbon dioxide is not mandatory.

  Routine monitoring of carbon dioxide, although not mandatory during conscious sedation, is highly recommended as it is a reliable indicator for spontaneous airway management and breathing. In addition, other parameters must be regularly assessed including heart rate, respiratory rate, blood pressure, and oxygen saturation. One member of staff needs to be responsible for monitoring the patient while another is performing the treatment.

  Fasting guidelines for conscious sedation are the same as for general anesthetic. However, surgical management of the airway is not required as the key concept is that the patients are able to maintain their own airway throughout. The rationale for maintenance of starvation times in spite of this is twofold. First, in case there is an airway issue and sufficient loss of consciousness where a risk of aspiration is incurred. Second, in case conversion to a general anesthetic is required due to failure of the procedure to advance without it.

  ASA status does need to be considered in relation to conscious sedation; however, it is only limited to ASA 1 and 2 patients when performed in the office setting. Clearly conscious sedation does not negate the need for local anesthetic as some form of analgesic is also required.[1,2]

REFERENCES

1. A Report by the American Society of Anesthesiologists Task Force on Moderate Procedural Sedation and Analgesia, the American Association of Oral and Maxillofacial Surgeons, American College of Radiology, American Dental Association, American Society of Dentist Anesthesiologists, and Society of Interventional Radiology. Practice Guidelines for Moderate Procedural Sedation and Analgesia 2018: A Report by the American Society of Anesthesiologists Task Force on Moderate Procedural Sedation and Analgesia, the American Association of Oral and Maxillofacial Surgeons, American College of Radiology, American Dental Association, American Society of Dentist Anesthesiologists, and Society of Interventional Radiology. Anesthesiology 2018;128(3):437–479
2. Green SM, Leroy PL, Roback MG, et al; International Committee for the Advancement of Procedural Sedation. An international multidisciplinary consensus statement on fasting before procedural sedation in adults and children. Anaesthesia 2020;75(3):374–385

TOPICAL LOCAL ANESTHETIC AGENTS

18. Topical local anesthetics are useful preoperatively, especially in the pediatric population. *Which one of the following is a topical anesthetic that contains lidocaine and prilocaine in equal concentrations?*

  A. EMLA

  There are a number of topical local anesthetic agents in common use, the vast majority of which contain lidocaine in varying concentrations between 2.5 and 5%. EMLA contains 2.5% prilocaine and 2.5% lidocaine. EMLA stands for **E**utectic **M**ixture of **L**ocal **A**nesthetic which refers to the situation where two chemical compounds solidify at a lower temperature when mixed together than they do separately. In practical terms, this means that EMLA is a convenient consistency at room temperature for topical use.

  Key points to remember when using EMLA are that it takes 1 hour to provide an anesthetic effect which then lasts for a further 2 hours, and that it requires placement of an occlusive dressing over the cream once it has been applied.

  Topical local anesthetics with just lidocaine include LMX-4 and LMX-5 (the number refers to the percentage of lidocaine), betacaine, and topicaine. Tetracaine contains 4% tetracaine only without lidocaine.[1-4]

REFERENCES

1. Kumar M, Chawla R, Goyal M. Topical anesthesia. J Anaesthesiol Clin Pharmacol 2015;31(4):450–456
2. Butterworth J. Clinical pharmacology of local anesthetics. In: Hadzic A, ed. Textbook of Regional Anesthesia and Acute Pain Management. New York: McGraw-Hill; 2007
3. British National Formulary. Available at www.bnf.org
4. Moore PA, Hersh EV. Local anesthetics: pharmacology and toxicity. Dent Clin North Am 2010;54(4):587–599

GENERAL ANESTHETIC STARVATION TIMES

19. You are producing a patient information leaflet for general anesthetic guidance. *When considering the presurgical starvation times, which one of the following would normally be advised prior to the planned start time for anesthesia?*

  D. Avoidance of food for 6 hours and clear fluids for 2 hours

  It is generally accepted that starvation times for general anesthetic, regional blocks, and conscious sedation are all kept to a 6-hour time free of food and a 2-hour time free of clear fluids. This is to minimize the risk of aspiration during induction of anesthetic, prior to complete airway control.

In the emergency setting, a rapid sequence induction of anesthesia can be performed without adherence to these starvation times. In this setting, cricoid pressure is applied by an assistant once the patient is asleep and until full airway control is achieved with endotracheal intubation.

In some settings, these starvation times are being reduced. In particular, in pediatric patients, some centers will reduce the clear fluid restriction to minimize the risk of dehydration. The rationale for this is that clear fluids are rapidly absorbed from the stomach and therefore present a low risk of subsequent vomiting and aspiration.[1-4]

REFERENCES

1. Wilson GR, Dorrington KL. Starvation before surgery: is our practice based on evidence? BJA Educ 2017;17(8):275–282
2. Thomas M, Morrison C, Newton R, Schindler E. Consensus statement on clear fluids fasting for elective pediatric general anesthesia. Paediatr Anaesth 2018;28(5):411–414
3. Brunet-Wood K, Simons M, Evasiuk A, et al. Surgical fasting guidelines in children: are we putting them into practice? J Pediatr Surg 2016;51(8):1298–1302
4. Maltby JR. Fasting from midnight—the history behind the dogma. Best Pract Res Clin Anaesthesiol 2006;20(3):363–378

13. Pain Management in Plastic Surgery

See *Essentials of Plastic Surgery*, third edition, pp. 159–169

PAIN MANAGEMENT

1. *With regards to pain and its management, which one of the following is true?*
   A. Acute and chronic pain share largely similar physiological pathways.
   B. Acute pain is intended to be physiologically useful as a protective mechanism.
   C. Chronic pain is categorized as either nociceptive or inflammatory.
   D. When treating severe postoperative pain, the adverse effects of analgesics are of secondary importance.
   E. A key role of the chronic pain response is to protect tissues in the later stages of healing.

POSTSURGICAL PAIN MANAGEMENT

2. *Which one of the following is true regarding analgesia in the surgical setting?*
   A. Opioids should form part of the postoperative discharge prescription in most cases.
   B. Medical practitioners are responsible for minimizing diversion and abuse of prescriptions.
   C. Patients do not become opioid dependent after undergoing a minor surgical procedure.
   D. Development of postsurgical opioid dependency would not be considered a postoperative complication.
   E. Intravenous acetaminophen is generally preferred postoperatively for its superior analgesic qualities even in patients taking medication orally.

CONSEQUENCES OF OVERTREATING OF POSTSURGICAL PAIN

3. *Which one of the following would be associated with overtreatment rather than undertreatment of postsurgical pain with opiates?*
   A. Anxiety and depression
   B. Poor wound healing
   C. Respiratory depression
   D. Myocardial ischemia
   E. Chronic persistent surgical pain

PERSISTENT OPIOID USE

4. *What does the term "new persistent use of opioid medications" mean?*
   A. That patients will continue to use opiates for more than 2 weeks following surgery.
   B. That patients will continue to use opiates for more than 6 weeks following surgery.
   C. That previously opioid naïve patients will need to use opiates beyond the time healing is complete.
   D. That previously opioid naïve patients will continue to use opioids 90 days post surgery.
   E. That previously opioid naïve patients will continue to use opioids permanently following surgery.

RISK FACTORS FOR OPIOID USE

5. *When taking history from patients planned for surgery, which one of the following represents the greatest increased risk of their developing reliance on opioids post surgery?*
   A. Female sex
   B. History of alcohol dependency
   C. Higher socioeconomic status
   D. Nonpsychiatric comorbidities
   E. Planned revision surgery

PERSISTENT OPIATE USE

6. *What percentage of opiate naive patients continue to use opioids beyond 90 days following surgery?*
   A. <1%
   B. 1–2%
   C. 5–13%
   D. 21–29%
   E. 33–45%

OPIATE WASTAGE

7. What percentage of opiates are thought to be over-prescribed following surgery?
- A. <10%
- B. 15–20%
- C. 25–30%
- D. 35–40%
- E. >40%

OPIATE PRESCRIPTION AND STORAGE

8. When considering what happens to opioid medications following their prescription in the surgical setting, which one of the following is true?
- A. The vast majority of opioid medications will be safely stored.
- B. Diversion refers specifically to the resale of opioid medications.
- C. Friends and family are key sources of the supply of illicit opioids.
- D. All unused medications must be flushed down the toilet.
- E. Surgeons' contribution to opioid prescription is less than 1%.

ENHANCED RECOVERY PATHWAYS

9. What is the primary emphasis on an enhanced recovery after surgery protocol?
- A. To decrease recovery time
- B. To decrease hospital stay
- C. To improve pain control
- D. To decrease infection rates
- E. To decrease complications

ENHANCED RECOVERY IN BREAST SURGERY

10. When considering the enhanced recovery after surgery (ERAS) protocol for breast reconstruction, which of the following is correct before surgery?
- A. Smoking cessation should be commenced 3 months prior to surgery.
- B. A target body mass index (BMI) of <35 kg/m^2 needs to be met.
- C. Clear fluids should be continued until the time of surgery to avoid dehydration.
- D. Carbohydrate loading with maltodextrin drinks 2 hours before surgery is advocated.
- E. All patients should receive preoperative pharmacological venous thromboembolism (VTE) prophylaxis.

ENHANCED RECOVERY IN BREAST RECONSTRUCTION

11. When considering the enhanced recovery after surgery (ERAS) protocol for breast reconstruction, which of the following is correct during surgery?
- A. Iodine based skin preparation should be used.
- B. Intravenous (IV) antibiotics should be administered at induction of anesthesia.
- C. A preference is given to IV based anesthesia.
- D. Patient's core temperature should be maintained above a minimum of 37° C.
- E. Avoid vasopressors when reconstructing with free flaps.

ENHANCED RECOVERY IN BREAST RECONSTRUCTION

12. When considering the enhanced recovery after surgery (ERAS) protocol for breast reconstruction, which of the following is correct following surgery?
- A. Use a carefully selected and individualized multimodal analgesic regimen.
- B. Avoid an oral diet for the first 24 hours post surgery in case of a return to the operating room (OR).
- C. Use standard protocols for fluid management.
- D. Mobilization should be commenced on day 2 post surgery.
- E. Physiotherapy and exercise programs should be instigated on discharge.

MULTIMODAL ANALGESIA (MMA)

13. Which one of the following medications targets the N-methyl-D-aspartate (NMDA) receptor and is used as part of a multimodality pain management approach?
- A. Celecoxib
- B. Naproxen
- C. Acetaminophen
- D. Ketamine
- E. Gabapentin

Answers

PAIN MANAGEMENT

1. With regards to pain and its management, which one of the following is true?

B. Acute pain is intended to be physiologically useful as a protective mechanism.

Acute pain is physiologically useful to protect individuals from injury and allow healing to occur. It can be either nociceptive and/or inflammatory and limit activities that may predispose to poor outcomes after surgery. In contrast, chronic pain is maladaptive and exceeds beyond the period of healing. This can be a real problem for patients with 1 in 10 adults being newly diagnosed with this annually in the US. Chronic pain is therefore is not to protect tissues while healing, even in the later stages. The focus of postoperative pain management should be not only to minimize physiologic consequences of untreated pain, but also to minimize adverse effects of analgesic medications. In this way, effective pain control can help patient recovery and optimize outcomes following surgery through the rehabilitation phase. Even where there is severe pain, side effects of medication must be considered and there must be a compromise or balance reached between the positive analgesic effects and the unwanted side effects of any regimen.[1]

REFERENCE

1. Fong A, Schug SA. Pathophysiology of pain: a practical primer. Plast Reconstr Surg 2014;134(4, Suppl 2):8S–14S

POSTSURGICAL PAIN MANAGEMENT

2. Which one of the following is true regarding analgesia in the surgical setting?

B. Medical practitioners are responsible for minimizing diversion and abuse of prescriptions.

All doctors and prescribing nurse practitioners owe a duty of care to their patients to take responsibility for safe and value based prescribing. The mainstay of postoperative medication should be nonopioid based as these medications are generally sufficiently effective for pain management and carry reduced adverse effects and risk for addiction. For example, acetaminophen and nonsteroidal anti-inflammatory drugs (NSAIDs) are often effective without the addition of opioids. Patients can become opioid dependent even after minor surgery where medications are unnecessarily prescribed, so their prescription is discouraged. Indeed, development of postsurgical opioid dependency would be considered a surgical complication.[1-5] According to a systematic review in 2015, acetaminophen efficacy is similar whether IV or oral delivery is undertaken in spite of the increased bioavailability of the former. Therefore, in patients who are able to take oral medication, acetaminophen should be preferentially prescribed orally.[6]

REFERENCES

1. Cozowicz C, Olson A, Poeran J, et al. Opioid prescription levels and postoperative outcomes in orthopedic surgery. Pain 2017;158(12):2422–2430
2. Funk RD, Hilliard P, Ramachandran SK. Perioperative opioid usage: avoiding adverse effects. Plast Reconstr Surg 2014;134(4, Suppl 2):32S–39S
3. Brummett CM, Waljee JF, Goesling J, et al. New persistent opioid use after minor and major surgical procedures in US adults. JAMA Surg 2017;152(6):e170504
4. Clarke H, Soneji N, Ko DT, Yun L, Wijeysundera DN. Rates and risk factors for prolonged opioid use after major surgery: population based cohort study. BMJ 2014;348:g1251
5. Johnson SP, Chung KC, Zhong L, et al. Risk of prolonged opioid use among opioid-naïve patients following common hand surgery procedures. J Hand Surg Am 2016;41(10):947–957.e3
6. Jibril F, Sharaby S, Mohamed A, Wilby KJ. Intravenous versus oral acetaminophen for pain: systematic review of current evidence to support clinical decision-making. Can J Hosp Pharm 2015;68(3):238–247

CONSEQUENCES OF OVERTREATING OF POSTSURGICAL PAIN

3. Which one of the following would be associated with overtreatment rather than undertreatment of postsurgical pain with opiates?

C. Respiratory depression

Respiratory depression is a significant risk for patients who have been given an excess of opioids. In the extreme they can lose consciousness and control of their airway. On the other hand, anxiety and depression, poor wound healing, myocardial ischemia and infarction, and chronic persistent surgical pain are sequelae each associated with failure to adequately manage pain postoperatively. Other potential problems of excess opioid use include impaired pulmonary function, ileus, and failure to progress. These can collectively lead to an increased hospital stay, and readmission to hospital.[1-3]

REFERENCES

1. Cozowicz C, Olson A, Poeran J, et al. Opioid prescription levels and postoperative outcomes in orthopedic surgery. Pain 2017;158(12):2422–2430
2. Funk RD, Hilliard P, Ramachandran SK. Perioperative opioid usage: avoiding adverse effects. Plast Reconstr Surg 2014;134(4, Suppl 2):32S–39S
3. Lee CW, Muo CH, Liang JA, Sung FC, Kao CH, Yeh JJ. Pulmonary embolism is associated with current morphine treatment in patients with deep vein thrombosis. Clin Respir J 2015;9(2):233–237

PERSISTENT OPIOID USE

4. *What does the term "new persistent use of opioid medications" mean?*

D. That previously opioid naïve patients will continue to use opioids 90 days post surgery.

The term *"new persistent use of opioid medications"* means that previously opioid naïve patients undergoing surgery who are prescribed opioids postoperatively will continue to use them for more than 90 days post surgery. For the vast majority of surgical procedures performed in plastic surgery, this would not be justified. Furthermore, this would be considered an avoidable postsurgical complication. As prescribers, it is the surgeon's responsibility to minimize opioid prescription and instead provide alternative solutions such as long-acting local and regional nerve blocks, in combination with appropriate splints or dressings, followed by multimodal therapy with nonopioid medications.[1,2] Surgeons are responsible for around 10% of total opioid prescriptions in the US so it has a significant impact on their use and may play a role in propagating the current addiction crisis.[3]

REFERENCES

1. Brummett CM, Waljee JF, Goesling J, et al. New persistent opioid use after minor and major surgical procedures in US adults. JAMA Surg 2017;152(6):e170504
2. Clarke H, Soneji N, Ko DT, Yun L, Wijeysundera DN. Rates and risk factors for prolonged opioid use after major surgery: population based cohort study. BMJ 2014;348:g1251
3. Levy B, Paulozzi L, Mack KA, Jones CM. Trends in opioid analgesic-prescribing rates by specialty, U.S., 2007–2012. Am J Prev Med 2015;49(3):409–413

RISK FACTORS FOR OPIOID USE

5. *When taking history from patients planned for surgery, which one of the following represents the greatest increased risk of their developing reliance on opioids post surgery?*

B. History of alcohol dependency

It is important to consider risk factors for patients undergoing surgery of developing reliance on analgesia following treatment. There are a number of predictable risk factors for patients developing reliance on opioids. These include a history of previous substance abuse including alcohol, prescription and nonprescription medications as well as smoking. Other risk factors include male sex (not female), low socioeconomic status (not high), and previous psychiatric comorbidities. Patients who already have established substance abuse disorders should ideally have surgery postponed until these have been resolved, unless it is a surgical emergency or really cannot be safely avoided.[1,2]

REFERENCES

1. Sun EC, Darnall BD, Baker LC, Mackey S. Incidence of and risk factors for chronic opioid use among opioid-naive patients in the postoperative period. JAMA Intern Med 2016;176(9):1286–1293
2. Zhao S, Chen F, Feng A, Han W, Zhang Y. Risk factors and prevention strategies for postoperative opioid abuse. Pain Res Manag 2019;2019:7490801

PERSISTENT OPIATE USE

6. *What percentage of opiate naive patients continue to use opioids beyond 90 days following surgery?*

C. 5–13%

There is currently an epidemic crisis in the US of addiction and excessive use of opioid medications. Current figures suggest that between 5 and 13% of previously opioid naïve patients continue to use opioids 90 days after both major and minor surgery including 13% for hand surgery patients. This high figure highlights the importance of minimizing opioid prescription across all types of surgery.[1-3] In the setting of hand surgery it is especially important to avoid such high rates of unnecessary opiate use as they should not normally be required except in more complex injuries. Given the high number of hand injuries, which occur each year inappropriate prescription can have a dramatic lasting effect. This can be managed preemptively by ensuring there is early access to physiotherapy, that splintage and immobilization are not unduly excessive in duration, and that early active and passive mobilization are both enhanced as soon as possible. Desensitization exercises can be taught to patients by therapists and surgeons to help them return to normal function. Where there may be early signs of chronic regional pain syndrome (CRPS) this should be targeted early with appropriate multimodal interventions.[4]

REFERENCES

1. Johnson SP, Chung KC, Zhong L, et al. Risk of prolonged opioid use among opioid-naïve patients following common hand surgery procedures. J Hand Surg Am 2016;41(10):947–957.e3
2. Brummett CM, Waljee JF, Goesling J, et al. New persistent opioid use after minor and major surgical procedures in US adults. JAMA Surg 2017;152(6):e170504
3. Clarke H, Soneji N, Ko DT, Yun L, Wijeysundera DN. Rates and risk factors for prolonged opioid use after major surgery: population based cohort study. BMJ 2014;348:g1251
4. Winston P. Early treatment of acute complex regional pain syndrome after fracture or injury with prednisone: why is there a failure to treat? A case series. Pain Res Manag 2016;2016:7019196

OPIATE WASTAGE

7. What percentage of opiates are thought to be over-prescribed following surgery?

   E. >40%

   Opioid wastage through over-prescription can be either where the medication is simply not used by anyone and ends up in cupboards stored for longer term or flushed down the toilet, or misused by individuals for whom it was never prescribed. Diversion is the term used for the transfer of prescription medications from their intended use to an illicit alternative. Doctors and patients can both help to minimize waste through education and common sense. Reducing prescriptions and exchanging opioid medications for less addictive but effective alternatives is the first step in this process. The second step is patient education to ensure that unused medications are returned or safely disposed of.[1]

REFERENCE

1. Bicket MC, Long JJ, Pronovost PJ, Alexander GC, Wu CL. Prescription opioid analgesics commonly unused after surgery: a systematic review. JAMA Surg 2017;152(11):1066–1071

OPIATE PRESCRIPTION AND STORAGE

8. When considering what happens to opioid medications following their prescription in the surgical setting, which one of the following is true?

   C. Friends and family are key sources of the supply of illicit opioids.

   Most people with prescription opioid abuse disorder get their medications from friends and family and this is termed diversion. Diversion broadly means that the "wrong" or unintended person receives the prescribed medication. Diversion does not mean that money has changed hands in the exchange. Unfortunately, a vast majority of medications are not safely stored. Figures suggest that up to 90% of medications are not safely stored in a locked location.[1,2]

   Most patients are not educated on proper storage or disposal of medications, which will also contribute to diversion. Unused medications should either be taken back to the pharmacy or flushed down the toilet based on FDA guidance for each individual medication. Surgeons' contribution to opioid prescription is estimated to be at least 10% (not just 1%).[3]

REFERENCES

1. Bartels K, Mayes LM, Dingmann C, Bullard KJ, Hopfer CJ, Binswanger IA. Opioid use and storage patterns by patients after hospital discharge following surgery. PLoS One 2016;11(1):e0147972
2. Bicket MC, Long JJ, Pronovost PJ, Alexander GC, Wu CL. Prescription opioid analgesics commonly unused after surgery: a systematic review. JAMA Surg 2017;152(11):1066–1071
3. Levy B, Paulozzi L, Mack KA, Jones CM. Trends in opioid analgesic-prescribing rates by specialty, U.S., 2007–2012. Am J Prev Med 2015;49(3):409–413

ENHANCED RECOVERY PATHWAYS

9. *What is the primary emphasis on an enhanced recovery after surgery protocol?*

    A. To decrease recovery time

The main aim of the enhanced recovery program is to decrease patient recovery time after surgery. There has been much support for this in recent years as there are many knock-on effects of successfully reducing recovery times. First, there are financial benefits. These include shorter hospital stay and quicker time to full function and working life or social independence where appropriate. If recovery is enhanced, there may be a secondary benefit on overall better outcomes, reduced complications, and better pain control. Taking further steps, there has been emphasis on preoperative conditioning of patients such that they enter their surgical pathway in the best shape they can. Factors include optimization of cardiovascular performance, BMI, smoking cessation, and blood glucose control. Sometimes this process is termed "prehabilitation," i.e., preoperative rehabilitation. Things we can alter to enhance recovery include early ambulation, improved pain control, and early access to diet and fluids.[1–3]

REFERENCES

1. Soteropolos CE, Tang SYQ, Poore SO. Enhanced recovery after surgery in breast reconstruction: a systematic review. J Reconstr Microsurg 2019;35(9):695–704
2. Ljungqvist O, Scott M, Fearon KC. Enhanced recovery after surgery: a review. JAMA Surg 2017;152(3):292–298
3. Parks L, Routt M, De Villiers A. Enhanced recovery after surgery. J Adv Pract Oncol 2018;9(5):511–519

ENHANCED RECOVERY IN BREAST SURGERY

10. *When considering the enhanced recovery after surgery (ERAS) protocol for breast reconstruction, which of the following is correct before surgery?*

    D. Carbohydrate loading with maltodextrin drinks 2 hours before surgery is advocated.

There is a recognized ERAS protocol for breast reconstruction patients. There are three phases to the protocol advice: preoperative factors, intraoperative factors, and postoperative factors.

The main preoperative factors include carbohydrate loading 2 hours before surgery, smoking cessation 1 month before surgery, a target BMI of <30 kg/m^2, adequate hydration with clear fluids up to 2 hours before surgery, and venous thromboembolism (VTE) prophylaxis according to risk stratification. This may involve chemoprophylaxis and/or compression stockings.[1,2]

REFERENCES

1. Soteropolos CE, Tang SYQ, Poore SO. Enhanced recovery after surgery in breast reconstruction: a systematic review. J Reconstr Microsurg 2019;35(9):695–704
2. Temple-Oberle C, Shea-Budgell MA, Tan M, et al; ERAS Society. Consensus review of optimal perioperative care in breast reconstruction: Enhanced Recovery after Surgery (ERAS) Society recommendations. Plast Reconstr Surg 2017;139(5):1056e–1071e

ENHANCED RECOVERY IN BREAST RECONSTRUCTION

11. *When considering the enhanced recovery after surgery (ERAS) protocol for breast reconstruction, which of the following is correct during surgery?*

    C. A preference is given to IV based anesthesia.

There is a recognized ERAS protocol for breast reconstruction patients. There are three phases to the protocol advice: preoperative factors, intraoperative factors, and postoperative factors. Within the intraoperative phase, a preference is given to total IV anesthesia where possible as this has many perceived advantages over inhalational anesthesia.

Surgical site infection is minimized by using chlorhexidine skin preparation in alcohol base, IV antibiotics are given 30–60 minutes before surgery not at induction, maintenance of core body temperature should be at least 36° C (not 37° C), and use of vasopressors as required even in the setting of free tissue transfer.[1,2]

REFERENCES

1. Soteropolos CE, Tang SYQ, Poore SO. Enhanced recovery after surgery in breast reconstruction: a systematic review. J Reconstr Microsurg 2019;35(9):695–704
2. Temple-Oberle C, Shea-Budgell MA, Tan M, et al; ERAS Society. Consensus review of optimal perioperative care in breast reconstruction: Enhanced Recovery after Surgery (ERAS) Society recommendations. Plast Reconstr Surg 2017;139(5):1056e–1071e

ENHANCED RECOVERY IN BREAST RECONSTRUCTION

12. *When considering the enhanced recovery after surgery (ERAS) protocol for breast reconstruction, which of the following is correct following surgery?*

    A. Use a carefully selected and individualized multimodal analgesic regimen.

       There is a recognized ERAS protocol for breast reconstruction patients. There are three phases to the protocol advice: preoperative factors, intraoperative factors, and postoperative factors. Postoperatively it is vital to ensure adequate pain relief to optimize rehabilitation and minimize adverse effects of uncontrolled pain such as myocardial ischemia, venous thromboembolism, anxiety, and depression. Therefore, a multimodal approach to pain relief is advocated. Other factors that need consideration include early diet and fluids, early mobilization, and supportive physiotherapy programs prior to and beyond hospital discharge.[1,2]

REFERENCES

1. Soteropulos CE, Tang SYQ, Poore SO. Enhanced recovery after surgery in breast reconstruction: a systematic review. J Reconstr Microsurg 2019;35(9):695–704
2. Temple-Oberle C, Shea-Budgell MA, Tan M, et al; ERAS Society. Consensus review of optimal perioperative care in breast reconstruction: Enhanced Recovery after Surgery (ERAS) Society recommendations. Plast Reconstr Surg 2017;139(5):1056e–1071e

MULTIMODAL ANALGESIA (MMA)

13. *Which one of the following medications targets the N-methyl-D-aspartate (NMDA) receptor and is used as part of a multimodality pain management approach?*

    D. Ketamine

       Ketamine is an example of an N-methyl-D-aspartate (NMDA) receptor antagonist that can be a useful component of multimodal analgesic therapy. The NMDA receptor is activated in response to intense and sustained painful stimuli so is implicated in both acute and chronic pain. Ketamine uniquely preserves respiratory drive and hemodynamic stability under anesthesia and is often used as an anesthetic adjunct in a multimodal pain management approach because it reduces opioid requirements and enhances analgesia. It is limited by its potential neuropsychiatric side effects, which include dysphoria, hallucinations, vivid unpleasant dreams, catatonia, or psychoses. Furthermore, it can have addictive qualities and is involved in substance misuse.

       Nonsteroidal anti-inflammatory medications such as naproxen and ibuprofen play an important role in multimodal pain therapy. They inhibit cyclooxygenase enzymes, either COX-2 selectively or both COX-1 and COX-2 nonselectively, which in turn inhibits the synthesis of prostaglandins and thromboxanes. Not only do they have analgesic qualities, but also have antipyretic and anti-inflammatory qualities as well. Unfortunately, they can cause gastrointestinal irritation and bleeding. They are contraindicated in patients with a history of coronary artery disease (CAD) or renal failure and may be contraindicated in asthmatics. Celecoxib is an example of a COX-2-specific inhibitor. It is better tolerated in terms of gastrointestinal side effects than nonselective nonsteroidal anti-inflammatory drugs (NSAIDs), but still should be avoided in patients with a history of CAD or renal failure.

       Acetaminophen is a very useful medication that has both analgesic and antipyretic qualities. The specific mechanism of action is unknown though it is thought it may also function as a COX inhibitor. It is contraindicated in patients with liver disease and those who have excessive alcohol intake. Both oral and intravenous preparations are available and efficacy is similar between the two in patients able to take their medications orally. Intravenous acetaminophen can be helpful in the anesthetized patient and in the recovery room.

       Gabapentin and its derivative pregabalin are examples of alpha-2-agonists. They bind to calcium channels causing the release of glutamate, norepinephrine, and substance P. These activate pathways in the dorsal horn that regulate pain. They can be very helpful in managing nerve pain but have side effects of somnolence and dizziness. They are contraindicated in patients on continuous positive airway pressure (CPAP) therapy as they can exacerbate obstructive sleep apnea. They should be used with caution in elderly patients.

       Multimodal analgesia (MMA) with a selective COX-2 inhibitor and gabapentin decreases postanesthesia care opioid use and pain scores in outpatient breast plastic surgery by 40%.[1] Nonopioid regimens with a selective COX-2 inhibitor and gabapentin decrease rescue opioid, rescue anti-emetic, and postanesthesia care unit (PACU) length-of-stay in aesthetic surgery.[2] The addition of a COX-2 inhibitor decreases pain scores, decreases opioid consumption, expedites return of bowel function and activities of daily living, and improves patient satisfaction in core plastic surgery procedures.[3]

REFERENCES

1. Barker JC, DiBartola K, Wee C, et al. Preoperative multimodal analgesia decreases postanesthesia care unit narcotic use and pain scores in outpatient breast surgery. Plast Reconstr Surg 2018;142(4):443e–450e
2. Nguyen TC, Lombana NF, Zavlin D, Moliver CL. Transition to nonopioid analgesia does not impair pain control after major aesthetic plastic surgery. Aesthet Surg J 2018;38(10):1139–1144
3. Sun T, Sacan O, White PF, Coleman J, Rohrich RJ, Kenkel JM. Perioperative versus postoperative celecoxib on patient outcomes after major plastic surgery procedures. Anesth Analg 2008;106(3):950–958

14. Photography for the Plastic Surgeon

See *Essentials of Plastic Surgery*, third edition, pp. 170–193

BENEFITS OF PHOTOGRAPHY IN PLASTIC SURGERY

1. *Which function of clinical photographs is probably the most useful from a patient's perspective?*
   A. Medicolegal protection
   B. Education and research
   C. Measurement of outcomes and enhanced communication
   D. Marketing
   E. Optimization of clinical care

THE CLINICAL PHOTOGRAPHY PROCESS

2. *When performing clinical photography, which one of the following is the most important aspect of the setup to ensure consistency and reproducibility?*
   A. To use a straight on flash
   B. To use a digital camera device
   C. To use a standardized series
   D. To use a wide-angle lens
   E. To use a 35-mm camera

STANDARDIZED PHOTOGRAPHY

3. *When taking photographs of patients before and after surgery, which one of the following is correct?*
   A. Digital zoom gives superior image quality to optical zoom.
   B. A change in background can be corrected for by white balancing the camera.
   C. Saving the image as a JPEG file preserves image quality better than TIFF format.
   D. A straight on flash angle is best for facial views.
   E. The same focal length should be used for comparative images.

PHOTOGRAPHIC TERMINOLOGY

4. *When using photographic terminology, which one of the following is described by the term "focal range"?*
   A. Aperture
   B. Depth of field
   C. Shutter speed
   D. Focal length
   E. Lens type

DIGITAL PHOTOGRAPHY TERMINOLOGY

5. *Which one of the following is true regarding image resolution in clinical images?*
   A. Resolution is specifically measured by the total number of pixels present.
   B. Required resolution is consistent across planned image uses.
   C. Increasing resolution will consistently improve the quality of clinical images.
   D. Retina display devices have a lower requirement for resolution than regular devices.
   E. Required resolution needs to be matched to the planned output type.

DIGITAL PHOTOGRAPHY TERMINOLOGY

6. *When setting up a PowerPoint presentation on cosmetic surgery, what is the suggested resolution for clinical images?*
   A. 72 pixels per square inch (PPI)
   B. 96 PPI
   C. 150 PPI
   D. 300 PPI
   E. 450 PPI

STANDARDIZED FACE AND NECK VIEWS

7. *When taking photographs before a face lift, which one of the following statements is correct?*
   A. The full series of images are normally taken as close-ups.
   B. The Frankfort plane provides the most accurate image of the submental tissue.
   C. A true lateral image can be ensured by viewing across the oral commissures.
   D. The lateral and oblique views are best obtained with the neck in extension.
   E. It is important to include worm's-eye (basal) and bird's-eye (cephalic) views.

CLINICAL PHOTOGRAPHY OF THE LIPS

8. *When photographing lips prior to injecting nonpermanent fillers, how should the lips be placed for the majority of the series?*
   A. Gently pressed together
   B. Smiling gently
   C. Pouting gently
   D. Parted and relaxed
   E. Firmly pressed together

CLINICAL IMAGING FOR SKIN RESURFACING

9. *Which one of the following is a specific difference between photographing a standard facial series and that which is required when undertaking laser resurfacing or chemical peels?*
   A. The removal of makeup
   B. The removal of jewelry
   C. The subject distance from camera
   D. The orientation of the images
   E. The level of facial animation

STANDARD PHOTOGRAPHIC RHINOPLASTY VIEWS

10. *When taking preoperative images for a patient seeking a rhinoplasty, which one of the following might conceal an underlying dynamic problem?*
    A. Taking a standardized oblique view
    B. Keeping the patient's face relaxed throughout
    C. Aligning the nasal tip with the eyebrows in full basal view
    D. Using a cephalic view to record deviation
    E. Taking close-ups in a landscape (horizontal) format

STANDARD PHOTOGRAPHIC BODY VIEWS

11. *Which one of the following statements is correct when taking photographs of the trunk before an abdominoplasty?*
    A. Patients should stand with their feet together.
    B. Patients should raise their arms above the head.
    C. Patients should wear their own choice of underwear.
    D. The camera should be level with the xiphisternum.
    E. The diver's view should be taken in the oblique plane.

STANDARD BREAST SERIES

12. *When performing a standard breast series prior to augmentation, which one of the following is true?*
    A. The patient's hands should be placed on the hips throughout.
    B. The photographs should be taken vertically in portrait view.
    C. The camera should be positioned vertically at the level of the clavicle.
    D. Both shoulders and navel should be included within the image.
    E. Lateral views with the arms elevated above the head are required.

STORAGE OF PATIENT'S PHOTOGRAPHIC DATA

13. *When storing photographic images of patients, which one of the following is advised?*
    A. The images should be stored on memory cards.
    B. The images should be stored in alphabetical order based on patient's surname.
    C. The images should be stored with encryption software and password protection.
    D. The images can be safely reviewed in public places using a screen guard.
    E. The image metadata should be left on all images to increase security.

PHOTOGRAPHIC CONSENT

14. *Which one of the following statements is correct regarding patient consent for photographs according to the Health Insurance Portability and Accountability Act (HIPAA)?*

   A. Key elements of protected health information are limited to name, date of birth, place of birth, home address, and social security number.

   B. The requirements for consent to photography are consistent for both treatment and nontreatment purposes.

   C. Written patient consent for the treatment photographs will cover their use in educational settings for other medical practitioners to view.

   D. It is considered that satisfactory anonymity on facial views is achieved by blacking out the eyes.

   E. Best practice should be to obtain formal consent from patients for any images taken although if for treatment purposes, this is not required by HIPAA.

Answers

BENEFITS OF PHOTOGRAPHY IN PLASTIC SURGERY

1. *Which function of clinical photographs is probably the most useful from a patient's perspective?*

C. Measurement of outcomes and enhanced communication

All of these options are useful reasons for photography before and after treatment in plastic surgery. The most useful function *from a patient's perspective* is probably to help measure outcomes and improve communication. For example, patients can be shown photographs of other patients to help them better understand likely outcomes, including scarring and cosmesis. They can also review their own preoperative and postoperative photographs with their surgeon to see positive and negative aspects of their outcome.

Clinical photography in plastic surgery is very important for education and research among clinicians. This should help to improve clinical care. Medicolegal protection may apply to both surgeon and patient. The use of patient photographs in marketing carries a high risk and is not advisable. Courts have imposed liability in cases in which the provider has exploited the patient for commercial benefit.[1-3]

REFERENCES

1. Grom RM. Clinical and operating room photography. Biomed Photogr 1992;20:251–301
2. Roos O, Cederblom S. A standardized system for patient documentation. J Audiov Media Med 1991;14(4):135–138
3. DiBernardo BE, Adams RL, Krause J, Fiorillo MA, Gheradini G. Photographic standards in plastic surgery. Plast Reconstr Surg 1998;102(2):559–568

THE CLINICAL PHOTOGRAPHY PROCESS

2. *When performing clinical photography, which one of the following is the most important aspect of the setup to ensure consistency and reproducibility?*

C. To use a standardized series

Standardized approaches must be used when performing clinical photography to ensure accuracy, reproducibility, and consistency across all images taken for any given individual, such that they show a fair representation of the person at any given stage of his or her treatment. This facilitates a comparison of pre- and postoperative images to help assess progress and outcomes. Such an approach also means that images from different patients can be compared or contrasted when required, and that when images are used for education and research purposes, the audience are able to view them in the context of a standardized setting. Often, when patients take their own photos such as "selfies" or have their family members/friends do so, there is significant distortion, and this means reliable analysis and interpretation of the images is difficult.

The standardization process not only considers the precise views which typically include frontal, lateral, and oblique or quarter views for most body areas (as well as more specific views for any given procedure series), it also includes the method for obtaining the images. For example, the type of camera used, its placement in relation to the patient, the lighting, background, and specific camera factors such as lens type, magnification, and focal length and depth. Patient factors should also be standardized including clothing worn, makeup, and jewelry removal.

The use of a flash or standard lighting setup should be standardized across any given series, but the type of flash will depend on the camera type and setting. For example, a separate bounce flash with a swivel head is recommended for photographs of the face and body so as to allow the consistent lighting without harsh flattened effect of a straight on flash. Clinical photographs can be taken well with either traditional or digital cameras and there are pros and cons to each. Camera lenses are categorized as normal, wide angle, and telephoto. Lens selection will need to be adjusted to suit the series being undertaken and will most often be a normal lens.[1-3]

REFERENCES

1. Grom RM. Clinical and operating room photography. Biomed Photogr 1992;20:251–301
2. Roos O, Cederblom S. A standardized system for patient documentation. J Audiov Media Med 1991;14(4):135–138
3. DiBernardo BE, Adams RL, Krause J, Fiorillo MA, Gheradini G. Photographic standards in plastic surgery. Plast Reconstr Surg 1998;102(2):559–568

STANDARDIZED PHOTOGRAPHY

3. *When taking photographs of patients before and after surgery, which one of the following is correct?*

E. The same focal length should be used for comparative images.

It is important to use the same focal length for comparative images (e.g., before and after rhinoplasty). A change in focal length can have dramatic distorting effects (**Fig. 14.1**). This can be achieved by using the same lens on a camera with interchangeable lenses, or by fixing the focal distance on a single lens camera and physically moving the camera to achieve focus.

Optical zoom gives a superior image as digital zoom simply mimics a greater zoom without gaining image detail. A consistent background and white balancing should be used but one cannot compensate for errors in the other. Saving an image in JPEG format uses lossy compression (i.e., image data is reduced each time it is saved), whereas TIFF format preserves image data but can be less practical for file storage. A separate bounce flash angled 45 degrees upwards is recommended for consistent lighting and less flattening than a straight on flash in facial views.[1–3]

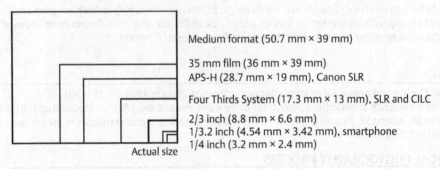

Medium format (50.7 mm × 39 mm)

35 mm film (36 mm × 39 mm)
APS-H (28.7 mm × 19 mm), Canon SLR

Four Thirds System (17.3 mm × 13 mm), SLR and CILC

2/3 inch (8.8 mm × 6.6 mm)
1/3.2 inch (4.54 mm × 3.42 mm), smartphone
1/4 inch (3.2 mm × 2.4 mm)

Actual size

Fig. 14.1 Comparison of digital camera sensor sizes, which affects quality of digital photographs.

REFERENCES

1. Grom RM. Clinical and operating room photography. Biomed Photogr 1992;20:251–301
2. Roos O, Cederblom S. A standardized system for patient documentation. J Audiov Media Med 1991;14(4):135–138
3. DiBernardo BE, Adams RL, Krause J, Fiorillo MA, Gheradini G. Photographic standards in plastic surgery. Plast Reconstr Surg 1998;102(2):559–568

PHOTOGRAPHIC TERMINOLOGY

4. *When using photographic terminology, which one of the following is described by the term "focal range"?*

B. Depth of field

Depth of field refers to the distance between the closest and farthest in-focus area of a photograph. It is also known as the focal range. The depth of field is affected by some of the other options described including aperture size and focal length. The aperture refers to the size of the adjustable opening (iris) of a camera lens. This determines the amount of light falling onto the film or sensor. The smaller the aperture, the greater the depth of field.

Shutter speed determines how long the iris of the camera is open to expose the film or sensor to light. In essence, it represents how long the camera spends taking a photo and therefore can affect both the brightness and crispness of a photo with shorter shutter speeds potentially freezing movement within an image and longer shutter speeds tending to emphasize or create an appearance of motion within an image. The focal length is the distance in millimeters from the optical center of the lens to the focal point, which is located on the sensor or film. The longer the length, the narrower the field of view. Lens types can be categorized as normal, wide angle, or telephoto according to focal length and film size. Normal lenses are most frequently used for clinical images.[1]

REFERENCE

1. Grom RM. Clinical and operating room photography. Biomed Photogr 1992;20:251–301

DIGITAL PHOTOGRAPHY TERMINOLOGY

5. *Which one of the following is true regarding image resolution in clinical images?*

E. Required resolution needs to be matched to the planned output type.

Resolution is a measurement of the pixel count of an image and is given either as pixels per square inch (PPI) or total number of pixels. The choice of resolution should be matched to the planned output type. It is, therefore, not consistent across all planned image uses. In general, a higher resolution is required for print uses compared with digital uses. Increasing resolution does not always improve image quality and can become excessively large with negative effects on software applications and file transfer times. Lower resolution, however, can lead to pixilation if the image is overly enlarged. High-resolution retina display devices require higher, not lower, resolution images than regular display devices.[1,2]

REFERENCES

1. Long B, ed. Complete Digital Photography. 7th ed. Boston: Course Technology; 2013
2. Young S. Maintaining standard scales of reproduction in patient photography using digital cameras. J Audiov Media Med 2001;24(4):162–165

DIGITAL PHOTOGRAPHY TERMINOLOGY

6. **When setting up a PowerPoint presentation on cosmetic surgery, what is the suggested resolution for clinical images?**
   C. **150 PPI**

   Resolution is a measurement of the pixel count of an image. When considering the resolution required for any given photograph, the planned output use for the image must be considered. There will be a balance to be met regarding resolution of the image in terms of quality and clarity versus image size and usability. Increased resolution is not always better and as resolution increases, so too does the image file size which can impact on file transfer times and storage.

   In general, it is recommended that lower resolution is used for digital images compared with those to be printed. The recommended resolution for a PowerPoint image is 150 PPI compared with 72–96 PPI for internet and email, and 300 PPI for print publications.[1,2]

REFERENCES

1. Sheridan P. Practical aspects of clinical photography: part 1—principles, equipment and technique. ANZ J Surg 2013;83(3):188–191
2. Long B, ed. Complete Digital Photography. 7th ed. Boston: Course Technology; 2013

STANDARDIZED FACE AND NECK VIEWS

7. **When taking photographs before a face lift, which one of the following statements is correct?**
   C. **A true lateral image can be ensured by viewing across the oral commissures.**

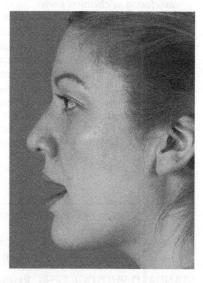

   A true lateral image can be ensured by viewing across the oral commissures (**Fig. 14.2**). This can be achieved by asking the patients to open their mouth to check alignment. It is important as under-rotation and over-rotation may markedly distort the appearance. Avoiding head tilt in the anterior view is also important and comparing the position of the earlobes can help with this. A face-lift series should include anterior, lateral, and oblique views. Images should be taken from both a distance and close-up to aid with scale, perspective, and proportion. The oblique view can either show the nasal tip touching the far cheek, or the nasal dorsum touching the medial canthus according to surgeon's preference. The Frankfort plane tends to exaggerate submental fullness compared to the natural horizontal facial plane. Therefore, this natural plane is generally preferred for face and neck images. To exaggerate the submental tissues, a reading view is used, which flexes the neck. Having the head held in extension will improve the appearance of the neck contour and must be avoided. Additional views with the teeth gritted will demonstrate platysmal banding (see **Fig. 14.9**, *A* and *B*, *Essentials of Plastic Surgery*, third edition). Bird's-eye and worm's-eye views are more typical of a rhinoplasty or midface/facial fracture series (see **Fig. 14.13**, *Essentials of Plastic Surgery*, third edition).[1–3]

Fig. 14.2   A true lateral image may be obtained by viewing straight across the two oral commissures to verify correct rotation.

REFERENCES

1. Grom RM. Clinical and operating room photography. Biomed Photogr 1992;20:251–301
2. Thomas JR, Tardy ME Jr, Przekop H. Uniform photographic documentation in facial plastic surgery. Otolaryngol Clin North Am 1980;13(2):367–381
3. Sommer DD, Mendelsohn M. Pitfalls of nonstandardized photography in facial plastic surgery patients. Plast Reconstr Surg 2004;114(1):10–14

CLINICAL PHOTOGRAPHY OF THE LIPS

8. *When photographing lips prior to injecting nonpermanent fillers, how should the lips be placed for the majority of the series?*

D. Parted and relaxed

The use of lip filler with hyaluronic acid has become very popular during the past decade both in the aging lip to restore volume and also in the youthful lip to augment the natural lip fullness. In this setting it is very important to have consistent images before and after treatment. The standardized lip series includes seven images, six of which will be taken with the lips slightly parted and relaxed. A seventh image is taken in the frontal view when smiling. The series includes close-ups in frontal, lateral, and oblique views. It is important to remove lipstick and liners for the images and treatment, and when photographing the oblique view, the inferior philtral column should intersect the cheek on the opposite side (**Fig. 14.3**).[1–3]

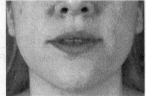

Fig. 14.3 Close-ups of the lips are photographed at 0.6 m with a 105 mm lens, whereas the full face is photographed at 1 m.

REFERENCES

1. Sommer DD, Mendelsohn M. Pitfalls of nonstandardized photography in facial plastic surgery patients. Plast Reconstr Surg 2004;114(1):10–14
2. Galdino GM, DaSilva And D, Gunter JP. Digital photography for rhinoplasty. Plast Reconstr Surg 2002;109(4):1421–1434
3. Davidson TM. Photography in facial plastic and reconstructive surgery. J Biol Photogr Assoc 1979;47(2):59–67

CLINICAL IMAGING FOR SKIN RESURFACING

9. *Which one of the following is a specific difference between photographing a standard facial series and that which is required when undertaking laser resurfacing or chemical peels?*

C. The subject distance from camera

When taking images for the purpose of skin resurfacing, additional views are required to try and capture the close-up appearance of the skin quality and texture. In a standard facial series, the camera is placed at 1 m with a 105-mm lens. In contrast, when performing a resurfacing series, a close-up at 0.6 m is required of the oblique cheek and also lateral photographs taken further back at 0.8 m. These are intended to show tonal changes in the skin if any from cheek to jaw (**Fig. 14.4**). The other elements are consistent across both series such as makeup and jewelry removal, image orientation (vertical) and the absence of facial animation.[1,2]

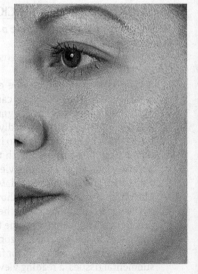

Fig. 14.4 Laser/chemical peel series. These photographs are taken in addition to the standard face/neck lift series. Close-ups are photographed at 0.6 and 0.8 m with a 105-mm lens.

REFERENCES

1. Long B, ed. Complete Digital Photography. 7th ed. Boston: Course Technology; 2013
2. Thomas JR, Tardy ME Jr, Przekop H. Uniform photographic documentation in facial plastic surgery. Otolaryngol Clin North Am 1980;13(2):367–381

STANDARD PHOTOGRAPHIC RHINOPLASTY VIEWS

10. *When taking preoperative images for a patient seeking a rhinoplasty, which one of the following might conceal an underlying dynamic problem?*

B. Keeping the patient's face relaxed throughout

The rhinoplasty series is difficult and often needs minor adjustment.
Keeping the patient's face relaxed throughout may misrepresent preoperative problems when release of depressor septi is required. To demonstrate this, additional anterior and lateral views are required with the patient smiling.

The oblique view may either have the nasal tip touching the cheek or the dorsum touching the medial canthus (see **Fig. 14.5**, *Essentials of Plastic Surgery*, third edition). Also see **Figs. 14.13–14.15**, *Essentials of Plastic Surgery*, third edition for additional rhinoplasty views and note that while the full-face views are portrait (see **Fig. 14.8**, *Essentials of Plastic Surgery*, third edition) close-up images are better taken as landscape (horizontal) views.[1]

REFERENCE

1. Galdino GM, DaSilva And D, Gunter JP. Digital photography for rhinoplasty. Plast Reconstr Surg 2002;109(4):1421–1434

STANDARD PHOTOGRAPHIC BODY VIEWS

11. *Which one of the following statements is correct when taking photographs of the trunk before an abdominoplasty?*

   E. The diver's view should be taken in the oblique plane.

   The diver's view is taken in the oblique plane and demonstrates abdominal skin laxity by asking the patient to lean forward with the abdomen relaxed (**Fig. 14.5**). The standard body series is described in Box 14.6 and Figs. 14.16 and 14.17, *Essentials of Plastic Surgery*, third edition, and should include the patient standing with the feet parallel at hip width. The patient should wear standardized undergarments, the camera should be at level with the umbilicus and the patient's arms should be no higher than breast level.[1–3]

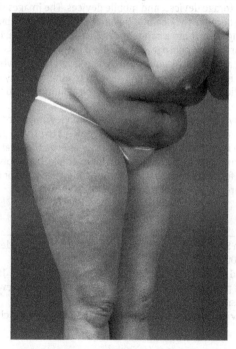

Fig. 14.5   The diver's view is an oblique view with the patient folded over while relaxing the abdomen.

REFERENCES

1. Sheridan P. Practical aspects of clinical photography: part 1—principles, equipment and technique. ANZ J Surg 2013;83(3):188–191
2. Gherardini G, Matarasso A, Serure AS, Toledo LS, DiBernardo BE. Standardization in photography for body contour surgery and suction-assisted lipectomy. Plast Reconstr Surg 1997;100(1):227–237
3. DiBernardo BE, Adams RL, Krause J, Fiorillo MA, Gheradini G. Photographic standards in plastic surgery. Plast Reconstr Surg 1998;102(2):559–568

STANDARD BREAST SERIES

12. *When performing a standard breast series prior to augmentation, which one of the following is true?*

   D. Both shoulders and navel should be included within the image.

   When performing the standard breast series, both shoulders and navel should be included in the views to achieve reference and proportion. The images should be taken horizontally (landscape) with a 50-mm lens at a distance of 1 m. The camera should be at level with the areolae rather than the clavicle. Patients should have their hands placed by their side with shoulders relaxed for the majority of the images. These will include frontal, oblique, and lateral views. In addition, a frontal image with hands on hips to show pectoralis major activation is also included. When performing reductions, mastopexies, and reconstructions, the arms may be positioned behind the body and when performing latissimus dorsi reconstruction, the back should also be imaged and a lateral view taken with arms above the head.[1]

REFERENCE

1. DiBernardo BE, Adams RL, Krause J, Fiorillo MA, Gheradini G. Photographic standards in plastic surgery. Plast Reconstr Surg 1998;102(2):559–568

STORAGE OF PATIENT'S PHOTOGRAPHIC DATA

13. *When storing photographic images of patients, which one of the following is advised?*
    C. The images should be stored with encryption software and password protection.
        When storing patient data in the form of clinical photographs, it is important to use both encryption software and password protection in order to prevent unauthorized access in the event of theft or loss. This includes desktop and laptop computers, external storage devices, and mobile devices. The images should not be saved on memory cards for any extended duration because they cannot be encrypted. It is advisable to transfer the images from a memory card, shortly after taking them, onto a computer with a backup system. It is also advisable to destroy or erase any memory cards used for patient photographs when no longer in use.
        It is advisable to avoid adding any patient information to the saved images when storing them and ideally an alternative method such as saving by date taken can be helpful to eliminate any patient information. Of course, facial images will remain identifiable even without name, hospital number, or date of birth being listed, but the patient details should still not be saved within the file.
        The use of a screen guard may be helpful to avoid unintended viewing of images. However, patient images should not be reviewed in public settings. Their review should be kept to private places such as the office or clinic.
        It is better to remove metadata from photographs in most cases as even the location taken for the image may not be desired, and beware as such metadata can often be seen, for example, by simply "mousing over" digital images on the computer or web if used for that purpose. When taking photographs for patients they should complete written consent to include the precise usage for and storage of their images.[1-4]

REFERENCES

1. US Department of Health and Human Services. Standards for privacy of individually identifiable health information (45 CFR parts 160 and 164). Fed Regist 2000:65
2. Roach WH Jr, ed. Medical Records and the Law. Gaithersburg, MD: Aspen Publishers; 1994
3. Reisman N. Scrub your commercial photographs for metadata. Plastic Surgery News, American Society of Plastic Surgeons, 2012. Available at http://psnextra.org/Columns/OLG-June-12.html
4. Ong CT, Yap JF, Wai YZ, Ng QX. A review of oculoplastic photography: a guide for clinician photographers. Cureus 2016;8(8):e733

PHOTOGRAPHIC CONSENT

14. *Which one of the following statements is correct regarding patient consent for photographs according to the Health Insurance Portability and Accountability Act (HIPAA)?*
    E. Best practice should be to obtain formal consent from patients for any images taken although if for treatment purposes, this is not required by HIPAA.
        The U.S. Department of Health and Human Services has published standards to protect the privacy of patients' identifiable health information. This comprises many elements, ranging from telephone number and IP address to credit card number and fingerprints or voiceprints. The standards are documented as the Health Insurance Portability and Accountability Act (HIPAA).[1] According to these guidelines, patient's authorization is not always required for photographs to be taken. However, best practice should be to always obtain written consent for images and have the agreement for use clearly documented. From a HIPAA perspective, the purpose of obtaining photographs is categorized into two groups, namely, treatment or nontreatment, and the need for consent differs between the two groups. Nontreatment purposes include education, research, or patient education. Treatment purposes do not technically require patient authorization; however, nontreatment purposes do. According to HIPAA, a situation in which all identifiable information is removed from the photograph is an exception. It is important to recognize that all identifiable information cannot be removed from a face, and merely blacking out the eyes is not acceptable. Facial views therefore will always require formal consent specific to the required

use. A safe approach to patient images is to obtain written consent and then to store images safely without any patient identifying information and ideally offline on a secure device. Care should be taken when taking and processing images to ensure that identifying features such as named jewelry and tattoos are hidden if possible. Unfortunately, because it is not really possible to anonymize full facial images, patients must accept the risk that if viewed, then this will identify them.[1-4]

REFERENCES

1. US Department of Health and Human Services. Standards for privacy of individually identifiable health information (45 CFR parts 160 and 164). Fed Regist 2000:65
2. https://www.hhs.gov/hipaa/index.html
3. Roach WH Jr, ed. Medical Records and the Law. Gaithersburg, MD: Aspen Publishers; 1994
4. Reisman N. Scrub your commercial photographs for metadata. Plastic Surgery News, American Society of Plastic Surgeons; 2012

15. Decreasing Complications in Plastic Surgery

See *Essentials of Plastic Surgery*, third edition, pp. 194–211

REDUCING COMPLICATIONS AND OPTIMIZING OUTCOMES

1. *When preparing a patient for elective plastic surgery, which one of the following is true with regard to minimizing complications and optimizing outcomes?*
   A. Meticulous preoperative surgical planning will reliably eliminate postoperative complications.
   B. Postoperative wound healing problems will be minimized where blood glucose levels are between 200 and 300 g/dL preoperatively.
   C. Preoperative hematologic consultation is advisable for the majority of elective plastic surgery patients to minimize venous thromboembolism risk.
   D. Even for low-risk ambulatory plastic surgery patients, preoperative laboratory tests are highly recommended to reduce postsurgical complications.
   E. Optimizing patient outcomes in terms of satisfaction begins at the time of consultation and continues well into the postoperative period.

MANAGEMENT OF SMOKING IN ELECTIVE PLASTIC SURGERY

2. *When planning elective plastic surgery in a long-term smoker, which one of the following is true?*
   A. Permanent smoking cessation would be mandated prior to undergoing surgery.
   B. Only pharmacologic smoking cessation therapies are likely to be helpful.
   C. No reliable biomarker tests currently exist to assess compliance with smoking cessation.
   D. A 4-week period of cessation before and after surgery is advised when proceeding with surgery.
   E. The perceived negative effects of tobacco smoking on healing have most likely been overstated.

DECOLONIZATION AND SKIN ANTISEPSIS

3. *In a patient undergoing elective abdominoplasty who has previously been found to be methicillin-resistant S. aureus (MRSA) positive, which one of the following is recommended?*
   A. Groin swabs should be taken 1 week prior to the planned date of surgery.
   B. Vancomycin should be given intravenously 15 minutes before surgery.
   C. Hibiclens scrub should be used as a shower gel for a 4-week period before surgery.
   D. Mupirocin ointment applied to the bilateral nares twice daily for 5 days preop is recommended.
   E. Cefazolin should be prescribed orally for 5 days post surgery.

PERIOPERATIVE VENOUS THROMBOEMBOLISM (VTE) RISK MANAGEMENT

4. *When considering prevention of venous thromboembolism (VTE) in a patient undergoing autologous breast reconstruction surgery, which one of the following is true?*
   A. A score of 8 or more using the Caprini risk assessment model indicates postoperative chemoprophylaxis should be considered.
   B. Administration of low dose prophylactic enoxaparin is likely to increase the risk of a postoperative hematoma.
   C. Compression stockings, intermittent calf compression devices, and venous foot pumps should be combined intraoperatively.
   D. VTE risk is increased by the use of intravenous anesthesia techniques.
   E. Early ambulation during the first 48 hours must be restricted in this setting.

INTRAOPERATIVE MEASURES TO REDUCE COMPLICATIONS

5. *When performing the World Health Organization (WHO) surgical checklist, which one of the following is true?*
   A. There are two key stages comprising pre- and postsurgical checks.
   B. The check listings for each stage are undertaken by the surgeon.
   C. The patient's identity is checked in all stages.
   D. The checklist protocol is only applicable to general anesthetic cases.
   E. The surgical procedure type is identified in all stages.

THE WHO PRESURGICAL CHECKLIST

6. *When performing the "time out" phase of the WHO surgical checklist, what is the first action undertaken?*
   A. Confirmation of patient identity
   B. Team member introduction
   C. Confirmation of planned surgical procedure
   D. Review of patient allergy status
   E. Confirmation of correct site and side of surgery

ANTIBIOTIC ADMINISTRATION

7. *When administering antibiotics in the perioperative period, which one of the following is true?*
   A. The optimal time for administration of most prophylactic antibiotics for abdominoplasty is immediately prior to making the surgical incision.
   B. When used intraoperatively for prophylaxis in facelifting, Ancef (cefazolin) should be redosed every 1–2 hours.
   C. Prophylactic dosing for clindamycin is 900 mg intravenous (IV) and should not need to be re-administered even in prolonged plastic surgical cases.
   D. Withholding postoperative antibiotics in prosthetic breast reconstruction is encouraged by the Surgical Care Improvement Project.
   E. Postoperative antibiotic prophylaxis is not routinely indicated for septorhinoplasty.

SURGICAL SITE PREP

8. *When selecting a skin preparation for elective plastic surgery, which one is most likely to be effective?*
   A. 1% chlorhexidine in alcohol base
   B. 2% chlorhexidine in aqueous base
   C. 4% chlorhexidine in alcohol base
   D. Povidone iodine in aqueous base
   E. A combination of chlorhexidine and iodine

PATIENT POSITIONING FOR SURGERY

9. *When considering patient positioning in operating theater, which position is associated with an increased risk of developing increased ocular pressure and subsequent visual problems?*
   A. Supine   D. Trendelenberg
   B. Prone   E. Lithotomy
   C. Lateral decubitus

POSTOPERATIVE STEROID ADMINISTRATION

10. *After which of the following types of surgery are steroids most likely to be indicated?*
    A. Facelift   D. Rhinoplasty
    B. Neck lift   E. Otoplasty
    C. Blepharoplasty

SCAR MANAGEMENT

11. A patient is undergoing breast reduction with a Wise pattern scar. She has previously developed poor-quality scars on the torso. *Which one of the following topical wound healing adjuncts would be most beneficial for her following this surgery?*
    A. Cyanoacrylate glue
    B. Silicone gel ointment
    C. Silicone gel sheeting
    D. Topical vitamin E with cocoa butter
    E. Glycosaminoglycan gel

NORMOTHERMIA

12. It is important to maintain normothermia during surgery. *Which one of the following is true regarding hypothermia in the perioperative period?*
    A. Hypothermia is defined as a core body temperature of <35° C.
    B. Hypothermia is strongly associated with hypercoagulability.
    C. Hypothermia is associated with an increase in wound infections.
    D. Shivering and vasoconstriction are good markers of hypothermia.
    E. Warmed fluids are the mainstay of reducing hypothermia during anesthesia.

Answers

REDUCING COMPLICATIONS AND OPTIMIZING OUTCOMES

1. **When preparing a patient for elective plastic surgery, which one of the following is true with regard to minimizing complications and optimizing outcomes?**

   E. Optimizing patient outcomes in terms of satisfaction begins at the time of consultation and continues well into the postoperative period

   Levels of patient satisfaction before and after surgery are highly dependent on the patient's experience throughout the entire clinical journey commencing from the initial consultation through to the final postsurgical consultation. It is vital, therefore, that the surgeon develops a good rapport with the patient from the outset in the first consultation. The strength of this early interaction provides the foundations for ongoing trust and understanding between the doctor and patient. Involving patients in their own management before surgery promotes understanding, empowers them to invest in their own results, and may help to manage expectations as well as deal more robustly with complications should they arise.[1,2]

   Meticulous attention to detail during preoperative planning through surgery and beyond can help minimize complications; however, complications cannot be completely avoided. It is often said that only the surgeon who does not operate will have no complications. Complications may be inherent to a specific procedure, individual patients and their comorbidities, or a particular systems-based issue. There are general principles that may be applied preoperatively, intraoperatively, and postoperatively to decrease the potential complications. One such area is the strict management of blood glucose levels in diabetic patients as poor control is associated with increased risk of surgical site infection and delayed wound healing. A perioperative serum glucose of over 200 mg/dL results in higher rates of wound healing complications and so should be avoided.[3,4]

   Other key risks to avoid are venous thromboembolic events (VTE) which include deep vein thrombosis (DVT) and pulmonary embolism (PE). All patients should be considered for VTE prophylaxis; however, only those considered to be at high risk, such as a strong history of previous embolic events, need preoperative review by a hematologist. Likewise, although preoperative blood tests are useful in many cases, low risk ambulatory patients probably do not benefit from routine preoperative laboratory tests and these only serve to increase costs and burden the health service.[5]

REFERENCES

1. Ho AL, Klassen AF, Cano S, Scott AM, Pusic AL. Optimizing patient-centered care in breast reconstruction: the importance of preoperative information and patient-physician communication. Plast Reconstr Surg 2013;132(2):212e–220e
2. McLafferty RB, Williams RG, Lambert AD, Dunnington GL. Surgeon communication behaviors that lead patients to not recommend the surgeon to family members or friends: analysis and impact. Surgery 2006;140(4):616–622, discussion 622–624
3. Endara M, Masden D, Goldstein J, Gondek S, Steinberg J, Attinger C. The role of chronic and perioperative glucose management in high-risk surgical closures: a case for tighter glycemic control. Plast Reconstr Surg 2013;132(4):996–1004
4. Guyuron B, Raszewski R. Undetected diabetes and the plastic surgeon. Plast Reconstr Surg 1990;86(3):471–474
5. Fischer JP, Shang EK, Nelson JA, Wu LC, Serletti JM, Kovach SJ. Patterns of preoperative laboratory testing in patients undergoing outpatient plastic surgery procedures. Aesthet Surg J 2014;34(1):133–141

MANAGEMENT OF SMOKING IN ELECTIVE PLASTIC SURGERY

2. **When planning elective plastic surgery in a long-term smoker, which one of the following is true?**

   D. A 4-week period of cessation before and after surgery is advised when proceeding with surgery.

   Smoking is one of the key lifestyle factors that can specifically increase the risk of postoperative complications including wound healing problems secondary to tissue hypoxia and ischemia.[1] In addition, general anesthetic complications are more likely, such as postoperative pulmonary complications. Therefore, in the elective setting, smoking cessation is strongly advised prior to aesthetic or reconstructive surgery and for a sustained period afterwards. Although from an overall health perspective it may be ideal for a patient to stop smoking permanently, it would not be absolutely necessary for the purposes of surgery alone. Instead, smoking abstinence for a 4-week period both before and after surgery is generally accepted as a reasonable compromise to safely proceed with elective plastic surgery from a wound healing perspective (pulmonary is longer).[2,3] Procedures most at risk of complications in smokers include face lifts with large areas of undermining, skin-sparing mastectomy, and abdominoplasty where large skin flaps are elevated reliant on altered blood supply.

   Patients willing to stop smoking can get benefits from both pharmacological and nonpharmacological interventions. Pharmacological interventions include nicotine replacement medicines and bupropion, which is a medication primarily used to treat major depressive disorder, but one that can help reduce cravings and withdrawal effects of smoking cessation. Nonpharmacological modalities include counseling, behavioral therapy, hypnosis, and psychotherapy. There are a number of reliable tests to assess for patient compliance with smoking cessation. These include urinary cotinine which is a byproduct of nicotine, or blood test measurement of multiple nicotine metabolites including cotinine, anabasine, and nornicotine. These tests can be performed preoperatively to ensure satisfactory compliance and allow for deferment of surgery if compliance is inadequate. As stated above, the negative effects of smoking are well described and not overstated. Hence, surgeons should routinely advise patients that smoking should be minimized or completely stopped in order to optimize postoperative outcomes and minimize complications.[4]

REFERENCES

1. Jensen JA, Goodson WH, Hopf HW, Hunt TK. Cigarette smoking decreases tissue oxygen. Arch Surg 1991;126(9):1131–1134
2. Sørensen LT. Wound healing and infection in surgery: the pathophysiological impact of smoking, smoking cessation, and nicotine replacement therapy: a systematic review. Ann Surg 2012;255(6):1069–1079
3. Sørensen LT. Wound healing and infection in surgery. The clinical impact of smoking and smoking cessation: a systematic review and meta-analysis. Arch Surg 2012;147(4):373–383
4. Harrison B, Khansa I, Janis JE. Evidence-based strategies to reduce postoperative complications in plastic surgery. Plast Reconstr Surg 2016;137(1):351–360

DECOLONIZATION AND SKIN ANTISEPSIS

3. *In a patient undergoing elective abdominoplasty who has previously been found to be methicillin-resistant S. aureus (MRSA) positive, which one of the following is recommended?*

   D. Mupirocin ointment applied to the bilateral nares twice daily for 5 days preop is recommended.
   Surgical site infection can be a devastating complication in aesthetic and reconstructive surgery, particularly where an implant is used. *Staphylococcus aureus* is the leading cause of surgical site infection, and the prevalence of community-acquired methicillin-resistant *S. aureus* (MRSA) surgical site infection is increasing. Therefore, presurgical decolonization, skin antisepsis, and systemic antibiotic use perioperatively should be utilized in order to minimize risk of surgical site infections.

   In patients who have a history of previous MRSA infection and those who are carriers should receive vancomycin 1 g 60 minutes before surgery.

   All other patients (notwithstanding those with allergy status issues) should be prescribed IV cefazolin 30–59 minutes before surgery, but not specifically postoperatively in oral formulation. Alternatively, some surgeons/centers may prefer to use flucloxacillin or amoxicillin/clavulanate instead.

   Most centers will routinely perform MRSA screening swabs on all patients prior to their undergoing elective surgery. Those who have a previous positive MRSA status or are at high risk, e.g., immunocompromised or a health care worker, must all be screened. Screening should normally be undertaken between 2 and 4 weeks before surgery. It involves taking swabs from the nasal mucosa bilaterally to assess nasal carriage, rather than groin swabs which were common previously. Both nares are swabbed with a single swab as the association with nasal carriage and subsequent infection is well established.[1,2] Those patients who grow positive MRSA cultures are instructed to apply 2% mupirocin nasal ointment twice daily (not once) to both nares and to bathe with chlorhexidine (40 mg/mL Hibiscrub) daily for 5 days (not 1 month) immediately before the scheduled surgery. Patients who are not MRSA positive do not require these eradication therapies.

REFERENCES

1. Bode LG, Kluytmans JA, Wertheim HF, et al. Preventing surgical-site infections in nasal carriers of Staphylococcus aureus. N Engl J Med 2010;362(1):9–17
2. Wenzel RP, Perl TM. The significance of nasal carriage of Staphylococcus aureus and the incidence of postoperative wound infection. J Hosp Infect 1995;31(1):13–24

PERIOPERATIVE VENOUS THROMBOEMBOLISM (VTE) RISK MANAGEMENT

4. *When considering prevention of venous thromboembolism (VTE) in a patient undergoing autologous breast reconstruction surgery, which one of the following is true?*

   A. A score of 8 or more using the Caprini risk assessment model indicates postoperative chemoprophylaxis should be considered.
   The Caprini risk assessment model has been developed to help guide clinicians on the appropriate use of venous thromboembolism (VTE) prophylaxis in surgical patients. A range of key risk factors are included within the assessment, which is downloadable as a form (**Fig. 15.1**).[1,2,3] A number of these risk factors are allocated a single

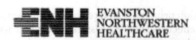

Thrombosis Risk Factor Assessment

Joseph A. Caprini, MD, MS, FACS, RVT
Louis W. Biegler Professor of Surgery,
Northwestern University
The Feinberg School of Medicine;
Professor of Biomedical Engineering,
Northwestern University;
Director of Surgical Research,
Evanston Northwestern Healthcare
Email: j-caprini@northwestern.edu
Website: venousdisease.com

Patient's Name:_____ Age: _____ Sex: _____ Wgt: ____lbs

Choose All That Apply

Each Risk Factor Represents 1 Point
☐ Age 41-60 years
☐ Minor surgery planned
☐ History of prior major surgery (< 1 month)
☐ Varicose veins
☐ History of inflammatory bowel disease
☐ Swollen legs (current)
☐ Obesity (BMI > 25)
☐ Acute myocardial infraction
☐ Congestive heart failure (< 1 month)
☐ Sepsis (< 1 month)
☐ Serious lung disease incl. pneumonia (< 1 month)
☐ Abnormal pulmonary function (COPD)
☐ Medical patient currently at bed rest
☐ Other risk factors_____

Each Risk Factor Represents 2 Points
☐ Age 60-74 years
☐ Arthroscopic surgery
☐ Malignancy (present or previous)
☐ Major surgery (> 45 minutes)
☐ Laparoscopic surgery (> 45 minutes)
☐ Patient confined to bed (> 72 hours)
☐ Immobilizing plaster cast (< 1 month)
☐ Central venous access

Each Risk Factor Represents 5 Points
☐ Elective major lower extremity arthroplasty
☐ Hip, pelvis or leg fracture (< 1 month)
☐ Stroke (< 1 month)
☐ Multiple trauma (< 1 month)
☐ Acute spinal cord injury (paralysis)(< 1 month)

Each Risk Factor Represents 3 Points
☐ Age over 75 years
☐ History of DVT/PE
☐ **Family history of thrombosis***
☐ Positive Factor V Leiden
☐ Positive Prothrombin 20210A
☐ Elevated serum homocysteine
☐ Positive lupus anticoagulant
☐ Elevated anticardiolipin antibodies
☐ Heparin-induced thrombocytopenia (HIT)
☐ Other congenital or acquired thrombophilia
If yes: Type_____
*most frequently missed risk factor

For Women only (Each Represents 1 Point)
☐ Oral contraceptives or hoemone replacement therapy
☐ Pregnancy or postpartum (<1 month)
☐ History of unexplained stillborn infant, recurrent spontaneous abortion (≥ 3), premature birth with toxemia or growth-restricted infant

Total Risk Factor Score ☐

Fig. 15.1   Caprini risk assessment model.[1,2]

point while others are allocated two, three, or five points according to risk level, before summing them to provide a total individualized risk score for the patient. There are more than 30 risk factors considered and these include patient age, type of surgery planned, and the patient's associated background of medical comorbidities including obesity, varicose veins, cardiopulmonary disease, proven coagulopathy, malignancy, sepsis, swollen legs, and stroke. In addition, postoperative immobilization and the need for plaster casts are considered. For females there are additional hormonal risk factors to be considered including use of oral contraceptives, pregnancy or recent pregnancy, and previous history of spontaneous abortion. The calculated score places patients into risk categories as shown in Fig. 15.1. A score of 0–1 is low risk, a score of 2 is moderate risk, a score of 3–4 is high risk, and a score of 5 or more is highest risk. A study looking at risk in more detail specifically for plastic surgery patients[4] has demonstrated a notable risk reduction in VTE in patients administered enoxaparin postoperatively where the Caprini score was 7 or 8. According to risk, the use of elastic stockings, intermittent pneumatic calf compression, low molecular weight heparin (LMWH), and factor Va inhibitors may be indicated.

Intermittent pneumatic compression, graduated compression stockings, and venous foot pumps are generally applied to all patients undergoing surgery, regardless of their risk. There is probably little to choose between them in terms of efficacy although evidence would suggest a slight benefit for pneumatic calf compression over the stockings alone.

The proposed mechanisms for each differ; stockings are meant to prevent distension of the veins, while intermittent calf compression or foot compression is meant to help physically empty the veins and also stimulate tissue thromboplastin. There is, therefore, no reason why the two approaches should not be combined during surgery to benefit from both mechanisms of action. However, there is only limited evidence to support such a practice in terms of flow velocity augmentation and reduced deep vein thrombosis (DVT) outcomes.[5,6] A major and frequently quoted study by Scurr et al[7] has shown a reduction in rates of DVT in general surgery patients when graded compression stockings were combined with graded sequential intermittent compression, as opposed to intermittent compression alone. However, one or the other is generally accepted as good practice and foot compression and calf compression would not be used simultaneously as each is aimed at achieving the same outcome. One caveat of compression is that it may be contraindicated in patients with peripheral vascular disease, cardiac failure, peripheral neuropathy, and some skin conditions (**Fig. 15.2**).

Prophylaxis Regimen

Total Risk Factor Score	Incidence of DVT	Risk level	Prophylaxis Regimen	Legend
0-1	<10%	Low Risk	No specific measures; early ambulation	**ES** - Elastic Stockings
2	10-20%	Moderate Risk	ES or IPC or LDUH, or LWMH	**IPC** - Intermittent Pneumatic Compression
3-4	20-40%	High Risk	IPC or LDUH, or LMWH alone or in combination with ES or IPC	**LDUH** - Low Dose Unfractionated Heparin
5 or more	40-80% 1-5% mortality	Highest Risk	Pharmacological; LDUH, LMWH*, Warfarin*, or Fac Xa* alone or in combination with ES or IPC	**LMWH** - Low molecular Weight Heparin **Fac Xa** - Factor X Inhibitor

Prophylaxis Safety Considerations: Check box if answer is 'YES'

Anticoagulants: Factors Associated with Increased Bleeding
☐ Is patient experiencing any active bleeding?
☐ Does patient have (or has had history of) heparin-induced thromnocytopenia?
☐ Is patient's platelet count <100,000/mm³?
☐ Is patient taking oral anticoagulants, platelet inhibitors (e.g. NSAIDS, Cloidigrel, Salicylates)?
☐ Is patient's creatinine clearance abnormal? If yes, please indicate value _____
If any of the above boxes are checked, the patient may not be a candidate for anticoagulant therapy and should consider alternative prophylactic measures.

Intermittent Pneumatic Compression (IPC)
☐ Does patient have severe peripheral arterial disease?
☐ Does patient have congestive heart failure?
☐ Does patient have an acute superficial/deep vein thrombosis?
If any of the above boxes are checked, the patient may not be a candidate for intermittent compression therapy and should consider alternative prophylactic measures.

Based on Geerts WH et al: Prevention of Venous Thromboembolism. Chest 2001; 119:132S-175S; Nicolaides AN et al: 2001 International Consensus Statement: Prevention of Venous Thromboembolism, Guidelines According to Scientific Evidence; Caprini JA, Arcelus JI et al: State-of-the-Art Venous Thromboembolism Prophylaxis. Scope 2001; 8: 228-240; and Oger E: Incidence of Venous Thromboembolism: A Community-based Study in Western France. Thromb Haemost 2000; 657-860. Turpie AG, Bauer KA, Eriksson BI, et al. Fondaparinux vs. Enoxaparin for the Prevention of Venous Thromboembolism in Major Orthopedic Surgery. A Meta-analysis of 4 Randomized Double-Blind Studies. Arch Intern Med 2002; 162(16):1833-40. Ringley et al. Evaluation of pulmonary - intermittent pneumatic compression boots in congestive heart failure. American Surgeon 2002; 68(3): 286-9. Morris et al. Effects of supine intermittent compression on arterial inflow to the lower limb. Archives of Surgery 2002: 137(11):1269-73. © 2001 Evanston Northwestern Healthcare, all rights reserved.

Examining Physician's Signature: _____ Date: _____

Fig. 15.2 Prophylaxis regimen and safety considerations.

The choice of chemoprophylaxis in terms of agent used and duration prescribed can be adjusted. In some cases, a short course of enoxaparin is administered solely when the patient has reduced mobility in hospital, and in other cases for 7–30 days. One concern that some surgeons have had is the increased risk for reoperative hematoma where LMWH is prescribed. A recent paper reviewed this in more than 3000 plastic surgery patients and found no evidence to support an increase in reoperative hematoma following enoxaparin administration.[8] The type of anesthesia used can potentially affect VTE risk. For example, the use of intravenous anesthesia and SAFE (spontaneous breathing, avoid gas, face up, extremities mobile) anesthesia methods may also decrease risk for thromboembolic disease.[8,9]

Early ambulation is key to minimizing postoperative complications such as VTE as well as atelectasis, chest infection, and pressure damage. In this case of autologous breast reconstruction, the patient should mobilize early after surgery and maintain adequate hydration with a view to early postoperative discharge as extended hospital stay is also associated with increased complication risk.

REFERENCES

1. Caprini JA. Thrombosis risk assessment as a guide to quality patient care. Dis Mon 2005;51(2-3):70–78
2. Caprini JA, Arcelus JI, Hasty JH, Tamhane AC, Fabrega F. Clinical assessment of venous thromboembolic risk in surgical patients. Semin Thromb Hemost 1991;17(Suppl 3):304–312
3. Caprini JA, Arcelus JI, Reyna JJ. Effective risk stratification of surgical and nonsurgical patients for venous thromboembolic disease. Semin Hematol 2001;38(2, Suppl 5):12–19
4. Pannucci CJ, Dreszer G, Wachtman CF, et al. Postoperative enoxaparin prevents symptomatic venous thromboembolism in high-risk plastic surgery patients. Plast Reconstr Surg 2011;128(5):1093–1103
5. Morris RJ, Woodcock JP. Evidence-based compression: prevention of stasis and deep vein thrombosis. Ann Surg 2004;239(2):162–171
6. Morris RJ, Woodcock JP. Intermittent pneumatic compression or graduated compression stockings for deep vein thrombosis prophylaxis? A systematic review of direct clinical comparisons. Ann Surg 2020;251(3):393–396
7. Scurr JH, Coleridge-Smith PD, Hasty JH. Regimen for improved effectiveness of intermittent pneumatic compression in deep venous thrombosis prophylaxis. Surgery 1987;102(5):816–820
8. Pannucci CJ, Wachtman CF, Dreszer G, et al. The effect of postoperative enoxaparin on risk for reoperative hematoma. Plast Reconstr Surg 2012;129(1):160–168
9. Swanson E. The case against chemoprophylaxis for venous thromboembolism prevention and the rationale for SAFE anesthesia. Plast Reconstr Surg Glob Open 2014;2(6):e160

INTRAOPERATIVE MEASURES TO REDUCE COMPLICATIONS

5. *When performing the World Health Organization (WHO) surgical checklist, which one of the following is true?*
   E. The surgical procedure type is identified in all stages.
   The WHO checklist has been designed to reduce the risk of accidental error, mistakes, and adverse events occurring during surgery.[1] In particular, things such as wrong site, wrong side, or wrong type of surgery, inadvertent drug administration where allergies are present, and other errors associated with surgery and anesthesia are targeted. It serves to ensure the team members caring for the patient understand the procedure planned and are all on the same page in terms of equipment required, potential or unusual risks specific to either the patient or surgery type, and key steps and duration of surgery. The implementation of this check-listing system has been shown to decrease both perioperative morbidity and mortality.[2,3]

   The WHO procedure has 19 steps incorporated into three stages, not two, and the surgical procedure is described in each of the three stages. The first stage is the *"sign in"* phase and is undertaken prior to anesthesia, usually by the anesthesiologist and supporting team. The patient's identity is confirmed in both this stage and the second stage which follows it, but not specifically the final stage as the identity has already been confirmed repeatedly by this time. The second stage is called the *"time out"* phase and is performed once the patient is anesthetized in the operating room (OR) prior to commencement of surgery. The *"time out"* is generally led and conducted by the lead surgeon with the intention of everyone pausing to focus that the correct procedure is being undertaken and that all team members are onboard with the surgical plan. The WHO checklist applies not only to general anesthetic cases, but also to both regional blocks and local anesthetic cases too. The third stage is the *"sign out"* phase. This is usually performed by one of the nursing team prior to the patient leaving the theater. In this phase, the procedure is again confirmed as is the postoperative plan and any concerns for the recovery team. Confirmation of needle, sponge, and instrument counts is made at this time, as well as correct labeling of specimens. Knowledge of the WHO checklist is vital for any surgeon and the team in order to minimize risks during and following surgery.

REFERENCES

1. https://www.who.int/patientsafety/safesurgery/checklist/en/
2. Haynes AB, Weiser TG, Berry WR, et al; Safe Surgery Saves Lives Study Group. A surgical safety checklist to reduce morbidity and mortality in a global population. N Engl J Med 2009;360(5):491–499
3. Haynes AB, Edmondson L, Lipsitz SR, et al. Mortality trends after a voluntary checklist-based surgical safety collaborative. Ann Surg 2017;266(6):923–929

THE WHO PRESURGICAL CHECKLIST

6. *When performing the "time out" phase of the WHO surgical checklist, what is the first action undertaken?*

B. Team member introduction

The second phase of the WHO checklist is performed as a *"time out"* once the patient is anesthetized, if having a general anesthetic, or once the patient arrives in the OR prior to delivery of local anesthetic if having a local anesthetic. The time out is undertaken prior to commencement of surgery.

The first action is to repeat the team member introduction to ensure all team members know each other and understand their respective roles. This can be particularly relevant where staff members have changed or have been added following the initial preoperative briefing. Once this introduction has been done, the patient's identity is checked once more using the name band and cross referencing with the provided documentation. The surgical site, procedure, and consent are each checked and confirmed. Most teams will also recheck the patient's allergy status at this time although it is not formally documented as part of the original WHO time out. A review of the critical or nonroutine steps is made by the lead surgeon, including anticipated blood loss and expected duration of surgery. The anesthetic team reviews any specific concerns the patient may have. Then the nursing team confirms the sterility and availability of instruments/equipment, and any other anticipated concerns. Antibiotic prophylaxis is confirmed to have been administered prior to making the first incision. All essential imaging results are confirmed to be present and correct. Once completed the procedure may be commenced.[1]

REFERENCE

1. https://www.who.int/patientsafety/safesurgery/checklist/en/

ANTIBIOTIC ADMINISTRATION

7. *When administering antibiotics in the perioperative period, which one of the following is true?*

E. Postoperative antibiotic prophylaxis is not routinely indicated for septorhinoplasty.

Routine postoperative prescription of antibiotics following septorhinoplasty is not indicated, even though intuitively it can be, given the potential for intranasal organisms to cause problems. A number of publications have explored the evidence for routine prophylactic antibiotics in rhinoplasty, including a recent systematic review and meta-analysis. Each of these have concluded there is no justification for routine postoperative antibiotic use in such cases based on the low incidence of infection. In those that compared patients having been given postoperative antibiotics and those who had not, there was no difference in the observed outcome. There may, however, still be an indication for their use in select cases such as more complex revision procedures particularly where infection has been an issue in the past, where nasal packs are left in situ for an extended time, or where patients have reduced immune system reserve.[1-3]

There is a role for prophylactic antibiotic use in the perioperative period for many different types of plastic surgery and in most cases, a single dose of intravenous antibiotic is administered 30–60 minutes prior to commencement of surgery. The precise timing of this will depend on the antibiotic chosen. For example, Ancef (cefazolin) and many others should be administered 30–60 minutes prior, whereas vancomycin and fluoroquinolones should be administered no less than 1 hour before surgery (typically 1–2 hours before incision). In some cases, it is acceptable to administer antibiotics postoperatively; however, many guidelines and protocols including those produced by the Surgical Care Improvement Project (SCIP) encourage clinicians to avoid prescription of antibiotics where not clinically indicated beyond the first 24 hours of surgery. The consensus position of the working group involved in SCIP concluded that infusion of the first antimicrobial dose should begin within 60 minutes before surgical incision and that prophylactic antimicrobial agents should be discontinued within 24 hours of the end of surgery. There is however no specific reference by SCIP to the use of postoperative antibiotics following breast implant use in either primary augmentation or reconstructive surgery settings.[4]

One study looked at the effects of changing antibiotic protocol to comply with the SCIP protocol (as described above) in breast reconstruction patients, and found that when postoperative antibiotics were omitted, the rate of postoperative infection increased.[5] Therefore, the authors concluded that postoperative antibiotics should be used after augmentation surgery. Overall, there remains a paucity of robust evidence to guide the use of antibiotic prophylaxis in breast reconstruction and implant surgery and there is no specific consensus on this.

In one systematic review of breast reconstruction patients, the infection rate was higher where no antibiotics were given, but there was no difference in infection rates where less than or more than 24 hours of antibiotics were prescribed. Therefore, it would seem that prophylaxis of up to 24 hours would be adequate.[6] In contrast, another study compared the use of antibiotics (single dose cephalosporin before induction of anesthesia) with no antibiotics in primary breast augmentation and found no significant difference in infection rates or complications between the two groups. Although this was a smaller single operator study with 90 patients in each arm, it provides evidence to suggest that antibiotic use may not be indicated in primary augmentation.[7]

Intraoperatively, for longer procedures IV antibiotics may need to be redosed. The timings for this depend on the antibiotic. For example, Ancef should be redosed every 4 hours and clindamycin every 6 hours.

REFERENCES

1. Georgiou I, Farber N, Mendes D, Winkler E. The role of antibiotics in rhinoplasty and septoplasty: a literature review. Rhinology 2008;46(4):267–270
2. Nuyen B, Kandathil CK, Laimi K, Rudy SF, Most SP, Saltychev M. Evaluation of antibiotic prophylaxis in rhinoplasty: a systematic review and meta-analysis. JAMA Facial Plast Surg 2019;21(1):12–17
3. Kullar R, Frisenda J, Nassif PS. The more the merrier? Should antibiotics be used for rhinoplasty and septorhinoplasty? a review. Plast Reconstr Surg Glob Open 2018;6(10):e1972
4. Bratzler DW, Houck PM; Surgical Infection Prevention Guideline Writers Workgroup. Antimicrobial prophylaxis for surgery: an advisory statement from the National Surgical Infection Prevention Project. Am J Surg 2005;189(4):395–404
5. Clayton JL, Bazakas A, Lee CN, Hultman CS, Halvorson EG. Once is not enough: withholding postoperative prophylactic antibiotics in prosthetic breast reconstruction is associated with an increased risk of infection. Plast Reconstr Surg 2012;130(3):495–502
6. Phillips BT, Bishawi M, Dagum AB, Khan SU, Bui DT. A systematic review of antibiotic use and infection in breast reconstruction: what is the evidence? Plast Reconstr Surg 2013;131(1):1–13
7. Keramidas E, Lymperopoulos NS, Rodopoulou S. Is antibiotic prophylaxis in breast augmentation necessary? A prospective study. Plast Surg (Oakv) 2016;24(3):195–198

SURGICAL SITE PREP

8. *When selecting a skin preparation for elective plastic surgery, which one is most likely to be effective?*

C. 4% chlorhexidine in alcohol base

The combination of a 4% chlorhexidine gluconate (CHG) preparation with a 70% isopropyl alcohol (IPA) has the highest probability of being effective in minimizing surgical site infections (SSI) according to a recent Cochrane review.[1]

Another recent review of common skin preparation agents demonstrated that 2% chlorhexidine gluconate (CHG) and 4% CHG (Hibiclens) had inferior antimicrobial activity to isopropyl alcohol (IPA) (70%) or 2% CHG combined with IPA (ChloraPrep).[2] In general, alcohol-based antiseptics are currently thought to be more effective than those with an aqueous base as the alcohol itself has antimicrobial qualities. This may be a factor of equal importance to the prep type itself. A further thing to consider when interpreting this evidence is that little of this actually relates to plastic and reconstructive surgical procedures, but is instead based on other specialty procedures such as general surgery and orthopedics. If it is accepted that alcohol-based skin preps are more effective and they are selected for use, caution must be taken when using them as if they are not completely dry, they risk ignition when using electrocautery leading to fires in the OR and patients with burn injuries. Chloroprep has a good evidence base to support its use and is marketed as a unit with a sponge applicator included. Although this may be advantageous for reducing SSI, it is a more expensive way of delivering the skin preparation and is limited in some regards by the small applicator sponge size and shape. Combining iodine and chlorhexidine has no proven antimicrobial benefits; however, it can be useful to perform a first prep with iodine before applying a second prep of alcohol bases chlorhexidine where detailed preoperative markings have been made (e.g., breast reduction/mastopexy) as this seems to limit the removal of the marking ink.

REFERENCES

1. Dumville JC, McFarlane E, Edwards P, Lipp A, Holmes A, Liu Z. Preoperative skin antiseptics for preventing surgical wound infections after clean surgery. Cochrane Database Syst Rev 2015;CD003949(4):CD003949
2. Hibbard JS. Analyses comparing the antimicrobial activity and safety of current antiseptic agents: a review. J Infus Nurs 2005;28(3):194–207

PATIENT POSITIONING FOR SURGERY

9. *When considering patient positioning in operating theater, which position is associated with an increased risk of developing increased ocular pressure and subsequent visual problems?*

B. Prone

Safe patient positioning is key to minimizing complications during surgery and a number of key points must be considered. There is potential risk in each of the positions described above, if due care is not taken. It is the teams' responsibility to ensure the patient is well protected during this time. Positioning patients in the prone position is required for a number of procedures in plastic and reconstructive surgery, for example, debridement and reconstruction of sacral pressure sores, excision of tumors from the dorsal surface of the thorax, and reconstruction of perianal wounds with gluteal flaps after laparoscopic abdominoperineal resection. Placing patients in the prone position increases intraoperative risks compared with other positions, including raised intraocular pressure, vertebral artery dissection, and increased pressure on the knees, chest, and pubis, which can each place strain on the shoulders, elbows, hips, and knees. In addition, it is more challenging to safely maintain the airway and ensure adequate respiratory function as well as avoid nerve injury to the upper limbs and neck. When placing patients in this position, great care must be taken to ensure pressure areas are well padded with gel rolls, foam crates, or pillows such that body weight is evenly distributed and pressure avoided on the abdomen, knees, and face. The eyes should be protected with padded goggles.

In all positions, the same approach should be applied with care taken to examine pressure areas prior to starting the procedure, ensuring they are well padded with gel pads during the procedure, and then checking them at the end of the procedure. In extended procedures, it may be prudent to move or turn the patient intraoperatively to minimize pressure damage and postoperative stiffness.

An important consideration when moving and positioning the anesthetized patient is to consider potential nerve damage either due to poor manipulation or poor positioning. For example, arms and legs should be well supported throughout with joints in neutral, comfortable positions and areas such as the elbow and knee well-padded to avoid pressure damage where nerves are at risk of compression, e.g., ulnar nerve or common perineal nerve. A 1990 analysis of the American Society of Anesthesiologists Closed Claims Project database showed that 15% of claims were for nerve injuries and this highlights this point well.[1,2]

REFERENCES

1. Bund M, Heine J, Jaeger K. [Complications due to patient positioning: anaesthesiological considerations]. Anasthesiol Intensivmed Notfallmed Schmerzther 2005;40(6):329–339
2. Shermak M, Shoo B, Deune EG. Prone positioning precautions in plastic surgery. Plast Reconstr Surg 2006;117(5):1584–1588, discussion 1589

POSTOPERATIVE STEROID ADMINISTRATION

10. *After which of the following types of surgery are steroids most likely to be indicated?*

D. Rhinoplasty

For patients undergoing rhinoplasty, perioperative corticosteroids can be indicated as they decrease postoperative edema and ecchymosis. Evidence suggests that preoperative use is superior to postoperative use, and extended dosing is superior to singular.[1–4]

The evidence that perioperative corticosteroids decrease facial swelling and ecchymosis following facelift remains anecdotal and unsubstantiated. Steroids may be associated with increased cost and risk of complications, including exacerbation of hypertension, deterioration of glucose control, increased rate of infection, and potential for avascular osteonecrosis.[5–8] There is no evidence to support the use of steroids following otoplasty or blepharoplasty.

REFERENCES

1. Hatef DA, Ellsworth WA, Allen JN, Bullocks JM, Hollier LH Jr, Stal S. Perioperative steroids for minimizing edema and ecchymosis after rhinoplasty: a meta-analysis. Aesthet Surg J 2011;31(6):648–657
2. Hoffmann DF, Cook TA, Quatela VC, Wang TD, Brownrigg PJ, Brummett RE. Steroids and rhinoplasty. A double-blind study. Arch Otolaryngol Head Neck Surg 1991;117(9):990–993, discussion 994
3. Kargi E, Hoşnuter M, Babucçu O, Altunkaya H, Altinyazar C. Effect of steroids on edema, ecchymosis, and intraoperative bleeding in rhinoplasty. Ann Plast Surg 2003;51(6):570–574
4. Totonchi A, Guyuron B. A randomized, controlled comparison between arnica and steroids in the management of postrhinoplasty ecchymosis and edema. Plast Reconstr Surg 2007;120(1):271–274
5. Pulikkottil BJ, Dauwe P, Daniali L, Rohrich RJ. Corticosteroid use in cosmetic plastic surgery. Plast Reconstr Surg 2013;132(3):352e–360e

6. Echavez MI, Mangat DS. Effects of steroids on mood, edema, and ecchymosis in facial plastic surgery. Arch Otolaryngol Head Neck Surg 1994;120(10):1137–1141

7. Owsley JQ, Weibel TJ, Adams WA. Does steroid medication reduce facial edema following face lift surgery? A prospective, randomized study of 30 consecutive patients. Plast Reconstr Surg 1996;98(1):1–6

8. Rapaport DP, Bass LS, Aston SJ. Influence of steroids on postoperative swelling after facialplasty: a prospective, randomized study. Plast Reconstr Surg 1995;96(7):1547–1552

SCAR MANAGEMENT

11. A patient is undergoing breast reduction with a Wise pattern scar. She has previously developed poor-quality scars on the torso. *Which one of the following topical wound healing adjuncts would be most beneficial for her following this surgery?*

   C. Silicone gel sheeting

   There are a number of adjuncts which may be used to help scar quality post surgery. Of these, silicone is the most widely accepted modality for high-risk patients such as this woman who is having surgery to a high-risk area for poor scars on the background of previous poor scarring. Steroid gel sheeting should be started once the wounds have fully epithelialized (i.e., at 1–2 weeks post surgery) and continued for at least 1 month. The sheets should be worn for a minimum of 12 hours per day. Although silicone gels may be effective, evidence supports the preferential use of the sheets over gel.[1,2] Application of microporous tape onto wounds after closure in the OR has been shown to help improve scar quality. It most likely achieves this by supporting the wound externally during the healing phase and reducing swelling.[3,4] It may be worthwhile using for the first few weeks following surgery for this patient, but a switch to silicone is probably indicated once epithelialization is complete. Topical vitamin E, cocoa butter, onion extract cream (e.g., Mederma), and glycosaminoglycan gel have not been shown to consistently improve scar appearance as single agents.[5]

   Using skin glue can have benefits in terms of avoiding external sutures and providing a wound dressing that allows patients to shower the area; however, it is not proven to help the scars in the long term. Overall, the benefits of many topical agents could result from massage associated with their application and so firm wound massage therapy is commonly recommended by surgeons.

   The product used for the massage may have less impact on outcome than the massage procedure itself.

REFERENCES

1. Mustoe TA, Cooter RD, Gold MH, et al; International Advisory Panel on Scar Management. International clinical recommendations on scar management. Plast Reconstr Surg 2002;110(2):560–571

2. Khansa I, Harrison B, Janis JE. Evidence-based scar management: how to improve results with technique and technology. Plast Reconstr Surg 2016; 138(3, Suppl):165S–178S

3. Atkinson JA, McKenna KT, Barnett AG, McGrath DJ, Rudd M. A randomized, controlled trial to determine the efficacy of paper tape in preventing hypertrophic scar formation in surgical incisions that traverse Langer's skin tension lines. Plast Reconstr Surg 2005;116(6):1648–1656, discussion 1657–1658

4. Reiffel RS. Prevention of hypertrophic scars by long-term paper tape application. Plast Reconstr Surg 1995;96(7):1715–1718

5. Havlik RJ; Plastic Surgery Educational Foundation DATA Committee. Vitamin E and wound healing. Plast Reconstr Surg 1997;100(7):1901–1902

NORMOTHERMIA

12. It is important to maintain normothermia during surgery. *Which one of the following is true regarding hypothermia in the perioperative period?*

   C. Hypothermia is associated with an increase in wound infections.

   Hypothermia can result in increased wound infections by impairing immune defenses and decreasing local oxygen tension.[1] Hypothermia is defined as a core body temperature of <36° C (not 35° C). Standards of the Surgical Care Improvement Project (SCIP) require that patients have at least one documented temperature of ≥36° C within 30 minutes before or 15 minutes after the documented anesthesia end time. Mild hypothermia may also affect coagulation, recovery time, and the rate of perioperative myocardial events.[2] Very mild hypothermia (down to 35° C) doesn't seem to affect any part of the coagulation cascade. In some patients, hypothermia below 35° C may cause a mild drop in platelet count and cause mild platelet dysfunction. Below 33° C, other steps in the coagulation cascade can also be affected and this is dramatic below 33° C.[3] Anesthetic agents disrupt the body's natural thermoregulatory mechanisms and can inhibit shivering, vasoconstriction, and sweating. Therefore, these signs cannot be relied upon during surgery as markers of body temperature. Instead, temperature can be accurately measured using thermometers contained within the endotracheal tube or passed intranasally or transrectally. Patient temperature can be maintained passively through blankets, surgical drapes, and humidified respiratory gases.

REFERENCES

1. Hernandez M, Cutter TW, Apfelbaum JL. Hypothermia and hyperthermia in the ambulatory surgical patient. Clin Plast Surg 2013;40(3):429–438
2. Polderman KH. Hypothermia and coagulation. Crit Care 2012;16(Suppl 2):A20
3. Ruzicka J, Stengl M, Bolek L, Benes J, Matejovic M, Krouzecky A. Hypothermic anticoagulation: testing individual responses to graded severe hypothermia with thromboelastography. Blood Coagul Fibrinolysis 2012;23(4):285–289

PART II

Skin and Soft Tissue

16. The Basics of Skin

See *Essentials of Plastic Surgery, third* edition, pp. 215–222

CELLULAR CONTENT OF THE SKIN

1. *Which one of the following represents an epidermal cell involved in the immune response?*
   A. Langerhans cell
   B. Mast cell
   C. Merkel cell
   D. Keratinocyte
   E. Schwann cell

CELLULAR CONTENT OF THE SKIN

2. *Which one of the following represents an epidermal cell that provides ultraviolet (UV) protection and pigmentation to the skin?*
   A. Keratinocyte
   B. Melanocyte
   C. Fibroblast
   D. Macrophage
   E. Adipocyte

SENSORY RECEPTORS OF THE SKIN

3. *Which one of the following is found in the dermis and is tested by assessing light touch and dynamic two-point discrimination?*
   A. Naked nerve fiber
   B. Meissner's corpuscle
   C. Merkel cell
   D. Pacinian corpuscle
   E. Ruffini ending

APPENDAGES OF THE DERMIS

4. *Which one of the following represents a dermal appendage with a primary function of thermoregulation?*
   A. Ruffini ending
   B. Eccrine sweat gland
   C. Apocrine sweat gland
   D. Bulb of Krause
   E. Sebaceous gland

LAYERS OF THE EPIDERMIS

5. *Which one of the following statements is correct regarding the epidermis?*
   A. The stratum corneum and stratum lucidum contain viable keratinocytes.
   B. The stratum granulosum is the only layer containing both viable and nonviable cells.
   C. The stratum basale is multilayered and has mitotically active keratinocytes.
   D. The stratum spinosum contains melanocytes, tactile cells, and granular dendrocytes.
   E. The stratum lucidum is translucent and tends to be thicker in the axilla and scalp.

LAYERS OF THE EPIDERMIS

6. *Which one of the following epidermal layers is only found in the hands and feet?*
   A. Stratum basale
   B. Stratum spinosum
   C. Stratum granulosum
   D. Stratum lucidum
   E. Stratum corneum

STRUCTURE AND FUNCTION OF THE DERMIS

7. *Which one of the following statements is correct regarding the dermis?*
A. The ratio of collagen types I to III is uniform throughout the dermis.
B. The dermis has a consistent thickness throughout the body.
C. The papillary dermis represents 30% of total dermal thickness.
D. Mature elastic fibers are present throughout the entire dermis.
E. Ground substance facilitates diffusion of metabolites within the dermis.

COLLAGEN SUBTYPES

8. *In which anatomic location is collagen subtype II most likely to be found?*
A. Bone
B. Tendon
C. Hyaline cartilage
D. Ligament
E. Blood vessels

SKIN DISORDERS AND WOUND HEALING

9. *In which one of the following conditions it is generally acceptable to proceed with elective surgery?*
A. Iron deficiency
B. Cutis laxa
C. Cutis hyperelastica
D. Hutchinson-Gilford syndrome
E. Werner's syndrome

CLINICAL DIAGNOSIS OF SOFT TISSUE ABNORMALITY

10. A 12-year-old girl presents with joint hypermobility; thin, fragile tissue; and subcutaneous hemorrhages. *What is the most likely diagnosis?*
A. Cutis laxa
B. Parkes-Weber syndrome
C. Ehlers-Danlos syndrome
D. Progeria
E. Pseudoxanthoma elasticum

CLINICAL DIAGNOSIS OF SOFT TISSUE ABNORMALITY

11. A 20-year-old patient presents with skin laxity, yellow plaques, and cardiopulmonary problems but has normal wound healing. *What is the most likely diagnosis?*
A. Hutchinson-Gilford Syndrome
B. Cutis laxa
C. Cutis Hyperelastica
D. Werner's syndrome
E. Pseudoxanthoma elasticum

Answers

CELLULAR CONTENT OF THE SKIN

1. Which one of the following represents an epidermal cell involved in the immune response?

A. Langerhans cell

A number of different cells are found within the skin, with functions ranging from provision of structure through sensation, protection, and immunity. Langerhans cells are part of the macrophage/monocyte cell lineage and are antigen-presenting cells involved in immunity. Mast cells are found in the dermis and function as part of an allergic response. They are derived from bone marrow precursor cells. Activation of mast cells leads to histamine release and activation of various cytokines including interleukins, leukotrienes, and prostaglandins. These serve to increase vascular permeability, smooth muscle contraction and tissue inflammation. Merkel cells are found in the epidermis, and provide constant touch and pressure sensation. They are thought to be of neuroendocrine origin and are clinically relevant in that they can undergo malignant change resulting in an aggressive form of skin cancer.

The keratinocyte is the predominant cell of the epidermis and provides a protective physical barrier and UV protection by the uptake of melanin produced by melanocytes. Schwann cells are found covering myelinated nerves and these tend to run within the subcutis, but may be found in the dermis. They serve to increase nerve conduction velocity.[1]

REFERENCE

1. Burkitt HG, Young B, Heath JW. Wheater's Functional Histology: A Text and Colour Atlas. London: Churchill Livingstone; 2003

CELLULAR CONTENT OF THE SKIN

2. Which one of the following represents an epidermal cell that provides UV protection and pigmentation to the skin?

B. Melanocyte

Melanocytes are derived from the neural crest and have a key role in UV protection and skin pigmentation. They are responsible for the production of melanin which is a pigment produced in melanosomes. A common misunderstanding is that melanocytes retain the melanin pigment and are solely responsible for the increased skin pigmentation with tanning. However, it is the increased uptake by keratinocytes, following increased production by the melanocytes, that provides the increased skin pigmentation. The keratinocyte is the predominant cell of the epidermis and provides a protective physical barrier and UV protection by the uptake of melanin produced by melanocytes. Fibroblasts are the building blocks of the dermis and are responsible for collagen production. Macrophages are specialized cell types derived from blood monocytes that leave the circulation to differentiate in different tissues.

They are involved in the detection, phagocytosis, and destruction of bacteria and other harmful organisms. In addition, they can also present antigens to T cells and initiate inflammation by releasing cytokines that activate other cells. Adipocytes are fat cells found within the subcutis. Their main role is lipid storage but also have roles within endocrine, nervous, and immune system function.[1]

REFERENCE

1. Burkitt HG, Young B, Heath JW. Wheater's Functional Histology: A Text and Colour Atlas. London: Churchill Livingstone; 2003

SENSORY RECEPTORS OF THE SKIN

3. Which one of the following is found in the dermis and is tested by assessing light touch and dynamic two-point discrimination?

B. Meissner's corpuscle

All of the options are involved in skin sensation. The Meissner's corpuscle is involved in light touch and dynamic two-point discrimination. It represents a type of unmyelinated nerve ending most commonly found in the fingertips and lips. A reduction in the number of Meissner's corpuscles is observed with increasing age and may be partly responsible for age-related changes in manual dexterity.[1]

Naked nerve fibers or free nerve endings are the simplest of sensory receptors and are located along the dermoepidermal junction. They consist of multiple small terminal branches of afferent nerves and provide a primitive function for temperature, touch, and pain sensation. Merkel cells are associated with free nerve endings, particularly in thicker skin. They are also involved with constant touch and pressure sensation, providing a static two-point discrimination. Pacinian corpuscles are large sensory receptors involved in pressure, coarse touch, vibration, and tension. They are located in the deeper layers of the skin as well as in ligaments and joint capsules and have the appearance of an onion on microscopy. Pacinian corpuscles can be recognized when operating around nerve fibers and can be useful to guide dissection when trying to identify damaged or divided nerves, particularly in the palm and digits. Ruffini corpuscles are spindle shaped structures on microscopy found most often in the foot soles. They are associated with pressure and touch sensation.[2]

REFERENCES

1. Cauna N, Ross LL. The fine structure of Meissner's touch corpuscles of human fingers. J Biophys Biochem Cytol 1960;8:467–482
2. Burkitt HG, Young B, Heath JW. Wheater's Functional Histology: A Text and Colour Atlas. London: Churchill Livingstone; 2003

APPENDAGES OF THE DERMIS

4. *Which one of the following represents a dermal appendage with a primary function of thermoregulation?*

B. **Eccrine sweat gland**

Eccrine sweat glands are found within the skin throughout the body and are involved in thermoregulation by the production of watery hypotonic fluid, whereas apocrine glands produce thickened secretions in the axilla and groin. These are involved in conditions such as hidradenitis suppurativa where patients have recurrent infective episodes affecting the axilla or groin.

Ruffini endings are slow adapting mechanoreceptors found in the skin and are high in density in the nail bed region and foot sole. The bulb of Krause are bulbous capsules in the skin containing sensory nerve endings, which may be mechanoreceptors, but which are also thought to be thermoreceptors specifically sensitive to cold. They become activated by temperatures less than 20° C. They occur more superficially in the skin than heat receptors. Sebaceous glands are usually found in association with hair follicles, the so-called "pilosebaceous unit" and are responsible for the secretion of sebum. Ectopic sebaceous glands without attached follicles may be found as tiny yellow papules near mucocutaneous junctions, particularly the upper lip, and in the buccal mucosa (Fordyce's spots). They may also be found in the areolae of the breasts, where they are known as Montgomery's tubercles. Like Fordyce's spots, the sebaceous gland in a Montgomery's tubercle opens directly onto the surface.[1]

REFERENCE

1. Burkitt HG, Young B, Heath JW. Wheater's Functional Histology: A Text and Colour Atlas. London: Churchill Livingstone; 2003

LAYERS OF THE EPIDERMIS

5. *Which one of the following statements is correct regarding the epidermis?*

B. **The stratum granulosum is the only layer containing both viable and nonviable cells.**

The epidermis consists of four or five layers, depending on the anatomic location. The layers from superficial to deep may be remembered using the mnemonic "come let's get some beer." The layers are as follows: stratum corneum, stratum lucidum, stratum granulosum, stratum spinosum, and stratum basale. The upper two layers contain nonviable keratinocytes, while the deepest two layers consist only of viable keratinocytes. The stratum granulosum is the transition zone and is three to four layers thick. It contains both viable and nonviable cells. It has clinical relevance in melanomas as the Breslow thickness is measured from this layer to the deepest part of the tumor. The stratum corneum and stratum lucidum do not contain viable cells. The stratum basale is a single layer and contains melanocytes, tactile cells, granular dendrocytes, and mitotically active keratinocytes. The stratum spinosum contains only viable keratinocytes. The stratum lucidum is translucent but is not present in the axilla or face (**Fig. 16.1**).[1]

REFERENCE

1. Burkitt HG, Young B, Heath JW. Wheater's Functional Histology: A Text and Colour Atlas. London: Churchill Livingstone; 2003

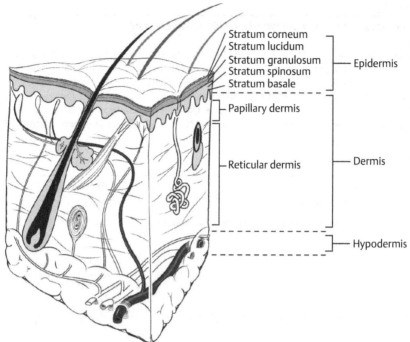

Fig. 16.1   Layers of the skin with adnexal structures.

LAYERS OF THE EPIDERMIS

6. *Which one of the following epidermal layers is only found in the hands and feet?*
   E. **Stratum corneum**
   The stratum corneum or cornified layer of the skin is only found in glabrous areas which are the sole of the foot and palm. These areas represent the thickest areas of skin and provide excellent protective function.
   Sometimes these areas are used as skin graft donor sites when palm or foot sole defects are being reconstructed. Two passes are required with the dermatome. The first pass removes the superficial layer of keratinocytes and the second removes a deeper layer used as a graft. The original layer is then replaced on the donor site.

STRUCTURE AND FUNCTION OF THE DERMIS

7. *Which one of the following statements is correct regarding the dermis?*
   E. **Ground substance facilitates diffusion of metabolites in the dermis.**
   Ground substance is an amorphous transparent material with a semifluid gel consistency. It allows metabolite diffusion and comprises glycosaminoglycans in the form of hyaluronic acid and proteoglycans. Hyaluronic acid is an important component of ground substance and is used as an injectable filler to plump out the dermis for management of rhytids, for filling contour deformities or replacing volume loss with age. The dermis comprises two layers: the more superficial papillary dermis and the deeper reticular dermis. The ratio of collagen types I to III differs according to dermal layer, with the papillary dermis having a higher concentration of type III collagen. Dermal thickness has significant variability according to the anatomic location. The scalp, back, palms, and foot soles are generally thickest and the eyelids are thinnest. The papillary dermis is much thinner than the reticular dermis (approximately 1/20th) and has a thickness more similar to the epidermis. Mature elastic fibers are only present in the reticular dermis. Understanding of the different skin layers and being able to recognize them clinically is useful when managing trauma injuries such as burns. Burns are classified according to depth and can be first degree, second degree, or third degree. First degree burns do not involve the dermis and heal quickly. Third degree burns involve the entire dermis and adnexal structures and have a prolonged healing time that means they are usually excised and skin grafted. Second degree burns can be either superficial or deep and will involve different levels of the dermis. In general, the more superficial dermal burns can heal within a few weeks because the dermal appendages are present and facilitate re-epithelialization. In deeper dermal burns this will not be possible and they are generally treated the same as full-thickness burns.

COLLAGEN SUBTYPES

8. In which anatomic location is collagen subtype II most likely to be found?

C. Hyaline cartilage

Collagen is a protein that forms the key building blocks for skin, bone, cartilage, and tendon. The basic structure consists of three left-handed polypeptide helices wound together to form a right-handed helix. Collagen comprises of two alpha-1 and one alpha-2 chains; each of these are formed by amino acid sequences, glycine-prolene-X and glycine-X-hydroxyprolene. There are more than 20 types of collagen and of these, type I represents 90% of the body total. Type II is found in the cornea and hyaline cartilage. Other important types are III and IV. Type III predominates in immature wounds, vessel, and bowel walls. Type IV is found in the basement membrane (**Table 16.1**).

Table 16.1   *Five Types of Collagen*

Type	Structure	Distribution
Type I	Hybrid of two chains	Bone
	Low in hydroxyzine and glycosylated hydroxyzine	Tendon Skin Dentin Ligament Fascia Arteries Uterus
Type II	Relatively high in hydroxyzine and glycosylated hydroxyzine	Hyaline cartilage
		Eye tissues
Type III	High in hydroxyzine	Skin
	Contains interchain disulfide bonds	Arteries
		Uterus
		Bowel wall
Type IV	High in hydroxyzine and glycosylated hydroxyzine	Basement membrane
	May contain large globular regions	
Type V	Similar to type IV	Basement membrane

SKIN DISORDERS AND WOUND HEALING

9. In which one of the following conditions it is generally acceptable to proceed with elective surgery?

B. Cutis laxa

Cutis laxa is a very rare condition associated with degeneration of elastic fibers in the dermis. The name is derived from Latin meaning "loose skin" as it results in hyperextensible skin with the appearance of premature aging. It can be autosomal dominant, recessive, or crosslinked and in general recessive inheritance results in the most severe form. It is often most noticeable on the face, neck, axilla, and groin. It can also affect connective tissues of the lungs, heart, vessels, and joints. In spite of this, wound healing is normal and it is considered safe to proceed with surgery.

In contrast, the other options are all associated with abnormal wound healing. Deficiencies in iron, copper, and vitamin C all interfere with collagen production. Cutis hyperelastica is also known as Ehlers-Danlos syndrome and is a connective tissue disorder with abnormal collagen cross-linking resulting in poor wound healing and thin friable skin. Hutchinson-Gilford and Werner's syndromes are both types of progeria (premature aging conditions) and wound healing is impaired.

CLINICAL DIAGNOSIS OF SOFT TISSUE ABNORMALITY

10. A 12-year-old girl presents with joint hypermobility; thin, fragile tissue; and subcutaneous hemorrhages. *What is the most likely diagnosis?*

C. Ehlers-Danlos syndrome

Ehlers-Danlos syndrome is also known as *Cutis hyperelastica*. It has an incidence of 1:400,000, with variable inheritance patterns. It is a connective tissue disorder with an abnormality of collagen cross-linking. This results in hypermobile joints and thin, friable, and hyperextensive skin. Patients have poor wound healing and a tendency for hypertrophic scarring. Surgery should be avoided when possible.

Cutis laxa is a rare connective tissue disorder in which the skin becomes inelastic and hangs loosely due to degeneration of elastic fibers, but healing is normal. Parkes-Weber syndrome is characterized by an extremity port-wine stain with a deeper venous and lymphatic malformation and an arteriovenous fistula.

Pseudoxanthoma elasticum is a condition with a combination of cutaneous, ocular, and cardiac manifestations. Skin manifestations include yellow plaques that typically involve the neck, first appearing in adolescence.

Progeria is a rare autosomal recessive condition with features of premature aging in children. Patients first present with signs such as failure to thrive and retarded growth.

They display abnormal skin laxity and loss of subcutaneous fat associated with poor wound healing.

CLINICAL DIAGNOSIS OF SOFT TISSUE ABNORMALITY

11. A 20-year-old patient presents with skin laxity, yellow plaques, and cardiopulmonary problems but has normal wound healing. *What is the most likely diagnosis?*

    E. Pseudoxanthoma elasticum

Pseudoxanthoma elasticum is a progressive disorder characterized by the accumulation of deposits of calcium and other minerals (mineralization) within elastin fibers. A common finding is the presence of yellow colored plaques to the neck, axillae, and flexor surfaces of joints, which first appear in adolescence. Because the mineralization can affect elastin fibers throughout the body, the manifestations of pseudoxanthoma elasticum include ocular, cardiovascular, and gastrointestinal problems.

Hutchinson-Gilford syndrome is also known as progeria, an autosomal recessive condition associated with premature aging in children. It is very rare with an incidence of 1:1,000,000 and patients first present with signs such as failure to thrive, retarded growth, craniosynostoses, micrognathia, baldness, and prominent ears. They display abnormal skin laxity and loss of subcutaneous fat associated with poor wound healing.

Cutis laxa is also known as *elastolysis* and is extremely rare with only a few hundred cases reported worldwide. It is a hypoelastic condition with degeneration of elastin fibers so the skin loses its elastic recoil and becomes hyperextensible. This gives an appearance of premature aging and is associated with an increased risk of ventral hernia and cardiopulmonary problems. However, hound healing remains normal.

Werner's syndrome (also known as adult progeria) is also a rare autosomal recessive condition with features of premature aging. Other associated features include altered skin pigmentation, microangiopathy, diabetes, scleroderma-like skin, and a high-pitched voice. Wound healing is affected by this condition and elective surgery should be preferentially avoided.

17. Basics of Plastic Surgery Wound Closure

See *Essentials of Plastic Surgery*, third edition, pp. 223–237

ACHIEVING HEMOSTASIS WITHIN WOUNDS

1. *When closing a small tension-free wound following surgery, how best should dermal bleeding be managed?*
   A. Meticulous hemostasis with bipolar forceps
   B. Meticulous hemostasis with monopolar forceps
   C. Wound closure with standard sutures
   D. Closure with multiple horizontal mattress sutures
   E. Compression bandaging after closure

WOUND CLOSURE IN INFLAMMED TISSUES

2. *In a situation where the soft tissues surrounding an open wound are inflamed, how best should the wound be managed?*
   A. Direct closure with interrupted sutures   D. Closure with a full-thickness graft
   B. Direct closure with mattress sutures   E. Allow healing by secondary intent
   C. Closure with a split skin graft

WOUND CLOSURE WITH SUTURES

3. *When closing a wound with sutures, which one of the following is true?*
   A. A set number of sutures are required per unit wound length.
   B. In general, more sutures are preferable to fewer sutures.
   C. Suture placement is unlikely to compromise tissue perfusion.
   D. Within 1 week, single layer sutures can reliably be removed.
   E. Suture tension should be set to offset tension but avoid strangulation.

SUTURE REMOVAL

4. *Following elective plastic surgery, in which one of the following body sites can sutures be safely removed earliest?*
   A. Scalp   D. Trunk
   B. Back   E. Thigh
   C. Face

WOUND HEALING

5. *What is the maximum peak tensile strength expected for a wound to reach following direct closure at 1 year?*
   A. 50%   D. 80%
   B. 60%   E. 90%
   C. 70%

MANAGEMENT OF BITE INJURIES

6. *A patient comes to the emergency (ER) department with a history of cat bite in the right hand 3 hours previously. Which one of the following is true regarding management of this injury?*
   A. This mechanism of injury carries a relatively low risk of infection.
   B. The wound edges should ideally be approximated after first debridement.
   C. A total of three doses of intravenous antibiotic should be prescribed.
   D. The wounds are likely to require multiple daily washout procedures.
   E. Such wounds are likely to need early skin grafting for wound closure.

APPROACHES TO WOUND CLOSURE

7. *Which one of the following is correct regarding delayed primary wound closure?*
   A. Final healing tends to be inferior to primary closure techniques.
   B. It most often involves application of a negative pressure dressing.
   C. It is purely indicated in cases where infection is being treated with antibiotics.
   D. The main contraindication is in the setting of a chronic wound.
   E. It generally involves sharp debridement followed by direct closure.

APPROACHES TO WOUND CLOSURE

8. *Which one of the following is true of healing by secondary intention?*
   A. It generally involves use of skin sutures or staples.
   B. It most often requires a split skin graft.
   C. It can often result in significant contraction and tissue distortion.
   D. It results in the lowest rates of overall scarring.
   E. It would be unsuitable for closure of primary surgical incisions.

SURGICAL DEBRIDEMENT

9. *When debriding a wound following trauma, in which anatomic area can the surgeon be more conservative with the debridement margins, if there is some doubt about the vascularity of the tissues?*
   A. Chest
   B. Back
   C. Face
   D. Foot
   E. Hand

WOUND MANAGEMENT

10. You have a patient in the operating room undergoing first debridement of an open limb fracture. *Which one of the following factors is probably the most important component of the wound irrigation process to optimize outcome?*
    A. The type of irrigation fluid used
    B. The surgical skin preparation used
    C. The use of loupe magnification
    D. The use of a syringe with a blunt needle
    E. The overall technique and volume of irrigation

WOUND DEBRIDEMENT

11. *When surgically debriding a wound, which one of the following tools should be avoided during the debridement process?*
    A. Scalpel
    B. Tenotomy scissors
    C. Curette
    D. Versajet
    E. Monopolar

WOUND CLOSURE WITH SUTURES

12. When supervising wound closure by new residents, you advise them to ensure the skin edges are everted. *What is the key reason for doing this?*
    A. To improve the early postoperative scar appearance
    B. To increase the dermal contact surfaces
    C. To reduce the effects of tissue strangulation
    D. To selectively deepen the final scar appearance
    E. To minimize overall tissue edge handling

BRAIDED VERSUS MONOFILAMENT SUTURES

13. *In which one of the following scenarios would a multifilament (braided) suture be indicated rather than a monofilament alternative?*
    A. When closing a wound following a dog bite injury to the limb
    B. Where suture loosening would be detrimental to final outcomes
    C. Where operating room (OR) time is restricted and the most rapid wound closure is needed
    D. Where tension distribution across the wound needs to be optimized
    E. Where long-term cosmesis is of the highest priority

WOUND CLOSURE

14. *When closing a scalp wound in a 35-year-old lady with blonde hair, which one of the following sutures would be best in terms of postoperative wound care?*
    A. Undyed Vicryl
    B. Clear Monocryl
    C. Clear prolene
    D. Blue polypropylene
    E. Black silk

WOUND CLOSURE DURING ABDOMINOPLASTY

15. *When performing wound closure during an abdominoplasty, which one of the following is true?*
    A. The choice of Monocryl versus Vicryl for the buried dermal sutures makes no difference to outcomes in terms of suture extrusion risk.
    B. Repairs of the rectus fascia (i.e., rectus plication) should ideally be performed with an absorbable suture material such as polydiaxone (PDS).
    C. Silk should be used to secure the drains as it represents the ideal suture material for this purpose due to its high friction coefficient.
    D. The transverse skin wound should be closed in two layers using a combination of absorbable sutures.
    E. When insetting the umbilicus using a monofilament permanent suture, the knots should be loose to allow for postsurgical tissue swelling.

SUTURE TECHNIQUES

16. *Which one of the following suture techniques would be most suitable when trying to partially close a circular defect to the cheek following wide excision of a skin cancer?*
    A. Three-point suture
    B. Purse string suture
    C. Figure-of-eight suture
    D. Progressive tension suture
    E. Running horizontal mattress suture

WOUND CLOSURE WITH STAPLES

17. *Which one of the following represents a key advantage of using external skin staples for final wound closure following abdominoplasty?*
    A. They decrease surgical operating time.
    B. They accommodate for postoperative swelling.
    C. They reduce patient discomfort at first wound check.
    D. They obviate the need for deeper suture placement.
    E. They result in improved scar cosmesis.

Answers

ACHIEVING HEMOSTASIS WITHIN WOUNDS

1. **When closing a small tension-free wound following surgery, how best should dermal bleeding be managed?**
   C. Wound closure with standard sutures

   Ensuring hemostasis prior to wound closure is important to minimize risk of postoperative hematoma and complications with wound healing. However, although the visible deeper tissue vessels will require meticulous hemostasis with either bipolar or monopolar forceps, the skin edge dermal bleeding does not usually require this. Instead, dermal bleeding usually stops once the dermal edges are reapproximated. Excessive cautery to the dermal edge can lead to unnecessary tissue damage and subsequent wound healing problems. Where bleeding from the wound edges persists such as in anticoagulated patients, or specific body sites such as the scalp, use of hemostatic sutures can be helpful. These include horizontal mattress sutures which serve to evert the wound edges more effectively, or running sutures which more effectively seal the entire wound edge. However, care must be taken when using such suture techniques not to strangulate the tissues and cause necrosis.

WOUND CLOSURE IN INFLAMMED TISSUES

2. **In a situation where the soft tissues surrounding an open wound are inflamed, how best should the wound be managed?**
   E. Allow healing by secondary intent

   When soft tissues are inflamed, they tend to be more fragile and less resilient to manipulation and even careful tissue handling. Prolonged or intense inflammation can cause injury to viable tissues, resulting in failure for the wound to progress in terms of healing.[1] Furthermore, independent of etiology, local edema impedes cell signaling and cell migration, thereby disrupting normal immunological processes essential to wound healing. It is generally accepted that meticulous tissue handling is vital, especially in such circumstances, and that where tissue is inflamed, direct wound closure should be avoided or postponed.

REFERENCE

1. Janis JE, Kwon RK, Lalonde DH. A practical guide to wound healing. Plast Reconstr Surg 2010;125(6):230e–244e

WOUND CLOSURE WITH SUTURES

3. **When closing a wound with sutures, which one of the following is true?**
   E. Suture tension should be set to offset tension but avoid strangulation.

   When suturing wounds, there is a fine balance to be achieved between the provision of adequate support for the healing wound, and avoiding an excess of sutures which may cause vascular compromise or scarring to the wound edges. In addition, the duration of support must be sufficient to facilitate wound healing. For this reason, a safe guide is to adequately offset tension with enough sutures and avoid either overtightening them or placing too many of them such that vascular compromise at the wound edge occurs. There are no set numbers of sutures required to close a given wound length although there may be rules of thumb. In most delicate areas such as the face, placement of sutures 5–10 mm apart is usually satisfactory. They may be placed slightly further apart in the trunk and limbs. Placing them closer will only serve to restrict wound edge blood supply. If there remains obvious gapping, then additional sutures may be selectively placed to address this. When considering timing for suture removal, wound strength needs to be considered. For example, at 1 week it is estimated that the newly healing wound will only have 3% of its previous strength and should therefore be supported further with sutures. The exception to this rule is where deeper sutures have also been placed and this can facilitate early removal of the superficial external sutures. Unwisely placed sutures can cause local tissue damage and ischemia. Avoiding excessive compression at the wound edge is especially critical when reapproximating a "tip" or "corner" of a skin flap or where there is pre-existing vascular compromise. Sutures should not be overtightened as this can further compromise wound edge vascularity.

SUTURE REMOVAL

4. **Following elective plastic surgery, in which one of the following body sites can sutures be safely removed earliest?**
   C. Face

   The timing of suture removal following surgery will be dependent on a number of factors including wound type (size, location, chronicity, vascularity, wound tension) and general patient factors (systemic disease, age, nutrition, recent infection, and smoking history). Furthermore, it will depend on sutures used, for example, whether deeper dermal sutures have been placed or not. However, it is generally accepted that sutures may be removed at fairly consistent times post wound closure with predictable results.

Sutures are normally removed earlier from areas where vascularity is highest and where cosmesis is most critical such as the central face. For this reason, sutures can be removed from the periorbital, cheek, lip, and chin areas early, e.g., 4–7 days post surgery. Ideally, there will be deeper absorbable sutures supporting the wound beyond this timeframe unless the skin is particularly thin like the upper eyelid, where a single layer closure is safe and effective. Sutures in the scalp can also be removed fairly early and 7–10 days is typical for this body site, although again deeper support may still be required. Sutures are left longer in other areas such as the trunk and limbs (2–3 weeks typically). The downside to leaving them longer is that suture marks are left on the skin. For this reason, many plastic surgeons have a preference for using buried sutures, such as a running subcuticular, on the trunk and limbs (**Table 17.1**).

Table 17.1   *Timing for Suture Removal*

Location	Timing
Scalp	1–2 weeks
Face	4–7 days
Trunk	2 weeks
Extremities	2 weeks

WOUND HEALING

5. *What is the maximum peak tensile strength expected for a wound to reach following direct closure at 1 year?*
   D. 80%
   Following wound closure, there ensues a process of scar maturation and remodeling as collagen fibers realign and progressively change in ratio of type III to type I subtypes. By 3 months the wound should have reached a fairly steady state in terms of new collagen formation and turnover, but may still undergo further maturation until 1 year. Peak tensile strength is normally reached at approximately 90 days (80% preinjury strength) and ultimately determined by the quality and quantity of collagen. It never reaches 100% of the preinjury of presurgery status.

MANAGEMENT OF BITE INJURIES

6. A patient comes to the emergency (ER) department with a history of cat bite in the right hand 3 hours previously. *Which one of the following is true regarding management of this injury?*
   D. The wounds are likely to require multiple daily washout procedures.
   All bite injuries should be thoroughly debrided as early as possible due to the fact that animals and humans carry a high volume of bacteria within the mouth so bite injuries have a high chance of developing wound infection. Although in some carefully debrided human and dog bite wounds loose approximation of the wound edges is an acceptable practice, this is not appropriate in cat bites which tend to be small, but deeply penetrating injuries that have a high risk of associated infection. For this reason, they warrant aggressive early intervention with formal debridement, copious irrigation, and should then be left open to heal by secondary intent. Cat bites can be quite resistant to treatment and daily review with wound irrigation and continued antibiotics are the mainstay of treatment. Due to the small wound size (as feline teeth are small), it would be extremely unusual to require skin grafting. Human and dog bites should also be debrided and irrigated early after presentation to the ER, and antibiotics commenced immediately. Bites affecting the face which are well vascularized (and also cosmetically sensitive) should generally be closed directly, if possible, at the time of initial debridement. Many surgeons prefer leaving bite injuries elsewhere on the body, such as the trunk and limbs, open with at most some loose tacking sutures or none at all to minimize the risk of infection.

APPROACHES TO WOUND CLOSURE

7. *Which one of the following is correct regarding delayed primary wound closure?*
   E. It generally involves sharp debridement followed by direct closure.
   Delayed primary closure is where a wound, which may be subacute or chronic, is converted to an acute wound by sharp debridement back to healthy viable tissues. Following this delayed debridement, the wound can be treated as an acute wound and closed directly, providing there is sufficient tissue laxity to do so. This approach may be indicated in wounds which are edematous at presentation, or those which have been contaminated or recently infected. For example, during limb fasciotomies in a trauma setting, the wounds can be left open for a few days until soft tissue swelling has reduced, then closed directly. Sometimes in the situation where a leg has a medial

and lateral wound, the medial wound can be closed by delayed primary closure, but the lateral wound will still require a split skin graft. This will depend on many factors related to both the wounds themselves and the patient. Other wounds that may be treated well with delayed primary closure are those where infection has been present, but is no longer active. This can be undertaken providing there is sufficient soft tissue laxity and the tissues are sufficiently pliable. Otherwise allowing to heal by secondary intention or skin grafting may be required.

The final outcome following delayed primary healing is comparable to primary closure of a wound and is generally a preferable approach to flap or graft closure in terms of long-term function and cosmesis.

Negative pressure dressings are useful to temporize larger wounds after their initial debridement until definitive wound closure is performed. Therefore, they sometimes have a role in the process of delayed primary closure, for example, in open tibial fractures where primary closure is delayed to allow soft tissues to recover from the initial injury and swelling to reduce. The benefit of the negative pressure dressing in this setting is that it maintains a closed wound environment in the interim between first debridement and final closure.

APPROACHES TO WOUND CLOSURE

8. *Which one of the following is true of healing by secondary intention?*

C. It can often result in significant contraction and tissue distortion.

Healing by secondary intention is where a wound is allowed to heal on its own by contraction, granulation, and epithelialization. It does not involve sutures or skin grafts. This modality can be very useful in some cases where there is insufficient tissue laxity for direct closure or where there has been tissue damage and/or infection where it is not ideal to seal the wound early. It is therefore used for closure of primary surgical wounds as well as wounds in the emergency setting. In some situations, healing by secondary intent will give a good cosmetic outcome and one which is superior to skin grafting. For example, small wounds on the scalp tend to do well with healing by secondary intent as do some on the lower limb after removal of small skin cancers. The classic example of good healing by secondary intent is the donor site of a paramedian forehead flap when used for nasal reconstruction. The main reason this is preferable to a graft in the longer term is that the use of a graft leaves a depression where the graft is inset. In contrast, during the process of secondary intent, the healing wound fills with granulation tissue such that there is usually no contour defect once healing is complete. The other obvious benefit for allowing healing by secondary intent is that it avoids a donor graft site. However, not all cases are well suited to healing by secondary intention because it results in contraction of the wound edges and can lead to quite significant distortion of tissues. This can be quite marked in areas such as the lower eyelid where an ectropion can develop, or around the nose where distortion of the alar and nostrils can occur. It is important to explain to patients before surgery that the process will be quite drawn out and their wound is likely to take at least 6–8 weeks to fully heal depending on site and size.

SURGICAL DEBRIDEMENT

9. *When debriding a wound following trauma, in which anatomic area can the surgeon be more conservative with the debridement margins, if there is some doubt about the vascularity of the tissues?*

C. Face

When surgically managing a wound following trauma, it is important to ensure removal of all potentially nonviable/damaged tissue as well as foreign material. Therefore, the surgeon should sharply debride grossly nonviable tissue and ragged skin edges prior to reapproximation of the wound edges. For facial wounds and cosmetically sensitive areas, one should err on the side of leaving marginal appearing tissue behind. This is because the scalp and face have a rich vascular supply and the skin and soft tissues tend to tolerate insult better than within other anatomic regions. Furthermore, there tends to be less excess tissue (except in the elderly patient) and also the tissue can be quite specialized (e.g., lips, nose and eyelids); so it should be preserved, if at all possible. This is particularly important when taking infants and children to operating theater even for animal bite injuries.

WOUND MANAGEMENT

10. You have a patient in the operating room undergoing first debridement of an open limb fracture. *Which one of the following factors is probably the most important component of the wound irrigation process to optimize outcome?*

E. The overall technique and volume of irrigation

Ensuring thorough wound irrigation is key to the proper management of traumatic soft tissue wounds prior to definitive wound closure. The most important element of this process is the technique used by the operating surgeon, rather than choice of irrigation fluid. This means that sufficient irrigation volume needs to be used with adequate pressure to facilitate satisfactory removal of foreign bodies and gross contamination. Of course, irrigation alone is not a substitute for surgical debridement in the presence of necrotic tissue or biofilm. The two processes go together.

The fluid options for irrigation include sterile water, normal saline, hydrogen peroxide, chlorhexidine and iodine-based products. However, there is little evidence to support the use of one lavage fluid over another. By tradition, surgeons tend to use normal saline as the lavage fluid of choice, although sterile water or iodine-based substances are also each regularly used for wound irrigation.

In terms of skin preparation, both iodine- and chlorhexidine-based skin preparations are effective, although there is conflicting evidence on which is superior. What is known definitively is that alcohol-based skin preparations are superior to those that are not alcohol based. For this reason, many units will use this as their first-line skin preparation agent in open fracture management.[1,2] (Note that care should be taken when using hydrogen peroxide or chlorhexidine close to the eyes as these can potentially cause ocular damage.)

The use of loupe magnification is standard practice for plastic surgeons and this helps the surgeon to identify small foreign body particles and accurately assess the viability of wound margins. However, this alone is not the most important factor in irrigation or debridement.

For small wounds, using a blunt tipped needle on a syringe is sometimes favored for irrigation to increase driving pressure of the irrigate, but again, this alone is not the key factor in optimizing the outcome. Indeed, it should not be assumed that higher pressures will necessarily improve wound irrigation as one study has shown. In this multicenter randomized control trial, a low pressure lavage was effective in reducing infection, wound healing problems, and nonunion in open fracture wounds.[3]

REFERENCES

1. Global Guidelines for the Prevention of Surgical Site Infection. Geneva: World Health Organization; 2018. Web Appendix 8, Summary of a systematic literature review on surgical site preparation. Available from: https://www.ncbi.nlm.nih.gov/books/NBK536434/
2. Davies BM, Patel HC. Systematic review and meta-analysis of preoperative antisepsis with combination chlorhexidine and povidone-iodine. Surg J (NY) 2016;2(3):e70–e77
3. Petrisor B, Sun X, Bhandari M, et al; FLOW Investigators. Fluid lavage of open wounds (FLOW): a multicenter, blinded, factorial pilot trial comparing alternative irrigating solutions and pressures in patients with open fractures. J Trauma 2011;71(3):596–606

WOUND DEBRIDEMENT

11. *When surgically debriding a wound, which one of the following tools should be avoided during the debridement process?*

    E. Monopolar

Debridement is a term used to describe the removal of all nonviable tissue and foreign material from a wound to return it to a healthy wound bed that should be suitable for wound closure. Surgical debridement is performed either in operating theater or in the ward using a range of different surgical instruments. These include a scalpel, scissors, curette, rongeur, or hydrosurgical device, such as a Versajet. The aim is to achieve the following end points:

- Healthy skin edges with bleeding, dense dermis
- Viable, soft, yellow subcutaneous fat
- Solid tendon substance
- Red bleeding muscle
- Hard, healthy bone with pinpoint bleeding, or "paprika sign"

Debridement should ideally be performed with no tourniquet (if working on a limb) and with sharp, progressive, tissue removal so that continued assessment of viability is possible. If viability of the tissue is in question, either more should be resected or reconstruction should be delayed to allow time for demarcation of nonviable tissue. For this reason, monopolar is not recommended for debridement as this will mask dermal and wound edge bleeding, thereby making accurate assessment of tissue viability more difficult. Furthermore, the electrocautery can further damage wound edges secondary to thermal injury. Instead, sharp debridement should be performed and once done, electrocautery can be used to control bleeding as required. It should also be remembered that debridement does not only need to be surgical, but can be chemical or mechanical and in some cases these approaches are favored.

WOUND CLOSURE WITH SUTURES

12. *When supervising wound closure by new residents, you advise them to ensure the skin edges are everted. What is the key reason for doing this?*

    B. To increase the dermal contact surfaces

When closing skin wounds, it is important to ensure that the wound edges are everted. This serves to increase the amount of dermal contact, i.e., surface area for skin healing. Eversion can be achieved by both buried and epidermal sutures, whether simple or mattress techniques are used. This is achieved by passing the needle in such a way that more dermal tissue is captured at the depths than at the surface. Eversion of the skin edges will, however, result in a poorer early cosmetic result as it leaves a ridged appearance often described as a "pasty" or "Cornish pasty" look where pastry is squeezed into a ridge. This is only a temporary finding and will settle with time. It is important therefore to advise patients of this prior to and following surgery that it is intended and will settle. This can help reduce their anxiety about early wound appearances. This ridge should ultimately lead to less dehiscence, less scar widening, and better cosmesis. An important consideration when closing skin wounds is to minimize strangulation of tissues and thus disrupting local blood supply. Eversion, per se, does not cause strangulation of tissues but certain techniques such as mattress sutures can increase strangulation as can poor or excessive suture placement. Creating wound eversion will not affect the tissue handling providing it is done carefully with respect to the tissues. In cases where it is desirable to deepen the final scar appearance as may be the case in some nasolabial fold closures, the use of an inverting suture would be preferable, but everting would not help in this situation.

BRAIDED VERSUS MONOFILAMENT SUTURES

13. *In which one of the following scenarios would a multifilament (braided) suture be indicated rather than a monofilament alternative?*
    B. Where suture loosening would be detrimental to final outcomes

    There are a number of advantages and disadvantages to both monofilament and braided sutures, so it is important that surgeons have a good understanding of these in order to select the most appropriate suture material for a given situation. In general, braided or multifilament sutures have good handling characteristics, with good pliability, low memory, and secure knot strength. Therefore, in the situation described they would be ideal where loosening of knots would be detrimental to overall outcome. In contrast, monofilament sutures are more likely to have slippage of knots due to their smooth surface. That does not mean that monofilament sutures will be unsuitable for permanent repairs, although in theory, the knots will be less secure. For example, monofilament sutures remain popular in flexor tendon repair, but in this situation a high number of throws are passed on the knot to minimize slippage post surgery.

    The disadvantages of braided sutures include a higher coefficient of friction and hence increased drag and tissue damage with each pass of the thread, and a theoretical increase in risk of infection due to their higher surface area, capillarity, and inflammatory potential. For this reason, they would be best avoided in the context of a dog bite wound closure to the limb. Usually, there is no significant difference in terms of wound closure speed with a monofilament versus a multifilament suture. This probably is affected only by surgeon's preference and experience. If more rapid wound closure is required or where more even tension distribution is required, a barbed suture may be advantageous as it can potentially achieve both.

WOUND CLOSURE

14. *When closing a scalp wound in a 35-year-old lady with blonde hair, which one of the following sutures would be best in terms of postoperative wound care?*
    D. Blue Polypropylene

    When placing sutures, it is important to consider postoperative wound management and general aftercare. Often surgeons may place sutures without giving much thought to their subsequent removal. Therefore, when placing sutures in long hair of the scalp, it is wise to select a color that will be easily visible for both the surgeon placing them and the individual removing them down the line. In addition, it is helpful to leave the sutures longer than usual to facilitate this. Therefore, a colored suture such as blue polypropylene is well suited to this scenario. Although silk is easily visible, it is not a good choice for skin closure due to its reactivity.

WOUND CLOSURE DURING ABDOMINOPLASTY

15. *When performing wound closure during an abdominoplasty, which one of the following is true?*
    D. The transverse skin wound should be closed in two layers using a combination of absorbable sutures.

    When closing skin wounds, it is normally recommended to do so with a two-layer approach involving a series of sutures placed in the dermis with deep buried knots (sometimes called deep dermal) followed by either a subcutaneous continuous suture (which can be either absorbable or nonabsorbable), or an external suture (which again can be either absorbable or nonabsorbable). This helps to distribute tension across the wound and allows for nonabsorbable sutures to be removed early and thereby reduce the risk of suture track marks. Although Monocryl and Vicryl have similar qualities and are often used in similar settings, there is some evidence that deep absorbable sutures with Monocryl demonstrate less extrusion than polyglactin 910 (Vicryl). Sutures placed in the deep fascia, tendons, or cartilage are preferentially made with nonabsorbable suture material. In the setting of a rectus plication, it is best to use either long-acting resorbable or permanent suture, as use of a rapidly absorbable suture will not provide the desired long-term outcome in terms of soft tissue support. In contrast, buried skin sutures and superficial fascial sutures should be of an absorbable type.

Although the use of silk sutures for securing drains to the skin is a widely practiced technique among surgeons in all disciplines (because of its high friction coefficient and grip on materials), it increases the local inflammatory response and the surface can harbor more bacteria. With proper technique, monofilament suture material (Nylon, polypropylene, etc.) will reliably secure drains, so consideration of these for drain fixation should be given. When insetting the umbilicus using a monofilament permanent or braided nonpermanent sutures, the knots should be tightened to be snug, but not loose nor overly tight as it is important to allow for postoperative soft tissue swelling without compromising wound edge vascularity. Furthermore, it may be beneficial to use a half-buried mattress in this setting as this will enable the knots to be buried on the inside of the umbilicus and therefore any scarring from the suture will be less visible post surgery.[1]

REFERENCE

1. ElHawary H, Abdelhamid K, Meng F, Janis JE. A comprehensive, evidence-based literature review of the surgical treatment of rectus diastasis. Plast Reconstr Surg 2020;146(5):1151–1164

SUTURE TECHNIQUES

16. *Which one of the following suture techniques would be most suitable when trying to partially close a circular defect to the cheek following wide excision of a skin cancer?*

    B. **Purse string suture**

    A purse string suture is used to reduce the size of a circular defect that cannot be closed directly. It involves using a continuous subcuticular suture around the edge of the defect and tightening it to reduce the overall internal wound length. Such an approach is useful to allow healing by secondary intention or reduce the size of skin graft required.

    A three-point suture is indicated for use as a corner suture in many situations. One example is when closing a Wise pattern breast reduction. The lower medial and lateral skin flap corners are sutured to one another and then sutured to the inframammary fold as a single suture. This is usually performed as a buried dermal suture. A figure-of-eight suture is typically indicated for closure of fascia, muscle, or tendon, rather than skin. There is less chance of cutting through the tissues with such a suture compared with a standard interrupted suture of similar equivalent material. It is also effective at obtaining hemostasis, for example, where bleeding is through a muscle and the precise bleeding point is not easily identified. Progressive tension sutures are useful when closing large subcutaneous skin flaps such as an abdominoplasty as they distribute tension to multiple points and help obliterate dead space. The horizontal mattress suture is used to close the skin where significant eversion is required, such as when closing the palm after fasciectomy. The running horizontal mattress distributes the coaptive tension of the suture along a greater length of the wound and is indicated where the wound edges are friable.

WOUND CLOSURE WITH STAPLES

17. *Which one of the following represents a key advantage of using external skin staples for final wound closure following abdominoplasty?*

    A. **They decrease surgical operating time.**

    Externally placed skin staples have a number of potential advantages for wound closure. First, they are rapid to use and can therefore help reduce operating times compared with suture placement, particularly in long wounds such as abdominoplasty or brachioplasty. They are also useful as they evert the wound edges well and therefore should result in good healing due to dermal apposition and are also hemostatic, so are well suited for use in the scalp. In addition, they have a high tensile strength and low reactivity with low rates of infection. The downside to using skin clips is that their removal in clinic following surgery is time consuming and patients can find them uncomfortable or painful to remove. This is often the case where wounds are slightly inflamed or swollen or where the staples are not fully opened before attempted removal. In contrast, buried subcuticular continuous sutures such as Monocryl for the same closure would have taken longer time in the OR, but will avoid the need for any removal in clinic, saving time and completely avoiding patient discomfort. Furthermore, if staples are left for too long, they will leave permanent markings on the skin as do skin sutures (i.e., railroad track). This is in part because of their shape and the fact that there is no give in the metal staple to allow for expansion secondary to swelling.

    Skin staples have an excellent place in plastic surgery for "tailor tacking" temporary wound closure in procedures such as breast reduction, reconstruction, and mastopexy as they provide a rapid means of closure for the operating surgeon to trial close wounds intraoperatively. Otherwise they are probably best reserved for use in the scalp for definitive wound closure.[1-4]

REFERENCES

1. Cochetti G, Abraha I, Randolph J, et al. Surgical wound closure by staples or sutures? Systematic review. Medicine (Baltimore) 2020;99(25):e20573
2. Regula CG, Yag-Howard C. Suture products and techniques: what to use, where, and why. Dermatol Surg 2015;41(Suppl 10):S187–S200
3. Khan AN, Dayan PS, Miller S, Rosen M, Rubin DH. Cosmetic outcome of scalp wound closure with staples in the pediatric emergency department: a prospective, randomized trial. Pediatr Emerg Care 2002;18(3):171–173
4. Krishnan R, MacNeil SD, Malvankar-Mehta MS. Comparing sutures versus staples for skin closure after orthopaedic surgery: systematic review and meta-analysis. BMJ Open 2016;6(1):e009257

18. Scars and Scar Management

See *Essentials of Plastic Surgery*, third edition, pp. 238–245

FETAL WOUND HEALING

1. *What is the key difference between the processes of fetal versus adult wound healing?*
   A. Healing occurs by regeneration
   B. Healing occurs by maturation
   C. Healing occurs by repair
   D. Healing occurs with inflammation
   E. Healing occurs with epithelialization

FETAL WOUND HEALING

2. *Which one of the following growth factors is found in high concentration within the fetal healing process and is believed to be key to the scarless repairs seen in utero?*
   A. Interleukin-8 (IL-8)
   B. Interleukin-10 (IL-10)
   C. Vascular endothelial growth factor (VEGF)
   D. Transforming growth factor beta (TGF-β1)
   E. Transforming growth factor beta (TGF-β3)

HYPERTROPHIC AND KELOID SCARRING

3. *What is the key clinical finding which will differentiate a keloid from a hypertrophic scar?*
   A. The color relative to the surrounding skin
   B. The overall size of the scar
   C. The chronicity of the scar
   D. The growth relative to the original scar border
   E. The mechanism of injury preceding the scar

SCAR ASSESSMENT

4. You have been asked to assess a scar in clinic with either the Vancouver scar score, or the Patient and Observer Scar Assessment Scale (POSAS). *What would be the key advantage of using the POSAS score in this instance?*
   A. It considers scar pigmentation
   B. It considers scar vascularity
   C. It considers scar thickness
   D. It considers scar pliability
   E. It considers the patient's opinion

SCAR IMPROVEMENT

5. A patient is seen in clinic with poor early scarring following plastic surgery 3 weeks previously. *Which one of the following topical agents would be most likely to help improve scar quality?*
   A. Vitamin E
   B. Onion extract (Quercetin)
   C. Silicone
   D. Anti-transforming growth factor-β1 (anti-TGF-β1) antibodies
   E. 5-Fluocouracil

SCAR MANAGEMENT

6. *Which one of the following treatment modalities may be particularly useful for improving scar appearance and contour in irradiated fields?*
   A. Steroid injection
   B. Fat transfer
   C. Bleomycin
   D. Scar massage
   E. Hyaluronic acid

POSTSURGICAL SCAR MANAGEMENT

7. *Which one of the following adjunctive treatment modalities is used to improve scar quality by causing destruction of small blood vessels leading to tissue ischemia and altered fibroblast activity?*
   A. Pulsed dye laser
   B. CO_2 laser
   C. Intense pulsed light (IPL)
   D. Anti-TGF-β1 antibodies
   E. Alexandrite laser

POSTSURGERY SCAR MANAGEMENT

8. *Which one of the following should patients be advised to undertake following surgery to help them optimize their final scar quality?*
   A. To wear sunscreen from day 5 post surgery
   B. To avoid sunscreen for the first 6 months post surgery
   C. To commence regular scar massage from 2–3 weeks post surgery
   D. To wear sunscreen 18 months post surgery
   E. To wear a pressure garment daily for 6 months post surgery

KELOID TREATMENT

9. *Which one of the following is true regarding keloid scar management?*
   A. Steroid treatment alone would be completely ineffective at reducing scar appearance.
   B. Surgical excision alone has recurrence rate of 90%.
   C. Surgical excision with steroid injection has recurrence rate of 75%.
   D. Surgical excision with postoperative radiation therapy has recurrence rate of 5%.
   E. Radiation therapy dosage for keloid scars is typically 15–30 Gy over 3 doses.

Answers

FETAL WOUND HEALING

1. *What is the key difference between the processes of fetal versus adult wound healing?*

  A. Healing occurs by regeneration

  The process of wound healing differs markedly in utero compared with life after birth. In the first and second trimesters, fetal wounds heal by regeneration and without scarring. In contrast adult healing occurs via a series of processes starting with hemostasis, followed by inflammation, cellular proliferation, and remodeling. This process results in the formation of scar tissue to replace lost or damaged tissue. At the skin level this is seen as a visible linear scar, for example, after direct wound closure. As a result of this knowledge, there has been much research into the process of fetal wound healing in order to help adults ultimately achieve scarless wound healing. Thus far, however, this objective has never been met and we have, at best, approaches that minimize scar tissue formation by reducing inflammation, tissue loss, and improving the remodeling phase. Such modalities include steroid injection, scar massage, laser therapy, and radiotherapy.[1]

REFERENCE

1. Rolfe KJ, Grobbelaar OA. A review of fetal scarless healing. ISRN Dermatol 2012;1–9:698034

FETAL WOUND HEALING

2. *Which one of the following growth factors is found in high concentration within the fetal healing process and is believed to be key to the scarless repairs seen in utero?*

  E. Transforming growth factor (TGF)-β3

  The process of wound healing in fetal tissue differs significantly from adult healing in a number of ways. Research into the differences to identify the reason/s has shown that there are different ratios of TGF-β subtypes, namely, that TGF-β3 is seen in much higher quantities in fetal tissue compared with adults. Furthermore, TGF-β1 and TGF-β2 are found in low concentration in fetal wounds whereas they are increased in adult healing wounds. The TGF-β family has multiple functions in both tissue repair and scarring. The addition of TGF-β3 to a wound model has been shown to decrease scar formation.[1,2] It has roles in both fibroblast migration and proliferation. In contrast, TGF-β1 and TGF-β2 are considered to be profibrotic.

  Fetal healing displays many other differences including reduced immune cell activation, and lower cytokine and growth factor levels, which lead to lower inflammation. Specifically, there is decreased expression of interleukins, interleukin (IL)-6, -8, and -10. In addition, there is a higher expression of hyaluronic acid, altered collagen cross linking, and increased levels of matrix metalloproteinases (MMPs). Myofibroblasts are present but have a transitory appearance. The role that angiogenesis and vascular endothelial growth factor (VEGF) have in scar formation remains unclear but it is generally accepted that both are reduced in fetal scarless repair. VEGF is important in endothelial cell proliferation.

REFERENCES

1. Rolfe KJ, Grobbelaar OA. A review of fetal scarless healing. ISRN Dermatol Volume, 2012;1–9:698034
2. Shah M, Foreman DM, Ferguson MW. Neutralisation of TGF-beta 1 and TGF-beta 2 or exogenous addition of TGF-beta 3 to cutaneous rat wounds reduces scarring. J Cell Sci 1995;108(Pt 3):985–1002

HYPERTROPHIC AND KELOID SCARRING

3. *What is the key clinical finding which will differentiate a keloid from a hypertrophic scar?*

  D. The growth relative to the original scar border

  Following injury and complete healing, the ideal scar will be subtle to visualize, be soft, smooth, and similarly colored and textured to the adjacent uninjured tissues. Ideally scars will be barely visible. In reality scarring can be considered to be on a spectrum with model scarring at one end and extremely poor scarring at the other. Poor scarring may involve tissue thickening or thinning, scar stretch, abnormal pigmentation (either hypo- or hyperpigmentation), and patient discomfort leading to functional as well as aesthetic concerns. At one extreme there lies keloid scarring, where poor features are seen as just described extending beyond the original zone of injury. Further along the scar spectrum lies hypertrophic scarring, which may too have many of the poor features described within the confines of injured tissue. It is this key finding that differentiates keloid from hypertrophic scarring, the extension of the keloid scar beyond the initial scar edge. Keloids grow like a soft tissue tumor and are thus essentially scar growths rather than poor scars alone. They can continue to grow for weeks, months, or even years after the original injury. In contrast, a hypertrophic scar may have many similar features of a keloid clinically but will remain within the borders of the original scar and will not grow further over time.

Keloid scars tend to occur on specific body sites including the sternum following chest wall surgery, and on the ear after ear piercing or surgery. Hypertrophic scars tend to occur on the knees, ankles, and other areas of high tension wound closure, or following burn injury treated with skin grafting or secondary intention healing.

SCAR ASSESSMENT

4. You have been asked to assess a scar in clinic with either the Vancouver scar score, or the Patient and Observer Scar Assessment Scale (POSAS). *What would be the key advantage of using the POSAS score in this instance?*

    E. It considers the patient's opinion

    Being able to evaluate a scar using a scoring system can be useful for a given scar to compare the effects before and after treatment, and also to compare scars between patients and different treatment modalities within a research setting. There are a number of different scoring systems described, including the Vancouver score and the Patient and Observer Scar Assessment Scale (POSAS). The Vancouver score involves a clinician's assessment of the following points: vascularity, pigmentation, pliability, and thickness or height. The POSAS also considers vascularity, pigmentation, pliability, and thickness or height from the clinician's perspective, as well as surface area and overall opinion on scar. The patient assessment considers pain, itching, color, stiffness, thickness, irregularity, and overall opinion. Other commonly used scar assessment tools include the Visual Analog Scale (VAS) and Stony Brook Scar Evaluation Scale (SBSES).[1,2]

REFERENCES

1. Fearmonti R, Bond J, Erdmann D, Levinson H. A review of scar scales and scar measuring devices. Eplasty 2010;10:e43
2. Draaijers LJ, Tempelman FR, Botman YA, et al. The patient and observer scar assessment scale: a reliable and feasible tool for scar evaluation. Plast Reconstr Surg 2004;113(7):1960–1965, discussion 1966–1967

SCAR IMPROVEMENT

5. A patient is seen in clinic with poor early scarring following plastic surgery 3 weeks previously. *Which one of the following topical agents would be most likely to help improve scar quality?*

    C. Silicone

    Silicone is used topically for scar management in either sheet or gel forms. The medical form used for scars is polydimethylsiloxane. Application should ideally be started 1–2 weeks after surgery once the wound has completely epithelialized, and continued for at least 3 months following this. It is thought that silicone works by improving scar hydration and can decrease fibroblast activity. In addition, it may act by scar warming, leading to increased collagenase activity and by applying a static negative charge leading to tissue polarization. It is proven to decrease the formation of hypertrophic scar after surgery and help improve established hypertrophic scars too.[1,2,3] Vitamin E causes mild inhibition of collagen synthesis but most studies show no real efficacy in scar improvement.[4,5,6] Onion extract is the main active ingredient in Mederma (Merz Pharmaceuticals, Raleigh, NC). This is thought to inhibit fibroblast proliferation, inhibit histamine, and upregulate matrix metalloproteinase with improved collagen organization. However, clinical evidence on effectiveness for hypertrophic scar prevention and scar improvement is mixed.[7,8,9] Anti-TGF-β1 antibodies do not represent a topical agent but are injected into the scar. Although they have been effective in animal models, they have not been shown to be effective in humans.[10,11,12] 5-Fluocouracil inhibits fibroblast proliferation and can be effective in the treatment of hypertrophic scars and keloids when combined with steroids and pulsed dye laser (PDL) as well as in its role in treatment of actinic keratosis. However, it can lead to skin ulceration and pain.[13]

REFERENCES

1. Gold MH, Foster TD, Adair MA, Burlison K, Lewis T. Prevention of hypertrophic scars and keloids by the prophylactic use of topical silicone gel sheets following a surgical procedure in an office setting. Dermatol Surg 2001;27(7):641–644
2. Kim SM, Choi JS, Lee JH, Kim YJ, Jun YJ. Prevention of postsurgical scars: comparsion of efficacy and convenience between silicone gel sheet and topical silicone gel. J Korean Med Sci 2014;29(Suppl 3):S249–S253
3. Chan KY, Lau CL, Adeeb SM, Somasundaram S, Nasir-Zahari M. A randomized, placebo-controlled, double-blind, prospective clinical trial of silicone gel in prevention of hypertrophic scar development in median sternotomy wound. Plast Reconstr Surg 2005;116(4):1013–1020, discussion 1021–1022
4. Ehrlich HP, Tarver H, Hunt TK. Inhibitory effects of vitamin E on collagen synthesis and wound repair. Ann Surg 1972;175(2):235–240
5. Baumann LS, Spencer J. The effects of topical vitamin E on the cosmetic appearance of scars. Dermatol Surg 1999;25(4):311–315

6. Khoo TL, Halim AS, Zakaria Z, Mat Saad AZ, Wu LY, Lau HY. A prospective, randomised, double-blinded trial to study the efficacy of topical tocotrienol in the prevention of hypertrophic scars. J Plast Reconstr Aesthet Surg 2011;64(6):e137–e145

7. Chanprapaph K, Tanrattanakorn S, Wattanakrai P, Wongkitisophon P, Vachiramon V. Effectiveness of onion extract gel on surgical scars in asians. Dermatol Res Pract 2012;2012:212945

8. Jenwitheesuk K, Surakunprapha P, Jenwitheesuk K, Kuptarnond C, Prathanee S, Intanoo W. Role of silicone derivative plus onion extract gel in presternal hypertrophic scar protection: a prospective randomized, double blinded, controlled trial. Int Wound J 2012;9(4):397–402

9. Cho JW, Cho SY, Lee SR, Lee KS. Onion extract and quercetin induce matrix metalloproteinase-1 in vitro and in vivo. Int J Mol Med 2010;25(3):347–352

10. Saulis AS, Mogford JH, Mustoe TA. Effect of Mederma on hypertrophic scarring in the rabbit ear model. Plast Reconstr Surg 2002;110(1):177–183, discussion 184–186

11. Denton CP, Merkel PA, Furst DE, et al; Cat-192 Study Group; Scleroderma Clinical Trials Consortium. Recombinant human anti-transforming growth factor beta1 antibody therapy in systemic sclerosis: a multicenter, randomized, placebo-controlled phase I/II trial of CAT-192. Arthritis Rheum 2007;56(1):323–333

12. Walmsley GG, Maan ZN, Wong VW, et al. Scarless wound healing: chasing the holy grail. Plast Reconstr Surg 2015;135(3):907–917

13. Asilian A, Darougheh A, Shariati F. New combination of triamcinolone, 5-Fluorouracil, and pulsed-dye laser for treatment of keloid and hypertrophic scars. Dermatol Surg 2006;32(7):907–915

SCAR MANAGEMENT

6. Which one of the following treatment modalities may be particularly useful for improving scar appearance and contour in irradiated fields?

   B. Fat transfer

   Fat transfer has become very popular in a number of body sites for increasing tissue volume and contour irregularities, particularly within breast tissue and the reconstructed breast. Fat is obtained from a distant body site, most commonly the abdomen, flanks, or thighs, and reinjected at the recipient site. This approach has found widespread use in breast after wide local excision and radiotherapy for breast cancer. Initially it was intended as a contour filler, but it has been found that the scar quality also improves following this treatment. The precise mechanism for this is not known, but it is thought that the fat cell solution also contains adipose derived stem cells which induce neoangiogenesis. Both fat grafts and adipose derived stem cells have been shown to improve scar pliability in irradiated fields as well as their volumetric effect on depressed scars.[1] Corticosteroids have a major role in scar management but not specifically in irradiated tissue. They are often part of a multimodality approach to scar management. Bleomycin is an antineoplastic agent that causes DNA damage, leading to fibroblast apoptosis. It has many clinical uses including treatment of vascular malformations and scar management. Bleomycin is a particularly good option for hypertrophic scars and keloids in patients with dark skin at risk of depigmentation with steroids. Scar massage is regularly recommended to patients following surgery to facilitate remodeling of the scar and soften the feel and appearance. Hyaluronic acid is used to volumize the face in the aesthetic setting. It is a synthetic nonpermanent filler that helps draw fluid into the injected site and reduce static rhytids, deep nasolabial folds, and enhance the lips, cheeks, and nose.

REFERENCE

1. Garza RM, Paik KJ, Chung MT, et al. Studies in fat grafting: Part III. Fat grafting irradiated tissue—improved skin quality and decreased fat graft retention. Plast Reconstr Surg 2014;134(2):249–257

POSTSURGICAL SCAR MANAGEMENT

7. Which one of the following adjunctive treatment modalities is used to improve scar quality by causing destruction of small blood vessels leading to tissue ischemia and altered fibroblast activity?

   A. Pulsed dye laser

   Pulsed dye laser (PDL) can be a useful adjunct to scar management in order to reduce scar pigmentation and vascularity, i.e., pinkness, by destruction of small blood vessels. During the early phases of wound healing there is increased vascularity within a wound and this serves to improve blood supply to the area and allow delivery of key cells and growth factors required for healing. In a normal wound this vascularity will subside later in the healing process. This increased vascularity is why immature scars are pink and mature ones tend to be pale. In cases where the paling process is not occurring, laser treatment with PDL may be helpful. The most likely mechanism is the destruction of small blood vessels. In addition to the color change, scar hypoxia with PDL can also lead to decreased fibroblast activity which can help a treated scar to become less active and reduce the appearance of hypertrophic scars. For this reason, it has been used on both new and pre-existing scars to determine whether hypertrophic or keloid scarring can be avoided or treated once established. Studies on the use of PDL early after surgery have shown mixed results in the prevention of hypertrophic scars, but PDL has been shown to be effective in the treatment of established hypertrophic scars,[1,2,3]

CO_2 laser and erbium-doped yttrium aluminum garnet (Er:YAG) lasers are both ablative lasers used most commonly for skin resurfacing in the cosmetic setting. These lasers can also be used to thin hypertrophic scars and improve their pliability by induction of collagen remodeling. Intense pulsed light (IPL) is a nonlaser modality that is also used for cosmetic surgical applications. For scars it can be helpful to treat scar dyschromia. Treatment modalities which modulate TGF-β should, in theory, help modify scar development given that fetal wound healing is scarless in contrast to healing after birth, and that one factor in this is the different ratios of TGF-β1, TGF-β2, and TGF-β3. In fetal wounds there is a proportionally higher amount of TGF-β3.[1] However, anti-TGF-β1 antibodies and human recombinant TGF-β3 have only shown to be effective in animal models rather than in humans.[4] Scar massage can be helpful to optimize scar quality outcomes and may work by reducing fibroblast activity or helping collagen remodeling. There is no evidence to suggest it works by reducing vascularity of the tissues by destruction of small blood vessels. Alexandrite laser has a target chromophore of oxyhemoglobin and is therefore useful in the management of tattoos, hair removal, and treating pigmented skin lesions.

REFERENCES

1. Parrett BM, Donelan MB. Pulsed dye laser in burn scars: current concepts and future directions. Burns 2010;36(4):443–449
2. Davari P, Gorouhi F, Hashemi P, et al. Pulsed dye laser treatment with different onset times for new surgical scars: a single-blind randomized controlled trial. Lasers Med Sci 2012;27(5):1095–1098
3. de las Alas JM, Siripunvarapon AH, Dofitas BL. Pulsed dye laser for the treatment of keloid and hypertrophic scars: a systematic review. Expert Rev Med Devices 2012;9(6):641–650
4. Shah M, Foreman DM, Ferguson MW. Neutralisation of TGF-beta 1 and TGF-beta 2 or exogenous addition of TGF-beta 3 to cutaneous rat wounds reduces scarring. J Cell Sci 1995;108(Pt 3):985–1002

POSTSURGERY SCAR MANAGEMENT

8. *Which one of the following should patients be advised to undertake following surgery to help them optimize their final scar quality?*

   C. To commence regular scar massage from 2–3 weeks post surgery

   Patients should be advised to start firm scar massage several times a day starting 2–3 weeks after surgery to help improve the scar pliability and appearance. Scar massage probably works in a number of ways to help the remodeling phase of healing in terms of collagen formation and alignment, and one particular aspect of the mechanism is to cause fibroblast apoptosis.

   Many patients will ask about the effectiveness of one massage product over another, e.g., oil, cream, and emollient, and it is most likely that the product used has less importance than the massage process itself.[1,2,3]

   Following surgery, it is important to protect the new scar from ultraviolet (UV) radiation both with physical barriers such as clothing or dressings and sun block because UV exposure to immature scars leads to hyperpigmentation which can be difficult to correct subsequently. Sunscreen should be worn from the second or third week following surgery once the wound has epithelialized and continued for 18 months.

   Application of pressure to scars can help flatten them and improve their appearance. However, pressure therapy is not routinely indicated for most scars. It is used most commonly in burn scars in children and adults, where grafting has been performed or where healing has occurred by secondary intention. Pressure therapy can also be helpful for keloid scars, particularly those on the ear. One of the most challenging aspects to pressure garment use is achieving patient compliance as pressure needs to be maintained for 24 hours each day in most circumstances.[4]

REFERENCES

1. Shin TM, Bordeaux JS. The role of massage in scar management: a literature review. Dermatol Surg 2012;38(3):414–423
2. Renò F, Sabbatini M, Lombardi F, et al. In vitro mechanical compression induces apoptosis and regulates cytokines release in hypertrophic scars. Wound Repair Regen 2003;11(5):331–336
3. Field T, Peck M, Scd, et al. Postburn itching, pain, and psychological symptoms are reduced with massage therapy. J Burn Care Rehabil 2000;21(3):189–193
4. Anzarut A, Olson J, Singh P, Rowe BH, Tredget EE. The effectiveness of pressure garment therapy for the prevention of abnormal scarring after burn injury: a meta-analysis. J Plast Reconstr Aesthet Surg 2009;62(1):77–84

KELOID TREATMENT

9. Which one of the following is true regarding keloid scar management?

E. Radiation therapy dosage for keloid scars is typically 15–30 gray (Gy) over 3 doses.

Keloid scars are notoriously challenging to treat as although there are a number of potentially effective treatment options, there is also a high risk of recurrence. Multimodality treatment is most likely to provide a meaningful and lasting result. The two main approaches are steroid and surgery or radiotherapy and surgery. Evidence suggests that the combination of radiotherapy and surgery has the lowest recurrence rates. When surgery and radiotherapy are combined, surgery can either be performed first and then radiotherapy is commenced on postoperative day 2, in three fractions or doses with a total dose of 15–30 Gy. Alternatively, radiotherapy may be commenced on the day of surgery. In general radiotherapy is ideally done within 3 days of surgery. Reported recurrence rates with such treatment are 10–30% compared to recurrence rates of 40–50% for surgery and steroid.[1,2]

Steroid therapy alone is not completely ineffective, but it is unlikely to help even a small keloid to resolve fully. The effects of steroid injection on a keloid can be seen within a week or two following injection. The clinical signs include softening of the keloid and some reduction in size.

The key point to communicate to patients when selecting treatment is that treatment may not be effective particularly in the longer term and recurrence is a potential risk so that they enter the treatment plan with realistic expectations.

REFERENCES

1. Kal HB, Veen RE. Biologically effective doses of postoperative radiotherapy in the prevention of keloids. Dose-effect relationship. Strahlenther Onkol 2005;181(11):717–723

2. Ogawa R, Miyashita T, Hyakusoku H, Akaishi S, Kuribayashi S, Tateno A. Postoperative radiation protocol for keloids and hypertrophic scars: statistical analysis of 370 sites followed for over 18 months. Ann Plast Surg 2007;59(6):688–691

19. Skin Grafting

See *Essentials of Plastic Surgery*, third edition, pp. 246–253

SKIN ANATOMY

1. **When considering the anatomy of the skin, which one of the following is true?**
   A. The epidermis represents one quarter of the total skin thickness.
   B. The dermis consists of four distinct layers incorporating different strata.
   C. The stratum corneum is a consistent finding throughout the body.
   D. Total skin depth is governed by dermal thickness in any given anatomic location.
   E. The main skin appendages are located beneath the dermis in the subcutis.

GRAFT CLASSIFICATION

2. **What type of graft best describes a split-thickness skin graft taken from a cadaver and used in a patient with a large body surface area burn?**
   A. Autograft
   B. Allograft
   C. Xenograft
   D. Composite graft
   E. Alloplast

CONTRAINDICATIONS TO SKIN GRAFTING

3. **Which one of the following scenarios represents a contraindication to proceeding with split skin grafting?**
   A. In a patient with significant medical comorbidities
   B. Where there is a large body surface area skin defect
   C. Where a local flap is being used to close a defect
   D. Where there is tendon devoid of paratenon at the wound base
   E. Where there is a treated recent wound bed infection

POSTOPERATIVE GRAFT CARE

4. **Following application of a skin graft to a radial forearm donor site, what is the most important element of the process to help graft take?**
   A. To immobilize the hand and wrist in a splint for 1–2 weeks
   B. To use a compression, tie over with Jelonet, and foam for 5 days
   C. To leave the wound open to the air to help re-epithelialization
   D. To commence a 5-day course of oral antibiotics
   E. To inspect the wound on a daily basis

SPLIT SKIN GRAFT TAKE

5. **What is the correct order of events for successful skin graft take?**
   A. Fibrin deposition, imbibition, inosculation, revascularization
   B. Inosculation, fibrin deposition, imbibition, revascularization
   C. Revascularization, imbibition, fibrin deposition, inosculation
   D. Fibrin deposition, inosculation, imbibition, revascularization
   E. Imbibition, fibrin deposition, inosculation, revascularization

HARVEST AND APPLICATION OF SΔPLIT-THICKNESS SKIN GRAFT (STSG)

6. **Which one of the following is true regarding split-thickness skin grafts?**
   A. Split-thickness grafts are harvested between 5 and 30/10,000 of an inch thick.
   B. Sheet graft is mainly indicated over meshed graft to increase chances of graft take.
   C. A meshed graft at 1:1.5 will provide 50% more surface area graft than unmeshed.
   D. Recipient wound contraction is greater than if a full-thickness graft was used.
   E. The scalp should be avoided as a split skin graft donor site in most cases.

TYPES OF SKIN GRAFT

7. *Which one of the following represents an advantage of using a split-thickness graft over that of a full-thickness skin graft?*
   A. The donor site is more easily managed.
   B. The cosmetic outcome is better.
   C. Graft take is more reliable.
   D. Total healing time is reduced.
   E. Innervation is more robust.

CLINICAL APPEARANCES POST SKIN GRAFTING

8. You see a patient in an examination setting and are asked whether a split-thickness or full-thickness graft has been used to reconstruct a small scalp defect. *Which one of the following would most likely guide you to the correct answer?*
   A. The absence of any obvious donor scar
   B. The presence of hair in the graft
   C. The presence of wound contracture
   D. A poor skin color match
   E. Evidence of graft failure

POSTOPERATIVE WOUND CARE

9. An open tibial fracture has been managed with a free latissimus dorsi flap and split skin graft. *Which would be the most appropriate wound dressing in this scenario for the recipient site?*
   A. Negative pressure dressing for the first 48 hours
   B. A tie over bolster dressing with a nonadherent layer and cotton wool
   C. Alginate covered with an occlusive dressing for the first week
   D. Loose nonadherent and absorptive layers with a window to view the flap
   E. Left open with no dressings applied

FULL-THICKNESS SKIN GRAFTING

10. You review patient outcomes of head and neck skin cancer patients using full-thickness skin grafts to reconstruct the defect which have been harvested from the groin. They seem to have had a higher than expected proportion of graft failures across different patient groups. *Which one of the following may represent the most likely reason for the high graft failure rates in this scenario?*
   A. The use of a bolster dressing
   B. Poor wound bed vascularity
   C. Excessive graft thickness
   D. Failure to mesh the graft
   E. Inadequate tumor excision

Answers

SKIN ANATOMY

1. *When considering the anatomy of the skin, which one of the following is true?*

    D. Total skin depth is governed by dermal thickness in any given anatomic location.

    The skin comprises the epidermis and dermis, and beneath these layers lies the subcutis or subcutaneous fat layer. Skin thickness ranges throughout the body and is thinnest on areas such as the eyelids, and thickest on areas such as the scalp and back. The variation in skin thickness according to anatomic location is primarily due to differences in dermal depth or thickness. This can be helpful to note when training residents new to surgery who are first developing their surgical skills. For example, suturing on the back is generally easier and the added depth of tissue facilitates practice of deep dermal buried sutures for the resident.

    The epidermis (not the dermis) has four or five layers or strata (depending on anatomic location). From deep to superficial these are: the stratum basale, stratum spinosum, stratum granulosum, stratum lucidum, and stratum corneum. Only the deeper three layers have live cells, with the lucidum and corneum having dead or cornified keratinocytes present. The epidermis provides the protective outer layer for the skin and typically represents around 5% of total skin depth, not 25%. The stratum corneum is only found in glabrous skin which is present on the foot soles and palms. The main skin appendages are found in the dermis although they can extend into the subcutis, and this is relevant when transferring full-thickness grafts as the appendages will be transferred too. For example, hair follicles may be transferred to the recipient site resulting in hair growth, so donor sites are generally selected to avoid this transfer from happening.[1]

REFERENCE

1. Burkitt HG, Young B, Heath JW. Wheater's Functional Histology: A Text and Colour Atlas. London: Churchill Livingstone; 2003

GRAFT CLASSIFICATION

2. *What type of graft best describes a split-thickness skin graft taken from a cadaver and used in a patient with a large body surface area burn?*

    B. Allograft

    Grafts are generally classified according to their composition or origin into autografts, allografts, xenografts, composite grafts, and alloplasts. The most commonly used grafts are from the patient themselves and these are termed autografts. They represent the benchmark against which all grafts and other biomaterials are compared because of their high tolerance, and host incorporation. Their main disadvantage is the requirement for a donor site.

    Allografts in contrast are derived from another donor of the same species, so all cadaveric tissues used in clinical practice represent allografts. There are many of these in common use including skin for burn patients, and tendon, bone, or fascia for more complex reconstructions. There is generally no limitation to such tissue availability; however, skin, for example, has only a short-term use as it will subsequently be rejected and an alternative cover will still be required. Xenografts are derived from a different species. Again these sources can be plentiful but integration with host tissues may be less reliable than with autologous grafts. Composite grafts are most commonly autologous in nature and a key example would be a skin and cartilage graft harvested from the ear for nasal alar reconstruction. Alloplasts are synthetic grafts or implants such as silicone breast prostheses or joint replacements. They are associated with a foreign body response and never truly integrate with the donor in the way that biological tissue does.[1,2]

REFERENCES

1. Thorne CH, ed. Grabb and Smith's Plastic Surgery. 7th ed. Philadelphia: Lippincott Williams & Wilkins; 2014
2. Hallock GG, Morris SF. Skin grafts and local flaps. Plast Reconstr Surg 2011;127(1):5e–22e

CONTRAINDICATIONS TO SKIN GRAFTING

3. *Which one of the following scenarios represents a contraindication to proceeding with split skin grafting?*

    D. Where there is tendon devoid of paratenon at the wound base

    Split skin grafting is indicated in large wounds where direct closure is not possible providing the wound bed is clean, infection free, and well vascularized. There should be healthy viable tissue at the wound base without avascular structures being present such as exposed tendon, bone, or cartilage. This is because these structures do not have sufficient vascularity to support the graft successfully. If they are covered with granulation tissue, or paratenon, periosteum, or perichondrium, however, then skin grafting is a viable option. For this reason, in cases where there are exposed structures, a period of treatment with negative pressure wound therapy can be beneficial as this can condition the wound to take a graft by creation of new granulation tissue, thereby avoiding more complex reconstructive processes such as flap surgery. One exception to this rule is the cranium where if the outer calvarial layer is burred, it is possible to successfully utilize a skin graft. This is because the process improves the vascularity and adherence of the wound base.

Split skin grafting is, of course, best performed in patients where health status is good and significant comorbidities are absent. However, having comorbidities is not a specific contraindication as grafts can be performed under local anesthetic and can avoid more complex intervention. Bear in mind that donor site healing may be poor in patients with multiple medical problems (which can be painful and inconvenient for many weeks) and the risk of graft failure is increased, so a careful discussion about risks and benefits is particularly important in this setting. Grafting in the presence of active infection is contraindicated; however, once infection is treated, grafting is entirely appropriate. In some cases, it is advisable to have evidence of negative wound cultures prior to grafting (e.g., group A streptococcus); however, in most cases clinical assessment is sufficient particularly where a final wound debridement is performed at the time of grafting. Grafts are often used in combination with flap surgery to close donor site defects such as scalp transposition, radial forearm fasciocutaneous, or fibula osseocutaneous flaps.[1,2]

REFERENCES

1. Hallock GG, Morris SF. Skin grafts and local flaps. Plast Reconstr Surg 2011;127(1):5e–22e
2. Brown DL, Borschel GB, Levi B. Michigan Manual of Plastic Surgery. 2nd ed. Philadelphia. Lippincott Williams & Wilkins; 2014

POSTOPERATIVE GRAFT CARE

4. *Following application of a skin graft to a radial forearm donor site, what is the most important element of the process to help graft take?*

A. **To immobilize the hand and wrist in a splint for 1–2 weeks**

There are a number of reasons why grafts fail to take and the most common reasons include hematoma which stops the graft from adhering to the recipient site and obtaining a blood supply, infection resulting in the inability for the graft to take, or a physical/mechanical reason, such as shearing of the graft.

For this reason, care is taken to ensure adequate hemostasis before graft placement, ensure absence of infection, and secure the graft to the recipient site.

When raising a radial forearm flap, it is important to retain paratenon over the long flexor tendons so that a viable graft bed is preserved. Once the graft is secured it is important to minimize movement beneath the graft where it lies on the flexor tendons. For this reason, it is important to splint the hand and wrist to stop this movement in the early phases of graft take. Usually a period of immobilization of 1–2 weeks is sufficient.

Compression is not usually required in this scenario although many surgeons will still use a low adherence dressing on the graft followed by gauze or foam to secure and contour the graft. Few surgeons would recommend leaving this site exposed until the graft has taken at 1–2 weeks as it would be likely to sustain inadvertent damage. Daily wound inspection would serve no useful purpose and antibiotics would not normally be indicated.

SPLIT SKIN GRAFT TAKE

5. *What is the correct order of events for successful skin graft take?*

A. **Fibrin deposition, imbibition, inosculation, revascularization**

Skin graft survival, or "take," is based upon the ability of the graft to adhere to a recipient site, receive nutrients from the underlying wound bed, and progress to vascular ingrowth and maturity. Split-thickness skin grafts initially adhere to the wound with formation of a fibrin layer over the first 24 hours. Over the next 24–48 hours, the graft swells and obtains nutrients from the wound bed by diffusion. This process is called *serum imbibition*. During the following days, recipient and donor site vessels align. This process is called *inosculation* and occurs in nature when tree branches join together. The final process is called *revascularization*, which involves full ingrowth of host capillaries into the graft. Once revascularization has occurred, there is continued ingrowth of fibrous tissue and vessels producing a long-term permanent adherence and tissue integration. The process of skin graft take is often discussed in clinical examinations.[1,2]

Timings for the various processes are as follows:

- **0–24 hours: Fibrin adherence**
- **24–48 hours: Serum imbibition**
- **48–72 hours: Inosculation**
- **4–6 days: Revascularization**

REFERENCES

1. Thorne CH, ed. Grabb and Smith's Plastic Surgery. 7th ed. Philadelphia: Lippincott Williams & Wilkins; 2014
2. Hallock GG, Morris SF. Skin grafts and local flaps. Plast Reconstr Surg 2011;127(1):5e–22e

HARVEST AND APPLICATION OF SPLIT-THICKNESS SKIN GRAFT (STSG)

6. *Which one of the following is true regarding split-thickness skin grafts?*

D. **Recipient wound contraction is greater than if a full-thickness graft was used.**

There are two types of skin graft contraction: primary and secondary. Primary contraction occurs intraoperatively when a graft is harvested. Secondary contraction occurs later in the healing phase. The greater the amount of dermis present, the greater will be the primary contraction and conversely there will be less secondary contraction. Primary contraction is thought to be related to elastin content within the dermis, whereas secondary contraction is thought to be related to myofibroblast activity.

It is standard practice to mesh split-thickness grafts where there are large areas of defect to be covered such as in large total body surface area (TBSA) burn injuries. Common meshing ratios include 1.5:1, 2:1, and 3:1. This will allow for greater surface coverage while minimizing donor site size. However, meshing ratios have been shown to be inaccurate representations of final graft size where, for example, a 1.5:1 meshing resulted in 1.36× expansion, and a 3:1 mesh resulted in 1.8× expansion. This is important to consider when deciding whether to mesh or not and also to gauge how much donor skin needs to be harvested for any given defect. In addition, when going ahead with meshing of the graft, this process may improve graft take over sheet graft as fluids such as blood and serum can escape from the wound bed, which may otherwise compromise the graft take. The downside to meshing is that the cosmetic outcome is poorer than with sheet graft so it should be avoided in cosmetically sensitive areas, and also the functional outcome can be worse so, for example, sheet should be preferentially used around joints in the hand.

When using a dermatome to harvest skin the settings are measured in 1000ths of an inch and not 10,000ths of an inch. A typical graft harvest will be at 10–12/1000ths of an inch. This should harvest all of the epidermis and part of the dermis. Although the most common donor site is the thigh, the scalp should be considered as a potential donor site in head and neck reconstruction, particularly in the setting of burns. The benefits include a better color match, a more rapid donor healing, and better long-term donor site aesthetics due to camouflage and hair regrowth.[1,2]

REFERENCES

1. Thorne CH, ed. Grabb and Smith's Plastic Surgery. 7th ed. Philadelphia: Lippincott Williams & Wilkins; 2014
2. Hallock GG, Morris SF. Skin grafts and local flaps. Plast Reconstr Surg 2011;127(1):5e–22e

TYPES OF SKIN GRAFT

7. *Which one of the following represents an advantage of using a split-thickness graft over that of a full-thickness skin graft?*

C. **Graft take is more reliable.**

Split-thickness and full-thickness skin grafts each have their own advantages and disadvantages and consequent indications for use. The main advantages of split-thickness grafts are that they have a higher chance of graft survival due to the decreased dermal component, greater availability of donor sites, an ability to reharvest from the same site, and faster reinnervation. Furthermore, the surgical time can be reduced compared with full-thickness grafts especially as donor site closure is not required. In contrast, full-thickness grafts provide a better color and texture match with more robust reinnervation, they display less secondary contraction, and the donor site can be closed directly. Downsides are more limited availability, a lower chance of graft survival, and increased surgical time. Given the above, split-thickness grafts are indicated in larger areas of noncosmetically sensitive regions and full-thickness grafts are indicated in smaller defects where aesthetics and function are paramount (**Table 19.1**).[1–3]

REFERENCES

1. Janis JE. Essentials of Plastic Surgery. New York: Thieme Publishers; 2021
2. Tanner JC Jr, Vandeput J, Olley JF. The mesh skin graft. Plast Reconstr Surg 1964;34:287–292
3. Henderson J, Arya R, Gillespie P. Skin graft meshing, over-meshing and cross-meshing. Int J Surg 2012;10(9):547–550

Table 19.1 *STSG versus FTSG*

	Advantages	Disadvantages
STSG All epidermis and part of dermis: Thin: 5–12/1000 inch Medium: 12–16/1000 inch Thick: >16/1000 inch	- Higher chance of graft survival due to decreased dermis - Ability to reharvest from prior donor site - Greater availability of donor sites - Faster reinnervation	- Greater secondary contracture - Poor color/texture match - Hair growth not possible
FTSG Includes all of dermis and epidermis	- Less secondary contracture - Ability to close donor site - Better color/texture match - Dermal appendages more likely to regenerate - More robust reinnervation (pain, touch, then temperature)	- Lower chance of graft survival - Need to close donor site limits size of harvested graft

FTSG, full-thickness skin grafts; *STSG*, split-thickness skin grafts.

CLINICAL APPEARANCES POST SKIN GRAFTING

8. **You see a patient in an examination setting and are asked whether a split-thickness or full-thickness graft has been used to reconstruct a small scalp defect. *Which one of the following would most likely guide you to the correct answer?***

   B. **The presence of hair in the graft**

   One of the key differences in split-thickness versus full-thickness skin grafts is that only full-thickness grafts will transfer the skin appendages which include hair follicles. Therefore, in this scenario it is possible to conclude that a full-thickness graft has been used. The absence of any obvious donor site is not a reliable guide to surgery performed. Both split- and full-thickness donor sites can be discretely placed and well concealed, especially if the graft size is small. Wound contracture will be present in both full-thickness or split-thickness grafts and this, too, will be influenced by how well the graft took. If there was partial graft loss, then some of the wound would heal by secondary intention with associated scarring. This could cancel the benefits of reduced secondary contracture by a full-thickness graft. In general, skin color match is better in full-thickness grafts, but only where due consideration has been given to donor site selection to optimize the match, e.g., cheek or preauricular donor sites for central face reconstruction. Evidence of graft failure may make it more likely that a full-thickness graft was used but as both can fail, it would not exclude one or the other.

POSTOPERATIVE WOUND CARE

9. **An open tibial fracture has been managed with a free latissimus dorsi flap and split skin graft. *Which would be the most appropriate wound dressing in this scenario for the recipient site?***

   D. **Loose nonadherent and absorptive layers with a window to view the flap**

   Negative pressure wound therapy (NPWT) can be a very effective dressing for a split skin graft recipient site because it ensures uniform pressure across graft, minimizes shear, splints the wound, and can accelerate the process of inosculation. A bolster is commonly used following skin grafting in order to apply external pressure to the graft and maintain a clean moist environment. This can be achieved with a nonadherent base layer and either cotton wool balls or foam. The pressure effect is, however, very short-lived. However, neither of these approaches should normally be used on free tissue muscle flaps with split-thickness skin grafts as this would result in undue pressure on the flap and an inability to assess flap viability. The ideal dressing is therefore one which is nonadherent and allows for fluid egress from the wound and yet has some ability to absorb fluid, while allowing for regular flap monitoring. For this reason, a simple nonadherent dressing such as Mepitel™ in combination with gauze is ideal for this purpose and a viewing window in the flap is readily created. Alginate or Duoderm™ dressings are more commonly used for donor site dressings and can be left in situ for 1 week. Aquacel AG™ is a silver-impregnated antimicrobial absorbent nonocclusive dressing that again may be used for split-thickness donor site wounds. Duoderm™ is a hydrocolloid dressing that absorbs exudate to form a soft gel. It promotes a moist environment, is occlusive, is waterproof, and can improve epithelialization. It is used for some donor site dressings and may also be useful as a sealant at the interface of normal skin and wound where a negative pressure dressing is used (**Table 19.2**).[1-3]

Table 19.2 *Common Donor Site Dressings*

Xeroform (Covidien, Dublin, Ireland)	Mepitel (Molnlycke, Norcross, Georgia)	Aquacel Burn (ConvaTec, Bridgewater, NJ)	DuoDERM (ConvaTec, Bridgewater, NJ)
Bismuth tribromophenate-impregnated petroleum gauze	Transparent breathable silicone film	Silver-impregnated hydrofiber	Hydrocolloid
- Common dressing - Widely available - Inexpensive - Antimicrobial - Becomes dry dressing, forming eschar - May demonstrate increased donor site pain	- Nonadherent - Moist wound environment - Nonocclusive, allowing fluid egress - Persistent drainage until epithelialization - Can remain in place for 14 days	- Antimicrobial - Absorbent - Nonocclusive - Can remain in place for up to 21 days - Forms dry eschar similar to Xeroform that is peeled off the donor site	- Hydrocolloid absorbs exudate to form soft gel -Promotes moist environment - Occlusive, waterproof - Improved degree of epithelialization - Dressing can remain in place for 7 days

REFERENCES

1. Brown DL, Borschel GB, Levi B. Michigan Manual of Plastic Surgery. 2nd ed. Philadelphia. Lippincott Williams & Wilkins; 2014
2. Llanos S, Danilla S, Barraza C, et al. Effectiveness of negative pressure closure in the integration of split thickness skin grafts: a randomized, double-masked, controlled trial. Ann Surg 2006;244(5):700–705
3. Janis JE. Essentials of Plastic Surgery. New York: Thieme Publishers, 2021.

FULL-THICKNESS SKIN GRAFTING

10. You review patient outcomes of head and neck skin cancer patients using full-thickness skin grafts to reconstruct the defect which have been harvested from the groin. They seem to have had a higher than expected proportion of graft failures across different patient groups. *Which one of the following may represent the most likely reason for the high graft failure rates in this scenario?*

C. Excessive graft thickness

There are a number of pitfalls to avoid when taking full-thickness skin grafts. Of these one of the most important is to ensure that the graft is sufficiently thinned and contains no residual subcutaneous fat on the undersurface, as this can lead to an increased graft failure rate. Skin grafts are avascular once harvested and need to obtain nutrition and a new blood supply from the recipient bed. If the graft is too thick, it is more difficult for it to successfully achieve this in the early phases of healing. The other key elements of graft failure should also be borne in mind and these include infection, inadequate hemostasis, inadequate debridement or tumor excision, and inadequate graft fixation. Full-thickness grafts are usually harvested in an elliptical design with a scalpel ideally just beneath the dermis with no fat. If there is residual fat on the undersurface, this should be debulked or removed to promote survival. Where the dermis is thick, this should be thinned. The use of a bolster dressing is the standard of many surgeons although others choose to leave the graft exposed with little more than petroleum jelly covering it. The use of a bolster is unlikely to be the cause of graft failure in this scenario and even the absence of one may well not be the primary cause. Where grafts are left exposed, it is important to remember that they display a cyanotic discoloration during revascularization, which can be disconcerting for both patient, nurse, and surgeon if not anticipated.

Full-thickness grafts are not meshed but may be fenestrated to allow fluid egress. In this scenario, there would have to be a significant volume of residual tumor for incomplete tumor excision to be the cause of graft failure.

20. Basal Cell Carcinoma, Squamous Cell Carcinoma, and Melanoma

See *Essentials of Plastic Surgery*, third edition, pp. 254–275

DEMOGRAPHICS OF BASAL CELL CARCINOMA

1. *Which one of the following statements is correct regarding basal cell carcinoma basal cell carcinoma (BCC)?*
   A. Incidence has recently plateaued.
   B. It more commonly affects females.
   C. It usually affects the trunk and limbs.
   D. The most commonly affected single site is the upper lip.
   E. It is the most common eyelid malignancy.

RISK FACTORS FOR BASAL CELL CARCINOMA

2. *Which one of the following is a risk factor more typical of squamous cell carcinoma (SCC) rather than basal cell carcinoma (BCC)?*
   A. Immune suppression
   B. Human papilloma virus
   C. Fitzpatrick skin types I and II
   D. Sun exposure
   E. Advancing age

GORLIN'S SYNDROME

3. You are referred a patient with a diagnosis of Gorlin's syndrome. *Which one of the following is a typical feature of this condition?*
   A. Recurrent dental abscesses
   B. Posterior plagiocephaly
   C. Yellowish plaques on the scalp
   D. Multiple small pits on the palm or sole
   E. Coffee-colored patches in the axilla

BASAL CELL CARCINOMA (BCC) SUBTYPES

4. *When considering the differences between different BCC subtypes, which one of the following is true?*
   A. Superficial spreading is the most common subtype.
   B. Micronodular is often mistaken for psoriasis or fungal infection.
   C. Nodular subtypes are best treated nonsurgically.
   D. Infiltrative subtypes are often confused clinically with melanomas.
   E. Morpheaform tumors are the most aggressive subtype.

RISK STRATIFICATION FOR BASAL CELL CARCINOMA

5. *Which one of the following represents a low-risk BCC?*
   A. A 10 mm diameter infiltrative BCC on the genitals
   B. A 9 mm diameter nodular BCC on the nasal tip
   C. A 6 mm diameter morpheaform BCC on the hand
   D. An 18 mm diameter superficial BCC on the trunk
   E. A 9 mm diameter micronodular BCC on the thigh

NONSURGICAL MANAGEMENT OF BASAL CELL CARCINOMA

6. *Which one of the following is correct?*
   A. Photodynamic therapy (PDT) uses 5-aminolevulinic acid to create free radicals that destroy target cells but its use should be limited to treating superficial BCCs.
   B. Radiation therapy can be used for most types of BCC, is administered as a single treatment dose, and avoids surgery.
   C. Topical treatment of BCCs with Imiquimod or 5-fluorouracil (5-FU) is uniformly effective because these agents are able to penetrate deep into the reticular dermis.
   D. Standard cryotherapy involves cooling cells to –40° C and is indicated for tumors up to 5 mm deep.
   E. Vismodegib has received FDA approval as a first-line BCC treatment as an alternative to surgery or radiation therapy.

SURGICAL MANAGEMENT OF BASAL CELL CARCINOMA

7. You have a patient in the operating room (OR) with a 5-mm diameter pearly nodular lesion on the forehead which you suspect to be a BCC. It has well-defined borders and visible telangiectasia. *What peripheral excision margin should you use?*
   A. 2 mm
   B. 4 mm
   C. 6 mm
   D. 8 mm
   E. 10 mm

SURGICAL MANAGEMENT OF BASAL CELL CARCINOMA

8. *What is the major advantage of Mohs surgery for BCC management?*
   A. The intraoperative time is reduced.
   B. Complex reconstruction is avoided.
   C. Completeness of excision is confirmed intraoperatively.
   D. Cure rates are 100%.
   E. Excision and reconstruction are completed in a single stage.

RISK FACTORS FOR SQUAMOUS CELL CARCINOMA

9. *Which one of the following factors most increases the risk of developing an SCC?*
   A. Fitzpatrick skin types I and II
   B. Sun exposure
   C. Arsenic and hydrocarbons
   D. Human papilloma virus
   E. Immune suppression after transplant surgery

SQUAMOUS CELL CARCINOMA–RELATED DEATHS

10. *An SCC in which one of the following sites will is associated with the highest overall mortality risk?*
    A. Ear
    B. Lip
    C. Trunk
    D. Limb
    E. Scalp

RISK FACTORS FOR RECURRENCE OF SQUAMOUS CELL CARCINOMA

11. *Which one of the following describes a low-risk SCC?*
    A. A tumor with depth of invasion of 4.5 mm
    B. A recurrent tumor
    C. A 2.5 cm diameter tumor
    D. A tumor on the upper lip
    E. A verrucous tumor subtype

PREMALIGNANT SKIN LESIONS

12. A patient is referred to clinic by his or her general practitioner with an 8-week history of a dome-shaped keratotic lesion to the forearm that displayed initial rapid growth followed by spontaneous partial regression after 7 weeks. *What is the most likely diagnosis?*
    A. Actinic keratosis
    B. Bowen's disease
    C. Leukoplakia
    D. Keratoacanthoma
    E. Erythroplasia of Queyrat

TREATMENT OF CUTANEOUS SQUAMOUS CELL CARCINOMA

13. You see an 85-year-old otherwise healthy patient with a thick, necrotic, 2-cm diameter SCC involving the left cheek and preauricular region. There is no obvious palpable lymphadenopathy present and the lesion remains mobile over deeper tissues. *Which one of the following is correct regarding management of this patient?*
    A. The lesion should be excised with a 4-mm margin and closed directly.
    B. Radiotherapy is the best modality for management in this case.
    C. The patient is unlikely to benefit from elective nodal dissection.
    D. The lesion should be treated with Mohs micrographic surgery.

E. Posttreatment follow-up will be every 3 months for 5 years.

MELANOMA SUBTYPES

14. *Which one of the following is the most common cutaneous melanoma subtype?*
    A. Superficial spreading
    B. Nodular
    C. Lentigo maligna
    D. Acral-lentiginous
    E. Desmoplastic

MELANOMA SUBTYPES

15. You see a 45-year-old white patient in your office who has evidence of a new-onset, single-digit, linear, pigmented nail streak. You are concerned that this may be melanoma, and you perform a biopsy. *With which melanoma subtype may this presentation be associated?*
    A. Desmoplastic
    B. Amelanotic
    C. Ocular
    D. Superficial spreading
    E. Acral-lentiginous

MELANOMA SUBTYPES

16. *When assessing a patient in clinic with a suspected melanoma, which one of the following would be most in keeping with development of a nodular subtype?*
    A. Development within a long-standing mole
    B. Development de novo
    C. Development from a Hutchinson freckle
    D. Development within a sun-protected site
    E. Development from a spitz nevus

MELANOMA PROGNOSIS

17. *When reviewing the histopathology report of a melanoma specimen, what is the single most important histologic prognostic factor for the patient?*
    A. Mitotic count
    B. Ulceration
    C. Perineural invasion
    D. Breslow thickness
    E. Clark's level

AMERICAN JOINT COMMITTEE ON CANCER MELANOMA STAGING CLASSIFICATION (AJCC)

18. You discuss a patient at the weekly multidisciplinary team meeting to plan treatment. The patient has a melanoma of Breslow thickness (BT) 2.5 mm, three positive regional lymph nodes, and metastases involving the skin. *What would be the correct melanoma staging for this patient according to the classification of the American Joint Committee on Cancer (AJCC)?*
    A. T1bN1M1
    B. T2cN0M0
    C. T2N1M1b
    D. T3N2M1a
    E. T4N1M1a

SURGICAL MANAGEMENT OF MELANOMA

19. *Which one of the following is correct regarding the surgical management of melanoma?*
    A. A full-thickness excision biopsy is required for all suspected melanomas.
    B. Long-term survival is improved by excision of the deep fascial layer during a wide local excision.
    C. Amputation proximal to the proximal interphalangeal joint is recommended for subungual melanomas of the digit.
    D. Sentinel lymph node biopsy is only indicated in stage II and III patients.
    E. A positive Cloquet's node is not the only indication for pelvic dissection.

NONSURGICAL MANAGEMENT OF MELANOMA

20. *Which one of the following is correct regarding nonsurgical management of melanoma?*
    A. Sentinel lymph node biopsy is a useful therapeutic treatment for melanoma.
    B. Elective lymph node dissection shows a survival benefit only with melanomas greater than 4 mm.
    C. The use of dacarbazine or cisplatin may help to reduce the tumor burden.
    D. Radiation therapy is often indicated as a primary treatment for cutaneous melanoma.

E. Interferon alpha-2 can give a disease-free survival benefit in early

WIDE EXCISION MARGINS IN MELANOMA

21. *What would be the recommended wide excision margin for a primary melanoma with a Breslow thickness of 3.2 mm once it had been completely excised for diagnosis?*
    A. 1 mm
    B. 5 mm
    C. 1 cm
    D. 2 cm
    E. 3 cm

TREATMENT IN ADVANCED-STAGE MELANOMA

22. *In a patient with stage IV melanoma who has tested positive for BRAF, which one of the following treatment modalities is specifically indicated?*
    A. Radiotherapy
    B. Dacarbazine
    C. Cisplatin
    D. Vemurafenib
    E. Vinblastin

ADVANCED-STAGE MELANOMA

23. *Which one of the following is a monoclonal antibody directed to the receptor CTLA-4, approved by the FDA for patients with unresectable melanoma?*
    A. Ipilimumab
    B. MAGE-A3
    C. Imatinib
    D. Interleukin-2
    E. Canvaxin

MELANOMA FOLLOW-UP

24. *Following complete resection of a 2.5-mm Breslow thickness melanoma from the calf, for how long should patients be followed (in the US), assuming they have no palpable lymph nodes?*
    A. 1 year
    B. 2 years
    C. 5 years
    D. 10 years
    E. Lifelong

CLINICAL SCENARIOS IN SKIN CANCER

25. A 65-year-old patient presents with multiple raised verrucous papules with varied deep pigmentation affecting the back. His normal medical practitioner refers him with concern of melanoma in one of the lesions as it appears darker than the others. *Which one of the following represents the most likely diagnosis?*
    A. Junctional nevus
    B. Seborrheic keratosis
    C. Compound nevus
    D. Blue nevus
    E. Lentigo

Answers

DEMOGRAPHICS OF BASAL CELL CARCINOMA

1. *Which one of the following statements is correct regarding basal cell carcinoma (BCC)?*
   E. It is the most common eyelid malignancy.
   BCC is a malignant tumor of the skin arising from the basal cells of the epidermis and it represents the most common type of eyelid malignancy. It is the most common type of skin cancer with more than 1.2 million cases reported annually in the US. Its incidence is rapidly rising which is probably due to a combination of increasing population age, increased sun exposure, and better detection. Males are affected more commonly than females. At least 80% of BCCs occur in the head and neck region with the most common sites being the nose, eyelid, and ear. Other sites that are often affected include the cheek, lip, neck, and brow.[1–5]

REFERENCES

1. Habif TP, ed. Clinical Dermatology: A Color Guide to Diagnosis and Therapy. 4th ed. St Louis: Mosby-Year Book; 2004
2. Shanoff LB, Spira M, Hardy SB. Basal cell carcinoma: a statistical approach to rational management. Plast Reconstr Surg 1967;39(6):619–624
3. Miller S, Alam M, Anderson J, et al. NCCN Guidelines. Clinical practice guidelines in oncology: basal cell and squamous cell skin cancers version 2. 2012. DOI: 10.6004/jnccn.2004.0001
4. American Cancer Society. Medical and editorial content team. www.cancer.org/cancer/melanoma-skin-cancer/about/key-statistics.html
5. Netscher DT, Leong M, Orengo I, Yang D, Berg C, Krishnan B. Cutaneous malignancies: melanoma and nonmelanoma types. Plast Reconstr Surg 2011;127(3):37e–56e

RISK FACTORS FOR BASAL CELL CARCINOMA

2. *Which one of the following is a risk factor more typical of squamous cell carcinoma (SCC) rather than basal cell carcinoma (BCC)?*
   B. Human papilloma virus
   Human papilloma virus (HPV) is not associated with development of BCCs. It is however associated with SCC of the skin and mucous membranes such as the oropharynx and oral cavity. It is also implicated in cervical cancer. Risk factors for BCC include skin type and color (Fitzpatrick types I and II), increasing age, male sex, sun exposure, immune compromise (e.g., human immunodeficiency virus [HIV], steroid, or organ transplant medication), genetic predisposition, and carcinogen exposure (e.g., UV and ionizing radiation, hydrocarbons). Risk factors for SCC generally parallel those of BCC but also include chronic wounds, psoralen and ultraviolet A light (PUVA) treatment for psoriasis, and irradiation.[1–7]

REFERENCES

1. Rowe DE, Carroll RJ, Day CL Jr. Prognostic factors for local recurrence, metastasis, and survival rates in squamous cell carcinoma of the skin, ear, and lip. Implications for treatment modality selection. J Am Acad Dermatol 1992;26(6):976–990
2. Bichakjian CK, Olencki T, Aasi SZ, et. Al. NCCN Clinical Practice Guidelines in Oncology: Squamous Cell Skin Cancer. 2018:2. NCCN.org
3. Telfer NR, Colver GB, Morton CA; British Association of Dermatologists. Guidelines for the management of basal cell carcinoma. Br J Dermatol 2008;159(1):35–48
4. Veness MJ. High-risk cutaneous squamous cell carcinoma of the head and neck. J Biomed Biotechnol 2007;2007(3):80572
5. Miller S, Alam M, Anderson J, et al. NCCN Guidelines. Clinical practice guidelines in oncology: basal cell and squamous cell skin cancers version 2, 2012. Available at http://www.nccn.org/professionals/ physician_gls/f_guidelines.asp#nmsc
6. Immerman SC, Scanlon EF, Christ M, Knox KL. Recurrent squamous cell carcinoma of the skin. Cancer 1983;51(8):1537–1540
7. Motley RJ, Preston PW, Lawrence CM. Multi-professional Guidelines for the Management of the Patient with Primary Cutaneous Squamous Cell Carcinoma. London, United Kingdom: British Association of Dermatology; 2009

GORLIN'S SYNDROME

3. You are referred a patient with a diagnosis of Gorlin's syndrome. *Which one of the following is a typical feature of this condition?*
   D. Multiple small pits on the palm or sole
   A common finding in patients with Gorlin's syndrome is the presence of multiple small red pits on the palm or sole. They appear as small depressions and are caused by partial or complete absence of the stratum corneum.

They are typically 2–3 mm diameter with a similar depth. They are present in up to one-third of patients by the start of the second decade, and almost all patients by age 20.[1] Although the presence of three or more palmar pits constitutes a major diagnostic criterion in Gorlin's syndrome, pits may also be seen in patients with other conditions, such as psoriasis.[2]

Gorlin's syndrome (nevoid basal cell syndrome) is an autosomal dominant condition affecting chromosome 9 that is characterized by multiple BCCs at an early age. These patients will require lifelong review and multiple procedures for tumor excision. Another common feature associated with Gorlin's syndrome is development of odontogenic keratocysts, which show as radiolucent areas on panorex. Recurrent dental abscesses are not a specific finding. There are often cranial abnormalities, which include absence of the falx cerebri, hypertelorism, and a broad nasal root. Neither posterior plagiocephaly or recurrent dental abscesses are typical findings. A yellowish plaque on the skin may represent a sebaceous nevus which itself is benign but has the potential for transformation to BCC in around 10% of cases. Coffee-colored patches are more typical of neurofibromatosis.

REFERENCES

1. Lo Muzio L. Nevoid basal cell carcinoma syndrome (Gorlin syndrome). Orphanet J Rare Dis 2008;3:32
2. Kimonis VE, Goldstein AM, Pastakia B, et al. Clinical manifestations in 105 persons with nevoid basal cell carcinoma syndrome. Am J Med Genet 1997;69(3):299–308

BASAL CELL CARCINOMA (BCC) SUBTYPES

4. *When considering the differences between different BCC subtypes, which one of the following is true?*

E. Morpheaform tumors are the most aggressive subtype.

More than 20 subtypes of BCC have been described. The most common subtype is nodular (50–60%) and other common subtypes are micronodular (15%), superficial spreading (9–15%), infiltrative (7%), and morpheaform (2–3%). Subtypes differ in their behavior and the most aggressive is morpheaform, which has a high incidence of positive margins following excision. These tend to present as an "enlarging scar" without history of trauma and have a flat or slightly elevated scarlike appearance. Infiltrative subtypes are also aggressive, whereas nodular and superficial subtypes are fairly low risk. Despite this, nodular subtypes are still best treated surgically. The classic described appearance of a BCC is a raised lesion with a rolled edge, visible telangiectasia, and central ulceration. This appearance is most in keeping with a nodular subtype, which was traditionally referred to as a "rodent ulcer." Superficial spreading BCCs are located in the epidermis with no dermal invasion. They are pink, flat scaly patches with ulceration and crusting rather than the classic nodular appearances described above. Accordingly, they can be confused with fungal infections or eczema. Pigmented subtypes represent 6% of all BCCs and are most likely to be confused with melanomas.[1-4]

REFERENCES

1. Telfer NR, Colver GB, Morton CA; British Association of Dermatologists. Guidelines for the management of basal cell carcinoma. Br J Dermatol 2008;159(1):35–48
2. Miller S, Alam M, Anderson J, et al. NCCN Guidelines. Clinical practice guidelines in oncology: basal cell and squamous cell skin cancers version 2.2012. DOI: 10.6004/jnccn.2004.0001
3. Breuninger H, Dietz K. Prediction of subclinical tumor infiltration in basal cell carcinoma. J Dermatol Surg Oncol 1991;17(7):574–578
4. Wolf DJ, Zitelli JA. Surgical margins for basal cell carcinoma. Arch Dermatol 1987;123(3):340–344

RISK STRATIFICATION FOR BASAL CELL CARCINOMA

5. *Which one of the following represents a low-risk BCC?*

D. An 18 mm diameter superficial BCC on the trunk

Risk factors for the recurrence of BCCs depend on many factors including the subtype, diameter, depth, anatomic site, clarity of borders, rate of growth, and histopathologic findings and whether they are primary or recurrent lesions. BCCs less than 2 cm diameter on the trunk or proximal limbs are generally considered to be low-risk lesions. Low-risk subtypes are nodular and superficial. High-risk subtypes are morpheaform, sclerosing, infiltrative, and micronodular. High-risk lesions based on size (diameter) are larger than 2 cm on the trunk or proximal limbs; larger than 1 cm on the cheek, forehead, neck, or scalp; and larger than 6 mm on the central face, genitalia, hands, or feet. Other factors suggestive of high risk include poor differentiation, perineural/lymphovascular invasion, rapid growth, and recurrent tumors. In a standard histopathological report key features should be detailed such as subtype, diameter, depth, completeness of excision (mm), perineural or perivascular involvement, and tumor growth/regression in order to determine further treatment and the risk of recurrence.[1-6]

REFERENCES

1. Miller S, Alam M, Anderson J, et al. NCCN Guidelines. Clinical practice guidelines in oncology: basal cell and squamous cell skin cancers version 2.2012. DOI: 10.6004/jnccn.2004.0001
2. Quazi SJ, Aslam N, Saleem H, Rahman J, Khan S. Surgical margin of excision in basal cell carcinoma: a systematic review of literature. Cureus 2020;12(7):e9211
3. Nahhas AF, Scarbrough CA, Trotter S. A review of the global guidelines on surgical margins for nonmelanoma skin cancers. J Clin Aesthet Dermatol 2017;10(4):37–46
4. Wolf DJ, Zitelli JA. Surgical margins for basal cell carcinoma. Arch Dermatol 1987;123(3):340–344
5. Telfer NR, Colver GB, Morton CA; British Association of Dermatologists. Guidelines for the management of basal cell carcinoma. Br J Dermatol 2008;159(1):35–48
6. Kimyai-Asadi A, Alam M, Goldberg LH, Peterson SR, Silapunt S, Jih MH. Efficacy of narrow-margin excision of well-demarcated primary facial basal cell carcinomas. J Am Acad Dermatol 2005;53(3):464–468

NONSURGICAL MANAGEMENT OF BASAL CELL CARCINOMA

6. **Which one of the following is correct?**

   A. **Photodynamic therapy (PDT) uses 5-aminolevulinic acid to create free radicals that destroy target cells but its use should be limited to treating superficial BCCs.**

   Photodynamic therapy (PDT) uses the light-activated photosensitizing drug 5-aminolevulinic acid to create oxygen free radicals that selectively destroy target cells. It can be used in premalignant or superficial lesions, but should not be used in deeper or high-risk lesions. Radiation therapy provides an alternative to surgery and can be effective for most BCCs. It tends to be reserved for older patients (age 60 and older) and has cure rates >90%. One of the caveats of radiation therapy is that multiple treatments are required over a 4- to 6-week period and it requires a diagnostic biopsy to be obtained before treatment. Furthermore, completeness of excision cannot be confirmed and subsequent surgery to the area is more challenging. Topical treatments with either Imiquimod or 5-fluorouracil (5-FU) can be effective in low-risk superficial lesions because they can destroy the surface cells. They should not be used in deeper lesions because they cannot destroy deeper cells and risk growth recurrence due to residual tumor cell presence. Standard cryotherapy involves cooling the tissues to –40° C during repeated freeze–thaw cycles, but it is not indicated for tumors deeper than 3 mm. It has a more useful role in management of early actinic keratosis. Vismodegib is a hedgehog inhibitor with FDA approval for use in locally advanced BCC when other treatment forms have been exhausted, and therefore is not a first-line treatment. Unfortunately, it is an expensive drug and no longer has approval in UK National Health Service because of this in relation to its perceived benefits. Adverse effects include muscle spasm, alopecia, ageusia, and fatigue.[1-5]

REFERENCES

1. Telfer NR, Colver GB, Morton CA; British Association of Dermatologists. Guidelines for the management of basal cell carcinoma. Br J Dermatol 2008;159(1):35–48
2. Wong TH, Morton CA, Collier N, et al. British Association of Dermatologists and British Photodermatology Group guidelines for topical photodynamic therapy 2018. Br J Dermatol 2019;180(4):730–739
3. Sekulic A, Migden MR, Basset-Seguin N, et al; ERIVANCE BCC Investigators. Long-term safety and efficacy of vismodegib in patients with advanced basal cell carcinoma: final update of the pivotal ERIVANCE BCC study. BMC Cancer 2017;17(1):332
4. Peris K, Fargnoli MC, Garbe C, et al; European Dermatology Forum (EDF), the European Association of Dermato-Oncology (EADO) and the European Organization for Research and Treatment of Cancer (EORTC). Diagnosis and treatment of basal cell carcinoma: European consensus-based interdisciplinary guidelines. Eur J Cancer 2019;118:10–34
5. https://www.nice.org.uk/guidance/ta489/documents/final-appraisal-determination-document

SURGICAL MANAGEMENT OF BASAL CELL CARCINOMA

7. You have a patient in the operating room (OR) with a 5-mm diameter pearly nodular lesion on the forehead which you suspect to be a BCC. It has well-defined borders and visible telangiectasia. *What peripheral excision margin should you use?*

   B. **4 mm**

   Excision margins required for well-defined BCCs are commonly 4 mm, while those for infiltrative subtypes are significantly greater. Studies have been undertaken using Mohs techniques to assess completeness of excision in BCCs with increasing margins. These studies have shown that excision of small (<20 mm), well-defined lesions using a 3-mm peripheral margin will result in complete removal in 85% of cases. Increasing this margin to 4 mm will increase complete excision rates to around 95%. This suggests that around 5% of well-defined BCCs will have tumor extension beyond 4 mm that cannot be identified clinically. Morpheaform and large BCCs will require peripheral margins of 13–15 mm to achieve 95% complete excision. Margins of 3 and 5 mm provide clearance in only 66 and 82% of these cases, respectively. Depth of excision is less well guided but in general taking a cuff of subcutaneous fat with the specimen is believed to be sufficient. In cases where completeness of excision is uncertain at the time of surgery, a further deeper specimen should be taken and carefully labeled. If excision is still uncertain then the wound should be temporized with a dressing and histological confirmation of completeness should be obtained before proceeding with reconstruction.

Mohs micrographic surgery involves sequential horizontal excision using a topographic map of the lesion and repeated excision until all positive tumor margins are clear. Reported cure rates are higher than standard excision at 99%. In addition, tissue conservation is increased. For this reason, Mohs is indicated not only in recurrent tumors but also in primary tumors in cosmetically sensitive areas, aggressive tumor subtypes such as morpheaform and sclerosing variants, and those with poorly delineated peripheral margins.[1-7]

REFERENCES

1. Breuninger H, Dietz K. Prediction of subclinical tumor infiltration in basal cell carcinoma. J Dermatol Surg Oncol 1991;17(7):574–578
2. Wolf DJ, Zitelli JA. Surgical margins for basal cell carcinoma. Arch Dermatol 1987;123(3):340–344
3. Kimyai-Asadi A, Alam M, Goldberg LH, Peterson SR, Silapunt S, Jih MH. Efficacy of narrow-margin excision of well-demarcated primary facial basal cell carcinomas. J Am Acad Dermatol 2005;53(3):464–468
4. Quazi SJ, Aslam N, Saleem H, Rahman J, Khan S. Surgical margin of excision in basal cell carcinoma: a systematic review of literature. Cureus 2020;12(7):e9211
5. Nahhas AF, Scarbrough CA, Trotter S. A review of the global guidelines on surgical margins for nonmelanoma skin cancers. J Clin Aesthet Dermatol 2017;10(4):37–46
6. Telfer NR, Colver GB, Morton CA; British Association of Dermatologists. Guidelines for the management of basal cell carcinoma. Br J Dermatol 2008;159(1):35–48
7. Miller S, Alam M, Anderson J, et al. NCCN Guidelines. Clinical practice guidelines in oncology: basal cell and squamous cell skin cancers version 2. 2012. DOI: 10.6004/jnccn.2004.0001

SURGICAL MANAGEMENT OF BASAL CELL CARCINOMA

8.   *What is the major advantage of Mohs surgery for BCC management?*

   C.   Completeness of excision is confirmed intraoperatively.

Mohs micrographic surgery involves sequential horizontal excision using a topographic map of the lesion with repeated excision until all positive tumor margins are clear. The main benefits are that completeness can be confirmed because tissue is assessed at every margin and this is confirmed at the time of surgery. In contrast, standard histological analysis does not sample every margin so completeness cannot be guaranteed. Furthermore, the procedure would need to be staged if confirmation of excision is required before reconstruction. Reported cure rates are higher than standard excision at 99%, but 100% cure is still not achieved. A further benefit is that tissue conservation is increased because only involved margins are re-excised in contrast to the standard surgical approach where an arbitrary margin is taken. For this reason, Mohs is indicated in both primary and recurrent tumors, particularly those in cosmetically sensitive areas. It is also useful in treating aggressive tumor subtypes such as morpheaform and sclerosing variants and those with poorly delineated peripheral margins. The problem with Mohs is that it takes significantly longer to treat each patient and the patients must wait for the analysis to be performed at each excision stage. Patients still require complex reconstruction in many cases with flaps or grafts. Some Mohs surgeons can and do reconstruct the defects created, but many will return the patient back to the reconstructive plastic surgeon once excision is complete. Therefore, many patients still have a staged procedure with regard to reconstruction.[1-4]

REFERENCES

1. Mohs FE. Chemosurgery: a microscopically controlled method of cancer excision. Arch Surg 1941;42(2):279–295
2. Rowe DE, Carroll RJ, Day CL Jr. Long-term recurrence rates in previously untreated (primary) basal cell carcinoma: implications for patient follow-up. J Dermatol Surg Oncol 1989;15(3):315–328
3. Samarasinghe V, Madan V, Lear JT. Focus on Basal cell carcinoma. J Skin Cancer 2011;2011:328615
4. Rowe DE, Carroll RJ, Day CL Jr. Mohs surgery is the treatment of choice for recurrent (previously treated) basal cell carcinoma. J Dermatol Surg Oncol 1989;15(4):424–431

RISK FACTORS FOR SQUAMOUS CELL CARCINOMA

9.   *Which one of the following factors most increases the risk of developing an SCC?*

   E.   Immune suppression after transplant surgery

All of the options represent risk factors for SCC. However, the risk of developing an SCC after immunosuppression for renal transplant is increased by 253 times, making this the most significant single-risk factor Immunosuppression after transplant usually involves combination therapy with steroids (prednisolone) and immunomodulators such as mycophenolate mofetil (MMF) and tacrolimus.

Patients with lighter skin tones (Fitzpatrick I to II) have an increased risk. Overall lifetime sun exposure, episodes of sunburn, and the use of tanning beds can further increase the risk. Carcinogens implicated include pesticides, arsenic, and organic hydrocarbons. Viruses such as HPV and herpes are also implicated. This emphasizes the importance of assessing these areas during history taking in patients with suspected SCCs and providing prevention advice.[1-7]

REFERENCES

1. Veness MJ. High-risk cutaneous squamous cell carcinoma of the head and neck. J Biomed Biotechnol 2007;2007(3):80572
2. Miller S, Alam M, Anderson J, et al. NCCN Guidelines. Clinical practice guidelines in oncology: basal cell and squamous cell skin cancers version 2, 2012. Available at http://www.nccn.org/professionals/ physician_gls/f_guidelines.asp#nmsc
3. Immerman SC, Scanlon EF, Christ M, Knox KL. Recurrent squamous cell carcinoma of the skin. Cancer 1983;51(8):1537–1540
4. Motley RJ, Preston PW, Lawrence CM. Multi-professional Guidelines for the Management of the Patient with Primary Cutaneous Squamous Cell Carcinoma. London, United Kingdom: British Association of Dermatology; 2009
5. Vitaliano PP, Urbach F. The relative importance of risk factors in nonmelanoma carcinoma. Arch Dermatol 1980;116(4):454–456
6. Gallagher RP, Hill GB, Bajdik CD, et al. Sunlight exposure, pigmentation factors, and risk of nonmelanocytic skin cancer. II. Squamous cell carcinoma. Arch Dermatol 1995;131(2):164–169
7. American Cancer Society. Medical and editorial content team. www.cancer.org/cancer/melanoma-skin-cancer/about/key-statistics.html

SQUAMOUS CELL CARCINOMA–RELATED DEATHS

10. An SCC in which one of the following sites will is associated with the highest overall mortality risk?

A. **Ear**

SCCs arising on the external ear are particularly high-risk lesions that can spread through the lymphatics to the parotid gland and neck. Of all the head and neck skin SCC sites, the ear is considered to be the most likely site to result in death. Other high-risk sites include the temple, forehead, scalp, and lower lip. In each of these sites, metastatic spread can occur in the neck or parotid nodes. Other high-risk factors for metastases should also be considered such as tumor diameter (>2 cm), depth (>4 mm), poor differentiation, incomplete margins, and perineural invasion as a tumor spread can proceed along nerves.[1-4]

REFERENCES

1. Veness MJ. High-risk cutaneous squamous cell carcinoma of the head and neck. J Biomed Biotechnol 2007;2007(3):80572
2. Habif TP, ed. Clinical Dermatology: A Color Guide to Diagnosis and Therapy. 4th ed. St Louis: Elsevier; 2004
3. Miller S, Alam M, Anderson J, et al. NCCN Guidelines. Clinical practice guidelines in oncology: basal cell and squamous cell skin cancers version 2, 2012. Available at http://www.nccn.org/professionals/ physician_gls/f_guidelines.asp#nmsc
4. Immerman SC, Scanlon EF, Christ M, Knox KL. Recurrent squamous cell carcinoma of the skin. Cancer 1983;51(8):1537–1540

RISK FACTORS FOR RECURRENCE OF SQUAMOUS CELL CARCINOMA

11. Which one of the following describes a low-risk SCC?

E. **A verrucous tumor subtype**

Many factors are used to classify SCCs as low risk or high risk.[1] Factors that characterize low-risk lesions include the following: sun-exposed sites, excluding the lip and the ear, diameter less than 2 cm, depth less than 4 mm, tumor confined to the dermis, well-differentiated or verrucous subtypes, and no evidence of host immune suppression. Factors that characterize high-risk lesions are the following: involvement of the ear or lip, diameter greater than 2 cm, depth greater than 4 mm, moderate or poor differentiation, host immune suppression, recurrence, and sites not exposed to the sun such as the perineum (**Table 20.1**).[1-3]

REFERENCES

1. Motley RJ, Preston PW, Lawrence CM. Multi-professional Guidelines for the Management of the Patient with Primary Cutaneous Squamous Cell Carcinoma. London, United Kingdom: British Association of Dermatology; 2009
2. Miller S, Alam M, Anderson J, et al. NCCN Guidelines: Clinical Practice Guidelines in Oncology: Basal Cell and Squamous Cell Skin Cancers Version 2.2012. DOI: 10.6004/jnccn.2004.0001
3. Immerman SC, Scanlon EF, Christ M, Knox KL. Recurrent squamous cell carcinoma of the skin. Cancer 1983;51(8):1537–1540

Table 20.1   *Risk Factors for Recurrence of BCC and SCC*

	Low Risk	High Risk
Location/size	<20 mm trunk/ext	≥20 mm trunk/ext
	≥10 mm cheek, forehead, scalp, neck	>10 mm cheek, forehead, scalp, neck
	<6 mm central face, genitalia, hands, feet	>6 mm central face, genitalia, hands, feet
Defined borders	Well defined	Poorly defined
Primary vs. recurrent	Primary	Recurrent
Immunosuppression	–	+
Prior radiotherapy	–	+
Pathology	Nodular, superficial, keratotic, infundibulocystic	Morpheaform, sclerosing, micronodular, mixed infiltrative, adenoid,* desmoplastic*
Perineural involvement	–	+
Rapidly growing*	–	+
Depth*	<2 mm, Clark I–III	>2 mm, Clark IV and V
Lymphovascular invasion*	–	+
Degree of differentiation*	Well differentiated	Poorly differentiated

BCC, basal cell carcinoma; *SCC*, squamous cell carcinoma
*SCC only.
(Adapted from Miller S, Alam M, Anderson J, et al. NCCN Guidelines: Clinical Practice Guidelines in Oncology: Basal Cell and Squamous Cell Skin Cancers Version 2.2012. Available at nccn.org.)

PREMALIGNANT SKIN LESIONS

12. A patient is referred to clinic by his or her general practitioner with an 8-week history of a dome-shaped keratotic lesion to the forearm that displayed initial rapid growth followed by spontaneous partial regression after 7 weeks. *What is the most likely diagnosis?*

    D. Keratoacanthoma

    Keratoacanthomas are premalignant skin lesions with a typical domed-shaped appearance and a keratin plug. Their clinical and histologic appearance closely resembles a well-differentiated SCC and it can be difficult to differentiate between the two. They usually progress rapidly over a number of weeks before spontaneous regression begins. They are frequently excised to exclude an SCC diagnosis as the initial history and clinical appearances are so similar. Treatment is complete once full excision is achieved. Actinic keratosis represents such damage leading to dry crusting of the skin in sun-exposed sites such as the scalp, face, ears, and limbs. Malignant transformation to SCC can occur and so more progressive lesions are often biopsied. Nonsurgical management of actinic keratoses includes cryotherapy and topical agents such as 5-FU or Imiquamod. Bowen's disease presents with an erythematous plaque with sharp borders and slight scaling. It represents in situ SCC and has a 10% chance of malignant transformation. Erythroplasia of Queyrat is Bowen's disease of the glans penis, vulva, or oral mucosa and is associated with a 30% malignant transformation. Leukoplakia is a premalignant condition affecting the oral mucosa. There are mucosal changes with a visible white patch. Malignant transformation occurs in around 15% of cases.[1–5]

REFERENCES

1. Morton CA, Birnie AJ, Eedy DJ. British Association of Dermatologists' guidelines for the management of squamous cell carcinoma in situ (Bowen's disease) 2014. Br J Dermatol 2014;170(2):245–260
2. Keratoacanthoma. https://www.bad.org.uk/shared/get-file.ashx?id=96&itemtype=document
3. Gibbons M, Ernst A, Patel A, Armbrecht E, Behshad R. Keratoacanthomas: a review of excised specimens. J Am Acad Dermatol 2019;80(6):1794–1796

4. Moss M, Weber E, Hoverson K, Montemarano AD. Management of keratoacanthoma: 157 tumors treated with surgery or intralesional methotrexate. Dermatol Surg 2019;45(7):877–883
5. van der Waal I, Schepman KP, van der Meij EH, Smeele LE. Oral leukoplakia: a clinicopathological review. Oral Oncol 1997;33(5):291–301

TREATMENT OF CUTANEOUS SQUAMOUS CELL CARCINOMA

13. You see an 85-year-old otherwise healthy patient with a thick, necrotic, 2-cm diameter SCC involving the left cheek and preauricular region. There is no obvious palpable lymphadenopathy present and the lesion remains mobile over deeper tissues. *Which one of the following is correct regarding management of this patient?*
    C. The patient is unlikely to benefit from elective nodal dissection.
    Wide local excision is the most suitable management for this patient and a peripheral margin greater than 6 mm is required. Many surgeons would opt for a 1-cm margin in this case given the size and thickness of the tumor and its anatomic location. Cure rates for primary surgery are around 95%. Wound closure in patients of this age group is usually achieved with local flap techniques given the skin laxity in the cheek and neck at this age. Primary radiotherapy has a cure rate of 90% and is reserved for patients in whom surgery is not advisable, or as adjuvant therapy in high-stage large or recurrent tumors.

    Elective lymph node dissection is not advocated for cutaneous SCC, in contrast to an equivalently sized intraoral tumor. The technique is, however, indicated in cases where there is evidence of tumor spread to the parotid capsule or contiguous nodal basin drainage as may be suggested by adherence of the tumor to underlying deep structures. Sentinel lymph node biopsy (SLNB) is sometimes indicated for node-negative patients with high-risk tumors. Mohs surgery is not required in this case given the high cure rates with standard surgical techniques. Following surgical excision, the patient should be followed up in clinic for an extended period. This should be on a 3–6 months basis for 2 years, then every 6–12 months for 3 years, then annually thereafter.[1-4]

REFERENCES

1. Kim JYS, Kozlow JH, Mittal B, Moyer J, Olenecki T, Rodgers P; Work Group; Invited Reviewers. Guidelines of care for the management of cutaneous squamous cell carcinoma. J Am Acad Dermatol 2018;78(3):560–578
2. Motley R, Kersey P, Lawrence C; British Association of Dermatologists; British Association of Plastic Surgeons; Royal College of Radiologists, Faculty of Clinical Oncology. Multiprofessional guidelines for the management of the patient with primary cutaneous squamous cell carcinoma. Br J Dermatol 2002;146(1):18–25
3. National Comprehensive Cancer Center. NCCN clinical practice guidelines in oncology; squamous cell carcinoma (V1.2015). Available at: www.nccn.org
4. Jennings L, Schmults CD. Management of high-risk cutaneous squamous cell carcinoma. J Clin Aesthet Dermatol 2010;3(4):39–48

MELANOMA SUBTYPES

14. *Which one of the following is the most common cutaneous melanoma subtype?*
    A. Superficial spreading
    There are a number of different melanoma subtypes and the most common cutaneous variant is superficial spreading, representing more than half of all melanomas (50–70%). Nodular subtypes are the next most common, representing 15–30% of all cases. Lentigo maligna and acral-lentiginous usually each represent less than 10% of all melanomas, and desmoplastic subtypes are least common, representing around 1% of all cases.[1-5]

REFERENCES

1. Coricovac D, Dehelean C, Moaca EA, et al. Cutaneous melanoma–a long road from experimental models to clinical outcome: a review. Int J Mol Sci 2018;19(6):1566
2. Marsden JR, Newton-Bishop JA, Burrows L, et al; British Association of Dermatologists (BAD) Clinical Standards Unit. Revised UK guidelines for the management of cutaneous melanoma 2010. J Plast Reconstr Aesthet Surg 2010;63(9):1401–1419
3. Bichakjian CK, Halpern AC, Johnson TM, et al; American Academy of Dermatology. Guidelines of care for the management of primary cutaneous melanoma. J Am Acad Dermatol 2011;65(5):1032–1047
4. National Comprehensive Cancer Network. NCCN clinical practice guidelines in oncology: melanoma (version 1.2018). October 11, 2017. Available at: https://www.nccn.org/guidelines/guidelines-detail?category=1&id=1492
5. Dummer R, Hauschild A, Guggenheim M, Keilholz U, Pentheroudakis G; ESMO Guidelines Working Group. Cutaneous melanoma: ESMO Clinical Practice Guidelines for diagnosis, treatment and follow-up. Ann Oncol 2012;23(Suppl 7):vii86–vii91

MELANOMA SUBTYPES

15. You see a 45-year-old white patient in your office who has evidence of a new-onset, single-digit, linear, pigmented nail streak. You are concerned that this may be melanoma, and you perform a biopsy. *With which melanoma subtype may this presentation be associated?*

    E. Acral-lentiginous

        Acral-lentiginous melanoma can occur on the palms and soles, subungually, or in other sun-protected sites. Melanonychia represents a linear pigmented streak within the nail and is associated with this melanoma subtype. Although melanonychia is often a benign finding, if it involves a single digit and has a recent onset, it should raise concerns. In this situation, the entire nail should be examined closely with magnification or dermatoscopy. The skin borders surrounding the nail must also be carefully reviewed. In the event that concern remains following clinical examination, further investigation with removal of the nail plate and biopsy of the nailbed and/or eponychium would be indicated.[1,2]

REFERENCES

1. Krementz ET, Feed RJ, Coleman WP III, Sutherland CM, Carter RD, Campbell M. Acral lentiginous melanoma. A clinico-pathologic entity. Ann Surg 1982;195(5):632–645
2. Nakamura Y, Fujisawa Y. Diagnosis and management of acral lentiginous melanoma. Curr Treat Options Oncol 2018;19(8):42

MELANOMA SUBTYPES

16. *When assessing a patient in clinic with a suspected melanoma, which one of the following would be most in keeping with development of a nodular subtype?*

    B. Development de novo

        Development of melanoma commonly differs between subtypes. For example, nodular melanoma typically arises de novo in normal skin. It appears as a dome-shaped pigmented lesion that may resemble a blood blister. It displays a lack of horizontal growth so keeps sharp demarcation. Nodular melanomas are aggressive and more commonly affect men. Superficial spreading subtypes tend to arise from long-standing junctional or compound nevi, and patients may have noticed a change in the color, size, or borders of the lesion. These tumors tend to have a prolonged horizontal growth before vertical growth commences. A Hutchinson freckle is also known as a senile freckle or lentigo maligna and this is an in situ melanoma. It can progress to form lentigo maligna melanoma, which is the least aggressive subtype and is related to sun exposure. The Hutchinson freckle represents the horizontal growth phase and the vertical growth phase represents the transition to melanoma. Melanomas in sun-protected sites tend to be acral-lentiginous and are seen on the soles or palms. They have a long radial growth phase followed by transition to a vertical growth phase. A spitz nevus is a smooth dome-shaped benign lesion seen in children or young adults that represents a proliferation of enlarged spindle melanocytes. It does not represent a precursor to melanoma, although there is a melanoma subtype call spitzoid melanoma that has a similar histologic appearance to a spitz nevus.[1–3]

REFERENCES

1. Marsden JR, Newton-Bishop JA, Burrows L, et al; British Association of Dermatologists (BAD) Clinical Standards Unit. Revised UK guidelines for the management of cutaneous melanoma 2010. J Plast Reconstr Aesthet Surg 2010;63(9):1401–1419
2. Bichakjian CK, Halpern AC, Johnson TM, et al; American Academy of Dermatology. Guidelines of care for the management of primary cutaneous melanoma. J Am Acad Dermatol 2011;65(5):1032–1047
3. Kelly JW, Chamberlain AJ, Staples MP, McAvoy B. Nodular melanoma. No longer as simple as ABC. Aust Fam Physician 2003;32(9):706–709

MELANOMA PROGNOSIS

17. *When reviewing the histopathology report of a melanoma specimen, what is the single most important histologic prognostic factor for the patient?*

    D. Breslow thickness

        All of the options are important factors in melanoma, but Breslow thickness (BT) is the single most important factor. It represents the measurement of tumor depth from the granular layer of the epidermis to the deepest extension of the tumor. BT is used to stage the disease using the tumor, node and metastasis (TNM) classification system and to plan subsequent treatment. A number of key features will be displayed on a histological report for melanoma including those listed in answer options A, B, C, and E. For example, the mitotic rate (especially relevant to tumors less than 1 mm deep) and ulceration (relevant to all tumors), perineural or perivascular invasion, and Clark's level which relates to the anatomic depth of the tumor. Completeness of excision is also critical to plan further management, and subtype and growth phase are both important to provide information on prognosis.[1–5]

REFERENCES

1. Marsden JR, Newton-Bishop JA, Burrows L, et al; British Association of Dermatologists (BAD) Clinical Standards Unit. Revised UK guidelines for the management of cutaneous melanoma 2010. J Plast Reconstr Aesthet Surg 2010;63(9):1401–1419
2. Azzola MF, Shaw HM, Thompson JF, et al. Tumor mitotic rate is a more powerful prognostic indicator than ulceration in patients with primary cutaneous melanoma: an analysis of 3661 patients from a single center. Cancer 2003;97(6):1488–1498
3. Breslow A. Thickness, cross-sectional areas and depth of invasion in the prognosis of cutaneous melanoma. Ann Surg 1970;172(5):902–908
4. Scolyer RA, Mihm MC Jr, Cochran AJ, Busam KJ, McCarthy SW. Pathology of melanoma. In: Balch CM, Houghton Jr A, Sober A, Soong SJ, eds. Cutaneous Melanoma. 5th ed. St. Louis, Missouri: Quality Medical Publishing; 2009:205–248
5. Edge SE, Byrd DR, Compton CC, Fritz AG, Greene FL, Trotti A, eds. AJCC Cancer Staging Manual. 7th ed. New York, NY.: Springer; 2010

AMERICAN JOINT COMMITTEE ON CANCER MELANOMA STAGING CLASSIFICATION (AJCC)

18. You discuss a patient at the weekly multidisciplinary team meeting to plan treatment. The patient has a melanoma of Breslow thickness (BT) 2.5 mm, three positive regional lymph nodes, and metastases involving the skin. *What would be the correct melanoma staging for this patient according to the classification of the American Joint Committee on Cancer (AJCC)?*

    D. T3N2M1a

    The American Joint Committee on Cancer (AJCC) has produced guidelines for melanoma staging based on the TNM (tumor, node, metastasis) system. In this classification, tumors are initially classified by their Breslow depth as T1 to T4 lesions, with lesions less than 1 mm graded as T1, those between 1.01 and 2.0 mm as T2, those between 2.01 and 4.0 mm as T3, and those greater than 4 mm as T4. The presence of ulceration or mitotic rate greater than 1 will upgrade a T1a lesion to T1b. For T2, 3, and 4 tumors the presence of ulceration will upgrade them to T2b, 3b, and, 4b, respectively. The mitotic rate does not alter the T classification for these tumors.[1]

    Nodal status is N0 (no spread), N1 (spread to one nearby lymph node), N2 (spread to 2 or 3 nearby lymph nodes), and N3 (spread to 4 or more lymph nodes). Again, this is further altered by pathological information on micrometastases, in transit satellites, and macrometastases, which may be obtained following sentinel lymph node biopsy (SLNB) or excisional surgery.

    Metastatic spread is subclassified as M1a, b, or c, depending on the extent and type of metastases present.

    Once the T, N, and M groups have been determined, they are combined to give an overall stage called stage grouping. This provides prognostic information, which is also used to guide treatment (**Tables 20.2 and 20.3**).

Table 20.2 *AJCC TNM Melanoma Staging Classification, 2010*

Tumor Classification	Depth of Invasion
TX	Primary tumor cannot be assessed
Tis	Melanoma in situ
T1	<1.0 mm
T2	1.01–2.0 mm
T3	2.01–4.0 mm
T4	>4.0 mm

NOTE: a and b subcategories of T: a, without ulceration and mitosis < 1/mm²; b, with ulceration or mitoses >1/mm².

Node Classification	
NX	Cannot be assessed
N1	One node
N2	Two to three nodes
N3	Four or more nodes, matted, or in transit satellites with metastatic nodes

NOTE: a, b, and c subcategories of N: a, micrometastasis (diagnosed after sentinel lymph node biopsy); b, macrometastasis (clinically positive nodes); c, in transit satellites without nodes (N2 only).

Metastatic Classification	
M1a	Metastases to skin, subcutaneous, distant nodes
M1b	Metastases to lung
M1c	Metastases to other viscera or any distant site combined with elevated serum LDH

Table 20.3 *Pathologic Staging*

Stage	Tumor	Node	Metastasis
Stage 0	Tis	N0	M0
Stage IA	T1a	N0	M0
Stage IB	T1b	N0	M0
	T2a	N0	M0
Stage IIA	T2b	N0	M0
	T3a	N0	M0
Stage IIB	T3b	N0	M0
	T4a	N0	M0
Stage IIC	T4b	N0	M0
Stage IIIA	T(1–4)a	N1a	M0
	T(1–4)a	N2a	M0
Stage IIIB	T(1–4)b	N1a or N2a	M0
	T(1–4)a	N1b, N2b, or N2c	M0
Stage IIIC	T(1–4)b	N1b, N2b, or N2c	M0
	Any T	N3	M0
Stage IV	Any T	Any N	M1

REFERENCE

1. Available at. https://cancerstaging.org/references-tools/quickreferences/Documents/MelanomaSmall. pdf

SURGICAL MANAGEMENT OF MELANOMA

19. Which one of the following is correct regarding the surgical management of melanoma?

E. A positive Cloquet's node is not the only indication for pelvic dissection.

In patients with positive nodal disease or positive sentinel lymph nodes, therapeutic lymph node dissection is generally advocated. In patients with positive groin disease an extended procedure to include dissection of pelvic nodes is required in some cases. The indications include where multiple groin nodes are clinically palpable, where there is computed tomography (CT) or ultrasound evidence of multiple groin nodes involved, where multiple groin nodes are found to be positive during sentinel lymph node biopsy (SLNB), and where there is a conglomerate of groin nodes.

Full-thickness excision biopsies (1–3 mm margins) are required for the vast majority of suspected melanomas in order to confirm diagnosis, completely remove the lesion, and fully assess their histological features including Breslow thickness. However, full-thickness biopsies are not required for subungual melanoma as this offers no prognostic information. Incisional biopsies may be considered for low-suspicion lesions or cosmetically sensitive regions. Shave biopsies are not recommended.

Long-term survival is not improved by excising the deep fascial layer and recommendations are to perform the wide local excision down to the fascial layer only. Removal of the fascia may increase metastatic spread. Recommendations for subungual melanoma are that amputation is performed proximal to the distal interphalangeal joint, not the proximal interphalangeal joint. Sentinel lymph node biopsy is a staging procedure and is indicated in both stage Ib and stage II disease but not in stage III, as by definition nodal spread must have already taken place. Following a positive SLNB, patients will be offered the option of elective lymph node dissection or regular ultrasound of the lymphatic basin as part of the ongoing follow-up.[1-5]

REFERENCES

1. Morton DL, Thompson JF, Cochran AJ, et al; MSLT Group. Sentinel-node biopsy or nodal observation in melanoma. N Engl J Med 2006;355(13):1307–1317

2. Coit D, Andtbacka R, Anker C, et al. NCCN Guidelines. Clinical practice guidelines in oncology: melanoma version 2. 2013. https://www.nccn.org/guidelines/guidelines-detail?category=1&id=1492

3. Peach H, Board R, Cook M, et al. Current role of sentinel lymph node biopsy in the management of cutaneous melanoma: a UK consensus statement. J Plast Reconstr Aesthet Surg 2020;73(1):36–42

4. Sladden MJ, Nieweg OE, Howle J, Coventry BJ, Thompson JF. Updated evidence-based clinical practice guidelines for the diagnosis and management of melanoma: definitive excision margins for primary cutaneous melanoma. Med J Aust 2018;208(3):137–142

5. Marsden JR, Newton-Bishop JA, Burrows L, et al; British Association of Dermatologists (BAD) Clinical Standards Unit. Revised UK guidelines for the management of cutaneous melanoma 2010. J Plast Reconstr Aesthet Surg 2010;63(9):1401–1419

NONSURGICAL MANAGEMENT OF MELANOMA

20. *Which one of the following is correct regarding nonsurgical management of melanoma?*

C. The use of dacarbazine or cisplatin may help to reduce the tumor burden.

Dacarbazine and cisplatin are chemotherapy agents that may be considered in melanoma to reduce tumor burden, but they are generally only palliative. Sentinel lymph node biopsy is a staging procedure, not a therapeutic procedure that is used in patients with intermediate depth melanomas in order to identify whether the tumor has spread to the sentinel lymph node. If SLNB is positive, then progression to completion lymphadenectomy should proceed. There remains debate about the clinical benefits of SLNB as overall life expectancy does not appear to be improved, but local tumor recurrence may be; further evidence is awaited. Elective lymph node dissection appears to have a survival benefit only in intermediate melanoma (1–2 mm) and is not routinely performed because of the comorbidity involved unless the SLNB or clinical examination is positive for lymph node involvement. Radiation therapy is rarely indicated as a primary treatment of melanoma except for lentigo maligna or desmoplastic lesions. Interferon can be useful in patients with regional nodal disease or deep primary tumors.[1–3]

REFERENCES

1. Morton DL, Thompson JF, Cochran AJ, et al; MSLT Group. Sentinel-node biopsy or nodal observation in melanoma. N Engl J Med 2006;355(13):1307–1317

2. Coit D, Andtbacka R, Anker C, et al. NCCN Guidelines. Clinical practice guidelines in oncology: melanoma version 2. 2013. Available at http://www.nccn.org/professionals/physician_gls/f_guidelines. aspimelanoma

3. Peach H, Board R, Cook M, et al. Current role of sentinel lymph node biopsy in the management of cutaneous melanoma: a UK consensus statement. J Plast Reconstr Aesthet Surg 2020;73(1):36–42

WIDE EXCISION MARGINS IN MELANOMA

21. *What would be the recommended wide excision margin for a primary melanoma with a Breslow thickness of 3.2 mm once it had been completely excised for diagnosis?*

D. 2 cm

Evidence for the selection of excision margins in melanoma is provided by six key papers considering five major studies.[1–6]

Recommended peripheral margins for melanoma excision vary between different guidelines and this reflects the available evidence and differences in its interpretation (**Table 20.4**).

In situ disease is commonly excised with a 5-mm margin. Melanomas less than 1 mm in depth are commonly excised with a 1-cm margin. Thicker melanomas are excised with a 2-cm margin. Most evidence for peripheral margin selection relates to melanoma on the trunk and excludes the head, neck, and distal limbs. In clinical

Table 20.4 *United States Excision Margin Guidelines for Melanoma Excision*

Primary Tumor Type	Recommended Peripheral Excision Margin	Commonly Recommended Deep Excision Margin
In situ disease	5 mm	Cuff of subcutaneous tissue
Less than 1 mm Breslow depth	1 cm	To next fascial plane
1.01–2 mm Breslow depth	1–2 cm (wider is preferable if possible, depending on tumor site, patient, and surgeon preference)	To next fascial plane
2.01–4 mm Breslow depth	1–2 cm (wider is preferable if possible, depending on tumor site, patient, and surgeon preference)	To next fascial plane
Greater than 4.01 mm Breslow depth	2 cm	To next fascial plane

practice, margins should be tailored to patients on an individual basis depending on site, size, and tumor biology, ideally in a multidisciplinary team setting.[7]

REFERENCES

1. Veronesi U, Cascinelli N, Adamus J, et al. Thin stage I primary cutaneous malignant melanoma. Comparison of excision with margins of 1 or 3 cm. N Engl J Med 1988;318(18):1159–1162
2. Balch CM, Urist MM, Karakousis CP, et al. Efficacy of 2-cm surgical margins for intermediate-thickness melanomas (1 to 4 mm). Results of a multi-institutional randomized surgical trial. Ann Surg 1993;218(3):262–267, discussion 267–269
3. Cohn-Cedermark G, Rutqvist LE, Andersson R, et al. Long term results of a randomized study by the Swedish Melanoma Study Group on 2-cm versus 5-cm resection margins for patients with cutaneous melanoma with a tumor thickness of 0.8–2.0 mm. Cancer 2000;89(7):1495–1501
4. Khayat D, Rixe O, Martin G, et al; French Group of Research on Malignant Melanoma. Surgical margins in cutaneous melanoma (2 cm versus 5 cm for lesions measuring less than 2.1-mm thick). Cancer 2003;97(8):1941–1946
5. Balch CM, Soong SJ, Smith T, et al; Investigators from the Intergroup Melanoma Surgical Trial. Long-term results of a prospective surgical trial comparing 2 cm vs. 4 cm excision margins for 740 patients with 1–4 mm melanomas. Ann Surg Oncol 2001;8(2):101–108
6. Thomas JM, Newton-Bishop J, A'Hern R, et al; United Kingdom Melanoma Study Group; British Association of Plastic Surgeons; Scottish Cancer Therapy Network. Excision margins in high-risk malignant melanoma. N Engl J Med 2004;350(8):757–766
7. Marsden JR, Newton-Bishop JA, Burrows L, et al; British Association of Dermatologists (BAD) Clinical Standards Unit. Revised UK guidelines for the management of cutaneous melanoma 2010. J Plast Reconstr Aesthet Surg 2010;63(9):1401–1419

TREATMENT IN ADVANCED-STAGE MELANOMA

22. In a patient with stage IV melanoma who has tested positive for BRAF, which one of the following treatment modalities is specifically indicated?

D. Vemurafenib

Vemurafenib is a BRAF inhibitor with FDA approval for use in advanced-stage melanoma. It is indicated in patients who are BRAF-positive (i.e., those who have a mutation of the intracellular signaling kinase BRAF). Mutations in the BRAF gene are present in 40–70% of melanomas, leading to uncontrolled cell proliferation. Vemurafenib has been shown to increase overall survival and progression-free survival when compared with dacarbazine (a standard monochemotherapeutic agent).[1] Although the survival improvements have been statistically significant, the real benefits have been modest as lifespan was extended by just a few months in most cases. A further problem with BRAF inhibitors such as vemurafenib is that resistance can occur. For this reason, combination therapy is also being studied. Also, patients have an increased risk of developing SCC while taking this treatment. Furthermore, the financial implications of using this drug are significant with a course of treatment costing many thousands of dollars. Radiotherapy may be indicated as adjuvant treatment following lymphadectomy with more significant disease and can be used in palliation for metastatic disease. Dacarbazine, cisplatin, and vinblastin are standard chemotherapy agents used in combination rather than individually that are generally palliative only with modest response rates.[2]

REFERENCES

1. Chapman PB, Hauschild A, Robert C, et al; BRIM-3 Study Group. Improved survival with vemurafenib in melanoma with BRAF V600E mutation. N Engl J Med 2011;364(26):2507–2516
2. Maverakis E, Cornelius LA, Bowen GM, et al. Metastatic melanoma—a review of current and future treatment options. Acta Derm Venereol 2015;95(5):516–524

ADVANCED-STAGE MELANOMA

23. Which one of the following is a monoclonal antibody directed to the receptor CTLA-4, approved by the FDA for patients with unresectable melanoma?

A. Ipilimumab

Immune-based treatment options for patients with advanced-stage melanoma can be subclassified as immune agents such as interleukin-2, checkpoint inhibitors such as ipilimumab, or signal transduction inhibitors such as vemurafenib and trametinib. Ipilimumab is a monoclonal antibody that blocks the CTLA-4 receptor (a downregulator of T-cells). The resultant stimulation of T-cells may present a risk for immune-related reactions. It received FDA approval in 2011 for patients with advanced-stage melanoma. Imatinib (also known as *Glivec*) is a tyrosine kinase inhibitor that works by blocking growth pathways within a variety of tumors. Canvaxin and MAGE-A3 have been trialed as vaccines against melanoma in advanced disease, but results have not been particularly successful.[1–4]

REFERENCES

1. Coit D, Andtbacka R, Anker C, et al. NCCN Guidelines. Clinical practice guidelines in oncology: melanoma version 2. 2013. Available at http://www.nccn.org/professionals/physician_gls/f_guidelines. aspimelanoma
2. Maverakis E, Cornelius LA, Bowen GM, et al. Metastatic melanoma—a review of current and future treatment options. Acta Derm Venereol 2015;95(5):516–524
3. Wolchok JD, Rollin L, Larkin J. Nivolumab and ipilimumab in advanced melanoma. N Engl J Med 2017;377(25):2503–2504
4. Faries MB, Morton DL. Therapeutic vaccines for melanoma: current status. BioDrugs 2005;19(4):247–260

MELANOMA FOLLOW-UP

24. *Following complete resection of a 2.5-mm Breslow thickness melanoma from the calf, for how long should patients be followed (in the US), assuming they have no palpable lymph nodes?*

E. Lifelong

Standard follow-up for melanoma patients varies according to country but in the US, lifelong surveillance is currently advised by the National Comprehensive Cancer Network (NCCN) and American Academy of Dermatology (AAD). The German Cancer Society and German Dermatologic Society recommend 10-year follow-up for most stages as do the Swiss, while the British Association of dermatologists advise follow-up according to stage and this varies from 5 to 10 years. The Australian and New Zealand guidelines also vary according to stage with 5-year follow-up advised for stage I and lifelong for stages II and III.

Typical follow-up will involve clinical assessment with review of the primary site and nodal basins as well as review of other skin sites for new or changing pigmented lesions. Local recurrence usually occurs within 5 cm of the original lesion within the first 3–5 years. In the first 5 years patients are typically seen at 3- to 6-monthly intervals. Beyond 5 years patients are seen on an annual basis. Routine imaging beyond 5 years is not recommended.[1]

REFERENCE

1. Trotter SC, Sroa N, Winkelmann RR, Olencki T, Bechtel M. A global review of melanoma follow-up guidelines. J Clin Aesthet Dermatol 2013;6(9):18–26

CLINICAL SCENARIOS IN SKIN CANCER

25. A 65-year-old patient presents with multiple raised verrucous papules with varied deep pigmentation affecting the back. His normal medical practitioner refers him with concern of melanoma in one of the lesions as it appears darker than the others. *Which one of the following represents the most likely diagnosis?*

B. Seborrheic keratosis

Seborrheic keratoses are benign lesions commonly found on the trunk of older patients. They are slow growing and have a raised verrucous appearance with varying degrees of pigmentation. They may often be mistaken for melanomas but do not usually require excision.

Care must be taken to examine them fully as many older patients will have multiple seborrheic keratoses but if there is one which is changing or behaving differently to the other, an excision biopsy may still be warranted.

Junctional nevi are flat and are generally found on the palms, soles, genitalia, and mucosa. They tend to have a uniform color which ranges from pale to dark brown. They are smooth, macular, and sharply defined with first appearance in childhood.

Compound nevi are darker that junctional nevi and are palpable with a raised border. They may be smooth or rough and have hair within them.

Blue nevi are blue/black colored lesions often found on the hands, feet, head, neck, or buttocks. They are usually smaller than 5 mm diameter and in rare cases can progress to melanoma.

Lentigo are benign pigmented macular lesions most commonly seen in middle age and beyond. Lentiginous lesions that change in appearance may warrant a tissue biopsy as they can progress to melanoma in situ and melanoma itself.[1,2]

REFERENCES

1. Jackson JM, Alexis A, Berman B, Berson DS, Taylor S, Weiss JS. Current understanding of seborrheic keratosis: prevalence, etiology, clinical presentation, diagnosis, and management. J Drugs Dermatol 2015;14(10):1119–1125
2. Damsky WE, Bosenberg M. Melanocytic nevi and melanoma: unraveling a complex relationship. Oncogene 2017;36(42):5771–5792

21. Burns

See *Essentials of Plastic Surgery*, third edition, pp. 276–290

STAGES IN THE MANAGEMENT OF BURNS

1. When considering total burn management, we often consider the five R's to guide the most suitable therapy for each individual patient. *Which one is primarily focused on Advanced Trauma Life Support (ATLS) principles?*
   A. Rehabilitation
   B. Resuscitation
   C. Resurfacing
   D. Recovery
   E. Reconstruction

PROGNOSIS AFTER SEVERE BURN INJURY

2. *Which one of the following factors is a major predictor of survival used when calculating the Baux score in a patient with a severe, acute burn injury?*
   A. The depth of the burn
   B. The burn subtype
   C. The age of the patient
   D. The first aid treatment provided
   E. The patient's past medical history

PATHOPHYSIOLOGY OF BURNS

3. A 22-year-old patient with a thermal injury is referred to you. The referring unit described the injury as a second-degree burn. *Which one of the following is correct regarding second-degree burns?*
   A. Blistering is usually present.
   B. Sensation is usually absent.
   C. Capillary refill is rarely present.
   D. The entire dermis is normally involved.
   E. The skin appendages are completely destroyed.

BURN TISSUE HISTOLOGY

4. The early management of burn injuries is based on Jackson's burn model. *Which area of the burn is most likely to benefit from early aggressive resuscitation according to this model?*
   A. Zone of necrosis
   B. Zone of stasis
   C. Zone of infiltration
   D. Zone of coagulation
   E. Zone of hyperemia

TRANSFER TO A BURN CENTER

5. *Which one of the following adult burns should be managed locally by a well-equipped plastic surgery department without referral to a burn center?*
   A. A 4% third-degree burn involving the upper forearm and hand
   B. A 15% first-degree burn involving the trunk and upper limbs
   C. A 12% second-degree burn involving the lower limbs
   D. A 1% hydrofluoric acid burn to the hand
   E. A 4% second-degree flash burn to the face and neck in an enclosed space

MANAGEMENT OF INHALATION INJURY

6. *In a patient who has sustained an inhalational injury during a house fire, which one of the following is true?*
   A. Cyanide poisoning would be unlikely in this scenario.
   B. Cytotoxicity in cyanide poisoning is generally irreversible.
   C. Signs of cyanide poisoning will begin at levels of 2.0 µg/mL.
   D. Management of cyanide toxicity includes IV hydroxocobalamin.
   E. Delivery of 100% oxygen is the mainstay of treatment for cyanide poisoning.

MANAGEMENT OF ELECTRICAL BURNS

7. A 70 kg patient has sustained a high-voltage electrical burn to the left lower limb and is admitted acutely to the burn center. A normal electrocardiogram (EKG) was obtained on admission. Clinical observations are normal, but the involved limb is tense and painful, with intracompartmental pressures measured at 20 mm Hg. Urine output is 30 mL per hour but is colored dark brown. *Which one of the following is correct?*
    A. Urine output should be maintained above 75 mL per hour.
    B. Bicarbonate and mannitol are contraindicated.
    C. Fasciotomy is not indicated at present.
    D. No further cardiac monitoring is required.
    E. The urine discoloration indicates renal failure.

MANAGEMENT OF CHEMICAL BURNS

8. *Which one of the following is the most appropriate treatment for a patient after a chemical injury with phenol?*
    A. Application of calcium gluconate gel
    B. Copious irrigation and neutralization with a weak acid
    C. Copious irrigation with water alone
    D. Irrigation followed by application of polyethylene glycol
    E. Application of copper sulfate

BURN RESUSCITATION

9. *Which one of the following is the correct resuscitation volume for a 95 kg patient with 42% total body surface area (TBSA) burns (using the modified Parkland formula)? The patient had 3 L before arrival at the burn unit, and the burn occurred 4 hours ago.*
    A. 1250 mL per hour for 4 hours, then 500 mL per hour for 16 hours
    B. 1000 mL per hour for 8 hours, then 400 mL per hour for 16 hours
    C. 1000 mL per hour for 4 hours, then 500 mL per hour for 16 hours
    D. 1500 mL per hour for 4 hours, then 500 mL per hour for 16 hours
    E. 750 mL per hour for 12 hours, then 580 mL per hour for 12 hours

FLUID RESUSCITATION IN BURN INJURY

10. There has been a recent shift to the use of the modified Brooke formula from the modified Parkland formula during initial burn fluid resuscitation. *What is the proposed benefit of this change?*
    A. To simplify the resuscitation process
    B. To reduce the potential for under resuscitation
    C. To reduce the potential for over resuscitation
    D. To move away from the use of crystalloid-based resuscitation
    E. To commence the resuscitation at an earlier time point

ESTIMATION OF BURN EXTENT

11. You are asked to see an adult patient in the emergency room. On examination, the patient has a large burn to the left arm and thorax that involves almost all of the left upper limb and half of the anterior trunk. *What is your estimate of burn extent?*
    A. 12%   D. 28%
    B. 18%   E. 32%
    C. 24%

OPERATIVE MANAGEMENT OF BURNS

12. *When considering the operative management of a major burn–injured patient, which one of the following is correct?*
    A. Fascial excision increases blood loss.
    B. Tangential excision creates a more severe deformity.
    C. Volume of excision is limited by the availability of blood for transfusion.
    D. Typical blood loss for burn excision can be estimated as 0.5 mL per cm^2 burn.
    E. Allograft material is usually required for early wound cover.

POSTOPERATIVE MANAGEMENT

13. *Which one of the following statements is true regarding early postoperative management of acute burns?*
    A. Systemic antibiotics should be routinely prescribed for patients.
    B. The Curreri formula must be used to calculate precise caloric requirements.
    C. Total parenteral nutrition is preferred over enteral feeding to rest the gut.
    D. Metabolic demands are increased by 300% so nutritional intake should be tripled.
    E. A calorie/nitrogen ratio of 100:1 is recommended for optimal nutritional support.

NUTRITIONAL REQUIREMENTS IN BURN PATIENTS

14. *Which one of the following represents the Curreri formula for patients between the ages of 16 and 59 years?*
    A. 20 kcal/kg/day + 40 kcal/%TBSA/day
    B. 25 kcal/kg/day + 40 kcal/%TBSA/day
    C. 25 kcal/kg/day + 60 kcal/%TBSA/day
    D. 20 kcal/kg/day + 60 kcal/%TBSA/day
    E. 25 kcal/kg/day + 25 kcal/%TBSA/day

TOPICAL ANTIMICROBIALS IN BURN WOUNDS

15. A patient with a large burn treated with a topical antibacterial agent for *Pseudomonas* infection develops a metabolic acidosis and compensatory hyperventilation. *Which one of the following agents may be responsible for this clinical picture?*
    A. Silver sulfadiazine
    B. Mafenide acetate
    C. Sodium hypochlorite
    D. Silver nitrate
    E. Manuka honey

SIGNS OF SEPSIS

16. You see a 30-year-old woman in the burn unit as the staff is concerned she is becoming septic. She has a 20% TBSA second-degree burn that has been debrided and grafted. She weighs 45 kg and was previously fit and well. *Which one of the following observations would best support a diagnosis of sepsis?*
    A. A respiratory rate of 12 breaths per minute
    B. A core temperature of 35.5° C
    C. A random blood glucose of 85 mg/dL
    D. A systolic blood pressure of 95 mm Hg
    E. A urine output of 20 mL per hour

Answers

STAGES IN THE MANAGEMENT OF BURNS

1. When considering total burn management, we often consider the five R's to guide the most suitable therapy for each individual patient. *Which one is primarily focused on Advanced Trauma Life Support (ATLS) principles?*

   B. Resuscitation

   Burn management can be broken down to the 5R principles to guide the most suitable therapy for each individual patient. These are as follows:

   1. Resuscitation refers to the initial process to stabilize a patient following injury and includes keeping them warm, well perfused, and comfortable. The usual Advanced Trauma Life Support (ATLS) approaches apply with some specific adaptations pertinent to burn injury. Fluid resuscitation is required for most larger burn injury patients as such injuries are associated with fluid loss. Those with total body surface area (TBSA) burns over 10% should be formally resuscitated with one of the preferred formulae such as the modified Brooke or Parkland. In children with larger burns, additional maintenance fluids may also be warranted. In patients with smaller burns, oral fluid resuscitation alone can be sufficient.
   2. Resurfacing involves firstly removing burn tissue with either tangential or suprafascial excision, followed by coverage with either temporary dressings, biologic matrices, xenograft, allograft, autograft, or vascularized tissues.
   3. Reconstruction refers to the restoration of form and function following burn injury and can be divided in to acute, intermediate, and late reconstruction.
   4. Rehabilitation involves early mobilization, splinting, scar management, sensory re-education, strengthening, and conditioning.
   5. Recovery involves the return of self-esteem and self-worth, coupled with the confidence to move toward independence, enabling patients to return to school, work, and social functions.[1,2]

REFERENCES

1. Janis JE. Essentials of Plastic Surgery. NY: Thieme; 2021
2. Hultman CS, Neumeister MW. Burn care: rehabilitation, reconstruction, and recovery. Clin Plast Surg 2017;44(4):A1–A6, 695–948

PROGNOSIS AFTER SEVERE BURN INJURY

2. *Which one of the following factors is a major predictor of survival used when calculating the Baux score in a patient with a severe, acute burn injury?*

   C. The age of the patient

   The Baux score is a predictor of mortality after a burn injury. It takes into account the patient's age, the % total body surface area (TBSA) burn, and the presence or absence of inhalation injury. A Baux score is calculated by adding age and % TBSA burn. A score greater than 100 in the presence of an inhalation injury or 110 without an inhalation injury is associated with a 50% mortality. The other factors are also relevant to the prognosis—in particular the patient's preinjury status, the burn subtype, and burn depth, but do not form part of the Baux scoring system (**Fig. 21.1**).[1-3]

REFERENCES

1. Williams DJ, Walker JD. A nomogram for calculation of the revised Baux score. Burns 2015;41(1):85–90
2. American Burn Association National Burn Repository. Burn Incidence and Treatment in the United States: 2016. Burn Incidence Fact Sheet. Available at https://ameriburn.org/who-we-are/media/burn-incidence-fact-sheet
3. Advanced Burn Life Support Advisory Committee. Advanced Burn Life Support Course: Provider Manuel. Chicago, IL: American Burn Association; 2007. Available at http://ameriburn.org/ABLSProviderManual 20101018.pdf

PATHOPHYSIOLOGY OF BURNS

3. A 22-year-old patient with a thermal injury is referred to you. The referring unit described the injury as a second-degree burn. *Which one of the following is correct regarding second-degree burns?*

   A. Blistering is usually present.

   A characteristic finding in most second-degree burns is that blistering is present. Burn depth is classified as first degree, second degree, or third degree. First-degree burns involve the epidermis only, and third-degree burns

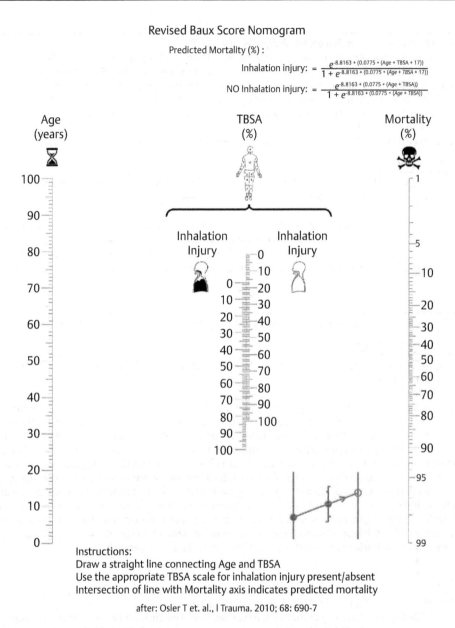

Revised Baux Score Nomogram

Predicted Mortality (%) :

Inhalation injury: $= \dfrac{e^{-8.8163 + (0.0775 \cdot (Age + TBSA + 17))}}{1 + e^{-8.8163 + (0.0775 \cdot (Age + TBSA + 17))}}$

NO Inhalation injury: $= \dfrac{e^{-8.8163 + (0.0775 \cdot (Age + TBSA))}}{1 + e^{-8.8163 + (0.0775 \cdot (Age + TBSA))}}$

Age (years)

TBSA (%)

Mortality (%)

Inhalation Injury

Inhalation Injury

Instructions:
Draw a straight line connecting Age and TBSA
Use the appropriate TBSA scale for inhalation injury present/absent
Intersection of line with Mortality axis indicates predicted mortality

after: Osler T et. al., I Trauma. 2010; 68: 690-7

Fig. 21.1   Nomogram for the revised Baux score for mortality following burns. (Reproduced with permission from Williams DJ and Walker JD. A nomogram for calculation of the Revised Baux Score. Burns 41(1), 2015.)

involve the entire dermis and adnexal structures. Second-degree burns can be superficial or deep, involving variable amounts of dermis and both types usually have blistering. Deeper second-degree and third-degree burns can be insensate, but superficial second-degree burns are characteristically painful. The clinical relevance of the adnexal structures being preserved in partial-thickness burns is that the ability for re-epithelialization is maintained as these epithelial-lined structures are able to provide a source of keratinocytes in the center of the wound. Burn appearance can guide clinical estimation of injury depth. More superficial second-degree burns will be pink and blanch with pressure. Deep second-degree burns may display fixed staining or pallor similar to a full-thickness injury. Sometimes it is not easy to determine the precise burn depth in a mixed partial-thickness burn. Such burns are referred to as indeterminate depth. In these circumstances serial clinical assessments over several days following injury may be required to determine potential treatment. In such cases laser Doppler imaging may be helpful.[1-4]

REFERENCES

1. Herndon DN, ed. Total Burn Care. 5th ed. Edinburg: Elsevier; 2018
2. Advanced Burn Life Support Advisory Committee. Advanced Burn Life Support Course: Provider Manuel. Chicago, IL: American Burn Association; 2018. http://ameriburn.org/wp-content/uploads/2019/08/2018-abls-providermanual.pdf
3. American College of Surgeons Committee on Trauma. Guidelines for the operation of burn centers. In: American College of Surgeons Committee on Trauma, ed. Resources for Optimal Care of the Injured Patient. Chicago, IL: American College of Surgeons; 2014. Available at https://www.facs.org/~/media/files/quality%20programs/trauma/vrc%20resources/resources%20for%20optimal%20care.ashx
4. Gill P. The critical evaluation of laser Doppler imaging in determining burn depth. Int J Burns Trauma 2013;3(2):72–77

BURN TISSUE HISTOLOGY

4. The early management of burn injuries is based on Jackson's burn model. *Which area of the burn is most likely to benefit from early aggressive resuscitation according to this model?*

   B. Zone of stasis

      The model for burn histology involves three areas. The central zone of coagulation is sometimes called the *zone of necrosis* and is nonviable. This is treated by excision and grafting. The surrounding zone of stasis is initially viable. High-quality, timely treatment can prevent necrosis in this zone and avoid the need for excision and grafting. The zone of hyperemia is sometimes called the *zone of inflammation* and is viable. No zone of infiltration is present.[1]

REFERENCE

1. Jackson DM. [The diagnosis of the depth of burning]. Br J Surg 1953;40(164):588–596 PubMed

TRANSFER TO A BURN CENTER

5. *Which one of the following adult burns should be managed locally by a well-equipped plastic surgery department without referral to a burn center?*

   B. A 15% first-degree burn involving the trunk and upper limbs

      First-degree burns involve the epidermis only and display erythema without blistering. They are commonly a result of sunburn. It is unusual to have to admit or refer a patient with a first-degree burn to the hospital or burn center, even at 15% total body surface area (TBSA) unless pain control is not being achieved. This may be more likely in the pediatric population. Criteria for transfer of patients to a burn center include partial-thickness burns greater than 10% TBSA, third-degree burns, and burns involving the hands, feet, genitalia, perineum, or major joints. Additional criteria include electrical burns, inhalation injury, burns in the context of associated trauma, burn-injured patients with significant preexisting medical disorders, and children, when the hospital does not have the facilities to care for them. Patients with chemical burns should also be referred to a burn center and in particular hydrofluoric acid burns even as small as 1% can be life threatening and hence require immediate referral. Lastly, patients who will require special social, emotional, or rehabilitative intervention who do not meet any of the above physical criteria may be better served by transfer to a burn center.[1–3]

REFERENCES

1. Herndon DN, ed. Total Burn Care. 5th ed. Edinburg: Elsevier; 2018
2. Advanced Burn Life Support Advisory Committee. Advanced Burn Life Support Course: Provider Manuel. Chicago, IL: American Burn Association; 2018. http://ameriburn.org/wp-content/uploads/2019/08/2018-abls-providermanual.pdf
3. American College of Surgeons Committee on Trauma. Guidelines for the operation of burn centers. In: American College of Surgeons Committee on Trauma, ed. Resources for Optimal Care of the Injured Patient. Chicago, IL: American College of Surgeons; 2014. Available at https://www.facs.org/~/media/files/quality%20programs/trauma/vrc%20resources/resources%20for%20optimal%20care.ashx

MANAGEMENT OF INHALATION INJURY

6. *In a patient who has sustained an inhalational injury during a house fire, which one of the following is true?*

   D. Management of cyanide toxicity includes intravenous (IV) hydroxocobalamin.

      Hydrogen cyanide (CN) is the gaseous form of cyanide and is generated by the combustion of nitrogen and carbon containing substances, such as wool, silk, cotton, and paper. Therefore, it is likely to occur in subjects exposed to house fires. The cytotoxicity is due to its reversible (not irreversible) inhibition of cytochrome c oxidase, which suppresses cellular respiration and causes tissue anoxia and metabolic acidosis. Elevated CN concentrations are directly related to the probability of death as it causes severe central nervous system (CNS), respiratory, and cardiovascular dysfunction. Toxicity occurs at a level of just 0.1 µg/mL (not 2.0 µg/mL) and by 2.0 µg/mL, death would likely have already occurred. Early administration of hydroxocobalamin 5–10 g intravenously for adults or

70 mg/kg for children is indicated if clinical suspicion of cyanide poisoning is high. This is sold as a preprepared medication (Cyanokit™). An alternative is sodium thiosulfate with sodium nitrite (Nithiodote™). The overall goal of therapy following inhalation injury is to maintain oxygenation while facilitating adequate ventilation. The use of high-flow oxygen is also important; however, 100% oxygen is most indicated in carbon monoxide (CO) poisoning to dissociate CO from hemoglobin (Hb) with which it binds. Other strategies for management of inhalation injury include prevention of barotrauma with low tidal volumes, permissive hypercapnia, high frequency percussive ventilation, and extracorporeal membranous oxygenation (ECMO).[1-3]

REFERENCES

1. Dries DJ, Endorf FW. Inhalation injury: epidemiology, pathology, treatment strategies. Scand J Trauma Resusc Emerg Med 2013;21:31
2. Advanced Burn Life Support Advisory Committee. Advanced Burn Life Support Course: Provider Manuel. Chicago, IL: American Burn Association; 2018. http://ameriburn.org/wp-content/uploads/2019/08/2018-abls-providermanual.pdf
3. American College of Surgeons Committee on Trauma. Guidelines for the operation of burn centers. In: American College of Surgeons Committee on Trauma, ed. Resources for Optimal Care of the Injured Patient. Chicago, IL: American College of Surgeons; 2014. Available at https://www.facs.org/~/media/files/quality%20programs/trauma/vrc%20resources/resources%20for%20optimal%20care.ashx

MANAGEMENT OF ELECTRICAL BURNS

7. A 70 kg patient has sustained a high-voltage electrical burn to the left lower limb and is admitted acutely to the burn center. A normal electrocardiogram (EKG) was obtained on admission. Clinical observations are normal, but the involved limb is tense and painful, with intracompartmental pressures measured at 20 mm Hg. Urine output is 30 mL per hour but is colored dark brown. *Which one of the following is correct?*

A. Urine output should be maintained above 75 mL per hour.

In this case the patient shows signs of myoglobinuria secondary to extensive muscle damage, but not renal dysfunction. This must be carefully treated with fluid therapy to ensure that urine output is maintained between 75 and 100 mL per hour. This aims to minimize myoglobin precipitation and subsequent renal damage. Bicarbonate and mannitol are not contraindicated and, in fact, may be useful in cases of myoglobinuria. The involved limb is at risk of compartment syndrome and a painful, tense limb in the setting of a high-voltage electrical injury should be considered for early fasciotomy. The threshold for fasciotomy is usually an intracompartmental pressure greater than 30 mm Hg, but a decision to operate is made on clinical factors and would be warranted in this case given the clinical presentation. Following a high-voltage injury, there is a significant risk of cardiac arrhythmia and in spite of a normal admission electrocardiogram (EKG), continued cardiac monitoring is required in the acute phase.[1-5]

REFERENCES

1. Kidd M, Hultman CS, Van Aalst J, Calvert C, Peck MD, Cairns BA. The contemporary management of electrical injuries: resuscitation, reconstruction, rehabilitation. Ann Plast Surg 2007;58(3):273–278
2. Herndon DN, ed. Total Burn Care. 5th ed. Edinburg: Elsevier; 2018
3. Chudasama S, Goverman J, Donaldson JH, van Aalst J, Cairns BA, Hultman CS. Does voltage predict return to work and neuropsychiatric sequelae following electrical burn injury? Ann Plast Surg 2010;64(5):522–525
4. Janis JE, Khansa I, Lehrman CR, Orgill DP, Pomahac B. Reconstructive management of devastating electrical injuries to the face. Plast Reconstr Surg 2015;136(4):839–847
5. Hultman CS, Neumeister MW. Burn care: rescue, resuscitation, and resurfacing. Clin Plast Surg 2017;44(4):A1–A6, 695–948

MANAGEMENT OF CHEMICAL BURNS

8. *Which one of the following is the most appropriate treatment for a patient after a chemical injury with phenol?*

D. Irrigation followed by application of polyethylene glycol

In general, chemical burns should initially be managed with copious irrigation. Some chemicals such as phenol require specific treatments such as topical application of polyethylene glycol. Phenol burns have severe local and systemic toxic effects that can result in death with relatively small volumes.

Hydrofluoric acid burns release fluoride ions that bind with calcium, leading to profound hypocalcemia. These burns should be treated with calcium gluconate to chelate the fluoride ions. Alkalis should be treated with copious water irrigation, but neutralization with weak acids should be avoided as this can cause an exothermic reaction. Phosphorus should be stained with 0.5% copper sulfate solution or detected with ultraviolet (UV) light and surgically removed. Acid, alkali, and ammonia burns should each generally be irrigated copiously with water only for 15–20 minutes.[1-3]

REFERENCES

1. Herndon DN, ed. Total Burn Care. 5th ed. Edinburg: Elsevier; 2018
2. Advanced Burn Life Support Advisory Committee. Advanced Burn Life Support Course: Provider Manuel. Chicago, IL: American Burn Association; 2018. http://ameriburn.org/wp-content/uploads/2019/08/2018-abls-providermanual.pdf
3. Friedstat J, Brown DA, Levi B. Chemical, electrical, and radiation injuries. Clin Plast Surg 2017;44(3):657–669

BURN RESUSCITATION

9. *Which one of the following is the correct resuscitation volume for a 95 kg patient with 42% total body surface area (TBSA) burns (using the modified Parkland formula)? The patient had 3 L before arrival at the burn unit, and the burn occurred 4 hours ago.*
   A. 1250 mL per hour for 4 hours, then 500 mL per hour for 16 hours

---

Box 21.1   *THE MODIFIED PARKLAND FORMULA*

4 mL/kg/%TBSA burn = Total fluid volume for the first 24 hours from the time of injury. Half of this volume is given in the first 8 hours, and the rest is given over the last 16 hours. 4 mL × 95 (kg) × 42 (%TBSA) = (15,960 mL) or 16 L total fluid volume. Therefore, 8 L is given in the first 8 hours, and 8 L is given over the next 16 hours. The burn occurred 4 hours ago and 3 L was already given. Therefore, the remaining fluid requirement in the next 4 hours is 5 L (1250 mL/hour), followed by 500 mL/hour for 16 hours.[1-5]

REFERENCES

1. Herndon DN, ed. Total Burn Care. 5th ed. Edinburg: Elsevier; 2018
2. Advanced Burn Life Support Advisory Committee. Advanced Burn Life Support Course: Provider Manuel. Chicago, IL: American Burn Association; 2018. http://ameriburn.org/wp-content/uploads/2019/08/2018-abls-providermanual.pdf
3. Baxter CR, Shires T. Physiological response to crystalloid resuscitation of severe burns. Ann N Y Acad Sci 1968;150(3): 874–894
4. Ete G, Chaturvedi G, Barreto E, Paul M K. Effectiveness of Parkland formula in the estimation of resuscitation fluid volume in adult thermal burns. Chin J Traumatol 2019;22(2):113–116
5. Jones AP, Barnard AR, Allison KP. Trauma: burns. In: Nutbeam T, Boylan M, eds. ABC of Prehospital Emergency Medicine. Oxford, UK: BMJ Books; 2013

FLUID RESUSCITATION IN BURN INJURY

10. There has been a recent shift to the use of the modified Brooke formula from the modified Parkland formula during initial burn fluid resuscitation. *What is the proposed benefit of this change?*
    C. To reduce the potential for over resuscitation
    Following burn injury, fluid loss occurs and in more significant injuries, the use of a formal fluid resuscitation process is advocated. The cut off for a resuscitation burn is usually over 10% total body surface area (TBSA) in children and 15% TBSA in adults. Burn shock is typically seen in adults where TBSA is greater than 20% and this will require formal resuscitation. There are a number of different formulae for fluid resuscitation and these include the Parkland formula, the Modified Parkland formula, the Brooke formula, the modified Brooke formula, and the Evans formula. Both the modified Parkland and modified Brooke use crystalloid for the initial 24 hour resuscitation process and are both commenced as soon as possible after the burn injury. The key difference is that the modified Brooke uses less total fluid in the formula calculation and hence reduces the potential for over resuscitation.
    The Brooke formula is 2 mL/kg/%TBSA, compared with the Parkland, which is 4 mL/kg/%TBSA. For each a total fluid volume is calculated and then this volume is delivered intravenously over the first 24 hours from the time of injury. Half is delivered in the first 8 hours following injury and the remaining half is delivered in the second 16 hours following injury. This means that if a patient arrives in hospital 7 hours after injury without resuscitation, half the total calculated volume would, in theory, need to be delivered in the first hour.[1-5]

REFERENCES

1. Herndon DN, ed. Total Burn Care. 5th ed. Edinburg: Elsevier; 2018
2. Advanced Burn Life Support Advisory Committee. Advanced Burn Life Support Course: Provider Manuel. Chicago, IL: American Burn Association; 2018. http://ameriburn.org/wp-content/uploads/2019/08/2018-abls-providermanual.pdf
3. Baxter CR, Shires T. Physiological response to crystalloid resuscitation of severe burns. Ann N Y Acad Sci 1968;150(3): 874–894
4. Baker RH, Akhavani MA, Jallali N. Resuscitation of thermal injuries in the United Kingdom and Ireland. J Plast Reconstr Aesthet Surg 2007;60(6):682–685
5. Ete G, Chaturvedi G, Barreto E, Paul M K. Effectiveness of Parkland formula in the estimation of resuscitation fluid volume in adult thermal burns. Chin J Traumatol 2019;22(2):113–116

ESTIMATION OF BURN EXTENT

11. You are asked to see an adult patient in the emergency room. On examination, the patient has a large burn to the left arm and thorax that involves almost all of the left upper limb and half of the anterior trunk. *What is your estimate of burn extent?*

    B. 18%

    Assessment of burn extent is commonly performed using Lund and Browder charts[1] or the rule of nines (**Fig. 21.2**). The approximate areas are as follows:
    - Head and neck: 9%
    - Anterior and posterior trunk: 18% (each)
    - Lower limbs: 18% (each)
    - Upper limbs: 9% (each)
    - Perineum: 1%

    Alternative ways to assess burn extent include the 1% rule and serial halving. The 1% rule is based on the assumption that the palm and fingers represent 1% of the total body surface area (TBSA). For smaller burns this is a useful approach. Serial halving is useful for a rapid estimation of a large burn and involves making repeated assessments of the burn area stating whether more than half or less than half is involved.[2]

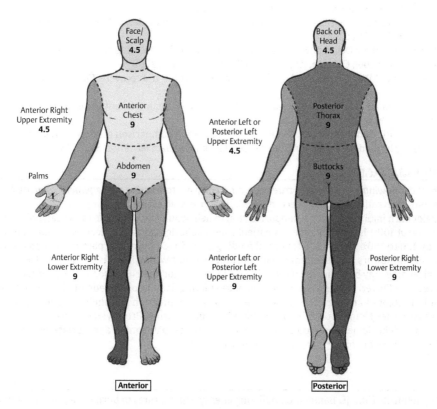

Fig. 21.2 "Rule of 9" for adults.

REFERENCES

1. Lund C, Browder N. The estimation of areas of burns. Surg Gynecol Obstet 1944;79:352–358
2. Jones AP, Barnard AR, Allison KP. Trauma: burns. In: Nutbeam T, Boylan M, eds. ABC of Prehospital Emergency Medicine. Oxford, UK: BMJ Books; 2013

OPERATIVE MANAGEMENT OF BURNS

12. *When considering the operative management of a major burn–injured patient, which one of the following is correct?*

    D. Typical blood loss for burn excision can be estimated as 0.5 mL per cm² burn.

    Blood loss during burn excision can be estimated at 0.5 mL loss for each cm² burn injury debrided. Potential blood loss and the amount of blood available for transfusion both need to be considered when deciding how much excision can be performed in one sitting. The volume of excision achievable will also, however, depend on many other factors and the amount of blood available is only one component. For example, the patient's premorbid status, the area and depth of burn, the timing in relation to the burn injury, the stability of the patient in the operating room (OR), and the tissue availability to cover the wound.

A benefit of fascial excision with respect to bleeding is that blood loss is reduced. However, it does leave a more severe contour deformity and may result in unnecessary removal of healthy tissue.

Tangential excision provides a better contour and depth control as tissue is excised until bleeding tissue is identified. However, blood loss is more difficult to control. When excising large burn areas, it is vital to keep the patient warm and resuscitated from a cardiovascular perspective. Systematic staged excision of individual areas can help to minimize heat and fluid loss intraoperatively.

The benchmark for grafting is to use the patient's own skin (autograft) rather than use a cadaver (allograft). This is because cadaveric grafts are only temporary and the graft is rejected 3–4 weeks after reconstruction. Autograft split-thickness skin graft (STSG) is then required at this stage. Other options for temporary burn cover include semisynthetic and synthetic materials such as Biobrane™, Transcyte™, and Integra™.[1-6]

REFERENCES

1. Herndon DN, ed. Total Burn Care. 5th ed. Edinburg: Elsevier; 2018
2. Marsden NJ, Van M, Dean S, et al. Measuring coagulation in burns: an evidence-based systematic review. Scars Burn Heal 2017;3:2059513117728201
3. Kagan RJ, Peck MD, Ahrenholz DH, et al. Surgical management of the burn wound and use of skin substitutes. American Burn Association White Paper. Chicago, IL: American Burn Association; 2009
4. Hultman CS, Neumeister MW. Burn care: rehabilitation, reconstruction, and recovery. Clin Plast Surg 2017;44(4):A1–A6, 695–948
5. Janis JE, Khansa I, Lehrman CR, Orgill DP, Pomahac B. Reconstructive management of devastating electrical injuries to the face. Plast Reconstr Surg 2015;136(4):839–847
6. Herndon DN, Barrow RE, Rutan RL, Rutan TC, Desai MH, Abston S. A comparison of conservative versus early excision. Therapies in severely burned patients. Ann Surg 1989;209(5):547–552, discussion 552–553

POSTOPERATIVE MANAGEMENT

13. Which one of the following statements is true regarding early postoperative management of acute burns?

E. A calorie/nitrogen ratio of 100:1 is recommended for optimal nutritional support.

After a major burn injury, nutritional support is vital to help wound healing. Due to the catabolic state, a caloric to nitrogen ratio of 100:1 is recommended. A patient's metabolic demands significantly increase after a major burn, but only by 120 to 150%, not by 300%. Enteral feeding is preferred over total parenteral feeds, and prophylactic proton pump inhibitors are recommended to protect the gut which is at risk of stress ulcer formation. Total parenteral feeding may be indicated if there is a sustained period of ileus or some other reason for absorption to be impaired. The Curreri formula is one method of calculating daily caloric needs, but it does not have to be used.

Systemic antibiotics are required in the presence of active infection and their selection should be guided by culture sensitivities from wounds, sputum, blood, tissue, or urine. Prophylactic antibiotics are not routinely required. Early debridement and topical antimicrobials are probably more appropriate. Minimizing antibiotics where possible is best in order to avoid bacterial resistance.[1-4]

REFERENCES

1. Turner WW Jr, Ireton CS, Hunt JL, Baxter CR. Predicting energy expenditures in burned patients. J Trauma 1985;25(1):11–16
2. Mendonça Machado N, Gragnani A, Masako Ferreira L. Burns, metabolism and nutritional requirements. Nutr Hosp 2011;26(4):692–700
3. Herndon DN, ed. Total Burn Care. 5th ed. Edinburg: Elsevier; 2018
4. Avni T, Levcovich A, Ad-El DD, Leibovici L, Paul M. Prophylactic antibiotics for burns patients: systematic review and meta-analysis. BMJ 2010;340:c241

NUTRITIONAL REQUIREMENTS IN BURN PATIENTS

14. Which one of the following represents the Curreri formula for patients between the ages of 16 and 59 years?

B. 25 kcal/kg/day + 40 kcal/%TBSA/day

The Curreri formula is one method of calculating the required caloric intake after a major burn injury.[1,2] **The standard calculation is 25 kcal per kg of body mass per day** plus **40 kcal per %TBSA per day.** The Curreri formula differs slightly for more elderly patients (over 60 years of age), and is reduced to 20 kcal per kg per day + 65 kcal per % total body surface area (TBSA) per day. Although formulas like this are useful tools to guide treatment, care should be taken when they are used because overestimation of caloric requirements is possible. The nutritional plan following burn injury is generally made on an individual patient basis, taking advice from dieticians and nutritionists.

REFERENCES

1. Turner WW Jr, Ireton CS, Hunt JL, Baxter CR. Predicting energy expenditures in burned patients. J Trauma 1985;25(1):11–16
2. Mendonça Machado N, Gragnani A, Masako Ferreira L. Burns, metabolism and nutritional requirements. Nutr Hosp 2011;26(4):692–700

TOPICAL ANTIMICROBIALS IN BURN WOUNDS

15. A patient with a large burn treated with a topical antibacterial agent for Pseudomonas infection develops a metabolic acidosis and compensatory hyperventilation. *Which one of the following agents may be responsible for this clinical picture?*

B. **Mafenide acetate**

Mafenide acetate is available in 5 and 8.5% forms and has a large amount of data to support its use as an effective topical antibacterial agent. It is particularly useful for treating wounds that are infected with *Pseudomonas*. Mafenide is a potent carbonic anhydrase inhibitor that can cause hyperchloremic metabolic acidosis and compensatory hyperventilation. In some cases, this can be fatal. Other caveats are that prolonged use of mafenide can promote growth of candida in the wound and it is painful for the patient on application.

Silver-containing agents are popular in burn dressings as they have a broad spectrum of cover for both gram-positive and gram-negative organisms. They include silver nitrate and silver sulfadiazine. Sodium hypochlorite also has a broad spectrum of cover, and at concentrations of 0.025% is bactericidal without inhibiting fibroblasts. Manuka honey is popular as a topical antibacterial agent in many wounds including burns. The antibacterial qualities derive in part from generation of bactericidal hydrogen peroxide. Honey has a low pH, creating an environment that also limits bacterial growth and its high sugar content interferes with bacterial cell division and the development of biofilms. Low toxicity of human keratinocytes and dermal fibroblasts has been demonstrated.[1–3]

REFERENCES

1. Herndon DN. Total Burn Care. 3rd ed. Philadelphia: Elsevier; 2012
2. Lee DS, Sinno S, Khachemoune A. Honey and wound healing: an overview. Am J Clin Dermatol 2011;12(3):181–190
3. Nímia HH, Carvalho VF, Isaac C, Souza FÁ, Gemperli R, Paggiaro AO. Comparative study of silver sulfadiazine with other materials for healing and infection prevention in burns: a systematic review and meta-analysis. Burns 2019;45(2):282–292

SIGNS OF SEPSIS

16. You see a 30-year-old woman in the burn unit as the staff is concerned she is becoming septic. She has a 20% total body surface area (TBSA) second-degree burn that has been debrided and grafted. She weighs 45 kg and was previously fit and well. *Which one of the following observations would best support a diagnosis of sepsis?*

B. **A core temperature of 35.5° C**

Patients with large burns are at high risk of developing sepsis and it is key to identify this early so that appropriate treatment can be instigated. The key signs include hyperventilation, hypothermia or hyperthermia, hyperglycemia, obtundation, ileus, hypotension, and oliguria. Core temperature should normally be around 37° C but can vary according to activity level, site of measurement, and time of day. The normal range for respiratory rate in an adult is 12–16 breaths per minute. A normal random blood glucose should be between 80 and 110 mg/dL (4.3 to 6.1 mmol/L). A systolic blood pressure of 90 mm Hg is normal in many young females, but this is patient specific and can represent a sign of sepsis in many patients. A urine output of approximately 0.5 mL per hour would be normal in this patient.

A retrospective review of more than 5000 pediatric patients with a burn injury showed that of the 144 patients who died and underwent autopsy, 47% had sepsis confirmed as the primary cause of death. A further 29% had respiratory compromise as the primary cause of death. Many patients subsequently developed multiorgan system failure as a result. This highlights the importance of recognizing and treating sepsis early following a burn injury.[1]

REFERENCE

1. Williams FN, Herndon DN, Hawkins HK, et al. The leading causes of death after burn injury in a single pediatric burn center. Crit Care 2009;13(6):R183

22. Vascular Anomalies

See *Essentials of Plastic Surgery*, third edition, pp. 291–300

EPIDEMIOLOGY OF HEMANGIOMAS

1. *Which one of the following statements regarding hemangiomas is correct?*
   A. They represent the most common tumor in infancy.
   B. They occur twice as often in males compared with females.
   C. 20% of hemangiomas occur in the head and neck region.
   D. All subtypes typically develop a few weeks after birth.
   E. Most patients have two or more concurrent lesions.

MANAGEMENT OF HEMANGIOMAS

2. A 3-month-old infant is seen in clinic with an enlarging vascular lesion to the buttock. It began as a small spot shortly after birth and has grown to measure 1.5 cm diameter. There had been some episodes of bleeding following minor trauma, but it has been stable for the past 3 weeks. *How best can this patient be managed?*
   A. Propranolol
   B. Steroids
   C. Laser
   D. Surgery
   E. Observation

CLINICAL COURSE OF HEMANGIOMAS

3. You are discussing long-term outcomes with the family of a 6-week-old infant with a 1-cm infantile hemangioma to the cheek. *Which one of the following should you tell them?*
   A. Involution is most likely to complete within a year.
   B. Involution is unlikely to occur without treatment.
   C. Further growth is unlikely.
   D. Involution occurs in 75% of cases by age 5.
   E. Involution may be incomplete, and the infant may require surgery.

DIAGNOSIS OF VASCULAR GROWTHS

4. A 5-year-old child presents with a new-onset rapidly growing vascular tumor that stabilizes after 1 month at a size of around 7-mm diameter. It is friable and bleeds regularly. There has been no history of trauma. *What is the most likely diagnosis?*
   A. Congenital hemangioma (RICH)
   B. Congenital hemangioma (NICH)
   C. Congenital hemangioma (PICH)
   D. Infantile hemangioma
   E. Lobular capillary hemangioma

MANAGEMENT OF HEMANGIOMAS

5. *Which one of the following characteristics do timolol and propranolol share in the management of infantile hemangiomas?*
   A. They are both nonselective beta-blockers.
   B. They both have similar dosing profiles.
   C. They are both administered orally.
   D. They are both administered topically.
   E. They are both used from birth onwards.

COMPLICATIONS OF HEMANGIOMAS

6. *What is the most common complication of a hemangioma?*
   A. Congestive cardiac failure
   B. Visual obstruction
   C. Ulceration
   D. Bleeding
   E. Infection

COMPLICATIONS WITH VASCULAR ANOMALIES

7. *Which one of the following describes a profound thrombocytopenia in conjunction with a hemangioma?*
   A. Osler-Weber-Rendu disease
   B. Klippel-Trenaunay syndrome
   C. Parkes-Weber syndrome
   D. Kasabach-Merritt phenomenon
   E. Blue rubber bleb nevus syndrome

VASCULAR MALFORMATIONS

8. *Which one of the following statements is correct regarding vascular malformations?*
   A. They are not present at birth and develop during the first year of life.
   B. They grow proportionally with the child and often subsequently regress.
   C. The autonomic nervous system has little influence on their development.
   D. They represent structural anomalies secondary to faulty embryonic morphogenesis.
   E. During embryonic development, capillaries develop from arterial and venous precursors.

PORT-WINE STAINS (CAPILLARY MALFORMATIONS)

9. *Which one of the following statements regarding port-wine stains is correct?*
   A. They affect 3 in 100 newborn babies.
   B. The neck is the most common anatomic location.
   C. They often correspond to the distribution of the facial nerve.
   D. Treatment is most effective after age 4 with a KTP laser and steroids.
   E. If left untreated, 70% will progress to a cobblestone ectasia.

CONDITIONS WITH ASSOCIATED VASCULAR MALFORMATIONS

10. An infant presents with a capillary malformation to the face involving the forehead, nose, and upper lip and cheeks. *Which one of the following conditions should be excluded?*
   A. PHACE syndrome
   B. Sturge-Weber syndrome
   C. Maffucci's syndrome
   D. von Hippel-Lindau disease
   E. CLOVES syndrome

VENOUS MALFORMATIONS

11. *Which one of the following statements is correct regarding venous malformations?*
   A. They increase in size when elevated.
   B. They are treated successfully with the Er:YAG laser.
   C. They are usually painless.
   D. They tend to enlarge in puberty and pregnancy.
   E. They are no longer treated with sclerotherapy.

LYMPHATIC MALFORMATIONS

12. *Which one of the following statements is correct regarding lymphatic malformations?*
   A. They have little effect on adjacent bone growth.
   B. They rarely occur in combination with venous abnormalities.
   C. Dermal involvement is indicated by the presence of clear cutaneous vesicles.
   D. They rarely require antibiotic therapy.
   E. Morbidity is consistently low following their surgical resection.

ARTERIOVENOUS MALFORMATIONS

13. *When managing arteriovenous malformations, which one of the following is correct?*
   A. Although pulsatile, they are generally low-flow lesions.
   B. Their vascular anatomy is best imaged using MRI.
   C. Embolization is indicated before surgical excision.
   D. Recurrence rates are low following complete excision.
   E. Consumptive coagulopathy is generally managed intraoperatively.

Answers

EPIDEMIOLOGY OF HEMANGIOMAS

1. *Which one of the following statements regarding hemangiomas is correct?*

   A. **They represent the most common tumor in infancy.**

   Hemangiomas are the most common tumor in infancy. They are abnormal endothelial proliferations and are considered to be true tumors. They are found more commonly in females, with a female/male ratio of 3:1. They are usually seen in the head and neck region (60%, not 20%) but may occur on the trunk, limbs, or intracranially. Hemangiomas can be divided into infantile and congenital subtypes. Most are infantile and these develop shortly after birth appearing as a small red spot. Congenital hemangiomas however are fully grown at birth and are classified into two forms, rapidly involuting (rapidly involuting congenital hemangioma [RICH]) or noninvoluting (noninvoluting congenital hemangioma [NICH]). Most patients with hemangiomas have a single lesion, although some do have more than one. Presentation of multiple hemangiomas is most often as part of a syndrome such as Maffucci's or PHACE syndrome.[1-3]

REFERENCES

1. Mulliken JB, Glowacki J. Hemangiomas and vascular malformations in infants and children: a classification based on endothelial characteristics. Plast Reconstr Surg 1982;69(3):412–422
2. Wassef M, Blei F, Adams D, et al; ISSVA Board and Scientific Committee. Vascular anomalies classification: recommendations from the International Society for the Study of Vascular Anomalies. Pediatrics 2015;136(1):e203–e214
3. Drolet BA, Esterly NB, Frieden IJ. Hemangiomas in children. N Engl J Med 1999;341(3):173–181

MANAGEMENT OF HEMANGIOMAS

2. A 3-month-old infant is seen in clinic with an enlarging vascular lesion to the buttock. It began as a small spot shortly after birth and has grown to measure 1.5 cm diameter. There had been some episodes of bleeding following minor trauma, but it has been stable for the past 3 weeks. *How best can this patient be managed?*

   E. **Observation**

   The mainstay of treatment for hemangiomas is conservative management given that the vast majority are self-limiting and resolve over time. This infant is at risk of further bleeding episodes and should be seen again in clinic, but does not require further intervention as present. Hemangiomas may be treated with surgery, laser therapy, steroids, or other injectable agents if they are causing visual or airway obstruction, or bleeding and ulceration that is difficult to control with conservative measures.[1,2] There has been recent interest in the use of beta-blocker medication in the form of systemic propranolol or topical timolol for treatment of ulcerated hemangiomas and results are promising. Starkey and Shahidullah[3] published a comprehensive review of evidence on this topic in 2011. Propranolol is thought to restrict growth in hemangiomas by causing vasoconstriction, inhibition of vascular endothelial growth factor (VEGF), and induction of apoptosis. Typical doses are 1–3 mg/kg/day for up to 12 months. Potential side effects include bradycardia, bronchoconstriction, and hypotension.

   Bleomycin is a chemotherapeutic agent that has also shown promising results in the management of ulcerated hemangiomas and other vascular malformations.[4] Steroids may be injected locally or given systemically to arrest growth of hemangiomas but do not cause regression. Laser therapy can be used for hemangiomas in the acute setting to help with ulceration, or in the later stages of regression to remove residual color from the area.[5]

REFERENCES

1. Chang LC, Haggstrom AN, Drolet BA, et al; Hemangioma Investigator Group. Growth characteristics of infantile hemangiomas: implications for management. Pediatrics 2008;122(2):360–367
2. Couto RA, Maclellan RA, Zurakowski D, Greene AK. Infantile hemangioma: clinical assessment of the involuting phase and implications for management. Plast Reconstr Surg 2012;130(3):619–624
3. Starkey E, Shahidullah H. Propranolol for infantile haemangiomas: a review. Arch Dis Child 2011;96(9):890–893
4. Sainsbury DCG, Kessell G, Fall AJ, Hampton FJ, Guhan A, Muir T. Intralesional bleomycin injection treatment for vascular birthmarks: a 5-year experience at a single United Kingdom unit. Plast Reconstr Surg 2011;127(5):2031–2044
5. Blei F, Guarini A. Current workup and therapy of infantile hemangiomas. Clin Dermatol 2014;32(4):459–470

CLINICAL COURSE OF HEMANGIOMAS

3. You are discussing long-term outcomes with the family of a 6-week-old infant with a 1-cm infantile hemangioma to the cheek. *Which one of the following should you tell them?*

    E. Involution may be incomplete, and the infant may require surgery.

    The vast majority of infantile hemangiomas will involute spontaneously and parents and other family members should be reassured about this. However, a number of patients will have residual fullness at the site of the hemangioma that may require surgical excision. Others may have residual discoloration that may benefit from laser therapy. Infantile hemangiomas appear shortly after birth and have an initial phase of rapid growth. This often lasts for 6–18 months before involution begins. Therefore, this child is likely to have further growth of the hemangioma before involution. Involution has traditionally been said to have occurred in 50% of patients by the age of 5, 70% by the age of 7, and 90% by the age of 9. However, this overestimates the duration of hemangioma involution as most often involution is complete by age 4. Congenital hemangiomas differ in their ability to spontaneously involute. They are of two types: RICH (rapidly involuting) and NICH (noninvoluting). Both are present at birth but only RICH involute spontaneously. They do so within the first year of life. NICH lesions do not respond well to pharmacotherapy and may need surgery if problematic.[1,2]

REFERENCES

1. Blei F, Guarini A. Current workup and therapy of infantile hemangiomas. Clin Dermatol 2014;32(4):459–470
2. Mulliken JB. Diagnosis and natural history of hemangiomas. In: Mulliken JB, Burrows PE, Fishman SJ, eds. Mulliken and Young's Vascular Anomalies: Hemangiomas and Malformations. Ch. 4. Oxford University Press; 2013

DIAGNOSIS OF VASCULAR GROWTHS

4. A 5-year-old child presents with a new-onset rapidly growing vascular tumor that stabilizes after 1 month at a size of around 7-mm diameter. It is friable and bleeds regularly. There has been no history of trauma. *What is the most likely diagnosis?*

    E. Lobular capillary hemangioma

    A lobular capillary hemangioma is more commonly known as a pyogenic granuloma. The latter is a misnomer as it is neither pyogenic nor a granuloma. A lobular capillary hemangioma is a rapidly growing skin lesion seen in infants and young children which develops over a short time interval such as just a few weeks. Growth tends to plateau within 1 month and the size remains static around 6–7 mm in diameter. Although it is often thought to occur following trauma, it is more likely to occur spontaneously. The main problem with such lesions is that they are friable and tend to bleed regularly. They are often therefore best treated with surgical excision and direct closure. In contrast, congenital hemangiomas are present at birth and do not further grow beyond this. They are subclassified into those which rapidly involute (RICH), those which do not involute (NICH), and those which partially involute (PICH). NICH and PICH lesions will generally be treated surgically, while RICH do not usually require this. Infantile hemangiomas do develop spontaneously; however, they do so much earlier in life than the pyogenic granuloma in this case (**Fig. 22.1**).[1]

REFERENCE

1. Mulliken JB. Diagnosis and natural history of hemangiomas. In: Mulliken JB, Burrows PE, Fishman SJ, eds. Mulliken and Young's Vascular Anomalies: Hemangiomas and Malformations. Ch. 4. Oxford University Press; 2013

MANAGEMENT OF HEMANGIOMAS

5. *Which one of the following characteristics do timolol and propranolol share in the management of infantile hemangiomas?*

    A. They are both nonselective beta-blockers.

    Timolol and propranolol are both nonselective beta-blocker agents used in the management of infantile hemangiomas. They are used in different ways; however, propranolol is used orally whereas timolol is used as a topical agent. Timolol is therefore indicated for use on more superficial lesions. One drop of 0.5% gel forming solution is used twice daily. It can be started from birth and continued while the lesion is in the proliferative phase of development. In contrast, propranolol is delivered as an oral syrup two to three times per day at doses of 1–3 mg/kg. It is reserved for infants over 2 months of age. As a systemic medication, it does carry some risks including hypotension and patients are seen on a monthly basis in clinic as dose changes will be required over the first months/years of life.[1,2]

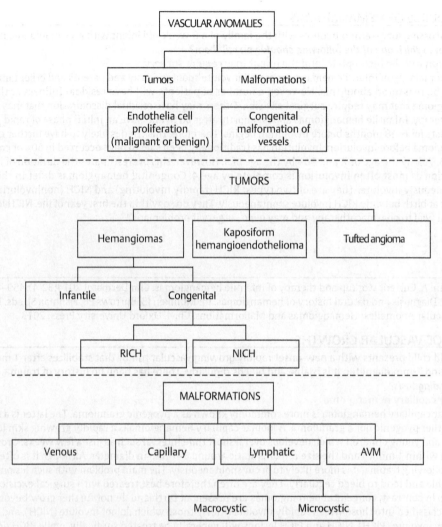

Fig. 22.1 Classifications. (*AVM*, Arteriovenous malformation; *NICH*, noninvoluting congenital hemangioma; *RICH*, rapidly involuting congenital hemangioma.)

REFERENCES

1. Blei F, Guarini A. Current workup and therapy of infantile hemangiomas. Clin Dermatol 2014;32(4):459–470
2. Drolet BA, Frommelt PC, Chamlin SL, et al. Initiation and use of propranolol for infantile hemangioma: report of a consensus conference. Pediatrics 2013;131(1):128–140

COMPLICATIONS OF HEMANGIOMAS

6. *What is the most common complication of a hemangioma?*
   C. Ulceration
      Ulceration is the most common complication of a hemangioma, but even this is relatively uncommon occurring in <5% of patients. Ulceration is one of the main reasons for clinical presentation and consideration during treatment of a hemangioma. Beta-blockers can be useful in this situation as can laser therapy or steroid injection. Other common complications include bleeding, infection, and emotional/psychological issues. Hemangiomas located close to the periorbital region risk visual obstruction that if untreated can lead to anisometropia, a condition where two eyes have significantly unequal refractive power. Each eye can be near sighted (myopic) or farsighted (hyperoptic) or a combination of both. This can cause problems with binocular vision. The patient will tend to see a smaller image in one eye and a larger one in the other or in development the brain may select to ignore the weaker eye and the neglected eye becomes progressively weaker (amblyopia). Hemangiomas located around the oral or

nasal cavities can affect feeding and risk airway obstruction. Hemangiomas in the perineum can cause problems with toileting and hygiene, with subsequent sores and infection. High output heart failure is associated with very large liver/visceral hemangiomas. Skeletal distortion can occur secondary to pressure from the hemangioma if the two are closely apposed.[1-5]

REFERENCES

1. Chang LC, Haggstrom AN, Drolet BA, et al; Hemangioma Investigator Group. Growth characteristics of infantile hemangiomas: implications for management. Pediatrics 2008;122(2):360–367
2. Couto RA, Maclellan RA, Zurakowski D, Greene AK. Infantile hemangioma: clinical assessment of the involuting phase and implications for management. Plast Reconstr Surg 2012;130(3):619–624
3. Bauland CG, Lüning TH, Smit JM, Zeebregts CJ, Spauwen PHM. Untreated hemangiomas: growth pattern and residual lesions. Plast Reconstr Surg 2011;127(4):1643–1648
4. Baselga E, Roe E, Coulie J, et al. Risk factors for degree and type of sequelae after involution of untreated hemangiomas of infancy. JAMA Dermatol 2016;152(11):1239–1243
5. Blei F, Guarini A. Current workup and therapy of infantile hemangiomas. Clin Dermatol 2014;32(4):459–470

COMPLICATIONS WITH VASCULAR ANOMALIES

7. *Which one of the following describes a profound thrombocytopenia in conjunction with a hemangioma?*

D. Kasabach-Merritt phenomenon

Kasabach-Merritt phenomenon involves platelet sequestration within vascular tumor cells which leads to life-threatening thrombocytopenia and coagulopathy. Although infrequent, it is potentially fatal in infants with rapidly growing vascular lesions, and early recognition with prompt management is essential. It occurs in half of all patients with kaposiform hemangioendothelioma (KHE) which is locally aggressive but does not metastasize. It is treated with combination therapy including vincristine (a chemotherapy agent) plus steroids with or without interferon, aspirin, or rapamycin (sirolimus—an antirejection/immunosuppressant medication). Osler-Weber-Rendu syndromes is also known as hereditary hemorrhagic telangiectasia and involves multiple ectatic postcapillary venules in the skin, mucous membranes, and viscera. It is associated with epistaxis and arteriovenous malformations. Klippel-Trenaunay syndrome involves limb overgrowth associated with capillary and venous malformations. There are enlarged lateral leg veins termed the "veins of Servelle."

Parkes-Weber syndrome involves multifocal capillary malformations and arteriovenous malformations and may have associated limb overgrowth.

Blue rubber bleb nevus syndrome involves multifocal venous malformations which are most often in the skin, soft tissues, and gastrointestinal tract. Chronic anemia is a common problem for these patients.[1-7]

REFERENCES

1. Mahajan P, Margolin J, Iacobas I. Kasabach-Merritt phenomenon: classic presentation and management options. Clin Med Insights Blood Disord 2017;10:X17699849
2. Maguiness SM, Liang MG. Management of capillary malformations. Clin Plast Surg 2011;38(1):65–73
3. Piram M, Lorette G, Sirinelli D, Herbreteau D, Giraudeau B, Maruani A. Sturge-Weber syndrome in patients with facial port-wine stain. Pediatr Dermatol 2012;29(1):32–37
4. Uller W, Fishman SJ, Alomari AI. Overgrowth syndromes with complex vascular anomalies. Semin Pediatr Surg 2014;23(4):208–215
5. Fishman SJ, Smithers CJ, Folkman J, et al. Blue rubber bleb nevus syndrome: surgical eradication of gastrointestinal bleeding. Ann Surg 2005;241(3):523–528
6. Guttmacher AE, Marchuk DA, White RI Jr. Hereditary hemorrhagic telangiectasia. N Engl J Med 1995;333(14):918–924
7. Banzic I, Brankovic M, Maksimović Ž, Davidović L, Marković M, Rančić Z. Parkes Weber syndrome—diagnostic and management paradigms: a systematic review. Phlebology 2017;32(6):371–383

VASCULAR MALFORMATIONS

8. *Which one of the following statements is correct regarding vascular malformations?*

D. They represent structural anomalies secondary to faulty embryonic morphogenesis.

Vascular malformations can be subdivided into **capillary, venous, arteriovenous,** and **lymphatic** subtypes. They occur because of faulty embryonic morphogenesis. They are always present at birth and grow proportionally with the child, but they do not regress. The autonomic nervous system influences vascular development. This explains why some abnormalities such as port-wine stains occur in specific nerve distributions. During embryonic development, the venous and arterial channels only appear after the initial capillary network has been formed. Errors in this developmental stage are thought to be responsible for development of vascular malformations.[1]

REFERENCE

1. Mulliken JB. Diagnosis and natural history of hemangiomas. In: Mulliken JB, Burrows PE, Fishman SJ, eds. Mulliken and Young's Vascular Anomalies: Hemangiomas and Malformations. Ch. 4. Oxford University Press; 2013

PORT-WINE STAINS (CAPILLARY MALFORMATIONS)

9. *Which one of the following statements regarding port-wine stains is correct?*

E. If left untreated, 70% will progress to a cobblestone ectasia.

Port-wine stains or capillary malformations affect 0.3% of newborn babies (not 3%) and most commonly occur on the face (80%). One of the main reasons for treating them early in life is to avoid development of a cobblestone appearance which can occur in adulthood if left untreated. They can correspond to the trigeminal nerve (V1–3) distribution, but not the facial nerve and are sometimes accompanied by ocular and central nervous system disorders. Females are affected three times as often as males. Treatment modalities include potassium titanyl phosphate (KTP), pulsed dye, or neodymium-doped yttrium aluminum garnet (Nd:YAG) laser which is best performed *before* age 4 (not after). Multimodality treatment is preferred and combines laser treatment with antiangiogenic agents such as imiquimod or rapamycin. Either way, multiple treatments will be required.[1]

REFERENCE

1. Maguiness SM, Liang MG. Management of capillary malformations. Clin Plast Surg 2011;38(1):65–73

CONDITIONS WITH ASSOCIATED VASCULAR MALFORMATIONS

10. An infant presents with a capillary malformation to the face involving the forehead, nose, and upper lip and cheeks. *Which one of the following conditions should be excluded?*

B. Sturge-Weber syndrome

Sturge-Weber syndrome is a condition in which there is a large capillary malformation seen in V1 and commonly V2 trigeminal nerve distribution associated with leptomeningeal malformations, neurologic impairment, seizures, developmental delay, and glaucoma. Therefore, in an infant with capillary malformations in the trigeminal nerve distribution, evaluation for Sturge-Weber syndrome should be made at 6 months of age with a magnetic resonance imaging (MRI) and ophthalmology review.

PHACES syndrome involves **P**osterior fossa malformations, facial **H**emangiomas, **A**rterial abnormalities, **C**oarctation of the aorta, **E**ye abnormalities, and anomalies of the **S**ternum, hence the term **"PHACES."** It is not associated with capillary malformations.

Maffucci's syndrome is a rare sporadic condition (less than 200 cases described) that involves enchondromas with multiple cutaneous hemangiomas and lymphangiomas. The enchondromas are benign but have the potential for malignant change leading to chondrosarcomas.

von Hippel-Lindau disease is another rare condition, this time inherited, that involves hemangiomas of the retina, hemangioblastomas of the cerebellum, and pancreatic, liver, and adrenal gland cysts. Seizures and mental retardation can also occur. Inheritance is autosomal dominant and results from a mutation in the von Hippel-Lindau tumor suppressor gene. It occurs in around 1 in 30,000 births and patients are at risk of developing various different malignant tumors including renal tumors as well as benign proliferations.

CLOVES syndrome is another extreme condition which involves vascular anomalies. It stands for: **C**ongenital, **L**ipomatous, **O**vergrowth, **V**ascular malformations, **E**pidermal nevi, and **S**keletal/**S**pinal/**S**coliosis anomalies. Often, there are large macrocystic lymphatic malformations with truncal fatty overgrowth and scoliosis.[1–5]

REFERENCES

1. Frieden IJ, Reese V, Cohen D. PHACE syndrome. The association of posterior fossa brain malformations, hemangiomas, arterial anomalies, coarctation of the aorta and cardiac defects, and eye abnormalities. Arch Dermatol 1996;132(3): 307–311
2. Piram M, Lorette G, Sirinelli D, Herbreteau D, Giraudeau B, Maruani A. Sturge-Weber syndrome in patients with facial port-wine stain. Pediatr Dermatol 2012;29(1):32–37
3. Martinez-Lopez A, Salvador-Rodriguez L, Montero-Vilchez T, Molina-Leyva A, Tercedor-Sanchez J, Arias-Santiago S. Vascular malformations syndromes: an update. Curr Opin Pediatr 2019;31(6):747–753
4. Singh B, Singla M, Singh R, Rathore SS, Gupta A. Von Hippel-Lindau syndrome: multi-organ involvement highlighting its diverse clinical spectrum in two adult cases. Cureus 2020;12(7):e9402
5. Uller W, Fishman SJ, Alomari AI. Overgrowth syndromes with complex vascular anomalies. Semin Pediatr Surg 2014;23(4):208–215

VENOUS MALFORMATIONS

11. *Which one of the following statements is correct regarding venous malformations?*

D. **They tend to enlarge in puberty and pregnancy.**

Venous malformations are present at birth (in contrast to congenital hemangiomas) and can grow significantly during pregnancy or puberty if they are hormone sensitive. They decrease in size when elevated and swell in a dependent position. Demonstrating this is a key part of the clinical examination of these lesions. They commonly cause aching when full, especially in the extremities such as where varicose veins are present. Sclerotherapy is a popular treatment modality, with a variety of different injectables, and laser therapy is successful with neodymium-doped yttrium aluminum garnet (Nd:YAG) rather than erbium-doped yttrium aluminum garnet (Re:YAG) laser.[1]

REFERENCE

1. Greene AK, Alomari AI. Management of venous malformations. Clin Plast Surg 2011;38(1):83–93

LYMPHATIC MALFORMATIONS

12. *Which one of the following statements is correct regarding lymphatic malformations?*

C. **Dermal involvement is indicated by the presence of clear cutaneous vesicles.**

Clear cutaneous vesicles signify a dermal lymphatic component in a lymphatic malformation. This is termed lymphangioma circumscriptum and is generally part of a microcystic subtype of lymphatic malformation. Bony overgrowth and simultaneous venous anomalies are common associations. Lymphatic malformations frequently become infected and require aggressive antibiotic therapy. Surgery for lymphatic malformations is associated with many complications, including delayed wound healing, infection, and prolonged drainage. Furthermore, surgery is associated with a high recurrence rate. Treating these with intralesional bleomycin has shown promising results.[1,2]

REFERENCES

1. Sainsbury DCG, Kessell G, Fall AJ, Hampton FJ, Guhan A, Muir T. Intralesional bleomycin injection treatment for vascular birthmarks: a 5-year experience at a single United Kingdom unit. Plast Reconstr Surg 2011;127(5):2031–2044
2. Greene AK, Perlyn CA, Alomari AI. Management of lymphatic malformations. Clin Plast Surg 2011;38(1):75–82

ARTERIOVENOUS MALFORMATIONS

13. *When managing arteriovenous malformations, which one of the following is correct?*

C. **Embolization is indicated before surgical excision.**

Arteriovenous malformations (AVMs) are high-flow pulsatile lesions that are difficult to treat surgically and require preoperative embolization to minimize risk of bleeding during resection. It is usual to embolize AVMs 24–72 hours before surgery. The main risk for patients undergoing resection of AVMs is bleeding due to the high-flow and consumptive coagulopathy. The latter must be addressed preoperatively with correction of any clotting dysfunction. Preoperative imaging consists of an MRI to determine the extent of the lesion and surrounding soft tissue involvement. Angiography is required to identify the feeding vessels and vascular anatomy. Recurrence rates are high after surgical excision and for this reason generous margins should be taken where possible. Patients may need not only hypotensive anesthesia but also cardiopulmonary bypass in some situations. Management of these malformations is a multidisciplinary task, given the complexity and high risks of morbidity and mortality.[1]

REFERENCE

1. Greene AK, Orbach DB. Management of arteriovenous malformations. Clin Plast Surg 2011;38(1):95–106

23. Congenital Melanocytic Nevi

See *Essentials of Plastic Surgery*, third edition, pp. 301–306

GIANT CONGENITAL MELANOCYTIC NEVI (CMN)

1. *When examining a patient with a giant congenital nevocytic nevus, which one of the following features is a consistent finding?*
   A. A bathing suit distribution
   B. Multiple satellite lesions
   C. Multiple neurofibromas
   D. A verrucous surface texture to the nevus
   E. A tan to brown coloration

HISTOLOGY OF CONGENITAL AND ACQUIRED NEVI

2. *Which one of the following statements is correct regarding congenital and acquired nevi?*
   A. Congenital nevi tend to be located more superficially within the dermis compared with acquired nevi.
   B. Small, medium, and large congenital nevi each has very different histological features.
   C. Congenital nevi differ from acquired nevi in their involvement with skin appendages.
   D. Growth of congenital nevi is often disproportionate to overall patient growth.
   E. Most types of congenital and acquired nevi generally have extension into muscle and bone.

RISK OF MALIGNANT TRANSFORMATION IN CONGENITAL MELANOCYTIC NEVI (CMN)

3. *Which one of the following statements regarding malignant transformation of congenital melanocytic nevi (CMN) is correct?*
   A. Management with respect to the potential for malignant transformation remains controversial.
   B. There is minimal lifetime risk of malignant transformation in smaller CMN.
   C. The most common age range for malignant transformation of giant CMN is 10–20 years.
   D. Transformation of giant CMN to melanoma occurs in more than a fifth of cases.
   E. Malignant transformation carries a better prognosis compared with other melanoma subtypes.

MANAGEMENT OF GIANT CONGENITAL MELANOCYTIC NEVI (CMN)

4. *Which one of the following is probably the most important indication to treat a giant congenital melanocytic nevi (CMN)?*
   A. Cosmetic appearance
   B. Parental request
   C. Psychological effects
   D. Risk of malignant change
   E. Site and size of lesion

MANAGEMENT OF CONGENITAL MELANOCYTIC NEVI (CMN)

5. *When planning management of congenital melanocytic nevi (CMN) which one of the following statements is correct?*
   A. Nongiant cell congenital nevi should be assessed three times per year.
   B. Early excision is not warranted in lesions just because they are difficult to monitor.
   C. Any atypical congenital nevi should be excised regardless of size.
   D. Reconstruction of giant CMN will require tissue expansion to achieve primary closure.
   E. Laser or curettage are recommended for smaller lesions and have low recurrence rates.

DIAGNOSIS OF PIGMENTED SKIN LESIONS

6. A baby is found to have a 3-cm-diameter, steel-blue macule in the lumbosacral region soon after birth. *Which one of the following is the most likely diagnosis?*
   A. Mongolian spot
   B. Blue nevus
   C. Spitz nevus
   D. Café au lait spot
   E. Halo nevus

CLINICAL PRESENTATION OF PIGMENTED SKIN LESIONS

7. A baby girl presents with a yellowish waxy plaque on the scalp. She is otherwise fit and well. *What is the most likely diagnosis?*
   - A. Dysplastic nevus
   - B. Sebaceous nevus
   - C. Nevus spilus
   - D. Epidermal nevus
   - E. Basal cell carcinoma

CONGENITAL MELANOCYTIC NEVI (CMN)

8. *What is the key difference between a tardive congenital nevus and a congenital nevus?*
   - A. The timing of first presentation
   - B. The rate of growth
   - C. The histological appearance
   - D. The surgical management
   - E. The color and texture

NEUROCUTANEOUS MELANOSIS

9. *When seeing an infant with a diagnosis of neurocutaneous melanosis, which one of the following would be most expected?*
   - A. Muscle weakness
   - B. Headache and photophobia
   - C. Microtia
   - D. More than five congenital nevi
   - E. Limb anomalies

CLINICAL PRESENTATION OF PIGMENTED SKIN LESIONS

10. An Asian newborn baby has a right-sided, blue-brown periocular macule of 2 cm diameter. *What is the most likely diagnosis?*
    - A. Nevus of Ito
    - B. Nevus of Ota
    - C. Spitz nevus
    - D. Tardive congenital nevus
    - E. Mongolian spot

CLINICAL PRESENTATION OF PIGMENTED SKIN LESIONS

11. An adolescent male is seen in clinic with a 10-cm-diameter, tan-colored, hairy lesion on the right shoulder. It has been present for 6 months. *What is the most likely diagnosis?*
    - A. Becker's nevus
    - B. Café au lait spot
    - C. Halo nevus
    - D. Dysplastic nevus
    - E. Spitz nevus

Answers

GIANT CONGENITAL MELANOCYTIC NEVI (CMN)

1. *When examining a patient with a giant congenital nevocytic nevus, which one of the following features is a consistent finding?*

    D. A verrucous surface texture to the nevus

    Giant cell nevi are characterized by a dark, hairy verrucous appearance, and although satellite lesions are commonly seen, they are not a consistent finding.[1] Giant cell nevi vary in their anatomic location and accordingly can be found in *bathing suit, stocking,* or *coat sleeve* distributions. Sometimes giant cell nevi are associated with neurofibromatosis, but not consistently so. Neurocutaneous manifestations include leptomeningeal extension, meningomyelocele, and spina bifida. Leptomeningeal melanosis is considered to be more likely in the presence of scalp or dorsal spinal cutaneous lesions. Suspicion of these warrants further investigation with magnetic resonance imaging (MRI).

REFERENCE

1. Foster RD, Williams ML, Barkovich AJ, Hoffman WY, Mathes SJ, Frieden IJ. Giant congenital melanocytic nevi: the significance of neurocutaneous melanosis in neurologically asymptomatic children. Plast Reconstr Surg 2001;107(4):933–941

HISTOLOGY OF CONGENITAL AND ACQUIRED NEVI

2. *Which one of the following statements is correct regarding congenital and acquired nevi?*

    C. Congenital nevi differ from acquired nevi in their involvement with skin appendages.

    Congenital nevi consist of nevus cells located in the deeper dermis and can invade skin appendages, vessels, and nerves. In contrast, acquired nevi tend to consist of nevus cells that are limited to the papillary and upper reticular dermis and do not involve skin appendages. The histologic appearance of all congenital nevi is largely similar but giant cell nevi differ in that they may have extension into muscle, bone, and dura. After birth, congenital melanocytic nevi (CMN) grow in proportion to the overall increase in body size.[1]

REFERENCE

1. Rhodes AR, Silverman RA, Harrist TJ, Melski JW. A histologic comparison of congenital and acquired nevomelanocytic nevi. Arch Dermatol 1985;121(10):1266–1273

RISK OF MALIGNANT TRANSFORMATION IN CONGENITAL MELANOCYTIC NEVI (CMN)

3. *Which one of the following statements regarding malignant transformation of congenital melanocytic nevi (CMN) is correct?*

    A. Management with respect to the potential for malignant transformation remains controversial.

    The risk of malignant transformation in congenital nevi and their preemptive management is a controversial topic on which there are many opinions. This is because many factors remain uncertain, such as the true lifetime risk of malignant change for any given lesion, and the impact of prophylactic excision in reducing development of subsequent cutaneous or noncutaneous malignancy.

    The lifetime risk of malignant change is probably 1–2% for small congenital nevi. The risk in medium congenital melanocytic nevi (CMN) is uncertain, and neither small- nor medium-sized CMN are likely to change before puberty. In contrast, giant CMN have a 5–10% risk of malignant transformation, and half of these will occur between the ages of 3 and 5 years. The size and site of a giant CMN as well as the number of satellite lesions appear to impact the risk of malignant transformation. Trunk lesions have a higher risk of malignant transformation as do those greater than 20 cm in diameter. When malignant transformation occurs in giant nevi, the prognosis is poor.[1,2] If a diagnosis of melanoma is found following removal of a CMN, screening should be undertaken for *NRSA* and *BRAF* mutations.[3]

REFERENCES

1. Krengel S, Marghoob AA. Current management approaches for congenital melanocytic nevi. Dermatol Clin 2012;30(3):377–387

2. Marghoob AA, Borrego JP, Halpern AC. Congenital melanocytic nevi: treatment modalities and management options. Semin Cutan Med Surg 2007;26(4):231–240
3. Kinsler VA, O'Hare P, Bulstrode N, et al. Melanoma in congenital melanocytic naevi. Br J Dermatol 2017;176(5):1131–1143

MANAGEMENT OF GIANT CONGENITAL MELANOCYTIC NEVI (CMN)

4. *Which one of the following is probably the most important indication to treat a giant congenital melanocytic nevi (CMN)?*

    D. Risk of malignant change

    All of the options are reasonable reasons for surgical removal of a congenital nevus. However, the most important reason for treatment is the potential risk of malignant change.

    Cosmesis will often be very important to parents and patients. It is particularly important to patients as they begin to develop social awareness. The presence of large congenital melanocytic nevi (CMN) can lead to both social and behavioral consequences. The site, size, and location of the lesion and availability of tissue for reconstruction play a significant role in decision-making, especially if this makes the lesion difficult to monitor accurately. Both scarring from surgery and the original nevus can carry significant potential psychological effects, so this must be discussed in depth prior to embarking on any treatment plan.[1,2]

REFERENCES

1. Price HN. Congenital melanocytic nevi: update in genetics and management. Curr Opin Pediatr 2016;28(4):476–482
2. Marghoob AA. Congenital melanocytic nevi. Evaluation and management. Dermatol Clin 2002;20(4):607–616, viii

MANAGEMENT OF CONGENITAL MELANOCYTIC NEVI (CMN)

5. *When planning management of congenital melanocytic nevi (CMN), which one of the following statements is correct?*

    C. Any atypical congenital nevi should be excised regardless of size.

    Early excision of small and medium congenital nevi is warranted if they are difficult to monitor (e.g., on the back or scalp) or if they have atypical features such as color variegation, abnormal borders, or growth. Nongiant nevi can be observed on an annual basis (not every 4 months) unless suspicious, in which case a diagnostic biopsy is performed instead. Giant congenital melanocytic nevi (CMN) should be excised completely as soon as possible after appropriate imaging. Reconstruction often requires a combination of tissue expansion, grafts, and flaps but is dependent on size and anatomic location. For example, giant CMN representing 1% total body surface area (TBSA) located on the trunk may be closed directly without expansion techniques. Laser and curettage are not recommended for managing CMN as they are associated with high recurrence rates.[1,2]

REFERENCES

1. Price HN. Congenital melanocytic nevi: update in genetics and management. Curr Opin Pediatr 2016;28(4):476–482
2. Marghoob AA. Congenital melanocytic nevi. Evaluation and management. Dermatol Clin 2002;20(4):607–616, viii

DIAGNOSIS OF PIGMENTED SKIN LESIONS

6. A baby is found to have a 3-cm-diameter, steel-blue macule in the lumbosacral region soon after birth. *Which one of the following is the most likely diagnosis?*

    A. Mongolian spot

    Mongolian spots are more common in races with darkly pigmented skin and can vary from a couple of centimeters to 20 cm. They are present at birth and usually disappear during childhood. In contrast, blue nevi usually appear in late adolescence and are small (less than 1 cm). They are typically blue or black and can be located on the hands, feet, head, or neck. A Spitz nevus is a red or pigmented dome-shaped papule that usually appears at birth and is commonly found on the head or neck. Excision is normally recommended. Café au lait spots are well-circumscribed, homogeneous, macular, coffee-colored lesions often seen with neurofibromatosis. A halo nevus has a white halo around the nevus due to a lymphocytic reaction and most commonly is found on the back during puberty.[1–3]

REFERENCES

1. Zhong CS, Huang JT, Nambudiri VE. Revisiting the history of the "Mongolian spot": the background and implications of a medical term used today. Pediatr Dermatol 2019;36(5):755–757
2. Marghoob AA. Congenital melanocytic nevi. Evaluation and management. Dermatol Clin 2002;20(4):607–616, viii
3. Kaushik A, Natsis N, Gordon SC, Seiverling EV. A practical review of dermoscopy for pediatric dermatology part I: Melanocytic growths. Pediatr Dermatol 2020;37(5):789–797

CLINICAL PRESENTATION OF PIGMENTED SKIN LESIONS

7. **A baby girl presents with a yellowish waxy plaque on the scalp. She is otherwise fit and well. *What is the most likely diagnosis?***

    B. Sebaceous nevus

    A sebaceous nevus is a solitary yellowish waxy congenital plaque usually found on the scalp. Alternatively, they can be located on the face, neck, or forehead. They consist of overgrown epidermis with hair follicles and sebaceous glands and are classified as a type of benign hair follicle tumor. However, they do also have a risk of malignant transformation to basal cell carcinoma (BCC) (10 or 15%) later in life and for this reason they are often treated surgically. Dysplastic (atypical) nevi often occur during or after puberty and are slightly odd-looking nevi with irregular edges, altered pigmentation, and are usually larger than 6 mm in diameter. They are often referred to as "changing moles" in order to exclude melanoma and are generally treated surgically with complete excision. Dysplastic nevi can be mild, moderate, or severely dysplastic according to their histologic appearance. Many centers will treat severely dysplastic nevi the same as in situ melanoma, i.e., with 5-mm wide excision.

    Nevus spilus (speckled lentiginous nevi) are tan colored macules that measure 1–4 cm in diameter and have speckling with dark brown papules or macules 1–6 mm in diameter. They usually present before age 2 as acquired lesions but may be congenital in some cases. They do not usually require intervention but may be removed surgically or treated with laser therapy.

    Epidermal nevi are skin lesions involving overgrowth of the epidermis. They include linear nevi which occur on the trunk and limbs, first appearing at birth or shortly after. They comprise of tan or brown colored warty macules or papules, without plaques or hair. Again surgery or laser treatment is often performed for these lesions. Basal cell carcinomas are slow-growing, nonmelanoma skin cancers seen in older age groups. They almost never metastasize and have an association with sebaceous nevi as described above. Their management may be surgical, topical, or with radiotherapy depending on their subtype.[1–4]

REFERENCES

1. Jiao L, Han X, Xu J, Sun J, Ma L. Four pediatric cases of secondary neoplasms arising in nevus sebaceous. Dermatol Ther (Heidelb) 2020;33(6):e13762
2. Constant E, Davis DG. The premalignant nature of the sebaceous nevus of Jadassohn. Plast Reconstr Surg 1972;50(3):2 57–259
3. Mehregan AH, Pinkus H. Life history of organoid nevi. Special reference to nevus sebaceus of Jadassohn. Arch Dermatol 1965;91:574–588
4. Cribier B, Scrivener Y, Grosshans E. Tumors arising in nevus sebaceus: a study of 596 cases. J Am Acad Dermatol 2000; 42(2 Pt 1):263–268

CONGENITAL MELANOCYTIC NEVI (CMN)

8. ***What is the key difference between a tardive congenital nevus and a congenital nevus?***

    A. The timing of first presentation

    Melanocytic nevi occurring in infancy or during the first 2 years of life are classified as *tardive congenital melanocytic nevi (CMN)* or *congenital nevus-like nevi (CNLN)*. They are clinically and histologically indistinguishable from CMN. Therefore, the two subtypes are treated in the same manner with regular observation or surgical excision. The rate of growth itself is not different; it is purely that presentation is later.[1,2]

REFERENCES

1. Schaffer JV. Update on melanocytic nevi in children. Clin Dermatol 2015;33(3):368–386
2. Moustafa D, Blundell AR, Hawryluk EB. Congenital melanocytic nevi. Curr Opin Pediatr 2020;32(4):491–497

NEUROCUTANEOUS MELANOSIS

9. ***When seeing an infant with a diagnosis of neurocutaneous melanosis, which one of the following would be most expected?***

    B. Headache and photophobia

    Melanocytic proliferation within the brain parenchyma or leptomeninges (the combined pia and arachnoid mater) is described as *neuromelanosis*. When seen in combination with congenital melanocytic nevi (CMN) this is called *neurocutaneous melanosis* and raised intracranial pressure can be a problem for such patients. Symptoms of this include headache, photophobia, lethargy, and recurrent vomiting. Ultimately this condition can result in seizures, developmental delay, cranial nerve palsies, sensorimotor deficits, and bladder and bowel dysfunction. Where there is central nervous system (CNS) involvement, patients are usually symptomatic by 2 years of age. Investigation with magnetic resonance imaging (MRI) is warranted in the first 4 months of life. Unfortunately, there is little treatment that can be offered other than managing intracranial pressure issues. In general, where neurologic symptoms are present, prognosis is very poor. The other options listed are not specifically related to this condition.[1-3]

REFERENCES

1. Lee JH, Jackson AB, Ren Y, Rao KI. Neurocutaneous melanosis: a rare manifestation of congenital melanocytic nevus. BMJ Case Rep 2019;12(8):e227621
2. Alikhan A, Ibrahimi OA, Eisen DB. Congenital melanocytic nevi: where are we now? Part I. Clinical presentation, epidemiology, pathogenesis, histology, malignant transformation, and neurocutaneous melanosis. J Am Acad Dermatol 2012;67(4):495.e1–495.e17, quiz 512–514
3. Fledderus AC, Franke CJJ, Eggen CAM, et al. Outcomes and measurement instruments used in congenital melanocytic naevi research: a systematic review. J Plast Reconstr Aesthet Surg 2020;73(4):703–715

CLINICAL PRESENTATION OF PIGMENTED SKIN LESIONS

10. An Asian newborn baby has a right-sided, blue-brown periocular macule of 2 cm diameter. *What is the most likely diagnosis?*

   B. Nevus of Ota

   The nevus of Ota has an onset at birth or within the first year of life and during puberty. It is especially common in Asians and blacks. It appears as a blue-brown unilateral periocular macule varying in size from a few centimeters to one which affects half of the face and follows the trigeminal nerve distribution.

   The nevus of Ito usually appears at birth and is typically seen in Asians and blacks. It appears as a large blue-brown lesion on the posterior shoulder innervated by the supraclavicular and lateral cutaneous brachial nerves.

   Spitz nevi are red or pigmented, smooth, dome-shaped papules with telangiectasia measuring about 8 mm in diameter. They usually appear at birth and are also called juvenile melanoma. They are best managed with surgical excision for both diagnostic and therapeutic purposes.

   Tardive congenital nevi are congenital nevi that develop within the first 2 years after birth. They are managed the same as other congenital nevi with either monitoring or removal as they carry a small risk of malignant transformation. A Mongolian spot is a steel-blue macula present at birth or during first few weeks of life located in the lumbosacral area. Size of these lesions ranges from a few centimeters to 20 cm or more. They are more common in darkly pigmented skin and usually disappear in early childhood.[1-4]

REFERENCES

1. Tse JY, Walls BE, Pomerantz H, et al. Melanoma arising in a nevus of Ito: novel genetic mutations and a review of the literature on cutaneous malignant transformation of dermal melanocytosis. J Cutan Pathol 2016;43(1):57–63
2. Krengel S, Scope A, Dusza SW, Vonthein R, Marghoob AA. New recommendations for the categorization of cutaneous features of congenital melanocytic nevi. J Am Acad Dermatol 2013;68(3):441–451
3. Price HN. Congenital melanocytic nevi: update in genetics and management. Curr Opin Pediatr 2016;28(4):476–482
4. Marghoob AA. Congenital melanocytic nevi. Evaluation and management. Dermatol Clin 2002;20(4):607–616, viii

CLINICAL PRESENTATION OF PIGMENTED SKIN LESIONS

11. An adolescent male is seen in clinic with a 10-cm-diameter, tan-colored, hairy lesion on the right shoulder. It has been present for 6 months. *What is the most likely diagnosis?*

   A. Becker's nevus

   A Becker's nevus (pigmented hairy epidermal nevus) is a late-onset birthmark which is first observed in adolescence as a tan to brown hairy lesion most commonly affecting one's shoulder. The hairs and pigmentation are often treated with laser therapy.

   Café au lait spots may be present at birth, but usually develop in childhood. They are well-circumscribed, oval macular lesions that have a homogenous milky coffee color. They are often associated with neurofibromatosis.

   Halo nevi are small, brown-colored nevi with a surrounding white halo. The white halo represents a lymphocytic reaction and such lesions are most commonly found on upper backs of teenagers.

   Dysplastic nevi most often develop after adolescence and appear as an irregular, brown-colored skin lesion with areas of different pigmentation, and are most commonly found on the trunk. They are usually larger than 6 mm and should be treated with surgical excision.

   Spitz nevi are red or pigmented, smooth, dome-shaped papules with telangiectasia measuring about 8 mm in diameter. They usually appear at birth and are also called juvenile melanoma. They are best managed with surgical excision for both diagnostic and therapeutic purposes.[1-4]

REFERENCES

1. Becker SW. Concurrent melanosis and hypertrichosis in distribution of nevus unius lateris. Arch Derm Syphilol 1949; 60(2):155–160
2. Patel P, Malik K, Khachemoune A. Sebaceus and Becker's nevus: overview of their presentation, pathogenesis, associations, and treatment. Am J Clin Dermatol 2015;16(3):197–204
3. Patrizi A, Medri M, Raone B, Bianchi F, Aprile S, Neri I. Clinical characteristics of Becker's nevus in children: report of 118 cases from Italy. Pediatr Dermatol 2012;29(5):571–574
4. Danarti R, König A, Salhi A, Bittar M, Happle R. Becker's nevus syndrome revisited. J Am Acad Dermatol 2004;51(6): 965–969

PART III

Head and Neck

24. Head and Neck Embryology

See *Essentials of Plastic Surgery*, third edition, pp. 309–314

HUMAN EMBRYOLOGY

1. *Which one of the following statements is correct regarding human embryological development?*
   A. The nervous system derives from the mesodermal layer.
   B. The endoderm forms both the gastrointestinal and genitourinary tracts.
   C. The heart and great vessels derive from both ectoderm and mesoderm.
   D. Bone, cartilage, muscle, dermis, and epidermis all derive from mesoderm.
   E. Hair follicles, sebaceous glands, and eccrine sweat glands derive from ectoderm.

PHARYNGEAL (BRANCHIAL) ARCHES

2. *Which one of the following statements is correct regarding the pharyngeal arches in embryological development?*
   A. The muscles of mastication are derived from the second arch.
   B. The digastric muscle develops from two separate arches.
   C. The facial nerve and facial musculature derive from different arches.
   D. Levator veli palatini and tensor veli palatini arise from the same arch.
   E. The ossicles derive from a single pharyngeal arch.

PHARYNGEAL (BRANCHIAL) GROOVES

3. *Which one of the following statements is correct regarding the pharyngeal grooves in embryological development?*
   A. Groove I develops into the internal auditory canal and tympanic membrane.
   B. The most common branchial groove sinus derives from cleft IV and runs from the sternocleidomastoid muscle to the tongue base.
   C. Branchial cleft abnormalities are most often detected in the fourth decade of life as discharging sinuses.
   D. The cervical sinus is formed from grooves II through IV, and incomplete obliteration is the cause of branchial sinus tracts.
   E. Branchial clefts from groove II differ from groove III by their relationship to the internal jugular vein.

PHARYNGEAL (BRANCHIAL) POUCHES

4. *Which one of the following statements is correct regarding the pharyngeal pouches in embryological development?*
   A. The first pouch gives rise to the external auditory canal.
   B. The second pouch gives rise to the lingual tonsil.
   C. The third pouch gives rise to the superior parathyroid and thymus.
   D. The fourth pouch gives rise to the ultimobranchial body and T-cells.
   E. The fourth pouch migrates above the third pouch.

HEAD AND NECK DEVELOPMENT

5. *Which one of the following statements is correct regarding embryology of the head and neck?*
   A. The tongue is formed from two different arches.
   B. The thyroid gland develops from the tongue.
   C. The external ear receives contribution from all arches.
   D. The facial skeleton forms by endochondral ossification.
   E. The face develops from paired frontonasal prominences.

EMBRYOLOGIC ORIGINS OF ADULT STRUCTURES

6. *When considering embryological development in the head and neck, what is the origin of the primary palate and central upper lip?*
   A. Frontonasal prominence
   B. Lateral nasal prominence
   C. Maxillary prominence
   D. Medial nasal prominence
   E. Mandibular prominence

EMBRYOLOGY OF THE TONGUE

7. *Which cranial nerve (CN) is responsible for taste in the anterior part of the tongue?*
   A. Trigeminal (CN V)
   B. Facial (CN VII)
   C. Glossopharyngeal (CN IX)
   D. Vagus (CN X)
   E. Hypoglossal (CN XII)

Answers

HUMAN EMBRYOLOGY

1. *Which one of the following statements is correct regarding human embryological development?*

   E. Hair follicles, sebaceous glands, and eccrine sweat glands derive from ectoderm.

   The ectoderm forms the epidermis, the epidermal appendages, and the nervous system. This has clinical relevance in the healing process in partial-thickness wounds as the ectodermally derived skin appendages such as hair follicles, eccrine and apocrine sweat glands, and sebaceous glands are lined with epithelium and provide a source of keratinocytes for re-epithelialization. This knowledge also helps to understand how certain conditions present. For example, the fact that skin and neural tissue share embryologic origin explains why patients with neurofibromatosis develop both skin and nerve tissue tumors. The mesodermal derivatives are also clinically relevant in plastic surgery as this embryologic layer forms bone, cartilage, muscle, connective tissue, and blood vessels. The endoderm has less applicability in plastic surgery as it forms the lining of the gastrointestinal and respiratory tracts and the digestive organ parenchyma. The endoderm does not however form the genitourinary tract. The heart and great vessels are derived from mesoderm, but not ectoderm.[1–3]

REFERENCES

1. Afshar M, Brugmann SA, Helms JA. Embryology of the craniofacial complex. In: Neligan PC, ed. Plastic Surgery. 3rd ed. London: Elsevier; 2013
2. Carlson BM, ed. Human Embryology and Developmental Biology. 5th ed. Philadelphia: Elsevier; 2013
3. Hopper RA. Cleft lip and palate: embryology, principles, and treatment. In: Thorne CH, Chung KC, Gosain A, Guntner GC, Mehrara BJ, eds. Grabb and Smith's Plastic Surgery. 7th ed. Philadelphia: Lippincott Williams & Wilkins; 2014

PHARYNGEAL (BRANCHIAL) ARCHES

2. *Which one of the following statements is correct regarding the pharyngeal arches in embryological development?*

   B. The digastric muscle develops from two separate arches.

   There are six pharyngeal arches and each comprises a mixture of endoderm, mesoderm, and ectoderm such that all layers of the head and neck can be formed (**Table 24.1**). Knowledge of the embryologic origins of the head and neck has clinical relevance to plastic surgery. For example, each of the digastric muscles has an anterior and a posterior belly, which have different embryologic origins. The anterior belly develops from the first arch along with the muscles of mastication and tensor veli palatini. The main nerve derived from this arch is the trigeminal (CN V) and this supplies these structures. The posterior belly develops from the second arch, which also forms the muscles of facial expression and the stapes. The main nerve derived from this arch is the facial nerve (CN VII) and this supplies these structures (**Fig. 24.1**).

   When the facial nerve is damaged, the muscles of facial expression become paralyzed but the trigeminally supplied muscles of mastication and anterior belly of digastric remain functional. Therefore, the digastric

Table 24.1 *Pharyngeal Arch Derivatives*

Arch	Nerve	Artery	Bone	Muscle
I	**CN V**	Maxillary	Greater wing of sphenoid, incus, malleus, **maxilla,** zygomatic, temporal (squamous), **mandible**	**Muscles of mastication,** anterior digastric, mylohyoid, tensor tympani, **tensor veli palatini**
II	**CN VII**	Stapedial (corticotympanic)	Stapes, styloid process, stylohyoid ligament, lesser horn, and upper body of hyoid	**Muscles of facial expression,** posterior digastric, stylohyoid stapedius
III	**CN IX**	Common carotid, proximal internal carotid	Greater horns and lower body of hyoid	Stylopharyngeus
IV/VI	**CN X**	Aortic arch, right subclavian, origin of pulmonary arteries, ductus arteriosus	Laryngeal cartilages	**Pharyngeal constrictors, levator veli palatini,** palatoglossus, striated upper esophageal muscles, **laryngeal muscles**

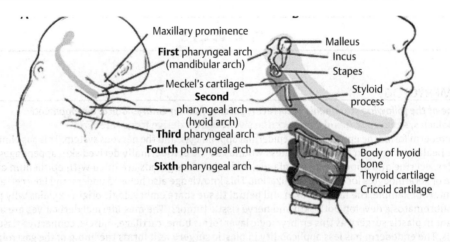

Fig. 24.1 ***A,*** Lateral view of pharyngeal arches. ***B,*** Cartilaginous and bony structures.

muscle can be transferred to the lower lip to compensate for marginal nerve branch weakness and the temporalis muscle can be transferred to compensate for buccal and zygomatic nerve branch weakness. Of further interest is that facial nerve paralysis also results in a loss of sound dampening and again this can be explained by embryologic development because the nerve to the stapedius, the stapedius itself, and the stapes are all derived from the second arch. The other two ossicles (incus and malleus) are derived from the first arch.

A common exam question relates to the innervation of the palatal musculature. All but one are innervated by the pharyngeal plexus as they are derived from arches four to six. The tensor veli palatini opens the Eustachian tube and is derived from the first arch and so is trigeminal innervation.[1-5]

REFERENCES

1. Afshar M, Brugmann SA, Helms JA. Embryology of the craniofacial complex. In: Neligan PC, ed. Plastic Surgery. 3rd ed. London: Elsevier; 2013
2. Carlson BM, ed. Human Embryology and Developmental Biology. 5th ed. Philadelphia: Elsevier; 2013
3. Hopper RA. Cleft lip and palate: embryology, principles, and treatment. In: Thorne CH, Chung KC, Gosain A, Guntner GC, Mehrara BJ, eds. Grabb and Smith's Plastic Surgery. 7th ed. Philadelphia: Lippincott Williams & Wilkins; 2014
4. Moore KL, Persaud TV, Torchia MD, eds. The Developing Human: Clinically Oriented Embryology. 10th ed. Philadelphia: Elsevier; 2016
5. Sadler TW, ed. Langman's Medical Embryology. 13th ed. Philadelphia: Wolters Kluwer Health; 2014

PHARYNGEAL (BRANCHIAL) GROOVES

3. *Which one of the following statements is correct regarding the pharyngeal grooves in embryological development?*

D. The cervical sinus is formed from grooves II through IV, and incomplete obliteration is the cause of branchial sinus tracts.

There are five pharyngeal grooves (also known as clefts), and the cervical sinus is formed from grooves II through IV. Failure of the sinus to obliterate leads to the formation of a branchial sinus tract, cyst, or fistula. These are often detected in the second (not fourth) decade of life as neck swellings and those formed from groove II (not IV) are most common. Groove I forms the external auditory meatus and tympanic membrane, not the **internal** auditory meatus, which is formed by the first pharyngeal pouch. Grooves II and III differ in their relationship to the internal and external **carotids** (not the **internal jugular vein**). A groove II anomaly runs **between** the external and internal carotid arteries toward the tonsillar fossa, and a groove III anomaly passes **under** the internal carotid. Knowledge of this anatomy can be useful intraoperatively when excising branchial sinuses.[1-5]

REFERENCES

1. Afshar M, Brugmann SA, Helms JA. Embryology of the craniofacial complex. In: Neligan PC, ed. Plastic Surgery. 3rd ed. London: Elsevier; 2013
2. Carlson BM, ed. Human Embryology and Developmental Biology. 5th ed. Philadelphia: Elsevier; 2013

3. Hopper RA. Cleft lip and palate: embryology, principles, and treatment. In: Thorne CH, Chung KC, Gosain A, Guntner GC, Mehrara BJ, eds. Grabb and Smith's Plastic Surgery. 7th ed. Philadelphia: Lippincott Williams & Wilkins; 2014
4. Moore KL, Persaud TV, Torchia MD, eds. The Developing Human: Clinically Oriented Embryology. 10th ed. Philadelphia: Elsevier; 2016
5. Sadler TW, ed. Langman's Medical Embryology. 13th ed. Philadelphia: Wolters Kluwer Health; 2014

PHARYNGEAL (BRANCHIAL) POUCHES

4. *Which one of the following statements is correct regarding the pharyngeal pouches in embryological development?*

E. **The fourth pouch migrates above the third pouch.**

There are five pharyngeal pouches which grow inward between the pharyngeal arches. The fourth pouch migrates above the third pouch during embryonic development. This explains why the third pouch forms the inferior parathyroid, and the fourth pouch forms the superior parathyroid. The first pouch forms the internal auditory canal (the first groove or cleft forms the external auditory canal), and the second pouch forms the palatine (not the lingual) tonsil. The ultimobranchial body forms from the fifth pouch and produces the thyroid C cells.[1-5]

REFERENCES

1. Afshar M, Brugmann SA, Helms JA. Embryology of the craniofacial complex. In: Neligan PC, ed. Plastic Surgery. 3rd ed. London: Elsevier; 2013
2. Carlson BM, ed. Human Embryology and Developmental Biology. 5th ed. Philadelphia: Elsevier; 2013
3. Hopper RA. Cleft lip and palate: embryology, principles, and treatment. In: Thorne CH, Chung KC, Gosain A, Guntner GC, Mehrara BJ, eds. Grabb and Smith's Plastic Surgery. 7th ed. Philadelphia: Lippincott Williams & Wilkins; 2014
4. Moore KL, Persaud TV, Torchia MD, eds. The Developing Human: Clinically Oriented Embryology. 10th ed. Philadelphia: Elsevier; 2016
5. Sadler TW, ed. Langman's Medical Embryology. 13th ed. Philadelphia: Wolters Kluwer Health; 2014

HEAD AND NECK DEVELOPMENT

5. *Which one of the following statements is correct regarding embryology of the head and neck?*

B. **The thyroid gland develops from the tongue.**

The clinical relevance of the thyroid developing from the foramen caecum of the tongue is that during embryologic development, the thyroid moves caudally to its final destination in the neck just below the cricoid cartilage. If a persistent connection is retained between these two structures, then a thyroglossal duct cyst may form and this presents as a painless midline neck swelling in the region of the hyoid bone. A cyst can develop anywhere along the path of the descending thyroid between the tongue base and thyroid, but cysts close to the tongue and floor of the mouth are uncommon. Clinical examination of a patient with a thyroglossal cyst will display swelling elevation on protrusion of the tongue. Treatment is by complete surgical excision under general anesthesia. Recurrence is likely to occur if excision is incomplete.

The tongue is formed from three arches (I, III, and IV), not just two. The anterior two-thirds originates from the first arch and receives sensory innervation from the lingual nerve (trigeminal nerve branch) and taste sensation from the facial nerve (CN VII) through the chordae tympani. The posterior third originates from arches III and IV, with sensory and taste innervation from the glossopharyngeal (CN IX) and vagus (CN X) nerves. The hypoglossal nerve (CN XII) supplies motor innervation to the tongue. The external ear is formed from arches I and II and develops in the neck region before passing cranially during the first trimester. This explains why microtia usually results in an inferiorly placed ear remnant.

The bones of the facial skeleton including the maxilla, mandible, frontal, squamous, and parietal bones are formed by the process of intramembranous ossification. In contrast, the bones of the skull base including the sphenoid, ethmoid, mastoid, and petrous temporal bone are formed by endochondral ossification from cartilage precursors. Meckel's cartilage is an exception to the rule as this forms the malleus and mandibular condyle via endochondral ossification.

The face develops from five prominences: the paired mandibular and maxillary prominences and the single frontonasal prominence. This has clinical relevance in the development of Tessier clefts and cleft lip/palate.[1-4]

REFERENCES

1. Afshar M, Brugmann SA, Helms JA. Embryology of the craniofacial complex. In: Neligan PC, ed. Plastic Surgery. 3rd ed. London: Elsevier; 2013
2. Moore KL, Persaud TV, Torchia MD, eds. The Developing Human: Clinically Oriented Embryology. 10th ed. Philadelphia: Elsevier; 2016
3. Sadler TW, ed. Langman's Medical Embryology. 13th ed. Philadelphia: Wolters Kluwer Health; 2014

4. Rice DP. Craniofacial genetics and dysmorphology. In: Guyuron B, Eriksson S, Persing J, eds. Plastic Surgery: Indications and Practice. Philadelphia: Saunders Elsevier; 2009

EMBRYOLOGIC ORIGINS OF ADULT STRUCTURES

6. ***When considering embryological development in the head and neck, what is the origin of the primary palate and central upper lip?***

D. **Medial nasal prominence**

The face develops from the paired maxillary and mandibular prominences along with the frontonasal prominence, which comprises the medial and lateral nasal prominences. The medial nasal prominence forms the primary palate, the midmaxilla, midlip, philtrum, central nose, and nasal septum. The lateral nasal prominence forms the nasal alae. The maxillary prominences form the secondary palate, lateral maxilla, and lateral lip. The mandibular prominences form the mandible, lower lip, and face. Knowledge of the embryologic development and fusion of these prominences provides the basis for understanding the concepts of cleft lip, cleft palate, and Tessier clefts. Unilateral cleft lips result from failure of fusion of a medial nasal prominence with the corresponding maxillary prominence (**Fig. 24.2**).[1,2]

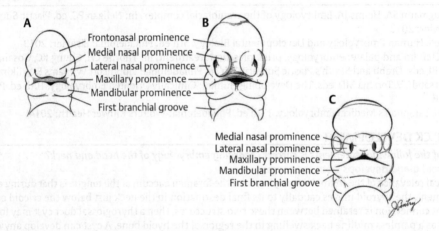

Fig. 24.2 Embryonic development of the human face. *A*, Week 5. *B*, Week 6. *C*, Week 7.

REFERENCES

1. Sadler TW, ed. Langman's Medical Embryology. 13th ed. Philadelphia: Wolters Kluwer Health; 2014
2. Tepper OM, Warren SM. Craniofacial embryology. In: Weinzwig J, ed. Plastic Surgery Secrets Plus. 2nd ed. Philadelphia: Elsevier; 2010

EMBRYOLOGY OF THE TONGUE

7. ***Which cranial nerve is responsible for taste in the anterior part of the tongue?***

B. **Facial (CN VII)**

The tongue has multiple embryologic origins and therefore has multiple different nerve supplies. These elements are often tested in written and clinical examinations. The anterior two-thirds of the tongue originates from the first pharyngeal arch and sensation is supplied by the lingual nerve from the trigeminal nerve (CN V_3). However, the innervation for taste comes from the chorda tympani branch of the facial nerve (CN VII). The posterior third of the tongue originates from the third and fourth pharyngeal arches and taste and sensation are supplied by the glossopharyngeal nerve (CN IX) and the vagus nerve (CN X). Motor innervation for the tongue is largely from the hypoglossal nerve (CN VII) with some innervation from the vagus (CN X).[1,2]

REFERENCES

1. Sadler TW, ed. Langman's Medical Embryology. 13th ed. Philadelphia: Wolters Kluwer Health; 2014
2. Tepper OM, Warren SM. Craniofacial embryology. In: Weinzwig J, ed. Plastic Surgery Secrets Plus. 2nd ed. Philadelphia: Elsevier; 2010

25. Surgical Treatment of Migraine Headaches

See *Essentials of Plastic Surgery*, third edition, pp. 315–328

MEDICAL THERAPY FOR MIGRAINES

1. *Which one of the following medications is used to stop a migraine attack once it has started?*
   A. Propranolol
   B. Gabapentin
   C. Diphenhydramine
   D. Sumatriptan
   E. Verapamil

TRIGGER ANATOMY IN MIGRAINE HEADACHES

2. *Peripheral compression of which one of the following cranial nerves may be indicated in development of migraine headaches?*
   A. Facial
   B. Trigeminal
   C. Olfactory
   D. Vagus
   E. Glossopharyngeal

TRIGGER ANATOMY IN MIGRAINE HEADACHES

3. *Which one of the following tissue types is not thought to be implicated as a source contributing to migraine headaches?*
   A. Muscle
   B. Fascia
   C. Tendon
   D. Bone
   E. Blood vessel

SURGICAL ANATOMY IN MIGRAINE HEADACHES

4. *During surgical exploration of the supraorbital nerve, what is the most likely anatomic arrangement causing compression at the supraorbital notch?*
   A. A bony spicule
   B. A fascial band
   C. A muscular band
   D. A narrow foramen
   E. A dilated artery

SURGICAL ANATOMY IN MIGRAINE HEADACHES

5. You are undertaking nerve decompression of the greater occipital nerve. *Which muscle does the greater occipital nerve usually pass through just before it enters the trapezius?*
   A. Splenius capitis
   B. Semispinalis capitis
   C. Rectus capitis
   D. Obliquus capitis inferior
   E. Medialis capitis superiori

SYMPTOMS RELATED TO DIFFERENT MIGRAINE HEADACHES

6. A patient who is generally fit and well presents with a history of morning migraine headaches. The patient was recently advised by a dentist to use a night mouthguard. *Which type of migraine is most likely?*
   A. Rhinogenic
   B. Occipital
   C. Temporal
   D. Frontal
   E. Parietal

SYMPTOMS RELATED TO DIFFERENT MIGRAINE HEADACHES

7. A 30-year-old surgeon presents with a history of migraines that occur most often after she works out at the gym. The attacks can be particularly bad after a full day of operating. *Which type of migraine is most likely?*
   A. Rhinogenic
   B. Temporal
   C. Occipital
   D. Frontal
   E. Parietal

DIAGNOSIS OF SURGICAL CANDIDATES IN MIGRAINE THERAPY

8. *When reviewing a new patient in clinic regarding the management of migraine headaches, which one of the following is likely to be the most appropriate initial part of the clinical interview?*
   A. Injection of lidocaine just above the brow and lateral canthal regions
   B. Performing an intranasal examination with a speculum
   C. Performing a handheld Doppler ultrasound of the forehead and temple
   D. Arranging for some radiologic imaging including plain films and computed tomography (CT)
   E. Asking the patient to place a single finger on the site of pain during an attack

MANAGEMENT OF PATIENTS WITH MIGRAINE HEADACHES

9. A 40-year-old patient has severe migraine headaches two or three times each week, with pain originating above the eyebrows, radiating into the forehead and scalp. Attacks are helped, but not arrested, by manual pressure on the brow. She has been prescribed sumatriptan and propanolol and also uses nonsteroidal anti-inflammatory drugs (NSAIDs). She has active forehead pain that has been present for 3 hours before seeing you in clinic. *What is the next best step in management of this patient?*
   A. Record a migraine journal for 1 month
   B. Add in zolmitriptan and elitriptan
   C. Inject local anesthetic into the supraorbital nerve (SON)/supratrochlear nerve (STN) trigger sites
   D. Inject botulinum toxin A into the SON/STN trigger sites
   E. Surgically decompress the SON and STN

DIAGNOSIS OF SURGICAL CANDIDATES FOR MIGRAINE SURGERY

10. *In which anatomic area is use of the handheld Doppler particularly useful for diagnosis of trigger points in migraine patients?*
    A. Brow
    B. Temple
    C. Occiput
    D. Neck
    E. Nose

EFFECTIVENESS OF BOTULINUM TOXIN IN MIGRAINE HEADACHES

11. *Which one of the following sensory nerves is most likely to be intentionally sacrificed in migraine surgery, resulting in an area of residual paresthesia?*
    A. Greater occipital nerve
    B. Lesser occipital nerve
    C. Supraorbital nerve
    D. Supratrochlear nerve
    E. Zygomaticotemporal nerve

12. *Which one of the following is correct regarding the surgical management of migraines?*
    A. Supraorbital nerve decompression requires an endoscopic approach.
    B. Greater occipital nerve decompression involves multipoint trigger release.
    C. Surgery should be considered the mainstay of treatment for most migraine patients.
    D. Most surgical approaches involve resection of bone or osteotomies.
    E. Correction of a deviated septum is first-line treatment for most cases.

OUTCOMES AFTER MIGRAINE SURGERY

13. *Following migraine surgery, what percentage of patients are likely to report an improvement in migraine symptoms?*
    A. 20%
    B. 40%
    C. 60%
    D. 80%
    E. 100%

Answers

MEDICAL THERAPY FOR MIGRAINES

1. *Which one of the following medications is used to stop a migraine attack once it has started?*

    D. Sumatriptan

    Having baseline knowledge of medications used to treat a migraine is important when assessing patients for migraine surgery. There are three main types of medication used to manage migraines: prophylactic agents, abortive agents, and acute analgesics. The triptans, including sumatriptan, represent an abortive type of therapy and are given to prevent a suspected early migraine or stop an attack once it has begun. They act on serotonin 5-HT receptors and inhibit release of neuropeptides. The frequency of triptan use is a useful guide to both the frequency and severity of migraine attacks. Recording a journal of triptan use is also helpful for comparison before and after intervention with botox injections or surgery.

    Prophylactic agents have the goal of reducing severity and frequency of migraine attacks. They are subclassified as beta-blockers (e.g., propranolol), calcium channel blockers (e.g., verapamil), antidepressants (e.g., amitriptyline), anticonvulsants (e.g., gabapentin or valproate), and antihistamines (e.g., diphenhydramine).

    Acute analgesics have the goal of relieving mild to moderate symptoms of migraine during an episode. These comprise nonsteroidal anti-inflammatory drugs (NSAIDs) such as ibuprofen, aspirin, or diclofenac. Another popular agent is acetaminophen.[1,2]

REFERENCES

1. Ong JJY, De Felice M. Migraine treatment: current acute medications and their potential mechanisms of action. [published correction appears in Neurotherapeutics, January 8, 2018] Neurotherapeutics 2018;15(2):274–290
2. Whyte CA, Tepper SJ. Adverse effects of medications commonly used in the treatment of migraine. Expert Rev Neurother 2009;9(9):1379–1391

TRIGGER ANATOMY IN MIGRAINE HEADACHES

2. *Peripheral compression of which one of the following cranial nerves may be indicated in development of migraine headaches?*

    B. Trigeminal

    Migraine headaches have traditionally been treated with medications including analgesics, such as acetaminophen, anti-inflammatory agents such as ibuprofen, serotonin agonists such as the triptans, beta-blockers such as propranolol, or calcium channel inhibitors such as verapamil. However, migraines persist in many patients in spite of these medical treatments and as a result, surgical approaches to their management have been developed. These are based on the theory that extracranial sensory branches of the trigeminal and cervical spinal nerves can be irritated, entrapped, or compressed at points throughout their anatomic course. Surgical treatments are aimed at addressing the compression sites in order to reduce compression and ultimately the frequency and severity of migraine attacks.[1]

    Specific compression of the facial, vagus, or glossopharyngeal nerves is not thought to be responsible for the development of migraines although patients can experience visual disturbances and abnormal smells or tastes before or during an attack. Nasal abnormalities such as a deviated septum may be implicated in migraines via irritation of the anterior and posterior ethmoid and nasopalatine nerves, which are branches of the trigeminal nerve, but the olfactory nerve, which is responsible for the sense of smell is not involved.

REFERENCE

1. Janis JE, Barker JC, Javadi C, Ducic I, Hagan R, Guyuron B. A review of current evidence in the surgical treatment of migraine headaches. Plast Reconstr Surg 2014;134(4, Suppl 2):131S–141S

TRIGGER ANATOMY IN MIGRAINE HEADACHES

3. *Which one of the following tissue types is not thought to be implicated as a source contributing to migraine headaches?*

    C. Tendon

    A number of different anatomic trigger points of the trigeminal nerve and cervical plexus have been implicated in the development of migraine headaches. A variety of tissue types have been attributed to the compression or irritation, but tendon is not one of them.

Tissues implicated in causing compression and/or irritation of the nerves include muscle, fascia, bone, and vessel. For example, supraorbital nerve triggers may be caused by the corrugator or procerus muscles, bone, and fascia at the supraorbital foramen, or by the adjacent supraorbital artery. In addition, cartilage may be implicated in intranasal compression by the effects of septal deviation on paranasal branches of the trigeminal nerve (branches of the sphenopalatine ganglion).[1-5]

REFERENCES

1. Khansa I, Barker JC, Janis JE. Sensory nerves of the head and neck. In: Watanabe K, ed. Anatomy for Plastic Surgery of the Face, Head and Neck. Thieme; 2016
2. Khansa I, Janis JE. Surgical anatomy of the frontal and occipital trigger sites. In: Guyuron B, ed. Migraine Surgery. Thieme; 2018
3. Fallucco M, Janis JE, Hagan RR. The anatomical morphology of the supraorbital notch: clinical relevance to the surgical treatment of migraine headaches. Plast Reconstr Surg 2012;130(6):1227–1233
4. Janis JE, Ghavami A, Lemmon JA, Leedy JE, Guyuron B. The anatomy of the corrugator supercilii muscle: part II. Supraorbital nerve branching patterns. Plast Reconstr Surg 2008;121(1):233–240
5. Janis JE, Hatef DA, Hagan R, et al. Anatomy of the supratrochlear nerve: implications for the surgical treatment of migraine headaches. Plast Reconstr Surg 2013;131(4):743–750

SURGICAL ANATOMY IN MIGRAINE HEADACHES

4. *During surgical exploration of the supraorbital nerve, what is the most likely anatomic arrangement causing compression at the supraorbital notch?*
   B. A fascial band

Compression of the supraorbital nerve is implicated in migraine headaches and can occur at a number of sites. In approximately 86% of cases there is a fascial band across the supraorbital notch that may be the cause of compression in this area. The anatomy of fascial compression is subclassified into the subgroups type I, type II, and type III, depending on the anatomic arrangement of fascia and bone.

Type I represents a single fascial band over a single foramen and is the most common type.

Type II bands have partial bony spicules that extend to the neurovascular bundle. Type III bands contain a horizontal *(A)* or vertical *(B)* septum that encases the nerve (**Fig. 25.1**). Muscular sites of compression beyond the supraorbital foramen include the corrugator and procerus muscles. Dilated arteries can cause irritation of nerves such as in the temple secondary to the action of the superficial temporal artery.[1-4]

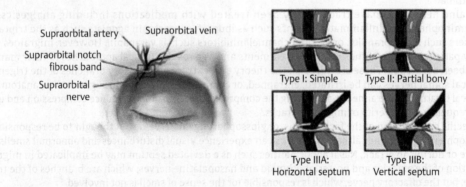

Fig. 25.1   Bony, fascial, and vascular compression of the supraorbital nerve.

REFERENCES

1. Khansa I, Janis JE. Surgical anatomy of the frontal and occipital trigger sites. In: Guyuron B, ed. Migraine Surgery. Thieme; 2018
2. Fallucco M, Janis JE, Hagan RR. The anatomical morphology of the supraorbital notch: clinical relevance to the surgical treatment of migraine headaches. Plast Reconstr Surg 2012;130(6):1227–1233
3. Janis JE, Ghavami A, Lemmon JA, Leedy JE, Guyuron B. The anatomy of the corrugator supercilii muscle: part II. Supraorbital nerve branching patterns. Plast Reconstr Surg 2008;121(1):233–240
4. Janis JE, Hatef DA, Hagan R, et al. Anatomy of the supratrochlear nerve: implications for the surgical treatment of migraine headaches. Plast Reconstr Surg 2013;131(4):743–750

SURGICAL ANATOMY IN MIGRAINE HEADACHES

5. You are undertaking nerve decompression of the greater occipital nerve. *Which muscle does the greater occipital nerve usually pass through just before it enters the trapezius?*

    B. Semispinalis capitis

The greater occipital nerve is the medial branch of the dorsal primary ramus of C2 (**Fig. 25.2**).

The trunk exits approximately 3 cm below and 1.5 cm lateral to the occipital protuberance. It passes around the obliquus capitis inferior and then the rectus capitis superior before piercing the semispinalis capitis medially. It finally passes through the trapezius, where it is closely associated with the occipital artery. Surgical access to this nerve is through a 5 cm long midline incision a few centimeters below the occipital protuberance.[1,2]

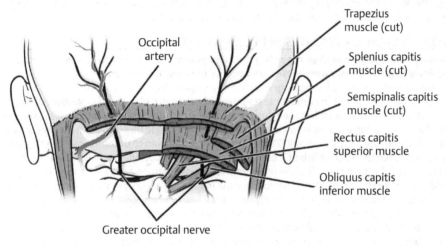

Occipital artery

Trapezius muscle (cut)

Splenius capitis muscle (cut)

Semispinalis capitis muscle (cut)

Rectus capitis superior muscle

Obliquus capitis inferior muscle

Greater occipital nerve

Fig. 25.2   Greater occipital nerve anatomy.

REFERENCES

1. Janis JE, Hatef DA, Ducic I, et al. The anatomy of the greater occipital nerve: Part II. Compression point topography. Plast Reconstr Surg 2010;126(5):1563–1572
2. Janis JE, Hatef DA, Reece EM, McCluskey PD, Schaub TA, Guyuron B. Neurovascular compression of the greater occipital nerve: implications for migraine headaches. Plast Reconstr Surg 2010;126(6):1996–2001

SYMPTOMS RELATED TO DIFFERENT MIGRAINE HEADACHES

6. A patient who is generally fit and well presents with a history of morning migraine headaches. The patient was recently advised by a dentist to use a night mouthguard. *Which type of migraine is most likely?*

    C. Temporal

Temporal migraine often occurs in the morning and is associated with bruxism (grinding of the teeth) overnight. Pain is often associated with the temporalis or masseter muscles and originates just lateral and cephalad to the lateral canthus. Patients with temporal headaches may describe improvement with manual pressure applied to the area of the superficial temporal artery during a migraine attack.[1] It is postulated that pulsation of the superficial temporal artery causes irritation to local sensory nerve fibers.[2] For this reason, some surgical treatments involve tying off the superficial temporal artery for such patients.

REFERENCES

1. Cianchetti C, Cianchetti ME, Pisano T, Hmaidan Y. Treatment of migraine attacks by compression of temporal superficial arteries using a device. Med Sci Monit 2009;15(4):CR185–CR188
2. Chim H, Okada HC, Brown MS, et al. The auriculotemporal nerve in etiology of migraine headaches: compression points and anatomical variations. Plast Reconstr Surg 2012;130(2):336–341

SYMPTOMS RELATED TO DIFFERENT MIGRAINE HEADACHES

7. A 30-year-old surgeon presents with a history of migraines that occur most often after she works out at the gym. The attacks can be particularly bad after a full day of operating. *Which type of migraine is most likely?*

    C. Occipital

Occipital migraines can be triggered by heavy exercise and stress. Patients often have tight posterior neck musculature. Pain originates just lateral to the midline, a few centimeters caudal to the occipital tuberosity and there is often a tender site on manual palpation close to the origin of trapezius. Irritation of the greater occipital nerve, which is a branch of C2 (**see Fig. 25.2**), is thought to be implicated in this type of migraine and may be due to muscle or fascial compression, or irritation from the occipital artery.[1,2]

REFERENCES

1. Liu MT, Armijo BS, Guyuron B. A comparison of outcome of surgical treatment of migraine headaches using a constellation of symptoms versus botulinum toxin type A to identify the trigger sites. Plast Reconstr Surg 2012;129(2):413–419
2. Janis JE, Hatef DA, Reece EM, McCluskey PD, Schaub TA, Guyuron B. Neurovascular compression of the greater occipital nerve: implications for migraine headaches. Plast Reconstr Surg 2010;126(6):1996–2001

DIAGNOSIS OF SURGICAL CANDIDATES IN MIGRAINE THERAPY

8. *When reviewing a new patient in clinic regarding the management of migraine headaches, which one of the following is likely to be the most appropriate initial part of the clinical interview?*
    E. Asking the patient to place a single finger on the site of pain during an attack
    When meeting a new patient in clinic for assessment of suitability of surgical treatment of migraine, there are a number of key steps that must be taken during the consultation. Of these, a really useful and simple approach to guide the consultation early on is to ask the patient to use a single finger to describe precisely where the pain originates from during a typical attack. This will guide the clinician to determine which trigger sites are likely to be involved. Once this is established it can be useful to inject lidocaine into suspected compression or trigger sites. This can only be done once all of the other information is obtained and examination is complete. The use of a handheld Doppler in clinic may also be useful once the main pain/trigger point location has been identified by the patient in order to see if it corresponds closely to arterial location. Imaging in the form of CT is sometimes useful for patients with migraine, although this is less commonly needed. Plain films are not part of the usual workup. Physical examination should include intranasal examination with a speculum to identify deviated septum, septal spur, or turbinate hypertrophy, particularly where patients describe migraines associated with pain behind the eye, rhinorrhea, or nasal obstruction.[1-3]

REFERENCES

1. Liu MT, Armijo BS, Guyuron B. A comparison of outcome of surgical treatment of migraine headaches using a constellation of symptoms versus botulinum toxin type A to identify the trigger sites. Plast Reconstr Surg 2012;129(2):413–419
2. Janis JE, Barker JC, Palettas M. Targeted peripheral nerve-directed Onabotulinumtoxin A injection for effective long-term therapy for migraine headache. Plast Reconstr Surg Glob Open 2017;5(3):e1270
3. Guyuron B, Reed D, Kriegler JS, Davis J, Pashmini N, Amini S. A placebo-controlled surgical trial of the treatment of migraine headaches. Plast Reconstr Surg 2009;124(2):461–468

MANAGEMENT OF PATIENTS WITH MIGRAINE HEADACHES

9. A 40-year-old patient has severe migraine headaches two or three times each week, with pain originating above the eyebrows, radiating into the forehead and scalp. Attacks are helped, but not arrested, by manual pressure on the brow. She has been prescribed sumatriptan and propanolol and also uses nonsteroidal anti-inflammatory drugs (NSAIDs). She has active forehead pain that has been present for 3 hours before seeing you in clinic. *What is the next best step in management of this patient?*
    C. Inject local anesthetic into the supraorbital nerve (SON)/supratrochlear nerve (STN) trigger sites
    If the patient's constellation of symptoms suggests a specific trigger site, and if the patient has active pain in this location at the time of presentation, a local nerve block can be performed to help confirm the diagnosis.
      She is already taking a triptan so there is no benefit in adding in other triptans in this case. Furthermore, manipulation of medications is best left to the treating neurologist. Injection of Botox to the trigger sites in question will also provide diagnostic information (and potentially therapeutic effect) but does not have immediate action and would require a separate visit, usually 1 month later, to review the migraine log and determine the benefit. Although this is a potential option, blocks are typically preferred over Botox if the patient has active pain. Moving to surgical decompression is only indicated for this patient once the diagnostic workup has been completed.[1]

REFERENCE

1. Janis JE, Barker JC, Palettas M. Targeted peripheral nerve-directed Onabotulinumtoxin A injection for effective long-term therapy for migraine headache. Plast Reconstr Surg Glob Open 2017;5(3):e1270

DIAGNOSIS OF SURGICAL CANDIDATES FOR MIGRAINE SURGERY

10. *In which anatomic area is use of the handheld Doppler particularly useful for diagnosis of trigger points in migraine patients?*

    B. Temple

        The auriculotemporal nerve is a branch of CN V_3 and extends through the parotid gland, then travels over the temporomandibular joint (TMJ) before dividing over the zygomatic arch and within the layers of the temporoparietal fascia. It provides sensation to the tragus, the anterior portion of the ear, and posterior temple. Compression may be caused by soft tissues of the temple or oftentimes the superficial temporal artery. Due to its intimate proximity to the superficial temporal vessels, Doppler is particularly useful in this location.[1,2]

REFERENCES

1. Janis JE, Hatef DA, Ducic I, et al. Anatomy of the auriculotemporal nerve: variations in its relationship to the superficial temporal artery and implications for the treatment of migraine headaches. Plast Reconstr Surg 2010;125(5):1422–1428
2. Chim H, Okada HC, Brown MS, et al. The auriculotemporal nerve in etiology of migraine headaches: compression points and anatomical variations. Plast Reconstr Surg 2012;130(2):336–341

EFFECTIVENESS OF BOTULINUM TOXIN IN MIGRAINE HEADACHES

11. *Which one of the following sensory nerves is most likely to be intentionally sacrificed in migraine surgery, resulting in an area of residual paresthesia?*

    E. Zygomaticotemporal nerve

        Temporal migraines can be triggered by compression of the zygomaticotemporal or auriculotemporal nerves which are branches of the trigeminal nerve. The zygomaticotemporal nerve arises from the maxillary division (V_2), and the auriculotemporal nerve arises from the mandibular division (V_3). The zygomaticotemporal nerve supplies a small patch of skin on the parietal scalp and is a nerve that is avulsed rather than decompressed in order to improve symptoms of migraine.[1]

REFERENCE

1. Janis JE, Hatef DA, Thakar H, et al. The zygomaticotemporal branch of the trigeminal nerve: Part II. Anatomical variations. Plast Reconstr Surg 2010;126(2):435–442

12. *Which one of the following is correct regarding the surgical management of migraines?*

    B. Greater occipital nerve decompression involves multipoint trigger release.

        Greater occipital nerve release is performed with either a vertical or horizontal approach. It involves release at a number of compression sites: Musculofascial release between obliquus capitis and semispinalis capitis muscles, partial resection of semispinalis capitis muscle, partial resection of trapezius muscle and fascial bands, and ligation/ablation of the occipital artery. Supraorbital nerve decompression (SON) may be achieved through endoscopic, open brow, or transpalpebral approaches. The transpalpebral approach is gaining favor due to ease of exposure.[1,2] This surgery involves complete or partial resection of the corrugators, foraminotomies if needed, and release of all compression points to release the trunk and all branches of the SON and supratrochlear nerve (STN).

        Surgery should not be the mainstay of treatment for most migraine patients. It is used for patients who have an established diagnosis of migraine by a neurologist and where traditional medication has failed. Most surgical approaches involve decompression of muscle, fascial bands, and ablation of blood vessels as the primary aim and do not require osteotomies or foraminotomies except on rare occasion.

REFERENCES

1. Guyuron B, Kriegler JS, Davis J, Amini SB. Five-year outcome of surgical treatment of migraine headaches. Plast Reconstr Surg 2011;127(2):603–608
2. Hagan RR, Fallucco MA, Janis JE. Supraorbital rim syndrome: definition, surgical treatment, and outcomes for frontal headache. Plast Reconstr Surg Glob Open 2016;4(7):e795

OUTCOMES AFTER MIGRAINE SURGERY

13. *Following migraine surgery, what percentage of patients are likely to report an improvement in migraine symptoms?*

    D. 80%

        Outcomes at 5 years after migraine surgery were described by Guyuron's team.[1] They found that more than 80% of patients who had surgery reported improvement in terms of reduced frequency of attacks and improved symptoms. They found that patients who had multiple trigger sites treated were more likely to have a successful outcome. This applied to targeting both frontal and temporal trigger sites together and targeting all four sites where appropriate (including nasal and occipital). In patients treated surgically at all trigger sites, 57% reported complete elimination of migraine headaches. Factors associated with better outcomes also included an older age at first onset of migraine symptoms, fewer baseline migraines per month, and daily use of over-the-counter medications. Factors associated with worse outcomes included a history of head or neck injury, increased intraoperative bleeding, and single-site surgery that could result in inadequate treatment of all trigger sites.

REFERENCE

1. Guyuron B, Kriegler JS, Davis J, Amini SB. Five-year outcome of surgical treatment of migraine headaches. Plast Reconstr Surg 2011;127(2):603–608

26. Craniosynostosis

See *Essentials of Plastic Surgery*, third edition, pp. 329–345

CRANIAL GROWTH AND DEVELOPMENT

1. *When considering the timing of normal cranial suture fusion, which one of the following suture lines is expected to close within the first year of life?*
   A. Metopic
   B. Sagittal
   C. Coronal
   D. Lambdoidal
   E. Squamosal

PATHOPHYSIOLOGY OF CRANIOSYNOSTOSIS

2. *Which one of the following statements is correct regarding craniosynostosis?*
   A. Most cases are syndromic and linked to the *FGFR* gene.
   B. Normal cranial growth occurs parallel to the suture lines.
   C. Virchow's law relates to changes in intracranial pressure (ICP) with untreated synostoses.
   D. Appositional growth is part of normal cranial development.
   E. Cranial base theory fully explains all types of craniosynostoses.

DIAGNOSIS OF RAISED INTRACRANIAL PRESSURE

3. *Which one of the following is expected in a craniosynostosis patient with elevated intracranial pressure (ICP)?*
   A. Normal fundoscopic examination
   B. Soft fontanelles on physical examination
   C. Decreased optic nerve sheath diameter on transorbital ultrasound
   D. Decreased latency on measurement of visual evoked potentials
   E. Headaches, irritability, and an altered developmental progression

ELEVATED INTRACRANIAL PRESSURE IN CRANIOSYNOSTOSIS

4. *Which one of the following is correct regarding the pediatric population?*
   A. The normal ICP value in children is well documented.
   B. Fundoscopy is an unreliable tool for assessment of ICP in young children.
   C. A Chiari malformation is a vascular malformation resulting in elevated ICP.
   D. Cephalocranial disproportion is the sole cause of raised ICP in syndromic craniosynostosis.
   E. Elevated ICP is most likely in a single-suture craniosynostosis.

IMAGING IN CRANIOSYNOSTOSIS

5. *Which one of the following is correct regarding imaging of a patient who has nonsyndromic craniosynostosis?*
   A. Cortical thickening, fingerprinting, and loss of cisternae are early radiologic findings that suggest raised ICP.
   B. A CT scan is usually required in all cases of craniosynostosis, because plain radiographic films are unhelpful.
   C. The absence of suture lines on plain radiographic films is evidence of suture fusion.
   D. A copper-beaten appearance on CT is highly specific for elevated intracranial pressure.
   E. Serial MRI assessment is helpful for most cases of craniosynostosis.

DIAGNOSIS OF CRANIOSYNOSTOSIS

6. The parents of a 12-week-old baby have concerns about their child's head shape. On examination the child has a misshapen head with a triangular appearance when viewed from above. The child's eyes are close together. *What is the most likely suture involved in this craniosynostosis?*
   A. Unilateral coronal
   B. Metopic
   C. Lambdoid
   D. Sagittal
   E. Bilateral coronal

CLASSIFICATION OF SYNOSTOSIS

7. **Which one of the following is the most common craniosynostosis?**
   A. Unilateral coronal
   B. Metopic
   C. Lambdoid
   D. Sagittal
   E. Bilateral coronal

HARLEQUIN DEFORMITY

8. **Which one of the following cranial sutures is associated with a harlequin deformity?**
   A. Unilateral coronal
   B. Metopic
   C. Lambdoid
   D. Sagittal
   E. Bilateral coronal

DEFORMATIONAL PLAGIOCEPHALY

9. A child is referred to clinic with a diagnosis of deformational plagiocephaly. **What head shape is typical of this condition?**
   A. Triangular
   B. Parallelogram
   C. Boat shaped
   D. Square
   E. Trapezoidal

DEFORMATIONAL PLAGIOCEPHALY

10. A child is referred with an abnormal head shape but normal physical development. **When trying to differentiate between a deformational plagiocephaly and a true craniosynostosis, which anatomic structure will be positioned normally in only the deformational condition?**
    A. Cheek
    B. Chin
    C. Brow
    D. Nasal root
    E. Ear

MORPHOLOGICAL VARIANTS IN CRANIOSYNOSTOSIS

11. You see a syndromic child who has an untreated bicoronal synostosis. **Which one of the following would you expect to see on examination?**
    A. Turribrachycephaly
    B. Oxycephaly
    C. Kleeblatschadel
    D. Posterior plagiocephaly
    E. Scaphocephaly

CROUZON SYNDROME

12. **Which one of the following is correct regarding Crouzon syndrome?**
    A. The inheritance pattern is autosomal recessive.
    B. Multiple different cranial sutures may be involved.
    C. Intracranial pressure (ICP) is rarely elevated.
    D. Class I malocclusion is consistently present.
    E. Extremity abnormalities are commonly observed.

APERT SYNDROME

13. A child who has been diagnosed with Apert syndrome presents to clinic. **Which one of the following features will differentiate this condition from other similar synostotic syndromes?**
    A. Normal intracranial pressure (ICP)
    B. Cleft palate
    C. Brachycephaly
    D. Complex syndactyly
    E. Midface hypoplasia

PFEIFFER SYNDROME

14. **Which one of the following is least expected during examination of a patient with Pfeiffer syndrome?**
    A. Broad thumbs and halluces
    B. Mild cutaneous syndactyly
    C. Tracheostomy in situ
    D. Mental impairment
    E. Turribrachycephaly

SAETHRE-CHOTZEN SYNDROME

15. *Which one of the following is correct regarding Saethre-Chotzen syndrome?*
   A. It has an incidence of 1:200,000.
   B. It is associated with a *TWIST-1* gene mutation.
   C. It involves symmetrical brachycephaly.
   D. Patients have a relative absence of upper eyelid skin.
   E. A high hairline is typically seen.

SURGERY FOR SYNOSTOSES

16. *When considering the role of surgery in craniosynostosis, which one of the following is correct?*
   A. The primary goal is to normalize head shape and appearance.
   B. The surgical approach is similar for both syndromic and nonsyndromic cases.
   C. Associated blood loss represents the greatest risk for patients undergoing surgery.
   D. Surgery is generally best performed shortly after the child's first birthday.
   E. Delaying surgery makes the bones easier to manipulate and reshape.

SURGICAL TECHNIQUES FOR SYNOSTOSES

17. *Which one of the following surgical techniques may be most useful for treating a patient with an isolated scaphocephaly?*
   A. Endoscopic strip craniectomy with helmet
   B. LeFort midface advancement
   C. Fronto-orbital advancement
   D. Posterior vault expansion with distraction osteogenesis
   E. Biparieto-occipital craniotomies

Answers

CRANIAL GROWTH AND DEVELOPMENT

1. *When considering the timing of normal cranial suture fusion, which one of the following suture lines is expected to close within the first year of life?*

   A. Metopic

   There are four key suture lines in the growing skull, namely, metopic, sagittal, coronal, and lambdoid. These are shown in **Fig. 26.1**. They allow progressive growth of the skull to accommodate rapid brain growth in the early years of life. In addition, there are two corresponding fontanelles, which are spaces between the bones of the skull where ossification is incomplete to facilitate birth passage. The fusion of cranial sutures occurs earliest in the metopic suture between the two frontal bones. This closes between 6 and 8 months of age. The remaining three sutures remain open until the third decade (sagittal 22 years, coronal 24 years, and lambdoid 26 years). The fontanelles usually close within the first 12 months with the posterior fontanelle closing between 3 and 6 months, and the anterior fontanelle closing between 9 and 12 months.[1,2]

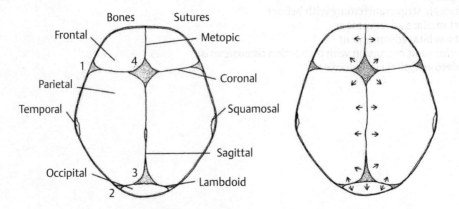

Fig. 26.1   Cranial sutures in the human fetus. Premature closure produces growth restriction perpendicular to the line of the suture and compensatory overgrowth parallel to it.

REFERENCES

1. Weinzweig J, Kirschner RE, Farley A, et al. Metopic synostosis: defining the temporal sequence of normal suture fusion and differentiating it from synostosis on the basis of computed tomography images. Plast Reconstr Surg 2003;112(5):1211–1218
2. Carson BS, Dufresne CR. Craniosynostosis and neurocranial asymmetry. In: Defresne CR, Carson BS, Zinreich SJ, eds. Complex Craniofacial Problems. New York: Churchill Livingstone; 1992

PATHOPHYSIOLOGY OF CRANIOSYNOSTOSIS

2. *Which one of the following statements is correct regarding craniosynostosis?*

   D. Appositional growth is part of normal cranial development.

   Cranial growth usually occurs through two processes, suture growth and appositional growth. Appositional growth involves bone resorption on the inner surface and deposition on the outer surface of the skull. Suture growth usually occurs perpendicular to the cranial sutures and premature suture fusion will result in predominantly parallel growth. This is known as Virchow's law and explains the deformities observed with fusion of a given suture.

   Only one-third of craniosynostoses are syndromic. In cases that are syndromic, genetic mutations in the *FGFR2*, *FGFR3*, and *TWIST1* genes may be identified. Various theories exist regarding abnormal suture fusion and include the cranial base theory and the intrinsic suture theory. The cranial base theory states that synostoses result from abnormal tension exerted by the cranial base through the dura, but this does not account for isolated synostoses. The intrinsic suture biology theory proposes that synostoses result from the osteoinductive properties of dura mater, which contains osteoblast-like cells.[1–3]

REFERENCES

1. Cohen MM Jr, MacLean RE. Anatomic, genetic, nosologic, diagnostic, and psychosocial considerations. In: Cohen MM Jr, MacLean RE, eds. Craniosynostosis: Diagnosis, Evaluation, and Management. 2nd ed. New York: Oxford University Press; 2000
2. Derderian CA, Bartlett SP. Craniosynostosis syndromes. In: Thorne C, ed. Grabb and Smith's Plastic Surgery. 7th ed. Philadelphia: Lippincott Williams & Wilkins; 2013
3. Knoll B, Persing JA. Craniosynostosis. In: Bentz ML, Bauer BS, Zuker RM, eds. Pediatric Plastic Surgery. 2nd ed. St Louis: Quality Medical Publishing; 2008

DIAGNOSIS OF RAISED INTRACRANIAL PRESSURE

3. *Which one of the following is expected in a craniosynostosis patient with elevated intracranial pressure (ICP)?*

E. **Headaches, irritability, and an altered developmental progression**

Elevated intracranial pressure (ICP) is associated with craniosynostosis either due to cephalocranial disproportion or other factors such as intracranial venous congestion, hydrocephalus, or upper airway obstruction. Early clinical findings that suggest a raised ICP include headache, irritability, nausea, vomiting, and sleeping difficulties. Later findings include mental impairment, delayed development, and visual disturbances. Fundoscopic examination may show papilledema and examination of the fontanelles may show tense bulging, sometimes known as the *volcano sign.*

Raised ICP may be measured directly or indirectly. Transorbital ultrasound can be used to measure optic nerve sheath diameter, which will increase (not decrease) with raised ICP. Visual evoked potentials measure the latency time of an encephalographic response to visual stimuli and will also be increased with raised ICP and axonal injury. Other modalities used to assess raised ICP include plain radiographs which may show late signs of a copper-beaten appearance or thumb printing from pressure of the gyri on the inner table.[1-4]

REFERENCES

1. Renier D, Sainte-Rose C, Marchac D, Hirsch JF. Intracranial pressure in craniostenosis. J Neurosurg 1982;57(3):370–377
2. Tuite GF, Chong WK, Evanson J, et al. The effectiveness of papilledema as an indicator of raised intracranial pressure in children with craniosynostosis. Neurosurgery 1996;38(2):272–278
3. Swanson JW, Aleman TS, Xu W, et al. Evaluation of optical coherence tomography to detect elevated intracranial pressure in children. JAMA Ophthalmol 2017;135(4):320–328
4. Xu W, Gerety P, Aleman T, Swanson J, Taylor J. Noninvasive methods of detecting increased intracranial pressure. Childs Nerv Syst 2016;32(8):1371–1386

ELEVATED INTRACRANIAL PRESSURE IN CRANIOSYNOSTOSIS

4. *Which one of the following is correct regarding the pediatric population?*

B. **Fundoscopy is an unreliable tool for assessment of ICP in young children.**

No universal definition exists for raised ICP in children. Fundoscopy is a useful tool for assessing raised ICP in many cases, but it should be interpreted with caution in children. Across all age groups it has a specificity of 98% and a sensitivity of 100%. However, in children younger than 8 years of age, the sensitivity is around 22%. A Chiari malformation is not a vascular malformation, but it can result in a raised ICP. It is present when the cerebellar tonsils are displaced downward through the foramen magnum. This malformation may be a cause of hydrocephalus and neurodevelopmental injury. It is commonly seen in patients with Crouzon or Pfeiffer syndrome. Cephalocranial disproportion refers to a decreased intracranial volume and restriction of brain growth. It is one cause of raised ICP; others include intracranial venous congestion, hydrocephalus, and airway obstruction. The incidence of elevated ICP is affected by the number of sutures involved in craniosynostosis. The incidence of elevated ICP with single suture involvement is 13 and 42% when multiple sutures are involved.[1-4]

REFERENCES

1. Renier D, Sainte-Rose C, Marchac D, Hirsch JF. Intracranial pressure in craniostenosis. J Neurosurg 1982;57(3):370–377
2. Tuite GF, Chong WK, Evanson J, et al. The effectiveness of papilledema as an indicator of raised intracranial pressure in children with craniosynostosis. Neurosurgery 1996;38(2):272–278
3. Swanson JW, Aleman TS, Xu W, et al. Evaluation of optical coherence tomography to detect elevated intracranial pressure in children. JAMA Ophthalmol 2017;135(4):320–328
4. Xu W, Gerety P, Aleman T, Swanson J, Taylor J. Noninvasive methods of detecting increased intracranial pressure. Childs Nerv Syst 2016;32(8):1371–1386

IMAGING IN CRANIOSYNOSTOSIS

5. *Which one of the following is correct regarding imaging of a patient who has nonsyndromic craniosynostosis?*

   C. **The absence of suture lines on plain radiographic films is evidence of suture fusion.**

      Plain radiographs are useful to show an absence of suture lines and are usually the only imaging modality required for patients with craniosynostoses. In syndromic cases, however, CT can be helpful to diagnose associated abnormalities, to plan surgery, and to monitor hydrocephalus. MRI is typically unnecessary except in patients with selected syndromes such as Apert or Pfeiffer, when associated brain abnormalities are suspected.

      Radiographs may show other signs of synostosis. For example, a copper-beaten appearance on radiograph is also known as *Luckenschadel* and is a characteristic late sign (with a low specificity) of raised ICP in craniosynostosis. Other late findings are cortical thickening, fingerprinting, and loss of cisternae.[1,2]

REFERENCES

1. Persing JA. MOC-PS(SM) CME article: management considerations in the treatment of craniosynostosis. Plast Reconstr Surg 2008;121(4, Suppl):1–11
2. Kim HJ, Roh HG, Lee IW. Craniosynostosis: updates in radiologic diagnosis. J Korean Neurosurg Soc 2016;59(3):219–226

DIAGNOSIS OF CRANIOSYNOSTOSIS

6. **The parents of a 12-week-old baby have concerns about their child's head shape. On examination the child has a misshapen head with a triangular appearance when viewed from above. The child's eyes are close together. *What is the most likely suture involved in this craniosynostosis?***

   B. **Metopic**

      The appearance described is known as *trigonocephaly* where the head shape is *"keel shaped"* or triangular. This is caused by premature fusion of the metopic suture. A spectrum of deformities occurs with this condition, including bitemporal narrowing, hypotelorism, bilateral supraorbital retrusion, medially slanted lateral orbital rims, and epicanthal folds. ICP elevation is present in up to 10% of such cases. Unilateral coronal synostosis is associated with ipsilateral frontal flattening and contralateral bossing. Lambdoid synostosis is associated with ipsilateral occipital flattening and a mastoid bulge with downward cant of the posterior skull base on the affected side. Sagittal synostosis is associated with a boat-shaped head rather than triangular. Bilateral coronal synostosis will result in a broad flat head termed "brachycephaly."[1,2]

REFERENCES

1. Beckett JS, Chadha P, Persing JA, Steinbacher DM. Classification of trigonocephaly in metopic synostosis. Plast Reconstr Surg 2012;130(3):442e–447e
2. Selber J, Reid RR, Gershman B, et al. Evolution of operative techniques for the treatment of single-suture metopic synostosis. Ann Plast Surg 2007;59(1):6–13

CLASSIFICATION OF SYNOSTOSIS

7. *Which one of the following is the most common craniosynostosis?*

   D. **Sagittal**

      Sagittal synostosis represents half of all synostoses. They are four times as common in males and clinically present with an increased anteroposterior (AP) cranial diameter and decreased biparietal width. This appearance is described as *scaphocephaly,* meaning "boat shaped." Coronal synostoses represent approximately one-third of all synostoses, and they are usually unilateral. Metopic synostoses are a little less common than coronal synostoses, and affected babies develop trigonocephaly. The least common form is lambdoid, which is extremely rare (**Fig. 26.2**).[1]

REFERENCE

1. Hubli EH. A functional aesthetic approach to correcting the sequelae of sagittal synostosis. Semin Plast Surg 2014;28(3):130–137

HARLEQUIN DEFORMITY

8. *Which one of the following cranial sutures is associated with a harlequin deformity?*

   A. **Unilateral coronal**

      A harlequin deformity results from a lack of descent of the greater wing of the sphenoid on the affected side. It is seen on radiographs of patients with a unilateral coronal synostosis. Physical findings in unilateral synostosis include an anterior plagiocephaly that involves ipsilateral frontal and occipitoparietal flattening, contralateral

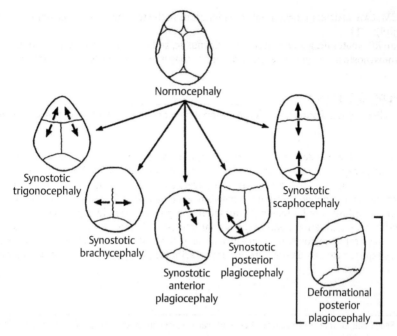

Fig. 26.2   Skull shapes and affected sutures in craniosynostosis.

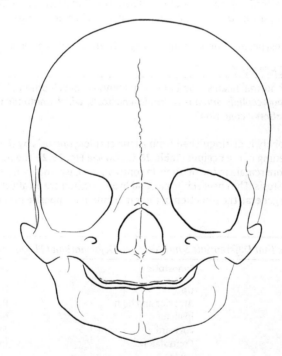

Fig. 26.3   Harlequin deformity.

frontal and parietal bossing, and posterior displacement of the ipsilateral ear (**Fig. 26.3**). The nasal root is constricted and deviated to the affected side. The chin tends to point to the contralateral side due to an anteriorly displaced ipsilateral glenoid fossa.[1-3]

REFERENCES

1. Kim HJ, Roh HG, Lee IW. Craniosynostosis: updates in radiologic diagnosis. J Korean Neurosurg Soc 2016;59(3):219–226

2. Persing JA. MOC-PS(SM) CME article: management considerations in the treatment of craniosynostosis. Plast Reconstr Surg 2008;121(4, Suppl):1–11
3. Cohen MM Jr, MacLean RE. Anatomic, genetic, nosologic, diagnostic, and psychosocial considerations. In: Cohen MM Jr, MacLean RE, eds. Craniosynostosis: diagnosis, evaluation, and management. 2nd ed. New York: Oxford University Press; 2000

DEFORMATIONAL PLAGIOCEPHALY

9. A child is referred to clinic with a diagnosis of deformational plagiocephaly. *What head shape is typical of this condition?*

B. **Parallelogram**

The characteristic head shape in deformational plagiocephaly is a parallelogram appearance (**see Fig. 26.2**).

Deformational plagiocephaly can be mistaken for either posterior (lambdoidal) or anterior (unilateral coronal) synostoses, but is not a true craniosynostosis. It is relatively common with an incidence of 1 in 300 and occurs secondary to external forces applied through the baby's head. It has recently become more common and this may be due to the fact that infants are increasingly nursed in a supine position in order to minimize risk of sudden infant death syndrome. A triangular head shape is characteristic of metopic synostosis. A boat-shaped head is associated with a sagittal synostosis. A square, broad head shape is associated with a bicoronal synostosis. A trapezoidal head shape is associated with anterior or posterior plagiocephaly (lambdoidal or coronal synostoses, respectively).[1–3]

REFERENCES

1. Persing JA. MOC-PS(SM) CME article: management considerations in the treatment of craniosynostosis. Plast Reconstr Surg 2008;121(4, Suppl):1–11
2. Cohen MM Jr, MacLean RE. Anatomic, genetic, nosologic, diagnostic, and psychosocial considerations. In: Cohen MM Jr, MacLean RE, eds. Craniosynostosis: Diagnosis, Evaluation, and Management. 2nd ed. New York: Oxford University Press; 2000
3. Kim HJ, Roh HG, Lee IW. Craniosynostosis: updates in radiologic diagnosis. J Korean Neurosurg Soc 2016;59(3):219–226

DEFORMATIONAL PLAGIOCEPHALY

10. A child is referred with an abnormal head shape but normal physical development. *When trying to differentiate between a deformational plagiocephaly and a true craniosynostosis, which anatomic structure will be positioned normally in only the deformational condition?*

D. **Nasal root**

Deformational plagiocephaly is distinguished from a true craniosynostosis by the presence of a parallelogram configuration with flattening of the occiput (**Table 26.1, also see Fig. 26.2**). The nasal root will be unaffected in this condition and therefore remain in the midline. In contrast, the nasal root will be moved toward the ipsilateral side in a true craniosynostosis. The cheek, chin, ear, and brow position are all affected in both deformational and synostotic conditions. In general, the direction of their movement is opposite in each of two conditions.[1,2]

Table 26.1 *Anatomic Features That Differentiate Synostotic and Deformational Plagiocephaly*

Anatomic Feature	Synostotic	Deformational
Ipsilateral superior orbital rim	Up	Down
Ipsilateral ear	Anterior and high	Posterior and low
Nasal root	Ipsilateral	Midline
Ipsilateral cheek	Forward	Backward
Chin deviation	Contralateral	Ipsilateral
Ipsilateral palpebral fissure	Wide	Narrow
Anterior fontanel deviation	Low contralateral	High none

REFERENCES

1. Morris LM. Nonsyndromic craniosynostosis and deformational head shape disorders. Facial Plast Surg Clin North Am 2016;24(4):517–530
2. Robinson S, Proctor M. Diagnosis and management of deformational plagiocephaly. J Neurosurg Pediatr 2009;3(4): 284–295

MORPHOLOGICAL VARIANTS IN CRANIOSYNOSTOSIS

11. You see a syndromic child who has an untreated bicoronal synostosis. *Which one of the following would you expect to see on examination?*

A. Turribrachycephaly

Turribrachycephaly is where there is excessive skull height and vertical forehead secondary to an untreated brachycephaly, such as can occur in bicoronal synostosis. *Oxycephaly* refers to a pointed head with a retroverted forehead secondary to a pansynostosis. *Kleeblatschadel* refers to a cloverleaf deformity secondary to involvement of all sutures except squamosal. Posterior *plagiocephaly* occurs secondary to lambdoid synostosis. *Scaphocephaly (or dolichocephaly)* is secondary to premature fusion of the sagittal suture.[1-4]

REFERENCES

1. Persing JA. MOC-PS(SM) CME article: management considerations in the treatment of craniosynostosis. Plast Reconstr Surg 2008; 121(4, Suppl):1–11
2. Derderian CA, Bartlett SP. Craniosynostosis syndromes. In: Thorne C, ed. Grabb and Smith's Plastic Surgery. 7th ed. Philadelphia: Lippincott Williams & Wilkins; 2013
3. Knoll B, Persing JA. Craniosynostosis. In: Bentz ML, Bauer BS, Zuker RM, eds. Pediatric Plastic Surgery. 2nd ed. St Louis: Quality Medical Publishing; 2008
4. Cohen MM Jr, MacLean RE. Anatomic, genetic, nosologic, diagnostic, and psychosocial considerations. In: Cohen MM Jr, MacLean RE, eds. Craniosynostosis: Diagnosis, Evaluation, and Management. 2nd ed. New York: Oxford University Press; 2000

CROUZON SYNDROME

12. *Which one of the following is correct regarding Crouzon syndrome?*

B. Multiple different cranial sutures may be involved.

Crouzon syndrome is the most common syndromic craniosynostosis that occurs in 1 in 25,000 live births. It most commonly involves the coronal sutures but may involve other sutures including the sagittal and metopic. It is an autosomal dominant condition and ICP is elevated in approximately 65% of cases. Crouzon patients have normal extremities and this is a key finding that helps to differentiate this condition from some other synostotic conditions. Midface hypoplasia with exorbitism and turribrachycephaly are typical findings. This results in a class III malocclusion (not I) in most cases, with an anterior open bite and high arched palate.[1-3]

REFERENCES

1. Derderian C, Seaward J. Syndromic craniosynostosis. Semin Plast Surg 2012;26(2):64–75
2. Katzen JT, McCarthy JG. Syndromes involving craniosynostosis and midface hypoplasia. Otolaryngol Clin North Am 2000;33(6):1257–1284, vi
3. Agochukwu NB, Solomon BD, Muenke M. Impact of genetics on the diagnosis and clinical management of syndromic craniosynostoses. Childs Nerv Syst 2012;28(9):1447–1463

APERT SYNDROME

13. A child who has been diagnosed with Apert syndrome presents to clinic. *Which one of the following features will differentiate this condition from other similar synostotic syndromes?*

D. Complex syndactyly

Apert syndrome is an autosomal dominant condition that affects 1:100,000 to 1:160,000 live births. The presence of a complex symmetrical syndactyly distinguishes this syndrome from other craniosynostoses which may have the other features described. Apert syndactyly has three distinct subtypes and was classified by Upton[1] in 1991. Type I is a spade hand with the thumb and little finger separate and a syndactyly of the second and third web spaces. Type II is a mitten hand with the thumb free and syndactyly between the second, third, and fourth web spaces. Type III is a rosebud hand with all digits involved in the syndactyly (**Fig. 26.4**).

Raised ICP is seen in more than three quarters of patients with Apert syndrome and ventriculoperitoneal (VP) shunts are often required. Many, but not all, patients have decreased intelligence. Apert syndrome is associated with bicoronal synostoses with significant turribrachycephaly and midface hypoplasia; therefore, patients have some features in keeping with both Crouzon and Pfeiffer syndromes.[2] Cleft palate is also a feature of many different craniosynostotic syndromes so it is not a good differentiating factor.

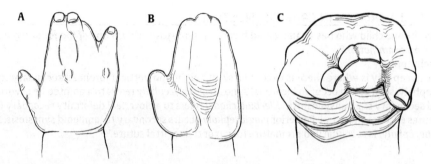

Fig. 26.4 *A,* Typical type I or spade-shaped hand. *B,* Type II or mitten hand. *C,* Type III or rosebud hand.

REFERENCES

1. Upton J. Apert syndrome. Classification and pathologic anatomy of limb anomalies. Clin Plast Surg 1991;18(2):321–355
2. Cohen MM Jr. Pfeiffer syndrome update, clinical subtypes, and guidelines for differential diagnosis. Am J Med Genet 1993;45(3):300–307

PFEIFFER SYNDROME

14. Which one of the following is least expected during examination of a patient with Pfeiffer syndrome?
  D. Mental impairment

Patients with Pfeiffer syndrome usually have a normal mental status, although this may be decreased in the most severe cases. Pfeiffer syndrome is a rare craniofacial condition involving synostoses in conjunction with extremity deformities and hydrocephalus. Incidence is 1:100,000 and is a result of mutations in the *FGFR* genes. Three different subtypes have been described according to clinical features and syndrome severity.[1]

Type I features include brachycephaly, midface hypoplasia, finger, toe abnormalities, and normal intelligence. Type 2 features a cloverleaf skull, proptosis, and major finger/toe abnormalities. Developmental delay may be present. Type 3 patients are similar to type 2 but without the cloverleaf skull.

REFERENCE

1. Cohen MM Jr. Pfeiffer syndrome update, clinical subtypes, and guidelines for differential diagnosis. Am J Med Genet 1993;45(3):300–307

SAETHRE-CHOTZEN SYNDROME

15. Which one of the following is correct regarding Saethre-Chotzen syndrome?
  B. It is associated with a *TWIST-1* gene mutation.

Saethre-Chotzen syndrome occurs in 1:25,000 to 1:50,000 live births. It was described by Saethre in 1931 and then by Chotzen the following year. It is inherited in an autosomal dominant fashion and is associated with the *TWIST-1* gene mutation. Patients have asymmetrical brachycephaly, eyelid ptosis, prominent crus helicis, deviated nasal septum, narrow palate, and a low hairline. Mental status is usually normal in these patients.[1]

REFERENCE

1. Foo R, Guo Y, McDonald-McGinn DM, Zackai EH, Whitaker LA, Bartlett SP. The natural history of patients treated for TWIST1-confirmed Saethre-Chotzen syndrome. Plast Reconstr Surg 2009;124(6):2085–2095

SURGERY FOR SYNOSTOSES

16. When considering the role of surgery in craniosynostosis, which one of the following is correct?
  C. Associated blood loss represents the greatest risk for patients undergoing surgery.

The greatest risk for infants undergoing craniosynostosis surgery is major bleeding, especially given the low circulating volume they have. This is typically just 70–80 mL per kg. So the total circulating volume for a 10-kg infant would, for example, be just 700 mL. There is a large surface area of raw bone following surgery which tends to bleed most in the initial 24 hours post surgery. Patients are, therefore, closely monitored following surgery with neurologic examination every 2 hours and hemoglobin/hematocrit and sodium reassessed every 6 hours for 24 hours. Transfusions are commonly given if hematocrit falls below 21%.

The primary goal of synostosis surgery is not to address the abnormal head shape and appearance, instead it is to facilitate normal or optimal brain growth, while minimizing risk of developing raised intracranial pressure (ICP) and its consequences. Improvements in appearance are secondary goals. The approach to treatment is significantly different for nonsyndromic than for syndromic patients because the number of sutures involved is usually different and there are other considerations that need to be taken into account.

Single-suture nonsyndromic patients usually require only a single open vault procedure, whereas syndromic patients typically have multiple sutures involved and hence require multiple complex procedures. Furthermore, they are at increased risk of other complications of craniosynostosis such as raised ICP.

The timing of surgery is controversial and there are advantages and disadvantages of early versus later scheduling for surgery. For example, early surgery (6–12 months) has the advantage of more malleable bones, faster bone regeneration, and spontaneous healing. However, there is risk of recurrence, needing repeated surgery further down the line. In contrast, later surgery (after 12 months) means that bones are stronger and better able to hold fixation devices solidly, but the deformity is more advanced, the bones are less malleable, and healing may be less effective.[1–3]

REFERENCES

1. Selber J, Reid RR, Gershman B, et al. Evolution of operative techniques for the treatment of single-suture metopic synostosis. Ann Plast Surg 2007;59(1):6–13
2. Tessier P. The definitive plastic surgical treatment of the severe facial deformities of craniofacial dysostosis. Crouzon's and Apert's diseases. Plast Reconstr Surg 1971;48(5):419–442
3. Persing JA. MOC-PS(SM) CME article: management considerations in the treatment of craniosynostosis. Plast Reconstr Surg 2008;121(4, Suppl):1–11

SURGICAL TECHNIQUES FOR SYNOSTOSES

17. Which one of the following surgical techniques may be most useful for treating a patient with an isolated scaphocephaly?

A. Endoscopic strip craniectomy with helmet

The management of an isolated scaphocephaly involves treating a sagittal suture craniosynostosis. This may be undertaken with an extended strip craniectomy, a spring-assisted cranioplasty, or open vault reconstruction. The extended strip craniectomy has the advantage of being able to be performed endoscopically thereby minimizing scar incision length, blood loss, operative time, and recovery. It is used primarily for isolated sagittal synostoses in infants younger than 4 months of age.[1] Wedge osteotomies are made adjacent to the coronal and lambdoid sutures to allow for transverse expansion. Helmet molding is used postoperatively for up to 18 months. The spring-assisted cranioplasty is another approach that can be useful for management of the sagittal suture or other sutures where there is symmetrical synostosis present. It uses continuous force generated by a spring across the osteotomy/craniectomy site. It does, however, require a second procedure for device removal.

LeFort midface advancement is part of the management of syndromic cases with multiple synostoses. It is used to advance the midface rather than address a sagittal suture synostosis. It may be performed in childhood or delayed until skeletal maturity. Fronto-orbital advancement is used to expand intracranial volume and reshape the cranial vault with advancement of the frontal bone. It is indicated for use in bilateral coronal synostoses (brachycephaly). It is also useful to protect the globes from compression and provide an aesthetic improvement of the face in such cases. Posterior vault expansion with or without distraction osteogenesis is also used to increase intracranial volume in syndromic cases of synostoses such as severe turribrachycephaly and occipital flattening.

Biparieto-occipital craniotomies are used for the management of lambdoid craniosynostoses.

REFERENCE

1. Barone CM, Jimenez DF. Endoscopic craniectomy for early correction of craniosynostosis. Plast Reconstr Surg 1999;104(7):1965–1973, discussion 1974–1975

27. Craniofacial Clefts

See *Essentials of Plastic Surgery*, third edition, pp. 346–356

CRANIOFACIAL EMBRYOLOGY

1. *Which one of the following statements is correct regarding facial embryology?*
   A. Development of the face occurs between weeks 2 and 10.
   B. The frontonasal prominence derives from the primitive forebrain.
   C. The lateral nasal prominence forms the nasal ala and premaxilla.
   D. The basic facial features are clearly recognizable by week 4.
   E. The external ear is formed mainly from the mandibular arch.

TESSIER CLEFTS

2. *Which one of the following statements is correct regarding Tessier clefts?*
   A. All clefts are numbered in increasing order according to their position relative to the midline.
   B. Cleft numbers 10–14 are described as *cranial clefts*.
   C. The lateral facial clefts are the most common subtypes.
   D. Fifteen different types of clefts are described in Tessier's classification.
   E. Oral-ocular clefts (numbers 4–6) usually disrupt nasal integrity.

TESSIER CLEFT TYPES

3. *Which one of the following is a midline oral-nasal cleft that can continue as cleft number 14?*
   A. Cleft number 0
   B. Cleft number 1
   C. Cleft number 2
   D. Cleft number 3
   E. Cleft number 4

TREACHER COLLINS SYNDROME

4. A patient is referred to clinic with a diagnosis of Treacher Collins syndrome. *Which one of the following is associated with this condition?*
   A. Bilateral oronasal Tessier clefts
   B. A mitochondrial inheritance pattern
   C. A genetic abnormality on chromosome 12
   D. An incidence of 1 in 1000 live births
   E. A high risk of airway compromise

TREACHER COLLINS SYNDROME

5. A patient with a diagnosis of Treacher Collins syndrome requests cosmetic reconstructive surgery to improve their facial appearance. *Which one of the following procedures is least likely to be required based on the clinical features of this condition?*
   A. Lower eyelid surgery
   B. Cheek reconstruction
   C. Ear reconstruction
   D. Rhinoplasty
   E. Upper eyelid blepharoplasty

GOLDENHAR'S SYNDROME

6. A patient presents to clinic with a diagnosis of Goldenhar's syndrome. On examination they have two polypoid soft tissue protuberances on the cheek which the parents would like removed. *What is the most likely diagnosis?*
   A. Pedunculated papillomas
   B. Epibulbar dermoids
   C. Colobomas
   D. Lipomas
   E. Auricular appendages

CRANIOFACIAL CLEFTS

7. *Which one of the following craniofacial clefts is postulated to arise secondary to disruption of the stapedial artery in embryogenesis?*
   A. Cleft number 5
   B. Cleft number 6
   C. Cleft number 7
   D. Cleft number 8
   E. Cleft number 9

TESSIER CLEFT NUMBER 14

8. *Which one of the following is expected in a patient with a Tessier cleft 14?*
   A. A normal life expectancy
   B. A coexisting cleft through the alar rim
   C. A short frontal midline hairline
   D. Midline herniation of the intracranial contents
   E. A decreased intraorbital distance

TESSIER CLEFT NUMBER 30

9. A 5-year-old child is noted to have a bifid tongue and notching of the lower lip. *Which one of the following findings would you also expect to note on examination of this child?*
   A. An absent thyroid
   B. An absent hyoid
   C. A hypoplastic thyroid
   D. Absence of the central incisors
   E. Notching of the upper lip

Answers

CRANIOFACIAL EMBRYOLOGY

1. *Which one of the following statements is correct regarding facial embryology?*

    B. The frontonasal prominence derives from the primitive forebrain.

Facial development occurs between weeks 3 and 8. Key facial features such as the mouth, ears, eyes, and nose are clearly recognizable by week 8 (not 4). They become progressively defined from week 6 onwards (**Fig. 27.1**). Facial embryological structures originate from the frontonasal prominence of the forebrain, which forms the forehead, nasal dorsum, and medial and lateral nasal prominences. The lateral nasal prominences then form the nasal alae, but the premaxilla (along with the nasal tip, columella, philtrum) is formed from the medial nasal prominences. The first pharyngeal arch bifurcates to form the mandibular and maxillary processes, which then form the upper lateral and lower parts of the mouth. The external ear is formed from both the mandibular (first) and hyoid (second) pharyngeal arches.[1-3]

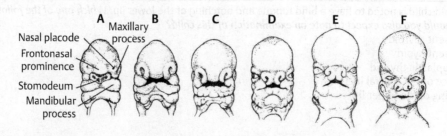

Fig. 27.1   Embryonic development of the human face. *A*, 4-week embryo. *B*, 5-week embryo. *C*, 6-week embryo. *D*, 6½-week embryo. *E*, 7-week embryo. *F*, 8-week embryo. (From Bentz ML, Bauer BS, Zuker RM. Principles & Practice of Pediatric Plastic Surgery. St Louis: Quality Medical Publishing, 2008.)

REFERENCES

1. Moore KL, Persaud TV, Torchia MD, eds. The Developing Human: Clinically Oriented Embryology. 10th ed. Philadelphia: Elsevier; 2016
2. Sadler TW, ed. Langman's Medical Embryology. 13th ed. Philadelphia: Wolters Kluwer Health; 2014
3. Tepper OM, Warren SM. Craniofacial embryology. In: Weinzwig J, ed. Plastic Surgery Secrets Plus. 2nd ed. Philadelphia: Elsevier; 2010

TESSIER CLEFTS

2. *Which one of the following statements is correct regarding Tessier clefts?*

    B. Cleft numbers 10–14 are described as *cranial clefts*.

Tessier described cleft numbers 0–14 relative to the midline and subgrouped them according to their location as oral-nasal, oral-ocular, lateral facial, and cranial. An additional cleft number 30 does not fit into this subcategorization. It passes inferiorly from the lower lip toward the neck and is not numbered according to the midline per se, although it is a midline cleft. Of this total 16 clefts the most common is a lateral cleft (number 7). The other lateral clefts (numbers 8 and 9), however, are rare. Oral-ocular clefts do not disrupt the integrity of the nose. They occur lateral to Cupid's bow and extend through the cheek and maxillary process. This is called *meloschisis* (**Fig. 27.2**).[1]

REFERENCE

1. Tessier P. Anatomical classification facial, cranio-facial and latero-facial clefts. J Maxillofac Surg 1976;4(2):69–92

TESSIER CLEFT TYPES

3. *Which one of the following is a midline oral-nasal cleft that can continue as cleft number 14?*

    A. Cleft number 0

The lower facial clefts (numbers 0–4) may continue as cranial clefts (numbers 14–10), respectively, totaling 14. Cleft numbers 0 to 3, termed oral-nasal clefts, occur between the midline and Cupid's bow, disrupting both the lip and nose. Cleft 4 is one of the oral-ocular clefts (4–6) which disrupt the mouth and eye but avoid disruption of the nose. Cleft number 0 can be tissue deficient or have an excess of tissue within midline structures. Deficiencies involve soft tissues of the upper lip and nose and absence of the premaxilla with partial or total absence of the

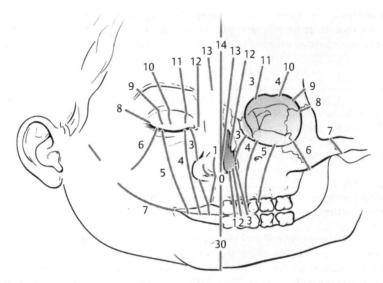

Fig. 27.2 Tessier classification of clefts. Paths of various clefts on the face (*left*); location of the clefts on the facial skeleton (*right*). (Adapted from Tessier P. Anatomical classification of facial, cranio-facial, and laterofacial clefts. J Maxillofac Surg 4:69–92, 1976.)

nasal bones. Cases of tissue excess can have a bifid nose and diastema of the upper incisors with broad nasal bones and septum. Cleft numbers 0 and 14 are both midline clefts, and 14 are associated with central nervous system (CNS) abnormalities, hypotelorism or hypertelorism, and frontonasal encephaloceles.[1]

REFERENCE

1. Tessier P. Anatomical classification facial, cranio-facial and latero-facial clefts. J Maxillofac Surg 1976;4(2):69–92

TREACHER COLLINS SYNDROME

4. A patient is referred to clinic with a diagnosis of Treacher Collins syndrome. *Which one of the following is associated with this condition?*

   E. A high risk of airway compromise

   Treacher Collins described this syndrome in 1900. It has an incidence of 1 in 10,000 to 1 in 50,000 live births. A genetic alteration occurs on chromosome 5, and the condition is inherited in an autosomal dominant pattern. Bilateral oral ocular and lateral facial clefts are typically seen, and the airway is a major priority in these patients, many of whom will require long-term tracheostomy placement. This is secondary to mandibular hypoplasia in combination with a narrow pharynx.[1–3]

REFERENCES

1. Treacher Collins E. Cases with symmetrical congenital notches in the outer part of each lower lid and defective development of the malar bones. Trans Opthalmol Soc UK 1900;20:190–192
2. Aljerian A, Gilardino MS. Treacher Collins syndrome. Clin Plast Surg 2019;46(2):197–205
3. Plomp RG, van Lieshout MJS, Joosten KFM, et al. Treacher Collins syndrome: a systematic review of evidence-based treatment and recommendations. Plast Reconstr Surg 2016;137(1):191–204

TREACHER COLLINS SYNDROME

5. A patient with a diagnosis of Treacher Collins syndrome requests cosmetic reconstructive surgery to improve their facial appearance. *Which one of the following procedures is least likely to be required based on the clinical features of this condition?*

   D. Rhinoplasty

   The clinical findings in Treacher Collins syndrome include upper and lower eyelid deformity, absence of the zygomatic arch with a malar deficiency, and varying degrees of microtia. Patients do, however, generally have normal nasal development and would be least likely to require a rhinoplasty given the other options listed.

   The lower eyelid has coloboma and retraction, which may require reconstruction and the lateral canthi are displaced inferiorly and therefore may benefit from canthal elevation. The lack of cheek projection due to absence of the zygomatic arch and malar bone hypoplasia may require cheek reconstruction using composite flaps or lipofilling techniques. Formal ear reconstruction may be required using costal cartilage and local flaps. Upper eyelid surgery may be required as patients have an excess of upper eyelid skin laterally giving a false impression of ptosis.[1-3]

REFERENCES

1. Treacher Collins E. Cases with symmetrical congenital notches in the outer part of each lower lid and defective development of the malar bones. Trans Opthalmol Soc UK 1900;20:190–192
2. Aljerian A, Gilardino MS. Treacher Collins syndrome. Clin Plast Surg 2019;46(2):197–205
3. Plomp RG, van Lieshout MJS, Joosten KFM, et al. Treacher Collins syndrome: a systematic review of evidence-based treatment and recommendations. Plast Reconstr Surg 2016;137(1):191–204

GOLDENHAR'S SYNDROME

6. A patient presents to clinic with a diagnosis of Goldenhar's syndrome. On examination they have two polypoid soft tissue protuberances on the cheek which the parents would like removed. *What is the most likely diagnosis?*

E. Auricular appendages

Goldenhar's syndrome is a type of hemifacial microsomia with sporadic occurrence in which patients have a constellation of abnormalities including bilateral accessory auricular appendages, varying degrees of microtia, epibulbar dermoids, vertebral anomalies, a low anterior hairline, and mandibular hypoplasia. The description in this patient is most in keeping with auricular appendages and these may well comprise of skin and underlying cartilage. They can safely be excised under general anesthetic on an elective basis. Pedunculated papillomas and subcutaneous lipomas can have a similar appearance but are not typical of Goldenhar's syndrome. Epibulbar dermoids and colobomas are characteristic of Goldenhar's syndrome but affect the eye, not the cheek.[1,2]

REFERENCES

1. Gorlin RJ, Pindborg JJ. Syndromes of the Head and Neck. New York: McGraw-Hill; 1964
2. Mellor DH, Richardson JE, Douglas DM. Goldenhar's syndrome. Oculoauriculo-vertebral dysplasia. Arch Dis Child 1973;48(7):537–541

CRANIOFACIAL CLEFTS

7. *Which one of the following craniofacial clefts is postulated to arise secondary to disruption of the stapedial artery in embryogenesis?*

C. Cleft number 7

Cleft number 7 is a lateral cleft that passes from the oral commissure toward the ear. It stops at the anterior border of the masseter. It is the most common overall cleft (1–6/8000 births) and may occur because of disruption of the stapedial artery. This cleft affects males more often than females and is bilateral in 10% of cases. It is associated with variable degrees of soft tissue and bony deformity including craniofacial microsomia, facial and trigeminal nerve paresis, microtia, and middle ear abnormalities.

Cleft numbers 8 and 9 are also lateral clefts but are far less common than cleft 7. Cleft 8 is associated with Goldenhar's syndrome and almost always exists in combination with another rare cleft. It is largely isolated to the orbital area with coloboma of the lateral commissure and absence of the lateral canthus. The zygoma is either hypoplastic or absent, and the lateral orbital wall is deficient. Cleft 9 is extremely rare and may be accompanied by encephaloceles. It is associated with soft tissue abnormalities of the lateral third of the upper eyelid and brow as well as hypoplasia of the greater wing of the sphenoid, which results in posterior displacement of lateral orbital rim.

Cleft numbers 5 and 6 are both oral-ocular clefts which connect the oral and orbital cavities without disrupting the nose. They occur lateral to Cupid's bow and extend through the soft tissue of the cheek and maxillary process. Cleft 5 is the rarest of the three oral-ocular clefts (Clefts 3, 4, and 5) and begins medial to the oral commissure and courses along the cheek lateral to the nasal ala to terminate in the lateral half of the lower eyelid. Cleft number 6 includes incomplete forms of Treacher Collins syndrome and represents a transition between oral-ocular and lateral facial clefts. The ear is normal but there is downslanting of the palpebral fissure as the lateral fissure and canthus are pulled inferiorly, creating an appearance of ectropion and colobomas of the lower eyelid. In addition, choanal atresia is common and the zygoma is hypoplastic.[1,2]

REFERENCES

1. Tessier P. Anatomical classification facial, cranio-facial and latero-facial clefts. J Maxillofac Surg 1976;4(2):69–92
2. David DJ, Moore MH, Cooter RD. Tessier clefts revisited with a third dimension. Cleft Palate J 1989;26(3):163–184, discussion 184–185

TESSIER CLEFT NUMBER 14

8. Which one of the following is expected in a patient with a Tessier cleft 14?

D. **Midline herniation of the intracranial contents**

Cleft 14 is one of the cranial clefts and has a very poor prognosis. It is a midline cleft with associated central nervous system abnormalities including a midline encephalocele, holoprosencephaly, and microcephaly. It is often paired with a facial midline cleft 0 (not a cleft 3, which would pass through the alar rim). Hypertelorism is present because the cleft increases the distance between the bony orbits. A Harlequin deformity may be seen on radiographs due to upslanting of the anterior cranial fossa (**Fig. 27.3**).[1–4]

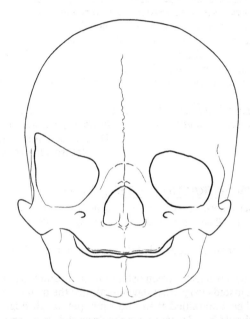

Fig. 27.3 Harlequin deformity.

REFERENCES

1. Tessier P. Anatomical classification facial, cranio-facial and latero-facial clefts. J Maxillofac Surg 1976;4(2):69–92
2. David DJ, Moore MH, Cooter RD. Tessier clefts revisited with a third dimension. Cleft Palate J 1989;26(3):163–184, discussion 184–185
3. Kawamoto HK Jr. The kaleidoscopic world of rare craniofacial clefts: order out of chaos (Tessier classification). Clin Plast Surg 1976;3(4):529–572
4. Alonso N, da Silva Freitas R. Craniofacial clefts and other related deformities. In: Guyuron B, Eriksson E, Persing JA, eds. Plastic Surgery: Indications and Practice. London: Elsevier; 2009

TESSIER CLEFT NUMBER 30

9. A 5-year-old child is noted to have a bifid tongue and notching of the lower lip. Which one of the following findings would you also expect to note on examination of this child?

B. **An absent hyoid**

Tessier described cleft 30 in his original 1976 publication.[1] It is a very rare anomaly, with fewer than 70 cases described in the literature. In its milder form it may be limited to a defect of soft tissue in the lower lip. In more severe forms it may involve a cleft of the mandibular symphysis, absence of the hyoid, and hypoplasia of the thyroid cartilage, or strap muscles. The tongue abnormality ranges from total absence to a bifid anterior portion or complete duplication. A cleft of the mandibular symphysis usually passes between the central incisors, which are present. The thyroid gland itself is not involved, although the thyroid cartilage can be hypoplastic.[1,2]

REFERENCES

1. Tessier P. Anatomical classification facial, cranio-facial and latero-facial clefts. J Maxillofac Surg 1976;4(2):69–92
2. Alonso N, da Silva Freitas R. Craniofacial clefts and other related deformities. In: Guyuron B, Eriksson E, Persing JA, eds. Plastic Surgery: Indications and Practice. London: Elsevier; 2009

28. Distraction Osteogenesis

See *Essentials of Plastic Surgery*, third edition, pp. 357–362

GENERAL PRINCIPLES OF DISTRACTION OSTEOGENESIS

1. *Which one of the following statements is correct regarding distraction osteogenesis?*
   A. It is a single-stage surgical technique used to generate new bone.
   B. It relies on the principle that growth is stimulated when compressive stress is placed across tissue.
   C. Successful outcome requires the application of a consistent, moderate increase in tension.
   D. It often causes atrophy to the surrounding soft tissues.
   E. It results in bone whose characteristics are different from those of normal, mature bone.

BONE PHYSIOLOGY IN DISTRACTION OSTEOGENESIS

2. *Which one of the following represents a single zone within the bony generate in distraction osteogenesis?*
   A. Cellular proliferation zone
   B. Mineralization front
   C. Zone of vasculogenesis
   D. Osteoid paracentral zone
   E. Mature bone zone

THE DISTRACTION PROCESS IN DISTRACTION OSTEOGENESIS

3. An 18-month-old infant has micrognathia secondary to Treacher Collins syndrome. *After performing an osteotomy and placement of a mandibular distractor, which one of the following strategies should be part of the distraction process?*
   A. The activation phase should begin immediately following placement of the distraction device and should last for 6 months.
   B. The latency period should be 3 weeks between osteotomy and commencement of distraction.
   C. The distractor should be adjusted every other day to optimize the quality and volume of new bone.
   D. The distraction rate should be maintained at around 1 mm per day throughout the distraction process.
   E. The consolidation period should be 16 weeks once the desired distraction has been achieved, with the distractor left in place.

APPROACHES TO DISTRACTION OSTEOGENESIS

4. *Which one of the following represents the main advantage of using an external distractor over an internal distractor on the mandible?*
   A. Multidirectional distraction can be achieved.
   B. Only one general anesthetic will be required.
   C. It is less likely to disrupt tooth buds.
   D. Cutaneous scarring will be reduced.
   E. Fewer postoperative complications are observed.

MANDIBULAR DISTRACTION

5. *Which one of the following is not achieved with distraction of the mandible?*
   A. Lengthening of the ramus/body
   B. Reconstruction of a mandibular defect
   C. Normalization of a retroplaced tongue base
   D. Correction of class III malocclusion
   E. Improvement of airway patency

COMPLICATIONS OF CRANIOFACIAL DISTRACTION OSTEOGENESIS

6. You are consenting the parents of a 1-year-old child for craniofacial distraction osteogenesis using a single-vector external device. *Which one of the following is the most common complication of craniofacial distraction?*
   A. Bleeding
   B. Pin tract infection
   C. Nerve damage
   D. Inappropriate vector
   E. Premature consolidation

Answers

GENERAL PRINCIPLES OF DISTRACTION OSTEOGENESIS

1. Which one of the following statements is correct regarding distraction osteogenesis?

C. Successful outcome requires the application of a consistent, moderate increase in tension.

Distraction osteogenesis is a staged procedure that takes many months to complete. It relies on the principle that tissue generation is stimulated when tissues are placed under consistent, moderate tensile forces. The application of these principles allows bone to be lengthened after an osteotomy or corticotomy by progressive distraction of the divided bone ends using a surgically placed device. Soft tissues respond well to the process and typically hypertrophy, not atrophy. The characteristics of bone formed during distraction osteogenesis are identical to those of normal mature bone. Not only are these principles applicable to patients with micrognathia such as hemifacial microsomia and Treacher Collins syndrome, they are useful for bone transport in long bones after segmental loss of the tibia or femur.[1-3]

REFERENCES

1. Yu JC, Fearon J, Havlik RJ, Buchman SR, Polley JW. Distraction osteogenesis of the craniofacial skeleton. Plast Reconstr Surg 2004;114(1):1E–20E
2. McCarthy JG, Stelnicki EJ, Mehrara BJ, Longaker MT. Distraction osteogenesis of the craniofacial skeleton. Plast Reconstr Surg 2001;107(7):1812–1827
3. Iacobellis C, Berizzi A, Aldegheri R. Bone transport using the Ilizarov method: a review of complications in 100 consecutive cases. Strateg Trauma Limb Reconstr 2010;5(1):17–22

BONE PHYSIOLOGY IN DISTRACTION OSTEOGENESIS

2. Which one of the following represents a single zone within the bony generate in distraction osteogenesis?

A. Cellular proliferation zone

Distraction osteogenesis (DO) generates vascularized bone with normal cortical and medullary features. An osteotomy is first made in the bone, thereby creating a bone gap, which is then progressively distracted. The tissue within the bone gap in DO is similar to callus, but it has collagen fibers that run parallel to the vector of distraction. This area is called the *generate*. It has the following five key components, all of which are duplicated except the central cellular proliferation zone (**Fig. 28.1**).

1. A **central zone** in which proliferation of mesenchymal cells occurs
2. Two **transitional zones** of vasculogenesis that sandwich the central zone
3. Two **paracentral zones** in which osteoid production occurs
4. Two **mineralization fronts** in which primary mineralization occurs
5. Two **mature bone zones** in which bone is progressively calcified to form cortical and cancellous elements

During the final phase of DO, the less mature central portions of the generate mature and merge with the mineralization fronts for union to create bone that is ultimately indistinguishable from natural mature bone.[1,2]

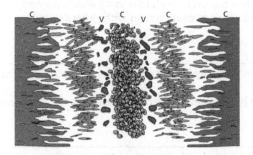

Fig. 28.1 Five zones and four transition areas are present in the generate during the activation phase of distraction osteogenesis (DO): a central zone of proliferating mesenchymal cells (*C*), two paracentral zones, and two zones where mature bone meets the generate. The four transitional areas comprise two areas of vasculogenesis (*v*) and two mineralization fronts. (Adapted from Yu JC, Fearon J, Havlik RJ, et al. Distraction osteogenesis of the craniofacial skeleton. Plast Reconstr Surg 114:1e–20e, 2004.)

REFERENCES

1. Yu JC, Fearon J, Havlik RJ, Buchman SR, Polley JW. Distraction osteogenesis of the craniofacial skeleton. Plast Reconstr Surg 2004;114(1):1E–20E
2. McCarthy JG, Stelnicki EJ, Mehrara BJ, Longaker MT. Distraction osteogenesis of the craniofacial skeleton. Plast Reconstr Surg 2001;107(7):1812–1827

THE DISTRACTION PROCESS IN DISTRACTION OSTEOGENESIS

3. An 18-month-old infant has micrognathia secondary to Treacher Collins syndrome. *After performing an osteotomy and placement of a mandibular distractor, which one of the following strategies should be part of the distraction process?*

   D. The distraction rate should be maintained at around 1 mm per day throughout the distraction process.

   The distraction process begins with an osteotomy and application of a distraction device. Distraction is delayed for about 1 week (not 3) after placement of the distractor to allow a callus to form at the fracture site. This is called the *latency period.* The latency period may be reduced to around 3 days in patients younger than 1 year of age. The period of active distraction is termed the *activation phase* and does not commence until the latency period is complete. Active distraction is usually complete within 6 weeks when distraction rates of 1 mm per day are used. Once distraction is complete, the distractor is left in situ for 8 weeks or until bone healing is evident clinically or radiologically. This is termed the *consolidation phase.* Distraction is usually increased at a rate of 1 mm per day because this avoids premature ossification or local ischemia. In neonates and infants less than 1 year of age it may be increased to 2–4 mm per day. The rhythm describes the number of times per day the distractor is increased. Usually this is done two to four times each day as this provides the best volume and quality of new bone formation.[1–4]

REFERENCES

1. Yu JC, Fearon J, Havlik RJ, Buchman SR, Polley JW. Distraction osteogenesis of the craniofacial skeleton. Plast Reconstr Surg 2004;114(1):1E–20E
2. McCarthy JG, Stelnicki EJ, Mehrara BJ, Longaker MT. Distraction osteogenesis of the craniofacial skeleton. Plast Reconstr Surg 2001;107(7):1812–1827
3. McCarthy JG, Schreiber J, Karp N, Thorne CH, Grayson BH. Lengthening the human mandible by gradual distraction. Plast Reconstr Surg 1992;89(1):1–8, discussion 9–10
4. Maheshwari S, Verma SK, Tariq M, Prabhat KC, Kumar S. Biomechanics and orthodontic treatment protocol in maxillofacial distraction osteogenesis. Natl J Maxillofac Surg 2011;2(2):120–128

APPROACHES TO DISTRACTION OSTEOGENESIS

4. *Which one of the following represents the main advantage of using an external distractor over an internal distractor on the mandible?*

   A. Multidirectional distraction can be achieved.

   The benefits of external craniofacial distractors are that they provide flexibility for alteration of distraction vectors and they can prevent formal reoperation to remove the device. However, a second general anesthetic is still often required to facilitate removal of the percutaneous pins. Furthermore, these pins will leave visible external scarring at the pin sites.

   In contrast, internal devices involve an intraoral approach, thus avoiding cutaneous scarring. However, they provide distraction only in a single vector that cannot be altered after insertion, and a second procedure will always be required for their removal. Careful planning should prevent disruption of the tooth buds in all distraction approaches. Complication rates are similar with either device.[1,2]

REFERENCES

1. Yu JC, Fearon J, Havlik RJ, Buchman SR, Polley JW. Distraction osteogenesis of the craniofacial skeleton. Plast Reconstr Surg 2004;114(1):1E–20E
2. McCarthy JG, Stelnicki EJ, Mehrara BJ, Longaker MT. Distraction osteogenesis of the craniofacial skeleton. Plast Reconstr Surg 2001;107(7):1812–1827

MANDIBULAR DISTRACTION

5. *Which one of the following is not achieved with distraction of the mandible?*

   D. Correction of class III malocclusion

   Mandibular distraction can help patients achieve proper occlusion, but it does not correct a class III deformity which is essentially where the mandibular dentition is prominent with respect to the maxillary dentition (i.e., the patient is prognathic).

Correction requires orthodontic intervention, resetting of the mandible posteriorly, or advancement of the maxilla, depending on the underlying pathology. Mandibular distraction is often performed to improve the airway in patients with disorders such as Pierre Robin sequence. It provides more space for the tongue and moves the tongue base more anteriorly.[1-3]

REFERENCES

1. Yu JC, Fearon J, Havlik RJ, Buchman SR, Polley JW. Distraction osteogenesis of the craniofacial skeleton. Plast Reconstr Surg 2004;114(1):1E–20E
2. McCarthy JG, Stelnicki EJ, Mehrara BJ, Longaker MT. Distraction osteogenesis of the craniofacial skeleton. Plast Reconstr Surg 2001;107(7):1812–1827
3. Zhang RS, Hoppe IC, Taylor JA, Bartlett SP. Surgical management and outcomes of Pierre Robin sequence: a comparison of mandibular distraction osteogenesis and tongue-lip adhesion. Plast Reconstr Surg 2018;142(2):480–509

COMPLICATIONS OF CRANIOFACIAL DISTRACTION OSTEOGENESIS

6. You are consenting the parents of a 1-year-old child for craniofacial distraction osteogenesis using a single-vector external device. *Which one of the following is the most common complication of craniofacial distraction?*

   D. Inappropriate vector

   A review of 3278 cases of craniofacial distraction published in 2001 showed that an inappropriate vector was the most common complication, occurring in almost 9% of cases in which a single vector device was used.[1] This complication occurred in 7.2% of cases in which multivector devices were used. Other complications included pin tract infection (5.2%), compliance problems (4.7%), and hardware failure (4.5%) (see **Table 28.1**).

Table 28.1   *Incidence of Complications in Craniofacial Distraction Osteogenesis*

Complication	Frequency (%)
Compliance problems	4.7
Hardware failure	4.5
Device dislodgement	3.0
Premature consolidation	1.9
Pain that prevents distraction	1.0
Fibrous nonunion	0.5
Inappropriate vector (single-vector device)	8.8
Inappropriate vector (multivector device)	7.2
Pin tract infection	5.2

(Adapted from Mofid MM, Manson PN, Robertson BC, et al. Craniofacial distraction osteogenesis: a review of 3278 cases. Plast Reconstr Surg 108:1103–1114; discussion 1115–1117, 2001.)

REFERENCE

1. Mofid MM, Manson PN, Robertson BC, Tufaro AP, Elias JJ, Vander Kolk CA. Craniofacial distraction osteogenesis: a review of 3278 cases. Plast Reconstr Surg 2001;108(5):1103–1114, discussion 1115–1117

29. Cleft Lip

See *Essentials of Plastic Surgery*, third edition, pp. 363–375

DEMOGRAPHICS OF CLEFT LIP AND/OR PALATE (CL/P)

1. *Which one of the following statements is correct regarding cleft lip/palate?*
   A. It most commonly affects the right side.
   B. The overall incidence is 1:350.
   C. CL/P is twice as common in males than females.
   D. Incidence is unaffected by race.
   E. One in three patients have an associated syndrome.

ANATOMY OF THE NORMAL UPPER LIP

2. *Which one of the following components of the normal upper lip is created by the dermal insertion of orbicularis oris?*
   A. Philtral column
   B. Philtral dimple
   C. White roll
   D. Vermilion
   E. Red line

CLEFT LIP ANATOMY

3. *Which one of the following statements regarding the anatomy of the unilateral cleft lip is correct?*
   A. Vertical lip height and projection are increased.
   B. The vermilion width is essentially normal.
   C. The prolabium usually contains orbicularis muscle fibers.
   D. Muscle continuity is maintained in a microform lip.
   E. A Simonart's band is a skin bridge devoid of muscle.

ANATOMY OF THE CLEFT NASAL DEFORMITY

4. You are examining the nose of a 2-month-old infant with a unilateral incomplete cleft lip deformity. *Which one of the following findings is expected to be present on the cleft lip side of this infant?*
   A. A more acute angle between the medial and lateral crura
   B. Flattening of the alar-facial angle
   C. Narrowing of the nostril floor
   D. Deviation of the tip toward this side
   E. A normal columellar length.

RISK OF FAMILIAL RECURRENCE IN CLEFT LIP/PALATE (CL/P)

5. You are advising a young couple in clinic who are planning to start a family. The lady has an isolated cleft lip that was repaired as a child. *What is the approximate risk of this couple having a child with a cleft lip/palate assuming the father is unaffected?*
   A. 1%
   B. 4%
   C. 12%
   D. 20%
   E. 33%

FEEDING CLEFT LIP INFANTS

6. *What is the best feeding modality for a patient with a cleft lip deformity?*
   A. A normal bottle with a Haberman nipple
   B. A squeezable bottle with a normal nipple
   C. A pigeon nipple with a normal bottle
   D. A pigeon nipple with a soft squeezable bottle
   E. A normal bottle/nipple or breast-feeding

PRESURGICAL ORTHOPEDICS IN CLEFT LIP

7. *Which one of the following is true regarding presurgical orthopedics?*
  A. A Latham device is a passive type of presurgical orthopedic device.
  B. Lip adhesion is a surgical alternative to presurgical orthopedics.
  C. Nasoalveolar molding is solely indicated for improving the nasal deformity.
  D. A Latham device can usually be inserted in the clinic setting.
  E. Active presurgical techniques help reduce the clinic's attendance burden.

TIMING OF CLEFT LIP REPAIR

8. *Which one of the following is performed at the time of primary lip repair?*
  A. Full rhinoplasty
  B. Tip rhinoplasty
  C. Palatoplasty
  D. Primary alveolar bone grafting
  E. Correction of a whistle tip deformity

TYPES OF CLEFT LIP REPAIR

9. *Which one of the following techniques is a commonly used rotation-advancement repair for unilateral cleft lip that incorporates a superiorly placed Z-plasty?*
  A. LeMesurier
  B. Rose-Thompson
  C. Randall-Tennison
  D. Millard
  E. Modified Manchester

THE MILLARD REPAIR FOR UNILATERAL CLEFT LIPS (BYRD MODIFICATION)

10. *When undertaking the Millard repair for unilateral cleft lip, which one of the following tissue flap components is used to close the nasal sill or lengthen the columella?*
  A. A flap
  B. C flap
  C. L flap
  D. M flap
  E. R flap

MILLARD AND FISHER TECHNIQUES IN CLEFT LIP REPAIR

11. *Which one of the following is part of both the Millard and Fisher techniques for cleft lip repair?*
  A. A Noordhoff flap
  B. A geometric design
  C. A McComb suture
  D. A skin triangle above the white roll
  E. Identical skin incisions

WHISTLING DEFORMITY AFTER CLEFT LIP

12. A patient who presents to clinic after a cleft lip repair has a whistling deformity. *Which one of the following structures is deficient?*
  A. Buccal sulcus
  B. Vermilion
  C. White roll
  D. Upper lip skin
  E. Cupid's bow

Answers

DEMOGRAPHICS OF CLEFT LIP AND/OR PALATE (CL/P)

1. *Which one of the following statements is correct regarding cleft lip/palate?*

C. **CL/P is twice as common in males than females.**

Cleft lip/palate (CL/P) is the most prevalent facial abnormality in the world. CL/P is more frequent in males with a 2:1 ratio, although isolated cleft lip is seen equally in both sexes. Left-sided cleft defects are more common than right-sided cleft defects, and the ratio is 9:4.5:1 in the order of unilateral left/unilateral right/bilateral. The overall incidence is around 1:750 and ranges from 0.2 to 2.3 per 1000 depending on race. Cleft lip/palate is significantly more common in patients of Asian and Native American descent (1 in 450) and is least common in Afro-Caribbeans (1 in 2000). The incidence among white individuals is 1:1000. An incidence of 1:350 is more in keeping with hypospadias rather than cleft lip/palate. Associated syndromes are seen in around 10% of patients with cleft lip/palate (not 33%).[1-5]

REFERENCES

1. Mitchell LE, Lupo PJ. Epidemiology of Cleft Lip and Palate. Vol. 1, 2nd ed. Boca Raton, FL: CRC Press; 2016.
2. Monson LA, Kirschner RE, Losee JE. Primary repair of cleft lip and nasal deformity. Plast Reconstr Surg 2013;132(6):1040e–1053e
3. Mossey PA, Little J, Munger RG, Dixon MJ, Shaw WC. Cleft lip and palate. Lancet 2009;374(9703):1773–1785
4. Bentz M, Bauer B, Zuker R. Principles and Practice of Pediatric Plastic Surgery. St Louis: Quality Medical Publishing; 2008
5. Parker SE, Mai CT, Canfield MA, et al; National Birth Defects Prevention Network. Updated national birth prevalence estimates for selected birth defects in the United States, 2004–2006. Birth Defects Res A Clin Mol Teratol 2010;88(12):1008–1016

ANATOMY OF THE NORMAL UPPER LIP

2. *Which one of the following components of the normal upper lip is created by the dermal insertion of orbicularis oris?*

A. **Philtral column**

The normal lip comprises a number of key anatomic components that are relevant not only to cleft lip, but more generally to the management of lip injuries and in the context of lip reconstruction. The lips comprise of mucosa, muscle, subcutaneous tissues, and skin. The orbicularis oris muscles form a concentric ring of muscle around the mouth and superiorly, in the midline, the superficial fibers insert into the dermis of the lip to create the paired philtral columns. The philtral dimple is the concavity between the columns created by a relative paucity of muscle fibers. In a cleft lip, the orbicularis muscle abnormally inserts into the nasal alar and the philtral column is abnormally formed. Reconstruction of the philtral column is one of the key aims of cleft lip repair.

The white roll is the prominent ridge between the skin of the lip and the vermilion which is the red mucosal portion. The vermilion itself is divided into wet and dry components, with the wet being within the mouth (nonkeratinized) and the dry being externally located (keratinized). The wet and dry vermilion are separated by the red line. Cupid's bow is the curvature of the central white roll and has two lateral peaks. There is fullness to the vermilion at the central inferior apex of Cupid's bow called the tubercle.[1-3]

REFERENCES

1. Bentz M, Bauer B, Zuker R. Principles and Practice of Pediatric Plastic Surgery. St Louis: Quality Medical Publishing; 2008
2. Burt JD, Byrd HS. Cleft lip: unilateral primary deformities. Plast Reconstr Surg 2000;105(3):1043–1055, quiz 1056–1057
3. Millard DR. The Unilateral Deformity. Vol. 1. Boston, MA: Little Brown; 1976

CLEFT LIP ANATOMY

3. *Which one of the following statements regarding the anatomy of the unilateral cleft lip is correct?*

E. **A Simonart's band is a skin bridge devoid of muscle.**

A cleft lip results in the projection and outward rotation of the premaxilla, with retropositioning of the lateral maxillary segment. The vertical lip height is reduced, and the philtrum is short. The vermilion width is decreased on the medial side of the cleft and increased laterally. The superficial part of orbicularis oris inserts into the alar base on the cleft side. The deep portion is interrupted but does not abnormally insert. Neither the prolabium in a bilateral cleft lip nor the Simonart's band contains muscle. The continuity of muscle is disrupted in a microform cleft.[1-4]

REFERENCES

1. Bentz M, Bauer B, Zuker R. Principles and Practice of Pediatric Plastic Surgery. St Louis: Quality Medical Publishing; 2008
2. Burt JD, Byrd HS. Cleft lip: unilateral primary deformities. Plast Reconstr Surg 2000;105(3):1043–1055, quiz 1056–1057
3. Millard DR. The Unilateral Deformity. Vol. 1. Boston, MA: Little Brown; 1976
4. Marcus JR, Allori AC, Santiago PE. Principles of cleft lip repair: conventions, commonalities, and controversies. Plast Reconstr Surg 2017;139(3):764e–780e

ANATOMY OF THE CLEFT NASAL DEFORMITY

4. You are examining the nose of a 2-month-old infant with a unilateral incomplete cleft lip deformity. *Which one of the following findings is expected to be present on the cleft lip side of this infant?*

   B. Flattening of the alar-facial angle

   The cleft nasal deformity comprises a collection of specific abnormalities. They can be remembered by considering anatomical subgroups as shown in Box 29.1

Box 29.1 *ANATOMIC CHARACTERISTICS OF CLEFT NASAL DEFORMITY*

Cartilaginous Deformities
The caudal septum is deviated to the noncleft side.
The posterior septum is convex on the cleft side and can block the cleft-side airway.
Lower lateral cartilages are attenuated and displaced caudally on the cleft side.
The medial crura are separated from one another at the dome.
The angle between medial and lateral crura is more obtuse on the cleft side.

Soft Tissue and Bone
The nasal tip and columellar base deviate to the noncleft side.
The cleft-side alar base is displaced laterally, posteriorly, and caudally.
The maxilla is hypoplastic with a posteriorly displaced piriform margin on the cleft side.
The nostril sill is deficient, and the nostril is widened on the cleft side.
The cleft alar-facial angle is flattened.
The vestibular lining is deficient on the cleft side.
The columella is shorter on the cleft side.

Flattening of the alar facial angle is a key finding on the cleft side. There is a more obtuse angle between the medial and lateral crura (not acute). There is widening of the cleft nostril with a deficiency of the sill. The nasal tip deviates away from (not toward) the cleft side. Columellar length is reduced on the cleft side (**Fig. 29.1**).[1–3]

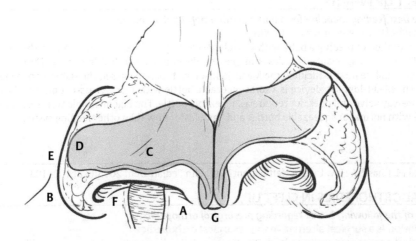

Fig. 29.1 Unilateral cleft nasal deformity. *A,* Nasal tip deviated. *B,* Alar cartilage displaced caudally. *C,* Angle between medial and lateral crura more obtuse. *D,* Buckling in the lateral crura. *E,* Flattened alar facial angle. *F,* Widened nostril floor. *G,* Columella and anterior caudal septal border deviated. Not shown: Deficiency in bony development, and posterior septum convex on cleft side causing varying degrees of obstruction. (Adapted from Spira M, Hardy SB, Gerow FJ. Correction of nasal deformities accompanying unilateral cleft lip. Cleft Palate J 7:112, 1970.)

REFERENCES

1. Burt JD, Byrd HS. Cleft lip: unilateral primary deformities. Plast Reconstr Surg 2000;105(3):1043–1055, quiz 1056–1057
2. Spira M, Hardy SB, Gerow FJ. Correction of nasal deformities accompanying unilateral cleft lip. Cleft Palate J 1970;7:112–123
3. Millard DR. The Unilateral Deformity. Vol. 1. Boston, MA: Little Brown; 1976

RISK OF FAMILIAL RECURRENCE IN CLEFT LIP/PALATE (CL/P)

5. You are advising a young couple in clinic who are planning to start a family. The lady has an isolated cleft lip that was repaired as a child. *What is the approximate risk of this couple having a child with a cleft lip/palate assuming the father is unaffected?*

   B. 4%

   If one parent is affected, the risk of cleft lip/palate in the first child is 3–5%. If an affected parent already has an affected child the risk increases to 17% for the second child. If unaffected parents have one affected child, the risk of having subsequent affected children is 4%. When unaffected parents have two affected children, the risk of having other affected children is 9%. It is important to have an idea of relative risk for cleft lip and palate development as patients and families are likely to ask about this during consultations (**Table 29.1**).[1–3]

Table 29.1   *Risk of Familial Recurrence in Cleft Lip with or without Cleft Palate*

Risk of Familial Recurrence	Percent
One affected parent	3–5
One affected child	4
Two affected children	9
Affected parent and affected child	17
Monozygotic twins	40–50
Dizygotic twins	5
Affected niece or nephew	1
Affected cousin	0.5

REFERENCES

1. Mitchell LE, Lupo PJ. Epidemiology of Cleft Lip and Palate. Vol 1. 2nd ed. Boca Raton, FL: CRC Press; 2016
2. Lees M. Familial risks of oral clefts. BMJ 2008;336(7641):399
3. Millard DR. The Unilateral Deformity. Vol. 1. Boston, MA: Little Brown; 1976

FEEDING CLEFT LIP INFANTS

6. *What is the best feeding modality for a patient with a cleft lip deformity?*

   E. A normal bottle/nipple or breast-feeding

   The best method of feeding a baby with an isolated cleft lip is either directly from the breast or with a regular bottle. The need for specialized bottles or nipples is only for infants with a cleft palate. Three types of bottles used to feed cleft palate infants include: the Mead-Johnson cleft palate nurser, the Haberman feeder, and the Pigeon nipple. The Mead-Johnson device is a soft squeezable bottle with a long cross-cut nipple. The Haberman feeder has a one-way valve and does not require a squeezable bottle. The Pigeon nipple works by compression and can be used with normal or squeezable bottles and has a faster flow than other feeding systems.[1]

REFERENCE

1. Kumar Jindal M, Khan SY. How to feed cleft patient? Int J Clin Pediatr Dent 2013;6(2):100–103

PRESURGICAL ORTHOPEDICS IN CLEFT LIP

7. *Which one of the following is true regarding presurgical orthopedics?*

   B. Lip adhesion is a surgical alternative to presurgical orthopedics.

   Presurgical approaches are used in cleft patients to help align and approximate maxillary segments, correct malposition of the nasal cartilages, and elongate the columella prior to definitive lip or palate repair. Lip adhesion is a surgical procedure used for wide cleft lips in which preliminary closure of the lip is performed around 2 months of age. The principal aim of this technique is to convert a complete cleft into an incomplete one with the hope that later definitive closure is facilitated and that the lip and nasal deformity are reduced by molding of the maxillary segments. The downsides are that an additional operation is required within the first 2 months of life and it risks damage to the tissues required for later definitive repair. To minimize this, the incisions are placed within tissue that will be discarded at final repair. In this procedure, the lateral lip and alar base are released from their attachments to the maxilla. A retention suture is placed to encircle the orbicularis muscle and a silicone nasal conformer is placed for columellar lengthening and to reshape the lower lateral cartilages.

Presurgical orthopedic devices may be used alternatively to narrow the cleft margin and improve arch alignment before surgery. They can be either active or passive. The Latham device is an active appliance that is placed and secured with pins while the patient is under general anesthetic. Screw activation will expand the plate and retract the premaxilla, but this process can adversely affect maxillary growth and should be reserved for severe deformities. An additional anesthetic will be required for its removal. Nasoalveolar molding (NAM) is a nonsurgical way to reshape the gums, lip, and nostrils with a plastic plate before cleft lip and palate surgery. Both Latham and NAM treatment will require multiple outpatient clinic visits which are usually weekly or biweekly for monitoring and adjustment and hence will not decrease the outpatient burden.[1-5]

REFERENCES

1. Marcus JR, Allori AC, Santiago PE. Principles of cleft lip repair: conventions, commonalities, and controversies. Plast Reconstr Surg 2017;139(3):764e–780e
2. Kirschner RE, Adetayo OA, Losee JE. Lip adhesion In: Losee JE, Kirschner RE, eds. Comprehensive Cleft Care. Vol. 2. Boca Raton, FL: CRC Press; 2016
3. Active Presurgical Infant Orthopedics for Unilateral Cleft Lip and Palate: Inter-Center Outcome Comparison of Latham, Modified McNeil, and Nasoalveolar Molding
4. Murthy PS, Deshmukh S, Bhagyalakshmi A, Srilatha K. Pre surgical nasoalveolar molding: changing paradigms in early cleft lip and palate rehabilitation. J Int Oral Health 2013;5(2):70–80
5. Millard DR Jr, Latham R, Huifen X, Spiro S, Morovic C. Cleft lip and palate treated by presurgical orthopedics, gingivo-periosteoplasty, and lip adhesion (POPLA) compared with previous lip adhesion method: a preliminary study of serial dental casts. Plast Reconstr Surg 1999;103(6):1630–1644

TIMING OF CLEFT LIP REPAIR

8. *Which one of the following is performed at the time of primary lip repair?*

B. Tip rhinoplasty

Primary repair of a cleft lip is performed around the age of 3 months. During this surgery the primary cleft nasal repair and gingivoperiosteoplasty are usually performed. A nasal repair involves release and repositioning of the cleft nasal components and alar cartilages (tip rhinoplasty). Tajima or McComb sutures may be used to support the lower lateral cartilage in primary cleft rhinoplasty. A gingivoperiosteoplasty involves the primary closure of an alveolar cleft using mucoperiosteal flaps.

Palatoplasty is typically performed at 9–12 months of age. Alveolar bone grafting involves harvesting cancellous bone from the iliac crest and is most successful between the ages of 8 and 12 years because this coincides with eruption of the canine teeth. Orthognathic surgery and secondary or full rhinoplasty are usually performed once facial growth and secondary dentition is complete (**Table 29.2**).[1,2]

Table 29.2 *Timings for Cleft Lip Repair and Associated Procedures*

Procedure	Age
Presurgical orthopedics	1 week–3 months
Cleft lip repair	3–6 months
Tip rhinoplasty	
Tympanostomy tubes	
Palatoplasty	9–18 months
T-tube placement	
Speech evaluation	3–4 years
Velopharyngeal insufficiency workup and surgery	4–6 years
Tip rhinoplasty	6–9 years
Phase I orthodontics	6–9 years
Alveolar bone grafting	6–9 years
Nasal reconstruction	12–18 years
Phase II orthodontics	14–18 years
Orthognathic surgery	Completion of mandibular growth (14–18 years)
Final touchup surgery	Early adulthood

REFERENCES

1. Shkoukani MA, Chen M, Vong A. Cleft lip—a comprehensive review. Front Pediatr 2013;1:53
2. Salyer KE, Rozen SM, Genecov ER, Genecov DG. Unilateral cleft lip—approach and technique. Semin Plast Surg 2005;19(4):313–328

TYPES OF CLEFT LIP REPAIR

9. *Which one of the following techniques is a commonly used rotation-advancement repair for unilateral cleft lip that incorporates a superiorly placed Z-plasty?*

    D. Millard

    A number of different techniques are available for cleft lip repair. The Millard repair is one of the most commonly used techniques and involves a superiorly placed Z-plasty. This is the one that is traditionally learned for clinical examinations in plastic surgery. The Randall-Tennison repair also uses a Z-plasty, but at the vermilion border, and can result in excessive vertical lip height. LeMesurier modified a quadrangular flap repair first described by Hagedorn. Techniques such as the Rose-Thompson technique involve a straight line and are no longer commonly used because they have been replaced with techniques involving Z-plasties to improve lip height. Bilateral cleft lip can be repaired using Millard or modified Manchester techniques. In the Millard technique the central skin of the prolabium is used to reconstruct the philtral dimple, but the white roll and vermilion are discarded. The modified Manchester technique preserves the white roll and vermilion from the prolabium to reconstruct Cupid's bow and tubercle.[1-9]

REFERENCES

1. Millard DR Jr. A radical rotation in single harelip. Am J Surg 1958;95(2):318–322
2. Manchester WM. The repair of double cleft lip as part of an integrated program. Plast Reconstr Surg 1970;45(3):207–216
3. Adenwalla HS, Narayanan PV. Primary unilateral cleft lip repair. Indian J Plast Surg 2009;42(Suppl):S62–S70
4. Monson LA, Kirschner RE, Losee JE. Primary repair of cleft lip and nasal deformity. Plast Reconstr Surg 2013;132(6):1040e–1053e
5. Rose W. On Harelip and Cleft Palate. London: H.K. Lewis; 1891
6. Thompson JE. An artistic and mathematically accurate method of repairing the defect in cases of harelip. Surg Gynecol Obstet 1912;14:498–505
7. Blair VP, Brown JB. Mirault operation for single harelip. Surg Gynecol Obstet 1930;51:81
8. Brown JB, McDowell F. Simplified design for repair of single cleft lips. Surg Gynecol Obstet 1945;80:12–26
9. LeMesurier AB. A method of cutting and suturing the lip in the treatment of complete unilateral clefts. Plast Reconstr Surg (1946) 1949;4(1):1–12

THE MILLARD REPAIR FOR UNILATERAL CLEFT LIPS (BYRD MODIFICATION)

10. *When undertaking the Millard repair for unilateral cleft lip, which one of the following tissue flap components is used to close the nasal sill or lengthen the columella?*

    B. C flap

    The markings and steps of the Millard rotation-advancement repair are shown in **Fig. 29.2,** *A* through *F.* The key flaps used in this repair are as follows: The C flap is known as the columellar flap and is a triangle of skin that begins inferiorly at the high point of Cupid's bow. It is used to close the nasal sill or lengthen the columella. The L flap is known as the lateral flap and is a superiorly based flap from the lateral lip that is used to line the lateral nasal vestibule. The M flap is known as the medial or mucosal flap and is a rectangular flap of mucosa from the medial lip. It is used to line the gingivobuccal sulcus. The R flap is the rotation flap based on the noncleft side (medial) lip that rotates into place during cleft lip repair to join with the cleft side lip (lateral). The A flap is the advancement flap based on the cleft side lip. It advances to join the R flap from the noncleft side.[1,2]

REFERENCES

1. Millard DR Jr. A radical rotation in single harelip. Am J Surg 1958;95(2):318–322
2. Byrd HS. Unilateral cleft lip. In: Aston SJ, Beasley RW, Thorne CHM, eds. Grabb and Smith's Plastic Surgery. 5th ed. Philadelphia: Lippincott-Raven; 1997

MILLARD AND FISHER TECHNIQUES IN CLEFT LIP REPAIR

11. *Which one of the following is part of both the Millard and Fisher techniques for cleft lip repair?*

    A. A Noordhoff flap

    The Noordhoff flap is a triangular flap of dry vermilion taken from the lateral lip element and rotated into an incision along the wet–dry junction of the medial lip element to even out heights of the medial and lateral labial

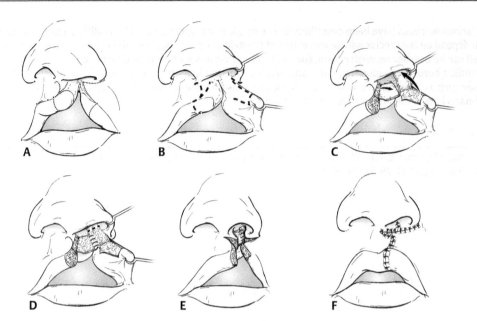

Fig. 29.2 **A,** Flaps are marked using the alar base, columella, lip margins, philtral columns, and Cupid's bow. **B** and **C,** The R, C, M, L, and A flaps are incised and elevated. **D,** The M and L flaps are sutured into place. **E** and **F,** Rotation-advancement is completed with interposition of C flap above A flap.

elements and help to prevent notching and development of a whistle deformity. It is incorporated into both the Millard and Fisher techniques.

The Millard repair has been the most popular approach to repair of cleft lips for a number of years. It involves rotation of the medial lip element downward and fills the resulting defect with the lateral lip. In doing so it places the scar along the proposed philtral column. Although it is well recognized and is associated with high-quality outcomes, some criticisms exist including the technical difficulty and challenges in dealing with wide clefts, wide soft tissue undermining, and tension across the nasal sill following closure.

The Fisher subunit repair is a geometric style technique which serves to address two perceived shortcomings in the rotation-advancement techniques. One issue is the complex scars created beneath the nose which may disrupt continuity of the columellar-labial crease and make future open rhinoplasty difficult. The other is the horizontal length of the lateral lip which is often shortened due to the Noordhoff point lying too laterally. In order to address these, the Fisher repair places the scars in the interfaces of anatomic subunits and incorporates a cutaneous triangle above the white roll to adjust the height of the medial labial element. The key differences in rotation-advancement (Millard) versus geometric style (Fisher) are therefore mostly related to the skin incisions and effect on symmetry. Both techniques allow for correction of mucosal, gingival, muscular, and nasal deformities.

A Tajima suture is a type of suture used in primary cleft rhinoplasty. The suture is placed through the caudal cleft side of the lower lateral cartilage to the contralateral upper lateral cartilage to provide support to the lower lateral cartilage. It is not specifically part of either the Fisher or Millard lip repair techniques.[1–3]

REFERENCES

1. Millard DR Jr. A radical rotation in single harelip. Am J Surg 1958;95(2):318–322
2. Fisher DM. Unilateral cleft lip repair: anatomic subunit approximation technique. In: Losee JE, Kirschner RE, eds. Comprehensive Cleft Care. Vol. 2. Boca Raton, FL: CRC Press; 2016
3. Tajima S, Maruyama M. Reverse-U incision for secondary repair of cleft lip nose. Plast Reconstr Surg 1977;60(2):256–261

WHISTLING DEFORMITY AFTER CLEFT LIP

12. A patient who presents to clinic after a cleft lip repair has a whistling deformity. *Which one of the following structures is deficient?*

B. Vermilion

The whistling or whistler deformity is normally secondary to a deficiency in the central part of the vermilion often in conjunction with abnormal orbicularis alignment.

Various methods have been described for the surgical management of this condition and technique selection will depend on the precise nature and extent of the deformity. For example, if the deficiency is mild, the upper lip itself can be used for reconstruction, such as Z-plasty, V-Y advancement, double pendulum flaps, bilateral lateral vermilion border transposition flaps, and bilobed mucosal flaps. If the deformity is more severe then adjacent tissue such as the tongue and lower lip (Abbe flap) may be required. More novel approaches include fat grafting, palmaris longus tendon grafting, and dermofat grafts.[1]

REFERENCE

1. Choi WY, Yang JY, Kim GB, Han YJ. Surgical correction of whistle deformity using cross-muscle flap in secondary cleft lip. Arch Plast Surg 2012;39(5):470–476

30. Cleft Palate

See *Essentials of Plastic Surgery*, third edition, pp. 376–388

EMBRYOLOGY OF THE PALATE

1. *Which one of the following is formed from the secondary palate?*
   A. Lip
   B. Nostril sill
   C. Alveolus
   D. Anterior hard palate
   E. Posterior hard palate

EMBRYOLOGY OF THE PALATE

2. *Which one of the following statements is correct regarding embryology of the palate?*
   A. The bony palate is formed entirely by the maxillary bone processes.
   B. Before 8 weeks of gestation, the palatal processes are horizontal.
   C. Embryologic development may explain a higher incidence of left-sided cleft palate.
   D. Rotation of the palatal processes is unaffected by tongue development.
   E. Both palatal processes become horizontal at the same time.

MUSCLES OF THE SOFT PALATE

3. *Which one of the velum muscles is innervated by the fifth cranial nerve?*
   A. Levator veli palatini
   B. Superior pharyngeal constrictor
   C. Palatopharyngeus
   D. Tensor veli palatini
   E. Palatoglossus

BLOOD SUPPLY TO THE PALATE

4. *Which one of the following is the main blood supply to the hard palate?*
   A. Nasopalatine artery from the maxillary artery
   B. Lesser palatine artery from the maxillary artery
   C. Greater palatine artery from the facial artery
   D. Greater palatine artery from the maxillary artery
   E. Ascending pharyngeal artery from the external carotid artery

SUBMUCOUS CLEFT PALATE

5. *Which one of the following represents the triad seen in submucous cleft palate?*
   A. Absent uvula, zona pellucida, and soft palate notch
   B. Absent uvula, zona pellucida, and hard palate notch
   C. Bifid uvula, lower lip pits, and hard palate notch
   D. Bifid uvula, lower lip pits, and zona pellucida
   E. Bifid uvula, hard palate notch, and zona pellucida

CLEFT PALATE DEFECTS

6. *Which one of the following is the most common palatal deformity?*
   A. Midline isolated cleft
   B. Complete primary palate cleft
   C. Complete secondary palate cleft
   D. Bifid uvula
   E. Submucous cleft

DEMOGRAPHICS OF FACIAL CLEFTS

7. *What is the approximate combined overall incidence of cleft lip, cleft palate, or cleft lip and palate?*
   A. 1:250 live births
   B. 1:500 live births
   C. 1:750 live births
   D. 1:1000 live births
   E. 1:1250 live births

RISK OF DEVELOPING AN ISOLATED CLEFT PALATE

8. A couple with no personal history of cleft palate have one child with a cleft palate. They are planning a second child. *What is the risk of their next child having a cleft palate?*
   A. 2%
   B. 6%
   C. 15%
   D. 30%
   E. 50%

RISK OF DEVELOPING CLEFT LIP/PALATE

9. You see a couple in clinic that have two children and are interested in having one more child. The father has a cleft lip/palate that was repaired as a child and the mother is unaffected. They have one unaffected child and one with a cleft lip/palate. *What is the risk of their next child having a cleft lip/palate deformity?*
   A. 2%
   B. 10%
   C. 17%
   D. 25%
   E. 42%

CLEFT SUBTYPES

10. *Which one of the following types of clefts is most commonly associated with another anomaly?*
    A. Unilateral cleft lip
    B. Bilateral cleft lip
    C. Isolated cleft palate
    D. Unilateral cleft lip and palate
    E. Bilateral cleft lip and palate

PIERRE ROBIN SEQUENCE

11. While on call for the pediatric plastic surgical team, you are referred an infant with a diagnosis of Pierre Robin sequence. *Which one of the following is the most likely reason for the infant to require an acute admission?*
    A. Failure to thrive
    B. Feeding issues
    C. Renal failure
    D. Airway compromise
    E. Chest infection

SYNDROMIC CLEFTS

12. A patient is referred with a syndromic cleft palate, ocular malformations, hearing loss, and arthropathies. They have a proven genetic mutation for type II collagen. *What syndrome does this specifically represent?*
    A. Stickler syndrome
    B. Shprintzen's syndrome
    C. Velocardiofacial syndrome
    D. Van der Woude syndrome
    E. Pierre Robin sequence

DEVELOPMENTAL RISK FACTORS IN CLEFT PALATE

13. *Which one of the following is most strongly associated with an increased risk of developing an isolated oral cleft?*
    A. Maternal smoking
    B. Maternal alcohol
    C. Maternal caffeine ingestion
    D. Increased paternal age
    E. Folic acid deficiency

CHALLENGES OF MANAGING INFANTS WITH ISOLATED CLEFT PALATE

14. *Which one of the following is a common problem for infants with cleft palate in the first few weeks of life?*
    A. Airway issues
    B. Recurrent chest infections
    C. Sleep difficulties
    D. Feeding difficulties
    E. Physical appearance concerns

SURGICAL REPAIR OF CLEFT PALATE

15. *Which one of the following techniques used in cleft patients involves reorientation of the levator veli palatini and palatopharyngeus muscles across the midline to reconstruct the levator sling?*
    A. von Langenbeck palatoplasty
    B. Intravelar veloplasty
    C. Veau-Wardill-Kilner pushback palatoplasty
    D. Double-opposing Z- plasty technique (Furlow)
    E. Pharyngeal flap

POSTOPERATIVE CARE OF CLEFT PALATE PATIENTS

16. *Which one of the following is often part of the postoperative regimen after cleft palate repair?*
    A. Discharge home on day of surgery
    B. The use of intranasal oxymetazoline
    C. Nursing supine without pillows
    D. Institution of a normal diet at day 3
    E. Heavy sedation for the first 48 hours

COMPLICATIONS OF CLEFT PALATE REPAIR

17. *Which one of the following statements is correct regarding cleft palate repairs?*
    A. Maxillary growth is normalized by cleft palate repair.
    B. Palatal fistulas should be surgically repaired.
    C. Fistula rates are consistent between series.
    D. Operative mortality risk remains above 2%.
    E. Fistulas most commonly form at the junction of the hard and soft palates.

Answers

EMBRYOLOGY OF THE PALATE

1. *Which one of the following is formed from the secondary palate?*

E. Posterior hard palate

The secondary palate forms the hard palate **posterior** to the incisive foramen and the soft palate. The primary palate forms the hard palate anterior to the incisive foramen as well as the lip, nostril sill, and alveolus. The primary palate is formed by the medial and lateral nasal prominences of the frontonasal process migrating and fusing with the maxillary prominence during **weeks 4–7** of gestation. The secondary palate is formed by migration and fusion of the lateral palatal processes of the maxillary prominence between **weeks 5 and 12** of gestation. Therefore, the hard palate is unusual as it develops from both the primary and secondary palates.[1-4]

REFERENCES

1. Moore KL, Persaud TV, Torchia MD, eds. The Developing Human: Clinically Oriented Embryology. 10th ed. Philadelphia: Elsevier; 2016
2. Sadler TW, ed. Langman's Medical Embryology. 13th ed. Philadelphia: Wolters Kluwer Health; 2014
3. Coleman JR Jr, Sykes JM. The embryology, classification, epidemiology, and genetics of facial clefting. Facial Plast Surg Clin North Am 2001;9(1):1–13
4. Marazita ML, Mooney MP. Current concepts in the embryology and genetics of cleft lip and cleft palate. Clin Plast Surg 2004;31(2):125–140

EMBRYOLOGY OF THE PALATE

2. *Which one of the following statements is correct regarding embryology of the palate?*

C. Embryologic development may explain a higher incidence of left-sided cleft palate.

The bony palate develops from the primary and secondary palates. The primary palate (anterior to the incisive foramen) is formed by the premaxillary portion of the maxilla. The secondary palate (posterior to the incisive foramen) is formed by the palatine processes of the maxilla and the palatine processes of the palatine bone. In week 8, the lateral palatal processes are vertical and progress to a horizontal position as the tongue moves caudally. The palatal processes rotate at different times, with the right moving before the left. This may explain the higher incidence of left-sided clefts. Fusion of the palatal processes takes longer in females (approximately 1 week), which may explain an increased incidence of cleft palate in females. Interruption of the migration or fusion steps may result in a cleft palate.[1-4]

REFERENCES

1. Moore KL, Persaud TV, Torchia MD, eds. The Developing Human: Clinically Oriented Embryology. 10th ed. Philadelphia: Elsevier; 2016
2. Sadler TW, ed. Langman's Medical Embryology. 13th ed. Philadelphia: Wolters Kluwer Health; 2014
3. Coleman JR Jr, Sykes JM. The embryology, classification, epidemiology, and genetics of facial clefting. Facial Plast Surg Clin North Am 2001;9(1):1–13
4. Marazita ML, Mooney MP. Current concepts in the embryology and genetics of cleft lip and cleft palate. Clin Plast Surg 2004;31(2):125–140

MUSCLES OF THE SOFT PALATE

3. *Which one of the velum muscles is innervated by the fifth cranial nerve?*

D. Tensor veli palatini

With the exception of the tensor veli palatini muscle, all of the muscles of the soft palate are innervated by the pharyngeal plexus, with contributions from cranial nerves IX, X, and XI. The tensor veli palatini muscle originates from the first pharyngeal arch and functions to open the Eustachian tube. This is logical embryologically because the first arch forms the second and third parts of the trigeminal nerve (**Fig. 30.1**).[1-4]

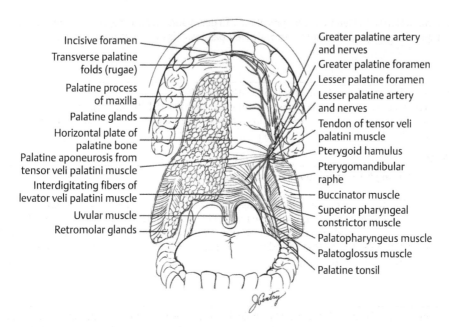

Incisive foramen
Transverse palatine folds (rugae)
Palatine process of maxilla
Palatine glands
Horizontal plate of palatine bone
Palatine aponeurosis from tensor veli palatini muscle
Interdigitating fibers of levator veli palatini muscle
Uvular muscle
Retromolar glands

Greater palatine artery and nerves
Greater palatine foramen
Lesser palatine foramen
Lesser palatine artery and nerves
Tendon of tensor veli palatini muscle
Pterygoid hamulus
Pterygomandibular raphe
Buccinator muscle
Superior pharyngeal constrictor muscle
Palatopharyngeus muscle
Palatoglossus muscle
Palatine tonsil

Fig. 30.1   Anatomy of the palate.

REFERENCES

1. Sadler TW, ed. Langman's Medical Embryology. 13th ed. Philadelphia: Wolters Kluwer Health; 2014
2. Moore KL, Dailey AF, Agur AMR. Clinically Oriented Anatomy. 7th ed. Philadelphia: Lippincott Williams & Wilkins; 2013
3. Ross RB, Johnston MC. Cleft Lip and Palate. Baltimore: Williams & Wilkins; 1972
4. Hopper RA, Cutting C, Grayson B. Cleft lip and palate. In: Thorne, CHea, eds. Grabb and Smith's Plastic Surgery. Philadelphia: Lippincott, Williams & Wilkins; 2007:201–225

BLOOD SUPPLY TO THE PALATE

4. *Which one of the following is the main blood supply to the hard palate?*

   D. Greater palatine artery from the maxillary artery

   The greater palatine artery passes through the greater palatine foramen to supply the hard palate. It originates from the maxillary artery via the descending palatine artery. The hard palate is also supplied by the nasopalatine artery and the anterior and posterior superior alveolar arteries, all of which arise from the maxillary artery. The soft palate is supplied by the lesser palatine artery (from the maxillary artery) and the ascending pharyngeal artery (from the external carotid artery) more laterally (see **Fig. 30.1**).[1–5]

REFERENCES

1. Sadler TW, ed. Langman's Medical Embryology. 13th ed. Philadelphia: Wolters Kluwer Health; 2014
2. Moore KL, Dailey AF, Agur AMR. Clinically Oriented Anatomy. 7th ed. Philadelphia: Lippincott Williams & Wilkins; 2013
3. Marks MW, Marks C. Cleft lip and palate. Philadelphia, PA: Saunders; 1997:156
4. Hopper RA, Cutting C, Grayson B. Cleft lip and palate. Philadelphia, PA: Lippincott, Williams & Wilkins; 2007:201–225
5. Kosowski TR, Weathers WM, Wolfswinkel EM, Ridgway EB. Cleft palate. Semin Plast Surg 2012;26(4):164–169

SUBMUCOUS CLEFT PALATE

5. *Which one of the following represents the triad seen in submucous cleft palate?*

   E. Bifid uvula, hard palate notch, and zona pellucida

   Submucous clefts have a triad of a posterior hard palate notch (not anterior), a bifid uvula, and a zona pellucida. The zona pellucida is a thin central area created by a diastasis of the soft palate musculature. It has a typical translucent appearance. The triad is sometimes referred to as Calnan's triad, as it was described by him in 1954.[1,2] Surgery is reserved for patients with velopharyngeal incompetence and may go unnoticed unless this is evident. Lower lip pits in conjunction with cleft palate is typical for Van der Woude syndrome, which is an autosomal dominant condition representing one-fifth of all syndromic cleft palates. It is not a feature of submucous cleft palate.[3]

REFERENCES

1. Calnan J. Submucous cleft palate. Br J Plast Surg 1954;6(4):264–282
2. Dreyer TM, Trier WC. A comparison of palatoplasty techniques. Cleft Palate J 1984;21(4):251–253
3. Coleman JR Jr, Sykes JM. The embryology, classification, epidemiology, and genetics of facial clefting. Facial Plast Surg Clin North Am 2001;9(1):1–13

CLEFT PALATE DEFECTS

6. *Which one of the following is the most common palatal deformity?*

D. **Bifid uvula**

A bifid uvula is effectively a partial cleft of the uvula and is traditionally regarded as a marker for submucous cleft palate. Submucous clefts are associated with the triad of bifid uvula, notching of the hard palate, and muscular diastasis of the soft palate.[1] Bifid uvula can however occur spontaneously in many healthy and otherwise normal individuals. In fact, it is estimated that a bifid uvula is present in around 2% of the population. The frequency of the other clefts is far less common.[1-3]

REFERENCES

1. Shprintzen RJ, Schwartz RH, Daniller A, Hoch L. Morphologic significance of bifid uvula. Pediatrics 1985;75(3):553–561
2. Lindemann G, Riis B, Sewerin I. Prevalence of cleft uvula among 2,732 Danes. Cleft Palate J 1977;14(3):226–229
3. Coleman JR Jr, Sykes JM. The embryology, classification, epidemiology, and genetics of facial clefting. Facial Plast Surg Clin North Am 2001;9(1):1–13

DEMOGRAPHICS OF FACIAL CLEFTS

7. *What is the approximate combined overall incidence of cleft lip, cleft palate, or cleft lip and palate?*

C. **1:750 live births**

The overall incidence of cleft lip with or without cleft palate, and isolated cleft palate is around 1:750 live births. The incidence of cleft lip with or without palate (CL/P) is affected by race and is highest in Asians at 1:500, but is less common in whites (1:1000) and blacks (1:2000). In contrast, the incidence of cleft palate (CP) is unaffected by race (1:2000 live births for all races). There is a gender difference in cleft lip and cleft palate. The male to female ratio for CL/P is 2:1, while the reverse is true for CP at 1:2.[1-5]

REFERENCES

1. Fraser F. Etiology of cleft lip and palate. In: Grabb WC, Rosenstein SW, Bzoch KR, eds. Cleft Lip and Palate: Surgical, Dental, and Speech Aspects. Boston: Little Brown; 1971
2. Christensen K, Mitchell LE. Familial recurrence-pattern analysis of nonsyndromic isolated cleft palate—a Danish registry study. Am J Hum Genet 1996;58(1):182–190
3. Mai CT, Cassell CH, Meyer RE, et al; National Birth Defects Prevention Network. Birth defects data from population-based birth defects surveillance programs in the United States, 2007 to 2011: highlighting orofacial clefts. Birth Defects Res A Clin Mol Teratol 2014;100(11):895–904
4. Tanaka SA, Mahabir RC, Jupiter DC, Menezes JM. Updating the epidemiology of cleft lip with or without cleft palate. Plast Reconstr Surg 2012;129(3):511e–518e
5. Hagberg C, Larson O, Milerad J. Incidence of cleft lip and palate and risks of additional malformations. Cleft Palate Craniofac J 1998;35(1):40–45

RISK OF DEVELOPING AN ISOLATED CLEFT PALATE

8. A couple with no personal history of cleft palate have one child with a cleft palate. They are planning a second child. *What is the risk of their next child having a cleft palate?*

A. **2%**

The standard risk for developing cleft palate is around 0.5% or 1 in 2000. The risk of having a child with an isolated cleft palate is significantly increased by either the parent or sibling having a cleft palate deformity. If unaffected parents have a child with a cleft palate, the risk of having another increases to 2%. If one parent has a cleft palate with no affected children, the risk for the first child is 6%. However, if an affected parent has one child with a cleft palate, the risk for the next child increases to 15%. These risks are relevant to clinical practice as parents will often wish to discuss risks during consultation.[1-4]

REFERENCES

1. Tanaka SA, Mahabir RC, Jupiter DC, Menezes JM. Updating the epidemiology of cleft lip with or without cleft palate. Plast Reconstr Surg 2012;129(3):511e–518e
2. Fraser F. Etiology of cleft lip and palate. In: Grabb WC, Rosenstein SW, Bzoch KR, eds. Cleft Lip and Palate: Surgical, Dental, and Speech Aspects. Boston: Little Brown; 1971
3. Jones MC. Facial clefting. Etiology and developmental pathogenesis. Clin Plast Surg 1993;20(4):599–606
4. Christensen K, Mitchell LE. Familial recurrence-pattern analysis of nonsyndromic isolated cleft palate—a Danish registry study. Am J Hum Genet 1996;58(1):182–190

RISK OF DEVELOPING CLEFT LIP/PALATE

9. You see a couple in clinic that have two children and are interested in having one more child. The father has a cleft lip/palate that was repaired as a child and the mother is unaffected. They have one unaffected child and one with a cleft lip/palate. *What is the risk of their next child having a cleft lip/palate deformity?*

   C. 17%

   The baseline risk for developing a cleft lip/palate (CL/P) deformity is dependent on race and varies between 0.05 and 0.2% (0.5:1000 to 2:1000). The risk of having a child with a CL/P is significantly increased by either a parent or sibling having a cleft deformity. If one parent has CL/P with no affected children, the risk is 4%. However, if an affected parent has one child with CL/P the risk increases to 17%. The risk for normal parents with two CL/P children increases to 9%. Risks of 30 and 50% do not relate to CL/P development.[1–4]

REFERENCES

1. Tanaka SA, Mahabir RC, Jupiter DC, Menezes JM. Updating the epidemiology of cleft lip with or without cleft palate. Plast Reconstr Surg 2012;129(3):511e–518e
2. Fraser F. Etiology of cleft lip and palate. In: Grabb WC, Rosenstein SW, Bzoch KR, eds. Cleft Lip and Palate: Surgical, Dental, and Speech Aspects. Boston: Little Brown; 1971
3. Jones MC. Facial clefting. Etiology and developmental pathogenesis. Clin Plast Surg 1993;20(4):599–606
4. Christensen K, Mitchell LE. Familial recurrence-pattern analysis of nonsyndromic isolated cleft palate—a Danish registry study. Am J Hum Genet 1996;58(1):182–190

CLEFT SUBTYPES

10. *Which one of the following types of clefts is most commonly associated with another anomaly?*

    C. Isolated cleft palate

    Cleft palate can be syndromic or nonsyndromic. Nonsyndromic clefts are characterized by one defect or multiple anomalies that are the result of a single initiating event or primary malformation. Syndromic clefts are characterized by more than one malformation involving more than one developmental field. Associated anomalies are most commonly seen with isolated cleft palates. This can be as high as 70% where Pierre Robin sequence is included. Anomalies are also higher in bilateral cleft patients. Syndromic clefts include syndromes such as Stickler, velocardiofacial, and Van der Woude.[1–3]

REFERENCES

1. Jones MC. Facial clefting. Etiology and developmental pathogenesis. Clin Plast Surg 1993;20(4):599–606
2. Hagberg C, Larson O, Milerad J. Incidence of cleft lip and palate and risks of additional malformations. Cleft Palate Craniofac J 1998;35(1):40–45
3. Coleman JR Jr, Sykes JM. The embryology, classification, epidemiology, and genetics of facial clefting. Facial Plast Surg Clin North Am 2001;9(1):1–13

PIERRE ROBIN SEQUENCE

11. While on call for the pediatric plastic surgical team, you are referred an infant with a diagnosis of Pierre Robin sequence. *Which one of the following is the most likely reason for the infant to require an acute admission?*

    D. Airway compromise

    The clinical features of Pierre Robin sequence are micrognathia/retrognathia and glossoptosis often with cleft palate. These can lead to significant airway problems, especially in young babies that require acute admission. The risk of airway compromise usually improves with age but in the acute setting needs meticulous care. Treatment includes lateral or prone positioning, and careful observation. In some cases, a nasopharyngeal airway or continuous positive airway pressure (CPAP) is required for a short duration. Occasionally tracheostomy is required. Infants with Pierre Robin sequence do not always have a cleft palate, but when one is present it tends to be wide and U-shaped as opposed to the normal V-shaped cleft.[1,2]

REFERENCES

1. Gangopadhyay N, Mendonca DA, Woo AS. Pierre Robin sequence. Semin Plast Surg 2012;26(2):76–82
2. Shprintzen RJ. The implications of the diagnosis of Robin sequence. Cleft Palate Craniofac J 1992;29(3):205–209

SYNDROMIC CLEFTS

12. A patient is referred with a syndromic cleft palate, ocular malformations, hearing loss, and arthropathies. They have a proven genetic mutation for type II collagen. *What syndrome does this specifically represent?*

A. Stickler syndrome

There are a number of syndromes associated with cleft palate (CP). The most common is Stickler syndrome, which represents 25% of all syndromic cases. This is an autosomal dominant condition with a mutation in the gene for type II collagen. The clinical presentation may include Pierre Robin sequence (but this is not specific to the other factors listed), ocular malformations, hearing loss, and arthropathies, each due to the collagen abnormality.[1,2]

Velocardiofacial and Shprintzen's syndrome are different terms used to describe the same condition and represent 15% of syndromic CP. This autosomal dominant condition is associated with a deletion on chromosome 22. It is also therefore known as 22q11 deletion. It involves cardiovascular abnormalities, abnormal facies, and developmental delay.[3,4] Van der Woude syndrome represents around 20% of all syndromic cleft palate cases. This is also autosomal dominant and is associated with lower lip pits.[5] Other syndromes associated with cleft palate include Apert syndrome and Crouzon syndrome.

REFERENCES

1. Stickler GB, Belau PG, Farrell FJ, et al. Hereditary progressive arthro-ophthalmopathy. Mayo Clin Proc 1965;40:433–455
2. Karempelis P, Hagen M, Morrell N, Roby BB. Associated syndromes in patients with Pierre Robin sequence. Int J Pediatr Otorhinolaryngol 2020;131:109842
3. Failla S, You P, Rajakumar C, Dworschak-Stokan A, Doyle PC, Husein M. Characteristics of velopharyngeal dysfunction in 22q11.2 deletion syndrome: a retrospective case-control study. J Otolaryngol Head Neck Surg 2020;49(1):54
4. Jackson OA, Paine K, Magee L, et al. Management of velopharyngeal dysfunction in patients with 22q11.2 deletion syndrome: a survey of practice patterns. Int J Pediatr Otorhinolaryngol 2019;116:43–48, 209
5. Rizos M, Spyropoulos MN. Van der Woude syndrome: a review. Cardinal signs, epidemiology, associated features, differential diagnosis, expressivity, genetic counselling and treatment. Eur J Orthod 2004;26(1):17–24

DEVELOPMENTAL RISK FACTORS IN CLEFT PALATE

13. *Which one of the following is most strongly associated with an increased risk of developing an isolated oral cleft?*

E. Folic acid deficiency

Folic acid and vitamin deficiencies are strongly associated with increased risk of cleft development. It is therefore really important to use oral folic acid and multivitamin supplements during early pregnancy. Doing so is also associated with a lower incidence of cleft lip or cleft lip and palate births in pregnant women with a family history of cleft lip/palate. The data on maternal smoking are inconsistent regarding the increased risk of clefts, but it probably does increase risk. Neither maternal alcohol nor caffeine ingestion is associated with increased risk. The risk of developing an isolated oral cleft increases with increased age of the parents, particularly if both are over the age of 30 years. Paternal age has the most profound effect.[1–3]

REFERENCES

1. Kelly D, O'Dowd T, Reulbach U. Use of folic acid supplements and risk of cleft lip and palate in infants: a population-based cohort study. Br J Gen Pract 2012;62(600):e466–e472
2. Butali A, Little J, Chevrier C, et al. Folic acid supplementation use and the MTHFR C677T polymorphism in orofacial clefts etiology: an individual participant data pooled-analysis. Birth Defects Res A Clin Mol Teratol 2013;97(8):509–514
3. Molina-Solana R, Yáñez-Vico RM, Iglesias-Linares A, Mendoza-Mendoza A, Solano-Reina E. Current concepts on the effect of environmental factors on cleft lip and palate. Int J Oral Maxillofac Surg 2013;42(2):177–184

CHALLENGES OF MANAGING INFANTS WITH ISOLATED CLEFT PALATE

14. *Which one of the following is a common problem for infants with cleft palate in the first few weeks of life?*

D. Feeding difficulties

A major challenge for infants with isolated cleft palate is early feeding as the presence of a cleft palate prevents them from achieving a negative pressure required for adequate suction. Most infants and their parents require assistance in feeding which necessitates squeezy bottle with large cross-section fissures or sometimes a palate obturator. Specialist nurse and dietician support are provided within the multidisciplinary team to new parents to support them. Regular assessment of weight gain should be undertaken to assess progress. Airway issues and recurrent chest infections are not generally a concern in isolated cleft palate. Sleeping difficulties may occur secondary to poor feeding and subsequent hunger but are not themselves a specific issue associated with cleft palate. Physical appearance is unaffected in isolated cleft palate unlike cleft lip patients. The social impact centers on speech issues later in life.[1]

REFERENCE

1. Miller CK. Feeding issues and interventions in infants and children with clefts and craniofacial syndromes. Semin Speech Lang 2011;32(2):115–126

SURGICAL REPAIR OF CLEFT PALATE

15. *Which one of the following techniques used in cleft patients involves reorientation of the levator veli palatini and palatopharyngeus muscles across the midline to reconstruct the levator sling?*

B. Intravelar veloplasty

The soft palate can be repaired using an intravelar veloplasty or a double-opposing Z-plasty, as described by Furlow. Both of these techniques should improve functional outcomes in terms of speech and feeding. The intravelar veloplasty involves reorientation of the levator veli palatini muscle and palatopharyngeus muscle complex transversely following their dissection from the abnormal insertion.[1,2] Furlow's technique uses double-opposing Z-plasties based on the cleft midline. The anteriorly based flaps contain only mucosa, while the posteriorly based flaps contain mucosa and levator muscle complex. Nasal mucosal flaps are transposed and closed, the levator sling is reoriented transversely, and the oral mucosal flaps are transposed and closed. Although the soft palate is lengthened, as per Z-plasty techniques in general, the transverse dimension is reduced, thereby making closure of wide clefts more difficult and increasing the risk of subsequent fistula formation. The hard palate can be repaired with the von Langenbeck technique, the Veau-Wardill-Kilner technique (V-Y pushback palatoplasty), or the Bardach technique (two-flap palatoplasty). Selection of technique is often based on personal preference.

The von Langenbeck palatoplasty uses bilateral bipedicled mucoperiosteal flaps with parallel incisions made along the cleft margin and lingual side of the alveolus. Nasal and oral mucosal flaps are mobilized and approximated in the midline. Poor speech outcomes have been attributed to the creation of a short immobile palate. These outcomes can be improved when combined with an intravelar veloplasty.[3] The V-Y pushback technique involves bilateral mucoperiosteal flaps based on the greater palatine arteries. It incorporates a V-Y closure anteriorly to lengthen the palate as well as fracture of the hamulus, levator muscle repair, and closure of the nasal and oral mucosa in separate layers. It has been associated with a high incidence of fistula formation and growth disturbances, and has fallen out of favor in many centers.[4] Vomer flaps can also be used to close hard palate defects. They can be either inferiorly or superiorly based and are useful in wide or bilateral clefts. Their use early in palatoplasty is controversial because of the risk of facial growth disturbance. Pharyngeal flaps are used to address poor speech in velopharygeal dysfunction.

REFERENCES

1. Kriens OB. An anatomical approach to veloplasty. Plast Reconstr Surg 1969;43(1):29–41
2. Marsh JL, Grames LM, Holtman B. Intravelar veloplasty: a prospective study. Cleft Palate J 1989;26(1):46–50
3. Dreyer TM, Trier WC. A comparison of palatoplasty techniques. Cleft Palate J 1984;21(4):251–253
4. Afifi GY, Kaidi AA, Hardesty RA. Cleft palate repair. In: Evans GR, ed. Operative Plastic Surgery. New York: McGraw-Hill; 2000

POSTOPERATIVE CARE OF CLEFT PALATE PATIENTS

16. *Which one of the following is often part of the postoperative regimen after cleft palate repair?*

B. The use of intranasal oxymetazoline

The key concerns after cleft palate repair are: (1) airway monitoring, (2) control of postoperative bleeding, and (3) encouragement of early feeding.

Bleeding can be controlled by meticulous intraoperative hemostasis and injection of local anesthetic that contains epinephrine, with packing of raw areas. Postoperative application of oxymetazoline (Afrin) can also reduce bleeding and is a popular adjunct. Oxymetazoline is a direct-acting sympathomimetic amine that acts on alpha-adrenergic receptors in the arterioles of the oronasal mucosa, resulting in decreased blood flow. Patients should be placed with the head gently elevated using pillows after cleft palate repair and not supine. Airway management involves continuous pulse oximetry and sedation is stopped as early as possible to minimize risk of respiratory compromise. Early feeding should be arranged, with liquid for the first 24 hours followed by a soft diet until day 10. Often, feeding can be the determining factor in discharge timing and all patients will stay overnight after surgery.[1-4]

REFERENCES

1. Fisher DM, Sommerlad BC. Cleft lip, cleft palate, and velopharyngeal insufficiency. Plast Reconstr Surg 2011;128(4): 342e–360e
2. Woo A. Evidence-based medicine: cleft palate. Plast Reconstr Surg 2017;139(1):191e–203e
3. Nguyen PN, Sullivan PK. Issues and controversies in the management of cleft palate. Clin Plast Surg 1993;20(4):671–682
4. Goudy SL, Tollefson T. Complete Cleft Care: Cleft and Velopharyngeal Insufficiency Treatment in Children. 1st ed. Thieme; 2015

COMPLICATIONS OF CLEFT PALATE REPAIR

17. *Which one of the following statements is correct regarding cleft palate repairs?*

    E. **Fistulas most commonly form at the junction of the hard and soft palates.**

      Palatal fistulas by definition occur posterior to the incisive foramen. They most often occur at the junction of the soft and hard palates. The most common long-term complication after cleft palate repair is development of a palatal fistula, but rates are diverse (5–60%).[1] They are likely to depend on many factors, including cleft severity, previous surgery, and surgical technique. The most common anatomic site is the junction of hard and soft palates.[2] Fistulas can be treated surgically (with local or distant flaps) but alternatively may be managed nonsurgically with or without an obturator. The operative mortality in cleft palate repair is approximately 0.5%. Cleft palate repair can interfere with maxillary growth and does not normalize it. This can display as midface hypoplasia or problems with occlusion.[3-5]

REFERENCES

1. Hardwicke JT, Landini G, Richard BM. Fistula incidence after primary cleft palate repair: a systematic review of the literature. Plast Reconstr Surg 2014;134(4):618e–627e
2. Nguyen PN, Sullivan PK. Issues and controversies in the management of cleft palate. Clin Plast Surg 1993;20(4):671–682
3. Afifi GY, Kaidi AA, Hardesty RA. Cleft palate repair. In: Evans GR, ed. Operative Plastic Surgery. New York: McGraw-Hill; 2000
4. Scheuermann M, Vanreusel I, Van de Casteele E, Nadjmi N. Spontaneous bone regeneration after closure of the hard palate cleft: a literature review. J Oral Maxillofac Surg 2019;77(5):1074.e1–1074.e7
5. Reddy RR, Gosla Reddy S, Vaidhyanathan A, Bergé SJ, Kuijpers-Jagtman AM. Maxillofacial growth and speech outcome after one-stage or two-stage palatoplasty in unilateral cleft lip and palate. A systematic review. J Craniomaxillofac Surg 2017;45(6):995–1003

31. Velopharyngeal Dysfunction

See *Essentials of Plastic Surgery*, third edition, pp. 389–399

VELOPHARYNGEAL DYSFUNCTION

1. *Which one of the following is correct regarding velopharyngeal dysfunction?*
   A. It will be due to incomplete closure of the velum against the pharynx.
   B. It can be exacerbated by adenoidectomy.
   C. It rarely presents after satisfactory cleft palate repair.
   D. It is usually associated with a small nasopharynx.
   E. It is most often due to an abnormal bow-tie sphincter closure pattern.

TERMINOLOGY OF VELOPHARYNGEAL ABNORMALITIES

2. *What is the most accurate term to describe impaired neuromotor control of the velum or pharyngeal wall resulting in abnormal velopharyngeal function?*
   A. Velopharyngeal disproportion
   B. Velopharyngeal insufficiency
   C. Velopharyngeal mislearning
   D. Velopharyngeal incompetence
   E. Velopharyngeal dysfunction

SPEECH ASSESSMENT IN VELOPHARYNGEAL DYSFUNCTION

3. *Which one of the following is associated with abnormal production of vowels during speech in a patient with velopharyngeal dysfunction?*
   A. Nasal substitution
   B. Compensatory substitution
   C. Sibilant distortion
   D. Hypernasality
   E. Nasal emission

SPEECH ASSESSMENT IN VELOPHARYNGEAL DYSFUNCTION

4. A speech and language therapist is testing specific speech sounds with a child in the cleft palate clinic. *Which one of the following is described as a "plosive"?*
   A. f
   B. v
   C. s
   D. sh
   E. t

FACIAL MOVEMENTS IN ABNORMAL SPEECH DEVELOPMENT

5. You observe abnormal facial movements in an isolated cleft palate patient during speech. *What are they trying to achieve by doing this?*
   A. Prevent abnormal nasal airflow by constricting the nares
   B. Seal the lips and achieve oral competence
   C. Close the palatal defect by moving the tongue to the roof of the mouth
   D. Facilitate lift of the soft palate against the posterior pharyngeal wall
   E. Trying to convey their words by expression

CLEFT SPEECH ERRORS

6. When listening to a patient with velopharyngeal dysfunction you note that when trying to say "b" an "m" sound is heard instead. *What is the term used to describe this problem?*
   A. Nasal rustle
   B. Nasal turbulence
   C. Sibilant distortion
   D. Nasal substitution
   E. Compensatory articulation

EVALUATION OF VELOPHARYNGEAL DYSFUNCTION

7. You have a 2-year-old child in clinic with velopharyngeal dysfunction. *Which one of the following modalities will provide a noninvasive, instrumented assessment of both the type and extent of velopharyngeal closure?*
   A. Nasometry
   B. Nasoendoscopy
   C. Magnetic resonance imaging (MRI)
   D. Videofluoroscopy
   E. Perceptual speech evaluation

TREATMENT OPTIONS FOR VELOPHARYNGAL DYSFUNCTION

8. *According to commonly accepted algorithms, what is the recommended surgical intervention in moderate to large gap (noncoronal) velopharyngeal dysfunction?*
   A. Furlow double-opposing Z-plasty
   B. Sphincter pharyngoplasty
   C. Intravelar veloplasty
   D. Pharyngeal flap
   E. Posterior pharyngeal wall augmentation

TREATMENT OPTIONS FOR VELOPHARYNGAL DYSFUNCTION

9. *Which one of the following has a limited success and a high complication rate in treating velopharyngeal dysfunction?*
   A. Furlow double-opposing Z-plasty
   B. Sphincter pharyngoplasty
   C. Intravelar veloplasty
   D. Pharyngeal flap
   E. Posterior pharyngeal wall augmentation

SURGICAL TECHNIQUES IN VELOPHARYNGEAL DYSFUNCTION

10. *What do the Hynes and Orticochea pharyngoplasty techniques have in common?*
    A. The number of flaps utilized
    B. The muscle included within the flaps
    C. The point of insertion of the flaps
    D. The creation of a sphincter at the velopharyngeal port
    E. The use of Z-plasties

SURGICAL TECHNIQUES FOR VELOPHARYNGEAL DYSFUNCTION

11. *Which one of the following techniques for velopharyngeal dysfunction represents an obstructive technique and creates a permanent tissue bridge between the velum and posterior pharyngeal wall?*
    A. Pharyngeal flap
    B. Pharyngoplasty
    C. Furlow double-opposing Z-plasty
    D. Straight line palate re-repair
    E. Posterior pharyngeal wall augmentation

POSTOPERATIVE CARE VELOPHARYNGEAL DYSFUNCTION

12. *In which patient group is postoperative airway management particularly important?*
    A. Secondary palate repair
    B. Post adenoidectomy
    C. Pierre Robin sequence
    D. Velocardiofacial syndrome
    E. Stickler syndrome

COMPLICATIONS IN SPEECH SURGERY

13. A 6-year-old girl has velopharyngeal insufficiency with poor speech in spite of continued speech therapy. Velopharyngeal surgery is subsequently planned. *When taking consent from the parents, which one of the following complications is particularly important to discuss?*
    A. Dysphagia
    B. Sleep apnea
    C. Odynophagia
    D. Gastric reflux
    E. Chest infection

Answers

VELOPHARYNGEAL DYSFUNCTION

1. *Which one of the following is correct regarding velopharyngeal dysfunction?*
   B. **It can be exacerbated by adenoidectomy.**

   Velopharyngeal dysfunction occurs in any situation in which air passes inappropriately through the nasal airway during speech. The causes can be categorized as cleft related or noncleft related. Situations which are not cleft related include adenoidectomy, neuromuscular disorders, or where there is an oronasal fistula. Velopharyngeal dysfunction can specifically occur when closure of the velum against the nasopharyngeal walls is incomplete. Normal velopharyngeal function involves composite movements of the velum posterosuperiorly, posterior pharyngeal wall ventrally, and the lateral pharyngeal wall medially. Dysfunction can be caused by a short or immobile velum or a large nasopharynx with poor function. It leads to poor speech quality and nasal regurgitation of food and is seen in patients following cleft palate repair and LeFort I/II midface advancement. Other patients at risk of velopharyngeal dysfunction are those with a relatively large nasopharynx. Normal closure patterns of the velopharyngeal sphincter are classified as coronal, sagittal, circular, or bow tie. Any of these patterns can be involved in dysfunction of the sphincter, but a bow tie is not the most common (**Fig. 31.1**).[1-3]

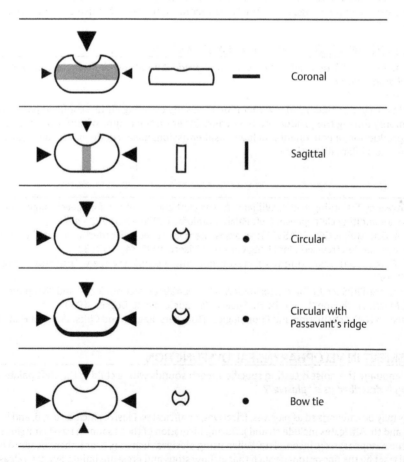

Fig. 31.1   Bird's-eye view of the velopharynx illustrating directional movements of the representative closure. (From Bentz ML, Bauer BS, Zuker RM. Principles & Practice of Pediatric Plastic Surgery. St Louis: Quality Medical Publishing, 2007.)

REFERENCES

1. Perry JL. Anatomy and physiology of the velopharyngeal mechanism. Semin Speech Lang 2011;32(2):83–92
2. Kummer AW, Strife JL, Grau WH, Creaghead NA, Lee L. The effects of Le Fort I osteotomy with maxillary movement on articulation, resonance, and velopharyngeal function. Cleft Palate J 1989;26(3):193–199, discussion 199–200
3. Kummer AW, Marshall JL, Wilson MM. Non-cleft causes of velopharyngeal dysfunction: implications for treatment. Int J Pediatr Otorhinolaryngol 2015;79(3):286–295

TERMINOLOGY OF VELOPHARYNGEAL ABNORMALITIES

2. *What is the most accurate term to describe impaired neuromotor control of the velum or pharyngeal wall resulting in abnormal velopharyngeal function?*

    D. Velopharyngeal incompetence

    Velopharyngeal dysfunction is a general descriptive term to describe any abnormal velopharyngeal function regardless of the cause. A more accurate description for a neuromotor control problem is velopharyngeal incompetence. In contrast, velopharyngeal insufficiency describes a structural abnormality resulting in dysfunction. Velopharyngeal dysfunction can result from a learned response that is neither structural nor neuromotor and this is termed velopharyngeal mislearning. Velopharyngeal disproportion describes a situation where the velum is small relative to the nasopharyngeal space as may be seen in patients with velocardiofacial syndrome.[1,2]

REFERENCES

1. Trost-Cardamone JE. Coming to terms with VPI: a response to Loney and Bloem. Cleft Palate J 1989;26(1):68–70
2. Loney RW, Bloem TJ. Velopharyngeal dysfunction: recommendations for use of nomenclature. Cleft Palate J 1987;24(4):334–335

SPEECH ASSESSMENT IN VELOPHARYNGEAL DYSFUNCTION

3. *Which one of the following is associated with abnormal production of vowels during speech in a patient with velopharyngeal dysfunction?*

    D. Hypernasality

    Hypernasality occurs secondary to reverberation of nasally escaping air in a confined postnasal space. It occurs most commonly during the production of vowels. Other distinct signs of abnormal speech associated with abnormal production of consonants include nasal emission, nasal rustle, nasal substitution, compensatory articulation, and sibilant distortion.[1-6]

REFERENCES

1. John A, Sell D, Sweeney T, Harding-Bell A, Williams A. The cleft audit protocol for speech-augmented: a validated and reliable measure for auditing cleft speech. Cleft Palate Craniofac J 2006;43(3):272–288
2. Sell D, Harding A, Grunwell P. GOS.SP.ASS.'98: an assessment for speech disorders associated with cleft palate and/or velopharyngeal dysfunction (revised). Int J Lang Commun Disord 1999;34(1):17–33
3. Kummer AW. Perceptual assessment of resonance and velopharyngeal function. Semin Speech Lang 2011;32(2):159–167
4. https://www.asha.org/PRPSpecificTopic.aspx?folderid=8589942918&section=Signs_and_Symptoms#Articulation
5. McWilliams BJ, Morris H, Shelton R. Cleft Palate Speech. Philadelphia: BC Decker; 1990
6. Bernthal JE, Bankson NW. Articulation and Phonological Disorders. Englewood Cliffs: Prentice Hall; 1988

SPEECH ASSESSMENT IN VELOPHARYNGEAL DYSFUNCTION

4. A speech and language therapist is testing specific speech sounds with a child in the cleft palate clinic. *Which one of the following is described as a "plosive"?*

    E. t

    Consonants may be categorized as plosives, fricatives, or affricates. Plosives include b, t, d, and k. Fricatives include f, v, s, z, sh, and th. Affricates include ch and j. During formation of these sounds, nasal emissions may be evident if closure of the nasopharynx is incomplete. When using plosives such as p, b, or t, there needs to be initial occlusion of the vocal tract by the lips or tongue such that airflow stops and pressure builds. Sudden release of the occlusion then produces the sound. Fricatives such as f and v require air being forced through a narrow channel made by placing two articulators such as the lower lip against the teeth. Sibilants are a subset of fricatives in which the tongue directs air over the edge of the teeth, resulting in high pitch sounds such as s or sh. Affricates such as ch represent sounds that start as a plosive and continue as a fricative.[1-6]

REFERENCES

1. John A, Sell D, Sweeney T, Harding-Bell A, Williams A. The cleft audit protocol for speech-augmented: a validated and reliable measure for auditing cleft speech. Cleft Palate Craniofac J 2006;43(3):272–288
2. Sell D, Harding A, Grunwell P. GOS.SP.ASS.'98: an assessment for speech disorders associated with cleft palate and/or velopharyngeal dysfunction (revised). Int J Lang Commun Disord 1999;34(1):17–33
3. Kummer AW. Perceptual assessment of resonance and velopharyngeal function. Semin Speech Lang 2011;32(2):159–167
4. Zajac DJ. The nature of nasal fricatives: articulatory-perceptual characteristics and etiologic considerations. Perspect Speech Sci Orofac Disord 2015;25:17–28
5. McWilliams BJ, Morris H, Shelton R. Cleft Palate Speech. Philadelphia: BC Decker; 1990
6. Bernthal JE, Bankson NW. Articulation and Phonological Disorders. Englewood Cliffs: Prentice Hall; 1988

FACIAL MOVEMENTS IN ABNORMAL SPEECH DEVELOPMENT

5. You observe abnormal facial movements in an isolated cleft palate patient during speech. *What are they trying to achieve by doing this?*

    A. Prevent abnormal nasal airflow by constricting the nares

    Clear phonation involves the generation of a column of air pressure passing from the subglottis into the upper airway. This airflow passes through the oral cavity for most sounds in the English language and nasal air emission is necessarily restricted. Exceptions are the sounds m, n, and ng, which require nasal airflow. When velopharyngeal closure is impaired, air can escape through the nose, when generating consonant sounds such as p, b, and t, clarity of speech is therefore impaired. Grimacing represents a subconscious attempt by the patient to inhibit abnormal nasal airflow and is evidenced by aberrant facial muscle movements during speech.[1–4]

REFERENCES

1. John A, Sell D, Sweeney T, Harding-Bell A, Williams A. The cleft audit protocol for speech-augmented: a validated and reliable measure for auditing cleft speech. Cleft Palate Craniofac J 2006;43(3):272–288
2. Sell D, Harding A, Grunwell P. GOS.SP.ASS.'98: an assessment for speech disorders associated with cleft palate and/or velopharyngeal dysfunction (revised). Int J Lang Commun Disord 1999;34(1):17–33
3. McWilliams BJ, Morris H, Shelton R. Cleft Palate Speech. Philadelphia: BC Decker; 1990
4. Bernthal JE, Bankson NW. Articulation and Phonological Disorders. Englewood Cliffs: Prentice Hall; 1988

CLEFT SPEECH ERRORS

6. When listening to a patient with velopharyngeal dysfunction you note that when trying to say "b" an "m" sound is heard instead. *What is the term used to describe this problem?*

    D. Nasal substitution

    When a patient with velopharyngeal dysfunction tries to produce an oral consonant with appropriately positioned articulators the sound is converted into its nasal equivalent. In this case a "b" becomes an "m" and a "d" becomes an "n." This is termed nasal substitution. Nasal rustle and nasal turbulence are equivalent to each other. They refer to a distinct fricative sound on the voiced pressure consonants b, d, and g. Sibilant distortion is the production of sounds "s" and "z" with incorrect tongue placement and often is secondary to malocclusion. Compensatory articulation is the production of plosives or fricatives in spite of velopharyngeal dysfunction by inappropriately positioned articulators and closure at the glottal or pharyngeal level.[1–4]

REFERENCES

1. Kosowski TR, Weathers WM, Wolfswinkel EM, Ridgway EB. Cleft palate. Semin Plast Surg 2012;26(4):164–169
2. Zajac DJ. The nature of nasal fricatives: articulatory-perceptual characteristics and etiologic considerations. Perspect Speech Sci Orofac Disord 2015;25:17–28
3. McWilliams BJ, Morris H, Shelton R. Cleft Palate Speech. Philadelphia: BC Decker; 1990
4. Bernthal JE, Bankson NW. Articulation and Phonological Disorders. Englewood Cliffs: Prentice Hall; 1988

EVALUATION OF VELOPHARYNGEAL DYSFUNCTION

7. You have a 2-year-old child in clinic with velopharyngeal dysfunction. *Which one of the following modalities will provide a noninvasive, instrumented assessment of both the type and extent of velopharyngeal closure?*

    D. Videofluoroscopy

    Instrumental assessment of velopharyngeal dysfunction is directed at identification of the cause and severity of the speech problem. Multiview videofluorscopy is a useful modality for semiquantitatively assessing both the type and extent of velopharyngeal closure. It involves static and dynamic frontal and lateral views of the velopharynx. It can be performed at an early age (usually from age 2 onward) and avoids the need for an invasive approach. Nasometry is performed from age 3 onward and involves placement of air pressure transducers inside the nostril and mouth. This enables measurement of oral and nasal air pressure, nasal airflow, and also facilitates calculation of the velopharyngeal port size. Nasoendoscopy can be performed from age 4 onward and allows qualitative assessment of velopharyngeal closure patterns and port size. MRI is used as an adjunct to velopharyngeal dysfunction and provides only static rather than dynamic views. Perceptual speech evaluation is not an instrumented assessment. It is undertaken by the speech and language therapist. Both spontaneous speech and provocative speech samples are assessed.[1-3]

REFERENCES

1. Croft CB, Shprintzen RJ, Rakoff SJ. Patterns of velopharyngeal valving in normal and cleft palate subjects: a multi-view videofluoroscopic and nasendoscopic study. Laryngoscope 1981;91(2):265–271
2. Perry JL, Sutton BP, Kuehn DP, Gamage JK. Using MRI for assessing velopharyngeal structures and function. Cleft Palate Craniofac J 2014;51(4):476–485
3. Siegel-Sadewitz VL, Shprintzen RJ. Nasopharyngoscopy of the normal velopharyngeal sphincter: an experiment of biofeedback. Cleft Palate J 1982;19(3):194–200

TREATMENT OPTIONS FOR VELOPHARYNGAL DYSFUNCTION

8. *According to commonly accepted algorithms, what is the recommended surgical intervention in moderate to large gap (noncoronal) velopharyngeal dysfunction?*

   D. Pharyngeal flap

   Some authorities propose an algorithmic approach to the surgical management of velopharyngeal dysfunction. This is dependent on the location and size of the velopharyngeal port closure deficiency:

   - Small to moderate gap and anterior midpalate velar musculature—re-repair palate and retroposition muscle (straight line or Furlow)
   - Small to moderate gap and posterior velar musculature—consider palatal lengthening with buccal myomucosal flaps or pharyngoplasty (for touch closure—consider velar fat grafting or re-repair of palate)
   - Large gap and short but highly mobile palate—consider palatal lengthening with buccal myomucosal flaps
   - Large gap and coronal closure pattern—consider pharyngoplasty
   - Large gap and noncoronal closure pattern—pharyngeal flap

   However, a recent meta-analysis refutes the effectiveness of this theoretical approach and suggests that a pharyngeal flap is the superior choice in most cases.[1-3]

REFERENCES

1. Naran S, Ford M, Losee JE. What's new in cleft palate and velopharyngeal dysfunction management? Plast Reconstr Surg 2017;139(6):1343e–1355e
2. Abyholm F, D'Antonio L, Davidson Ward SL, et al; VPI Surgical Group. Pharyngeal flap and sphincterplasty for velopharyngeal insufficiency have equal outcome at 1 year postoperatively: results of a randomized trial. Cleft Palate Craniofac J 2005;42(5):501–511
3. Collins J, Cheung K, Farrokhyar F, Strumas N. Pharyngeal flap versus sphincter pharyngoplasty for the treatment of velopharyngeal insufficiency: a meta-analysis. J Plast Reconstr Aesthet Surg 2012;65(7):864–868

TREATMENT OPTIONS FOR VELOPHARYNGAL DYSFUNCTION

9. *Which one of the following has a limited success and a high complication rate in treating velopharyngeal dysfunction?*

   E. Posterior pharyngeal wall augmentation

   Posterior wall augmentation creates a static posterior obstruction and can be achieved using injectable substances such as fat, collagen, or Teflon. Although it is quick and relatively simple, it is less effective than other surgical techniques and there is a risk of migration, extrusion, or embolization of the injected material. This is of particular concern where the internal carotid arteries are medialized and lie just deep to the posterior pharyngeal wall as can occur in velocardiofacial syndrome. It can also result in obstructive sleep apnoea.[1,2]

REFERENCES

1. Woo AS. Velopharyngeal dysfunction. Semin Plast Surg 2012;26(4):170–177
2. Mehendale FV, Sommerlad BC. Surgical significance of abnormal internal carotid arteries in velocardiofacial syndrome in 43 consecutive Hynes pharyngoplasties. Cleft Palate Craniofac J 2004;41(4):368–374

SURGICAL TECHNIQUES IN VELOPHARYNGEAL DYSFUNCTION

10. *What do the Hynes and Orticochea pharyngoplasty techniques have in common?*

D. The creation of a sphincter at the velopharyngeal port

The Hynes and Orticochea procedures are both types of sphincter pharyngoplasty. Although they are based on the same principle of raising pharyngeal wall flaps to create a sphincter at the velopharyngeal port, they differ in a number of ways. The Hynes technique involves bilateral superiorly based salpingopharyngeus musculomucosal flaps whereas the Orticochea technique involves bilateral superiorly based palatopharyngeus musculomucosal flaps. In addition, the Orticochea technique utilizes a third, inferiorly based, posterior pharyngeal wall flap. The flaps from the Orticochea technique are attached in an overlapped fashion to the posterior pharyngeal wall and covered by the third flap. Neither technique involves Z-plasties.[1,2]

REFERENCES

1. Hynes W. Pharyngoplasty by muscle transplantation. Br J Plast Surg 1950;3(2):128–135
2. Orticochea M. Construction of a dynamic muscle sphincter in cleft palates. Plast Reconstr Surg 1968;41(4):323–327

SURGICAL TECHNIQUES FOR VELOPHARYNGEAL DYSFUNCTION

11. *Which one of the following techniques for velopharyngeal dysfunction represents an obstructive technique and creates a permanent tissue bridge between the velum and posterior pharyngeal wall?*

A. Pharyngeal flap

Surgical procedures to treat velopharyngeal dysfunction can be categorized as either obstructive or nonobstructive. Obstructive techniques include the pharyngeal flap and pharyngoplasty. Nonobstructive techniques include the double opposing Z-plasty, straight line palate repair, palatal lengthening using buccal flaps, velar fat grafting, and posterior pharyngeal wall augmentation. Pharyngeal flap surgery involves raising a flap of mucosa and pharyngeal constrictor from the posterior pharyngeal wall and insetting this into the soft palate. This results in a permanent tissue bridge from the velum to the posterior pharyngeal wall and nasal airflow is achieved through the created two lateral ports. Velopharyngeal function is achieved by movement of the lateral pharyngeal walls medially to close the ports. The flap may be either superiorly or inferiorly based and varied in terms of size and inset (**Fig. 31.2**).[1–5]

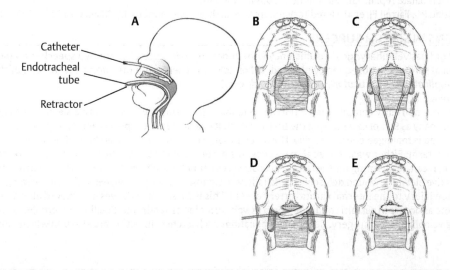

Fig. 31.2   Sphincter pharyngoplasty. *A,* A catheter is passed transnasally and attached to the uvula. *B,* Proposed incisions (*dashed lines*) are shown. *C,* Both tonsillar pillar flaps are elevated. *D,* Palatopharyngeal fl aps are rotated through 90 degrees. They are ready for attachment to the posterior pharyngeal wall. *E,* Completed sphincter pharyngoplasty. The flaps are overlapped and sutured to each other and to the posterior pharyngeal wall. (From Bentz ML, Bauer BS, Zuker RM. Principles & Practice of Pediatric Plastic Surgery. St Louis: Quality Medical Publishing, 2007.)

REFERENCES

1. Hogan VM. A clarification of the surgical goals in cleft palate speech and the introduction of the lateral port control (l.p.c.) pharyngeal flap. Cleft Palate J 1973;10:331–345
2. Naran S, Ford M, Losee JE. What's new in cleft palate and velopharyngeal dysfunction management? Plast Reconstr Surg 2017;139(6):1343e–1355e
3. Jackson IT, Silverton JS. The sphincter pharyngoplasty as a secondary procedure in cleft palates. Plast Reconstr Surg 1977;59(4):518–524
4. Hynes W. Pharyngoplasty by muscle transplantation. Br J Plast Surg 1950;3(2):128–135
5. Woo AS. Velopharyngeal dysfunction. Semin Plast Surg 2012;26(4):170–177

POSTOPERATIVE CARE VELOPHARYNGEAL DYSFUNCTION

12. In which patient group is postoperative airway management particularly important?

    C. Pierre Robin sequence

The most significant complication following velopharyngeal surgery is airway obstruction and this occurs in approximately 10% of patients. Approximately 1% will require reintubation. The risk will be affected by other factors such as mandibular size, age at surgery, and respiratory function. Therefore, airway monitoring is vital in all postoperative patients undergoing velopharyngeal surgery. However, Pierre Robin patients are particularly at risk because the sequence includes the triad of micrognathia/retrognathia, glossoptosis, and airway obstruction that can be exacerbated by speech surgery. Adenoidectomy can exacerbate velopharyngeal dysfunction (VPD), as it can increase the physical distance required to achieve velopharyngeal (VP) closure during speech. Velocardiofacial syndrome may be associated with VPD in conjunction with abnormal facies and cardiovascular abnormalities. Stickler syndrome often involves cleft palate in conjunction with a collagen gene mutation, leading to ocular malformations, hearing loss, and arthropathies. VPD may also be present. These conditions do not specifically predispose to airway issues.[1-5]

REFERENCES

1. Gangopadhyay N, Mendonca DA, Woo AS. Pierre Robin sequence. Semin Plast Surg 2012;26(2):76–82
2. Shprintzen RJ. The implications of the diagnosis of Robin sequence. Cleft Palate Craniofac J 1992;29(3):205–209
3. Saunders NC, Hartley BEJ, Sell D, Sommerlad B. Velopharyngeal insufficiency following adenoidectomy. Clin Otolaryngol Allied Sci 2004;29(6):686–688
4. Jackson OA, Kaye AE, Lee A, et al. Orofacial manifestations of Stickler syndrome: an analysis of speech outcome and facial growth after cleft palate repair. Ann Plast Surg 2020;84(6):665–671
5. Stickler GB, Belau PG, Farrell FJ, et al. Hereditary progressive arthro-ophthalmopathy. Mayo Clin Proc 1965;40:433–455

COMPLICATIONS IN SPEECH SURGERY

13. A 6-year-old girl has velopharyngeal insufficiency with poor speech in spite of continued speech therapy. Velopharyngeal surgery is subsequently planned. When taking consent from the parents, which one of the following complications is particularly important to discuss?

    B. Sleep apnea

The most common early complication following velopharyngeal surgery is obstructive sleep apnea and this can occur in as many as 90% of cases during the first 1–2 days. It usually resolves spontaneously as postoperative edema decreases and is managed conservatively. However, in some circumstances (less than 1%) intubation is required in the short term. Either way, it is vital to discuss this preoperatively as the effects can be life threatening and even if not, it can be alarming for the family to observe. Other potential complications include intraoperative and postoperative bleeding, wound dehiscence, and failure to significantly improve speech. Life-threatening bleeds can occur when injury to the internal carotid artery occurs. This is a risk when the vessel is placed aberrantly toward the midline as occurs in certain conditions such as velocardiofacial syndrome. Swallowing problems are unlikely following velopharyngeal surgery. General complications such as chest infection are also unlikely in most cases.[1-4]

REFERENCES

1. Abyholm F, D'Antonio L, Davidson Ward SL, et al; VPI Surgical Group. Pharyngeal flap and sphincterplasty for velopharyngeal insufficiency have equal outcome at 1 year postoperatively: results of a randomized trial. Cleft Palate Craniofac J 2005;42(5):501–511
2. Ettinger RE, Oppenheimer AJ, Lau D, et al. Obstructive sleep apnea after dynamic sphincter pharyngoplasty. J Craniofac Surg 2012;23(7, Suppl 1)1974–1976
3. Valnicek SM, Zuker RM, Halpern LM, Roy WL. Perioperative complications of superior pharyngeal flap surgery in children. Plast Reconstr Surg 1994;93(5):954–958
4. Fraulin FO, Valnicek SM, Zuker RM. Decreasing the perioperative complications associated with the superior pharyngeal flap operation. Plast Reconstr Surg 1998;102(1):10–18

32. Microtia

See *Essentials of Plastic Surgery*, third edition, pp. 400–414

DEMOGRAPHICS OF MICROTIA

1. *Which one of the following statements is correct regarding microtia demographics?*
   A. Males and females are equally affected.
   B. There are only subtle racial differences in incidence.
   C. It most commonly affects the left ear.
   D. Risk increases in a mother's fifth child.
   E. The incidence is approximately 1:2500 births worldwide.

EMBRYOLOGY AND PATHOPHYSIOLOGY OF MICROTIA

2. *Which one of the following statements is correct regarding the embryology of external ear development?*
   A. The ear develops from the second and third branchial arches.
   B. Nine identifiable hillocks are involved in normal ear development.
   C. The "free ear fold model" suggests there are no hillocks in ear development.
   D. Teratogens that are present in the second trimester have most profound effects on microtia.
   E. The tragus, helical root, and superior helix are formed from three anterior hillocks.

ASSOCIATED HEARING ABNORMALITIES WITH MICROTIA

3. *Which one of the following statements is correct regarding microtia?*
   A. Middle ear and external auditory canal defects are not usually involved.
   B. The severity of the external ear deformity is inversely related to hearing function.
   C. Sensorineural hearing deficits are more common than conductive deficits.
   D. CT imaging is strongly indicated in microtia patients with aural atresia.
   E. The cochlear, semicircular canals, and ossicles are usually preserved.

CURRENT CLASSIFICATION OF MICROTIA

4. A child presents with a remnant ear lobule that has a concha, acoustic meatus, and tragus. *What type of microtia does this represent when using current terminology?*
   A. Anotia type
   B. Conchal type
   C. Lobular type
   D. Small conchal type
   E. Atypical type

CONSIDERATIONS FOR RECONSTRUCTION IN MICROTIA

5. *When considering approaches to ear reconstruction, which one of the following statements is correct?*
   A. Middle ear surgery should be performed before autologous ear reconstruction.
   B. Silastic frameworks are a popular, reliable alternative to autologous reconstruction.
   C. Porous polyethylene has acceptable short-term results, but longer term outcomes are unproven.
   D. Osseointegrated prosthetic reconstruction should only be considered after failed reconstruction.
   E. Bone-anchored hearing devices have a key role for microtia patients with hearing loss.

THE MARX CLASSIFICATION SYSTEM FOR MICROTIA

6. You have been asked to present a case of microtia on the morning ward round and have selected to use the Marx/Rogers classification system to help you describe the deformity. *What is the key advantage of using this classification system?*
   A. It accurately guides surgical management.
   B. It is simple and straightforward to use.
   C. It considers the finer details about the ear deformity.
   D. It considers the hearing disability.
   E. It gives consideration to prominent ear deformity.

THE NAGATA TECHNIQUE FOR EAR RECONSTRUCTION

7. You are performing a Nagata technique autologous ear reconstruction. *Which one of the following statements is correct?*
   A. Reconstruction can begin at a younger age than with a porous polyethylene technique.
   B. The process will typically require three separate surgical stages.
   C. The preferred rib donors are the contralateral 4th and 5th.
   D. Perichondrium is included when harvesting the costal graft.
   E. Both the lobule and tragus are reconstructed in the first stage.

HIGH DENSITY POROUS POLYETHEYLENE EAR RECONSTRUCTION

8. You are performing ear reconstruction for microtia using a polyethylene construct. *Which one of the following is correct regarding this type of reconstruction according to Reinisch's approach?*
   A. Total implant coverage must be achieved with a temporoparietal fascial flap.
   B. A two-piece polyethylene ear prosthesis is linked together using permanent sutures.
   C. Suction drains should be avoided as they risk skin necrosis and implant extrusion.
   D. Skin is provided by recycling the microtic ear and combining with scalp split graft.
   E. A custom, premanufactured foam splint is used for 5 days following surgery.

COMPLICATIONS OF AUTOLOGOUS EAR RECONSTRUCTION

9. You are consenting the parents of a 9-year-old child for autologous ear reconstruction. *Which one of the following statements is correct?*
   A. Risk of chest wall deformity could be reduced by delaying the first stage of surgery.
   B. If skin loss develops over the construct, a further surgical procedure will be required.
   C. The procedure carries a relatively high risk of postoperative infection.
   D. Hematoma formation is rare and is usually self-limiting.
   E. The reconstructed ear will remain a static size as the child continues to grow.

Answers

DEMOGRAPHICS OF MICROTIA

1. Which one of the following statements is correct regarding microtia demographics?

D. Risk increases in a mother's fifth child.

The risk of microtia increases with maternal parity beyond four pregnancies, especially with anotia (the most severe form). Males are twice as likely to have microtia compared with females of the same race. Microtia displays significant racial variance with increased incidence in people of Japanese and Hispanic descent compared with whites. Some nonpopulation studies have shown exceptionally high risk in Navajo Native American, Chileans, and Ecuadorians. Unilateral microtia is far more common than bilateral, representing between 75 and 93% of cases. Right-sided microtia is most common (60%). The overall incidence varies from 8 to 43:100,000 births. Other risk factors include advanced maternal age, maternal insulin dependent diabetes mellitus (IDDM), advanced paternal age, multiple births, low birth weight, acute maternal illness, and teratogens such as alcohol and Accutane.[1–4]

REFERENCES

1. Harris J, Källén B, Robert E. The epidemiology of anotia and microtia. J Med Genet 1996;33(10):809–813
2. Luquetti DV, Heike CL, Hing AV, Cunningham ML, Cox TC. Microtia: epidemiology and genetics. Am J Med Genet A 2012;158A(1):124–139
3. Castilla EE, Orioli IM. Prevalence rates of microtia in South America. Int J Epidemiol 1986;15(3):364–368
4. Jaffe BF. The incidence of ear diseases in the Navajo Indians. Laryngoscope 1969;79(12): 2126–2134

EMBRYOLOGY AND PATHOPHYSIOLOGY OF MICROTIA

2. Which one of the following statements is correct regarding the embryology of external ear development?

E. The tragus, helical root, and superior helix are formed from three anterior hillocks.

The traditional theory of ear development suggests that the ear develops from the first and second branchial (pharyngeal) arches (not the second and third). It arises from six buds of mesenchyme, known as the hillocks of His. These were originally described by Wilheim His, hence the name. These are numbered from 1 to 6 with the first three formed by the first arch and the second three formed by the second arch. Each hillock relates to an adult component of the ear:

Hillock 1: Tragus
Hillock 2: Helical root
Hillock 3: Ascending helical rim
Hillock 4: Superior scapha and helical rim
Hillock 5: Inferior scapha and conchal bowl
Hillock 6: Lobule

The external auditory canal is formed by the first branchial (pharyngeal) cleft. The first 6–8 weeks of gestation (i.e., the first trimester) are the most significant with regard to development of microtia so teratogens would have impact at this stage of development.[1–3]

There have been newer concepts described regarding human auricular development. One suggestion is that the contribution of the posterior hillocks is limited to the concha, the body of antihelix, the triangular fossa, and the inferior crus. In this model, the helix, scapha, and superior crus are derived from the "free ear fold' that develops separately from the second pharyngeal arch hillocks from tissue immediately caudal to the second arch. This theory therefore does not suggest hillocks do not exist (**Fig. 32.1**).[4]

REFERENCES

1. Streeter GL. Development of the auricle in the human embryo. Carnegie Instn. Wash. Publ. 277, Contrib Embryol 1922;14:111–138.
2. Moore KL, Persaud TV, Torchia MD, eds. The Developing Human: Clinically Oriented Embryology. 10th ed. Philadelphia: Elsevier; 2016
3. Sadler TW, ed. Langman's Medical Embryology. 13th ed. Philadelphia: Wolters Kluwer Health; 2014
4. Porter CJ, Tan ST. Congenital auricular anomalies: topographic anatomy, embryology, classification, and treatment strategies. Plast Reconstr Surg 2005;115(6):1701–1712

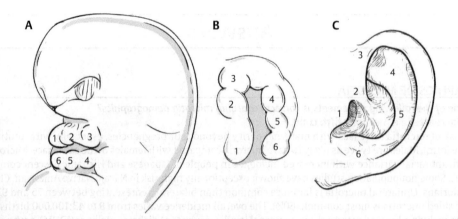

Fig. 32.1   Embryology of the external ear. *A,* Hillock formation in an 11-mm human embryo. *B,* Hillock configuration in a 15-mm embryo at 6 weeks of gestation. *C,* Adult auricle with hillock derivations. (Adapted from Beahm EK, Walton RL. Auricular reconstruction for microtia. Part I: Anatomy, embryology and clinical evaluation. Plast Reconstr Surg 109:2473–2782, 2002.)

ASSOCIATED HEARING ABNORMALITIES WITH MICROTIA

3.   Which one of the following statements is correct regarding microtia?

   D.   CT imaging is strongly indicated in microtia patients with aural atresia.

   Many patients with microtia also have aural atresia which itself is associated with hearing loss and canal cholesteatoma. Patients with aural atresia should undergo CT imaging as part of their workup. CT findings form part of the Jahrsdoerfer criteria which can help predict the likely hearing outcomes following surgery in patients with aural atresia. The Jahrsdoerfer grading system[1,2] is based on the appearance of the external ear and the findings on temporal CT including the appearance of the stapes. The grade assigned preoperatively has been shown to correlate well with the patient's chance of successful outcome in terms of postoperative speech reception. Knowledge of these specifics is highly relevant to plastic surgeons working with microtia patients and highlights the multidisciplinary approach required for such patients.

   Middle ear and external auditory canal defects are very commonly associated with microtia. There seems to be correlation between the severity of the external defect and severity of middle ear dysfunction. The most common type of hearing loss is conductive (>90% of cases), not sensorineural (10–15% of cases). Conductive loss can be caused by absence or fusion of the ossicles/ossicular chain. The ossicles are frequently absent as they are embryologically related to external ear development. In contrast, the cochlea and semicircular canals have a distinctly different embryological origin as they develop from the otic placode which is an ectodermal thickening not associated with the pharyngeal arches.[3]

REFERENCES

1. Jahrsdoerfer RA, Yeakley JW, Aguilar EA, Cole RR, Gray LC. Grading system for the selection of patients with congenital aural atresia. Am J Otol 1992;13(1):6–12
2. Kountakis SE, Helidonis E, Jahrsdoerfer RA. Microtia grade as an indicator of middle ear development in aural atresia. Arch Otolaryngol Head Neck Surg 1995;121(8):885–886
3. Sadler TW, ed. Langman's Medical Embryology. 13th ed. Philadelphia: Wolters Kluwer Health; 2014

CURRENT CLASSIFICATION OF MICROTIA

4.   A child presents with a remnant ear lobule that has a concha, acoustic meatus, and tragus. *What type of microtia does this represent when using current terminology?*

   B.   Conchal type

   The currently favored classification system for microtia is based on the surgical correction of the deformity as described by Nagata.[1] The classification system is as follows:

   Anotia: Absence of auricular tissue

   Lobular type: A remnant ear with a lobule and helix but without a concha, acoustic meatus, or tragus

   Conchal type: A remnant ear and lobule with a concha, acoustic meatus, and tragus

   Small conchal type: A remnant ear and lobule with a small indentation of the concha

   Atypical microtia: Cases that do not fall into the previous categories

A further classification worth knowing for exam purposes is that described by Tanzer[2] who previously classified auricular deformities into five types, some of which are then further subclassified. Type IV is subdivided into a, b, and c. The constricted ear is IVa, cryptocia (buried ear) is type IVb, and a hypoplastic upper one-third is IVc. The full classification is as follows:

Type I: Anotia
Type IIa: Microtia with atresia of the external auditory meatus
Type IIb: Microtia without atresia of the external auditory meatus
Type III: Hypoplasia of the middle third of the ear
Type IVa: Constricted ear
Type IVb: Cryptocia
Type IVc: Hypoplasia of the entire upper third of the ear
Type V: Prominent ear

In clinical practice, it is entirely reasonable to accurately describe the appearance of the microtia and support this pictorially with photographic images rather than try to use one of the classification schemes.

REFERENCES

1. Nagata S. A new method of total reconstruction of the auricle for microtia. Plast Reconstr Surg 1993;92(2):187–201
2. Tanzer RC, ed. Reconstructive Plastic Surgery. 2nd ed. Philadelphia: WB Saunders; 1977

CONSIDERATIONS FOR RECONSTRUCTION IN MICROTIA

5. *When considering approaches to ear reconstruction, which one of the following statements is correct?*

   E. Bone-anchored hearing devices have a key role for microtia patients with hearing loss.

   Conductive hearing loss affects around 90% of patients with microtia and therefore bone-anchored conductive hearing devices have a key role in management of these patients. This is important to consider in the multidisciplinary setting as the type of surgery and the order of surgery both need to be discussed by the otologist and plastic surgeon. For example, middle ear surgery is usually performed after autologous auricular reconstruction whereas if alloplastic reconstruction is planned, the canal is reconstructed first. Either way, it is important to liaise with the otologist to plan access so that flap and skin vascularity are not compromised, and optimal aesthetic positioning can be achieved.[1] Silastic frameworks as described by Cronin[2] have high extrusion rates, so they are not currently used in spite of the early excellent aesthetic appearance. In contrast, porous polyethylene implants for ear reconstruction were also shown to have good short-term aesthetic results and low rates of extrusion, and now, longer term results have proven to be good.[3,4] Osseointegrated prosthetic reconstruction has a role in many cases and should not be reserved solely for cases in which autologous reconstruction has failed. Although outcomes will be affected by the availability of skilled anaplastologists and manufacturing procedures, prostheses can provide very good aesthetic outcomes. They are particularly useful following trauma, cancer, irradiation, and in the elderly.[5]

REFERENCES

1. Mandelbaum RS, Volpicelli EJ, Martins DB, et al. Evaluation of 4 outcomes measures in microtia treatment: exposures, infections, aesthetics, and psychosocial ramifications. Plast Reconstr Surg Glob Open 2017;5(9):e1460
2. Cronin TD. Use of a silastic frame for total and subtotal reconstruction of the external ear: preliminary report. Plast Reconstr Surg 1966;37(5):399–405
3. Reinisch J, Tahiri Y. Polyethylene ear reconstruction: a state-of-the-art surgical journey. Plast Reconstr Surg 2018;141(2):461–470
4. Reinisch J. Ear reconstruction in young children. Facial Plast Surg 2015;31(6):600–603
5. Giot JP, Labbé D, Soubeyrand E, et al. Prosthetic reconstruction of the auricle: indications, techniques, and results. Semin Plast Surg 2011;25(4):265–272

THE MARX CLASSIFICATION SYSTEM FOR MICROTIA

6. You have been asked to present a case of microtia on the morning ward round and have selected to use the Marx/Rogers classification system to help you describe the deformity. *What is the key advantage of using this classification system?*

   B. It is simple and straightforward to use.

   The Marx/Rogers classification system is popular because it is simple and straightforward to use. It has just four classification grades and considers the appearance in simple descriptive terms only. It does not accurately guide surgical management, nor consider the finer anatomic details of the ear.[1,2] The Weerda[3] and Tanzer[4,5] classifications provide far greater detail and the Nagata[6] classification is said to help guide surgical management. None of the classifications consider the hearing disability. Both the Tanzer and Weerda classifications consider prominent ear, but the Marx classification does not do so (**Table 32.1**).

Table 32.1　*Classification Systems for Microtia*

Marx/Rogers	
Grade I features of an ear	A smaller than normal auricle with all others normal
Grade II structures	An abnormal auricle with some recognizable normal
Grade III structures	An abnormal auricle with some nonrecognizable normal
Grade IV	Anotia

REFERENCES

1. Marx H. Die Missbildungen des ohres. In: Denker AK, ed. Handbuch der Spez Path Anatomie Histologie. Berlin: Springer; 1926
2. Meurman Y. Congenital microtia and meatal atresia; observations and aspects of treatment. AMA Arch Otolaryngol 1957;66(4):443–463
3. Weerda H. Classification of congenital deformities of the auricle. Facial Plast Surg 1988;5(5):385–388
4. Tanzer RC. Total reconstruction of the external ear. Plast Reconstr Surg Transplant Bull 1959;23(1):1–15
5. Tanzer RC. Microtia. Clin Plast Surg 1978;5(3):317–336
6. Nagata S. A new method of total reconstruction of the auricle for microtia. Plast Reconstr Surg 1993;92(2):187–201

THE NAGATA TECHNIQUE FOR EAR RECONSTRUCTION

7. You are performing a Nagata technique autologous ear reconstruction. *Which one of the following statements is correct?*
   E. Both the lobule and tragus are reconstructed in the first stage.
   The Nagata[1] technique for ear reconstruction is a two-stage procedure (not three) that uses ipsilateral costal cartilage from ribs five through nine. It cannot usually be performed until 10 years of age because cartilage volume is insufficient before this time. In contrast, reconstruction with porous polyethylene can be undertaken at age 5. The first stage of the Nagata technique involves creation of a cartilage construct from ipsilateral ribs six to nine. Most but not all of the perichondrium is left in the chest wall to minimize residual deformity. The construct is placed in a subcutaneous pocket, and simultaneous lobule transposition is performed. Tragal reconstruction is also performed during this stage. The second stage is usually performed 6 months later, and further cartilage is harvested from the fifth rib (unless it has already been banked) to provide a wedge underneath the main cartilage construct. A temporoparietal fascial flap is elevated and inset to cover the grafts. This is then covered with split-skin graft from the scalp.[1–5]

REFERENCES

1. Nagata S. A new method of total reconstruction of the auricle for microtia. Plast Reconstr Surg 1993;92(2):187–201
2. Nagata S. Modification of the stages in total reconstruction of the auricle: Part I. Grafting the three-dimensional costal cartilage framework for lobule-type microtia. Plast Reconstr Surg 1994;93(2):221–230, discussion 267–268
3. Nagata S. Modification of the stages in total reconstruction of the auricle: Part II. Grafting the three-dimensional costal cartilage framework for concha-type microtia. Plast Reconstr Surg 1994;93(2):231–242, discussion 267–268
4. Nagata S. Modification of the stages in total reconstruction of the auricle: Part III. Grafting the three-dimensional costal cartilage framework for small concha-type microtia. Plast Reconstr Surg 1994;93(2):243–253, discussion 267–268
5. Nagata S. Modification of the stages in total reconstruction of the auricle: Part IV. Ear elevation for the constructed auricle. Plast Reconstr Surg 1994;93(2):254–266, discussion 267–268

HIGH DENSITY POROUS POLYETHEYLENE EAR RECONSTRUCTION

8. You are performing ear reconstruction for microtia using a polyethylene construct. *Which one of the following is correct regarding this type of reconstruction according to Reinisch's approach?*
   A. Total implant coverage must be achieved with a temporoparietal fascial flap.
   The key to successful outcome with high-density porous polyethylene ear reconstruction is to achieve total implant cover with a robust temporoparietal fascial flap. Reinisch found that extrusion rates were reduced from

44 to 7.3% by obtaining this complete coverage. During this procedure, a two-piece prosthesis is used. However, Reinisch prefers to avoid suturing the construct together and instead solders it with high temperature ophthalmic cautery. Following surgery suction drains are used under the implant and at the flap donor site, but these are removed the following day. Skin is provided by the microtic ear as well as from the mastoid and the contralateral posterior ear skin. These are used to graft the anterior aspect of the new ear over the temporoparietal flap. Further full-thickness graft is harvested from the groin and used to resurface the posterior aspect of the construct. A splint is used following surgery, but it is made from silicone, not foam. Furthermore, it is not premade, but is instead made on table using dental impression material. This is sutured to the scalp and left for 2 weeks and exchanged for a night splint that is worn for 6 months.[1-3]

REFERENCES

1. Reinisch J. Ear reconstruction in young children. Facial Plast Surg 2015;31(6):600–603
2. Reinisch J, Tahiri Y. Polyethylene ear reconstruction: a state-of-the-art surgical journey. Plast Reconstr Surg 2018;141(2):461–470
3. Reinisch JF, Lewin S. Ear reconstruction using a porous polyethylene framework and temporoparietal fascia flap. Facial Plast Surg 2009;25(3):181–189

COMPLICATIONS OF AUTOLOGOUS EAR RECONSTRUCTION

9. You are consenting the parents of a 9-year-old child for autologous ear reconstruction. *Which one of the following statements is correct?*

   A. **Risk of chest wall deformity could be reduced by delaying the first stage of surgery.**
   The most common late complication in ear reconstruction is chest wall deformity, which occurs in approximately two-thirds of cases. It is affected by age at the time of surgery and is reduced when surgery is performed after the age of 10. It is also reduced by leaving perichondrium at the donor site.[1,2] The most significant early complications are skin loss, infection, and hematoma, all of which are rare. However, each must be identified early and managed accordingly to prevent extrusion of the cartilage framework. Areas of skin loss should be debrided and only reconstructed if the area is greater than 1 cm. Smaller defects can be managed with dressings. Avoiding pressure dressings and replacing them with small suction drains has been shown to reduce skin-related complications from 33 to 1% in Brent's series.[1] Hematomas are not self-limiting and must be drained immediately to minimize risk of skin loss. Reconstructed ears commonly remained the same size over time (48%) but many increased in size as the child developed (42%) in Brent's series.[1]

REFERENCES

1. Brent B. Auricular repair with autogenous rib cartilage grafts: two decades of experience with 600 cases. Plast Reconstr Surg 1992;90(3):355–374, discussion 375–376
2. Nagata S. A new method of total reconstruction of the auricle for microtia. Plast Reconstr Surg 1993;92(2):187–201

33. Prominent Ear

See *Essentials of Plastic Surgery*, third edition, pp. 415–429

NORMAL EAR ANATOMY

1. *Which one of the following is true regarding the anatomy of the external ear?*
   A. The medial skin is dense, adherent, and thin.
   B. The ear grows to 95% of adult size by 2 years of age.
   C. Mature size is achieved in both sexes at the same age.
   D. Cartilage becomes less malleable with age and may calcify.
   E. Final ear length and height are reached the same time.

VASCULARITY OF THE EAR

2. *In addition to the posterior auricular artery, which other branch of the external carotid artery contributes a significant vascular supply to the ear?*
   A. Maxillary
   B. Facial
   C. Occipital
   D. Superficial temporal
   E. Deep temporal

INNERVATION TO THE EAR

3. *If a patient experiences numbness to most of the external ear following surgery, with preservation of the tragus, external auditory meatus, and helical root, which one of the following nerves is most likely to be affected?*
   A. Auriculotemporal
   B. Great auricular
   C. Facial
   D. Greater occipital
   E. Vagus

ASSESSMENT OF PROMINENT EARS

4. *Which one of the following is probably least relevant during the clinical assessment of a patient with prominent ears?*
   A. Depth and size of the conchal bowl
   B. Strength and spring of the auricular cartilage
   C. The angle between helical rim and mastoid plane
   D. Posterior inclination of the ear from the vertical plane
   E. Deformity of the lobule

CLINICAL FINDINGS IN PROMINENT EARS

5. *Which one of the following is a typical finding in a patient with prominent ears?*
   A. Overdevelopment of the antihelical fold
   B. A small diameter conchal bowl
   C. A conchoscaphal angle of more than 90 degrees
   D. A helical rim to mastoid distance of 10–20 mm
   E. Antihelical fold projection beyond the helical rim

TECHNIQUES FOR CORRECTION OF PROMINENT EARS

6. *Which one of the following represents a suture-based technique that is used for patients with upper pole prominence caused by a poorly defined antihelical fold?*
   A. Mustarde technique
   B. Furnas technique
   C. Converse-Wood technique
   D. Wood-Smith technique
   E. Chongchet

PERFORMING PINNAPLASTY SURGERY

7. **When performing otoplasty with a suture-based technique, which one of the following is true?**
   A. PDS is the preferred choice for the conchoscaphal sutures.
   B. The posterior skin incision should be placed at the level of the antihelical fold.
   C. The postauricular muscle attachments should be preserved.
   D. Conchomastoid sutures should take full-thickness bites of the cartilage.
   E. The new antihelical fold should follow a straight line cranially.

GIBSON'S PRINCIPLE

8. **Which one of the following pinnaplasty techniques is specifically based on Gibson's principle of interlocking stresses?**
   A. Cartilage scoring
   B. Cartilage molding
   C. Cartilage resection
   D. Cartilage breaking
   E. Cartilage reconstruction

PERFORMING OTOPLASTY

9. **When performing an otoplasty with anterior closed scoring in combination with a posterior approach suture technique, which one of the following surgical instruments is most likely to be particularly useful to help recreate the antihelical fold?**
   A. #11 blade scalpel
   B. Sharp Iris scissors
   C. 25-gauge hypodermic needle
   D. Freer elevator
   E. Otobrader

EAR ABNORMALITY IN CLINICAL PRACTICE

10. A patient is reviewed in clinic with concerns about the appearance of the right ear. On examination, the following findings are noted: From behind, the helix to mastoid distance is 12 mm superiorly and 20 mm inferiorly. From the front, the helix extends just beyond the antihelix all the way down. From the side, the ear is angled posteriorly at 30 degrees and there is a pointed thickening at the anterior junction of the upper and middle third of the helix. **What is the diagnosis in this case?**
    A. A normal ear
    B. A prominent ear
    C. A Stahl's ear
    D. A mastoid prominence
    E. A Darwin's tubercle

STAHL'S EAR DEFORMITY

11. **What is probably the most predictable and effective way to treat the Stahl's ear deformity?**
    A. A cartilage scoring otoplasty
    B. A cartilage molding otoplasty
    C. Lobule reduction surgery
    D. Cartilage excision surgery
    E. Local skin flaps

POSTOPERATIVE CARE AFTER OTOPLASTY

12. **Which one of the following is correct following otoplasty?**
    A. Dressings should be minimal and suture lines covered with antibiotic ointment.
    B. Hematomas are easily missed in the first 24 hours as they are usually pain free.
    C. The most common overall complication is infection leading to chondritis.
    D. Patients should be instructed to wear a headband at night for 3 months.
    E. Recurrence of prominence is the sole reason for needing surgical reoperation.

Answers

NORMAL EAR ANATOMY

1. *Which one of the following is true regarding the anatomy of the external ear?*

   D. Cartilage becomes less malleable with age and may calcify.

   The cartilage of the external ear is much softer and more malleable in infants and young children. This knowledge can be useful to guide treatment for prominent or misshapen ears. In the newborn baby, it may be possible to mold the ear with external splints comprised of tape, glue, and silicone.[1,2] Surgical correction of prominent ear is also ideally performed while the cartilage remains soft and hence surgery around the age of 5 represents a good time for this in terms of striking a balance between patient compliance, cartilage malleability, and schooling. With increasing age, it is more likely that cartilage weakening will be required as part of the surgical technique. Elderly patients my have calcification of the cartilage and this may have relevance where cartilage grafts are required for reconstruction of other areas such as the nose. The medial skin of the ear is loose fibrofatty and thick, whereas the lateral skin is more dense, adherent, and thinner. The ear grows to 85% of adult size by 3 years of age. Timing of ear development differs between the sexes. Ear development is complete 1 year earlier in girls. Maximum height and width occur at different developmental stages. In boys, maximum width typically occurs at the age of 7 years and maximum height at the age of 13 years. In girls, these occur at ages 6 and 12 years, respectively.[3-6]

REFERENCES

1. Tan ST, Abramson DL, MacDonald DM, Mulliken JB. Molding therapy for infants with deformational auricular anomalies. Ann Plast Surg 1997;38(3):263–268
2. Tan ST, Shibu M, Gault DT. A splint for correction of congenital ear deformities. Br J Plast Surg 1994;47(8):575–578
3. Allison GR. Anatomy of the external ear. Clin Plast Surg 1978;5(3):419–422
4. Adamson JE, Horton CE, Crawford HH. The growth pattern of the external ear. Plast Reconstr Surg 1965;36(4): 466–470
5. Farkas LG, Posnick JC, Hreczko TM. Anthropometric growth study of the ear. Cleft Palate Craniofac J 1992;29(4): 324–329
6. Janis JE, Rohrich RJ, Gutowski KA. Otoplasty. Plast Reconstr Surg 2005;115(4):60e–72e

VASCULARITY OF THE EAR

2. *In addition to the posterior auricular artery, which other branch of the external carotid artery contributes a significant vascular supply to the ear?*

   D. Superficial temporal

   The external ear receives its vascular supply from terminal branches of the external carotid artery. These are the posterior auricular (dominant supply) and the superficial temporal arteries. The occipital artery also contributes in a small number (7%) of patients.[1,2] The other branches of the external carotid artery can be remembered with a number of different mnemonics such as **S**ome **A**natomists **L**ove **F**acilitating **O**ur **P**recious **M**edical students. The branches are therefore:

   - **S**uperior thyroid
   - **A**scending pharyngeal
   - **L**ingual
   - **F**acial
   - **O**ccipital
   - **P**osterior auricular
   - **M**axillary
   - **S**uperficial temporal

REFERENCES

1. Allison GR. Anatomy of the external ear. Clin Plast Surg 1978;5(3):419–422
2. Farkas LG. Anthropometry of normal and anomalous ears. Clin Plast Surg 1978;5(3): 401–412

INNERVATION TO THE EAR

3. *If a patient experiences numbness to most of the external ear following surgery, with preservation of the tragus, external auditory meatus, and helical root, which one of the following nerves is most likely to be affected?*

B. Great auricular

A number of nerves supply sensation to the skin of the external ear and the main one is the great auricular nerve, which is a branch of the cervical plexus C2/C3. This runs up the superficial surface of sternocleidomastoid in the neck to supply the lower two-thirds of the lateral aspect including the lobule as well as most of the medial surface with the exception of the conchal bowl and the anterior-most aspect of the upper third which includes the tragus, the helical root, and the first part of the helical rim. This nerve is at risk of injury during surgical procedures involving the neck. The auriculotemporal nerve is a branch of the trigeminal nerve (V_3) that supplies sensation to the tragus, helical root, and first part of the ascending helical rim. The glossopharyngeal, vagus, and facial nerves contribute to Arnold's nerve, which supplies sensation to the external auditory canal. The greater and lesser occipital nerves originate from the cervical plexus. The lesser occipital nerve supplies the area to the superior surface of the ear, whereas the greater occipital supplies the scalp above the ear.[1,2]

REFERENCES

1. Allison GR. Anatomy of the external ear. Clin Plast Surg 1978;5(3):419–422
2. Farkas LG. Anthropometry of normal and anomalous ears. Clin Plast Surg 1978;5(3): 401–412

ASSESSMENT OF PROMINENT EARS

4. *Which one of the following is probably least relevant during the clinical assessment of a patient with prominent ears?*

D. Posterior inclination of the ear from the vertical plane

A full assessment of the characteristics of the external ear should be made in clinic when assessing a patient for otoplasty. All abnormalities need to be identified and documented and photographed preoperatively as they will have bearing on surgical approach and likely outcome in terms of patient satisfaction. Of all the factors described, the inclination in the vertical plane is probably least important with specific reference to ear prominence, but this should still be noted and highlighted to the patient if abnormal. Although not usually addressed with surgery, some techniques will allow the lateral prominence and the inclination in the vertical plane to be altered. For example, if a postauricular pocket (mastoid region) is created then the conchal bowl can be rotated posterosuperiorly into this, thereby decreasing prominence and posterior inclination. It can then be secured with a conchomastoid suture. The depth of the conchal bowl will affect ear prominence and needs to be assessed so it may be reduced or set back if required. The strength and spring of the auricular cartilage will guide the surgical decision-making process as stiff cartilage is unlikely to respond well to suture molding alone. The angle between the helical rim and mastoid plane is relevant and should ideally be less than 30 degrees. A lobule deformity may be addressed during otoplasty surgery and must be identified preoperatively.[1,2]

REFERENCES

1. Ellis DA, Keohane JD. A simplified approach to otoplasty. J Otolaryngol 1992;21(1):66–69
2. Janis JE, Rohrich RJ, Gutowski KA. Otoplasty. Plast Reconstr Surg 2005;115(4):60e–72e

CLINICAL FINDINGS IN PROMINENT EARS

5. *Which one of the following is a typical finding in a patient with prominent ears?*

C. A conchoscaphal angle of more than 90 degrees

The main causes of prominent ears are underdevelopment of the antihelical fold and conchal bowl excess. Often patients have a combination of both abnormalities. This results in conchoscaphal angles of more than 90 degrees and an increased helical–mastoid distance. Techniques used for prominent ear correction aim to address these issues. The distance between the mastoid and the helical rim differs at the top, middle, and bottom of the ear and ranges between 10 and 20 mm depending on location.

In the frontal view, a normal ear will have projection of the helical rim 2–5 mm beyond the antihelical fold. This is often exaggerated in prominent ears due to the underdevelopment of the antihelical fold. However, care must be taken when undertaking pinnaplasty to avoid overcorrection as having the antihelical fold as the most prominent part of the ear will look unnatural.[1–4]

REFERENCES

1. Ellis DA, Keohane JD. A simplified approach to otoplasty. J Otolaryngol 1992;21(1):66–69
2. Janis JE, Rohrich RJ, Gutowski KA. Otoplasty. Plast Reconstr Surg 2005;115(4):60e–72e
3. Adamson PA, Strecker HD. Otoplasty techniques. Facial Plast Surg 1995;11(4):284–300
4. McDowell AJ. Goals in otoplasty for protruding ears. Plast Reconstr Surg 1968;41(1):17–27

TECHNIQUES FOR CORRECTION OF PROMINENT EARS

6. *Which one of the following represents a suture-based technique that is used for patients with upper pole prominence caused by a poorly defined antihelical fold?*

   A. **Mustarde technique**

   Techniques for the correction of prominent ears can be classified as those involving sutures, cartilage scoring, cartilage breaking, or cartilage resection. Techniques can be combined in a single procedure, for example, scoring and suturing. The Mustarde technique[1] is a suture technique that is used to correct an underdeveloped antihelical fold. Mattress sutures are placed on either side of the planned fold to recreate it (**Figs. 33.1, A and** B). The Furnas technique[2] is a suture technique that is used to reduce conchal bowl prominence. Sutures are placed between

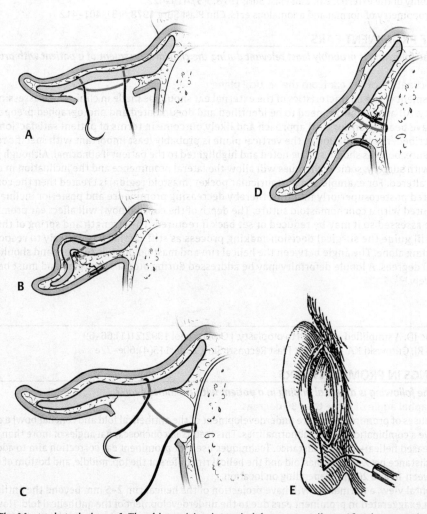

Fig. 33.1 The Mustarde technique: **A,** The skin excision is carried down to cartilage. After hemostasis is obtained, several sutures are placed through the full thickness of cartilage. Usually, two or three well-placed sutures are all that are required. **B,** The sutures are tied simultaneously. A subcuticular 4-0 nylon suture is used for closure. The Furnas technique: **C** and **D,** Several mattress sutures are used to attach conchal cartilage to the mastoid fascia. The mattress sutures should be placed through the full thickness of conchal cartilage. The sutures are tied simultaneously. Modified fishtail excision: **E,** A V-extension of the posterior auricular incision is drawn on the posterior surface of the lobule.

the mastoid and conchal bowl to reset the ear closer to the head (**Figs. 33.1, C and** D). The Converse-Wood-Smith[3] is a cartilage-breaking technique for correction of prominence of the entire ear. It also involves recreation of the antihelical fold with mattress sutures. Correction of the lobule can be combined with any of the techniques described by using a fishtail excision of skin from the posterior aspect of the lobule using the Wood-Smith technique (**Fig. 33.1,** E). Chongchet's technique[4] involves anterior blade scoring without sutures and is rarely used.[4]

REFERENCES

1. Mustarde JC. The correction of prominent ears using simple mattress sutures. Br J Plast Surg 1963;16:170–178
2. Furnas DW. Correction of prominent ears by conchamastoid sutures. Plast Reconstr Surg 1968;42(3):189–193
3. Converse JM, Wood-Smith D. Technical details in the surgical correction of the lop ear deformity. Plast Reconstr Surg 1963;31:118–128
4. Chongchet V. A method of antihelix reconstruction. Br J Plast Surg 1963;16:268–272

PERFORMING PINNAPLASTY SURGERY

7. *When performing otoplasty with a suture-based technique, which one of the following is true?*

D. Conchomastoid sutures should take full-thickness bites of the cartilage.

When placing sutures to set back the ear, it is important to ensure that the suture passes through the full thickness of the cartilage, without piercing the skin. The best way to achieve this is to feel the needle pass through the cartilage until there is slight give. Pausing for a moment with the needle in situ will allow for a check that it has not breached the skin anteriorly. Then the needle pass may be continued. When performing the deep suture placement in conchomastoid sutures, the suture should pass deep into mastoid fascia. The suture used should be permanent in most cases as this is less likely to result in recurrence of prominence. When performing otoplasty by a posterior approach, the incision should be placed close to or just in front of the posterior helical sulcus over the conchal cartilage. This is to minimize subsequent scar visibility post surgery. Many surgeons will remove a small width of skin at the same time via this incision, but this is not always necessary. When set back of the conchal bowl is planned, dissection of the ear posteriorly toward the mastoid is necessary to create a pocket in which the conchal bowl can sit. It is also necessary to gain access to the mastoid such that the scaphoconchal sutures can be placed. In order to do this, the postauricular muscles and ligaments will need to be divided or excised. This may be performed effectively with electrocautery. It is important to note that the antihelical fold is not a straight line, but actually follows a curve so scaphoconchal sutures must be placed to respect this.[1-5]

REFERENCES

1. Furnas DW. Correction of prominent ears by conchamastoid sutures. Plast Reconstr Surg 1968;42(3):189–193
2. Thorne CH. Otoplasty. Plast Reconstr Surg 2008;122(1):291–292
3. Sinno S, Chang JB, Thorne CH. Precision in otoplasty: combining reduction otoplasty with traditional otoplasty. Plast Reconstr Surg 2015;135(5):1342–1348
4. Mustarde JC. The correction of prominent ears using simple mattress sutures. Br J Plast Surg 1963;16:170–178
5. Janis JE, Rohrich RJ, Gutowski KA. Otoplasty. Plast Reconstr Surg 2005;115(4):60e–72e

GIBSON'S PRINCIPLE

8. *Which one of the following pinnaplasty techniques is specifically based on Gibson's principle of interlocking stresses?*

A. Cartilage scoring

Gibson's principle is based on the observation that cartilage will curl away from a cut surface because interlocking stresses are released when perichondrium is incised.[1] This is analogous to scoring cardboard on one side to allow it to fold. Gibson and Davis[1] published this work in 1958. Techniques that employ scoring are based on these principles. Cartilage is known to maintain its position because of the balancing forces of perichondrium on each side. When the perichondrium is incised on one side, the balance of forces is no longer equal, and the cartilage moves away from the incision. For this reason, anterior rather than posterior scoring has been more commonly performed and is generally advised for addressing antihelical fold underdevelopment. Suture techniques are termed cartilage molding procedures. For example, the Mustarde and Furnas techniques[2,3] rely solely on the ability of sutures to overpower the interlocking stresses within the cartilage construct, rather than break or unbalance them. Cartilage breaking or resection techniques such as the Converse–Wood-Smith approach[4] will obviously disrupt both sides of the perichondrium and the cartilage itself rather than release a single side of the perichondrium.

REFERENCES

1. Gibson T, Davis WB. The distortion of autogenous cartilage grafts: its cause and prevention. Br J Plast Surg 1958;10: 257–274
2. Mustarde JC. The correction of prominent ears using simple mattress sutures. Br J Plast Surg 1963;16:170–178
3. Furnas DW. Correction of prominent ears by conchamastoid sutures. Plast Reconstr Surg 1968;42(3):189–193
4. Converse JM, Wood-Smith D. Technical details in the surgical correction of the lop ear deformity. Plast Reconstr Surg 1963;31:118–128

PERFORMING OTOPLASTY

9. *When performing an otoplasty with anterior closed scoring in combination with a posterior approach suture technique, which one of the following surgical instruments is most likely to be particularly useful to help recreate the antihelical fold?*

   E. Otobrader

   When performing cartilage scoring otoplasty, it is generally accepted that scoring the anterior aspect of the cartilage is preferred to release perichondrium and allow recreation of the antihelical fold. This is often now combined with a suture technique involving a posterior approach with scaphoconchal mattress sutures. It is also accepted that minimizing the anterior skin dissection is best and therefore performing anterior scoring with minimal access is the goal. In order to facilitate this an otobrader can be used via either a small cartilage fenestration or a small anterior skin incision 3–4 mm in width. Otobraders are curved instruments paired for left and right that allow progressive and controlled removal of the anterior perichondrium along the line of the planned new antihelical fold. Their use helps avoid full-thickness scoring and cartilage damage. Many of the anterior scoring techniques have traditionally involved a full-thickness cartilage incision via a posterior skin approach which may be best avoided, meaning that a closed approach would be attractive.[1-4] In order to create a pocket for an anterior approach a small incision (3–4 mm) can be placed high up the ear under the helical rim, thereby leaving a well-disguised small scar. A #15 blade is ideal for this incision and tenotomy scissors can be used to dissect subcutaneously along the antihelical fold area. A 25- or 27-gauge needle is used to inject local anesthetic to the ear, while a 23- or 25-gauge needle is often used to mark the proposed antihelical fold using methylene blue. A bent 21-gauge injection needle has been used to score the cartilage anteriorly with minimal access but risks the needle tip breaking internally as the tip needs to be bent at a right angle. We have seen this occur in clinical practice.[5] A Freer elevator is used to lift perichondrium from cartilage during rhinoplasty.

REFERENCES

1. Salgarello M, Gasperoni C, Montagnese A, Farallo E. Otoplasty for prominent ears: a versatile combined technique to master the shape of the ear. Otolaryngol Head Neck Surg 2007;137(2):224–227
2. Hafiz R, Philandrianos C, Casanova D, Chossegros C, Bertrand B. Technical refinement of Stenström otoplasty procedure. Rev Stomatol Chir Maxillofac Chir Orale 2016;117(3): 147–150
3. Thorne CH, Wilkes G. Ear deformities, otoplasty, and ear reconstruction. Plast Reconstr Surg 2012;129(4): 701e–716e
4. Smittenberg MN, Marsman M, Veeger NJGM, Moues CM. Comparison of cartilage-scoring and cartilage-sparing otoplasty: a retrospective analysis of complications and aesthetic outcome of 1060 ears. Plast Reconstr Surg 2018;141(4): 500e–506e
5. Koul AR, Patil RK. An effective technique of helical cartilage scoring for correction of prominent ear deformity. Indian J Plast Surg 2011;44(3):505–508

EAR ABNORMALITY IN CLINICAL PRACTICE

10. A patient is reviewed in clinic with concerns about the appearance of the right ear. On examination, the following findings are noted: From behind, the helix to mastoid distance is 12 mm superiorly and 20 mm inferiorly. From the front, the helix extends just beyond the antihelix all the way down. From the side, the ear is angled posteriorly at 30 degrees and there is a pointed thickening at the anterior junction of the upper and middle third of the helix. *What is the diagnosis in this case?*

    E. A Darwin's tubercle

    Darwin's tubercle is a pointed thickening at the junction of the upper and middle third of the helix present in 1 in 10 individuals. This can be surgically treated with a full-thickness excision of the skin and the underlying prominent cartilage (**Fig. 33.2**). Because it is such a common finding with variation in severity, it may actually need no treatment at all. Aside from the description of Darwin's tubercle, the other measurements are all in keeping with a normal ear (**Box 33.1** and **Fig. 33.3**).[1,2]

    Stahl's ear refers to the presence of a third and/or horizontal superior crus with a pointed upper helix. Sometimes this is termed "Spock ears" and is associated with upper and mid-third helical prominence. A mastoid prominence will alter the appearance of the postauricular valley and can be surgically managed with either soft tissue or bone resection of this area.

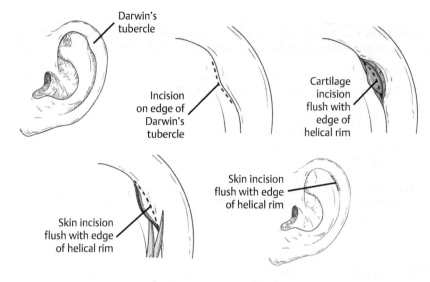

Fig. 33.2 Darwin's tubercle.

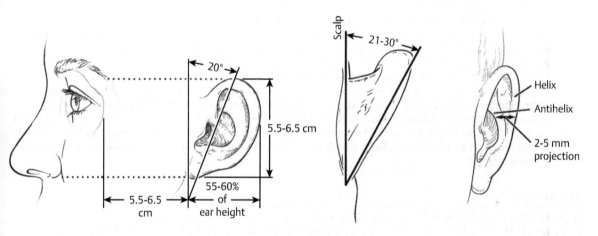

Fig. 33.3 Correct placement of ear.

Box 33.1 *Basic Goals of Otoplasty*

- Correction of all upper third protrusion
- Visibility of the helix beyond the antihelix when viewed from the front
- Smooth and regular helix
- No marked distortion or decrease in the depth of the postauricular sulcus
- Correct placement of the ear

The helix-to-mastoid distance falls in the normal range of 10–12 mm at the top, 16–18 mm in the middle, and 20–22 mm in the lower third.

- Bilateral symmetry

The position of the lateral ear border to the head matches within 3 mm at any point between the ears.

- Smooth, rounded, and well-defined antihelical fold
- Conchoscaphal angle of 90 degrees
- Conchal reduction or reduction of the conchomastoidal angle
- Helical rim that projects laterally farther than the lobule

REFERENCES

1. Millard DR, Pickard RE. Darwin's tubercle belongs to Woolner. Arch Otolaryngol 1970;91(4):334–335
2. Loh TY, Cohen PR. Darwin's tubercle: review of a unique congenital anomaly. Dermatol Ther (Heidelb) 2016;6(2):143–149

STAHL'S EAR DEFORMITY

11. *What is probably the most predictable and effective way to treat the Stahl's ear deformity?*

D. Cartilage excision surgery

Stahl's ear involves the presence of a third and/or horizontal superior crus with a pointed upper helix. This results in a pointy prominence in the upper and middle third of the ear ("Spock ear"). This has been traditionally felt to be challenging to correct. However, the most predictable and effective approach to treat Stahl's ear deformity is complete excision of the third crus through the helical rim.[1] The excised superior crus can then also be used as an onlay graft to create a superior crus if it is absent. The incision for this is within the scapha, similar to scapha reduction and a small scaphal cartilage excision may be used to facilitate forward rotation of the helical rim. The third crus is excised completely with a wedge excision of the helical rim skin extending onto the back of the ear. When closed, the wedge excision aids in forward rotation of the helical rim (**Fig. 33.4**).

REFERENCE

1. Thorne CH, Wilkes G. Ear deformities, otoplasty, and ear reconstruction. Plast Reconstr Surg 2012;129(4):701e–716e

POSTOPERATIVE CARE AFTER OTOPLASTY

12. *Which one of the following is correct following otoplasty?*

D. Patients should be instructed to wear a headband at night for 3 months.

Following otoplasty, most surgeons will advise patients to wear a headband at night for 3 months to protect the ears from mechanical trauma leading to recurrence of prominence. Although this is not evidence based, it makes sense in terms of wound healing and tissue remodeling. Following surgery, it is standard practice to protect the ears with layered dressings and a head bandage or similar. This is removed sometime between 4 and 7 days.

Hematomas probably represent the most common early complication and present with increasing pain in the first 24 hours after surgery. They should be treated swiftly with evacuation and hemostasis to reduce the risk of skin necrosis. Infection is a rare complication and is most likely due to *Staphylococcus*. It can in some circumstances lead to chondritis, which may need surgical debridement. Reoperation may be required following otoplasty, but this may not be solely due to recurrence of prominence. For example, it may be associated with suture problems such as sinuses, foreign body reaction, or extrusion. It may be for scar revision or adjustment for asymmetry.[1,2]

REFERENCES

1. Janis JE, Rohrich RJ, Gutowski KA. Otoplasty. Plast Reconstr Surg 2005;115(4):60e–72e
2. Thorne CH, Wilkes G. Ear deformities, otoplasty, and ear reconstruction. Plast Reconstr Surg 2012;129(4):701e–716e

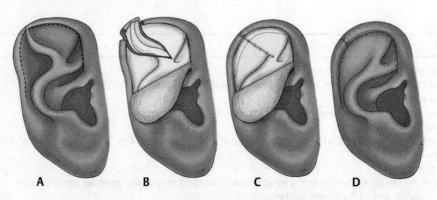

Fig. 33.4 Stahl's ear.

34. Facial Soft Tissue Trauma

See *Essentials of Plastic Surgery*, third edition, pp. 430–443

GENERAL PRINCIPLES IN THE MANAGEMENT OF SOFT TISSUE FACIAL WOUNDS

1. *When managing patients with soft tissue facial wounds, which one of the following is correct?*
   A. Formal assessment begins with administration of local anesthetic.
   B. Tetanus boosters are required for all patients with contaminated wounds.
   C. Abrasions are full-thickness skin defects, often managed with dressings.
   D. Permanent tattooing may be the result of inadequate debridement.
   E. Local flaps are often useful for closing wounds in the acute setting.

MANAGEMENT OF BITE WOUNDS

2. *In a patient with a human bite wound to the face, which one of the following is correct?*
   A. The wound should be debrided and left to heal by secondary intention.
   B. A course of amoxicillin should be prescribed for 7 days.
   C. *Pasteurella multocida* is the most likely pathogen to cause infection.
   D. Antibiotic coverage should target *Eikenella* and *Streptococcus*.
   E. The risk of developing infection is greater than with animal bites.

MANAGING SCALP WOUNDS

3. *Which one of the following methods of wound closure is recommended for the skin of the hair-bearing scalp to minimize alopecia?*
   A. Absorbable monofilament sutures
   B. Absorbable braided sutures
   C. Nonabsorbable monofilament sutures
   D. Nonabsorbable braided sutures
   E. Skin staples

WOUNDS TO THE PERIORAL AREAS

4. *You see a patient with a soft tissue injury involving the lip, cheek, and tongue. Which one of the following is correct?*
   A. Wharton's duct may be injured and should be repaired with microsurgical techniques.
   B. Divisions of the facial nerve close to the oral commissure require neurosyntheses.
   C. The parotid papilla should be located intraorally at the level of the canine to assess duct injury.
   D. The white roll should be marked with methylene blue following local anesthetic infiltration.
   E. Smaller lacerations of the tongue heal satisfactorily without surgical intervention.

ANATOMY OF THE FACIAL DUCTAL SYSTEMS

5. *Which one of the following structures drains directly into the common canaliculus and is often damaged in lower eyelid injuries?*
   A. Lacrimal gland
   B. Inferior canaliculus
   C. Lacrimal sac
   D. Superior canaliculus
   E. Valve of Hasner

CLINICAL SCENARIOS IN SOFT TISSUE FACIAL TRAUMA

6. *A 30-year-old man sustains an avulsion flap injury to the scalp in a motor vehicle accident. To what depth is the injury most likely to extend to?*
   A. Temporal bone
   B. Periosteum
   C. Frontalis
   D. Subcutaneous tissue
   E. Skin

NERVE INJURY IN SOFT TISSUE TRAUMA

7. A young male presents after an altercation in a bar. He was struck with a broken glass bottle and has a soft tissue wound that passes vertically from the zygomatic arch to the mandibular body. The wound does not breach the oral mucosa. *Which one of the following is least likely to be present on examination?*

    A. Weakness of the frontalis muscle
    B. Paresthesia to the ipsilateral ear helical root and lobule
    C. Weakness of the corrugator and procerus
    D. Saliva in the wound
    E. Loss of oral competence

SKIN PREPARATION

8. *Which one of the following is recommended for use as a facial skin preparation prior to surgery?*

    A. Chlorhexidine-gluconate
    B. Povidone-Iodine
    C. Hydrogen peroxide
    D. Normal saline
    E. Water

NERVE BLOCKS IN FACIAL TRAUMA SURGERY

9. *When providing nerve blocks in the head and neck region, which one of the following is true?*

    A. The midpupillary line will guide nerve blocks of the forehead, cheeks, and lips.
    B. A single point injection is effective at achieving a complete external ear block.
    C. Blocks to the three branches of the trigeminal nerve will completely anesthetize the face.
    D. Blocking the zygomaticotemporal nerve requires the use of a larger caliber needle.
    E. A mental nerve block should be administered at the mesial gum surface at the base of the 3rd molar.

Answers

GENERAL PRINCIPLES IN THE MANAGEMENT OF SOFT TISSUE FACIAL WOUNDS

1. When managing patients with soft tissue facial wounds, which one of the following is correct?

D. Permanent tattooing may be the result of inadequate debridement.

The principles of soft tissue wound management are careful examination of the patient and assessment of the injury, followed by meticulous sharp debridement, irrigation, and defect closure with repair of any specialized structures such as nerves and ducts. Inadequate debridement can lead to permanent tattooing of the skin. An example is road rash in a partial-thickness abrasion, where gravel left in the wound will be permanently visible as black pigment. Although local anesthetic is useful to helpfully assess and treat many wounds, it must not be used until nerve function has been assessed as it may mask underlying injury.

Although all patients should have their tetanus status checked, not all will need further tetanus doses. Current guidelines differ, with some advocating a booster every 10 years or at the time of an injury if no booster has been given within a 5-year period.[1] Even patients with tetanus-prone injuries do not require boosters, providing they have undergone complete immunization and received a booster within 5 years. There is often confusion regarding descriptions for soft tissue wounds. An abrasion is a scraped area of skin but may be partial or full thickness. Partial-thickness abrasions are generally treated with dressings, while full-thickness abrasions may require formal excision and direct closure, skin grafting, or flap coverage depending on size and location. Local flaps are not generally recommended for use in the acute setting, especially in wounds with crush components and should therefore be preserved for secondary reconstruction.[2,3]

REFERENCES

1. Mayo Clinic. Tetanus: prevention. Available at http://www.mayoclinic.com/health/tetanus/DS00227/DSECTION5prevention
2. Centers for Disease Control and Prevention (CDC). Deferral of routine booster doses of tetanus and diphtheria toxoids for adolescents and adults. MMWR Morb Mortal Wkly Rep 2001;50(20):418, 427
3. Update on adult immunization. Recommendations of the Immunization Practices Advisory Committee (ACIP). MMWR Recomm Rep 1991;40(RR-12):1–94

MANAGEMENT OF BITE WOUNDS

2. In a patient with a human bite wound to the face, which one of the following is correct?

D. Antibiotic coverage should target Eikenella and Streptococcus.

The most common pathogens implicated in infection in human bites are *Eikenella corrodens* and *Streptococcus viridans,* so antibiotics should be selected to target these organisms. Amoxicillin alone is not a suitable antibiotic for bite injuries and needs to be combined with clavulanate (Augmentin) to provide extended spectrum beta lactam coverage.

Most bite injuries should be left open to heal after debridement, but bites to the face should be closed primarily after debridement. An exception to this rule is where there is evidence of active infection. In this case, delayed primary closure is indicated after debridement and antibiotic treatment. *Pasteurella canis* and *Pasteurella multocida* are frequently associated with canine and feline bites, respectively. Although human bites can lead to severe infections, cat bites are most commonly associated with infection because of the deep, puncture type wounds and the virulent bacteria involved.[1-4]

REFERENCES

1. Talan DA, Citron DM, Abrahamian FM, Moran GJ, Goldstein EJ; Emergency Medicine Animal Bite Infection Study Group. Bacteriologic analysis of infected dog and cat bites. N Engl J Med 1999;340(2):85–92
2. Stefanopoulos PK. Management of facial bite wounds. Oral Maxillofac Surg Clin North Am 2009;21(2):247–257, vii
3. Talan DA, Abrahamian FM, Moran GJ, Citron DM, Tan JO, Goldstein EJ; Emergency Medicine Human Bite Infection Study Group. Clinical presentation and bacteriologic analysis of infected human bites in patients presenting to emergency departments. Clin Infect Dis 2003;37(11):1481–1489
4. Looke D, Dendle C. Bites (mammalian). BMJ Clin Evid 2015; 2015: 0914. Published online December 4, 2015

MANAGING SCALP WOUNDS

3. *Which one of the following methods of wound closure is recommended for the skin of the hair-bearing scalp to minimize alopecia?*

    E. Skin staples

    When closing scalp defects a layered approach is advised so the galea is approximated with interrupted absorbable sutures before skin closure. Skin closure can then be achieved with any of the above sutures; however, staples may cause the least tissue necrosis, provide adequate wound-edge eversion, and less subsequent scalp alopecia than other forms of closure.[1,2] Another advantage to staples is the ease and speed with which they can be placed. This is particularly useful in reducing bleeding from scalp wound edges. A disadvantage is that some patients find it painful when they are being removed. This can be minimized by ensuring the clips are fully opened before attempting to remove them. Alopecia may be further minimized by careful use of cautery at the wound edges. When planned incisions are made in the scalp, beveling the blade may also help reduce alopecia as this allows hair regrowth through the scar.

REFERENCES

1. Ritchie AJ, Rocke LG. Staples versus sutures in the closure of scalp wounds: a prospective, double-blind, randomized trial. Injury 1989;20(4):217–218
2. Brickman KR, Lambert RW. Evaluation of skin stapling for wound closure in the emergency department. Ann Emerg Med 1989;18(10):1122–1125

WOUNDS TO THE PERIORAL AREAS

4. You see a patient with a soft tissue injury involving the lip, cheek, and tongue. *Which one of the following is correct?*

    E. Smaller lacerations of the tongue heal satisfactorily without surgical intervention.

    Larger lacerations of the tongue notoriously break down because of the strength of the tongue musculature. For this reason layered closure is advocated in larger lacerations. However, smaller lacerations can be left to heal by secondary intention.[1,2]

    Although microsurgical repair of the parotid duct (Stensen's duct) is advocated, lacerations to Wharton's ducts, which are found on the floor of the mouth draining the submandibular gland, are usually managed with marsupialization. The parotid duct opens into the oral cavity at the level of the upper second molar (not canine) and should be identified in cases involving cheek or intraoral injury. Once the opening is identified, the duct can be stented with a 24-gauge angiocatheter and extravasation of saline indicates an injury that warrants repair.[3] When managing lip injuries, it is vital to ensure that close approximation of the white roll is achieved, as even small malalignments of 1 mm can be noticeable at short distances. For this reason, marking the white roll with methylene blue or a skin marking pen before (not after) infiltration with local anesthesia is recommended.[4] Once the local anesthetic has been infiltrated, distortion occurs that may limit the ability to accurately identify the white roll. Facial nerve lacerations medial to the lateral canthus do not usually require repair because of the significant arborization of the buccal and zygomatic branches.

REFERENCES

1. Lamell CW, Fraone G, Casamassimo PS, Wilson S. Presenting characteristics and treatment outcomes for tongue lacerations in children. Pediatr Dent 1999;21(1):34–38
2. Seiler M, Massaro SL, Staubli G, Schiestl C. Tongue lacerations in children: to suture or not? Swiss Med Wkly 2018;148:w14683
3. Lazaridou M, Iliopoulos C, Antoniades K, Tilaveridis I, Dimitrakopoulos I, Lazaridis N. Salivary gland trauma: a review of diagnosis and treatment. Craniomaxillofac Trauma Reconstr 2012;5(4):189–196
4. Thorne CH, Gosain A, et al, eds. Grabb and Smith's Plastic Surgery. Philadelphia, PA: Lippincott Williams & Wilkins; 2014

ANATOMY OF THE FACIAL DUCTAL SYSTEMS

5. *Which one of the following structures drains directly into the common canaliculus and is often damaged in lower eyelid injuries?*

    B. Inferior canaliculus

    The lacrimal apparatus is clinically relevant to soft tissue facial trauma as it can be damaged during periorbital injuries. Tears drain from the upper and lower eyelids through puncta and then pass along the superior or inferior canaliculus respectively to the common canaliculus and on toward the lacrimal sac. The lacrimal sac drains into the lacrimal duct and then enters the nasal cavity at the valve of Hasner. Injury to the ductal system is most commonly seen with lower medial eyelid injuries and will result in epiphora. It can be managed with surgical repair over a stent by the ophthalmology team. Dacryocystorhinostomy (DCR) may be necessary if cannulation is impossible and injury leads to persistent and problematic epiphora (**Fig. 34.1**).[1,2]

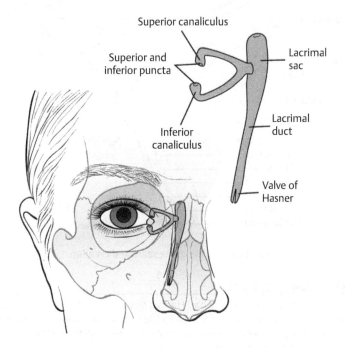

Fig. 34.1 The lacrimal system is made up of superior and inferior canaliculi that coalesce into the common canaliculus. This empties into the lacrimal sac, which drains into the nose through the lacrimal duct. The upper system is composed of the superior/inferior puncta through the common canaliculus, and the lower system consists of the lacrimal sac and duct. (From Marcus JR. Essentials of Craniomaxillofacial Trauma. St Louis: Quality Medical Publishing, 2012.)

REFERENCES

1. Marcus JR. Essentials of Craniomaxillofacial Trauma. St Louis: Quality Medical Publishing; 2012
2. Huang J, Malek J, Chin D, et al. Systematic review and meta-analysis on outcomes for endoscopic versus external dacryocystorhinostomy. Orbit 2014;33(2):81–90

CLINICAL SCENARIOS IN SOFT TISSUE FACIAL TRAUMA

6. A 30-year-old man sustains an avulsion flap injury to the scalp in a motor vehicle accident. *To what depth is the injury most likely to extend to?*

    B. Periosteum

    Avulsion injuries of the scalp are common and often referred to plastic surgery for evaluation and management. The soft tissues of the scalp have five layers: skin, subcutaneous tissue, galea, loose areolar tissue, and pericranium. Avulsion injuries most commonly occur at the level of the scalping plane between the galea and pericranium.[1,2] Other common injury types in the scalp are burst injuries in young children. With this mechanism of injury the patient falls onto the head and bangs it on a furniture corner or the floor. Wounds are deep and often pass down to the frontal bone, stripping a small amount of pericranium just above the brow. In some instances, these injuries cause an underlying fracture, and this should be excluded. Scalping injuries down to the temporal bone are rare because this anatomic area has multiple robust layers of soft tissue including temporalis, deep, and superficial temporal fascia as well as skin and subcutaneous fat. Wounds should be examined under anesthesia, debrided, and closed in layers with absorbable sutures (**Fig. 34.2**).

REFERENCES

1. Tolhurst DE, Carstens MH, Greco RJ, Hurwitz DJ. The surgical anatomy of the scalp. Plast Reconstr Surg 1991;87(4):603–612, discussion 613–614
2. Anderson JE, ed. Grant's Atlas of Anatomy. 8th ed. Baltimore: Williams & Wilkins; 2011

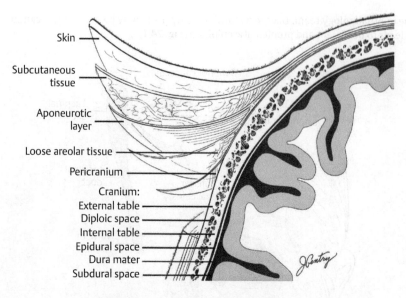

Fig. 34.2 Layers of the scalp and cranium.

NERVE INJURY IN SOFT TISSUE TRAUMA

7. A young male presents after an altercation in a bar. He was struck with a broken glass bottle and has a soft tissue wound that passes vertically from the zygomatic arch to the mandibular body. The wound does not breach the oral mucosa. *Which one of the following is least likely to be present on examination?*

   B. Paresthesia to the ipsilateral ear helical root and lobule

   This patient is at risk of damage to any of the five main branches of the facial nerve and therefore can have symptoms ranging from mild to complete unilateral facial paralysis. The paralysis can account for a loss in oral competence, which may be amplified by damage to the buccinator muscle itself.[1] Although the wound is not full thickness, saliva can be present because of injury to the parotid gland or division of the parotid duct (Stensen's duct).[2] The auriculotemporal branch of the trigeminal nerve is at risk of injury. This supplies the superior lateral aspect of the ear. Sensation to the lobule should be spared because this is supplied by the great auricular nerve.[3]

REFERENCES

1. Seckel BR, ed. Facial Danger Zones: Avoiding Nerve Injury in Facial Plastic Surgery. New York, NY: Thieme; 2010
2. Lazaridou M, Iliopoulos C, Antoniades K, Tilaveridis I, Dimitrakopoulos I, Lazaridis N. Salivary gland trauma: a review of diagnosis and treatment. Craniomaxillofac Trauma Reconstr 2012;5(4):189–196
3. Allison GR. Anatomy of the external ear. Clin Plast Surg 1978;5(3):419–422

SKIN PREPARATION

8. *Which one of the following is recommended for use as a facial skin preparation prior to surgery?*

   B. Povidone-Iodine

   Use of skin preparations prior to surgery should be undertaken with care, particularly when working on the head, neck, and face. The safest preparation to use is aqueous iodine as this clearly marks the areas prepared, and is virucidal and bactericidal yet is nontoxic to the eyes.

   Chlorhexidine is also bactericidal but is toxic to the cornea so care must be taken to avoid the eyes. Hydrogen peroxide is weakly bactericidal, but is not used as a skin preparation. Many surgeons like to use it to clean wounds and, in particular, the skin as it effectively removes dried blood. The use of saline or water will be most effective as irrigation agents to dilute and wash contaminated wounds as they are obviously both safe to use around the face. However, they do not possess bactericidal qualities and are therefore not effective skin preparations to form a sterile field.[1]

REFERENCE

1. Trott AT. Wound cleansing and irrigation. In: Wounds and Lacerations: Emergency Care and Closure. Philadelphia, PA: Elsevier; 2012

NERVE BLOCKS IN FACIAL TRAUMA SURGERY

9. *When providing nerve blocks in the head and neck region, which one of the following is true?*

A. The midpupillary line will guide correct placement of nerve blocks of the forehead, cheeks, and lips.

The use of nerve blocks to facilitate facial surgery can be very useful in both the emergency and elective settings. Nerve blocks allow larger areas of anesthesia with fewer needle sticks and less volume and consequent swelling compared with field blocks. This is important for patient's comfort and experience as well as minimizing swelling so that tissues can be accurately apposed or reconstructed.

Sensation to the face is provided by the three divisions of the trigeminal nerve (cranial nerve [CN] V) as well as C2–C4 cervical roots of the cervical plexus. Therefore, even with blockage of CN V there will be some sensation remaining. The midpupillary line is a useful anatomic landmark for nerve blocks because it guides the horizontal position of the supraorbital, infraorbital, and mental nerve foramina.

The ear requires a field block rather than a single nerve block because it has multiple innervations from the great auricular, auriculotemporal, lesser occipital, vagus, and facial nerves. The zygomaticotemporal nerve is best blocked using a small needle such as a 30 gauge with 1-inch length to be passed deep-to-deep temporal facia and will provide anesthesia to the temple region. It is generally combined with a zygomaticofacial nerve block.

A mental nerve block targets the mental nerve and is directed intraorally in the buccal sulcus at the level of the second premolar (not 3rd molar). It provides anesthesia to the lower lip and chin with minor modification.[1,2]

REFERENCES

1. Zide BM, Swift R. How to block and tackle the face. Plast Reconstr Surg 1998;101(3): 840–851
2. Hadzic A, ed. Hadzic's Textbook of Regional Anesthesia and Acute Pain Management. 2nd ed. New York, NY: McGraw-Hill; 2017

35. Facial Skeletal Trauma

See *Essentials of Plastic Surgery*, third edition, pp. 444–471

FACIAL FRACTURES

1. *Which one of the following facial bones requires the greatest force to fracture?*
    A. Mandible
    B. Nasal bone
    C. Maxilla
    D. Frontal bone
    E. Zygoma

MANAGEMENT AFTER SEVERE HEAD TRAUMA

2. *Which one of the following is correct regarding life-threatening hemorrhage after a major facial injury?*
    A. The external maxillary artery is the most common source of severe hemorrhage in facial fractures.
    B. Angiography and embolization are recommended for uncontrolled bleeding in an unstable patient.
    C. Ligation of the common carotid artery may be required.
    D. Nasal packing and immediate fracture reduction are key steps to control hemorrhage.
    E. Ligation of the external carotid artery risks ischemia to ipsilateral facial structures.

FRONTAL SINUS ANATOMY

3. *Which one of the following is correct regarding the frontal sinus?*
    A. It is normally present at birth.
    B. Drainage typically occurs through the nasofrontal duct.
    C. Adult size is achieved by age 5.
    D. It may be easily identified radiologically in all age groups.
    E. It usually drains into the inferior meatus.

DUCTAL INJURY IN FRONTAL SINUS FRACTURES

4. A patient is seen in the emergency department with a suspected frontal sinus fracture after an assault with a baseball bat to the forehead. A CT head scan is performed to confirm the diagnosis. *Which one of the following cannot be directly assessed by a standard CT scan?*
    A. Involvement of the anterior and posterior tables
    B. The presence of a nasofrontal duct injury
    C. Evidence of pneumocephalus
    D. The degree of posterior table involvement
    E. The injury level relative to the superior orbital rim

MANAGEMENT OF FRONTAL SINUS FRACTURES

5. A patient presents with a suspected frontal sinus fracture. Imaging reveals anterior and posterior table fractures with significant displacement of the posterior wall (more than one width of the table). A cerebrospinal fluid (CSF) leak is also present. *What is the recommended treatment in this case?*
    A. No operative intervention
    B. No operative intervention for 1 week, then reassess
    C. Reduce and stabilize anterior wall, but preserve the sinus
    D. Reduce and stabilize anterior wall, but obliterate the sinus
    E. Reduce and stabilize the anterior wall and perform cranialization

OPERATIVE MANAGEMENT OF FRONTAL SINUS FRACTURES

6. *When undertaking surgical reduction of a frontal sinus fracture, which one of the following is correct?*
    A. Surgical access should only be through a bicoronal approach.
    B. Dissection should proceed in the subperiosteal plane.
    C. Sinus obliteration should be achieved with either bone/fat grafts or bone cement.
    D. Cranialization simply involves removing mucosa and obliterating the ducts.
    E. When cranialization is required, the nasal and cranial cavities are separated with a pericranial flap.

NASOORBITAL ETHMOID FRACTURES

7. *For management of patients with nasoorbital ethmoidal fractures, which one of the following applies?*
   A. These are technically simple fractures to repair but commonly affect facial appearance.
   B. Thermoplastic splints should be used postoperatively to reduce soft tissue thickening.
   C. The Markowitz classification is used and is based on movement of the superior bony fragment.
   D. Surgical fixation is usually satisfactorily achieved with plates and bone graft alone.
   E. Bone grafts are favored in pediatric patients to minimize future growth disturbances.

MANAGEMENT OF NASAL FRACTURES

8. A patient is seen in clinic following an assault when the patient was punched in the face. The patient's nose is now deviated and flattened at the nasal bridge. The left airway is no longer patent and the septum appears abnormally positioned. There is no evidence of septal hematoma and only minimal swelling. *What is the next step in the management of this case in order to optimize long-term outcome?*
   A. Elevation and ice with reassessment in 5 days.
   B. Order a CT scan with 3-mm slices.
   C. Request a radiographic series of the skull base.
   D. Proceed with manipulation under anesthesia.
   E. Perform an open rhinoplasty.

ANATOMY OF THE BONY ORBIT

9. The lamina papyracea is the thinnest part of the orbital floor. *Which bone is it formed by?*
   A. Palatine
   B. Ethmoid
   C. Sphenoid
   D. Frontal
   E. Lacrimal

ORBITAL FRACTURES

10. You see a patient with a suspected orbital fracture. *Which one of the following statements is correct?*
    A. Increased intraorbital volume would be the sole cause of enophthalmos in this patient.
    B. Nausea and vomiting with limited eye excursion are highly suggestive of extraocular muscle entrapment.
    C. Dystopia most commonly refers to horizontal globe malposition.
    D. Entrapment of the extraocular muscles is most common in adults and leads to diplopia.
    E. Surgical access should be obtained through a subciliary approach.

ANATOMY OF THE ZYGOMA

11. *Which one of the following bones does not articulate with the zygoma?*
    A. Frontal
    B. Maxilla
    C. Sphenoid
    D. Temporal
    E. Ethmoid

ZYGOMATICOMAXILLARY COMPLEX FRACTURES (ZMC)

12. For management of a patient with an unstable zygomaticomaxillary complex (ZMC) fracture, which one of the following statements is correct?
    A. All four articulations must be reduced and stabilized with monocortical miniplates and screws.
    B. The patient is likely to have permanent deformity even if accurate reduction and stabilization are achieved.
    C. Fixation of the zygomaticofrontal articulation should ideally be performed first following reduction.
    D. The best surgical approach is through a combination of intraoral and lower blepharoplasty incisions.
    E. Accurate reduction of the zygomaticotemporal articulation is most important.

MAXILLARY FRACTURES

13. *Which one of the following statements is correct regarding maxillary fractures?*
    A. The maxilla contains three vertical and four horizontal buttresses.
    B. Dentoalveolar and LeFort I fractures are essentially the same.
    C. Their management in children follows different principles.
    D. Closed reduction and maxillomandibular fixation are recommended for LeFort fractures.
    E. Rowe forceps are useful for management of impacted fractures.

SURGICAL MANAGEMENT OF PANFACIAL FRACTURES

14. *When operating on a patient with panfacial fractures, which one of the following fracture sites should normally be stabilized first?*
    A. Maxilla
    B. Zygoma
    C. Mandible
    D. Orbital floor
    E. Nasal bone

TEMPORAL BONE FRACTURES

15. A patient presents with a transverse temporal bone fracture. *What is the most likely finding on clinical examination?*
    A. Trigeminal neuralgia
    B. Facial nerve paresis
    C. CSF otorrhea
    D. Hearing loss
    E. Vestibular dysfunction

OPHTHALMIC CONSEQUENCES OF FACIAL FRACTURES

16. Following a motor vehicle accident, a patient is found to have sustained significant facial fractures. Examination shows ptosis of the left upper eyelid, proptosis, ophthalmoplegia, numbness to the forehead and nose, and a dilated ipsilateral pupil. Normal vision is preserved. *What is the most likely diagnosis?*
    A. Superior orbital fissure syndrome
    B. Orbital apex syndrome
    C. Traumatic carotid–cavernous sinus fistula
    D. Traumatic optic neuropathy (TON)
    E. Sympathetic ophthalmia

EMERGENCIES IN FACIAL FRACTURES

17. *Which one of the following conditions ideally needs treatment within minutes?*
    A. Corneal abrasion
    B. Iridodialysis
    C. Traumatic mydriasis
    D. Hyphema
    E. Central retinal artery occlusion

CLINICAL ASSESSMENT IN FACIAL TRAUMA

18. You see a patient with suspected frontal bone fracture and CSF leak from the ears. *Which test is most helpful to confirm the diagnosis?*
    A. Alpha transferrin
    B. Beta transferrin
    C. Glucose
    D. Albumin
    E. Prealbumin

CLINICAL ASSESSMENT IN FACIAL TRAUMA

19. A patient sustains a high-impact trauma to the face and trunk. A CT confirms a maxillary fracture involving the frontonasal junction with movement of the upper jaw and nasal bones as a single unit. *What type of fracture does this represent?*
    A. LeFort I
    B. LeFort II
    C. LeFort III
    D. Dentoalveolar
    E. Alveolar

CLINICAL ASSESSMENT IN FACIAL TRAUMA

20. You are asked to assist your head and neck colleague with reduction and stabilization of a facial fracture using Gillies approach. *What type of fracture is involved?*
    A. Frontal
    B. Zygomatic
    C. Nasal
    D. Maxilla
    E. Mandible

CLINICAL ASSESSMENT IN FACIAL TRAUMA

21. A patient presents with bruising over the mastoid process with persistent headache 2 days following facial trauma. A CT scan of the head demonstrates a fracture. *Injury to which bone is associated with this bruising pattern?*
    A. Maxilla
    B. Mandible
    C. Zygoma
    D. Temporal
    E. Parietal

LONG-TERM COMPLICATIONS FOLLOWING FACIAL INJURY

22. A patient presents to clinic with bilateral inflammation of the uvea 3 months following a severe soft tissue injury to the right eye. *Which one of the following is the most likely diagnosis?*
    A. Sympathetic ophthalmia
    B. Vitreous hemorrhage
    C. Traumatic optic neuropathy
    D. Iridodialysis
    E. Orbital apex syndrome

Answers

FACIAL FRACTURES

1. Which one of the following facial bones requires the greatest force to fracture?

D. Frontal bone

In 1975 Nahum[1] presented the forces necessary to fracture various bones in the facial skeleton. The forces required to fracture the frontal bone were three times greater than those required to fracture the zygoma, maxilla, or mandible. The force required was 800–1600 pounds for the frontal sinus versus 300–750 pounds for the mandibular angle, 550–900 pounds for the mandibular symphysis, 200–400 pounds for the zygomatic arch, and 150–300 pounds for the maxilla. Frontal bone fractures therefore illustrate the high-energy trauma that has occurred and are likely to be associated with other coexisting injuries.

REFERENCE

1. Nahum AM. The biomechanics of maxillofacial trauma. Clin Plast Surg 1975;2(1):59–64

MANAGEMENT AFTER SEVERE HEAD TRAUMA

2. Which one of the following is correct regarding life-threatening hemorrhage after a major facial injury?

D. Nasal packing and immediate fracture reduction are key steps to control hemorrhage.

Significant facial fractures, especially those involving the midface, can be associated with uncontrolled hemorrhage, airway compromise, and intracranial and C-spine injury. Each of these elements must be assessed and managed at initial presentation as part of the advanced life support protocol. The internal maxillary artery is the most common source of bleeding in facial fractures although skin or mucosal tears and bone can all cause bleeding that is challenging to control. Uncontrolled bleeding in these cases should be initially managed with posterior nasal packing followed by early fracture reduction. Angiography and selective embolization are normally only recommended once a patient has been stabilized. If a patient is hemodynamically unstable, ligation of the external carotid artery or urgent embolization may be indicated. Neither ligation or embolization risk ischemia to the ipsilateral facial structures because of the considerable overlapping arterial networks in the head and neck.[1-4]

REFERENCES

1. Khanna S, Dagum AB. A critical review of the literature and an evidence-based approach for life-threatening hemorrhage in maxillofacial surgery. Ann Plast Surg 2012;69(4): 474–478
2. Vujcich N, Gebauer D. Current and evolving trends in the management of facial fractures. Aust Dent J 2018;63(Suppl 1):S35–S47
3. Ardekian L, Samet N, Shoshani Y, Taicher S. Life-threatening bleeding following maxillofacial trauma. J Craniomaxillofac Surg 1993;21(8):336–338
4. Bynoe RP, Kerwin AJ, Parker HH III, et al. Maxillofacial injuries and life-threatening hemorrhage: treatment with transcatheter arterial embolization. J Trauma 2003;55(1):74–79

FRONTAL SINUS ANATOMY

3. Which one of the following is correct regarding the frontal sinus?

B. Drainage typically occurs through the nasofrontal duct.

The focal point of frontal sinus drainage is commonly the osteomeatal complex, which comprises the maxillary, frontal, and anterior ethmoid ostia and is located in the middle meatus.[1] Drainage is usually through the nasofrontal ducts into the middle meatus, but this can occur directly. There is some evidence that the frontal sinus may have an independent drainage pattern in some patients. The frontal sinus does not develop until after birth. Development begins at about age 2, and it typically reaches adult size after age 12. It may be visible radiographically from age 8 onward.

REFERENCE

1. Wallace R, Salazar JE, Cowles S. The relationship between frontal sinus drainage and osteomeatal complex disease: a CT study in 217 patients. AJNR Am J Neuroradiol 1990;11(1):183–186

DUCTAL INJURY IN FRONTAL SINUS FRACTURES

4. A patient is seen in the emergency department with a suspected frontal sinus fracture after an assault with a baseball bat to the forehead. A CT head scan is performed to confirm the diagnosis. *Which one of the following cannot be directly assessed by a standard CT scan?*

    B. **The presence of a nasofrontal duct injury**

        A CT scan is an important imaging tool for suspected frontal sinus fractures. It allows assessment of the bony injury in terms of the table involved, the level of injury, and the degree of fracture displacement. All of these are important factors in the management algorithm. It also helps to identify associated neurologic injuries and pneumocephalus. A CT scan will only provide indirect evidence of a ductal injury, and injury should be assumed unless the CT shows transverse anterior and posterior table fractures above the sinus floor or an isolated anterior table fracture. Nasofrontal outflow tract can be evaluated by high-resolution CT.[1]

REFERENCE

1. Rodriguez ED, Stanwix MG, Nam AJ, et al. Twenty-six-year experience treating frontal sinus fractures: a novel algorithm based on anatomical fracture pattern and failure of conventional techniques. Plast Reconstr Surg 2008;122(6): 1850–1866

MANAGEMENT OF FRONTAL SINUS FRACTURES

5. A patient presents with a suspected frontal sinus fracture. Imaging reveals anterior and posterior table fractures with significant displacement of the posterior wall (more than one width of the table). A CSF leak is also present. *What is the recommended treatment in this case?*

    E. **Reduce and stabilize the anterior wall and perform cranialization**

        Frontal sinus fractures are high-energy injuries that present with upper-face edema and bruising. There is often a palpable deformity of the frontal bone with paresthesias of the supraorbital and supratrochlear nerves. CSF leak rhinorrhea may occur where dural laceration is present. The globe may be displaced forward and inferiorly. Management of frontal sinuses depends on a number of key factors built into the algorithm shown in **Figs. 35.1 and 35.2.**

        These will depend on the skull wall involved, the degree of fracture displacement, the presence or absence of CSF leak, and whether the nasofrontal duct is involved.[1,2]

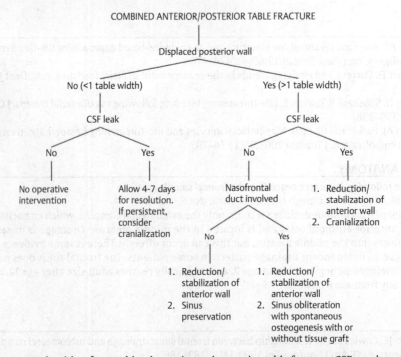

Fig. 35.1 Management algorithm for combined anterior and posterior table fracture. CSF, cerebrospinal fluid. (Adapted from Rohrich RJ, Hollier LH. Management of frontal sinus fractures: changing concepts. Clin Plast Surg 19:219, 1992.)

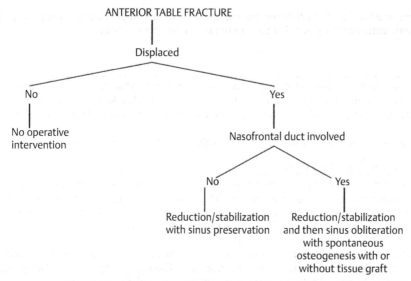

ANTERIOR TABLE FRACTURE

Displaced

No — No operative intervention

Yes — Nasofrontal duct involved

No — Reduction/stabilization with sinus preservation

Yes — Reduction/stabilization and then sinus obliteration with spontaneous osteogenesis with or without tissue graft

Fig. 35.2   Management algorithm for anterior table fracture. (Adapted from Rohrich RJ, Hollier LH. Management of frontal sinus fractures: changing concepts. Clin Plast Surg 19:219, 1992.)

REFERENCES

1. Rodriguez ED, Stanwix MG, Nam AJ, et al. Twenty-six-year experience treating frontal sinus fractures: a novel algorithm based on anatomical fracture pattern and failure of conventional techniques. Plast Reconstr Surg 2008;122(6):1850–1866
2. Rohrich RJ, Hollier LH. Management of frontal sinus fractures. Changing concepts. Clin Plast Surg 1992;19(1):219–232

OPERATIVE MANAGEMENT OF FRONTAL SINUS FRACTURES

6.   *When undertaking surgical reduction of a frontal sinus fracture, which one of the following is correct?*

   E.   **When cranialization is required, the nasal and cranial cavities are separated with a pericranial flap.**
   Although access is commonly through a bicoronal approach, access through existing lacerations may be used. Subgaleal dissection is performed to preserve a pericranial flap in case the sinus requires obliteration or cranialization. Obliteration of the sinus may be achieved with bone or fat grafts as alternatives to a pericranial flap, but bone cement should not be used because of potential complications from infection. Cranialization not only involves removal of mucosa and obliteration of the ducts, but also includes removal of the posterior table. The nasal cavity is isolated from the cranial cavity by interposing a pericranial flap, and the anterior table is then reconstructed.[1,2]

REFERENCES

1. Rodriguez ED, Stanwix MG, Nam AJ, et al. Twenty-six-year experience treating frontal sinus fractures: a novel algorithm based on anatomical fracture pattern and failure of conventional techniques. Plast Reconstr Surg 2008;122(6):1850–1866
2. Rohrich RJ, Hollier LH. Management of frontal sinus fractures. Changing concepts. Clin Plast Surg 1992;19(1):219–232

NASOORBITAL ETHMOID FRACTURES

7.   *For management of patients with nasoorbital ethmoidal fractures, which one of the following applies?*

   B.   **Thermoplastic splints should be used postoperatively to reduce soft tissue thickening.**
   Nasoethmoidal fractures are complex to manage and are associated with changes in postinjury facial appearance due to their involvement of the nasal dorsum, nasoorbital valley, and medial canthus. Use of either bolsters or thermoplastic nasal splints postoperatively is advised to help optimize soft tissue outcomes.
   Nasoethmoidal fractures have been classified by Markowitz into three groups according to the involvement of a central bony fragment.[1]
   The relevance of this is that the central fragment is the site of attachment of the medial canthal tendon. Disruption of this tendon results in telecanthus. Type I fractures do not involve telecanthus as they represent simple fractures of the central fragment without disruption of the canthal tendon. In type II fractures, there is comminution of the central fragment, but the tendon is not disrupted and may or may not involve telecanthus. Type III fractures involve severe comminution and disruption of the medial canthal tendon. These will display telecanthus. Treatment involves either a direct or bicoronal approach and stabilization requires a combination of

plates, wires, and bone graft. In children, bone grafts are avoided where possible and these patients are at high risk of growth disturbances, given that the septum is a major growth center.[2,3]

REFERENCES

1. Markowitz BL, Manson PN, Sargent L, et al. Management of the medial canthal tendon in nasoethmoid orbital fractures: the importance of the central fragment in classification and treatment. Plast Reconstr Surg 1991;87(5):843–853
2. Marcus JR, Erdmann D, Rodriguez ED, eds. Essentials of Craniomaxillofacial Trauma. St Louis: Quality Medical Publishing; 2012
3. Ellis E III. Sequencing treatment for naso-orbito-ethmoid fractures. J Oral Maxillofac Surg 1993;51(5):543–558

MANAGEMENT OF NASAL FRACTURES

8. A patient is seen in clinic following an assault when the patient was punched in the face. The patient's nose is now deviated and flattened at the nasal bridge. The left airway is no longer patent and the septum appears abnormally positioned. There is no evidence of septal hematoma and only minimal swelling. *What is the next step in the management of this case in order to optimize long-term outcome?*

D. Proceed with manipulation under anesthesia.

Isolated nasal fractures are the most common fracture of the facial skeleton and early accurate management is essential to minimize long-term deformity and morbidity. The key to achieving good long-term outcomes is to ensure accurate reduction of both the nasal bones and septum in the acute period.

Manipulation should therefore be performed in a controlled environment to ensure accuracy of reduction, particularly as in this case where the septum is disrupted. Therefore, a general anesthetic is advised. Where there is minimal swelling as in this case, the reduction is best performed as soon as possible. If there is significant swelling, then elevation and ice should be used, and the patient reassessed in 3–5 days. Imaging is not required for isolated nasal bone fractures. A CT scan, however, is warranted in cases of suspected nasoorbital ethmoid (NOE) fractures or other head injury. Open rhinoplasty is reserved for cases with residual problems after manipulation under anesthesia.

Rohrich and Adams[1] describe an algorithm for the management of nasal fractures which may be a useful guide in clinical practice. Fractures are classified from I through V, where I through III represents isolated nasal bone fractures, type IV has additional septal disruption (as in this case), and type V corresponds to NOE fractures.

Septal fractures (type IV injuries) may require specific attention with reduction, with or without reconstruction/resection. Septal hematomas are associated with type IVa injuries and require early intervention to avoid necrosis to the septum.[1]

REFERENCE

1. Rohrich RJ, Adams WP Jr. Nasal fracture management: minimizing secondary nasal deformities. Plast Reconstr Surg 2000;106(2):266–273

ANATOMY OF THE BONY ORBIT

9. The lamina papyracea is the thinnest part of the orbital floor. *Which bone is it formed by?*

B. Ethmoid

The orbit consists of seven bones that also include the maxilla and zygoma. The thinnest area is the lamina papyracea, and this is part of the ethmoid. It is so named as it is paper thin. Isolated fractures of the orbital floor and medial wall may occur (without associated fracture of the orbital rim) and these are postulated to occur either from increased pressure that develops within the orbit (from posterior displacement of orbital tissues) or when deformation of the orbital bones occurs from a blow, resulting in fractures of thin portions of the floor without fracture of the orbital rim.[1]

REFERENCE

1. Waterhouse N, Lyne J, Urdang M, Garey L. An investigation into the mechanism of orbital blowout fractures. Br J Plast Surg 1999;52(8):607–612

ORBITAL FRACTURES

10. You see a patient with a suspected orbital fracture. *Which one of the following statements is correct?*

B. Nausea and vomiting with limited eye excursion are highly suggestive of extraocular muscle entrapment.

Enophthalmos and dystopia may occur following an orbital fracture. Enophthalmos is posterior displacement of the globe and occurs either from an increase in the bony orbital volume or a decrease in volume of the globe and surrounding structures. Dystopia refers to a vertical globe malposition. Entrapment of the periocular muscles is rare in adults and is more common in children because of the elastic characteristics of pediatric bone. Entrapment will cause limited eye excursion and diplopia and is a surgical emergency because of potential ischemic muscle damage. Nausea and vomiting in association with pain and limited eye excursion are highly suggestive of entrapment.[1,2] Surgical access for orbital fractures is best achieved through subtarsal or transconjunctival approaches. A subciliary approach should be avoided because of a risk of lower eyelid deformity.[3,4]

REFERENCES

1. Marcus JR, Erdmann D, Rodriguez ED, eds. Essentials of Craniomaxillofacial Trauma. St Louis: Quality Medical Publishing; 2012
2. Harris GJ, Garcia GH, Logani SC, Murphy ML, Sheth BP, Seth AK. Orbital blow-out fractures: correlation of preoperative computed tomography and postoperative ocular motility. Trans Am Ophthalmol Soc 1998;96:329–347, discussion 347–353
3. North America AO. Review of surgical approaches to the cranial skeleton, 2010. Available at www.aona.org
4. Ridgway EB, Chen C, Colakoglu S, Gautam S, Lee BT. The incidence of lower eyelid malposition after facial fracture repair: a retrospective study and meta-analysis comparing subtarsal, subciliary, and transconjunctival incisions. Plast Reconstr Surg 2009;124(5): 1578–1586

ANATOMY OF THE ZYGOMA

11. Which one of the following bones does not articulate with the zygoma?

E. Ethmoid

The zygoma is an irregular-shaped bone of the skull that forms the lateral cheek and orbital rim. It also contributes to the zygomatic arch, the floor of the orbit, and the infratemporal fossa. The zygoma has four articulations; these are with the frontal, maxilla, sphenoid, and temporal bones. There are left and right zygomas that each comprise the cheek and malar regions. The zygoma is a commonly fractured bone that may be reduced for functional reasons such as correcting enophthalmos or dystopia, eyelid malposition, and trismus. Fractures of the arch are more commonly for cosmetic rather than functional benefits. For example, a fractured zygoma can often result in a flattened appearance to the upper/lateral cheek without any other disability. The exception is when the fracture impedes mandibular excursion by interfering with the coronoid process. When reducing and stabilizing zygoma fractures, it is usual to stabilize three of the articulations.[1,2]

REFERENCES

1. Ellis E III, Kittidumkerng W. Analysis of treatment for isolated zygomaticomaxillary complex fractures. J Oral Maxillofac Surg 1996;54(4):386–400, discussion 400–401
2. Buck DW II, Heyer K, Lewis VL Jr. Reconstruction of the zygomatic arch using a mandibular adaption plate. J Craniofac Surg 2009;20(4):1193–1196

ZYGOMATICOMAXILLARY COMPLEX FRACTURES (ZMC)

12. For management of a patient with an unstable zygomaticomaxillary complex (ZMC) fracture, which one of the following statements is correct?

C. Fixation of the zygomaticofrontal articulation should ideally be performed first following reduction.

Although the zygomaticomaxillary complex has four articulations, it is common practice to stabilize just three of these. When treated properly, these fractures do not leave deformities. The AO foundation guidelines recommend that the zygomaticofrontal articulation is plated first, as this allows more control to accurately reduce the remaining articulations.[1] It should also ensure the zygomaticosphenoid (not zygomaticotemporal) suture is well aligned and this is the most important to assess.

Surgical access will depend on the complexity of the fracture, but a common approach involves intraoral and upper blepharoplasty (not lower) incisions. Wide exposure using a bicoronal approach may be indicated.[2,3] The Carroll-Girard screw is a percutaneous T-bar–shaped device that can be used as a joystick to reduce and control the fracture.

REFERENCES

1. Foundation AO. Available at https://www2.aofoundation.org/wps/portal/surgery
2. Ellis E III, Reddy L. Status of the internal orbit after reduction of zygomaticomaxillary complex fractures. J Oral Maxillofac Surg 2004;62(3):275–283
3. Ellis E III, Kittidumkerng W. Analysis of treatment for isolated zygomaticomaxillary complex fractures. J Oral Maxillofac Surg 1996;54(4):386–400, discussion 400–401

MAXILLARY FRACTURES

13. *Which one of the following statements is correct regarding maxillary fractures?*

E. Rowe forceps are useful for management of impacted fractures.

Rowe forceps are used to facilitate disimpaction of maxillary fractures during surgery. The maxilla contains three vertical and three (not four) horizontal (AP) buttresses. An additional horizontal (AP) buttress is provided by the mandible, not related to the maxilla. Dentoalveolar and LeFort fractures are different. Dentoalveolar fractures pass through the dentition whereas LeFort fractures separate the entire alveolus and dentition from the midface. The fracture line is above the dentition. Malocclusion of the maxilla is commonly seen as an anterior open bite and this is secondary to posteroinferior displacement of the maxilla. LeFort fractures should be reduced and fixed with miniplates and screws through an open approach. Closed reduction and fixation to the mandible are not recommended because this leads to facial lengthening from the downward pull of the mandible.[1-3] Treatment considerations for maxillofacial fractures are the same as for adults but may be technically more difficult and some principles in management do differ. For example, arch bars are difficult to place in pediatric patients because of mixed dentition, missing teeth, and unfavorable dental anatomy of the primary teeth. Difficulty can also be encountered in placing fixation systems because of developing tooth buds.[4,5]

REFERENCES

1. Manson PN. Facial fractures. In: Aston SJ, Grabb WC, eds. Grabb and Smith's Plastic Surgery. New York: Lippincott-Raven; 1997:398–401
2. Cornelius CP, Audigé L, Kunz C, Buitrago-Téllez CH, Rudderman R, Prein J. The comprehensive AOCMF classification system: midface fractures—level 3 tutorial. Craniomaxillofac Trauma Reconstr 2014;7(Suppl 1):S068–S091
3. Louis M, Agrawal N, Truong TA. Midface fractures II. Semin Plast Surg 2017;31(2):94–99
4. Braun TL, Xue AS, Maricevich RS. Differences in the management of pediatric facial trauma. Semin Plast Surg 2017;31(2):118–122
5. Mukherjee CG, Mukherjee U. Maxillofacial trauma in children. Int J Clin Pediatr Dent 2012; 5(3):231–236

SURGICAL MANAGEMENT OF PANFACIAL FRACTURES

14. *When operating on a patient with panfacial fractures, which one of the following fracture sites should normally be stabilized first?*

C. Mandible

Panfacial fractures involve the upper and midfacial skeleton in association with fractures of the mandible. Management of these injuries is challenging because there is no stable reference from which to begin reduction and stabilization. It may be useful to begin with the mandible to provide a stable base from which to reconstruct the midface. Reconstruction of the zygomas should then be undertaken to provide normal facial projection. Reconstruction then proceeds inferiorly from the stable frontal process to the level of the maxilla. Fixation of the maxilla as a LeFort fracture is the last to be stabilized.[1-3]

REFERENCES

1. Marcus JR, Erdmann D, Rodriguez ED, eds. Essentials of Craniomaxillofacial Trauma. St Louis: Quality Medical Publishing; 2012
2. Curtis W, Horswell BB. Panfacial fractures: an approach to management. Oral Maxillofac Surg Clin North Am 2013;25(4):649–660
3. Gruss JS, Bubak PJ, Egbert MA. Craniofacial fractures. An algorithm to optimize results. Clin Plast Surg 1992;19(1): 195–206

TEMPORAL BONE FRACTURES

15. A patient presents with a transverse temporal bone fracture. *What is the most likely finding on clinical examination?*

D. Hearing loss

Temporal bone fractures can result in hearing loss, facial nerve paresis, vestibular dysfunction, and CSF leak. Of these, hearing loss is the most common complication, occurring in the vast majority of patients with temporal bone fractures. The risk is related to the fracture configuration with all transverse fractures resulting in hearing loss compared with half of longitudinal fractures. Hearing loss is either sensorineural or conductive. Sensorineural hearing loss does not improve, whereas conductive hearing loss may, unless there is disruption of the ossicular chain. Fracture pattern is also relevant to the risk of developing facial nerve paresis. Loss of facial nerve function is more likely when the fracture pattern is transverse (**Table 35.1**).[1]

Vestibular dysfunction can result in vertigo and nystagmus. This has a varied incidence and usually resolves spontaneously once the patient is mobilizing normally. CSF leaks occur in approximately 25% of cases following

Table 35.1 *Fracture Patterns and Complications in Temporal Bone Fractures*

Fracture Pattern	Representative Proportion of All Cases	Facial Nerve Involvement as a Proportion of Fracture Subtype	Hearing Loss as a Proportion of Fracture Subtype
Longitudinal	80–90%	20%	67%
Transverse	10–20%	40%	100%

temporal bone fracture and settle spontaneously within 24 hours. Involvement of the trigeminal nerve is unusual.[1,2]

REFERENCES

1. Tos M. [Practura ossi temporalis. The course and sequelae of 248 fractures of the temporal bones]. Ugeskr Laeger 1971;133(30):1449–1456
2. Patel A, Groppo E. Management of temporal bone trauma. Craniomaxillofac Trauma Reconstr 2010;3(2):105–113

OPHTHALMIC CONSEQUENCES OF FACIAL FRACTURES

16. Following a motor vehicle accident, a patient is found to have sustained significant facial fractures. Examination shows ptosis of the left upper eyelid, proptosis, ophthalmoplegia, numbness to the forehead and nose, and a dilated ipsilateral pupil. Normal vision is preserved. *What is the most likely diagnosis?*

A. **Superior orbital fissure syndrome**

Superior orbital fissure syndrome occurs in association with LeFort II/III or zygomatic orbital fractures. It involves the oculomotor, trochlear, abducens, and trigeminal nerves and the ophthalmic vein. It therefore results in the constellation of signs as described above. With reduction of fractures, recovery typically occurs over weeks. Orbital apex syndrome is similar, but also includes a loss of vision, because the optic nerve is involved at the apex.[1,2]

Traumatic cavernous sinus fistula occurs with arterial bleeding so blood shunts from the internal carotid artery to the cavernous sinus. Signs include proptosis, an ocular bruit, injection, chemosis of the affected eye, and ophthalmoplegia of CN II, IV, or VI. Angiography will provide the diagnosis with evidence of a dilated ophthalmic vein. Fistulas typically close spontaneously. Treatment may include surgical ligation of the carotid artery or placement of coils by an interventional radiologist.[3]

Traumatic optic neuropathy (TON) is a traumatic loss of vision without external or initial ophthalmoscopic evidence of injury to the eye or the optic nerve. It may occur secondary to globe injury, retinal vascular occlusion, or orbital compartment syndrome. The only objective finding is the presence of a relative afferent pupillary defect.[4,5] Sympathetic ophthalmia is a bilateral granulomatous inflammation of the uvea occurring as a complication of penetrating trauma.

REFERENCES

1. Rai S, Rattan V. Traumatic superior orbital fissure syndrome: review of literature and report of three cases. Natl J Maxillofac Surg 2012;3(2):222–225
2. Shokri T, Zacharia BE, Lighthall JG. Traumatic orbital apex syndrome: an uncommon sequela of facial trauma. Ear Nose Throat J 2019;98(10):609–612
3. Komiyama M, Nakajima H, Nishikawa M, Kan M. Traumatic carotid cavernous sinus fistula: serial angiographic studies from the day of trauma. AJNR Am J Neuroradiol 1998;19(9):1641–1644
4. Rajiniganth MG, Gupta AK, Gupta A, Bapuraj JR. Traumatic optic neuropathy: visual outcome following combined therapy protocol. Arch Otolaryngol Head Neck Surg 2003;129(11):1203–1206
5. Levin LA, Beck RW, Joseph MP, Seiff S, Kraker R. The treatment of traumatic optic neuropathy: the International Optic Nerve Trauma Study. Ophthalmology 1999;106(7):1268–1277

EMERGENCIES IN FACIAL FRACTURES

17. *Which one of the following conditions ideally needs treatment within minutes?*

E. **Central retinal artery occlusion**

There are three ocular emergencies that should have treatment commenced within minutes. They are central retinal artery occlusion, chemical burns, and retrobulbar hematoma. The other injuries listed should be assessed and treated quickly but less urgently.

Central retinal artery occlusion is caused by an embolic event, which occludes it. Essentially it is a cerebrovascular incident of the globe and may be transient or permanent depending on the cause and its longevity.

It is, in theory, a medical emergency yet there is no single proven treatment that will definitely help. For example, thrombolysis, hyperventilation, paracentesis, and ocular massage have all been trialled with no proven success. Often therefore management tends to be focused on prevention rather than cure.[1,2]

Chemical burns to the eye must be treated swiftly with copious irrigation, ideally commenced at the injury location with more formal treatment on arrival at hospital. Normal saline or water are most often indicated for the irrigation.[3]

Retrobulbar hematoma is associated with facial trauma and can occur following elective ocular surgery including blepharoplasty. Management is aimed at reducing ocular pressure and often takes the form of surgical decompression of the globe with a lateral canthotomy/cantholysis. Medical management can include oxygen therapy, intravenous mannitol, intravenous acetazolamide, steroids, and topical β-blockers.[4,5]

Corneal abrasions are treated conservatively. They usually re-epithelialize in 24 hours. Traumatic mydriasis is pupillary sphincter rupture resulting in a permanently dilated pupil. This is also treated nonoperatively. Hyphema is blood in the anterior eye chamber. This is treated by prevention of a rebleed, bed rest, and atropine to decrease iris movement.

REFERENCES

1. Dattilo M, Biousse V, Newman NJ. Update on the management of central retinal artery occlusion. Neurol Clin 2017;35(1):83–100
2. Chronopoulos A, Schutz JS. Central retinal artery occlusion—a new, provisional treatment approach. Surv Ophthalmol 2019;64(4):443–451
3. Soleimani M, Naderan M. Management strategies of ocular chemical burns: current perspectives. Clin Ophthalmol 2020;14:2687–2699
4. Wolfort FG, Vaughan TE, Wolfort SF, Nevarre DR. Retrobulbar hematoma and blepharoplasty. Plast Reconstr Surg 1999;104(7):2154–2162
5. Chen YA, Singhal D, Chen YR, Chen CT. Management of acute traumatic retrobulbar haematomas: a 10-year retrospective review. J Plast Reconstr Aesthet Surg 2012;65(10): 1325–1330

CLINICAL ASSESSMENT IN FACIAL TRAUMA

18. You see a patient with suspected frontal bone fracture and CSF leak from the ears. *Which test is most helpful to confirm the diagnosis?*

B. Beta transferrin

Diagnosis of CSF leak in patients following head injury is based on clinical examination of the nose and external ear, backed up by CT scanning or laboratory tests. Beta transferrin is a carbohydrate-free form of transferrin, which is almost exclusively found in the CSF. Beta transferrin is not present in blood, nasal mucus, tears, or mucosal discharge, so is specific to CSF even where the fluid is bloodstained and difficult to assess clinically. It has been shown to have a sensitivity of near 100% and a specificity of about 95% for CSF leak in a large retrospective study.[1]

Detection of glucose in the sample fluid using Glucostix test strips is another traditional test for CSF in nasal and ear discharge but is not recommended as a confirmatory test because of its lack of specificity and sensitivity.[2] Interpretation of the results is confounded by various factors such as contamination from glucose-containing fluid (tears, nasal mucus, blood in nasal mucus) or relatively low CSF glucose levels. The other tests listed do not relate to CSF leak tests. Albumin and prealbumin are used as markers of nutritional state.

REFERENCES

1. Skedros DG, Cass SP, Hirsch BE, Kelly RH. Sources of error in use of beta-2 transferrin analysis for diagnosing perilymphatic and cerebral spinal fluid leaks. Otolaryngol Head Neck Surg 1993;109(5):861–864
2. Chan DT, Poon WS, Ip CP, Chiu PW, goh KY. How useful is glucose detection in diagnosing cerebrospinal fluid leak? The rational use of CT and beta-2 transferrin assay in detection of cerebrospinal fluid fistula. Asian J Surg 2004;27(1):39–42

CLINICAL ASSESSMENT IN FACIAL TRAUMA

19. A patient sustains a high-impact trauma to the face and trunk. A CT confirms a maxillary fracture involving the frontonasal junction with movement of the upper jaw and nasal bones as a single unit. *What type of fracture does this represent?*

B. LeFort II

Maxillary fractures may be classified using the LeFort system. There are three types of LeFort fracture as shown in **Fig. 35.3, A through** C.

They differ in their extent. A LeFort I (**Fig. 35.3,** A) separates the tooth-bearing maxilla from the midface. It extends from the piriform aperture posteriorly through the nasal septum, lateral nasal walls, and maxillary

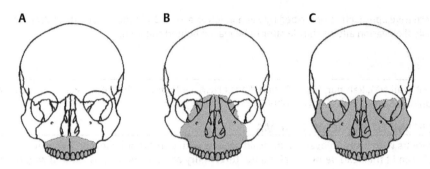

Fig. 35.3 LeFort midfacial fractures. ***A,*** LeFort I fracture separating the inferior portion of the maxilla in horizontal fashion, extending from the piriform aperture of the nose to the pterygoid maxillary suture area. ***B,*** LeFort II fracture involving separation of the maxilla and nasal complex from the cranial base, zygomatic orbital rim area, and pterygoid maxillary suture area. ***C,*** LeFort III fracture (i.e., craniofacial separation) is complete separation of the midface at the level of the nasoorbital ethmoid (NOE) complex and zygomaticomaxillary (ZM) suture area. It extends through the orbits bilaterally.

wall through the maxillary tuberosity or pterygoid plates. The LeFort II (**Fig. 35.3,** B) is a pyramidal fracture that extends through the frontonasal junction along the medial orbital wall, usually passing through the inferior orbital rim at the zygomaticomaxillary (ZM) suture. It continues posteriorly through the pterygoid plates. It leaves the upper jaw and nasal bones as a mobile solitary unit. The LeFort III (**Fig. 35.3,** C) fracture represents craniofacial disjunction extending through the frontonasal junction along the medial orbital wall and inferior orbital fissure and out the lateral orbital wall. Dentoalveolar fractures involve the teeth and supporting osseous structures only.[1]

REFERENCE

1. Louis M, Agrawal N, Truong TA. Midface fractures II. Semin Plast Surg 2017;31(2):94–99

CLINICAL ASSESSMENT IN FACIAL TRAUMA

20. You are asked to assist your head and neck colleague with reduction and stabilization of a facial fracture using Gillies approach. ***What type of fracture is involved?***

    B. Zygomatic

       A Gillies maneuver is an approach to elevate a zygomatic arch fracture through a temporal hairline incision. The elevator is passed beneath the deep temporal fascia under the arch and the arch is elevated, taking care not to lever against the underlying temporal bone (**Fig. 35.4**).

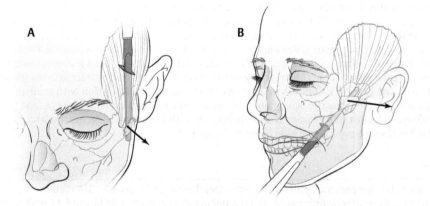

Fig. 35.4 Reduction maneuvers for an isolated zygomatic arch fracture. ***A,*** The Gillies approach involves a 2-cm incision placed 2 fingerbreadths above the helix and 2 fingerbreadths anterior. A blunt elevator is placed beneath the deep layer of deep temporal fascia, superficial to the temporalis muscle allowing the tip of the elevator to pass behind the arch without risking injury to the frontal branch of the facial nerve. ***B,*** In the intraoral approach (Keen), a 1- to 2-cm incision is made laterally in the buccal sulcus. Subperiosteal elevation allows the elevator to be placed behind the arch.

An alternative approach as described by Keen involves a 1- to 2-cm incision made lateral to the buccal sulcus. Subperiosteal elevation allows the elevator to be placed behind the arch.[1]

REFERENCE

1. Rahman RA, Ghazali NM, Rahman NA, Pohchi A, Razak NHA. Outcome of different treatment modalities of fracture zygoma. J Craniofac Surg 2020;31(4):1056–1062

CLINICAL ASSESSMENT IN FACIAL TRAUMA

21. A patient presents with bruising over the mastoid process with persistent headache 2 days following facial trauma. A CT scan of the head demonstrates a fracture. *Injury to which bone is associated with this bruising pattern?*

D. Temporal

This patient has *Battle's sign*, which is ecchymosis over the mastoid process and seen in conjunction with a skull base fracture. It is associated with temporal bone fractures but is not exclusive to them. For example, it is also seen in fractures of the occipital, sphenoid, and ethmoid bones. *Battle's sign* typically appears 2–3 days following injury and may be associated with other signs of skull base fracture such as otorrhea, rhinorrhea, facial nerve palsy, nystagmus, hemotympanum, and deafness. Raccoon eyes may also be present, which are black patches in the periorbital region secondary to ecchymosis.[1,2]

REFERENCES

1. Ishman SL, Friedland DR. Temporal bone fractures: traditional classification and clinical relevance. Laryngoscope 2004;114(10):1734–1741
2. Patel A, Groppo E. Management of temporal bone trauma. Craniomaxillofac Trauma Reconstr 2010;3(2):105–113

LONG-TERM COMPLICATIONS FOLLOWING FACIAL INJURY

22. A patient presents to clinic with bilateral inflammation of the uvea 3 months following a severe soft tissue injury to the right eye. *Which one of the following is the most likely diagnosis?*

A. Sympathetic ophthalmia

Sympathetic ophthalmia is a rare bilateral granulomatous inflammation of the uvea. It occurs as a consequence of penetrating trauma or a surgical insult to a single eye. The nontraumatized eye typically becomes inflamed within 1 year of injury, and a severely traumatized eye may be best treated early with enucleation early to prevent this. An alternative approach to treatment involves the use of immunosuppressive medical therapy. This may include locally injected or systemic steroids and infliximab. The precise pathophysiology is not known although recent developments in molecular biology and imaging technology are proving useful in elucidating the autoimmune processes involved.[1,2]

Vitreous hemorrhage is a condition where bleeding occurs within the vitreous humor of the globe. It can be secondary to trauma and associated with retinal detachment. Presenting signs and symptoms vary according to severity. In smaller bleeds patients may describe floaters, cobwebs, haze, or shadows in the eye. The most severe bleeds can cause complete visual loss. Traumatic optic neuropathy (TON) presents with loss of vision following trauma, without external or initial ophthalmoscopic evidence of injury to the eye or the optic nerve. It may occur secondary to globe injury, retinal vascular occlusion, or orbital compartment syndrome. The only objective finding is the presence of a relative afferent pupillary defect. Iridodialysis describes a traumatic separation between the iris root and ciliary body. It may be caused by nonpenetrating or penetrating trauma to the globe. Clinical features include pain and blurred vision. Orbital apex syndrome occurs in association with some midface or zygomatic orbital fractures. It involves the oculomotor, trochlear, abducens, and trigeminal nerves and the ophthalmic vein. It therefore results in a constellation of signs in keeping with damage to these nerves. It can lead to complete loss of vision because the optic nerve is involved at the apex.[3,4]

REFERENCES

1. Chang GC, Young LH. Sympathetic ophthalmia. Semin Ophthalmol 2011;26(4-5):316–320
2. Chu XK, Chan CC. Sympathetic ophthalmia: to the twenty-first century and beyond. J Ophthalmic Inflamm Infect 2013;3(1):49
3. Levin LA, Beck RW, Joseph MP, Seiff S, Kraker R. The treatment of traumatic optic neuropathy: the International Optic Nerve Trauma Study. Ophthalmology 1999;106(7):1268–1277
4. Roth FS, Koshy JC, Goldberg JS, Soparkar CNS. Pearls of orbital trauma management. Semin Plast Surg 2010;24(4):398–410

36. Mandibular Fractures

See *Essentials of Plastic Surgery*, third edition, pp. 472–485

ANATOMY OF THE MANDIBLE

1. *When considering the anatomy of the mandible, which one of the following represents the region between the mental foramen and the third molar?*
   A. Condyle
   B. Body
   C. Coronoid
   D. Ramus
   E. Angle

FRACTURE SITES OF THE MANDIBLE

2. A patient is involved in an assault and sustains a mandibular fracture. *What is the most commonly fractured site in this situation?*
   A. Condyle
   B. Coronoid
   C. Ramus
   D. Angle
   E. Body

CLINICAL FINDINGS IN MANDIBULAR FRACTURES

3. A patient comes to the emergency department following an assault. On examination the following findings are present. *Which one of them is pathognomonic of a mandibular fracture?*
   A. Malocclusion
   B. Mental nerve paresthesia
   C. Ecchymosis to the floor of mouth
   D. Trismus
   E. Loose teeth

IMAGING IN MANDIBULAR FRACTURES

4. *When requesting imaging of a patient after an isolated mandibular fracture, which one of the following is true?*
   A. A panoramic radiograph alone provides adequate views of the fractured mandible.
   B. CT imaging is commonly required to confirm the fracture sites involved prior to stabilization.
   C. MRI is preferable for imaging of the mandible in most cases.
   D. The single best radiograph for mandibular screening is the panoramic view.
   E. Imaging will confirm diagnosis of sensory nerve damage.

INDICATIONS FOR DENTAL EXTRACTION IN MANDIBULAR FRACTURES

5. *Which one of the following is not usually an indication for the removal of teeth in conjunction with a mandibular fracture?*
   A. Gross mobility with periodontal disease
   B. Periapical radiolucency
   C. Root fracture
   D. Exposure of the apices
   E. Complete bony impaction

FRACTURE STABILITY

6. *When considering surgical fixation of fractures, which one of the following most accurately describes a situation where primary bone healing can be achieved?*
   A. Load-bearing stability
   B. Load-sharing stability
   C. Absolute stability
   D. Functional stability
   E. Overall stability

THE CHAMPY SYSTEM

7. An 18-year-old male is admitted after a fall onto his chin during a vasovagal attack. Examination and imaging confirm the presence of an isolated symphyseal fracture. *Which one of the following statements is correct regarding the Champy system?*
   A. Open reduction and internal fixation (ORIF) will require the use of bicortical miniplates.
   B. ORIF will require a submental approach.
   C. Two miniplates will be required to stabilize the fracture.
   D. Temporary arch bars are likely to be required.
   E. The principles of fixation are based on neutralization of compression forces.

MANAGEMENT OF MANDIBULAR FRACTURES

8. *For the management of patients with mandibular fractures, which one of the following is correct?*
   A. Preoperative and postoperative broad-spectrum antibiotics should be prescribed.
   B. Oral chlorhexidine mouthwash should be used to reduce postoperative infections.
   C. Open reduction and internal fixation will uniformly be required.
   D. Principles of reduction, fixation, and early mobilization should be followed.
   E. Fracture reduction and stabilization should be achieved within 72 hours.

MANAGEMENT OF MANDIBULAR FRACTURES

9. A 25-year-old male is admitted following an alleged assault. Examination confirms tenderness and swelling over the left temporomandibular joint (TMJ). His mouth opening is reduced but normal occlusion is preserved. Radiographs show a unilateral extraarticular fracture of the left condyle. *How should this injury best be managed?*
   A. Application of arch bars
   B. Maxillomandibular fixation (MMF) screws and elastics
   C. Open reduction and internal fixation (ORIF) via a preauricular approach
   D. ORIF via an intraoral approach
   E. Soft diet and close observation

COMPLICATION RATES IN MANDIBULAR FRACTURES

10. *Which anatomic site is associated with the highest complication rate in mandibular fractures?*
    A. Angle   D. Condyle
    B. Body   E. Sigmoid notch
    C. Symphysis

SPECIAL CONSIDERATIONS IN MANDIBULAR FRACTURES

11. *Which one of the following is true regarding mandibular fracture management?*
    A. Bilateral fractures require rigid fixation at each of the fracture sites.
    B. Primary bone grafting in comminuted fractures is advocated.
    C. Fractures of the edentulous mandible should be treated conservatively.
    D. Pediatric mandibular fractures commonly involve the condyle and need close follow-up.
    E. Malocclusion is the single most common complication following mandibular fracture.

Answers

ANATOMY OF THE MANDIBLE

1. **When considering the anatomy of the mandible, which one of the following reresents the region between the mental foramen and the third molar?**

    B. Body

    The mandible has a number of discrete anatomic subunits and fracture sites are classified and treated according to these locations. The body forms the horizontal part of the mandible between the first or second premolar and the third molar. The angle forms the junction between these two subunits. The condyle forms part of the temporomandibular joint (TMJ) where it articulates with the glenoid fossa of the temporal bone. The coronoid is the site of attachment of the temporalis muscle. The sigmoid notch is found between these two points. The mandible also has muscle attachments from the masseter, pterygoids, digastric, stylohyoid, and geniohyoid. The symphysis is the midline region anteriorly between the central incisors. The parasymphysis is the region on either side of the symphysis between the midline and mental foramen. The alveolus is the site where dentition is located (**Fig. 36.1**).[1]

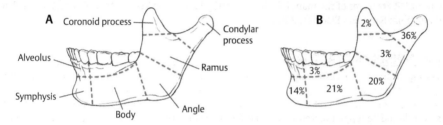

Fig. 36.1   A, Anatomic regions of the mandible. **B,** Frequency of fractures in those regions.

REFERENCE

1. Gray H. Anatomy of the Human Body. www.bartleby.com ed. New York: Bartleby.com; 2000

FRACTURE SITES OF THE MANDIBLE

2. **A patient is involved in an assault and sustains a mandibular fracture. *What is the most commonly fractured site in this situation?***

    D. Angle

    Mandibular fractures are a common injury especially in young adult males and are classified by anatomic location. The most common sites are the condyle, body, angle, and symphysis. The fracture site is dependent upon the mechanism of injury and is related to both the direction and magnitude of force. For example, assaults commonly result in angle fractures, while motor vehicle crashes more commonly result in body fractures. The mandible frequently fractures at two sites simultaneously (50% of cases). The coronoid is the least commonly fractured site in adults representing around 2% of cases.[1-3]

REFERENCES

1. Morrow BT, Samson TD, Schubert W, Mackay DR. Evidence-based medicine: mandible fractures. Plast Reconstr Surg 2014;134(6):1381–1390
2. Allareddy V, Allareddy V, Nalliah RP. Epidemiology of facial fracture injuries. J Oral Maxillofac Surg 2011;69(10): 2613–2618
3. Aston SJ, Beasley RW, Thorne CH, eds. Grabb and Smith's Plastic Surgery. 6th ed. Philadelphia: Lippincott-Raven; 2007

CLINICAL FINDINGS IN MANDIBULAR FRACTURES

3. A patient comes to the emergency department following an assault. On examination the following findings are present. *Which one of them is pathognomonic of a mandibular fracture?*

   C. Ecchymosis to the floor of mouth

   All of the above may be seen in conjunction with a mandibular fracture but ecchymosis to the floor of the mouth is said to be pathognomonic of this condition. When assessing patients with suspected mandibular fractures, external and internal examinations are required. A noticeable step-off is often visible between the teeth at the site of fracture in addition to the bruising. Asking patients whether their bite feels normal is a very useful and highly sensitive test. The mental nerve is a continuation of the inferior alveolar nerve that supplies sensation to the skin overlying the anterior mandible. Paresthesia in this region indicates that the fracture has resulted in damage to this nerve. This must be documented preoperatively. Trismus refers to a reduced ability to open the mouth and is often seen following a mandibular fracture as a result of pain, swelling, and muscle spasm. It may also be due to a mechanical problem where a displaced fracture is present and there is disruption of the normal mandibular U shape. Loose teeth are common following facial trauma and again this must be documented during initial assessment. Dental assessment is advised in such cases.[1,2]

REFERENCES

1. Ellis E III, Miles BA. Fractures of the mandible: a technical perspective. Plast Reconstr Surg 2007;120(7, Suppl 2):76S–89S
2. Kuang AA, Lorenz HP. Fractures of the mandible. In: McCarthy JG, Galiano RD, Boutros SG, eds. Current Therapy in Plastic Surgery. Philadelphia: Saunders Elsevier; 2006

IMAGING IN MANDIBULAR FRACTURES

4. *When requesting imaging of a patient after an isolated mandibular fracture, which one of the following is true?*

   D. The single best radiograph for mandibular screening is the panoramic view.

   Although the panoramic view of the mandible is excellent and will enable the vast majority of fractures to be diagnosed, it should be supplemented with a mandibular series. This will typically include a posteroanterior (PA) and lateral skull view, right and left lateral oblique views, Towne projection, and submental vertex views. CT scans are not usually required for isolated mandibular fractures, but they may be useful in situations where plain radiographs are inadequate, such as when cervical collars are still in place. MRI is better for imaging soft tissue than bone and is not required in mandibular fractures. Radiographs may be useful to identify the inferior alveolar nerve relationships, but nerve injury is best diagnosed during clinical examination.[1,2]

REFERENCES

1. Wilson IF, Lokeh A, Benjamin CI, et al. Prospective comparison of panoramic tomography (zonography) and helical computed tomography in the diagnosis and operative management of mandibular fractures. Plast Reconstr Surg 2001;107(6):1369–1375
2. Miloro M, Ghali GE, Larsen PE, et al, eds. Peterson's Principles of Oral and Maxillofacial Surgery, Vol. 1, 3rd ed. 2012

INDICATIONS FOR DENTAL EXTRACTION IN MANDIBULAR FRACTURES

5. *Which one of the following is not usually an indication for the removal of teeth in conjunction with a mandibular fracture?*

   E. Complete bony impaction

   There are five typical indications for tooth removal:

   1. Grossly mobile teeth in which *periapical* pathology or advanced periodontal disease is present
   2. Partially erupted third molars with an associated dental pathologic condition
   3. Teeth that prevent adequate reduction of the fracture
   4. Teeth with fractured roots
   5. Teeth with exposed root apices

   Nonrestorable teeth and bony impactions should be retained if this assists in reduction. For example, extraction of bony impactions can result in removal of excessive amounts of bone that may compromise both the fracture site and the potential placement points for plate or screw fixation.[1–3]

REFERENCES

1. Chidyllo SA, Marschall MA. Teeth in the line of a mandible fracture: which should be performed first, extraction or fixation? Plast Reconstr Surg 1992;90(1):135–136
2. Schneider SS, Stern M. Teeth in the line of mandibular fractures. J Oral Surg 1971;29(2): 107–109
3. Gerbino G, Tarello F, Fasolis M, De Gioanni PP. Rigid fixation with teeth in the line of mandibular fractures. Int J Oral Maxillofac Surg 1997;26(3):182–186

FRACTURE STABILITY

6. When considering surgical fixation of fractures, which one of the following most accurately describes a situation where primary bone healing can be achieved?

C. Absolute stability

There are a number of definitions of the stability required for optimal fracture healing to occur. Rigid or absolute stability means there is no movement occurring across the fracture site.

This allows for primary bone healing without callus formation. Rigid stability may be an ideal therapeutic principle in some situations, but in the mandible, it mandates the use of large reconstruction plates, multiple miniplates, or lag/locking screws. The lack of movement stimulation at the fracture ends may reduce the osteogenic healing process of the bone in some situations. Absolute stability is not usually achieved in mandibular fractures, as a subtle amount of movement at the fracture site is preferred.

Load-bearing stability occurs where all load is transmitted through the construct rather than the bone. This is required in situations where there is bony insufficiency either in terms of quality or quantity, such as extreme comminution or atrophic mandibles. Load-bearing stability is most often accomplished by large reconstruction plates such as those used when reconstructing segmental mandibular defects with free bone transfer. Load-sharing stability is where stability is achieved by the fixation system in conjunction with stabilizing forces provided by anatomic abutment of noncomminuted fracture segments. Some callous is likely to be formed with each of these approaches. Functional or nonrigid stability enables micromotion to occur across the fracture gap but is balanced by external forces and remains within limits so as to allow the fracture to progress satisfactorily to union. There will be formation of callus and secondary ossification. There are advantages and disadvantages of having rigid or semirigid fixations and the benefits of each will depend on factors including location and type of fracture/s and bone quality. In general load-sharing approaches with miniplates are still most often used in mandible fractures.[1]

REFERENCE

1. Morrow BT, Samson TD, Schubert W, Mackay DR. Evidence-based medicine: mandible fractures. Plast Reconstr Surg 2014;134(6):1381–1390

THE CHAMPY SYSTEM

7. An 18-year-old male is admitted after a fall onto his chin during a vasovagal attack. Examination and imaging confirm the presence of an isolated symphyseal fracture. Which one of the following statements is correct regarding the Champy system?

C. Two miniplates will be required to stabilize the fracture.

The Champy system was first described by Michelet et al[1] in 1973 and later validated by Champy et al[2] in 1978. It advocates the use of monocortical (not bicortical) miniplates and is based on the concept that only tensile stresses are harmful to fracture healing, as these tend to open up the fracture line. Compressive forces, however, tend to pull the fracture lines together and can be used to help fracture reduction and stabilization. The system involves placement of miniplates to counteract the tensile or opening forces and utilize the compressive forces. Anterior to the first premolar, two miniplates are required, one above the other, as there are multidirectional forces acting across this site. Fractures posterior to the first premolar normally only require single plate fixation. The standard approach to ORIF of a symphyseal fracture is intraoral (not submental) within the lower lip sulcus. Care should be taken to ensure that the incision is placed away from the attached gingiva to ensure there is sufficient nonadherent mucosa to facilitate tension-free soft tissue closure. Temporary arch bars are usually only required where there are two concomitant fractures such as a symphyseal, condyle, or angle.

REFERENCES

1. Michelet FX, Deymes J, Dessus B. Osteosynthesis with miniaturized screwed plates in maxillo-facial surgery. J Maxillofac Surg 1973;1(2):79–84
2. Champy M, Loddé JP, Schmitt R, Jaeger JH, Muster D. Mandibular osteosynthesis by miniature screwed plates via a buccal approach. J Maxillofac Surg 1978;6(1):14–21

MANAGEMENT OF MANDIBULAR FRACTURES

8. *For the management of patients with mandibular fractures, which one of the following is correct?*

  D. Principles of reduction, fixation, and early mobilization should be followed.

  Prophylactic antibiotic use in mandibular fractures has been proven to significantly reduce the incidence of postoperative infection. However, antibiotics only need to be prescribed until definitive fixation. Further antibiotic use (i.e., postoperative) does not affect infection rates, nor does the use of oral chlorhexidine, even though it can reduce bacterial counts. Not all fractures will require surgical fixation; for example, some condylar fractures may be managed conservatively with a soft diet and physical rehabilitation exercises. Some body fractures are amenable to maxillomandibular fixation (MMF) only. There is usually no great urgency to stabilize mandibular fractures if antibiotics and analgesics are being given.[1,2] The AO has comprehensive guidance on its website that includes approaches and fixation placement that can be a useful reference.[3]

REFERENCES

1. Mukerji R, Mukerji G, McGurk M. Mandibular fractures: historical perspective. Br J Oral Maxillofac Surg 2006;44(3): 222–228
2. Kelamis JA, Rodriguez ED. Mandible fractures. In: Marcus JR, Erdmann D, Rodriguez ED, eds. Essentials of Craniomaxillofacial Trauma. St Louis: Quality Medical Publishing; 2012
3. https://www.aofoundation.org/search-results#q=mandibular%20fracture

MANAGEMENT OF MANDIBULAR FRACTURES

9. A 25-year-old male is admitted following an alleged assault. Examination confirms tenderness and swelling over the left temporomandibular joint (TMJ). His mouth opening is reduced but normal occlusion is preserved. Radiographs show a unilateral extraarticular fracture of the left condyle. *How should this injury best be managed?*

  E. Soft diet and close observation

  Fractures of the condyle require early active range of motion (ROM) to rehabilitate TMJ articulation. In fractures such as this, where occlusion is maintained, soft diet and close observation represent the best treatment. If malocclusion subsequently develops, then arch bars or maxillomandibular fixation (MMF) should be placed and occlusion controlled with elastics. ORIF is indicated for some condylar fractures, such as bilateral cases or cases where there is significant displacement of the fracture and where occlusion cannot be established. Access to the TMJ and condyle are commonly through a preauricular approach and this can be difficult and risks damage to the facial nerve but would not be justified in this case.[1–3]

REFERENCES

1. Blitz M, Notarnicola K. Closed reduction of the mandibular fracture. Atlas Oral Maxillofac Surg Clin North Am 2009;17(1):1–13
2. Zide MF. Open reduction of mandibular condyle fractures. Indications and technique. Clin Plast Surg 1989;16(1):69–76
3. Stacey DH, Doyle JF, Mount DL, Snyder MC, Gutowski KA. Management of mandible fractures. Plast Reconstr Surg 2006;117(3):48e–60e

COMPLICATION RATES IN MANDIBULAR FRACTURES

10. *Which anatomic site is associated with the highest complication rate in mandibular fractures?*

  A. Angle

  The angle has the highest complication rate of any single region of the mandible. These fractures can also be difficult to reduce and stabilize accurately. Approaches include transbuccal, intraoral, and maxillomandibular fixation (MMF). Isolated fractures can be reliably treated with a single miniplate along the oblique ridge through an intraoral incision to provide functional stability. A second 2-mm miniplate can be added to the lower border if more rigid fixation is needed.[1,2]

REFERENCES

1. Ellis E 3rd. A prospective study of 3 treatment methods for isolated fractures of the mandibular angle. J Oral Maxillofac Surg 2010;68(11):2743–2754
2. Lee JH. Treatment of mandibular angle fractures. Arch Craniofac Surg 2017;18(2):73–75

SPECIAL CONSIDERATIONS IN MANDIBULAR FRACTURES

11. *Which one of the following is true regarding mandibular fracture management?*

    D. Pediatric mandibular fractures commonly involve the condyle and need close follow-up.

        A vast majority of mandibular fractures seen in children involve the condyle. Condylar fractures in this population must be followed very closely because they can lead to ankylosis and growth disturbances. Management of other mandibular fractures in children require additional care when managing them operatively as it is important to avoid damage to the developing tooth buds. Roughly half of all mandibular fractures are bilateral, and due to the increased instability these fractures display, at least one fracture should be fixated with more rigid plating. However, not all sites necessarily need rigid fixation. Common fracture patterns include a body/symphysis/angle fracture with a contralateral condylar/subcondylar fracture. The condyle is often treated nonoperatively while the body/symphysis/angle fracture is chosen for rigid fixation. In situations of comminution, it is best to have bridging of the area of comminution with load-bearing fixation using larger reconstruction plates. Where bone graft is required, it is preferable to delay this in heavily contaminated wounds or where there is poor soft tissue cover.

        Edentulous mandibles tend to have smaller and lesser quality bone stock; however, this does not mean they should always be treated conservatively. Accuracy of reduction is perhaps not as important as in the dentate mandible, as occlusion does not need to be restored, but approaches still include the use of reconstruction plates as alternatives to nonoperative treatment.

        Malocclusion is a potential risk factor following mandibular fracture and is almost always the result of a technical error intraoperatively. However, it is not the most common complication. Other potential problems include hardware failure, reinjury, infection, nonunion, and ongoing pain and jaw stiffness.[1-3]

REFERENCES

1. Morrow BT, Samson TD, Schubert W, Mackay DR. Evidence-based medicine: mandible fractures. Plast Reconstr Surg 2014;134(6):1381–1390
2. Gerbino G, Tarello F, Fasolis M, De Gioanni PP. Rigid fixation with teeth in the line of mandibular fractures. Int J Oral Maxillofac Surg 1997;26(3):182–186
3. Miloro M, Ghali GE, Larsen PE, et al, eds. Peterson's Principles of Oral and Maxillofacial Surgery, Vol. 1, 3rd ed. 2012

37. Basic Oral Surgery

See *Essentials of Plastic Surgery*, third edition, pp. 486–504

CRANIAL NERVE FORAMINA

1. *When considering the anatomy of the trigeminal nerve, where does the ophthalmic division (V1) exit from the skull base?*
   A. Foramen rotundum
   B. Superior orbital fissure
   C. Foramen ovale
   D. Inferior orbital fissure
   E. Foramen spinosum

CRANIAL NERVE FORAMINA

2. *When considering the anatomy of the facial nerve, through which foramen does it exit from the skull base?*
   A. Jugular foramen
   B. Stylomastoid foramen
   C. Optic foramen
   D. Hypoglossal foramen
   E. Superior orbital foramen

SURGICAL ANATOMY OF THE ORAL CAVITY

3. *When operating in the oral cavity, which one of the following is firmly adherent to the alveolus and should be preserved with some length attached when making incisions for access to the mandible?*
   A. Labial frenula
   B. Alveolar mucosa
   C. Gingiva proper
   D. Oral vestibule
   E. Wharton's duct

PRIMARY AND SECONDARY DENTITION

4. *Which one of the following is true regarding primary and secondary dentition?*
   A. The total number of teeth in primary dentition is 18.
   B. The total number of teeth in secondary dentition is 30.
   C. The reference number for the adult upper left central incisor is 9.
   D. The reference numbers for the adult lower first molars are 3 and 14.
   E. There are usually four premolars in adult dentition.

ERUPTION SEQUENCE FOR SECONDARY DENTITION

5. A 6-year-old child is seen in clinic following eruption of the first adult teeth, which are first molars. *Which tooth type would be most likely to erupt next?*
   A. Canine
   B. Incisor
   C. First molar
   D. Second premolar
   E. Second molar

DENTAL OCCLUSION

6. A patient is referred to the aesthetic clinic concerned about her lack of chin projection. On examination you note that the patient has excessive overjet with normal angulation of the incisors. *What type of occlusion does this likely represent?*
   A. Class I
   B. Class II
   C. Class III
   D. Class IV
   E. Normal occlusion

DENTAL TERMINOLOGY

7. *When using oral surgery terminology to describe a patient's dentition, what does the term distal refer to?*
   A. Away from the cheek
   B. Toward the feet
   C. Toward the midline
   D. Away from the tongue
   E. Away from the midline

CORRECTION OF FACIAL BONY DEFORMITY

8. A young adult patient who had Pierre Robin sequence as an infant presents with class II malocclusion and is concerned with regard to lack of chin prominence. *Which one of the following procedures may be most helpful in this scenario?*
   A. LeFort I osteotomy
   B. LeFort II osteotomy
   C. LeFort III osteotomy
   D. Bilateral sagittal split osteotomies
   E. Intraoral vertical ramus osteotomies

SENSORY NERVE BLOCKS

9. *Which one of the following nerve blocks may be given intraorally or extraorally to produce anesthesia of the upper lip, medial cheek, lower eyelid, nose, and buccal gingiva?*
   A. Infraorbital
   B. Inferior alveolar
   C. Greater palatine
   D. Buccal
   E. Mental

ODONTOGENIC INFECTIONS

10. A patient presents to the emergency department with a 24-hour history of facial swelling, trismus, and severe pain to the dentition. You suspect the symptoms are caused by an odontogenic infection. *Which one of the following is correct in this case?*
   A. The infection is most likely caused by a single organism.
   B. The infection is most likely to be periodontal in origin.
   C. The likely organism is anaerobic bacteria.
   D. The symptoms are consistent with a parapharyngeal space infection.
   E. Antibiotics are the mainstay of treatment in this case.

CYSTS AND TUMORS OF THE MANDIBLE

11. *In a patient with a significant history of basal cell carcinoma as a young adult, which one of the following intraoral pathologies would be most typical?*
   A. Periapical cyst
   B. Dentigerous cyst
   C. Odontogenic keratocyst
   D. Ameloblastic cyst
   E. Dental abscess

SOFT TISSUE CEPHALOMETRIC LANDMARKS

12. *Which one of the following soft tissue cephalometric points refers to the most anterior soft tissue point on the chin?*
   A. Pogonion
   B. Stomion superioris
   C. Menton
   D. Gnathion
   E. Labrale

BONY CEPHALOMETRIC LANDMARKS

13. *When reviewing a bony cephalogram, which one of the following is used as a guide to the external auditory meatus?*
   A. Sella turcica
   B. Porion
   C. Articulare
   D. Gonion
   E. Nasion

TEMPOROMANDIBULAR JOINT (TMJ)

14. You see a patient in clinic with chronic bilateral jaw pain just in front of the ears. She experiences problems with jaw locking and deviation on mouth opening. *Which one of the following is true regarding this condition?*
   A. This problem affects up to 15% of the US population.
   B. Males and females are equally affected.
   C. Articular joint involvement is nearly always attributable to rheumatoid arthritis.
   D. Treatment focuses on behavior modification with bite guards or splinting.
   E. Surgical treatment with joint replacement has become a popular option.

MANDIBULAR OSTEONECROSIS

15. **What do osteoradionecrosis (ORN) and osteonecrosis (ON) of the mandible have in common?**
    A. They share the same underlying pathological cause.
    B. The initial investigations should be identical.
    C. They can both occur following cancer treatment.
    D. They can both be avoided with dental clearance.
    E. Most cases will require wide resection and free tissue reconstruction.

ARCH BARS

16. A patient has a dentoalveolar fracture, which is unstable and displaced. **Which one of the following is correct when using arch bars in this scenario?**
    A. They should extend two teeth proximal and distal to the fracture line.
    B. The wires should normally be twisted anticlockwise to tighten.
    C. The first wires are usually placed posteriorly then progressively placed toward the midline.
    D. Normally, 5-gauge wires are used to secure the bar to the dentition.
    E. This is a more time efficient process than using intermaxillary screw fixation.

Answers

CRANIAL NERVE FORAMINA

1. When considering the anatomy of the trigeminal nerve, where does the ophthalmic division (V1) exit from the skull base?

B. Superior orbital fissure

The trigeminal nerve has three divisions: ophthalmic, maxillary, and mandibular. The ophthalmic and maxillary divisions are purely sensory, while the mandibular division is both motor and sensory. The ophthalmic division exits the cranial vault through the superior orbital fissure. It supplies sensation to the upper third of the face including the forehead, scalp, upper eyelid, nose conjunctiva, and cornea. The maxillary division exits the cranial vault through the foramen rotundum and supplies sensation to the lower eyelids, cheek, and upper dentition. The mandibular division exits the cranium through the foramen ovale and supplies sensation to the lower lip, chin, jaw, and lower dentition. It also supplies the muscles of mastication including the temporalis, masseter, and pterygoids. The inferior orbital fissure contains the infraorbital and zygomatic nerves which are branches of the maxillary division of the trigeminal nerve. In addition, the inferior ophthalmic vein and infraorbital artery also pass through this fissure. The foramen spinosum transmits the middle meningeal artery and vein and the meningeal branch of the mandibular nerve (**Fig. 37.1**).[1,2]

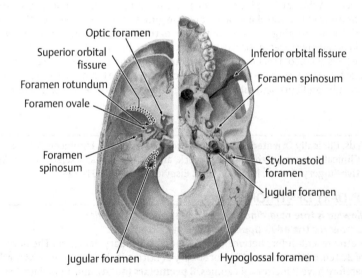

Fig. 37.1 Primary (pediatric) dentition. (From Gilroy AM, MacPherson BR. Atlas of Anatomy. 3rd ed. Thieme, 2016.)

REFERENCES

1. Moore KL, Dalley AF, eds. Clinically Oriented Anatomy. 4th ed. New York, NY: Lippincott, Williams, and Wilkins; 1999
2. Neligan PC, Sharaf B. Clinical anatomy of the head and neck, and recipient vessel selection. In: Wei FC, Mardini S, eds. Flaps and Reconstructive Surgery. 2nd ed. New York, NY: Elsevier Inc.; 2017:61–74

CRANIAL NERVE FORAMINA

2. When considering the anatomy of the facial nerve, through which foramen does it exit from the skull base?

B. Stylomastoid foramen

The facial nerve exits the skull base through the stylomastoid foramen. It has a number of motor and sensory functions. It supplies voluntary control of all muscles of facial expression, the stylohyoid muscle, the stapedius, and the posterior belly of digastric. It also supplies visceral motor function to the lacrimal and sublingual glands. It supplies general sensation to the external ear (concha and external auditory canal) as well as the tympanic membrane. It is involved in specialized taste in the anterior two-thirds of the tongue.

The glossopharyngeal nerve supplies sensation to the oropharynx and motor supply to the pharynx. It exits the cranium through the jugular foramen along with the vagus and accessory nerves and the sigmoid sinus, which becomes the internal jugular vein. The optic nerve supplies specialized sensation to the retina with information regarding brightness, contrast, and color. It exits the cranium through the optic foramen along with the ophthalmic artery. The hypoglossal nerve exits the skull base through the hypoglossal foramen and goes on to supply motor innervation to the tongue. The oculomotor nerve supplies motor function to the extraocular muscles: superior rectus, inferior rectus, medial rectus, inferior oblique, and the ciliary and sphincter muscles. It exits the cranium through the superior orbital fissure and can be compromised in conditions such as superior orbital fissure syndrome, leading to ptosis, proptosis, ophthalmoplegia, paresthesia, and dilated pupil (see **Fig. 37.1**).[1,2]

REFERENCES

1. Moore KL, Dalley AF, eds. Clinically Oriented Anatomy. 4th ed. New York, NY: Lippincott, Williams, and Wilkins; 1999
2. Neligan PC, Sharaf B. Clinical anatomy of the head and neck, and recipient vessel selection. In: Wei FC, Mardini S, eds. Flaps and Reconstructive Surgery. 2nd ed. New York, NY: Elsevier Inc.; 2017:61–74

SURGICAL ANATOMY OF THE ORAL CAVITY

3. *When operating in the oral cavity, which one of the following is firmly adherent to the alveolus and should be preserved with some length attached when making incisions for access to the mandible?*

   C. **Gingiva proper**

The mucosal covering on the alveolus of the mandible comprises the attached gingiva (gingiva proper) and mobile gingiva (alveolar mucosa). The gingiva proper is very tightly adherent to the alveolus whereas the alveolar mucosa is more loosely attached. When making incisions for access to the mandible, therefore, it is important to ensure that the length of the free end of the alveolar mucosa or loose gingiva is maximized such that there will be sufficient soft tissue to repair this to the gingiva proper at the end of the procedure. Otherwise, it is very difficult to suture the adherent and loose gingiva together because there is no space between the adherent tissue and bone. The labial frenula are midline folds of mucosa that may be incised during midline access, but preservation of tissue length is not specifically important. The oral vestibule refers to the space between the teeth and cheeks. Wharton's duct is the term used to describe the submandibular and sublingual salivary ducts, which enter the oral cavity on the floor of mouth.[1,2]

REFERENCES

1. Moore KL, Dalley AF, eds. Clinically Oriented Anatomy. 4th ed. New York, NY: Lippincott, Williams, and Wilkins; 1999
2. Neligan PC, Sharaf B. Clinical anatomy of the head and neck, and recipient vessel selection. In: Wei FC, Mardini S, eds. Flaps and Reconstructive Surgery. 2nd ed. New York, NY: Elsevier Inc.; 2017:61–74

PRIMARY AND SECONDARY DENTITION

4. *Which one of the following is true regarding primary and secondary dentition?*

   C. The reference number for the adult upper left central incisor is 9.

The number of teeth present differs between primary and secondary dentition. The normal primary dentition includes a total of **20 teeth** (10 per arch). The secondary dentition includes a total of **32 teeth** (16 per arch). Adult dentition will therefore have 8 incisors, 4 canines, **8 premolars (not 4)**, and 12 molars. In contrast children will only have eight molar teeth and the same number of other teeth as adults.[1]

There are different ways to number the teeth that are uniformly recognized internationally. These are the universal numbering system, the Palmer notation numbering system, and the Federation Dentaire Internationale (FDI) numbering system.[2]

The universal numbering system numbers the adult teeth from the right upper third molar to the left upper third molar then continues from the left lower third molar through to the third right lower molar from 1 through 32. So the left first upper incisor is the ninth tooth from the upper right. The first adult lower molars will be numbered 19 and 30 respectively. It would be the upper first molars that would be labelled 3 and 14.

The Palmer notation system uses four quadrants: right upper, left upper, right lower, and left lower, with each being given a different L notation. The left upper uses a standard L, while the right upper uses a mirror L. The left lower uses an upside down L, while the right lower uses an upside down mirrored L. Each tooth within a quadrant is then numbered 1 to 8 beginning at the midline. In this case the left upper incisor would be L1 instead of tooth 9 (**Figs. 37.2 and 37.3**).

The FDI system again uses four quadrants. In this case the quadrants are numbered 1 through 4 with the maxillary right being labelled 1, the maxillary left being labelled 2, the mandibular left being labelled 3, and the mandibular right being labelled 4. Again the teeth within each quadrant are labelled from the midline 1 through 8. So the left upper incisor would be 11.[1,2]

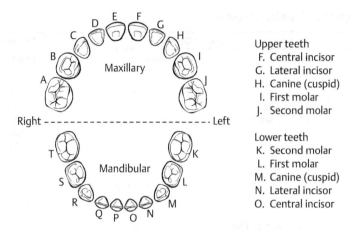

Upper teeth
  F. Central incisor
  G. Lateral incisor
  H. Canine (cuspid)
  I. First molar
  J. Second molar

Lower teeth
  K. Second molar
  L. First molar
  M. Canine (cuspid)
  N. Lateral incisor
  O. Central incisor

Fig. 37.2 Primary (pediatric) dentition.

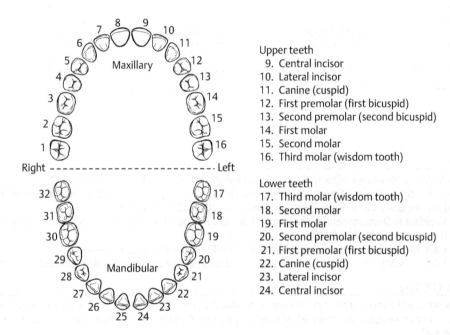

Upper teeth
  9. Central incisor
 10. Lateral incisor
 11. Canine (cuspid)
 12. First premolar (first bicuspid)
 13. Second premolar (second bicuspid)
 14. First molar
 15. Second molar
 16. Third molar (wisdom tooth)

Lower teeth
 17. Third molar (wisdom tooth)
 18. Second molar
 19. First molar
 20. Second premolar (second bicuspid)
 21. First premolar (first bicuspid)
 22. Canine (cuspid)
 23. Lateral incisor
 24. Central incisor

Fig. 37.3 Secondary (adult) dentition.

REFERENCES

1. Zohrabian VM, Poon CS, Abrahams JJ. Embryology and anatomy of the jaw and dentition. Seminars in Ultrasound, CT, and MRI 2015;36:397–406
2. Peck S, Peck L. A time for change of tooth numbering systems. J Dent Educ 1993;57(8): 643–647

ERUPTION SEQUENCE FOR SECONDARY DENTITION

5. A 6-year-old child is seen in clinic following eruption of the first adult teeth, which are first molars. *Which tooth type would be most likely to erupt next?*
    B. Incisor
       The adult eruption sequence is commonly first molars, central incisors, lateral incisors, first premolars, canines, and second then third molars. This can be remembered as an eight-digit code: 612 453 78. Each quadrant is labeled from one to eight, commencing with the central incisor (**Table 37.1**).[1–5]

Table 37.1 *Dental Eruption and Shedding Sequences*

	Primary Dentition		Permanent Dentition
	Erupt	Shed	Erupt
Maxillary Teeth			
Central incisor	8–12 months	6–7 years	7–8 years
Lateral incisor	9–13 months	7–8 years	8–9 years
Canine	16–22 months	10–12 years	**11–12 years (last before 3rd molar)**
First premolar			10–11 years
Second premolar			10–12 years
First molar	13–19 months	9–11 years	**6–7 years (first)**
Second molar	25–33 months	10–12 years	12–13 years
Third molar			17–21 years
Mandibular Teeth			
Central incisor	**6–10 months (first)**	6–7 years	6–7 years
Lateral incisor	10–16 months	7–8 years	7–8 years
Canine	17–23 months	9–12 years	9–10 years
First premolar			10–12 years
Second premolar			11–12 years
First molar	14–18 months	9–11 years	6–7 years
Second molar	23–31 months	10–12 years	11–13 years
Third molar			17–21 years

(Data from Zohrabian VM, Poon CS, Abrahams JJ. Embryology and anatomy of the jaw and dentition. Seminars in Ultrasound, CT, and MRI 2015;36:397–406.)

REFERENCES

1. Peck S, Peck L. A time for change of tooth numbering systems. J Dent Educ 1993;57(8): 643–647
2. Ekstrand KR, Christiansen J, Christiansen ME. Time and duration of eruption of first and second permanent molars: a longitudinal investigation. Community Dent Oral Epidemiol 2003;31(5):344–350
3. Logan WH, Kronfeld R. Development of the human jaws and surrounding structures from birth to the age of fifteen years. J Am Dent Assoc 1933;20:379–427
4. Schour I, Massler M. Development of human dentition. J Am Dent Assoc 1941;20:379–427
5. Tooth eruption: the permanent teeth. Available at www.ada.org/sections/scienceAndResearch/pdfs/ patient_58.pdf

DENTAL OCCLUSION

6. A patient is referred to the aesthetic clinic concerned about her lack of chin projection. On examination you note that the patient has excessive overjet with normal angulation of the incisors. *What type of occlusion does this likely represent?*

    B. Class II

    Occlusion refers to the relationship of the teeth to one another. Normal occlusion is based on the relationship of the upper and lower first permanent molars. It was described by Edward Angle who identified that in normal occlusion the mesiobuccal cusp of the maxillary first molar interfaces with the buccal groove of the mandibular first molar. Malocclusion is where this relationship is altered in some way and is split into three subtypes: classes I, II, and III. The descriptions of the three classes of malocclusion are:

    Class I: The mesiobuccal cusp of the first maxillary molar occludes in the buccal groove of the mandibular molar but the teeth are malpositioned or malrotated.

    Class II: The mandibular molar is distally positioned relative to the maxillary molar.

    Class III: The mandibular molar is mesially positioned relative to the maxillary molar.

    In general terms, patients with small or retruded mandibles have a class II occlusion and patients with prognathism have class III occlusion. The patient described in this scenario has class II malocclusion which can either be subdivided as division I or division II depending on the angulation of the incisors and the degree of overjet and overbite. Overjet refers to the amount of horizontal overlap of the incisal edges, while overbite refers to the amount of vertical overlap (**Fig. 37.4**).[1]

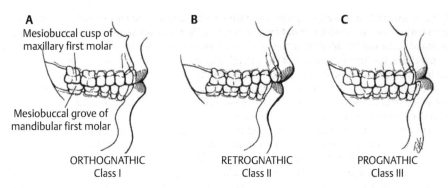

Fig. 37.4 Classes of malocclusion. (Used with permission from Facial Analysis in Cheney M, Hadlock T, ed. Facial Surgery. Plastic and Reconstructive. 1st ed. Thieme; 2014.)

REFERENCE

1. Türp JC, Greene CS, Strub JR. Dental occlusion: a critical reflection on past, present and future concepts. J Oral Rehabil 2008;35(6):446–453

DENTAL TERMINOLOGY

7. *When using oral surgery terminology to describe a patient's dentition, what does the term* distal *refer to?*

   E. Away from the midline

   In dental terminology *distal* means *away from the midline* and *mesial* means *toward the midline*. The term *buccal* means *toward the cheek and lingual means toward the tongue*. These terms can sometimes be confusing. For example, when describing teeth, the terms *distal* and *mesial are* applied to the dental arches, and as the arches are followed from the molars to the incisors, the teeth are becoming progressively more *mesial*. In more traditional anatomy we might describe this relationship as the incisors being more anterior and also more medial to the molars (**Fig. 37.5**).[1]

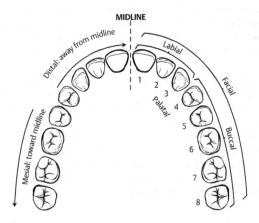

Fig. 37.5 Dental relationships. (From Marcus JR, Erdmann D, Rodriguez ED, eds. Essentials of Craniomaxillofacial Trauma. St Louis: Quality Medical Publishing, 2012.)

REFERENCE

1. Marcus JR, Erdmann D, Rodriguez ED, eds. Essentials of Craniomaxillofacial Trauma. St Louis: Quality Medical Publishing; 2012

CORRECTION OF FACIAL BONY DEFORMITY

8. A young adult patient who had Pierre Robin sequence as an infant presents with class II malocclusion and is concerned with regard to lack of chin prominence. *Which one of the following procedures may be most helpful in this scenario?*

   D. Bilateral sagittal split osteotomies

   Orthognathic surgery involves correction of the components of the facial skeleton to restore proper functional and aesthetic relationships such as occlusion and normal facial appearance. The *bilateral sagittal split osteotomy*

(BSSO) is a useful and commonly used orthognathic technique for the correction of dentofacial abnormalities such as in patients with mandibular deficiency who had Pierre Robin sequence as an infant. It can also be used to treat mandibular excess. BSSO is achieved through an intraoral approach with an incision made through the mucosa overlying the anterior border of the mandibular ramus. Extensive soft tissue dissection is performed at a subperiosteal level to adequately expose the angle, ramus, and body for the osteotomy and release of the soft tissues adequately to allow mandibular advancement (or set-back). Osteotomies are performed such that key neurovascular structures and dental roots are preserved. Once freed, the mandible can be advanced or set back as required and stabilized in place using plates and screws.[1]

A LeFort I osteotomy is typically performed to correct maxillary deficiency. This also involves an intraoral approach with a mucosal incision made in the upper buccal sulcus from first molar to first molar. An osteotomy is made to separate the tooth-bearing maxilla from the midface. This will extend from the piriform aperture through the anterior maxilla and posteriorly to the pterygoid plates. Again, preservation of key neurovascular structures and dental roots as well as the nasal mucosa must be ensured. Once adequate soft tissue and bone release have been achieved the desired position of the maxilla can be selected and fixation is performed with miniplates and screws.[2] LeFort II and III osteotomies are not used to correct mandibular deficiencies. Intraoral vertical ramus osteotomies may be used to correct mandibular excess in some cases.

REFERENCES

1. Monson LA. Bilateral sagittal split osteotomy. Semin Plast Surg 2013;27(3):145–148
2. Buchanan EP, Hyman CH. LeFort I osteotomy. Semin Plast Surg 2013;27(3):149–154

SENSORY NERVE BLOCKS

9. **Which one of the following nerve blocks may be given intraorally or extraorally to produce anesthesia of the upper lip, medial cheek, lower eyelid, nose, and buccal gingiva?**

   A. Infraorbital

   Local anesthetic blocks are very useful when performing intraoral surgery. Typically, a dental syringe is used, which gives good control for the injection and provides adequate reach for areas deeper in the oral cavity such as the posterior dentition. Lidocaine 2% is commonly used in small vials (2.2 mL each) that are combined with epinephrine 1:80,000. This concentration differs from the 1:200,000 dilution typically used and has the theoretical advantage of reducing bleeding while working in this highly vascular area.

   Local anesthetic blocks are not only useful for procedures where patients are fully conscious but are also useful combined with general anesthesia as they can reduce the requirements for anesthetic agents and systemic pain relief requirements such as opiates. They can also help reduce bleeding as discussed above and help with dissection of soft tissues. Knowledge of the main local anesthetic blocks, such as those described, is therefore useful in clinical practice.

   The infraorbital block is particularly useful when performing surgery on the nose under local anesthesia because injection at this site can reduce pain on subsequent external nasal injections. The inferior alveolar block is mainly used for dental procedures of the lower dentition, while the nasopalatine block is usually used for dental procedures of the upper dentition or in orthognathic surgery. The greater palatine block is injected into the hard palate at the level of the upper second molar to block the upper dentition and palate. A mental nerve block is also part of the inferior alveolar nerve block but can be given as an isolated block in the lower buccal sulcus at the level of the second premolar. It provides anesthesia of the buccal mucosa and gingiva anterior to the first premolar. A buccal block is performed at the mandibular ramus after withdrawing and confirming no aspiration of blood. It provides anesthesia of the buccal mucosa and gingiva anterior to the first premolar.[1,2]

REFERENCES

1. Zide BM, Swift R. How to block and tackle the face. Plast Reconstr Surg 1998;101(3): 840–851
2. Fedok F, Carniol P, eds. Minimally Invasive and Office-Based Procedures in Facial Plastic Surgery. 1st ed. Thieme; 2013

ODONTOGENIC INFECTIONS

10. A patient presents to the emergency department with a 24-hour history of facial swelling, trismus, and severe pain to the dentition. You suspect the symptoms are caused by an odontogenic infection. **Which one of the following is correct in this case?**

    D. The symptoms are consistent with a parapharyngeal space infection.

    When examining a patient with a suspected odontogenic infection, trismus may be the only indication of a parapharyngeal space abscess. Examination must include a thorough review of the oropharynx. Odontogenic infections can range from localized conditions to severe life-threatening infections. Almost all are polymicrobial and are not limited to anaerobic organisms alone. In more than half of cases, infections will be a mixed aerobic/anaerobic combination. Odontogenic infections arise from two major sources, namely, periapical and periodontal, of which the former is most common. Although antibiotics are a component of treatment, the main management is drainage of the abscess and this is undertaken by a dentally trained professional.[1]

REFERENCE

1. Flynn TR. What are the antibiotics of choice for odontogenic infections, and how long should the treatment course last? Oral Maxillofac Surg Clin North Am 2011;23(4): 519–536, v–vi

CYSTS AND TUMORS OF THE MANDIBLE

11. *In a patient with a significant history of basal cell carcinoma as a young adult, which one of the following intraoral pathologies would be most typical?*

C. Odontogenic keratocyst

Odontogenic keratocysts are aggressively destructive lesions that arise from dental lamina and contain parakeratin. They are associated with nevoid basal cell carcinoma syndrome which is also known as Gorlin's syndrome and have a high recurrence rate following surgical resection. On radiographs they appear with corticated, scalloped margins and expansion of cortical bone. Due to the high recurrence of these lesions, treatment may be more aggressive than simple excision and involve osseous resection with up to 1 cm bone margins. Alternatively, a two-stage decompression and enucleation may be preferred. Gorlin's syndrome is also associated with other abnormalities including palmar and plantar pits, calcification of the falx cerebri, bifid ribs, and hypertelorism.

Periapical cysts are the most common jaw cyst and occur in response to bacterial overgrowth, usually from caries or trauma. They appear as well-defined, confluent lesions on radiographs and require dental extraction and cyst enucleation if the tooth is nonviable. Dentigerous cysts are the second most common jaw cyst and arise from cystic degeneration around a tooth crown. They are well-corticated, radiolucent lesions located at the crown of a developing tooth. Treatment involves enucleation and histological analysis. Ameloblastoma is a neoplasm derived from ameloblasts. It is locally invasive and has metastatic potential. On imaging it is seen as a radiolucent uni- or multilocular lesion often with local bony distortion. It should be treated with wide resection to ensure clear margins. Major reconstruction is likely to be required with free tissue such as a fibula flap. Dental abscesses are common but are not specifically linked to Gorlin's syndrome.[1,2]

REFERENCES

1. Abaza NA, El-Mofty SK, Miller AD. Cysts of the oral and maxillofacial region. In: Fonseca RJ, ed. Oral and Maxillofacial Surgery. 3rd ed. New York, NY: Elsevier Inc.; 2018:338–390
2. Fujii K, Miyashita T. Gorlin syndrome (nevoid basal cell carcinoma syndrome): update and literature review. Pediatr Int 2014;56(5):667–674

SOFT TISSUE CEPHALOMETRIC LANDMARKS

12. *Which one of the following soft tissue cephalometric points refers to the most anterior soft tissue point on the chin?*

A. Pogonion

The most anterior soft tissue point on the chin is the soft tissue pogonion. The *menton* refers to the lowest point on the contour of the soft tissue chin, while the *gnathion* refers to the midpoint between the pogonion and menton. The *stomion superioris* refers to the lowest point of the lower lip vermilion and the *labrale* refers to the mucocutaneous border of the lip in the midsaggital plane. Cephalometrics are an important component of orthognathic and speech surgery. Both soft tissue and bony landmarks are used for a variety of analyses. Modern technology and imaging facilitates a fully automated approach to this (**Fig. 37.6**).[1]

REFERENCE

1. Lindner C, Wang CW, Huang CT, Li CH, Chang SW, Cootes TF. Fully automatic system for accurate localisation and analysis of cephalometric landmarks in lateral cephalograms. Sci Rep 2016;6:33581

BONY CEPHALOMETRIC LANDMARKS

13. *When reviewing a bony cephalogram, which one of the following is used as a guide to the external auditory meatus?*

B. Porion

Bony cephalometric landmarks may be useful for analysis of the facial and cranial skeleton with reference to orthodontics and mandibular/maxillary deformity. The *porion* is the most superior point of the external auditory meatus. The *sella turcica* represents the center of the pituitary fossa. The *articulare* represents the junction of the basisphenoid and the posterior part of the mandibular condyle. The *gonion* is the point at the angle of the mandible that is directed most inferiorly and posteriorly. The *nasion* is the most anterior point at the junction of the nasal and frontal bones in the midsagittal plane (see **Fig. 37.6**).[1,2]

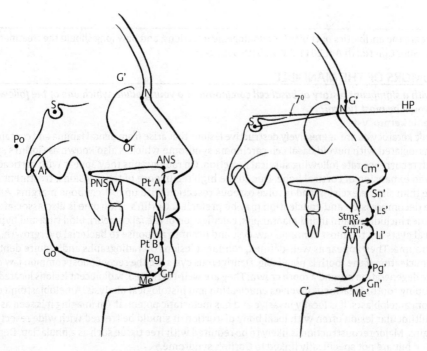

Fig. 37.6 Cephalometric landmarks.

REFERENCES

1. Kolokitha OE, Topouzelis N. Cephalometric methods of prediction in orthognathic surgery. J Maxillofac Oral Surg 2011;10(3):236–245
2. Lindner C, Wang CW, Huang CT, Li CH, Chang SW, Cootes TF. Fully automatic system for accurate localisation and analysis of cephalometric landmarks in lateral cephalograms. Sci Rep 2016;6:33581

TEMPOROMANDIBULAR JOINT (TMJ)

14. You see a patient in clinic with chronic bilateral jaw pain just in front of the ears. She experiences problems with jaw locking and deviation on mouth opening. *Which one of the following is true regarding this condition?*

    D. Treatment focuses on behavior modification with bite guards or splinting.

Temporomandibular (TMJ) disorders represent a spectrum of clinical problems involving the muscles of mastication, the TMJ itself or the surrounding soft tissues. They affect around 5% (not 15%) of the population and females are more commonly affected than males. Symptoms vary but can include decreased mandibular range of motion, pain in the muscles of mastication, pain in the ears or at the TMJ, joint crepitus, and jaw locking or deviation on mouth opening. TMJ problems can be subdivided into nonarticular and articular causes. Articular causes may be inflammatory or noninflammatory and include conditions such as rheumatoid arthritis (RA), ankylosing spondylitis, gout, and osteoarthritis, so are not solely attributed to RA. Nonarticular cases, which make up the majority of cases, are best treated with behavioral therapy, physical therapy, bite guards, and analgesia to try and reduce clenching and bruxism and improve symptoms. In some cases of articular causes, they are treated surgically, but this is not commonly undertaken.[1]

REFERENCE

1. De Rossi SS, Greenberg MS, Liu F, Steinkeler A. Temporomandibular disorders: evaluation and management. Med Clin North Am 2014;98(6):1353–1384

MANDIBULAR OSTEONECROSIS

15. What do osteoradionecrosis (ORN) and osteonecrosis (ON) of the mandible have in common?

    C. They can both occur following cancer treatment.

Osteoradionecrosis (ORN) and osteonecrosis (ON) of the mandible can both occur secondary to treatment for bony cancer. Radiotherapy is commonly used to treat head and neck tumors such as squamous cell carcinoma either as a primary treatment or after surgery. Radiotherapy can induce necrotic damage to the native mandible leading to soft tissue ulceration and bone exposure. Bisphosphonates can also cause necrosis of the mandible and overlying soft tissues and these are used to treat bone metastases. The underlying pathology is different as one is secondary to radiotherapy and the other to bisphosphonate use, although they may share some similarities. The initial investigations will differ and in particular it is important in ORN to exclude local tumor recurrence with a biopsy and imaging. Complete dental extraction clearance is sometimes offered to patients prior to undergoing radiotherapy of the head and neck as this can help reduce post-treatment problems with ORN. However, more often there is select dental extraction only. Prior to commencing bisphosphonates, it would be inappropriate to perform extractions for this potential risk alone. Treatment for either condition will depend on severity of symptoms and only more extreme cases will require wide resection and free tissue reconstruction. Initial treatment commences in both cases with conservative measures including maintenance of good oral hygiene and antibiotics. In some cases, debridement may be beneficial too. The use of hyperbaric oxygen therapy may be helpful in ORN or ON but still remains controversial in some circles.[1,2]

REFERENCES

1. Cheriex KCAL, Nijhuis THJ, Mureau MAM. Osteoradionecrosis of the jaws: a review of conservative and surgical treatment options. J Reconstr Microsurg 2013;29(2):69–75
2. Khan AA, Morrison A, Hanley DA, et al; International Task Force on Osteonecrosis of the Jaw. Diagnosis and management of osteonecrosis of the jaw: a systematic review and international consensus. J Bone Miner Res 2015;30(1):3–23

ARCH BARS

16. A patient has a dentoalveolar fracture, which is unstable and displaced. Which one of the following is correct when using arch bars in this scenario?

    A. They should extend two teeth proximal and distal to the fracture line.

Arch bars may be used to stabilize dentoalveolar fractures. They provide a stable base from which to institute maxillomandibular fixation (MMF) and control occlusion in the posttraumatic period. In mandibular fractures, arch bars ideally extend two teeth proximal and distal to a fracture line when possible. When using arch bars, they are usually placed from first molar to first molar and applied starting in the midline to prevent redundancy within the arch bar. Twenty-four-gauge wires (not 5-gauge) are used and are conventionally twisted clockwise to tighten. Proper occlusion and fracture reduction must be established before complete tightening of all wires within the quadrant of the fracture to prevent malreduction. This is facilitated by tightening the wires in the fracture segment after reducing the fracture. For this reason, complete tightening of each individual wire as it is placed is not performed. Alternatives to this technique include intermaxillary screw fixation and the SMARTLock system. Intermaxillary screw fixation is faster but less rigid than arch bars. The SMARTLock system involves self-locking screws and a plate design to eliminate the need for interdental wiring.[1]

REFERENCE

1. Neligan PC, Buck DW. Facial injuries. In: Neligan PC, Buck DW. Core Procedures in Plastic Surgery. New York, NY: Elsevier Inc.; 2014:91–109

38. Principles of Head and Neck Cancer: Staging and Management

See *Essentials of Plastic Surgery*, third edition, pp. 505–516

INCIDENCE OF HEAD AND NECK CANCER

1. *What is the most common tumor type in head and neck cancers?*
   A. Adenoid cystic
   B. Squamous cell
   C. Adenocarcinoma
   D. Lymphoma
   E. Melanoma

WORKUP IN SUSPECTED HEAD AND NECK CANCER

2. A 50-year-old male smoker presents with a 4-week history of a 3-cm diameter, left-sided neck mass without any other obvious signs or symptoms. *After the initial history and examination, what would the next most appropriate investigation be?*
   A. Excision biopsy of the mass
   B. Incision biopsy to the tongue base
   C. CT scan of the head, neck, and chest
   D. Panendoscopy to view the pharynx, larynx, esophagus, and bronchial tree
   E. Fine-needle aspiration cytology of the mass in the clinic

ANATOMIC LEVELS OF THE NECK

3. *When undertaking a selective neck dissection (I through III), which one of the following represents the inferior limit of the dissection?*
   A. Carotid bifurcation
   B. Clavicle
   C. Omohyoid
   D. Posterior belly of digastric
   E. Hyoid bone

ANATOMIC LEVELS OF THE NECK

4. You are undertaking a neck dissection for a patient with a floor-of-mouth squamous cell carcinoma (SCC). Your professor has asked you to include level IIa within the dissection but says that IIb can be preserved. *Which structure will subdivide these two areas?*
   A. Hypoglossal nerve
   B. Marginal mandibular nerve
   C. Phrenic nerve
   D. Spinal accessory nerve
   E. Vagus nerve

TYPES OF NECK DISSECTION

5. *What type of neck dissection removes levels I through V but sacrifices the sternocleidomastoid and internal jugular vein while preserving all other key structures?*
   A. Radical neck dissection
   B. Modified radical neck dissection
   C. Extended neck dissection
   D. Lateral neck dissection
   E. Selective neck dissection

TNM STAGING IN ORAL TUMORS

6. *What would the AJCC 8th edition staging be for a primary tumor of the oral cavity measuring 2.5 cm in diameter, with multiple positive ipsilateral nodes 3 cm in diameter, but no evidence of metastatic spread to distant organs?*
   A. T1N2bM0
   B. T2N2bM0
   C. T3N2cM0
   D. T4aN2aM0
   E. T4bN1M1

NODAL STAGING IN HEAD AND NECK CANCER

7. A patient with a supraglottic tumor of the larynx has a single ipsilateral neck node on imaging. *What is the nodal staging for this patient based on the current American Joint Committee on Cancer (AJCC) system?*
   A. N1
   B. N2a
   C. N2b
   D. N2c
   E. N3

PAROTID MALIGNANCY

8. A patient is discussed at the multidisciplinary team meeting (MDT) with a diagnosis of primary parotid malignancy. Examination and imaging show there is a 2-cm mass that does not have any evidence of extraparenchymal extension. *What would be the T staging for this tumor?*
   A. T1
   B. T2
   C. T3
   D. T4a
   E. T4b

SALIVARY GLAND TUMORS

9. *Which one of the following statements is true when considering salivary gland tumors?*
   A. Most salivary gland tumors can be managed nonsurgically.
   B. Half of all salivary gland tumors involve the parotid gland.
   C. Parotid gland pathology must be excluded in all preauricular masses.
   D. Minor salivary gland tumors are more likely to be benign than malignant.
   E. More than 90% of solid salivary gland tumors in children are benign.

SALIVARY GLAND TUMORS IN CHILDREN

10. A child is seen in clinic with confirmed salivary gland tumor. *Which one of the following statements is correct regarding salivary gland masses in children?*
    A. Most salivary gland masses are of vascular origin.
    B. Fewer than 10% of solid tumors are malignant.
    C. Lymphangiomas normally involute without treatment.
    D. Pleomorphic adenomas are rare in children.
    E. Most malignant tumor subtypes are adenoid cystic.

PLEOMORPHIC ADENOMAS

11. *Which one of the following statements is correct regarding pleomorphic adenomas?*
    A. They represent half of all benign parotid tumors in adults.
    B. They commonly present with facial paralysis and a palpable swelling.
    C. They have low rates of recurrence, even when completely excised.
    D. When adenomas recur, they tend to reappear as nodular tumor implants within extraglandular tissue.
    E. The responses to radiotherapy are consistently good.

HEAD AND NECK SALIVARY TUMORS

12. A patient is referred with a diagnosis of a low-grade malignant tumor of the parotid. *Which one of the following tumor subtypes is most likely to be a low-grade malignancy?*
    A. Adenoid cystic carcinoma
    B. Squamous cell carcinoma
    C. Adenocarcinoma
    D. Undifferentiated
    E. Acinic cell carcinoma

SALIVARY TUMOR MANAGEMENT

13. A patient is undergoing laryngectomy for a T4 tumor. *What is the benefit of performing intraoperative cricopharyngeal myotomy?*
    A. To optimize surgical margins
    B. To improve swallowing
    C. To reduce surgical time
    D. To avoid tracheostomy
    E. To improve airway patency

Answers

INCIDENCE OF HEAD AND NECK CANCER

1. *What is the most common tumor type in head and neck cancers?*

    B. Squamous cell

    The most common tumor subtype in head and neck cancer is the squamous cell carcinoma (SCC). This represents more than 90% of all head and neck cancers. Head and neck malignancies are increasingly common and represent around 3% of all cancers in the US. They represent around 2% of all US cancer deaths. Squamous cell carcinomas may originate from the skin or mucosal surfaces of the upper aerodigestive tract. Other common tumor types include adenocarcinoma, melanoma, adenoid cystic, lymphoma, and mucoepidermoid carcinoma. The incidence of human papillomavirus (HPV) related malignancies is increasing and is particularly important in the oropharynx and in younger patients who typically do not have the traditional risk factors for SCC.[1]

REFERENCE

1. Amin M, Edge S, Greene F, et al. AJCC Cancer Staging Manual. 8th ed. New York: Springer; 2017

WORKUP IN SUSPECTED HEAD AND NECK CANCER

2. A 50-year-old male smoker presents with a 4-week history of a 3-cm diameter, left-sided neck mass without any other obvious signs or symptoms. *After the initial history and examination, what would the next most appropriate investigation be?*

    E. Fine-needle aspiration cytology of the mass in the clinic

    New-onset neck masses should be considered malignant until proven otherwise. In this case the initial step would be to undertake fine-needle aspiration cytology to provide information on the nature of the mass. If this is inconclusive, or malignant cells are suspected, then a core biopsy could be considered either with or without ultrasound guidance. Only if this is unhelpful would an open or excision biopsy generally be offered at this stage. The subsequent steps would include baseline blood tests, panendoscopy, and a CT scan of the head, neck, chest, and abdomen. If malignancy is proven on the cytology sample, it may be appropriate to consider biopsies of the base of tongue and nasopharynx, or ipsilateral tonsillectomy. If the malignancy is suspected to be a lymphoma then excision biopsy may be indicated. Positron emission tomography (PET) is also a useful tool for evaluation of an unknown primary tumor as it highlights tissues displaying an increased metabolic rate.[1,2]

    This case would then require multidisciplinary team discussion. Once the primary diagnosis has been confirmed, a suitable management plan can be made such as surgical treatment with neck dissection or nonsurgical treatment with radiotherapy if malignancy is proven. This will be dependent upon many factors relating to both the individual patient and tumor location, size, and subtype.

REFERENCES

1. Smith OD, Ellis PD, Bearcroft PW, Berman LH, Grant JW, Jani P. Management of neck lumps—a triage model. Ann R Coll Surg Engl 2000;82(4):223–226
2. Pynnonen MA, Gillespie MB, Roman B, et al. Clinical practice guideline: evaluation of the neck mass in adults. Otolaryngol Head Neck Surg 2017;157(2_suppl, suppl):S1–S30

ANATOMIC LEVELS OF THE NECK

3. *When undertaking a selective neck dissection (I through III), which one of the following represents the inferior limit of the dissection?*

    C. Omohyoid

    There are seven levels used to describe the neck with reference to head and neck oncology. Primary tumors tend to metastasize in a predictable manner to specific areas of the neck. For example, floor of mouth and tongue tumors tend to spread to levels I through III, while laryngeal tumors tend to spread to levels II through IV. This means that treatment of neck disease can be targeted to specific levels. The levels of the neck are separated by key anatomical structures. The omohyoid is highly relevant to neck dissection as it crosses the lower part of the neck. It marks the junction between levels III and IV and is often included within the dissection specimen when undertaking a I through III dissection. As it passes into level V, it also subdivides this region into Va and Vb.

    The carotid bifurcation is the surgical landmark for the junction of levels II and III. The clavicle is the inferior border for both levels IV and V. The hyoid is an important landmark for many levels. It represents a boundary for levels I, II, III, and VI (**Fig. 38.1**).[1–3]

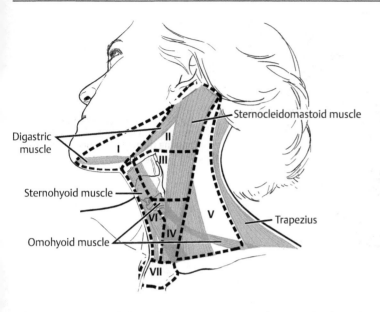

Fig. 38.1 Anatomic levels of the neck: The seven lymph node levels of the neck are described as I through VII.

REFERENCES

1. Lindberg R. Distribution of cervical lymph node metastases from squamous cell carcinoma of the upper respiratory and digestive tracts. Cancer 1972;29(6):1446–1449
2. Martin H, Del Valle B, Ehrlich H, Cahan WG. Neck dissection. Cancer 1951;4(3):441–499
3. Medina JE. A rational classification of neck dissections. Otolaryngol Head Neck Surg 1989;100(3):169–176

ANATOMIC LEVELS OF THE NECK

4. You are undertaking a neck dissection for a patient with a floor-of-mouth squamous cell carcinoma (SCC). Your professor has asked you to include level IIa within the dissection but says that IIb can be preserved. *Which structure will subdivide these two areas?*

D. Spinal accessory nerve

The boundaries of level II are the sternohyoid, the sternocleidomastoid (SCM), the skull base, and the carotid bifurcation.

The accessory nerve is a key structure to locate when undertaking a level II neck dissection. It should be preserved where possible, otherwise injury to it will result in weakness and subsequent wasting of the trapezius leading to chronic shoulder discomfort and instability.

It can be identified in levels II, III, and V. In level II it is identified by elevating the anterior border of the sternocleidomastoid, until it is seen passing obliquely into the muscle belly. Once identified, it is traced cranially to the posterior belly of digastric which marks the superior extent of a standard dissection. The internal jugular is also identified in this zone. The area below the nerve represents level IIa and the level above the nerve represents level IIb, which lies on the splenius capitis muscle. The accessory nerve is also seen during level V dissection after passing through SCM more caudally. It should be found in close proximity to the great auricular nerve at "Erbs point" where the former passes around SCM before travelling on its superficial surface to supply the ear. Caution must be taken when performing biopsies in level V of the neck as the accessory nerve travels superficially especially in slim individuals (**Fig. 38.2**).[1–5]

REFERENCES

1. Chen DT, Chen PR, Wen IS, et al. Surgical anatomy of the spinal accessory nerve: is the great auricular point reliable? J Otolaryngol Head Neck Surg 2009;38(3):337–339
2. Durazzo MD, Furlan JC, Teixeira GV, et al. Anatomic landmarks for localization of the spinal accessory nerve. Clin Anat 2009;22(4):471–475
3. Lloyd S. Accessory nerve: anatomy and surgical identification. J Laryngol Otol 2007; 121(12):1118–1125
4. Shah J, Patel S. Head and Neck surgery and oncology. 3rd ed. Edinburgh, London, New York, Toronto: Mosby; 2003: 353–394
5. Popovski V, Benedetti A, Popovic-Monevska D, Grcev A, Stamatoski A, Zhivadinovik J. Spinal accessory nerve preservation in modified neck dissections: surgical and functional outcomes [Preservazione del nervo accessorio spinale nelle dissezioni del collo: outcomes chirurgici e funzionali]. Acta Otorhinolaryngol Ital 2017;37(5):368–374

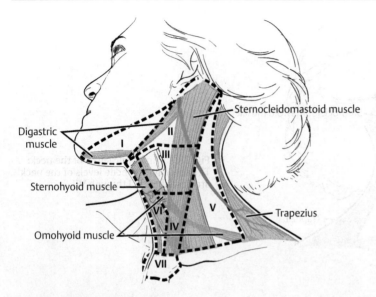

Fig. 38.2 The accessory nerve in the neck is found in both levels II and V passing through sternocleidomastoid between them.

TYPES OF NECK DISSECTION

5. *What type of neck dissection removes levels I through V but sacrifices the sternocleidomastoid and internal jugular vein while preserving all other key structures?*

B. Modified radical neck dissection

Neck dissections are commonly classified as selective or comprehensive. Comprehensive dissections involve resection of lymph node basins I through V. They include radical, modified radical, functional, and extended neck dissections. Modified radical nodal dissections (MRND) include three subtypes:

MRND I (preserves the spinal accessory nerve)
MRND II (preserves spinal accessory nerve and internal jugular vein)
MRND III (preserves spinal accessory nerve, internal jugular vein, and sternocleidomastoid)

A functional (Bocca) dissection is also called a *modified radical neck dissection type III.*

Selective neck dissections involve clearing some, but not all, of the lymphatic neck levels, and selection is according to the nature and site of the primary tumor. For example, in oral cavity cancers, levels I–III are commonly performed, whereas in oropharyngeal, hypopharyngeal, and laryngeal tumors, levels II–IV are most commonly performed. In selective neck dissections, the nonlymphatic structures are preserved unless otherwise stated.

Specific subtypes of selective neck dissections may also be described using the terms anterior, supraomohyoid, lateral, and posterolateral neck dissections. The anterior neck dissection includes level VI, the supraomohyoid neck dissection includes levels above omohyoid, that is, I through III. A lateral neck dissection includes levels II through IV. A posterolateral neck dissection includes levels II through V (**Fig. 38.3**).[1–4]

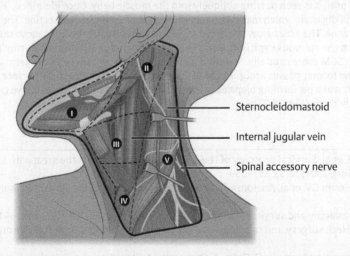

Fig. 38.3 Modified radical neck dissection showing removal of lymph node levels I–V with preservation of sternocleidomastoid, internal jugular vein, and spinal accessory nerve. Different subtypes of the modified radical neck relate to the preservation or sacrifice of the three key nonlymphatic structures.

REFERENCES

1. Robbins KT, Medina JE, Wolfe GT, Levine PA, Sessions RB, Pruet CW. Standardizing neck dissection terminology. Official report of the Academy's Committee for Head and Neck Surgery and Oncology. Arch Otolaryngol Head Neck Surg 1991;117(6):601–605

2. Spiro RH, Strong EW, Shah JP. Classification of neck dissection: variations on a new theme. Am J Surg 1994;168(5): 415–418

3. Suen JY, Goepfert H. Standardization of neck dissection nomenclature. [editorial] Head Neck Surg 1987;10(2):75–77

4. Shah JP. Patterns of cervical lymph node metastasis from squamous carcinomas of the upper aerodigestive tract. Am J Surg 1990;160(4):405–409

TNM STAGING IN ORAL TUMORS

6. *What would the AJCC 8th edition staging be for a primary tumor of the oral cavity measuring 2.5 cm in diameter, with multiple positive ipsilateral nodes 3 cm in diameter, but no evidence of metastatic spread to distant organs?*
    B. T2N2bM0

        The TNM classification is well known for many different tumor sites and types. The T stands for tumor size, the N stands for nodal disease, and the M stands for metastatic disease. The T grading will differ according to the site in question, although the general principles remain consistent. For example, a T1 lip tumor is less than 2 cm diameter. Although a nasopharyngeal T1 tumor is confined to the nasopharynx, no specific dimension is recorded. Tumors of the larynx are T1 if they are limited to one subsite. The full T stage description for intraoral and mucosal lip tumor types is shown in **Box 38.1a**. The tumor staging for the other head and neck tumors is shown in **Box 38.1b (Fig. 38.4)**.

BOX 38.1A   *TUMOR STAGING: AJCC 8TH EDITION, 2017*[1]

Lip and oral cavity

- ► Tx: No available information on primary tumor
- ► T0: No evidence of primary tumor
- ► Tis: Carcinoma in situ
- ► T1: Greatest diameter of primary tumor ≤2 cm
- ► T2: Greatest diameter of primary tumor >2 cm but ≤4 cm
- ► T3: Greatest diameter of primary tumor >4 cm
- ► T4a: Moderately advanced local disease:
  - ♦ Lip: Invades through cortical bone, inferior alveolar nerve, floor of mouth, skin of face
  - ♦ Oral cavity: Invades adjacent structures only (cortical bone of mandible/maxilla, deep extrinsic muscles of tongue—genioglossus, hyoglossus, palatoglossus, styloglossus—maxillary sinus, skin of face)
- ► T4b: Very advanced local disease that invades masticator space, pterygoid plates, skull base; encases internal carotid artery

---

BOX 38.1B   *TUMOR STAGING: AJCC 8TH EDITION, 2017*[1]

- ► T: Extent of primary tumor
- ► Nasopharynx
- ► T1: Tumor confined to nasopharynx
- ► T2: Parapharyngeal extension
- ► T3: Involves skull base or paranasal sinuses
- ► T4: Intracranial extension, involves cranial nerves, hypopharynx, orbit, infratemporal fossa/masticator space
  - • Oropharynx
- ► T1: Greatest diameter of tumor <2 cm
- ► T2: Tumor 2–4 cm in greatest dimension
- ► T3: Tumor >4 cm in greatest diameter or extension to lingual epiglottis
- ► T4a: Moderately advanced local disease:
  - ♦ Tumor invades larynx, tongue, medial pterygoid, hard palate, mandible
- ► T4b: Very advanced local disease:
  - ♦ Invades lateral pterygoid, pterygoid plates, lateral nasopharynx, skull base; encases internal carotid artery
    - • Larynx

- ► Supraglottis:
  - ♦ T1: Tumor limited to one subsite of supraglottis with normal vocal cord mobility
  - ♦ T2: Invades more than one adjacent subsite without fixation of larynx
  - ♦ T3: Limited to larynx with vocal cord fixation and/or invades postcricoid space, preepiglottic space, paraglottic space, and inner cortex of thyroid cartilage
  - ♦ T4a: Invades through thyroid cartilage and/or tissues beyond larynx
  - ♦ T4b: Invades prevertebral space; encases internal carotid artery and mediastinal structures
- ► Glottis:
  - ♦ T1a: Tumor limited to one vocal cord with normal mobility
  - ♦ T1b: Tumor involves both true vocal cords with normal mobility
  - ♦ T2: Extends to supraglottis or subglottis and/or impairs vocal cord mobility
  - ♦ T3: Limited to larynx with vocal cord fixation, invasion of paraglottic space and inner cortex of thyroid cartilage
  - ♦ T4a: Invades through outer cortex of thyroid cartilage and/or tissues beyond larynx
  - ♦ T4b: Invades prevertebral space; encases carotid artery and mediastinal structures
- ► Subglottis:
  - ♦ T1: Limited to subglottis
  - ♦ T2: Extends to vocal cords
  - ♦ T3: Limited to larynx with vocal cord fixation
  - ♦ T4a: Invades cricoid or thyroid cartilage or tissues beyond larynx
  - ♦ T4b: Invades prevertebral space and mediastinal structures; encases carotid artery
- ► Major salivary glands:
  - ♦ T1: Tumor ≤2 cm in greatest dimension without extraparenchymal extension
  - ♦ T2: Tumor 2–4 cm without extraparenchymal extension
  - ♦ T3: Tumor >4 cm and/or extraparenchymal extension
  - ♦ T4a: Moderately advanced disease that invades skin, mandible, ear canal, or facial nerve
  - ♦ T4b: Very advanced disease that invades skull base, pterygoid plates, or encases internal carotid artery

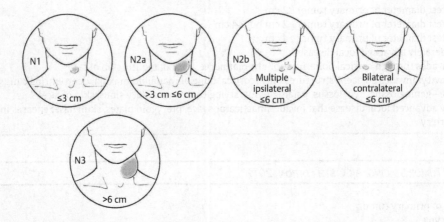

Fig. 38.4   The nodal staging system is generally the same for upper aerodigestive tumors (except those of the nasopharynx).

THE N STAGING IS CONSISTENT ACROSS ALL TUMOR TYPES EXCEPT FOR NASOPHARYNGEAL TUMORS:

- NX: Nodes cannot be assessed
- N0: No nodes containing metastasis
- N1: A single ipsilateral node metastasis, ≤3 cm in diameter
- N2a: A single ipsilateral positive node 3–6 cm in diameter
- N2b: Multiple positive ipsilateral nodes <6 cm in diameter
- N2c: Bilateral or contralateral positive nodes <6 cm in diameter
- N3: Nodes >6 cm in diameter

The M staging includes M0 (no distant metastases) and M1 (distant metastases).

REFERENCE

1. Amin M, Edge S, Greene F, et al. AJCC Cancer Staging Manual. 8th ed. New York: Springer; 2017

NODAL STAGING IN HEAD AND NECK CANCER

7. *A patient with a supraglottic tumor of the larynx has a single ipsilateral neck node on imaging. What is the nodal staging for this patient based on the current American Joint Committee on Cancer (AJCC) system?*
   A. N1

   The AJCC staging system is generally the same for all upper aerodigestive tumors except the nasopharynx. The presence of nodal metastasis has significant influence on survival, so it is a key component of the AJCC classification. The presence of nodes also directs treatment in terms of neck dissection and potential for radiotherapy (**Box 38.2** and **see Fig. 38.4**).

BOX 38.2 *TUMOR STAGING: AJCC 7TH EDITION, 2010[1]*

- ► Nx: Nodes cannot be assessed
- ► N0: No nodes containing metastasis
- ► N1: A single ipsilateral node metastasis, ≤3 cm in diameter
- ► N2a: A single ipsilateral positive node 3–6 cm in diameter
- ► N2b: Multiple positive ipsilateral nodes <6 cm in diameter
- ► N2c: Bilateral or contralateral positive nodes <6 cm in diameter
- ► N3: Nodes >6 cm in diameter

REFERENCE

1. Amin M, Edge S, Greene F, et al. AJCC Cancer Staging Manual. 8th ed. New York: Springer; 2017

PAROTID MALIGNANCY

8. A patient is discussed at the multidisciplinary team meeting (MDT) with a diagnosis of primary parotid malignancy. Examination and imaging show there is a 2-cm mass that does not have any evidence of extraparenchymal extension. *What would be the T staging for this tumor?*
   B. T2

   As with other head and neck TNM classifications, those for the salivary gland are unique to this condition. The AJCC staging of parotid tumors is as follows.[1]

   TX: Primary tumor cannot be assessed

   T0: No evidence of tumor

   T1: Less than 2 cm without extraparenchymal extension

   T2: 2–4 cm and without extraparenchymal extension

   T3: Greater than 4 cm and/or having extraparenchymal extension

   T4: Greater than 6 cm or extension into extraglandular tissues

   T4a: Invades the skin, mandible, ear canal, or facial nerve

   T4b: Invades the skull base and/or pterygoid plates and/or encases the carotid artery

   Therefore, this scenario represents a T2 lesion.

REFERENCE

1. Amin M, Edge S, Greene F, et al. AJCC Cancer Staging Manual. 8th ed. New York: Springer; 2017

SALIVARY GLAND TUMORS

9. *Which one of the following statements is true when considering salivary gland tumors?*
   C. Parotid gland pathology must be excluded in all preauricular masses.

   All preauricular masses are considered to be of parotid origin unless proven otherwise and should be thoroughly investigated. Most salivary gland tumors require surgical intervention. The most commonly involved gland is the parotid where 80% of all salivary gland tumors (benign and malignant) are located. The submandibular glands represent 10–15% of all salivary gland tumors. The sublingual or minor salivary glands constitute the remaining 5–10%. The ratio of benign to malignant salivary tumor type is related to gland size with a higher incidence of malignancy in smaller glands. Around half of all solid salivary gland tumors in children are malignant.[1,2]

REFERENCES

1. Thackray A, Lucas R, eds. Tumors of the Major Salivary Glands. Atlas of Tumor Pathology, Series 2. Washington, DC: Armed Forces Institute of Pathology; 1974
2. Witt R. Salivary gland diseases. In: Lee KJ, ed. Essential Otolaryngology: Head & Neck Surgery. 10th ed. New York: McGraw-Hill; 2012

SALIVARY GLAND TUMORS IN CHILDREN

10. A child is seen in clinic with confirmed salivary gland tumor. *Which one of the following statements is correct regarding salivary gland masses in children?*

    A. Most salivary gland masses are of vascular origin.

        Most salivary gland masses in children are vascular and hemangiomas represent the most common overall tumor type in children. Pleomorphic adenomas are the most common solid subtype in children, but are not the most common overall. Half of all solid salivary gland tumors are malignant and the most common subtype is mucoepidermoid, not adenoid cystic. Lymphangiomas present within the first year of life rarely involute. They are treated with surgery or sclerosing agents such as OK 432.[1-3]

REFERENCES

1. Bentz BG, Hughes CA, Lüdemann JP, Maddalozzo J. Masses of the salivary gland region in children. Arch Otolaryngol Head Neck Surg 2000;126(12):1435–1439
2. Schuller DE, McCabe BF. Salivary gland neoplasms in children. Otolaryngol Clin North Am 1977; 10: 399–412
3. Grasso DL, Pelizzo G, Zocconi E, Schleef J. Lymphangiomas of the head and neck in children. Acta Otorhinolaryngol Ital 2008;28(1):17–20

PLEOMORPHIC ADENOMAS

11. *Which one of the following statements is correct regarding pleomorphic adenomas?*

    D. When adenomas recur, they tend to reappear as nodular tumor implants within extraglandular tissue.

        Pleomorphic adenomas are the most common benign tumor of the parotid, representing 70% (not 55%) of all tumors. It is rare to have facial nerve involvement except in recurrent tumors, and most present as asymptomatic painless masses. Facial nerve palsy in the setting of a preauricular mass should raise concerns for malignancy. Treatment of pleomorphic adenomas involves surgical excision with parotidectomy. These tumors are radioresistant and tend to recur if surgical excision is incomplete. For this reason, enucleation is not recommended. All suspected pleomorphic adenomas need careful workup as misdiagnosis can cause multiple subsequent problems, particularly where the tumor cells are inadvertently seeded into the surrounding tissue or where lesions are only narrowly shelled out. Fine-needle aspiration cytology in clinic followed by magnetic resonance imaging (MRI) will confirm the diagnosis as well as the size and precise location of the lesion. Preservation of the facial nerve intraoperatively is paramount and patients must be counselled beforehand on the risk of temporary or permanent damage during surgery.[1-3]

REFERENCES

1. Thackray A, Lucas R, eds. Tumors of the Major Salivary Glands. Atlas of Tumor Pathology, Series 2. Washington, DC: Armed Forces Institute of Pathology; 1974
2. Witt R. Salivary gland diseases. In: Lee KJ, ed. Essential Otolaryngology: Head & Neck Surgery. 10th ed. New York: McGraw-Hill; 2012
3. Sood S, McGurk M, Vaz F. Management of salivary gland tumours: United Kingdom National Multidisciplinary Guidelines. J Laryngol Otol 2016;130(S2):S142–S149

HEAD AND NECK SALIVARY TUMORS

12. A patient is referred with a diagnosis of a low-grade malignant tumor of the parotid. *Which one of the following tumor subtypes is most likely to be a low-grade malignancy?*

    E. Acinic cell carcinoma

        Acinic cell carcinomas are low-grade tumors. In fact, they were previously considered to be benign tumors because of their behavioral characteristics of slow growth and a high degree of differentiation. The prognosis for acinic cell carcinomas is probably the best of all malignant salivary tumors. Conversely, high-grade tumors include:

        High-grade mucoepidermoid
        Adenoid cystic carcinoma
        Squamous cell carcinoma
        Adenocarcinoma
        Carcinoma ex-pleomorphic adenoma

        These will require more aggressive individualized management plans.[1,2]

REFERENCES

1. Thackray A, Lucas R, eds. Tumors of the Major Salivary Glands. Atlas of Tumor Pathology, Series 2. Washington, DC: Armed Forces Institute of Pathology; 1974
2. Witt R. Salivary gland diseases. In: Lee KJ, ed. Essential Otolaryngology: Head & Neck Surgery. 10th ed. New York: McGraw-Hill; 2012

SALIVARY TUMOR MANAGEMENT

13. A patient is undergoing laryngectomy for a T4 tumor. *What is the benefit of performing intraoperative cricophryngeal myotomy?*

    B. To improve swallowing

        The main purpose of performing a cricopharyngeal myotomy at the time of laryngectomy is to improve postoperative swallow. A secondary benefit may be observed with respect to speech when an implantable speech valve is used. It has no benefit in airway patency or surgical margins. The technique involves surgical sectioning of the cricopharyngeus muscle which normally acts as a sphincter to the upper esophagus from the distal pharynx. If left intact it can inhibit free flow of saliva and secretions into the upper esophagus post laryngectomy or total pharyngolaryngectomy and reconstruction. This may be helpful also in reducing fistula and wound healing problems.[1-4]

REFERENCES

1. Horowitz JB, Sasaki CT. Effect of cricopharyngeus myotomy on postlaryngectomy pharyngeal contraction pressures. Laryngoscope 1993;103(2):138–140
2. Op de Coul BMR, van den Hoogen FJA, van As CJ, et al. Evaluation of the effects of primary myotomy in total laryngectomy on the neoglottis with the use of quantitative videofluoroscopy. Arch Otolaryngol Head Neck Surg 2003;129(9): 1000–1005
3. Thackray A, Lucas R, eds. Tumors of the Major Salivary Glands. Atlas of Tumor Pathology, Series 2. Washington, DC: Armed Forces Institute of Pathology; 1974
4. Witt R. Salivary gland diseases. In: Lee KJ, ed. Essential Otolaryngology: Head & Neck Surgery. 10th ed. New York: McGraw-Hill; 2012

39. Scalp and Calvarial Reconstruction

See *Essentials of Plastic Surgery*, third edition, pp. 517–529

APPLIED ANATOMY OF THE SCALP

1. *Which component of the scalp provides most strength during layered repair?*
   - A. Epidermis
   - B. Dermis
   - C. Aponeurotic layer
   - D. Subgaleal fascia
   - E. Pericranium

VASCULARITY OF THE SCALP

2. *Which one of the following statements is correct regarding the blood supply to the scalp?*
   - A. The anterior scalp is supplied by the supraorbital and supratrochlear vessels from the external carotid artery.
   - B. The supratrochlear vessels are lateral to the supraorbital vessels.
   - C. The posterior territory is the largest area and is supplied by the occipital vessels.
   - D. The lesser occipital artery supplies the posterolateral scalp.
   - E. The lateral territory is supplied by the superficial temporal artery, which arises from the external carotid artery.

SCALP INNERVATION

3. *Which one of the following statements is correct regarding scalp innervation?*
   - A. The supraorbital nerve has both superficial and deep divisions.
   - B. The zygomaticofacial nerve is a branch of the ophthalmic division of trigeminal nerve.
   - C. The auriculotemporal nerve supplies the posterior and lateral scalp.
   - D. The lesser occipital nerve emerges from the semispinalis muscle, 3 cm below the occipital protuberance.
   - E. The muscles of the scalp are supplied by the facial and trigeminal nerves.

SKIN BIOMECHANICS

4. *Which one of the following specifically requires the application of a constant force intraoperatively in order to assist in closure of a tight scalp wound?*
   - A. Tissue creep
   - B. Stress relaxation
   - C. Galeal scoring
   - D. Undermining
   - E. Tissue expansion

TECHNIQUES FOR SCALP RECONSTRUCTION

5. *Which one of the following statements is correct regarding the use of Orticochea flaps to reconstruct a scalp defect?*
   - A. They are based entirely on the superficial temporal vessels.
   - B. They are useful for reconstructing large parietal defects.
   - C. Their classical description was for reconstruction of the frontal scalp.
   - D. Commonly, they involve elevation of three local pericranial flaps.
   - E. Modification of this technique to include more flaps can improve flap vascularity and reduce alopecia.

SOFT TISSUE RECONSTRUCTION OF THE PARIETAL SCALP

6. *Which one of the following statements is correct regarding parietal scalp defects?*
   - A. They are commonly reconstructed using flaps based on the terminal branch of the external carotid artery.
   - B. They are less likely to involve bone exposure compared with vertex defects.
   - C. They are at low risk of displacement of the sideburn and distortion of the hair pattern.
   - D. They are challenging to reconstruct given the limited scalp mobility.
   - E. They frequently require importation of distant tissue for closure.

SCALP RECONSTRUCTION

7. *In which scenario might the pinwheel flap be particularly useful to reconstruct a small scalp defect in a patient with a full head of hair?*
   A. A circular defect on the vertex
   B. A longitudinal defect on the occiput
   C. A triangular defect on the parietal area
   D. A rectangular defect on the forehead
   E. An elliptical defect on the temple

CALVARIAL RECONSTRUCTION

8. *When harvesting split calvarial bone for calvarial reconstruction, which anatomic area is normally preferred?*
   A. Occipital
   B. Frontal
   C. Parietal
   D. Temporal
   E. No specific region is preferred

CLINICAL SCENARIO IN SCALP RECONSTRUCTION

9. An 85-year-old woman has a 1.5 by 2 cm defect on her anterior scalp with exposed bone after excision of a basal cell carcinoma. The defect is within the hair-bearing skin. *Which one of the following is the best reconstructive option for this patient?*
   A. Leave to heal by secondary intention
   B. Direct layered closure with undermining
   C. Burring of the outer table and full-thickness skin graft
   D. Bilaminate neodermis reconstruction (Integra) and a split-thickness skin graft
   E. A posteriorly based scalp rotation flap

CLINICAL SCENARIO IN SCALP RECONSTRUCTION

10. A 4-year-old patient with a full head of hair requires reconstruction of a congenital nevus to the vertex of the scalp. The lesion covers 30% of the scalp. *Which one of the following is the best reconstructive option?*
    A. Serial excision and direct closure
    B. Tissue expansion and local flap reconstruction
    C. Transposition flap and skin graft to the donor site
    D. Free tissue muscle transfer and split-thickness skin graft
    E. Orticochea flaps with galeal scoring

SCALP RECONSTRUCTION IN ELDERLY PATIENTS

11. A frail, elderly bald man had a 3-cm squamous cell carcinoma excised from the vertex of his scalp. The pericranium is involved and the outer cortex is subsequently burred. *How might this defect best be managed?*
    A. Bilaminate neodermis reconstruction (Integra) and staged split-thickness skin grafting
    B. Full-thickness skin grafting
    C. Transposition flap and split skin graft to the donor site
    D. Tissue expansion and local flap reconstruction
    E. Free tissue transfer with radial forearm flap

RECONSTRUCTION OF LARGER SCALP DEFECTS

12. A 20-year-old patient has a near-total scalp defect after excision of an angiosarcoma. *How might this best be reconstructed?*
    A. Free tissue transfer with a radial forearm flap
    B. Free tissue transfer with a latissimus dorsi flap and split skin graft
    C. Tissue expansion and scalp rotation flap
    D. Bilaminate neodermis reconstruction (Integra) and split skin grafting
    E. An Orticochea flap and skin graft

SCALP REPLANTATION

13. *Which one of the following is true when considering scalp replantation following trauma?*
    A. Multiple arterial microvascular anastomoses will be required.
    B. There is no published evidence to show effectiveness of scalp replantation.
    C. Even with extended ischemia times, outcomes are favorable following replantation.
    D. Every attempt should be made to replant scalp defects greater than 75%.
    E. Studies suggest less than 50% success rates in scalp replantation.

CALVARIAL RECONSTRUCTION

14. *Which one of the following materials is particularly useful to reduce intraoperative time in cases of cranial bone reconstruction where complex shapes need to be reconstructed?*
    A. Autologous rib
    B. Methylmethacrylate
    C. Free scapula
    D. Hydroxyapatite
    E. Polyetheretherketone

Answers

APPLIED ANATOMY OF THE SCALP

1. **Which component of the scalp provides most strength during layered repair?**
   C. **Aponeurotic layer**
   The scalp comprises five layers, each of which can be remembered using the mnemonic *SCALP*: Skin, subCutaneous tissue, Aponeurotic layer, Loose areolar tissue, Pericranium.

   The aponeurotic layer is also known as the galea and connects the frontalis and occipitalis muscles. It is also contiguous with the superficial musculoaponeurotic system (SMAS) of the face and neck. It should be approximated during closure of scalp wounds as it provides deep support to the repair. The terms *subgaleal fascia* and *innominate fascia* are used interchangeably with the term *loose areolar layer* which provides scalp mobility rather than strength. It is at this layer that most injuries are sustained and it is described as the *scalping plane*. Skin thickness varies from 3 to 8 mm according to anatomic location on the scalp and provides additional strength to the repair. The pericranium is the deepest layer and is tightly adherent to the calvarium. It tends to be thin and can easily tear. Therefore, approximation does not add to the strength of a scalp repair.

   Skin comprises the dermis and the epidermis. Overall thickness varies from 3 to 8 mm according to anatomic location on the scalp, and placement of sutures or clips through the skin provides additional strength to the repair and reapproximates the wound edges, but does not represent the most strength (**Fig. 39.1**).[1-3]

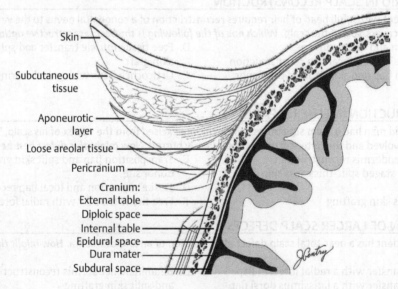

Skin
Subcutaneous tissue
Aponeurotic layer
Loose areolar tissue
Pericranium
Cranium:
External table
Diploic space
Internal table
Epidural space
Dura mater
Subdural space

Fig. 39.1   Anatomic layers of the scalp.

REFERENCES

1. Abul-Hassan HS, von Drasek Ascher G, Acland RD. Surgical anatomy and blood supply of the fascial layers of the temporal region. Plast Reconstr Surg 1986;77(1):17–28
2. Tolhurst DE, Carstens MH, Greco RJ, Hurwitz DJ. The surgical anatomy of the scalp. Plast Reconstr Surg 1991;87(4):603–612, discussion 613–614
3. Williams PL, Warwick R, eds. Gray's Anatomy. 36th British ed. Philadelphia: WB Saunders; 1980

VASCULARITY OF THE SCALP

2. **Which one of the following statements is correct regarding the blood supply to the scalp?**
   E. **The lateral territory is supplied by the superficial temporal artery, which arises from the external carotid artery.**
   The scalp derives its blood supply from both the internal and external carotid systems. It is divided into four zones: anterior, posterior, lateral, and posterolateral. Each zone has its own blood supply, with collateralization between zones. This is clinically relevant with respect to scalp reconstruction using local flaps and replantation.

The anterior scalp is supplied by the supraorbital and supratrochlear vessels. These derive from the internal carotid vessels (not the external carotid vessels). The supratrochlear vessels lie medial (not lateral) to the supraorbital vessels. The posterior territory is supplied by the occipital vessels and perforators from the splenius capitis and trapezius, but it is not the largest territory. The largest is the lateral territory, which is supplied by the superficial temporal arteries. A lesser occipital artery does not exist. The greater and lesser occipital nerves supply sensation to the occipital territory. The posterolateral scalp is the smallest territory and is supplied by the posterior auricular artery.[1-4] Knowledge of the impressive collateral circulation has been clinically proven with successful near-total scalp replantation based on a single anastomosed artery and vein such as the superficial temporal vessels. Although this can be enough to supply the scalp, multiple anastomoses are still advocated by many where technically possible (**Fig. 39.2**).[5]

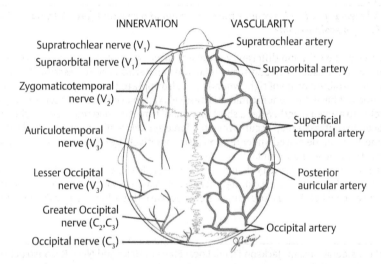

Fig. 39.2 Innervation and vascular anatomy of the scalp.

REFERENCES

1. Abul-Hassan HS, von Drasek Ascher G, Acland RD. Surgical anatomy and blood supply of the fascial layers of the temporal region. Plast Reconstr Surg 1986;77(1):17–28
2. Tolhurst DE, Carstens MH, Greco RJ, Hurwitz DJ. The surgical anatomy of the scalp. Plast Reconstr Surg 1991;87(4): 603–612, discussion 613–614
3. Taylor GI, Palmer JH. The vascular territories (angiosomes) of the body: experimental study and clinical applications. Br J Plast Surg 1987;40(2):113–141
4. Houseman ND, Taylor GI, Pan WR. The angiosomes of the head and neck: anatomic study and clinical applications. Plast Reconstr Surg 2000;105(7):2287–2313
5. Karibe J, Minabe T. Vascular consideration in repair of total scalp avulsion. BMJ Case Rep 2017, October 24;2017: bcr2017220605

SCALP INNERVATION

3. Which one of the following statements is correct regarding scalp innervation?

A. The supraorbital nerve has both superficial and deep divisions.

The supraorbital nerve has superficial and deep divisions. The superficial component supplies sensation to the forehead anterior to the hairline. The deep component supplies sensation posterior to the hairline. This has clinical relevance in brow-lift procedures, bicoronal cranial flaps, and trauma in which the nerves may be damaged, leaving an area of paresthesia. The zygomaticofacial nerve derives from the maxillary division (not the ophthalmic division) of the trigeminal nerve. It supplies a region of skin lateral to the brow. The auriculotemporal nerve derives from the mandibular division of the trigeminal nerve and supplies the lateral scalp. The greater and lesser occipital nerves supply the occipital territory, but it is the greater occipital nerve that emerges from the semispinalis 3 cm below the occipital protuberance. The facial nerve supplies the scalp muscles. The trigeminal nerve supplies the muscles of mastication and the tensor tympani (see **Fig. 39.2**).[1-5]

REFERENCES

1. Tolhurst DE, Carstens MH, Greco RJ, Hurwitz DJ. The surgical anatomy of the scalp. Plast Reconstr Surg 1991;87(4): 603–612, discussion 613–614
2. Williams PL, Warwick R, eds. Gray's Anatomy. 36th British ed. Philadelphia: WB Saunders; 1980
3. Janis JE, Hatef DA, Thakar H, et al. The zygomaticotemporal branch of the trigeminal nerve: Part II. Anatomical variations. Plast Reconstr Surg 2010;126(2):435–442
4. Janis JE, Hatef DA, Ducic I, et al. Anatomy of the auriculotemporal nerve: variations in its relationship to the superficial temporal artery and implications for the treatment of migraine headaches. Plast Reconstr Surg 2010;125(5): 1422–1428
5. Janis JE, Ghavami A, Lemmon JA, et al. The anatomy of the corrugator supercilii muscle revisited. Part 2. Supraorbital nerve topography. Plast Reconstr Surg 2008;121:233–240

SKIN BIOMECHANICS

4. *Which one of the following specifically requires the application of a constant force intraoperatively in order to assist in closure of a tight scalp wound?*

A. **Tissue creep**

The biomechanics of the skin and different viscoelastic properties of the scalp layers can be used to assist in closure of scalp defects. Tissue creep and stress relaxation are terms used to describe the viscoelastic properties of skin that enable on-table closure of tight wounds and also apply to tissue expansion techniques. The two terms are often confused but have different meanings. Stress relaxation occurs when a force is applied to the skin that causes it to stretch to a given length. After a short amount of time, the load required to achieve the desired length or stretch reduces. In contrast, creep occurs when the force applied remains constant and this causes a continued stretch over time. Skin can be placed under tension intraoperatively by either placing temporary sutures or using skin hooks to partially close the wound.

The skin has more stretch or elasticity than the underlying galea. Therefore, multiple perpendicular incisions or scores to the undersurface of the galea can significantly increase the amount of stretch within this layer. Simple undermining can also be helpful to close some defects because this allows redistribution of the available skin.[1]

REFERENCE

1. Jackson IT. General considerations. In: Jackson IT, ed. Local Flaps in Head and Neck Reconstruction. 2nd ed. St Louis: Quality Medical Publishing; 2007

TECHNIQUES FOR SCALP RECONSTRUCTION

5. *Which one of the following statements is correct regarding the use of Orticochea flaps to reconstruct a scalp defect?*

D. **Commonly, they involve elevation of three local pericranial flaps.**

The Orticochea technique uses either three or four subgaleal flaps to reconstruct large scalp defects. The three-flap technique comprises two lateral flaps based on the superficial temporal vessels, combined with a posterior flap based on the occipital vessels. This technique can improve flap vascularity and reduce alopecia, compared with the four-flap technique. Orticochea flaps were classically described for occipital defects and are not suitable for vertex or lateral defects (**Fig. 39.3**).[1-3]

REFERENCES

1. Arnold PG, Rangarathnam CS. Multiple-flap scalp reconstruction: Orticochea revisited. Plast Reconstr Surg 1982;69(4):605–613
2. Orticochea M. Four flap scalp reconstruction technique. Br J Plast Surg 1967;20(2): 159–171
3. Orticochea M. New three-flap reconstruction technique. Br J Plast Surg 1971;24(2): 184–188

SOFT TISSUE RECONSTRUCTION OF THE PARIETAL SCALP

6. *Which one of the following statements is correct regarding parietal scalp defects?*

B. **They are less likely to involve bone exposure compared with vertex defects.**

The parietal scalp has a high degree of mobility, which facilitates closure with direct suturing or local flap reconstruction. Bone exposure is less common because the temporalis muscle and fascia provide an additional layer of soft tissue cover anteriorly. Local flaps are at risk of changing the orientation of hair and affecting the hairline or sideburn. The parietal scalp is supplied by the superficial temporal artery, the terminal branch of the external carotid artery. The superficial temporal artery is unlikely to be the vascular supply to flaps used in reconstruction of this area because it is likely to have been sacrificed already. Because of the excellent mobility of local tissues, distant tissue use is limited.[1-4]

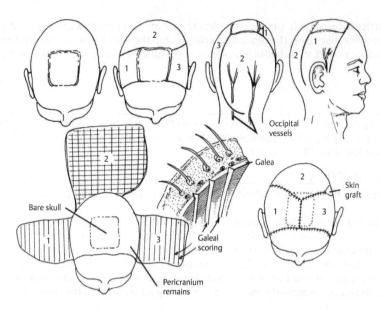

Fig. 39.3 Orticochea three-flap technique. (Adapted from Arnold PG, Rangarathnam CS. Multiple-flap scalp reconstruction: Orticochea revisited. Plast Reconstr Surg 69:607, 1982.)

REFERENCES

1. Leedy JE, Janis JE, Rohrich RJ. Reconstruction of acquired scalp defects: an algorithmic approach. Plast Reconstr Surg 2005;116(4):54e–72e
2. Jackson IT. Local flap reconstruction of defects after excision of nonmelanoma skin cancer. Clin Plast Surg 1997;24(4):747–767
3. Tolhurst DE, Carstens MH, Greco RJ, Hurwitz DJ. The surgical anatomy of the scalp. Plast Reconstr Surg 1991;87(4):603–612, discussion 613–614
4. Abul-Hassan HS, von Drasek Ascher G, Acland RD. Surgical anatomy and blood supply of the fascial layers of the temporal region. Plast Reconstr Surg 1986;77(1):17–28

SCALP RECONSTRUCTION

7. *In which scenario might the pinwheel flap be particularly useful to reconstruct a small scalp defect in a patient with a full head of hair?*

A. A circular defect on the vertex

The pinwheel flap is a type of local flap that uses three or four advancing triangular flaps which are arranged around a circular defect (**Fig. 39.4**).

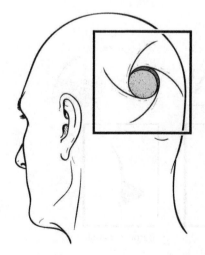

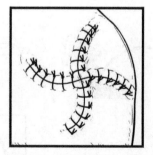

Fig. 39.4 The pinwheel flap for circular scalp defect closure. (Adapted from Lee S, Rafii AA, Sykes J. Advances in scalp reconstruction. Curr Opin Otolaryngol Head Neck Surg 14:249–253, 2006.)

It may be particularly useful in small defects less than 2 cm² on the vertex to recreate a whorl pattern at the patient's crown while disguising the remaining scars within the hair. It can be used in other sites on the scalp including nonhair-bearing areas but is probably less useful as the long flap limbs result in more noticeable scars.[1,2]

REFERENCES

1. Lee S, Rafii AA, Sykes J. Advances in scalp reconstruction. Curr Opin Otolaryngol Head Neck Surg 2006;14(4):249–253
2. Varnalidis I, Mantelakis A, Spiers HVM, Papadopoulou AN. Application of the pinwheel flap for closure of a large defect of the scalp. BMJ Case Rep 2019;12(8):e229420

CALVARIAL RECONSTRUCTION

8. ***When harvesting split calvarial bone for calvarial reconstruction, which anatomic area is normally preferred?***

   C. **Parietal**

Split calvarial bone graft is useful for reconstructing bony defects of the scalp as it has the same contour and can be harvested from the same operative site. Grafts are either taken full-thickness then split, or harvested at the level of the diploic space. The parietal region is the preferred donor site for calvarial bone harvest because it is thickest and minimizes risk of damage to dura or dural venous sinuses. Most split calvarial grafts are nonvascularized, and have a good take; however, it is possible to harvest a vascularized graft. This is based on the superficial temporal vessels by maintaining attachment to the superficial temporal fascia and pericranium.[1–3]

REFERENCES

1. Agrawal A, Garg LN. Split calvarial bone graft for the reconstruction of skull defects. J Surg Tech Case Rep 2011;3(1):13–16
2. Jackson IT. Local Flaps in Head and Neck Reconstruction. 2nd ed. St Louis: Quality Medical Publishing; 2007
3. Freund RM. Scalp, calvarium and forehead reconstruction. In: Aston SJ, Beasley RW, Thorne CH, eds. Grabb and Smith's Plastic Surgery. Philadelphia: Lippincott Williams & Wilkins; 1997

CLINICAL SCENARIO IN SCALP RECONSTRUCTION

9. An 85-year-old woman has a 1.5 by 2 cm defect on her anterior scalp with exposed bone after excision of a basal cell carcinoma. The defect is within the hair-bearing skin. ***Which one of the following is the best reconstructive option for this patient?***

   B. **Direct layered closure with undermining**

Small defects of the anterior scalp can often be closed directly with undermining of surrounding tissues. This avoids the need for a skin graft which will leave a bald patch and a contour defect at the surgical site. A scalp rotation flap is usually preserved for larger defects following triangulation of the defect **(Fig. 39.5)**. Small defects can be left to heal by secondary intention but are best for nonhair-bearing regions of the scalp such as the forehead when there is a deep layer of vascularized tissue covering bone. Bilaminate neodermis reconstruction (Integra) can be a useful adjunct when reconstructing scalp defects, as it adds tissue depth, but in this situation it would not provide any benefit.[1–6]

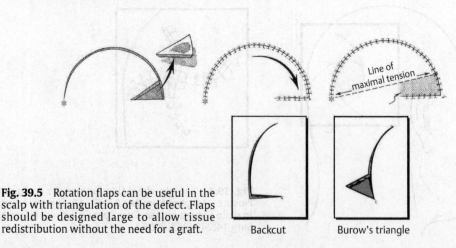

Fig. 39.5 Rotation flaps can be useful in the scalp with triangulation of the defect. Flaps should be designed large to allow tissue redistribution without the need for a graft.

Line of maximal tension

Backcut   Burow's triangle

REFERENCES

1. Freund RM. Scalp, calvarium and forehead reconstruction. In: Aston SJ, Beasley RW, Thorne CH, eds. Grabb and Smith's Plastic Surgery. Philadelphia: Lippincott Williams & Wilkins; 1997
2. Leedy JE, Janis JE, Rohrich RJ. Reconstruction of acquired scalp defects: an algorithmic approach. Plast Reconstr Surg 2005;116(4):54e–72e
3. Shestak KC, Ramasastry SS. Reconstruction of defects of the scalp and skull. In: Cohen M, ed. Mastery of Plastic and Reconstructive Surgery, Vol. 2. Philadelphia: Lippincott Williams & Wilkins; 1994
4. Magnoni C, De Santis G, Fraccalvieri M, et al. Integra in scalp reconstruction after tumor excision: recommendations from a multidisciplinary advisory board. J Craniofac Surg 2019;30(8):2416–2420
5. Schiavon M, Francescon M, Drigo D, et al. The use of Integra dermal regeneration template versus flaps for reconstruction of full-thickness scalp defects involving the calvaria: a cost-benefit analysis. Aesthetic Plast Surg 2016;40(6):901–907
6. Richardson MA, Lange JP, Jordan JR. Reconstruction of full-thickness scalp defects using a dermal regeneration template. JAMA Facial Plast Surg 2016;18(1):62–67

CLINICAL SCENARIO IN SCALP RECONSTRUCTION

10. A 4-year-old patient with a full head of hair requires reconstruction of a congenital nevus to the vertex of the scalp. The lesion covers 30% of the scalp. *Which one of the following is the best reconstructive option?*

    B. Tissue expansion and local flap reconstruction

    The primary aim in this case is to fully remove the nevus and provide soft tissue cover while retaining a full head of hair. Two approaches to the management of congenital nevi on the scalp are serial excision or excision and tissue expansion. Serial excision is best suited to smaller defects that can be excised within three or four sessions. A defect of 30% is best treated with tissue expansion and local flap closure. Defects up to 50% of the hair-bearing scalp can be closed with tissue expansion and avoid bald patches. A transposition flap and skin graft would create a large bald area and would not be aesthetically pleasing. Free tissue transfer would be reserved for near-total scalp defects, particularly where bone is exposed. The Orticochea flap is not well suited to vertex defects because the location does not allow a large third flap to cover the donor defect.[1–6]

REFERENCES

1. Manders EK, Graham WP III, Schenden MJ, Davis TS. Skin expansion to eliminate large scalp defects. Ann Plast Surg 1984;12(4):305–312
2. Leedy JE, Janis JE, Rohrich RJ. Reconstruction of acquired scalp defects: an algorithmic approach. Plast Reconstr Surg 2005;116(4):54e–72e
3. Shestak KC, Ramasastry SS. Reconstruction of defects of the scalp and skull. In: Cohen M, ed. Mastery of Plastic and Reconstructive Surgery, Vol. 2. Philadelphia: Lippincott Williams & Wilkins; 1994
4. McCauley RL. Tissue expansion reconstruction of the scalp. Semin Plast Surg 2005;19(2): 143–152
5. Lutz BS, Wei FC, Chen HC, Lin CH, Wei CY. Reconstruction of scalp defects with free flaps in 30 cases. Br J Plast Surg 1998;51(3):186–190
6. Pennington DG, Stern HS, Lee KK. Free-flap reconstruction of large defects of the scalp and calvarium. Plast Reconstr Surg 1989;83(4):655–661

SCALP RECONSTRUCTION IN ELDERLY PATIENTS

11. A frail, elderly bald man had a 3-cm squamous cell carcinoma excised from the vertex of his scalp. The pericranium is involved and the outer cortex is subsequently burred. *How might this defect best be managed?*

    A. Bilaminate neodermis reconstruction (Integra) and staged split-thickness skin grafting

    Several algorithms have been developed for scalp reconstruction. However, as with most reconstructions, the selection requires common sense and is based on each patient's needs. The goals are to reconstruct like with like tissue and to minimize deformity and alopecia. It is not always necessary to reconstruct the calvarium, provided that soft tissue cover is adequate.

    In this case, a simple and reliable approach is recommended due to the patient's frailty and the relatively small defect size. Although split skin graft cannot be usually placed directly onto bone, in the setting of burred calvarium it can be. The combined use of bilaminate neodermis reconstruction (Integra, LifeSciences, Plainsboro, NJ) and split skin grafting has been shown to be reliable for scalp defects like the one described, and may be as effective as a local flap option. It involves a two-stage approach with Integra placed at the first stage and graft placed at the second. It is well recommended in elderly patients as in this case for defects with exposed bone. It can add soft tissue bulk and contour with low rates of morbidity and short operative time.[1,2]

    Full-thickness skin grafting is generally not advised on full-thickness scalp defects as the chances of graft take are low even with burring. A skin and galea transposition flap leaving pericranium behind to accept a split skin graft is a reasonable alternative to Integra but is more likely to require a longer operative time and a general anesthetic which would ideally be avoided in this patient. Neither tissue expansion nor free tissue transfer would be warranted in this scenario, although both can be offered to elderly patients if their underlying medical health is good enough to withstand the impact of surgery.[3]

REFERENCES

1. Magnoni C, De Santis G, Fraccalvieri M, et al. Integra in scalp reconstruction after tumor excision: recommendations from a multidisciplinary advisory board. J Craniofac Surg 2019;30(8):2416–2420
2. Schiavon M, Francescon M, Drigo D, et al. The use of Integra dermal regeneration template versus flaps for reconstruction of full-thickness scalp defects involving the calvaria: a cost-benefit analysis. Aesthetic Plast Surg 2016;40(6):901–907 Dec.
3. Sosin M, Schultz BD, De La Cruz C, et al. Microsurgical scalp reconstruction in the elderly: a systematic review and pooled analysis of the current data. Plast Reconstr Surg 2015;135(3):856–866

RECONSTRUCTION OF LARGER SCALP DEFECTS

12. A 20-year-old patient has a near-total scalp defect after excision of an angiosarcoma. *How might this best be reconstructed?*

   B. **Free tissue transfer with a latissimus dorsi flap and split skin graft**
   The gold standard for near-total scalp reconstruction is free tissue transfer and the two most popular flaps for this are the latissimus dorsi and anterolateral thigh flaps. Of the two, the latissimus dorsi is generally preferred and harvested as a muscle-only flap because muscle flaps atrophy and contour well to the skull over time. The downside is that a large area requires split skin grafting and if they thin to excess, bone exposure can occur. Muscle flaps are also preferred in the setting of radiation. The other benefit of the latissimus dorsi is that the donor site can be closed directly and a long pedicle is standard to facilitate reach into the neck vessels. The radial forearm can be used for scalp reconstruction as it too has a long pedicle, but it will leave a major defect in the forearm which will require grafting if used for a large scalp defect as in this case. Tissue expansion would not work well here as there is little left to expand. Furthermore, immediate reconstruction is required. Integra and split skin grafting is best reserved for smaller defects in patients where free tissue transfer is contraindicated. The Orticochea flap is classically described for occipital scalp reconstruction. This flap is not well suited to large defects involving the vertex or near-total defects as there are no flaps to raise and reconstruct with.[1–3]

REFERENCES

1. Davison SP, Capone AC. Scalp reconstruction with inverted myocutaneous latissimus free flap and unmeshed skin graft. J Reconstr Microsurg 2011;27(4):261–266
2. Labow BI, Rosen H, Pap SA, Upton J. Microsurgical reconstruction: a more conservative method of managing large scalp defects? J Reconstr Microsurg 2009;25(8):465–474
3. Leedy JE, Janis JE, Rohrich RJ. Reconstruction of acquired scalp defects: an algorithmic approach. Plast Reconstr Surg 2005;116(4):54e–72e

SCALP REPLANTATION

13. *Which one of the following is true when considering scalp replantation following trauma?*

   D. **Every attempt should be made to replant scalp defects greater than 75%.**
   Scalp replantation of larger defects should be attempted in most traumatic amputations of the scalp providing the soft tissues to be replanted are in a reasonable condition to do so. For example, this should be avoided where there has been a severe shearing force, in association with an extended warm ischemia time, and in situations where there are other life- or limb-threatening injuries that may preclude this.
   There is actually a body of evidence to support replantation of the scalp following avulsion. One study of 20 patients who had replantation showed 100% survival in 16 patients, that is, 80% of cases.[1] Another systematic review which included 90 scalp replant cases found that overall success was above 70%.[2] It would be unlikely that more than one arterial anastomosis would be required due to the blood supply of the scalp, as there is extensive collateralization of the vascular territories within the scalp, so replantation can be reliably based on single arterial and venous anastomoses. Despite this some surgeons still recommend use of additional vascular anastomoses if possible.[3]

REFERENCES

1. Cheng K, Zhou S, Jiang K, et al. Microsurgical replantation of the avulsed scalp: report of 20 cases. Plast Reconstr Surg 1996;97(6):1099–1106, discussion 1107–1108

2. Efanov JI, Montoya IJ, Huang KN, et al. Microvascular replantation of head and neck amputated parts: a systematic review. Microsurgery 2017;37(6):699–706
3. Karibe J, Minabe T. Vascular consideration in repair of total scalp avulsion. BMJ Case Rep 2017, October 24;2017: bcr2017220605

CALVARIAL RECONSTRUCTION

14. *Which one of the following materials is particularly useful to reduce intraoperative time in cases of cranial bone reconstruction where complex shapes need to be reconstructed?*

E. Polyetheretherketone

Polyetheretherketone, or PEEK, has become a popular choice for reconstruction in the head and neck where complex shapes need reconstruction. It is advantageous because computer aided design based on CT imaging can be undertaken before surgery so that a custom implant is ready for immediate use after tumor resection. This increases accuracy of reconstruction and reduces intraoperative time, which would otherwise be needed to shape the construct. PEEK also has other advantages such as strength, durability, thermal conductivity, cost effectiveness, and radiolucency.[1]

However, tissue integration is still inferior to autologous bone which, in principle, remains the gold standard for reconstruction of bony defects. Autologous bone reconstruction for the cranium is generally nonvascularized with either split calvarial or rib graft being used. Free tissue transfer is less commonly used for the cranium but scapula bone may be well suited to create complex structures with relatively thin bone and a long vascular pedicle. It also has the advantage that soft tissue can be transferred with the harvested bone as a chimeric flap. However, shaping of bone, whether it is vascularized or nonvascularized, will add time to the surgical procedure, particularly for more complex shaped defects.

Of the alloplastic options for calvarial reconstruction, methylmethacrylate, titanium mesh, and hydroxyapatite all have a role to play. Methylmethacrylate has good strength and biocompatibility but can have poor integration and be prone to infection. Titanium mesh is easy to mold, inert, and fairly rigid. Hydroxyapetite is best used as an adjunct to refine scalp contour, for example, to fill craniotomy drill hole defects.[2,3]

REFERENCES

1. Hanasono MM, Goel N, DeMonte F. Calvarial reconstruction with polyetheretherketone implants. Ann Plast Surg 2009;62(6):653–655
2. Chim H, Schantz JT. New frontiers in calvarial reconstruction: integrating computer-assisted design and tissue engineering in cranioplasty. Plast Reconstr Surg 2005;116(6):1726–1741
3. Reddy S, Khalifian S, Flores JM, et al. Clinical outcomes in cranioplasty: risk factors and choice of reconstructive material. Plast Reconstr Surg 2014;133(4):864–873

40. Eyelid Reconstruction

See *Essentials of Plastic Surgery*, third edition, pp. 530–547

EYELID ANATOMY

1. *Which one of the following statements is correct regarding anatomy of the eyelids?*
   A. The outer lamella is known as the anterior lamella and consists of skin only.
   B. The middle lamella consists of orbital septum and capsulopalpebral fascia.
   C. The inner lamella includes the medial and lateral canthal tendons.
   D. Eyelid skin is usually thicker than postauricular skin at 1.5-mm depth.
   E. Hypertrophic scarring is a relatively common finding after eyelid surgery.

ORBICULARIS OCULI MUSCLE

2. *Which one of the following statements is correct regarding the orbicularis oculi?*
   A. This muscle has two components: orbital and pretarsal.
   B. This muscle is innervated by CN III.
   C. Pretarsal fibers are solely responsible for involuntary blinking.
   D. Orbital fibers overlie the bony rim and provide forceful voluntary contraction.
   E. Innervation is via the superficial surface of the muscle.

EYELID ANATOMY

3. *Which one of the following statements is correct regarding eyelid anatomy?*
   A. The terms "ROOF" and "SOOF" refer to the fat compartments between the orbicularis and the orbital septum.
   B. Both upper and lower eyelids contain three fat compartments separated by the extraocular muscles.
   C. The tarsal plate of the upper eyelid is slightly shorter in height and broader in length than that of the lower eyelid.
   D. The inferior margin of the upper eyelid tarsus is the attachment for Müller's muscle and the levator aponeurosis.
   E. The palpebral portion of the conjunctiva lines the sclera in order to protect and hydrate the globe.

EYELID RETRACTORS

4. *Which one of the following statements is correct regarding elevation of the upper eyelid?*
   A. Müller's muscle is innervated by CN III.
   B. Loss of Müller's muscle function typically results in 5–6 mm of upper eyelid ptosis.
   C. The levator palpebrae superioris originates from the greater wing of the sphenoid.
   D. The capsulopalpebral fascia is responsible for the formation of the supratarsal crease.
   E. Whitnall's ligament redirects the vector of the levator palpebrae superioris to provide superior eyelid retraction.

LACRIMAL APPARATUS

5. *Why do facial palsy patients primarily experience problems with epiphora?*
   A. The active mechanism for lacrimal sac filling is impaired.
   B. The lacrimal puncta are physically blocked.
   C. The lacrimal gland innervation is dysfunctional.
   D. The valve of Hesner fails due to loss of innervation.
   E. The lacrimal gland is stimulated to increase tear production.

BLOOD SUPPLY TO THE EYELIDS

6. *Which one of the following statements is correct regarding the vascular anatomy of the eyelid?*
   A. The upper eyelids are primarily supplied by branches of the facial artery.
   B. Contributions are made from the internal and external carotid arteries.
   C. The lower eyelids are primarily supplied by branches of the ophthalmic artery.
   D. The angular artery is a continuation of the zygomaticofacial artery.
   E. Only the marginal arcades provide blood supply to the eyelids.

GENERAL PRINCIPLES OF EYELID RECONSTRUCTION

7. *When considering eyelid reconstruction, which one of the following is true?*
   A. Selection of reconstructive technique is primarily based on the depth of defect.
   B. Selection of reconstructive technique is primarily based on the size of defect.
   C. Only defects of less than 20% can be closed directly, even in elderly patients.
   D. Canthal anchoring should be undertaken in newly reconstructed eyelids.
   E. The lower eyelid is best reconstructed using the upper eyelid as a donor site.

EYELID RECONSTRUCTION

8. *Which one of the following statements is correct regarding partial-thickness reconstruction of the eyelid?*
   A. The contralateral upper eyelid should not be used as a full-thickness skin graft donor site for eyelid reconstruction.
   B. Conjunctival losses are generally best replaced with advancement of adjacent conjunctiva.
   C. Buccal mucosal grafts are preferred over nasal mucosal grafts for conjunctival reconstruction because of their reduced rate of contraction.
   D. Skin grafts to the conjunctiva are a reasonable alternative to a mucosal graft.
   E. The only option for combined tarsal and conjunctival defects is to use palatal mucosal grafts.

FLAPS USED FOR EYELID RECONSTRUCTION

9. *When considering local flap options for eyelid reconstruction, which one of the following is true?*
   A. A Tenzel semicircular flap combines a lateral canthotomy and cantholysis with a laterally based skin flap.
   B. The Cutler-Beard flap is a single-stage technique useful for replacing upper eyelid tarsal plate and conjunctiva.
   C. A Fricke flap is a type of advancement flap that provides ideal tissue for upper or lower eyelid reconstruction.
   D. A paramedian forehead flap should only be used for eyelid reconstruction if there is a nasal element to the defect.
   E. The Hughes flap is indicated for reconstructing the outer lamella of the upper eyelid.

RECONSTRUCTION OF THE UPPER EYELID

10. You see an elderly patient with a partial-thickness defect of the upper eyelid following Mohs micrographic surgery. It measures 70% of the total eyelid width (2 cm) and measures 1.3 cm tall. The conjunctiva and tarsal plate are intact and most of the orbicularis oculi has been preserved. *Which one of the following would be the best reconstructive option in this case?*
    A. Split-thickness skin graft from the thigh
    B. Full-thickness skin graft from the contralateral upper eyelid
    C. Postauricular full-thickness skin graft from the ipsilateral neck
    D. Temporal forehead flap (Fricke)
    E. Primary closure

RECONSTRUCTION OF THE UPPER EYELID

11. A patient has a full-thickness defect of the upper eyelid (75% width) above the lash line which is preserved. *What is the best way to manage this defect?*
    A. Paramedian forehead flap
    B. Cutler-Beard flap
    C. Tenzel semicircular flap
    D. Fricke flap
    E. Tripier flap

RECONSTRUCTION OF THE LOWER EYELID

12. Following surgical excision of a basal cell carcinoma, a patient has a full-thickness defect of the lower eyelid that represents 65% of the eyelid width. *How best might this defect be reconstructed?*
    A. A Hughes flap and full-thickness skin graft
    B. A Tenzel semicircular flap and full-thickness skin graft
    C. Lateral canthotomy and cantholysis
    D. Paramedian forehead flap and septal cartilage graft
    E. Rotation cheek flap (Mustarde) and ear cartilage graft

Answers

EYELID ANATOMY

1. *Which one of the following statements is correct regarding anatomy of the eyelids?*

   C. **The inner lamella includes the medial and lateral canthal tendons.**

The eyelid can be considered to have three lamellae. The inner layer (posterior lamella) consists of the conjunctiva lining the globe and inner eyelid, the tarsal plates, (providing structural support) the medial and lateral canthal tendons, the retractor muscles, and the capsulopalpebral fascia. The middle layer includes the orbital septum and the pre- and postseptal fat compartments. The outer lamella (anterior lamella) consists of skin and orbicularis oculi. Knowledge of eyelid anatomy is key when considering reconstructive or aesthetic surgery in this area. The eyelid skin is the thinnest on the body, typically 1 mm, but this can range from as little as 0.3–1.3 mL. Postauricular skin is usually at least 1-mm thick but still can be a useful donor site for eyelid reconstruction where skin grafts are required. Hypertrophic scarring is seen typically in burns, sites of delayed healing, or undue tension on wounds. In contrast, surgery to the eyelids usually results in very high-quality scars.[1,2]

REFERENCES

1. Hollinshead WH, ed. Anatomy for Surgeons: The Head and Neck. 3rd ed. Philadelphia: Lippincott Williams & Wilkins; 1982
2. McCord CD, Codner MA, eds. Eyelid & Periorbital Surgery. St Louis: Quality Medical Publishing; 2008

ORBICULARIS OCULI MUSCLE

2. *Which one of the following statements is correct regarding the orbicularis oculi?*

   D. **Orbital fibers overlie the bony rim and provide forceful voluntary contraction.**

The orbicularis oculi acts as a sphincter around the eye and has three components (not two): orbital, pretarsal, and preseptal. Orbital fibers overlie the orbital rim and are responsible for voluntary closure of the eye such as winking and forceful squeezing. Pretarsal fibers overlie the tarsal plate and are responsible for involuntary blinking, but they are also assisted in this by the preseptal fibers which overly the orbital septum. The orbicularis oculi receive innervation from the facial nerve (CN VII) via its deep surface, as do most of the facial mimetic muscles. Only three of them are innervated via their superficial surfaces: the buccinator, levator anguli oris, and mentalis.[1,2]

REFERENCES

1. Hollinshead WH, ed. Anatomy for Surgeons: The Head and Neck. 3rd ed. Philadelphia: Lippincott Williams & Wilkins; 1982
2. McCord CD, Codner MA, eds. Eyelid & Periorbital Surgery. St Louis: Quality Medical Publishing; 2008

EYELID ANATOMY

3. *Which one of the following statements is correct regarding eyelid anatomy?*

   A. **The terms "ROOF" and "SOOF" refer to the fat compartments between the orbicularis and the septum.**

The eyelids contain preseptal and postseptal fat. The preseptal fat lies between the orbicularis oculi and the orbital septum. This can contribute to the aging process as it moves downward. In the upper eyelid it is known as the retro-orbicularis oculi fat (ROOF) and in the lower eyelid it is known as the suborbicularis oculi fat (SOOF). Behind the orbital septum there are further fat compartments. There are two in the upper eyelid (medial and central) which are separated by the trochlea and superior oblique extraocular muscles. There is no lateral fat compartment because this space is occupied by the lacrimal gland. In the lower eyelid there are three compartments (medial, central, and lateral). The medial and central fat pads are separated by the inferior oblique extraocular muscle. The tarsal plate is a dense cartilaginous structure located adjacent to the eyelid margin and provides structural support and rigidity to the eyelids. The tarsal plate of the upper eyelid has a greater vertical height (10 mm) than that of the lower eyelid (4 mm), but both have similar widths. The tarsus is separated from the orbital rim by the orbital septum. The superior margin of the upper eyelid tarsus is the attachment for Müller's muscle and the levator aponeurosis. The bulbar portion of the conjunctiva lines the sclera, and the palpebral portion lines the inner surface of the eyelids. The two join at the superior and inferior fornices.[1,2]

REFERENCES

1. Hollinshead WH, ed. Anatomy for Surgeons: The Head and Neck. 3rd ed. Philadelphia: Lippincott Williams & Wilkins; 1982
2. McCord CD, Codner MA, eds. Eyelid & Periorbital Surgery. St Louis: Quality Medical Publishing; 2008

EYELID RETRACTORS

4. Which one of the following statements is correct regarding elevation of the upper eyelid?

E. **Whitnall's ligament redirects the vector of the levator palpebrae superioris to provide superior eyelid retraction.**
The levator palpebrae superioris (LPS) is the primary upper eyelid elevator and is supported by Müller's muscle. The LPS is innervated by CN III and originates from the lesser wing of sphenoid (not greater) to insert the superior tarsus and dermis to create the supratarsal crease. It broadens as an aponeurosis at Whitnall's ligament which redirects the horizontal pull to a vertical one in order to elevate the eyelid effectively. Müller's muscle is innervated by the sympathetic nervous system, which is carried along with the ophthalmic nerve through the cavernous sinus. The fibers originate from the superior cervical ganglion. This muscle arises from the inferior surface of the LPS and inserts into the superior edge of the tarsal plate. Loss of Müller's muscle function results in 2–3 mm of ptosis. The lower eyelid also has retractors and these are the capsulopalpebral fascia and inferior tarsal muscle. These are analogous to the LPS and Müller's muscle, respectively.[1]

REFERENCE

1. McCord CD, Codner MA, eds. Eyelid & Periorbital Surgery. St Louis: Quality Medical Publishing; 2008

LACRIMAL APPARATUS

5. Why do facial palsy patients primarily experience problems with epiphora?

A. **The active mechanism for lacrimal sac filling is impaired.**
Tears produced by the lacrimal gland enter the external surface of the globe via the superior fornix. The tear film then coats the surface of the eye to provide lubrication, reduce risk of infection, mechanically remove foreign bodies, and increase the refractive power of incoming light. Following this, the normal passage of tears is to enter the lacrimal sac via the lacrimal puncta along the upper and lower eyelid margins. These puncta open into the superior and inferior canaliculi respectively. They join together to form the common canaliculus and empty into the lacrimal sac through the valve of Rosenmüller. From here the lacrimal sac empties into the nasolacrimal duct to drain tears into the nasal cavity.
In order for tears to move from the eye into the lacrimal sac, there needs to be a pressure difference with negative pressure within the lacrimal sac relative to the eye. Eye closure is required to create this negative pressure. On eye closure, the sac fills and then when the eyes reopen, the tears are expelled into the nasolacrimal duct. Therefore, the primary reason why patients with facial palsy have epiphora is that the negative pressure mechanism for filling the lacrimal sac is impaired due to the loss of innervation to the orbicularis oculi (usually innervated by CN VII) and consequent problems with reduced blinking. The lacrimal gland is not innervated by the facial nerve so is unaffected. It is innervated by the lacrimal nerve from CN V and has parasympathetic and sympathetic innervation from the pterygopalatine ganglion and superior cervical ganglion, respectively. The valve of Hesner is found between the nasolacrimal duct opening and the nose. It is a mechanical valve that stops reflux of air or nasal contents up the duct system.[1]

REFERENCE

1. McCord CD, Codner MA, eds. Eyelid & Periorbital Surgery. St Louis: Quality Medical Publishing; 2008

BLOOD SUPPLY TO THE EYELIDS

6. Which one of the following statements is correct regarding the vascular anatomy of the eyelid?

B. **Contributions are made from the internal and external carotid arteries.**
Blood supply contributions to the eyelid include the following:
Facial artery: This vessel forms the angular, lateral nasal, and inferior medial palpebral arteries.
Transverse facial artery: This vessel forms the zygomaticofacial and inferior palpebral arteries.
Superficial temporal artery: This vessel forms the superior medial palpebral artery (peripheral arcade).
Ophthalmic artery: This vessel forms the lacrimal, supraorbital, medial palpebral, and dorsal nasal vessels.
The upper eyelids are primarily supplied by branches of the ophthalmic artery (the first branch of the internal carotid). The lower eyelids are mainly supplied by branches of the facial artery (a branch of the external carotid). The angular artery is a continuation of the facial artery as it passes lateral to the nose. (This later becomes the lateral nasal artery, which anastomoses with the dorsal nasal artery from the ophthalmic artery.) Both marginal and peripheral arcades supply the eyelids (**Fig. 40.1**).[1]

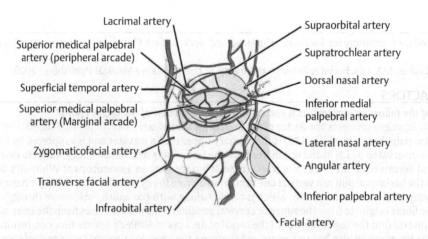

Lacrimal artery

Superior medical palpebral artery (peripheral arcade)

Superficial temporal artery

Superior medical palpebral artery (Marginal arcade)

Zygomaticofacial artery

Transverse facial artery

Infraobital artery

Supraorbital artery

Supratrochlear artery

Dorsal nasal artery

Inferior medial palpebral artery

Lateral nasal artery

Angular artery

Inferior palpebral artery

Facial artery

Fig. 40.1   Arterial supply to the eyelid. (Adapted from McCord CD Jr, Codner MA. Eyelid & Periorbital Surgery. St Louis: Quality Medical Publishing, 2008.)

REFERENCE

1. McCord CD, Codner MA, eds. Eyelid & Periorbital Surgery. St Louis: Quality Medical Publishing; 2008

GENERAL PRINCIPLES OF EYELID RECONSTRUCTION

7. When considering eyelid reconstruction, which one of the following is true?

   D. Canthal anchoring should be undertaken in newly reconstructed eyelids.

   When considering eyelid reconstruction, both size and depth of defect must be taken into account as this will affect reconstruction choice. Also during reconstruction, it is important to ensure satisfactory anchoring of the canthi or temporary closure of the eyelid margin with a "Frost stitch." In general, defects of up to 25 or 30% can usually be closed directly, but this depends on individual patient factors such as eyelid laxity, tissue quality, and age. In some elderly patients, it is possible to close defects of up to 40% directly. Defects between 25 and 50% can often be closed primarily with the addition of a lateral canthotomy and cantholysis (release of the lateral canthal tendon), but defects larger than this will still usually require additional importation of tissue from the opposite eyelid or adjacent regions such as the cheek, forehead, or temple.

   Although there are techniques that borrow tissue from the upper eyelid to reconstruct the lower eyelid, these should be performed with caution because the upper eyelid is a dynamic structure that contributes significantly to eyelid function.[1-4]

REFERENCES

1. Putterman AM. Reconstruction of the eyelids following resection for carcinoma. Clin Plast Surg 1985;12(3):393–410
2. Spinelli HM, Jelks GW. Periocular reconstruction: a systematic approach. Plast Reconstr Surg 1993;91(6):1017–1024, discussion 1025–1026
3. DiFrancesco LM, Codner MA, McCord CD. Upper eyelid reconstruction. Plast Reconstr Surg 2004;114(7):98e–107e
4. Codner MA, McCord CD, Mejia JD, Lalonde D. Upper and lower eyelid reconstruction. Plast Reconstr Surg 2010;126(5):231e–245e

EYELID RECONSTRUCTION

8. Which one of the following statements is correct regarding partial-thickness reconstruction of the eyelid?

   B. Conjunctival losses are generally best replaced with advancement of adjacent conjunctiva.

   There are a number of different approaches for reconstruction of conjunctival defects, depending on the size and whether the tarsus is also involved. Where possible it is preferable to reconstruct isolated conjunctival defects by advancing adjacent conjunctival tissue. In cases where this is not possible, grafts may be harvested from the buccal or nasal mucosa, and of these, nasal mucosa is generally preferred because there is less secondary contraction. Skin grafts are contraindicated for corneal reconstruction because they irritate the cornea. In contrast, for upper and lower eyelid skin reconstruction, full-thickness skin grafts from the contralateral upper eyelid work well and ensure good thickness and color match. Use of a lower eyelid graft to reconstruct the upper would, however, not be recommended as this may result in development of ectropion. Several options exist for reconstruction of the tarsal plate. These include palatal mucosa grafts, autologous cartilage, and allografts such as AlloDerm™.[1-4]

REFERENCES

1. Putterman AM. Reconstruction of the eyelids following resection for carcinoma. Clin Plast Surg 1985;12(3):393–410
2. Spinelli HM, Jelks GW. Periocular reconstruction: a systematic approach. Plast Reconstr Surg 1993;91(6):1017–1024, discussion 1025–1026
3. DiFrancesco LM, Codner MA, McCord CD. Upper eyelid reconstruction. Plast Reconstr Surg 2004;114(7):98e–107e
4. Codner MA, McCord CD, Mejia JD, Lalonde D. Upper and lower eyelid reconstruction. Plast Reconstr Surg 2010;126(5):231e–245e

FLAPS USED FOR EYELID RECONSTRUCTION

9. *When considering local flap options for eyelid reconstruction, which one of the following is true?*

    A. A Tenzel semicircular flap combines a lateral canthotomy and cantholysis with a laterally based skin flap.

The Tenzel semicircular flap is a single-stage, laterally based myocutaneous flap technique that is combined with lateral canthotomy and cantholysis to reconstruct upper eyelid defects.[1,2] The Cutler-Beard flap is a two-stage flap sharing technique used for full-thickness upper eyelid defect reconstruction. It involves advancement of a full-thickness lower eyelid flap that is passed under the lower eyelid margin and sutured into the upper eyelid defect. Division is usually performed at 3–6 weeks.[3] A Fricke flap is a type of transposition (not advancement) flap that is also known as a *temporal forehead flap*. It can be used to reconstruct partial-thickness upper or lower eyelid defects; however, the tissues of the brow from which it is harvested are different to the eyelid and these flaps tend to be rather bulky for eyelid reconstruction.[4] The paramedian forehead flap is primarily used for nasal reconstruction, but may be used in select cases of eyelid reconstruction where extensive defects are present. It can be useful for combined eyelid and nasal defects but is not limited purely to this. The Hughes flap is a tarsoconjunctival flap used in two stages to reconstruct the lower eyelid with the upper eyelid as a donor site. The flap is raised and inset into the defect to reconstruct the posterior lamella and covered with a full-thickness skin graft to reconstruct the anterior lamella (**Fig. 40.2**).[5]

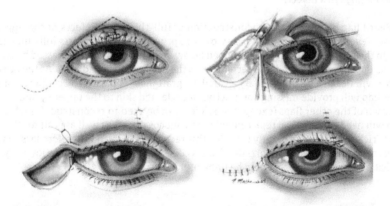

Fig. 40.2   The semicircular flap, or Tenzel flap, is used for defects involving up to 60% of the upper eyelid. Lateral canthotomy is required to rotate the flap. (Adapted from DiFrancesco LM, Codner MA, McCord CD Jr. Upper eyelid reconstruction. Plast Reconstr Surg 114:98e–107e, 2004.)

REFERENCES

1. Tenzel RR, Stewart WB. Eyelid reconstruction by the semicircle flap technique. Ophthalmology 1978;85(11):1164–1169
2. DiFrancesco LM, Codner MA, McCord CD. Upper eyelid reconstruction. Plast Reconstr Surg 2004;114(7):98e–107e
3. Fischer T, Noever G, Langer M, Kammer E. Experience in upper eyelid reconstruction with the Cutler-Beard technique. Ann Plast Surg 2001;47(3):338–342
4. Fricke JCG. Die Bildung neuer Augenlider (Blepharoplastik) nach Zerstorungen und dadurch hervorgebrachten Auswarts-wendungen derselben. Hamburg: Perthes and Bessler; 1929
5. Hughes WL. A new method for rebuilding a lower lid: report of a case. Arch Ophthalmol 1937;17(6):1008–1017

RECONSTRUCTION OF THE UPPER EYELID

10. You see an elderly patient with a partial-thickness defect of the upper eyelid following Mohs micrographic surgery. It measures 70% of the total eyelid width (2 cm) and measures 1.3 cm tall. The conjunctiva and tarsal plate are intact and most of the orbicularis oculi has been preserved.
    Which one of the following would be the best reconstructive option in this case?
    B. Full-thickness skin graft from the ipsilateral upper eyelid

    The general principles for eyelid reconstruction follow the principles common to most reconstructions: analyze the defect site and tissue structures involved, then reconstruct, replacing like with like where possible. The selection of a technique for eyelid reconstruction will therefore depend on the site; for example, upper versus lower eyelid, and the width, height, and depth of the defect. Partial-thickness defects such as this anterior lamella case can be reconstructed with a full-thickness skin graft, providing there is a well-vascularized recipient bed such as orbicularis oculi.

    A full-thickness graft is preferable to a split-thickness graft because there will be less secondary contraction which can risk development of ectropion. Many patients, particularly the elderly, will have an excess of upper eyelid skin and this can make a good graft donor site as the skin is thin and a good color match for the contralateral eyelid. Symmetry can be achieved between the sides with such an approach by taking a slightly undersized graft, and the donor and recipient sites are often difficult to identify in the longer term.

    The use of a graft from behind or just in front of the ear is a good alternative where there is insufficient upper eyelid skin as this also has a suitable color and thickness match. However, caution should be taken when using the ipsilateral preauricular area in case a local flap is later required from this side. The Fricke flap could be used in this case, but would provide tissue that will be unnecessarily thick. Primary closure would have been a good option if the defect was less tall, that is, up to 1 cm, but in this scenario, direct closure would likely result in lagophthalmos.[1,2]

REFERENCES

1. Putterman AM. Reconstruction of the eyelids following resection for carcinoma. Clin Plast Surg 1985;12(3):393–410
2. Spinelli HM, Jelks GW. Periocular reconstruction: a systematic approach. Plast Reconstr Surg 1993;91(6):1017–1024, discussion 1025–1026

RECONSTRUCTION OF THE UPPER EYELID

11. A patient has a full-thickness defect of the upper eyelid (75% width) above the lash line which is preserved. *What is the best way to manage this defect?*
    B. Cutler-Beard flap

    The Cutler-Beard flap is indicated in reconstruction of full-thickness defects of the upper eyelid using the ipsilateral lower eyelid as a donor site. It is a two-stage procedure that harvests full-thickness tissue from the lower eyelid. In the first stage, the flap is developed below the inferior tarsus and passed beneath the lower eyelid margin into the upper eyelid defect. It the second stage, the flap is divided and inset. As the tarsus is not harvested, eyelid support will need to be provided by a cartilage graft inset between the conjunctiva and muscle layers. However, this flap will provide missing conjunctiva, muscle, and skin to the upper eyelid.

    Although each of the other flaps (except the Tripier) can be used to reconstruct full-thickness upper eyelid defects, each will need conjunctival replacement with a mucosal graft as well as graft for the missing tarsus. The forehead and Fricke flaps will be unduly thick for this reconstruction and therefore less than ideal. The Tripier flap is a myocutaneous flap used for partial-thickness defect reconstruction in the lower eyelid. It is harvested from the ipsilateral upper eyelid, so would be unhelpful in this case (**Fig. 40.3**).[1,2]

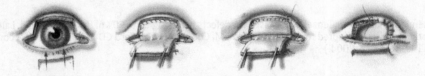

Fig. 40.3 The Cutler-Beard flap is used for total upper eyelid reconstruction. The flap is a biplanar flap passed beneath the lower eyelid margin. (Adapted from DiFrancesco LM, Codner MA, McCord CD Jr. Upper eyelid reconstruction. Plast Reconstr Surg 114:98e–107e, 2004.)

REFERENCES

1. Fischer T, Noever G, Langer M, Kammer E. Experience in upper eyelid reconstruction with the Cutler-Beard technique. Ann Plast Surg 2001;47(3):338–342
2. Rahmi D, Mehmet B, Ceyda B, Sibel O. Management of the large upper eyelid defects with cutler-beard flap. J Ophthalmol 2014;2014:424567

RECONSTRUCTION OF THE LOWER EYELID

12. Following surgical excision of a basal cell carcinoma, a patient has a full-thickness defect of the lower eyelid that represents 65% of the eyelid width. *How best might this defect be reconstructed?*
   A. **A Hughes flap and full-thickness skin graft**
   This represents a complex defect for reconstruction with all three lamellae deficient. The Hughes tarsoconjunctival flap represents a good option here because it provides both tarsus and conjunctiva for reconstruction of the posterior lamella and full-thickness graft can be applied to reconstruct the anterior lamella. The Tenzel flap is useful to reconstruct defects of the anterior lamella of up to 60% but will need a mucosal graft and cartilage graft for reconstruction of the posterior lamella. Lateral canthotomy and cantholysis are used for smaller defects. The paramedian forehead flap could in principle be used to reconstruct the outer lamella if combined with mucosa and tarsal reconstruction, but it is more normally indicated in upper eyelid and nasal reconstruction. The Mustarde cheek rotation flap is an ideal choice for reconstructing larger anterior lamella defects of the upper eyelid. However, it would not require a skin graft, but would again need a mucosal graft for the conjunctiva (**Fig. 40.4**).[1-3]

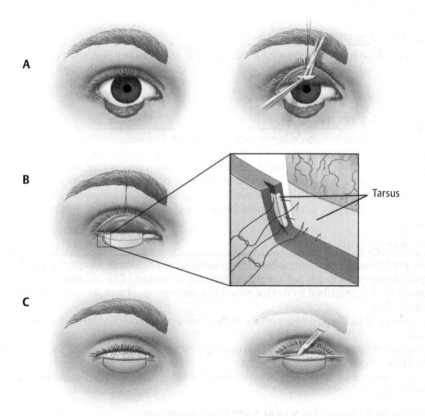

Fig. 40.4   Hughes tarsoconjunctival flap. *A,* The flap is elevated from the everted upper eyelid, closer to the margin than the free tarsoconjunctival graft. At least 4 mm of tarsus at the margin should be spared to preserve stability of the upper eyelid. The original Hughes procedure split the upper eyelid at the margin, which produced upper eyelid trichiasis. *B,* The flap should be as free of Müller's muscle as possible and sutured into the posterior lamellar defect. If tarsus remains on either edge, edge-to-edge approximation is needed. If the defect is toward the canthus, canthal fixation is needed. *C,* Since the tarsoconjunctival flap from the upper eyelid includes its own blood supply, a full-thickness skin graft can be used on its surface. A blepharoplasty or cheek-lift myocutaneous flap can be used if enough tissue is available. Separation usually takes place at 3 weeks, when the flap gains a new blood supply. Separation may be needed later if a full-thickness skin graft is used. (From McCord CD Jr, Codner MA. Eyelid & Periorbital Surgery. St Louis: Quality Medical Publishing, 2008.)

REFERENCES

1. Hughes WL. A new method for rebuilding a lower lid: report of a case. Arch Ophthalmol 1937;17(6):1008–1017
2. Bortz JG, Al-Shweiki S. Free tarsal graft and free skin graft for lower eyelid reconstruction. Ophthal Plast Reconstr Surg 2020;36(6):605–609
3. Jackson IT. General considerations. In: Jackson IT, ed. Local Flaps in Head and Neck Reconstruction. 2nd ed. St Louis: Quality Medical Publishing; 2007

41. Nasal Reconstruction

See Essentials of Plastic Surgery, third edition, pp. 548–567

BLOOD SUPPLY TO THE NOSE

1. *Which blood vessel represents the main vascular supply to the nasal sill and septum?*
   A. Angular artery
   B. Lateral nasal artery
   C. Maxillary artery
   D. Superior labial artery
   E. Ophthalmic artery

SENSORY INNERVATION OF THE NOSE

2. *Which one of the following parts of the nose is innervated by the maxillary division of the trigeminal nerve?*
   A. Radix
   B Rhinion
   C Cephalic portion of the nasal sidewalls
   D. Dorsal skin to the tip
   E. Columella

AESTHETIC SUBUNUITS OF THE NOSE

3. *When planning nasal reconstruction using an anatomic subunit approach, which one of the following is true?*
   A. There are seven key anatomic subunits in the nose when considering nasal reconstruction.
   B. The anatomic subunit approach to nasal reconstruction is universally accepted.
   C. A nasal defect should occupy more than 75% of a subunit to justify reconstruction of the entire subunit.
   D. The nasal tip is thought to represent the most challenging subunit to reconstruct.
   E. It relies on the premise that scar placement between nasal subunits will provide the most discreet long-term scars.

NASAL LINING RECONSTRUCTION

4. *Which one of the following statements is correct regarding reconstruction of a nasal lining defect?*
   A. Folding of an extranasal flap is only possible with staged forehead flap techniques.
   B. The septal door flap described by de Quervain involves removal of septal mucosa from the contralateral side to the defect.
   C. Skin grafts applied to the posterior surface of flaps are associated with high failure rates and stricture formation.
   D. Septal mucoperichondrial flaps involve harvesting a rectangle of mucosa with the underlying perichondrium from the ipsilateral septum.
   E. The mucosal advancement flap described by Burget and Menick involves a unipedicled advancement flap with a medial blood supply.

TECHNIQUES FOR PROVISION OF NASAL SKELETAL SUPPORT

5. *Which one of the following describes a composite flap that can be used to provide nasal lining and dorsal midline skeleton support and is based on a branch of the superior labial artery?*
   A. Hinged septal flap
   B. Rieger dorsal nasal flap
   C. Septal pivot flap
   D. Gillies strut technique
   E. Cantilever graft

TECHNIQUES FOR PROVISION OF ALAR SUPPORT

6. *Which one of the following techniques involves placement of a nonanatomic cartilage graft via an infracartilaginous incision into an alar vestibular pocket inferior and lateral to the rim of the lateral crus with the intention of reestablishing external valve function and normal alar shape?*
   A. Alar contour graft
   B. Alar batten graft
   C. Alar spreader graft
   D. Lateral crural strut graft
   E. Lateral crural turnover graft

SKELETAL AND CARTILAGINOUS SUPPORT FOR THE NOSE

7. A 37-year-old woman presents with a pinched-tip deformity of her nose and difficulty breathing at night. On examination she has a bilateral positive Cottle's test. *Which one of the following techniques is most likely to address both of her symptoms?*
   A. Alar batten graft
   B. Lateral crural strut graft
   C. Alar spreader graft
   D. Alar contour graft
   E. Cantilever graft

RECONSTRUCTION OF NASAL SKIN AND SOFT TISSUE

8. *Which one of the following flaps used in nasal reconstruction is normally based on the supratrochlear vessels?*
   A. Washio/Temporomastoid flap
   B. Frontotemporal flap
   C. Rieger dorsal nasal flap
   D. Forehead flap
   E. Converse scalping flap

NASAL RECONSTRUCTION AFTER MOHS SURGERY

9. A 56-year-old woman is referred by the local Mohs surgeon after excision of an infiltrative basal cell carcinoma from her nose 1 week earlier. On examination she has a full-thickness defect of her left ala measuring 2 by 1.5 cm. The nasal tip, dorsum, and caudal lateral sidewall are spared. *How might this best be reconstructed?*
   A. Single-stage paramedian forehead flap with full-thickness graft for lining
   B. Staged paramedian forehead flap and mucoperichondrial flap for lining
   C. Staged paramedian forehead flap with conchal cartilage and mucoperichondrial flap
   D. Staged nasalis flap with conchal cartilage and full-thickness graft
   E. Single-stage nasolabial flap with septal cartilage and mucoperichondrial flap

RECONSTRUCTION OF THE MEDIAL CANTHAL REGION

10. A 24-year-old woman develops a 3-mm nodular basal cell carcinoma on her medial canthus. The edges are well defined. You plan to excise this with a 3-mm margin. *How should this be addressed following excision?*
    A. Healing by secondary intention
    B. Full-thickness skin graft
    C. Split-thickness skin graft
    D. Banner flap
    E. Glabellar flap

RECONSTRUCTION OF THE PROXIMAL NASAL DORSUM

11. A 70-year-old man develops a 10-mm microcystic basal cell carcinoma on the dorsum of his nose, just below the nasal bridge. Following a staged excision with 4-mm margins, histology confirms complete excision. *How best should this defect be managed?*
    A. Banner flap
    B. Nasalis flap
    C. Cheek advancement flap
    D. Forehead flap
    E. Glabellar flap

SOFT TRIANGLE RECONSTRUCTION OF THE NOSE

12. A patient is referred with a soft triangle defect 3 months after a dog bite injury to the nose. The original injury was cleaned and sutured in the emergency department. On examination, an isolated, unilateral, soft triangle defect is present, with both mucosal and soft tissue deficiencies. There is no skin loss evident. *Which one of the following reconstructions is this patient most likely to require?*
    A. Composite conchal bowl graft
    B. Paramedian forehead flap
    C. Paramedian forehead flap, folded in for lining and cartilage graft
    D. Nasolabial flap
    E. Nasolabial flap and cartilage graft

NASAL DORSUM AND SIDEWALL RECONSTRCTION

13. *Which one of the following statements is correct when planning a bilobed flap for reconstruction of a circular alar tip defect that measures 1.3 cm in diameter?*
    A. The defect should be triangulated.
    B. The ideal rotation for each lobe is 90 degrees.
    C. The pivot point should be 1.3 cm from the defect.
    D. The vascular supply is the ipsilateral angular artery.
    E. All lobes should be of equal width.

RAISING A PARAMEDIAN FOREHEAD FLAP

14. *When elevating a paramedian forehead flap for nasal reconstruction, in which plane should flap elevation occur?*
    A. In a subcutaneous plane
    B. In a submuscular plane
    C. In a subgaleal plane
    D. In a subperiosteal plane
    E. In a number of different planes

RHINOPHYMA

15. A patient is examined in clinic with a diagnosis of rhinophyma. *Which one of the following statements is correct?*
    A. Rhinophyma is approximately twice as common in men as women.
    B. Patients carry a generalized increased risk of basal cell carcinoma (BCC) development.
    C. Dermabrasion is the gold standard for surgical management.
    D. Surgical treatment is the mainstay treatment for stage IV disease.
    E. Patients are likely to be heavy drinkers and smokers.

SKIN DISORDERS OF THE NOSE

16. A 63-year-old man presents with skin discoloration involving the tip of his nose and cheeks. He says that it has progressively worsened over the past 5 years and wishes to have it treated. On examination, multiple erythematous pustules and papules are present on his nasal tip and cheeks. *Which one of the following is part of the first-line treatment for this patient?*
    A. Topical metronidazole gel
    B. Retinoic acid
    C. Tetracycline
    D. Surgery
    E. Zinc oxide and sunscreen

Answers

BLOOD SUPPLY TO THE NOSE

1. **Which blood vessel represents the main vascular supply to the nasal sill and septum?**

   D. Superior labial artery

   The external nose is supplied by branches of the facial, ophthalmic, and maxillary arteries. The superior labial artery is a branch of the facial artery that supplies the nasal sill, the nasal septum, the columellar base, and the upper lip. The angular artery arises from the facial artery and supplies the lateral surface of the nose. The maxillary artery supplies the nasal dorsum and lateral sidewalls. The ophthalmic artery also supplies the nasal dorsum through the dorsal artery from the supratrochlear vessels.[1-3]

REFERENCES

1. Oneal RM, Beil RJ Jr, Schlesinger J. Surgical anatomy of the nose. Clin Plast Surg 1996;23(2):195–222
2. Anderson JE, ed. Grant's Atlas of Anatomy. 8th ed. Baltimore: Williams & Wilkins; 2011
3. Last RJ, ed. Anatomy, Regional and Applied. 12th ed. London: Churchill Livingstone; 1979

SENSORY INNERVATION OF THE NOSE

2. **Which one of the following parts of the nose is innervated by the maxillary division of the trigeminal nerve?**

   E. Columella

   The radix, rhinion, cephalic portion of the nasal sidewalls, nasal dorsum, and tip all receive their sensory nerve supply by the ophthalmic division of the trigeminal nerve (V_1). The columella and caudal portion of the lateral nasal sidewalls are supplied by the maxillary division of the trigeminal nerve (V_2). When performing surgery on the nose under local anesthesia, it is a painful area to inject. For this reason, it is helpful to begin with an intraoral injection of the infraorbital nerve. This is achieved by lifting the upper lip and passing a needle cranially in line with the pupil, just lateral to the lateral incisor. Slow injection here followed by a short pause can help to ensure patients remain comfortable during subsequent injections around the nose.[1,2]

REFERENCES

1. Oneal RM, Beil RJ Jr, Schlesinger J. Surgical anatomy of the nose. Clin Plast Surg 1996;23(2):195–222
2. Anderson JE, ed. Grant's Atlas of Anatomy. 8th ed. Baltimore: Williams & Wilkins; 2011

AESTHETIC SUBUNUITS OF THE NOSE

3. **When planning nasal reconstruction using an anatomic subunit approach, which one of the following is true?**

   E. It relies on the premise that scar placement between nasal subunits will provide the most discreet long-term scars.

   The anatomic subunit approach to nasal reconstruction has been described by Burget and Menick.[1] In this approach, there are considered to be nine key areas in the external nose:
   1. Dorsum
   2. Sidewalls (2)
   3. Tip
   4. Soft triangle (2)
   5. Alar lobule (2)
   6. Columella

   The premise of this approach is that reconstructing entire subunits helps to disguise scars by their anatomical placement and to provide the most discreet long-term aesthetic outcomes. Menick states:

   "If the scar is placed between topographic subunits, where it follows the normal lighted ridges and shadowed valleys of the nasal surface, it will be taken for normal."

   In this approach where there is more than 50% (not 75%) deficiency in a subunit, it should be removed and reconstructed in its entirety. Of the nine subunits, the soft triangle is generally considered to be the most difficult to reconstruct. Adopting the subunit approach is useful for both clinical decision-making and in examination scenarios, as it provides a foundation upon which to discuss cases and make decisions about their reconstruction. Applying the subunit to Mohs excision has also been considered to be a useful and valid approach.[2] However, it is not uniformly accepted, and some surgeons advocate a different approach where maximal conservation of native tissue is advocated and only the defect itself (not the subunit) is reconstructed.[3] Of course, some authors have a mixed stance and blend the two approaches. This may be a good approach as it takes strengths from each of the alternatives. At the end of the day, each patient and the nasal defect should be taken on a case-by-case basis and decisions made to optimize the outcome in a holistic manner.

REFERENCES

1. Burget GC, Menick FJ. The subunit principle in nasal reconstruction. Plast Reconstr Surg 1985;76(2):239–247
2. Jergensen ZR, Pezeshk RA, Thornton JF. Rationale and argument for subunit Mohs excision in nasal reconstruction. J Cutan Med Surg 2016;20(4):343–345
3. Rohrich RJ, Griffin JR, Ansari M, Beran SJ, Potter JK. Nasal reconstruction—beyond aesthetic subunits: a 15-year review of 1334 cases. Plast Reconstr Surg 2004;114(6):1405–1416, discussion 1417–1419

NASAL LINING RECONSTRUCTION

4. *Which one of the following statements is correct regarding reconstruction of a nasal lining defect?*
   D. **Septal mucoperichondrial flaps involve harvesting a rectangle of mucosa with the underlying perichondrium from the ipsilateral septum.**
   The mucosal surface of the nasal vestibule can be reconstructed in several different ways. When external tissue is used, such as a forehead or nasolabial flap, a full-thickness skin graft can be sutured to the underside of the flap before inset. These grafts are associated with good outcomes and are not prone to stricture formation. Alternatively, if the lining is deficient close to or at the alar rim, then the tip of the flap can be turned over and sutured to itself. This can be successful, but it requires thinning of the flap to attain closure. In most cases, a second procedure is needed to further thin the alar rim.
   Other reconstructive options include mucosal flaps harvested as composites with either cartilage or perichondrium. The septal door flap as described by de Quervain[1] involves removal and discarding of mucosa from the ipsilateral septum and then hinging of the septum and remaining contralateral mucosa to cover the mucosal defect.
   The mucosal advancement flap as described by Burget and Menick[2,3] involves a bipedicled (not unipedicled) mucosal flap based medially on the remaining septum and laterally at the piriform aperture. It is used to resurface small lining defects of the nasal ala.

REFERENCES

1. de Quervain F. Ueber partielle seitliche Rhinoplastik. Zentralbl Chir 1902;29:297
2. Burget GC, Menick FJ. Nasal support and lining: the marriage of beauty and blood supply. Plast Reconstr Surg 1989;84(2):189–202
3. Burget GC, Menick FJ. Nasal reconstruction: seeking a fourth dimension. Plast Reconstr Surg 1986;78(2):145–157

TECHNIQUES FOR PROVISION OF NASAL SKELETAL SUPPORT

5. *Which one of the following describes a composite flap that can be used to provide nasal lining and dorsal midline skeleton support and is based on a branch of the superior labial artery?*
   C. **Septal pivot flap**
   The septal pivot flap, described by Burget and Menick,[1,2] is used to reconstruct the nasal lining and can also be used to provide dorsal cartilage support (**Fig. 41.1**). The entire septum is pulled forward out of the nasal cavity on a narrow pedicle centered over the septal branch of the superior labial artery.

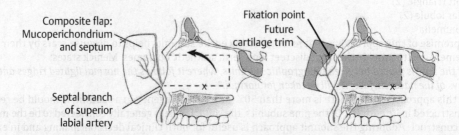

Fig. 41.1   The residual septum within the piriform aperture can be transposed on bilateral septal branches of the superior labial artery at the nasal spine to provide modest dorsal support and lining to the midvault and part of the ala. (Adapted from Burget GC, Menick FJ. Nasal support and lining: the marriage of beauty and blood supply. Plast Reconstr Surg 84:189, 1989.)

Millard's hinged septal flap is an L-shaped flap of septum that is hinged superiorly to augment the nasal angle. The septal flap is carved from the remaining septum and hinged on the caudal end of the nasal bones to pivot upward.[3] Rieger's dorsal nasal flap is a laterally based flap[4] used for reconstruction of external nasal lobule defects smaller than 2 cm in diameter. It is based on the angular arteries and allows the entire skin of the nasal dorsum to be rotated and advanced caudally.

The Gillies strut technique[5] is used to provide midline cartilaginous or skeletal support for the reconstructed nose. It involves placement of a longitudinal piece of bone or cartilage (often rib) onto the radix with extension along the nasal dorsum to the tip, where it is bent sharply to rest on the anterior nasal spine.

The cantilever graft as described by Converse[6] and Millard[7] is another technique used to provide midline nasal support. This involves placement of a longitudinal piece of bone (typically rib) fixed to the frontal or nasal bones. Unlike the strut technique it does not fix to the anterior nasal spine, hence the cantilever effect.

REFERENCES

1. Menick F, ed. Nasal Reconstruction: Art and Practice. Philadelphia: Saunders Elsevier; 2009
2. Burget GC, Menick FJ. The subunit principle in nasal reconstruction. Plast Reconstr Surg 1985;76(2):239–247
3. Millard DR Jr. Hemirhinoplasty. Plast Reconstr Surg 1967;40(5):440–445
4. Rieger RA. A local flap for repair of the nasal tip. Plast Reconstr Surg 1967;40(2):147–149
5. Gillies HD, ed. Plastic Surgery of the Face. London: Oxford University Press; 1920
6. Converse JM, ed. Reconstructive Plastic Surgery, Vol. 2. 2nd ed. Philadelphia: WB Saunders; 1977
7. Millard DR Jr. Total reconstructive rhinoplasty and a missing link. Plast Reconstr Surg 1966;37(3):167–183

TECHNIQUES FOR PROVISION OF ALAR SUPPORT

6. *Which one of the following techniques involves placement of a nonanatomic cartilage graft via an infracartilaginous incision into an alar vestibular pocket inferior and lateral to the rim of the lateral crus with the intention of reestablishing external valve function and normal alar shape?*

A. **Alar contour graft**

Alar support can be provided with anatomic or nonanatomic cartilage grafts, which either augment or replace native cartilage components of the upper and lower lateral cartilages. Alar contour grafts are nonanatomic grafts placed caudally at the alar rim to improve external nasal valve function and to provide support to the alar rim contour (**Fig. 41.2**).

Alar spreader grafts are placed between the lateral crura to push them apart and thereby reduce nasal valving. They are therefore also useful to correct a pinch tip deformity. Alar batten grafts are used to treat alar collapse and external valve obstruction. They are placed cephalad to the alar rim and fashioned to span the collapse. Lateral crural strut grafts prevent alar rim retraction and lateral crural malposition. Lateral crural turnover grafts are used to improve the strength and position/shape of the lateral crura. They involve a procedure where the cephalic portion of the lateral crura is turned over onto the remaining caudal lateral crura.

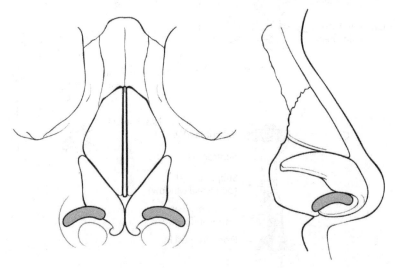

Fig. 41.2   Alar contour graft. (From Nahai F, ed. The Art of Aesthetic Surgery: Principles & Techniques. 2nd ed. St Louis: Quality Medical Publishing, 2011.)

SKELETAL AND CARTILAGINOUS SUPPORT FOR THE NOSE

7. A 37-year-old woman presents with a pinched-tip deformity of her nose and difficulty breathing at night. On examination she has a bilateral positive Cottle's test. *Which one of the following techniques is most likely to address both of her symptoms?*

   C. Alar spreader graft

   Nonanatomic cartilage grafts can help to stiffen the nasal ala and improve airway patency. Alar spreader grafts involve placement of cartilage between the vestibular surface and the undersurface of the lateral crura to force them apart. They help correct both pinched-tip deformities and internal valve collapse. Alar batten grafts involve placement of cartilage cephalad to the alar rim and can also improve alar collapse and external nasal valve obstruction. In lateral crural strut grafts, cartilage is placed between the deep surface of the lateral crus and then sutured to the crus. They help prevent rim retraction and lateral crural malposition. Alar contour grafts involve placement of cartilage into an alar vestibular pocket inferior and lateral to the rim of the crus. They are used to provide a natural alar contour and improve external nasal valving.[1]

REFERENCE

1. Gunter JP, Landecker A, Cochran CS. Nomenclature for frequently used grafts in rhinoplasty. Presented at the Twenty-second Annual Dallas Rhinoplasty Symposium, Dallas, TX, March 2005

RECONSTRUCTION OF NASAL SKIN AND SOFT TISSUE

8. *Which one of the following flaps used in nasal reconstruction is normally based on the supratrochlear vessels?*

   D. Forehead flap

   The forehead flap is a workhorse flap for nasal reconstruction. It may be midline or paramedian. The blood supply to this flap is normally from the supratrochlear vessels which run within it axially. These facilitate a long flap to width ratio such that nasal tip defects can be reliably reconstructed. When raising this flap, it can initially be raised at the level of pericranium to include the frontalis muscle. When dissection gets close to the base at the superior orbital rim, it is necessary to change plane and dissect deep to pericranium in order to preserve the blood supply. This flap defect can usually be closed directly with the exception of the most cranial part, which is left to heal by secondary intention. In the first stage of this reconstruction, the flap is inset but not usually thinned. In a subsequent stage the flap is reelevated, thinned, and replaced. Cartilage grafts may be placed during the second stage. The third stage typically involves division of the flap and reinset of the base to close the distal forehead region with minimal distortion of the brow (**Fig. 41.3**).

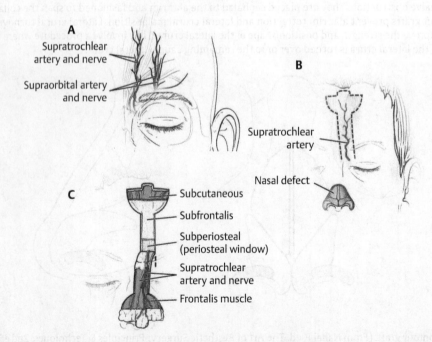

Fig. 41.3 *(A–C)* Forehead flap. (From Zenn MR, Jones G, eds. Reconstructive Surgery: Anatomy, Technique, and Clinical Applications, 2012.)

The temporomastoid flap is also known as the Washio flap.[1,2] It is based on the superficial temporal vessels to transfer mastoid and auricular skin. It is not a commonly used flap and more often dissected on cadaver dissection courses. The frontotemporal flap[3] is a tubular, bipedicled flap with an internal supraciliary pedicle carrying lateral forehead skin with embedded ear cartilage. The dorsal nasal flap as described by Rieger[4] is a useful flap for reconstructing some distal nasal skin defects. It is based on the angular artery and involves elevation of the nasal dorsal skin which is rotated and advanced caudally. The scalping flap described by Converse[5] may be used to reconstruct large nasal defects in elderly patients. It is based on the superficial temporal vessels and is elevated through a coronal incision just behind the superficial temporal artery, extending to a skin paddle in the contralateral forehead.

REFERENCES

1. Loeb R. Temporomastoid flap for reconstruction of the cheek. Rev Lat Am Chir Plast 1962;6:185
2. Washio H. Retroauricular temporal flap. Plast Reconstr Surg 2009;124:826
3. Meyer R. Aesthetic refinements in nose reconstruction. Aesthetic Plast Surg 2000;24(4):241–252
4. Rieger RA. A local flap for repair of the nasal tip. Plast Reconstr Surg 1967;40(2):147–149
5. Converse JM. A new forehead flap for nasal reconstruction. Proc R Soc Med 1942;35(12):811–812

NASAL RECONSTRUCTION AFTER MOHS SURGERY

9. A 56-year-old woman is referred by the local Mohs surgeon after excision of an infiltrative basal cell carcinoma from her nose 1 week earlier. On examination she has a full-thickness defect of her left ala measuring 2 by 1.5 cm. The nasal tip, dorsum, and caudal lateral sidewall are spared. *How might this best be reconstructed?*

C. Staged paramedian forehead flap with conchal cartilage and mucoperichondrial flap

This patient requires reconstruction of all three layers: skin, mucosa, and cartilage (support). A key element here is the need for a multistaged approach to optimize the cosmetic and functional result whichever techniques are adopted. Skin can be provided by a paramedian forehead flap or nasolabial flap. Mucosa can be provided by either a mucoperichondrial flap or a skin graft to the undersurface of the forehead flap. Cartilage support is required to reinforce the nasal ala and limit nasal valving and airway problems. This can be harvested from the conchal bowl with minimal morbidity and sandwiched between the reconstructed mucosa and skin layers. Alternatively, cartilage can be harvested from the nasal septum or ribs. If lining is provided by a mucoperichondrial flap, the cartilage can safely be placed in the first stage, otherwise it should be saved for the second stage. Although a nasolabial flap is an alternative option for this reconstruction scenario, it will blunt the nasojugal fold and may be undersized for this defect. A nasolabial flap will still require multiple stages to optimize aesthetic and functional outcomes in this scenario.[1–4]

REFERENCES

1. Converse JM. A new forehead flap for nasal reconstruction. Proc R Soc Med 1942;35(12):811–812
2. Reece EM, Schaverien M, Rohrich RJ. The paramedian forehead flap: a dynamic anatomical vascular study verifying safety and clinical implications. Plast Reconstr Surg 2008;121(6):1956–1963
3. Menick FJ. Neligan PC. Aesthetic nasal reconstruction. In: Plastic Surgery. 3rd ed. Vol. 3. New York, NY: Elsevier; 2013:134–186
4. Correa BJ, Weathers WM, Wolfswinkel EM, Thornton JF. The forehead flap: the gold standard of nasal soft tissue reconstruction. Semin Plast Surg 2013;27(2):96–103

RECONSTRUCTION OF THE MEDIAL CANTHAL REGION

10. A 24-year-old woman develops a 3-mm nodular basal cell carcinoma on her medial canthus. The edges are well defined. You plan to excise this with a 3-mm margin. *How should this be addressed following excision?*

A. Healing by secondary intention

This patient is likely to achieve the best cosmetic result if the area is left to heal without reconstruction. Some areas of the nose and surrounding areas of the face are best managed in this way, without formal reconstruction and instead allowing the area to heal by secondary intention. These include the glabellar, medial canthal regions, scalp, and forehead. Alternative options in this scenario are a small full-thickness skin graft or a local transposition flap, but in this case each of these will result in additional, unnecessary scarring. The full-thickness graft will tend to leave a contour defect, the local flap will give an extended scar line, and a split-thickness graft will accentuate the contour and color irregularities further. There is a balance to be achieved when dealing with these defects however, and defects that are too large to heal safely by secondary intent will distort the lower eyelid or upper eyelid and medial canthal area, so each case should be carefully assessed during the planning stage.[1]

REFERENCE

1. Lowry JC, Bartley GB, Garrity JA. The role of second-intention healing in periocular reconstruction. Ophthal Plast Reconstr Surg 1997;13(3):174–188

RECONSTRUCTION OF THE PROXIMAL NASAL DORSUM

11. A 70-year-old man develops a 10-mm microcystic basal cell carcinoma on the dorsum of his nose, just below the nasal bridge. Following a staged excision with 4-mm margins, histology confirms complete excision. *How best should this defect be managed?*

E. Glabellar flap

Following surgery, this patient will have a skin defect that measures at least 1.8 cm given the excision includes 4-mm margins. This defect can be reconstructed with a glabellar flap, which should provide a good cosmetic outcome with superior contour and skin color match to the defect area. The donor site will close easily leaving a linear scar running vertically. The only caveat with such flaps is that they can have a tendency to reduce the distance between the medial brows, but in this scenario that would be unlikely, and the donor scar should blend well with natural frown lines.

The banner flap is a useful skin flap typically indicated for reconstruction of small skin defects of the nasal dorsum using a triangular transposition flap from the adjacent nasal dorsum or cheek.[1]

The nasalis flap[2] is a useful flap for more caudal reconstruction over the alar region and tip. It involves elevation of a skin and muscle composite flap from the lateral aspect of the nose, which is advanced in a V-Y fashion medially with direct closure of the laterally placed donor defect. It would have insufficient reach in this scenario.

Cheek advancement flaps are useful for facial defect reconstruction, mostly of the cheek. In some defects that involve both cheek and nasal subunit reconstruction, a combination of a cheek rotation flap and a forehead flap works well to effectively reconstruct separate defects with scars hidden in the nasojugal and nasolabial folds. The forehead flap in this clinical scenario would be excessive and unnecessary for this defect. It is better suited to larger, more complex defects of the nasal dorsum, tip, lateral sidewall, and alar.

REFERENCES

1. Elliott RA Jr. Rotation flaps of the nose. Plast Reconstr Surg 1969;44(2):147–149
2. Rybka FJ. Reconstruction of the nasal tip using nasalis myocutaneous sliding flaps. Plast Reconstr Surg 1983;71(1):40–44

SOFT TRIANGLE RECONSTRUCTION OF THE NOSE

12. A patient is referred with a soft triangle defect 3 months after a dog bite injury to the nose. The original injury was cleaned and sutured in the emergency department. On examination, an isolated, unilateral, soft triangle defect is present, with both mucosal and soft tissue deficiencies. There is no skin loss evident. *Which one of the following reconstructions is this patient most likely to require?*

A. Composite conchal bowl graft

The soft triangle is a particularly difficult area to reconstruct because of its distal location on the nose and its complex shape, which is essentially quadrilateral with both convex and concave curvatures. Defects may be classified as type I, II, or III. Type I defects have intact skin but are deficient in soft tissue and mucosa. Type II defects have intact mucosa but are deficient in skin and soft tissue. Type III defects are deficient in all three layers. The patient described has a type I deformity. Constantine et al[1] have proposed an algorithm for reconstruction of soft triangle defects. According to this algorithm, the reconstruction of choice for this patient is a composite conchal bowl graft (**Fig. 41.4**).

REFERENCE

1. Constantine FC, Lee MR, Sinno S, et al. Soft tissue triangle reconstruction. Plast Reconstr Surg 2013;131:1045–1050

NASAL DORSUM AND SIDEWALL RECONSTRCTION

13. *Which one of the following statements is correct when planning a bilobed flap for reconstruction of a circular alar tip defect that measures 1.3 cm in diameter?*

D. The vascular supply is the ipsilateral angular artery.

A bilobed flap is a useful technique for reconstructing defects that involve the nasal lobule or tip (**Fig. 41.5**). Using the Zitelli modification,[1] some key principles should be followed. The defect does not need to be triangulated (as is the case for a large rotation flap), but it requires removal of a small triangle of tissue between the defect and the base of the first flap. This amounts to removal of a small dog-ear. The angle of rotation is a total of 90–100 degrees, split equally between the two transposing flaps. In this case the pivot point should be approximately 7 mm from the defect edge as this represents the defect radius. The blood supply for this flap will be from the

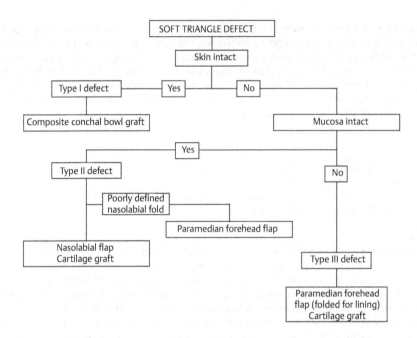

Fig. 41.4 Algorithm for the treatment of soft triangle defects.

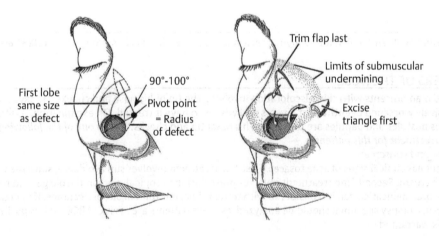

Fig. 41.5 Bilobed flap. (From Jackson IT. Local Flaps in Head and Neck Reconstruction. St Louis: Quality Medical Publishing, 2007.)

ipsilateral angular artery because the flap should be laterally based for tip reconstruction and medially based for alar reconstruction. It is usual to make the first flap equal in width to the defect and the second flap slightly narrower to facilitate direct closure.

REFERENCE

1. Zitelli JA. The bilobed flap for nasal reconstruction. Arch Dermatol 1989;125(7):957–959

RAISING A PARAMEDIAN FOREHEAD FLAP

14. When elevating a paramedian forehead flap for nasal reconstruction, in which plane should flap elevation occur?

    E. **In a number of different planes**

        The forehead flap is the gold standard flap for major nasal reconstruction cases. It is commonly elevated as a vertically oriented paramedian flap based on the supratrochlear vessels. It is customary to use the contralateral side for the flap as this helps to reach without twisting of the pedicle. This flap is usually raised in either two or three different planes according to surgeon's preference. The most cranial part of the flap (which becomes the most distal part of the flap after transposition) is usually raised either subcutaneously or submuscularly/subgaleally. Some surgeons start subcutaneously then change plane to the subgaleal plane one-third the way down the forehead. Others raise the first twothirds of the flap all submuscularly/subgaleally in a single plane. For the final part of the dissection, it is necessary to change plane and dissect deep to pericranium in order to preserve the blood supply and facilitate reach (see **Fig. 41.3**).[1,2]

REFERENCES

1. Correa BJ, Weathers WM, Wolfswinkel EM, Thornton JF. The forehead flap: the gold standard of nasal soft tissue reconstruction. Semin Plast Surg 2013;27(2):96–103
2. Menick FJ. A 10-year experience in nasal reconstruction with the three-stage forehead flap. Plast Reconstr Surg 2002;109(6):1839–1855, discussion 1856–1861

RHINOPHYMA

15. A patient is examined in clinic with a diagnosis of rhinophyma. *Which one of the following statements is correct?*

D. Surgical treatment is the mainstay treatment for stage IV disease.

Rhinophyma is a condition involving sebaceous hyperplasia of nasal skin with bulbous enlargement. It is typically seen in white men in their seventh decade. The male to female ratio is 12:1. Previously thought to be influenced by alcohol intake, this is no longer believed to be true.[1] Patients are at increased risk of developing basal cell carcinomas in the affected area only. Severe cases (such as stage IV disease) are treated surgically with blade excision, dermabrasion, dermaplaning, or CO_2 laser ablation. Outcomes appear to be similar for these various methods. Useful nonsurgical treatments for milder disease include tetracycline, isotretinoin, and metronidazole.

REFERENCE

1. Rohrich RJ, Griffin JR, Adams WP Jr. Rhinophyma: review and update. Plast Reconstr Surg 2002;110(3):860–869, quiz 870

SKIN DISORDERS OF THE NOSE

16. A 63-year-old man presents with skin discoloration involving the tip of his nose and cheeks. He says that it has progressively worsened over the past 5 years and wishes to have it treated. On examination, multiple erythematous pustules and papules are present on his nasal tip and cheeks. *Which one of the following is part of the first-line treatment for this patient?*

E. Zinc oxide and sunscreen

This patient has clinical signs of acne rosacea. First-line treatment involves sun avoidance, sunscreen, and topical zinc oxide cream. Second-line treatment involves prescription of topical metronidazole gel and retinoic acid. After this, oral medication can be considered with tetracycline, metronidazole, or Accutane. If malignant change is a concern, a biopsy specimen should be analyzed, as these patients are at risk of BCCs. If it is positive, surgical excision is warranted.[1–3]

REFERENCES

1. Rohrich RJ, Griffin JR, Adams WP Jr. Rhinophyma: review and update. Plast Reconstr Surg 2002;110(3):860–869, quiz 870
2. van Zuuren EJ, Fedorowicz Z, Carter B, van der Linden MM, Charland L. Interventions for rosacea. Cochrane Database Syst Rev 2015;2015(4):CD003262
3. Del Rosso JQ, Tanghetti E, Webster G, Stein Gold L, Thiboutot D, Gallo RL. Update on the management of rosacea from the American Acne & Rosacea Society (AARS). J Clin Aesthet Dermatol 2019;12(6):17–24

42. Cheek Reconstruction

See *Essentials of Plastic Surgery*, third edition, pp. 568–576

ANATOMY OF THE CHEEK

1. **Which one of the following is true regarding the anatomy of the cheek?**
   A. There are two main superficial fat compartments, the nasolabial and inferior orbital.
   B. The subcutaneous musculoaponeurotic system (SMAS) invests the facial mimetic muscles.
   C. The SMAS is continuous with the deep temporal fascia, galea, and platysma.
   D. Blood supply to the cheek is supplied almost entirely by the facial artery and facial vein.
   E. Sensory innervation to the cheek is provided solely by the maxillary and mandibular divisions of the trigeminal nerve.

SENSORY INNERVATION TO THE CHEEK

2. **Which one of the following nerves supplying the cheek arises from the maxillary division of the trigeminal nerve?**
   A. Buccal nerve
   B. Mental nerve
   C. Auriculotemporal nerve
   D. Great auricular nerve
   E. Zygomaticofacial nerve

AESTHETIC UNITS OF THE CHEEK

3. **Which one of the following is correct regarding the borders of the cheek?**
   A. A line between the tragus and midline chin represents the lower border.
   B. A line between the helical root, lateral canthus, and orbital rim represents the upper border.
   C. A line between the medial canthus, nasal tip, and midline chin represents the medial border.
   D. A line between the angle of mandible and the lateral canthus represents the posterior border.
   E. The superior and borders converge at the angle of the mandible.

RECONSTRUCTION OF THE CHEEK

4. **Which one of the following is most likely to produce the best cosmetic result when reconstructing a 2 by 2 cm, 6 mm deep defect of the central cheek?**
   A. Preauricular full-thickness skin graft
   B. Supraclavicular full-thickness skin graft
   C. Superiorly based rhomboid flap
   D. Cervicofacial flap
   E. Inferiorly based transposition flap

LOCAL FLAP RECONSTRUCTION OF THE CHEEK

5. You are planning a bilobed flap to reconstruct a central cheek skin defect. **What is the clinical significance of the Zitelli modification when designing this flap?**
   A. It increases the overall width ratios between the two flaps.
   B. It means that the flap can be completed in a single stage.
   C. It reduces the pivotal arc between each of the flaps.
   D. It changes the internal angles to those of a rhomboid flap.
   E. It means the flap will be superiorly based.

CERVICOFACIAL FLAP RECONSTRUCTION

6. **When reconstructing a suborbital cheek defect with a cervicofacial flap, which one of the following statements is correct?**
   A. The vertical incision is routinely placed in the preauricular sulcus.
   B. Flap elevation should remain in the subcutaneous plane throughout.
   C. The superior limit of the flap should be at level with the zygomatic arch.
   D. The flap should be anchored to the zygomatic arch and lateral orbital wall.
   E. Flap elevation should not continue beyond the lower border of the mandible.

TISSUE EXPANSION FOR CHEEK RECONSTRUCTION

7. You see a patient with a large nevus on the cheek which you are planning to excise and reconstruct using tissue expansion techniques. *Which one of the following is correct in this case?*
   A. The expander base area should be 2.5–3.5 times the defect area.
   B. The expander should ideally be placed deep to SMAS.
   C. Formal expansion should commence 4 weeks following initial surgery.
   D. Overexpansion is not usually required in this region of the face.
   E. Capsulectomy should be undertaken during the second stage.

LOCAL FLAPS FOR INTRAORAL RECONSTRUCTION

8. You are planning to reconstruct an intraoral defect of the cheek using a local flap following resection of a tumor. *Which one of the following flaps is supplied by a branch of the external carotid other than the facial artery?*
   A. Buccal fat pad flap
   B. Facial artery myomucosal (FAMM) flap
   C. Hemi-tongue flap
   D. Inferiorly based nasolabial flap
   E. Submental flap

RECONSTRUCTION OF LARGE INTRAORAL CHEEK DEFECTS

9. A 37-year-old woman presents with poor mouth opening (less than 2 cm intermaxillary distance) and a 3 by 4 cm ulcerated lesion involving the buccal mucosa. She regularly chews betel nut, is a nonsmoker, and is otherwise fit and well with a body mass index (BMI) of 23. Further investigations reveal a T4 squamous cell carcinoma involving the buccal mucosa and mandibular alveolus. Skin is not involved. Surgical excision of the tumor is planned with a mandibular rim resection and selective neck dissection. *Which one of the following is the most acceptable reconstructive approach for this patient, with the lowest donor site morbidity?*
   A. Pectoralis major pedicled flap
   B. Combined tongue and buccal pad flaps
   C. Free radial forearm flap
   D. Free fibular osseocutaneous flap
   E. Free anterolateral thigh (ALT) flap

SALVAGE FLAPS USED IN CHEEK RECONSTRUCTION

10. An elderly man has undergone a total parotidectomy and neck dissection for an aggressive, recurrent squamous cell carcinoma after radiotherapy. The overlying skin is involved. An 8 by 8 cm defect in the lower cheek and neck requires reconstruction. *Which one of the following potentially available flaps for reconstruction of this defect receives its major blood supply from the thoracoacromial vessels?*
    A. Deltopectoral
    B. Pectoralis major
    C. Sternocleidomastoid
    D. Trapezius
    E. Latissimus dorsi

RECONSTRUCTION OF THE CHEEK WITH FREE TISSUE TRANSFER

11. *When discussing complex reconstruction of the cheek with patients in clinic, which one of the following should they be advised of?*
    A. It is usual to need revision surgery 2 months after the initial procedure.
    B. That they should expect some form of subsequent revision surgery will be needed.
    C. That if revision is required, it would most likely involve liposuction techniques.
    D. That most patients require autologous fat grafting or hyaluronic acid fillers after the initial surgery.
    E. Revision is usually only required in cases where bony reconstruction has been performed.

Answers

ANATOMY OF THE CHEEK

1. Which one of the following is true regarding the anatomy of the cheek?

B. **The subcutaneous musculoaponeurotic system (SMAS) invests the facial muscles.**

The subcutaneous musculoaponeurotic system (SMAS) underlies the subcutaneous tissue and skin of the cheek to invest the facial muscles and is continuous superiorly with the superficial temporal fascia (not the deep) and inferiorly with the platysma. Motor nerves to the facial mimetic muscles run deep to the SMAS while sensory ones run superficial to it. The face has multiple superficial fat compartments that include the inferior orbital, nasolabial, medial, and lateral temporal zones. The cheek receives its blood supply from multiple vessels arising from branches of the external carotid artery. These include the facial artery, transverse facial artery (from superficial temporal artery), and infraorbital artery of the maxillary artery. Sensory innervation to the cheek is not only from the maxillary and mandibular divisions of the trigeminal nerve, but also from the cervical plexus.[1,2]

REFERENCES

1. Rohrich RJ, Pessa JE. The fat compartments of the face: anatomy and clinical implications for cosmetic surgery. Plast Reconstr Surg 2007;119(7):2219–2227
2. Mehara B. Cheek reconstruction. In: Grabb and Smith's Plastic Surgery. 6th ed. Philadelphia: Lippincott Williams & Wilkins; 2007

SENSORY INNERVATION TO THE CHEEK

2. Which one of the following nerves supplying the cheek arises from the maxillary division of the trigeminal nerve?

E. **Zygomaticofacial nerve**

The sensory innervation to the cheek arises from the second and third divisions of the trigeminal nerve and the cervical plexus. The only nerve listed above from the second (maxillary) division of the trigeminal nerve is the zygomaticofacial nerve which is the terminal branch of the zygomatic nerve. It passes along the inferolateral part of the bony orbit and exits the orbit at the zygomaticofacial foramen in the zygoma, then perforates the orbicularis oculi muscle to reach the malar skin which it innervates. The inferior orbital nerve is the other key branch of the maxillary division that innervates the skin of the cheek, nose, and upper lip. The buccal, mental, and auriculotemporal nerves are all branches of the mandibular division of the trigeminal nerve. The buccal nerve supplies the buccal mucosa, skin, and the second and third upper molars; the mental nerve supplies the lower cheek and chin, while the auriculotemporal nerve supplies the temple and upper part of the ear. The great auricular nerve is a branch of the cervical plexus C2/3 and supplies the preauricular region and the lower parts of the ear (**Fig. 42.1**).[1–3]

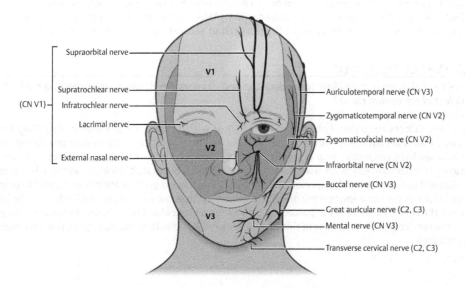

Fig. 42.1   Sensory nerve distribution to the face.

REFERENCES

1. Anderson JE, ed. Grant's Atlas of Anatomy. 8th ed. Baltimore: Williams & Wilkins; 2011
2. Last RJ, ed. Anatomy, Regional and Applied. 12th ed. London: Churchill Livingstone; 1979
3. Mehara B. Cheek reconstruction. In: Grabb and Smith's Plastic Surgery. 6th ed. Philadelphia: Lippincott Williams & Wilkins; 2007

AESTHETIC UNITS OF THE CHEEK

3. *Which one of the following is correct regarding the borders of the cheek?*

    B. A line between the helical root, lateral canthus, and orbital rim represents the upper border.

The cheek is the largest aesthetic unit of the face and has four borders, namely, upper, lower, medial, and lateral. The upper border is delineated by a line from the helical root to the lateral canthus which continues as the inferior orbital rim as far as the medial canthus. This border is also delineated by the zygomatic arch and inferior orbital rim. The lower border is delineated by the lower border of the mandible and passes from the mandibular angle to the chin. The posterior border is the junction between the pinna and the cheek, that is, the preauricular crease, passing from the zygomatic arch to the mandibular angle. The anterior or medial border is delineated by the nasojugal and nasolabial folds passing into the labiomandibular crease.

    The inferior and posterior borders therefore converge at the angle of the mandible.

    The cheek can be further subdivided into three or four overlapping subunits. These are the preauricular, infraorbital, and buccomandibular (**Fig. 42.2**).

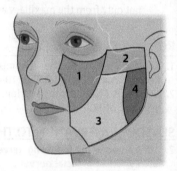

Fig. 42.2 Subunits of the cheek. (1. medial or infraorbital unit; 2. zygomatic unit; 3. buccomandibular unit; 4. lateral or preauricular unit)

    This has clinical relevance when reconstructing cheek defects. The main considerations are that the preauricular region overlies the parotid and facial nerve, the infraorbital region represents the junction between the lower eyelid and cheek, and the buccomandibular region includes the external mobile skin of the cheek and the internal lining of the oral cavity. From a reconstructive perspective, defects of the buccomandibular region may be full thickness and require more complex three-dimensional reconstructions with flaps or grafts for both internal and external lining. In contrast, the other areas are most often partial-thickness defects that can be managed with single layer flaps or grafts for external resurfacing.[1-5]

REFERENCES

1. Mehara B. Cheek reconstruction. In: Grabb and Smith's Plastic Surgery. 6th ed. Philadelphia: Lippincott Williams & Wilkins; 2007
2. Zide BM. Deformities of the lips and cheeks. In: McCarthy JR, ed. Plastic Surgery. Philadelphia: WB Saunders; 1990
3. Baker S. Local Flaps in Facial Reconstruction. 2nd ed. St Louis: Mosby-Elsevier Health Sciences; 2007
4. Pepper JP, Baker SR. Local flaps: cheek and lip reconstruction. JAMA Facial Plast Surg 2013;15(5):374–382
5. Başağaoğlu B, Bhadkamkar M, Hollier P, Reece E. Approach to reconstruction of cheek defects. Semin Plast Surg 2018;32(2):84–89

RECONSTRUCTION OF THE CHEEK

4. *Which one of the following is most likely to produce the best cosmetic result when reconstructing a 2 by 2 cm, 6 mm deep defect of the central cheek?*

    E. Inferiorly based transposition flap

Smaller cheek defects are generally best closed directly or with local flaps, particularly when they are deep, as in this case. This is because they provide superior color and texture match with avoidance of a contour defect. Inferiorly based flaps can reduce trap-door effect and postoperative edema because they facilitate flap drainage with gravity.[1,2] When skin grafts are used, full thickness is preferable to split thickness as there is less secondary contraction and the color match is superior. The optimal full-thickness graft location is probably the contralateral preauricular site as the color and texture match are good and the donor site may be well hidden at the junction of the ear and the cheek. Other sites are postauricular and supraclavicular. The location of this defect is not ideally suited to the cervicofacial flap and use of this flap is excessive for defects of this size, given the more conservative options available.

REFERENCES

1. Jackson IT. Local Flaps in Head and Neck Reconstruction. 2nd ed. St Louis: Quality Medical Publishing; 2007
2. Baker S. Local Flaps in Facial Reconstruction. 2nd ed. St Louis: Mosby-Elsevier Health Sciences; 2007

LOCAL FLAP RECONSTRUCTION OF THE CHEEK

5. *You are planning a bilobed flap to reconstruct a central cheek skin defect. What is the clinical significance of the Zitelli modification when designing this flap?*

    C. It reduces the pivotal arc between each of the flaps.

    The bilobed flap is a form of transposition flap that uses two flaps which share a common base area where the first advancing flap insets into the original defect and the second flap, which is smaller than the first, insets into the defect created by the movement of the first flap. In this way, the original defect is shared between the two donor areas (**Fig. 42.3**).

    The bilobed flap was traditionally described with internal angles of 90 degrees between the defect and each flap. However, the Zitelli modification reduces the entire internal angle to 90 degrees and the internal angle between each component to 45 degrees, which in most cases is more realistic given the characteristics of skin suppleness and the advancement required. The modification makes no change to the overall width ratios of the flaps and both descriptions are single-stage procedures anyway.[1] Other authors have made changes to the length of the leading limb to help avoid tissue distortion.[2] The internal angles of a rhomboid flap are 60 and 120 degrees, so are different to either description of the bilobed flap. Bilobed flaps can be superiorly or inferiorly based; however, inferiorly based flaps are generally preferred in the cheek as they facilitate lymphatic and venous flap drainage and minimize pin cushioning.[3]

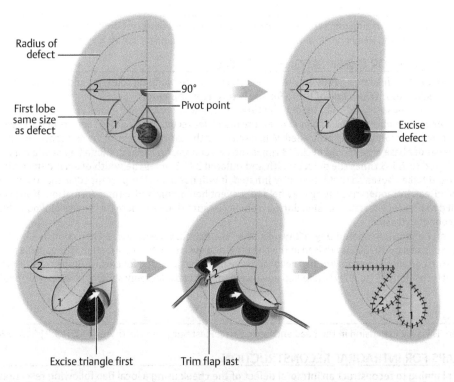

Fig. 42.3 The bilobed flap used for single-stage reconstruction with a total internal angle of 90 degrees between the defect and second flap. Note the defect should be triangulated to reduce standing cone or dog-ear, but care should be taken to avoid compromise to the flap base vascularity by doing so.

REFERENCES

1. Zitelli JA. The bilobed flap for nasal reconstruction. Arch Dermatol 1989;125(7):957–959
2. Cho M, Kim DW. Modification of the Zitelli bilobed flap: a comparison of flap dynamics in human cadavers. Arch Facial Plast Surg 2006;8(6):404–409, discussion 410
3. Jackson IT. Local Flaps in Head and Neck Reconstruction. 2nd ed. St Louis: Quality Medical Publishing; 2007

CERVICOFACIAL FLAP RECONSTRUCTION

6. *When reconstructing a suborbital cheek defect with a cervicofacial flap, which one of the following statements is correct?*
   D. The flap should be anchored to the zygomatic arch and lateral orbital wall.
   When insetting a cervicofacial flap, placement of anchor sutures to the periosteum of the lateral orbital wall and zygomatic arch is very important to minimize subsequent development of ectropion. This approach may also be combined with a lateral canthopexy if inadequate lower eyelid support remains a concern.

   A preauricular incision, as used in a face lift, can be ideal in some patients. However, in males the sideburn will be moved medially if this incision is performed. Therefore, it is preferable to place an incision along the medial aspect of the sideburn only passing to the preauricular sulcus beneath the tip of the sideburn. Furthermore, cervicofacial flaps can be either anteriorly or posteriorly based. The incisions will differ between the two. The incision for an anteriorly based flap starts at the superolateral aspect of the defect and is carried laterally across the lower eyelid and zygomatic arch then continued into the preauricular crease. In contrast, a posteriorly based flap starts at the medial aspect of the defect and continues along the nose–cheek junction, the nasolabial fold, and labiomental crease. The anteriorly based cervicofacial flap must be designed to extend above the zygomatic arch to ensure sufficient reach, as it has to both rotate and advance. The flap must be extensively undermined (often as far as the clavicle, when reconstructing large defects) to maximize reach and minimize tension during closure. The level of dissection should initially be in the subcutaneous plane, but should be subplatysmal in the neck to ensure adequate vascular supply to the flap. The marginal mandibular nerve must be carefully preserved during the dissection.[1,2]

REFERENCES

1. Mureau MA, Hofer SO. Maximizing results in reconstruction of cheek defects. Clin Plast Surg 2009;36(3):461–476
2. Jackson IT. Local Flaps in Head and Neck Reconstruction. 2nd ed. St Louis: Quality Medical Publishing; 2007

TISSUE EXPANSION FOR CHEEK RECONSTRUCTION

7. You see a patient with a large nevus on the cheek which you are planning to excise and reconstruct using tissue expansion techniques. *Which one of the following is correct in this case?*
   A. The expander base area should be 2.5–3.5 times the defect area.
   Tissue expansion offers the best color and texture match for reconstructing large defects of the cheek and multiple custom-made expanders may be needed. When selecting the expander device, the defect area must be considered. The expander base area should be 2.5–3 times the defect area. An expander for a flap over a curved area should be inflated to 2.5–3 times the defect width and inflated 2–3.5 times the width of a flat defect. Size and volume also need to be chosen so that when fully inflated, it will not distort important adjacent structures such as the eyelid or ear. Intraoperative filling may help to prevent hematoma and seroma formation. However, a balance is needed to prevent excessive tension during primary closure that will increase the risk of wound breakdown and subsequent extrusion.

   Formal expansion should begin 2 weeks after the primary surgery and then continue on a weekly basis. Overexpansion by 30–50% is advised in the cheek area to overcome flap contraction. The capsule is a very vascular structure and should remain within the local tissue flaps that are used for closure. If the capsule is tight, it can be scored (capsulotomy) to allow more flap advancement but capsulectomy should not be performed.[1]

REFERENCE

1. Hoffmann JF. Tissue expansion in the head and neck. Facial Plast Surg Clin North Am 2005;13(2):315–324, vii

LOCAL FLAPS FOR INTRAORAL RECONSTRUCTION

8. You are planning to reconstruct an intraoral defect of the cheek using a local flap following resection of a tumor. *Which one of the following flaps is supplied by a branch of the external carotid other than the facial artery?*
   C. Hemi-tongue flap
   Intraoral defects involving the cheek can be reconstructed using a number of different local flaps. Many of these receive blood supply from the facial artery. The hemi-tongue flap, however, is based on the lingual artery. It has many varied uses including resurfacing the buccal lining, and reconstructing the palate, the lips, and the floor of mouth.[1] Flaps based on the facial artery include the facial artery myomucosal flap (FAMM), the submental artery flap (from branches passing through the submandibular gland), and the random pattern nasolabial flap (predominantly from the angular branch of the facial artery).[2–4] The buccal fat pad is based on a subcapsular plexus formed by both the facial artery and the internal maxillary artery and has good reported outcomes in reconstructing smaller

intraoral defects.[5] The nasolabial region also receives blood supply from the infraorbital artery which is derived from the maxillary artery; however, this only supplies the superiorly based flap.

REFERENCES

1. Komisar A. The applications of tongue flaps in head and neck surgery. Bull N Y Acad Med 1986;62(8):847–853
2. Pribaz J, Stephens W, Crespo L, Gifford G. A new intraoral flap: facial artery musculomucosal (FAMM) flap. Plast Reconstr Surg 1992;90(3):421–429
3. Zhao Z, Li S, Yan Y, et al. New buccinator myomucosal island flap: anatomic study and clinical application. Plast Reconstr Surg 1999;104(1):55–64
4. Amin AA, Sakkary MA, Khalil AA, Rifaat MA, Zayed SB. The submental flap for oral cavity reconstruction: extended indications and technical refinements. Head Neck Oncol 2011, December 20;3:51
5. Chakrabarti J, Tekriwal R, Ganguli A, Ghosh S, Mishra PK. Pedicled buccal fat pad flap for intraoral malignant defects: a series of 29 cases. Indian J Plast Surg 2009;42(1):36–42

RECONSTRUCTION OF LARGE INTRAORAL CHEEK DEFECTS

9. A 37-year-old woman presents with poor mouth opening (less than 2 cm intermaxillary distance) and a 3 by 4 cm ulcerated lesion involving the buccal mucosa. She regularly chews betel nut, is a nonsmoker, and is otherwise fit and well with a BMI of 23. Further investigations reveal a T4 squamous cell carcinoma involving the buccal mucosa and mandibular alveolus. Skin is not involved. Surgical excision of the tumor is planned with a mandibular rim resection and selective neck dissection. *Which one of the following is the most acceptable reconstructive approach for this patient, with the lowest donor site morbidity?*

E. Free anterolateral thigh (ALT) flap

The defect created in this reconstruction is likely to be 5 by 6 cm in diameter and will require importation of distant soft tissue. Bone will not be required unless a segmental mandibular resection is planned. The pectoralis major can be tunneled under the neck dissection flaps and used for intraoral reconstruction, but reach will be difficult and the donor site is poor for young female patients. It tends to be used as a salvage flap in elderly patients, where free tissue transfer is contraindicated. Local flaps such as the tongue, FAMM, and buccal fat pads can be useful for smaller intraoral defects, and in this case may be sacrificed during tumor resection. Either free radial forearm or free anterolateral thigh (ALT) flaps can be used in this case. An ALT flap is favorable because of its hidden scarring. One problem with ALT flaps for intraoral reconstruction is that they can be bulky, causing functional difficulties with speech and eating. In a patient with a low BMI, this should not be a major problem. Other reconstructive options for this patient include the scapula, parascapular, lateral arm, or groin flaps.[1-4]

REFERENCES

1. Haddock NT, Saadeh PB, Siebert JW. Achieving aesthetic results in facial reconstructive microsurgery: planning and executing secondary refinements. Plast Reconstr Surg 2012;130(6):1236–1245
2. Wei FC, Jain V, Celik N, Chen HC, Chuang DC, Lin CH. Have we found an ideal soft-tissue flap? An experience with 672 anterolateral thigh flaps. Plast Reconstr Surg 2002;109(7):2219–2226, discussion 2227–2230
3. Klinkenberg M, Fischer S, Kremer T, Hernekamp F, Lehnhardt M, Daigeler A. Comparison of anterolateral thigh, lateral arm, and parascapular free flaps with regard to donor-site morbidity and aesthetic and functional outcomes. Plast Reconstr Surg 2013;131(2):293–302
4. Hsiao HT, Leu YS, Liu CJ, Tung KY, Lin CC. Radial forearm versus anterolateral thigh flap reconstruction after hemiglossectomy: functional assessment of swallowing and speech. J Reconstr Microsurg 2008;24(2):85–88

SALVAGE FLAPS USED IN CHEEK RECONSTRUCTION

10. An elderly man has undergone a total parotidectomy and neck dissection for an aggressive, recurrent squamous cell carcinoma after radiotherapy. The overlying skin is involved. An 8 by 8 cm defect in the lower cheek and neck requires reconstruction. *Which one of the following potentially available flaps for reconstruction of this defect receives its major blood supply from the thoracoacromial vessels?*

B. Pectoralis major

The blood supply to the flaps listed is as follows:

- Pectoralis major: Internal mammary perforators, thoracoacromial vessels, and lateral thoracic vessels
- Deltopectoral: Internal mammary perforators
- Trapezius: Transverse cervical, dorsal scapular, and posterior intercostal vessels
- Sternocleidomastoid:
    - Upper: Occipital artery
    - Middle: Superior thyroid or external carotid artery

- – Lower: Suprascapular artery from the transverse cervical artery
- • Latissimus dorsi: Thoracodorsal and posterior intercostal perforators

This defect can be reconstructed with a deltopectoral, pectoralis major, trapezius, or latissimus dorsi flap.[1] The sternocleidomastoid is unsuitable for this reconstruction because of its segmental blood supply and small size.[2,3] The pectoralis major muscle provides a reliable flap for reconstruction of the head and neck region. It can be muscle only or muscle and skin. The donor site can usually be closed directly by undermining adjacent tissue and rotating/advancing this into the donor defect. It will however distort the breast, particularly in women. The pedicle can be identified as it passes between the sternal and clavicular heads of the muscle, just below the clavicle. It is possible to dissect close to the vessel in this area in order to minimize bulk at the pivot point. The flap is then passed under a subcutaneous tunnel into the neck. The deltopectoral flap is usually reserved as a lifeboat flap and can be elevated and replaced during a pectoralis major flap harvest. The trapezius flap is particularly useful for posterior defects over the upper cervical spine as it has a reliable blood supply and easily reaches to provide muscle cover over the spinous processes. The donor site can usually be closed directly. A fasciocutaneous flap based on the transverse cervical vessels can be useful for head and neck reconstruction in both intraoral and skin defects. This is termed a supraclavicular artery perforator (a-SAP) flap.[4] The latissimus dorsi is not commonly used for head and neck reconstruction, although it may be incorporated into a free scapula flap when bone and soft tissue reconstruction is required (**Fig. 42.4**).

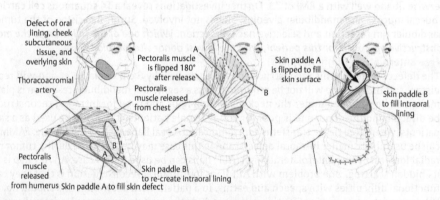

Fig. 42.4   Pectoralis major flap with two skin paddles: one for the intraoral defect and one for the cutaneous defect. (Although this was a common flap in years past, it is now mostly used as a salvage option.)

REFERENCES

1. Yang D, Morris SF. Trapezius muscle: anatomic basis for flap design. Ann Plast Surg 1998;41(1):52–57
2. Kierner AC, Aigner M, Zelenka I, Riedl G, Burian M. The blood supply of the sternocleidomastoid muscle and its clinical implications. Arch Surg 1999;134(2):144–147
3. Freeman JL, Walker EP, Wilson JS, Shaw HJ. The vascular anatomy of the pectoralis major myocutaneous flap. Br J Plast Surg 1981;34(1):3–10
4. Pallua N, Wolter TP. Moving forwards: the anterior supraclavicular artery perforator (a-SAP) flap: a new pedicled or free perforator flap based on the anterior supraclavicular vessels. J Plast Reconstr Aesthet Surg 2013;66(4):489–496

RECONSTRUCTION OF THE CHEEK WITH FREE TISSUE TRANSFER

11. When discussing complex reconstruction of the cheek with patients in clinic, which one of the following should they be advised of?

B. That they should expect some form of subsequent revision surgery will be needed.

A standard of care in free tissue transfer reconstruction is to preempt the need for revision procedures. Therefore, it is important to discuss this early with patients during consultations prior to undergoing the first part of the reconstructive process. In cases where there is already much other information to absorb, there remains a high chance that patients will not retain all of the information and so additional written information leaflets can be useful. The need for potential revision applies not only to facial reconstruction, but more broadly in many anatomic areas. The key is to ensure that patients are well informed and have realistic expectations at each stage of their care pathway.

The precise nature of and timing for revision will depend on each patient's individualized case. However, the principle is generally that revision is left for at least 6 months to allow the soft tissues to soften and mature. In addition, beyond this time point, most soft tissue flaps will have generated additional useful blood supply from the surrounding tissues and will no longer be purely reliant upon the vascular pedicle for their blood supply. This means that revisions can be more reliably and robustly undertaken. Common revisions include re-insetting and revising the skin elements of a flap, thinning bulky flaps such as the anterolateral thigh (ALT) with liposuction, and releasing scar tethering or adjusting tissue advancements particularly around the eye, nose, or mouth. Bony revision is less commonly needed as bone reconstruction in the cheek is less often needed anyway and bone inset is usually quite reliable and adequately placed in the first procedure. Contour defects can be managed with either permanent or nonpermanent fillers but are certainly not required in most cases.[1]

REFERENCE

1. Haddock NT, Saadeh PB, Siebert JW. Achieving aesthetic results in facial reconstructive microsurgery: planning and executing secondary refinements. Plast Reconstr Surg 2012;130(6):1236–1245

43. Ear Reconstruction

See *Essentials of Plastic Surgery*, third edition, pp. 577–589

ANATOMY OF THE EXTERNAL EAR

1. *What is the dominant arterial blood supply to the ear?*
   - A. Superficial temporal artery
   - B. Deep temporal artery
   - C. Posterior auricular artery
   - D. Occipital artery
   - E. Great auricular artery

SENSORY INNERVATION TO THE EXTERNAL EAR

2. *Which one of the following statements is correct regarding sensation to the external ear?*
   - A. The entire ear can be anesthetized with a circumferential ring block.
   - B. Sensation to the lobule is provided by the lesser occipital nerve.
   - C. The auriculotemporal nerve is the main nerve implicated in referred otalgia.
   - D. Arnold's nerve is formed by cranial nerves IX through XII.
   - E. The cervical plexus and trigeminal nerve supply the vast majority of the ear.

LYMPHATIC DRAINAGE OF THE EAR

3. *Which one of the following tumor sites is most likely to have lymphatic drainage to the parotid nodes?*
   - A. The antihelix
   - B. The antitragus
   - C. The lobule
   - D. The superior helix
   - E. The scapha

AESTHETIC RELATIONSHIPS OF THE EAR

4. *Which one of the following statements is correct regarding the normal position and size of the external ear?*
   - A. The ear is normally located one ear width posterior to the lateral orbital rim.
   - B. Ear height varies between 5.5 and 6.5 cm in adults.
   - C. Ear width is usually less than one-third the height.
   - D. Maximum projection from the mastoid to the helix occurs superiorly.
   - E. The long axis tilt is consistently within 1–2 degrees in all individuals.

ACUTE INJURIES TO THE EAR

5. *Which one of the following statements is correct regarding soft tissue injuries involving the ear?*
   - A. Dog bites in children frequently become infected secondary to viridans-group streptococci.
   - B. Hematomas are the most common complication after blunt trauma and should be evacuated early to prevent cauliflower ear.
   - C. Direct repair of the cartilage must be performed after debridement of a full-thickness ear laceration.
   - D. Frostbite involving the ear should be managed with gentle rewarming using warm water.
   - E. Thermal burns to the ear usually warrant aggressive debridement in the early phases to prevent burn progression and cartilage desiccation.

TUMORS OF THE EAR

6. *What is the most common site of a keloid tumor?*
   - A. The helix
   - B. The concha
   - C. The scapha
   - D. The lobule
   - E. The tragus

KELOID SCARRING TO THE EAR

7. *Which one of the following statements regarding keloid scarring is correct?*
   - A. Keloids involving the ear are five times more common in dark-skinned patients.
   - B. Recurrence after simple excision occurs in a third of cases.
   - C. Outcomes are unpredictable after combined steroid injection and excision.
   - D. The benefit of silicone therapy after excision is minimal.
   - E. Radiation is a reliable first-line treatment for keloids.

CHONDRODERMATITIS NODULARIS HELICIS (CDNH)

8. *Which one of the following is true of chondrodermatitis nodularis helicis (CDNH)?*
   A. It is a malignant condition of the ear.
   B. Patients are unlikely to notice the condition themselves.
   C. Recurrence after excision is unlikely.
   D. Males and females are equally affected.
   E. It is usually caused by a pressure effect.

AMPUTATION OF THE EAR

9. A young nonsmoker has a guillotine amputation of the superior two-thirds of the external ear. *How should this best be managed?*
   A. Wound closure and plan for subsequent bone-anchored prosthetic ear
   B. Dermabrasion and banking of ear cartilage under temporoparietal fascia
   C. Total ear reconstruction with rib cartilage and temporoparietal flap cover
   D. Early attempt at replantation onto the superficial temporal artery
   E. Reattachment with sutures as a nonvascularized composite graft

REPLANTATION OF THE EXTERNAL EAR

10. A 30-year-old woman is involved in a motor vehicle accident during which her ear is amputated. She is taken immediately to the operating room for debridement and replantation. *Which one of the following is most likely to be part of the postoperative regimen specific to this procedure?*
   A. Cartilage banking   D. Leech therapy
   B. Dextran   E. Aspirin
   C. Sulfamylon

RECONSTRUCTING EXTERNAL EAR DEFORMITIES

11. A patient has a partial-thickness, 2 by 2 cm defect in the anterior surface of the conchal bowl after excision of a basal cell carcinoma and the underlying cartilage. *How might this defect best be managed?*
   A. Left to heal by secondary intent   D. Preauricular transposition flap
   B. Split-thickness skin graft   E. Contralateral composite cartilage graft
   C. Full-thickness skin graft

RECONSTRUCTING EXTERNAL EAR DEFORMITIES

12. An elderly man has a full-thickness, 1.8-cm high defect involving the midportion of the helical rim that was created during excision of a squamous cell carcinoma. *How might this defect be best managed in a single stage?*
   A. Converse's tunnel technique   D. Antia-Buch flap
   B. Chondrocutaneous composite flap   E. Valaise handle technique
   C. Dieffenbach's flap

MANAGEMENT OF SPLIT OR CLEFT EARLOBES

13 A young woman has a 1.5-cm-long, vertically split earlobe caused by wearing heavy earrings. She wishes to wear earrings again in the future. *How would this defect normally be managed?*
   A. Lobule reduction
   B. Wedge excision of earlobe
   C. Composite graft from contralateral lobe
   D. Full-thickness skin graft
   E. Postauricular skin flap

RECONSTRUCTING EXTERNAL EAR DEFORMITIES

14. A patient has a 2.5 cm by 1.7 cm full-thickness defect in the middle third of the ear. It involves the helix, scapha, and antihelix but not the conchal bowl. *Which one of the following represents the best option for management of this defect?*
   A. Converse tunnel technique   C. Dieffenbach's flap
   B. Orticochea flap   D. Flip-flop flap
   E. Tubed pedicle flap

Answers

ANATOMY OF THE EXTERNAL EAR

1. **What is the dominant arterial blood supply to the ear?**
   C. Posterior auricular artery

   The external ear is supplied by three main arterial vessels: the posterior auricular (dominant supply), superficial temporal, and occipital. All three of these are branches of the external carotid artery. The other branches are the lingual, facial, superior thyroid, maxillary, and ascending pharyngeal. The deep temporal artery is a branch of the maxillary artery. The great auricular artery does not exist (although there is a great auricular nerve). Good interconnections exist between the main source vessels. The ear can be replanted on either the superficial temporal or posterior auricular vessels (**Fig. 43.1**).[1-3]

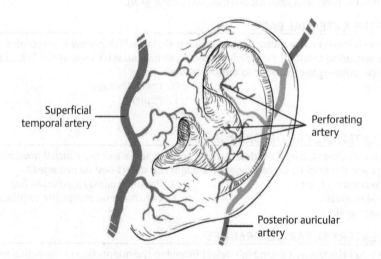

Superficial temporal artery

Perforating artery

Posterior auricular artery

Fig. 43.1   Vascular supply to the external ear.

REFERENCES

1. Allison GR. Anatomy of the external ear. Clin Plast Surg 1978;5(3):419–422
2. Park C, Lineaweaver WC, Rumly TO, Buncke HJ. Arterial supply of the anterior ear. Plast Reconstr Surg 1992;90(1):38–44
3. Brent B. Reconstruction of the auricle. In: McCarthy JG, ed. Plastic Surgery, Vol. 3. Philadelphia: WB Saunders; 1990

SENSORY INNERVATION TO THE EXTERNAL EAR

2. **Which one of the following statements is correct regarding sensation to the external ear?**
   E. The cervical plexus and trigeminal nerve supply the vast majority of the ear.

   The external ear receives sensory innervations from a number of nerves, but the main supply is from the cervical plexus (C2–C3) and the trigeminal nerve (CN V_3). Although most of the ear can be successfully anesthetized with a field block, the concha and external auditory meatus would remain spared by this approach. The auriculotemporal nerve (from CN V_3) supplies the superolateral surface of the ear and also contributes to the external auditory meatus. The lobule and lower part of the ear is supplied by the great auricular nerve (C2–C3). The lesser occipital nerve (C2–C3) supplies the superior cranial surface of the ear. Arnold's nerve receives contributions from the facial (CN VII), glossopharyngeal (CN IX), and vagus (CN X) nerves but not the eleventh or twelfth nerves. It supplies the external auditory canal and meatus as well as part of the conchal bowl. It is implicated in referred otalgia from other structures in the head and neck, and the initiation of coughing during manipulation of the ear canal.[1,2]

REFERENCES

1. Allison GR. Anatomy of the external ear. Clin Plast Surg 1978;5(3):419–422
2. Last RJ, ed. Anatomy, Regional and Applied. 12th ed. London: Churchill Livingstone; 1979

LYMPHATIC DRAINAGE OF THE EAR

3. *Which one of the following tumor sites is most likely to have lymphatic drainage to the parotid nodes?*

D. The superior helix

The lymphatic drainage of the ear corresponds to the embryologic origins. The tragus, helical root, and superior helix all originate from the first branchial arch and drain to the parotid nodes. The antihelix, antitragus, and lobule all arise from the second branchial arch and drain to the cervical nodes. When examining patients with squamous cell carcinoma or melanoma of the ear, it is vital that the parotid and neck nodes are thoroughly assessed, given the pathway of spread in metastatic disease. Often patients with metastatic disease originating from the ear will require both parotidectomy and neck dissection.[1-4]

REFERENCES

1. Allison GR. Anatomy of the external ear. Clin Plast Surg 1978;5(3):419–422
2. Last RJ, ed. Anatomy, Regional and Applied. 12th ed. London: Churchill Livingstone; 1979
3. Sadler TW, ed. Langman's Medical Embryology. 13th ed. Philadelphia: Wolters Kluwer Health; 2014
4. Pan WR, le Roux CM, Levy SM, Briggs CA. Lymphatic drainage of the external ear. Head Neck 2011;33(1):60–64

AESTHETIC RELATIONSHIPS OF THE EAR

4. *Which one of the following statements is correct regarding the normal position and size of the external ear?*

B. Ear height varies between 5.5 and 6.5 cm in adults.

The ear is located one ear height (not one width) posterior to the lateral orbital rim. The superior surface is usually at level with the eyebrow. Height varies between 5.5 and 6.5 cm in adults, and width is usually a little over half the height. Projection varies among individuals but is usually greatest inferiorly (approximately 2 cm) from the mastoid to the helix. The long axis tilts on average 20 degrees posteriorly, but this varies greatly.[1]

REFERENCE

1. Farkas LG. Anthropometry of normal and anomalous ears. Clin Plast Surg 1978;5(3):401–412

ACUTE INJURIES TO THE EAR

5. *Which one of the following statements is correct regarding soft tissue injuries involving the ear?*

B. Hematomas are the most common complication after blunt trauma and should be evacuated early to prevent cauliflower ear.

Cauliflower ear refers to a deformity that develops after a subperichondrial hematoma in the pinna. It results in devascularization of the cartilage with permanent fibrosis and scarring. Preventative management involves early evacuation of the hematoma and application of a pressure dressing.[1] Dog bites are commonly seen in children, but the pathogens involved in infection are most likely *Pasteurella multocida* or *P. canis*. Viridans-group streptococci are associated with human bites.[2,3] Ear lacerations should be carefully debrided and repaired with skin-only closure. Frostbite should be managed with rapid rewarming using saline-soaked dressings. To preserve maximal tissue, thermal burns are usually treated conservatively with dressings and later debrided once demarcation has occurred.

REFERENCES

1. Mudry A, Jackler RK. Tracing the origins of "cauliflower ear" and its earlier names over two millenia. Laryngoscope 2021;131(4):E1315–E1321
2. Talan DA, Citron DM, Abrahamian FM, Moran GJ, Goldstein EJ; Emergency Medicine Animal Bite Infection Study Group. Bacteriologic analysis of infected dog and cat bites. N Engl J Med 1999;340(2):85–92
3. Stefanopoulos PK. Management of facial bite wounds. Oral Maxillofac Surg Clin North Am 2009;21(2):247–257, vii

TUMORS OF THE EAR

6. *What is the most common site of a keloid tumor?*

D. The lobule

Keloids represent fibroproliferative disorders of the skin that grow beyond the boundaries of the original wound. They can occur spontaneously but commonly occur secondary to localized trauma. The most common anatomic site for development of a keloid is the lobule and this is frequently secondary to ear piercing. Other trauma or surgery to the ear such as otoplasty risks development of keloid scarring and this must be communicated to patients before proceeding with such techniques. Sites other than the head and neck that are affected include the anterior chest, lateral arm, and some flexor surfaces.[1,2]

REFERENCES

1. Ogawa R. The most current algorithms for the treatment and prevention of hypertrophic scars and keloids. Plast Reconstr Surg 2010;125(2):557–568
2. Ekstein SF, Wyles SP, Moran SL, Meves A. Keloids: a review of therapeutic management. Int J Dermatol 2021;60(6):661–671

KELOID SCARRING TO THE EAR

7. Which one of the following statements regarding keloid scarring is correct?

C. Outcomes are unpredictable after combined steroid injection and excision.

Ear piercing is the most common cause of keloids on the ear and may be associated with postpiercing infection or foreign body reaction. Keloids are 15 times (not 5 times) more frequent in dark-skinned individuals than in white individuals.[1] Keloids recur after simple excision in up to 100% of cases. Outcomes after combined excision and steroid therapy are still unpredictable and vary from 0 to 100% recurrence.[2] Continuous silicone therapy for 3 months after surgery can significantly decrease potential keloid formation. Radiation should be reserved for resistant lesions because of the side effects. Alternatively, it may be combined with surgical excision to provide a more reliable outcome.[1-3]

REFERENCES

1. Ogawa R. The most current algorithms for the treatment and prevention of hypertrophic scars and keloids. Plast Reconstr Surg 2010;125(2):557–568
2. Elsahy NI. Acquired ear defects. Clin Plast Surg 2002;29(2):175–186, v–vi
3. Ekstein SF, Wyles SP, Moran SL, Meves A. Keloids: a review of therapeutic management. Int J Dermatol 2021;60(6):661–671

CHONDRODERMATITIS NODULARIS HELICIS (CDNH)

8. Which one of the following is true of chondrodermatitis nodularis helicis (CDNH)?

E. It is usually caused by a pressure effect.

Chondrodermatitis nodularis helicis (CDNH) is a benign condition affecting the external ear resulting in a painful, chronic nodular, or ulcerative lesion. Patients notice these lesions because of the pain. This is in contrast to some asymptomatic ear lesions such as nodular basal cell carcinoma (BCC), where a patient's relatives often first notice the lesion. Males are four times more likely to develop CDNH, which is thought to be as a result of repeated external pressure being placed on the ear. When taking history, patients' sleeping position preference should be noted, as often they sleep lying on the affected side and this needs to be modified as part of the treatment plan. Lesions are treated surgically with a narrow margin excision. The key point is to remove the lesion while ensuring a smooth contour to the ear cartilage, such that no residual prominence remains. Recurrence rates vary between 10 and 30% according to series[1] and this can be affected by both surgical technique and subsequent pressure relief.[1,2]

REFERENCES

1. Wagner G, Liefeith J, Sachse MM. Clinical appearance, differential diagnoses and therapeutical options of chondrodermatitis nodularis chronica helicis Winkler. J Dtsch Dermatol Ges 2011;9(4):287–291
2. Shah S, Fiala KH. Chondrodermatitis nodularis helicis: a review of current therapies. Dermatol Ther (Heidelb) 2017;30(1)

AMPUTATION OF THE EAR

9. A young nonsmoker has a guillotine amputation of the superior two-thirds of the external ear. *How should this best be managed?*

D. Early attempt at replantation onto the superficial temporal artery

Successful replantation of the ear following an injury like this can provide a superior aesthetic result compared with secondary reconstruction. It requires arterial anastomosis with either the superficial temporal or posterior auricular artery. An additional venous anastomosis is preferable but not always technically possible, so venous drainage may be reliant on an external route into dressings or supplemented with other modalities.[1,2]

Prosthetic ears manufactured with a silicone elastomer can provide a very good aesthetic result for many patients and they are often, but not exclusively, bone-anchored devices. However, in this young patient with a clean-cut amputation, proceeding directly to prosthesis would not be indicated.[3,4] Cartilage banking can be a useful approach in cases where vascularized replantation is not feasible. The benefit of this approach is that the cartilage framework can be preserved and later inset under a vascularized skin or fascial flap such as the temporoparietal fascial flap.[5] The temporoparietal fascia should always be preserved for secondary ear reconstruction and not used for acute wound coverage. Autologous reconstruction of the ear may be considered in this patient if the replantation process failed. Ear reconstruction would not be performed in the acute setting though and is an elective, staged procedure. Reattachment of small composite grafts can be successful, but in a large area such as this case, the graft would fail.

REFERENCES

1. Lin PY, Chiang YC, Hsieh CH, Jeng SF. Microsurgical replantation and salvage procedures in traumatic ear amputation. J Trauma 2010;69(4):E15–E19
2. Momeni A, Liu X, Januszyk M, et al. Microsurgical ear replantation—is venous repair necessary?—A systematic review. Microsurgery 2016;36(4):345–350
3. Agarwal CA, Johns D, Tanner PB, Andtbacka RHI. Osseointegrated prosthetic ear reconstruction in cases of skin malignancy: technique, outcomes, and patient satisfaction. Ann Plast Surg 2018;80(1):32–39
4. Korus LJ, Wong JN, Wilkes GH. Long-term follow-up of osseointegrated auricular reconstruction. Plast Reconstr Surg 2011;127(2):630–636
5. Mladick RA, Horton CE, Adamson JE, Cohen BI. The pocket principle: a new technique for the reattachment of a severed ear part. Plast Reconstr Surg 1971;48(3):219–223

REPLANTATION OF THE EXTERNAL EAR

10. A 30-year-old woman is involved in a motor vehicle accident during which her ear is amputated. She is taken immediately to the operating room for debridement and replantation. *Which one of the following is most likely to be part of the postoperative regimen specific to this procedure?*

D. Leech therapy

During replantation of the ear, it may not be possible to achieve a satisfactory venous anastomosis. For this reason, leeches (*Hirudo medicinalis*) are commonly used as standard practice. They are typically used both in the presence or absence of a venous anastomosis. Sulfamylon (mafenide acetate) is used on ear burns as part of a conservative measure to minimize tissue loss and infection. Cartilage banking is performed in cases where replantation cannot be performed. Cartilage may be buried under a postauricular skin pocket or the forearm. The success of this approach is variable. Dextran and heparin are part of the treatment for frostbite to the ear. They are intended to limit thrombosis and tissue loss. Either may be used in ear replantation but are not a core part of treatment. Aspirin may help the arterial anastomosis but it is not evidence based.[1,2]

REFERENCES

1. Lin PY, Chiang YC, Hsieh CH, Jeng SF. Microsurgical replantation and salvage procedures in traumatic ear amputation. J Trauma 2010;69(4):E15–E19
2. Momeni A, Liu X, Januszyk M, et al. Microsurgical ear replantation—is venous repair necessary?—A systematic review. Microsurgery 2016;36(4):345–350

RECONSTRUCTING EXTERNAL EAR DEFORMITIES

11. A patient has a partial-thickness, 2 by 2 cm defect in the anterior surface of the conchal bowl after excision of a basal cell carcinoma and the underlying cartilage. *How might this defect best be managed?*

C. Full-thickness skin graft

Use of a full-thickness skin graft works well on the ear, particularly on the conchal bowl or scapha when the anterior or posterior skin remains intact and can accept a graft reliably. Providing the remainder of the ear construct is intact, there is no structural loss associated with conchal bowl defects (hence the suitability of this area for cartilage graft harvesting). Often the defect is difficult to see once the graft has healed well and matured for some months postoperatively. In contrast, if this defect was allowed to heal by secondary intent, there would be significant distortion and the aesthetic result would be poor. A split-thickness graft could be taken and provide a fair result; however, the contour and color would be worse than with the full-thickness graft and the donor site would need to be left to reepithelialize and such wounds can often be painful and more involved to manage than full-thickness donor sites. A preauricular transposition flap would work for this defect but would not add much to the aesthetics compared with a graft and actually would risk creating fullness at the flap base where the flap was transposed and inset. There is no rationale for using cartilage graft to reconstruct this defect as the structural and aesthetic outcomes are not affected by the absence of cartilage at this site. If a cartilage graft was to be used, a vascularized skin flap would also be required to cover it.[1,2]

REFERENCES

1. Brent B. Reconstruction of the auricle. In: McCarthy JG, ed. Plastic Surgery, Vol. 3. Philadelphia: WB Saunders; 1990
2. Elsahy NI. Reconstruction of the ear after skin and perichondrium loss. Clin Plast Surg 2002;29(2):187–200, vi

RECONSTRUCTING EXTERNAL EAR DEFORMITIES

12. An elderly man has a full-thickness, 1.8-cm high defect involving the midportion of the helical rim that was created during excision of a squamous cell carcinoma. *How might this defect be best managed in a single stage?*

    D. Antia-Buch flap

The Antia-Buch flap[1] is a very useful technique for reconstruction of helical rim defects up to approximately 2 cm in height (**Fig. 43.2**). An anterior incision is made in the helical sulcus through skin and cartilage and a posterior skin flap dissection is performed. This undermining allows advancement of the helix and lobule vertically toward the defect. The helical root is also released and advanced as a V-Y flap, although this part is not always required for smaller defects especially in elderly men with tall ears and long lobules. A variation of this is the swing flap which is based on the superior part of the Antia-Buch flap that can be used for larger defects of the helical rim. It involves raising a helical root and superior rim flap on a mesentery without the posterior skin (which is elevated thinly).

If the defect was greater than 2 cm tall then Converse's tunnel technique may be useful. This involves burying a piece of contralateral auricular cartilage under the postauricular skin and dividing and insetting the flap after 3 weeks.[2]

The chondrocutaneous composite flap is indicated for reconstructing superior third, full-thickness ear defects rather than the helical rim alone. It involves raising an anteriorly based flap on the root of the ear passing into the conchal bowl. This is transposed to the top of the ear and the donor site grafted as posterior skin is left in situ.

Dieffenbach's flap is used for combined middle third defects of the scapha and helical rim. It involves raising a postauricular skin flap placed over a contralateral auricular cartilage graft. This flap is also divided at 3 weeks.[2]

The *valise handle technique* is a staged reconstruction used for superior third defects of the ear rather than the helical rim alone. In the first stage, contralateral ear cartilage is implanted subcutaneously close to the defect. After 3 weeks the inferior helix is transposed to the cartilage graft. After a further 3 weeks, a bipedicled composite flap is elevated as a valise handle and skin graft is applied to the posterior sulcus to increase ear projection.

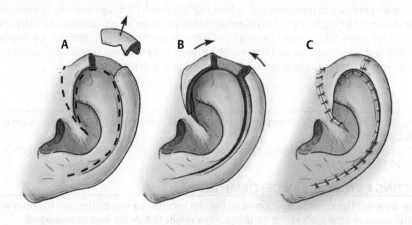

Fig. 43.2 The Antia-Buch procedure of helical rim advancement.

REFERENCES

1. Antia NH, Buch VI. Chondrocutaneous advancement flap for the marginal defect of the ear. Plast Reconstr Surg 1967;39(5):472–477
2. Aguilar EA. Traumatic total or partial ear loss. In: Evans GR, ed. Operative Plastic Surgery. New York: McGraw-Hill; 2000

MANAGEMENT OF SPLIT OR CLEFT EARLOBES

13. A young woman has a 1.5-cm-long, vertically split earlobe caused by wearing heavy earrings. She wishes to wear earrings again in the future. *How would this defect normally be managed?*

    B. Wedge excision of earlobe

There is a myriad of techniques described for the repair of a split earlobe or cleft lobe deformity,[1] but the most straightforward approach involves a wedge excision of the cleft and direct closure. This can be achieved with a linear vertical scar, or with incorporation of a Z-plasty within this line to reduce the risk of scar contraction and late lobule deformity. This may also help facilitate subsequent earring use in the future. An alternative is to preserve a thin flap from the edge of the cleft and roll this into the superior aspect of the wedge repair to provide a skin-lined channel for earrings.[2] Lobule reduction is indicated in patients with large lobules who wish to reduce the size of the lobules and the overall visual appearance of the ear. They are also indicated in patients who have used tissue expanding earrings for an extended time and want to return to a more anatomical appearance for their lobes. Composite grafts from the contralateral lobe and posteriorly based skin flaps are indicated for lobe reconstruction rather than split earlobe repair. Neither local flaps of grafts would normally be needed for surgery to the lobe.

REFERENCES

1. Park JK, Kim KS, Kim SH, Choi J, Yang JY. Reconstruction of a traumatic cleft earlobe using a combination of the inverted V-shaped excision technique and vertical mattress suture method. Arch Craniofac Surg 2017;18(4):277–281
2. Pardue AM. Repair of torn earlobe with preservation of the perforation for an earring. Plast Reconstr Surg 1973;51(4):472–473

RECONSTRUCTING EXTERNAL EAR DEFORMITIES

14. A patient has a 2.5 cm by 1.7 cm full-thickness defect in the middle third of the ear. It involves the helix, scapha, and antihelix but not the conchal bowl. *Which one of the following represents the best option for management of this defect?*

C. **Dieffenbach's flap**

Dieffenbach's flap is a two-stage reconstruction process of the ear that is well suited to reconstruct full-thickness defects of the middle section where the defect spans the helical rim and scapha as in this case. In the first stage, a contralateral ear graft is sutured into the defect and the postauricular skin is elevated and advanced over the cartilage graft to fill the defect. The postauricular skin is then divided at 3 weeks.[1] The Converse tunnel technique could potentially be useful here but tends to be used more for isolated helical rim reconstruction.[1] Orticochea has been associated with many different flaps in the head and neck including the scalp and speech surgery, but in this case the flap is a composite chondrocutaneous rotation flap for upper and middle third ear defects. It is based on the lateral helical rim.[2] The flip-flop flap is used to reconstruct conchal defects and involves a postauricular island flap that is elevated consisting the skin, postauricular muscle, and fascia. The flap is rotated anteriorly 180 degrees so that the posterior most aspect of the flap becomes anterior along the antihelix. The anterior most aspect of the donor flap is deep in the conchal bowl.[3] Staged tubed pedicle flaps using the postauricular skin work well for reconstruction of the helical rim. They require three stages: in the first stage the skin is tubed; in the second stage one end is divided and inset into the helical rim; and in the third stage the flap is detached posteriorly and inset into the helical rim. If the rim is subsequently droopy, it may be necessary to insert a small cartilage graft within the reconstructed soft tissue in order to provide additional support.

REFERENCES

1. Aguilar EA. Traumatic total or partial ear loss. In: Evans GR, ed. Operative Plastic Surgery. New York: McGraw-Hill; 2000
2. Orticochea M. Reconstruction of partial loss of the auricle. Plast Reconstr Surg 1970;46(4):403–405
3. Talmi YP, Wolf M, Horowitz Z, Bedrin L, Kronenberg J. "Second look" at auricular reconstruction with a postauricular island flap: "flip-flop flap". Plast Reconstr Surg 2002;109(2):713–715

44. Lip Reconstruction

See *Essentials of Plastic Surgery*, third edition, pp. 590–604

LIP ANATOMY

1. *Which one of the following represents the red mucosal portion of the lip that is divided into two parts?*
   A. Philtral column
   B. White roll
   C. Vermilion
   D. Red line
   E. Commissure

ANATOMY OF THE LIP

2. *Which one of the following is the same for both upper and lower lips?*
   A. The sensory innervation
   B. The blood supply
   C. The lymphatic drainage
   D. The number of subunit components
   E. The motor innervations to orbicularis

AESTHETICS OF THE LIP

3. *At conversational distances, what minimum amount of white roll mismatch is typically evident?*
   A. 1 mm
   B. 2 mm
   C. 3 mm
   D. 4 mm
   E. 5 mm

REPAIR OF VERMILION DEFECTS OF THE LIP

4. *Which one of the following statements is correct regarding defects of the vermilion?*
   A. Tongue flaps are useful single-stage procedures for defects that measure less than 50%.
   B. Total deficiency may be treated by advancing the buccal mucosa.
   C. Axial myomucosal advancement flaps are elevated superficial to the orbicularis.
   D. Vermilion lip switch is a single-stage procedure for subtotal defects.
   E. Tongue flaps provide the best aesthetic outcomes for vermilion reconstruction.

ALGORITHMIC APPROACH TO LIP RECONSTRUCTION

5. *Which one of the following statements is correct regarding lip reconstruction?*
   A. Upper and lower lip defects that are smaller than a third should be closed directly.
   B. Lower lip defects greater than 50% of total width require a two-stage reconstruction.
   C. A V-Y flap is the first choice for reconstruction of a lower lip defect involving the commissure.
   D. Perialar crescenteric advancement is a useful adjunct for the upper lip reconstruction.
   E. Full-thickness defects larger than two-thirds of the lip width require free flap reconstruction.

THE ABBE FLAP FOR LIP RECONSTRUCTION

6. *Which one of the following statements is correct when using an Abbe flap for lip reconstruction?*
   A. The flap should be designed to be the same width as the defect.
   B. The contralateral labial artery should be skeletonized during the dissection.
   C. Reconstruction of the commissure is the main indication of this flap.
   D. An advantage of this flap is that reconstruction is completed in a single stage.
   E. The flap is particularly well suited for reconstruction of the philtral dimple.

THE ESTLANDER FLAP FOR LIP RECONSTRUCTION

7. *Which one of the following statements is correct regarding an Estlander flap?*
   A. It is ideally suited to reconstruct central lip defects.
   B. It is only suitable for defects less than half the lip width.
   C. It is a two-stage process requiring flap division at 2 weeks.
   D. Blood supply is from the contralateral labial artery of the opposite lip.
   E. Postoperative commissure distortion is rarely observed.

THE KARAPANDZIC FLAP FOR LIP RECONSTRUCTION

8. *Which one of the following statements is correct regarding the Karapandzic flap?*
   A. It should only be used for lower lip reconstruction.
   B. Full-thickness dissection is required throughout.
   C. Some branches of the facial nerve will have to be divided.
   D. The flap is only full thickness medially.
   E. Oral competence is preserved without microstomia.

LOCAL FLAP RECONSTRUCTION OF LARGER LIP DEFECTS

9. *Which one of the following is the key advantage of the Karapandzic flap over the Bernard-Burow flap for lip reconstruction?*
   A. Larger defects may be reconstructed.
   B. It is better for reconstructing lateral defects including the oral commissure.
   C. Fewer stages are required for the reconstruction.
   D. Microstomia is avoided.
   E. Oral sphincter competence is better preserved.

TOTAL LIP RECONSTRUCTION

10. *When considering the radial forearm free flap for lower lip reconstruction, which one of the following is true?*
   A. Preoperative assessment with an Allen's test is rarely required.
   B. Tissue color match and aesthetics are generally excellent with this reconstruction.
   C. Sensory innervation can be achieved by coaptation of the antebrachial cutaneous nerve.
   D. Motor function is well preserved by harvest of flexor carpi radialis muscle.
   E. This flap should ideally be avoided when pre- or postoperative radiotherapy is required.

RECONSTRUCTIVE OPTIONS FOR LOWER LIP DEFECTS

11. A 70-year-old man presents with a 3.5-cm wide defect in his lower lip following an excision of a moderately differentiated squamous cell carcinoma. *Which one can best reconstruct this defect?*
   A. Abbe flap
   B. Estlander flap
   C. Karapandzic flap
   D. Bernard-Burow flap
   E. Direct closure with shield resection

RECONSTRUCTIVE OPTIONS FOR UPPER LIP DEFECTS

12. A 19-year-old woman is seen after a formal debridement of a facial dog bite. She has a full-thickness, centrally placed upper lip defect that measures 50% of the width. The commissure is preserved. *How best would this defect be managed once the risk of infection has been addressed?*
   A. Allowed to heal by secondary intent
   B. Reconstruction with a nasolabial flap and vermilion switch
   C. Reconstruction with an Abbe flap alone
   D. Reconstruction with an Abbe flap and perialar crescenteric excision
   E. Reconstruction with an Estlander flap alone

Answers

LIP ANATOMY

1. *Which one of the following represents the red mucosal portion of the lip that is divided into two parts?*

C. Vermilion

The lip is comprised of skin, fat, muscle, minor salivary glands, and mucosa. It begins superiorly beneath the nasal sill and passes inferiorly to the chin. The lateral borders are the nasolabial folds and marionette lines. The vermilion is the red part of the lip and has wet and dry components based on the presence or absence of surface keratinization. The red line is the junction between the wet and dry vermilion. The philtral column forms part of the upper central area where the superficial muscle inserts into the dermis. The philtral columns frame the central philtral dimple. Cupid's bow lies at the base of the philtral dimple between the two philtral columns. The white roll marks the interface between the skin and vermilion (**Fig. 44.1**).

The orbicularis oris forms the muscular component of the lips and has both deep and superficial components. The superficial component is involved with speech and facial expression, whereas the deep portion is involved with oral competence. The oral commissure is the point where the upper and lower lips join. Lateral to this is the modiolus, where muscle fibers from other mimetic muscles attach, such as the depressor anguli oris, levator anguli oris, risorius, and zygomaticus major.[1,2]

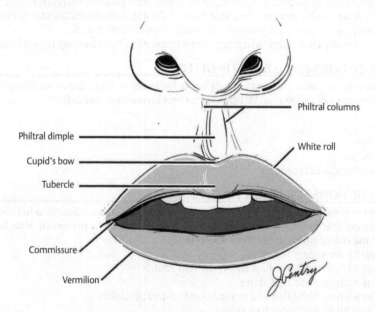

Fig. 44.1   The anatomy of the lip.

REFERENCES

1. Moore KL, Dalley AF, eds. Clinically Oriented Anatomy. 4th ed. New York, NY: Lippincott, Williams, and Wilkins; 1999
2. Williams PL, Warwick R, eds. Gray's Anatomy, 36th British ed. Philadelphia: WB Saunders; 1980

ANATOMY OF THE LIP

2. *Which one of the following is the same for both upper and lower lips?*

E. The motor innervations to orbicularis

The upper and lower lips differ in their vascular supply, sensory nerve supply, and their lymphatic drainage. However, orbicularis oris is innervated by the buccal branches of the facial nerve irrespective of whether the upper or lower lip is considered. The sensory innervation to the upper lip is from the second part of the trigeminal nerve (CN V₂) and the lower lip from the third part (CN V₃). The upper lip receives its main blood supply from the superior labial artery and the lower lip from the inferior labial artery. Each of these is a branch of the facial artery. The lower lip lymphatics drain to either the ipsilateral submandibular region (lateral part of the lip) or the submental and submandibular nodes (medial part of the lip). Drainage can be to either side so tumor spread can involve bilateral neck disease. In contrast, the upper lip primarily drains to the ipsilateral submandibular nodes and tends not to cross the midline. Drainage occasionally passes to the preauricular or parotid nodes.

Although the upper lip has three subunits (right, left, and philtral dimple), the lower lip is a single unit. This is relevant to lip surgery because it can increase the technical difficulty of upper lip reconstruction.[1,2]

REFERENCES

1. Moore KL, Dalley AF, eds. Clinically Oriented Anatomy. 4th ed. New York, NY: Lippincott, Williams, and Wilkins; 1999
2. Williams PL, Warwick R, eds. Gray's Anatomy, 36th British ed. Philadelphia: WB Saunders; 1980

AESTHETICS OF THE LIP

3. *At conversational distances, what minimum amount of white roll mismatch is typically evident?*

A. 1 mm

Malalignments of the white roll as small as 1 mm can be visualized at conversational distances. This highlights the importance of accurate lip repair after trauma or tumor resection. A good technical tip is to mark the white roll with ink *before* local anesthetic infiltration to ensure accurate alignment during reconstruction or repair. Clear contemporaneous documentation before and after lip repair surgery is really important to set patient expectations at a realistic level, whether having lip repair following tumor resection or trauma.[1]

REFERENCE

1. Thorne CH, Gurtner GC, Chung K, et al, eds. Grabb & Smith's Plastic Surgery. Philadelphia, PA: Lippincott Williams & Wilkins; 2013

REPAIR OF VERMILION DEFECTS OF THE LIP

4. *Which one of the following statements is correct regarding defects of the vermilion?*

B. Total deficiency may be treated by advancing the buccal mucosa.

Smaller vermilion defects may be reconstructed using axial myovermilion advancement flaps, V-Y advancement flaps, or a two-stage (not single-stage) lip switch procedure. Defects that are larger than 50% require either a tongue flap or advancement of the buccal mucosa. Aesthetic outcomes after a tongue flap are suboptimal compared with those of vermilion or oral mucosa flaps. The blood supply to an axial myovermilion flap is the labial artery; therefore, these flaps are elevated with the muscle deep to the arterial supply.[1–3]

REFERENCES

1. Kawamoto HK Jr. Correction of major defects of the vermilion with a cross-lip vermilion flap. Plast Reconstr Surg 1979;64(3):315–318
2. Spira M, Stal S. V-Y advancement of a subcutaneous pedicle in vermilion lip reconstruction. Plast Reconstr Surg 1983;72(4):562–564
3. Behmand RA, Rees R. Reconstructive lip surgery. In: Achauer BM, Eriksson E, Guyuron B, et al, eds. Plastic Surgery: Indications, Operations, and Outcomes. Maryland Heights, MO: Mosby; 2000

ALGORITHMIC APPROACH TO LIP RECONSTRUCTION

5. *Which one of the following statements is correct regarding lip reconstruction?*

D. Perialar crescenteric advancement is a useful adjunct for upper lip reconstruction.

Perialar crescenteric flaps are useful for reconstructing a range of defect sizes, particularly when combined with other procedures such as Abbe or Bernard-Burow flaps (**Fig. 44.2**).[1]

Although lower lip defects of less than a third are closed directly, the same is not true for upper lip defects because their reconstruction depends on the anatomic site. For example, lateral defects of the upper lip may be closed directly, but central defects may require perialar crescenteric excision, an Abbe flap, or both. Similarly, reconstruction of upper or lower lip defects that are larger than a half depends on the location of the defect. Some will require a two-stage procedure using an Abbe flap, but others can be reconstructed with single-stage techniques such as Estlander or Karapandzic flaps. The first choice for reconstruction of a commissure defect that involves the lower lip is usually an Estlander flap (not a V-Y flap). Local flaps can be used in combination to reconstruct defects that are larger than two-thirds of either lip. Free flaps are usually required in total lip reconstruction after radiation therapy or failed local flap reconstruction. However, free tissue transfer for lip reconstruction tends to give suboptimal functional and aesthetic results.

REFERENCE

1. Behmand RA, Rees R. Reconstructive lip surgery. In: Achauer BM, Eriksson E, Guyuron B, et al, eds. Plastic Surgery: Indications, Operations, and Outcomes. Philadelphia: Saunders-Elsevier; 2000

THE ABBE FLAP FOR LIP RECONSTRUCTION

6. *Which one of the following statements is correct when using an Abbe flap for lip reconstruction?*

   E. **The flap is particularly well suited for reconstruction of the philtral dimple.**

   Abbé[1] first described this flap for lip reconstruction in patients with double-hairlip deformities in 1898. It is particularly well suited for use in central defects of the upper lip. An Abbe flap is full thickness but not sensate and is not used for commissure defects. This flap is usually designed to be half the width of the original defect. It requires a two-stage process that requires division of the pedicle at 2–3 weeks. The flap receives its blood supply from the ipsilateral labial artery, which is within the orbicularis oris just deep to the white roll. To ensure safe preservation of the blood supply, a cuff of muscle should be maintained around the artery (see **Fig. 44.2**).

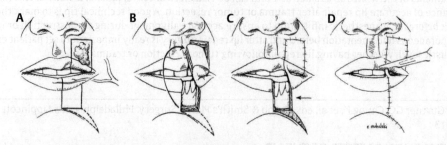

Fig. 44.2 The Abbe flap for upper lip reconstruction. The flap is designed to be smaller than the defect which it is reconstructing. The vascularity is maintained by elevating the flap full thickness but retaining a cuff of muscle around the ipsilateral labial artery. Division is performed at 3 weeks.

REFERENCE

1. Abbé RA. A new plastic operation for the relief of deformity due to double harelip. Med Rec 1898;53:477

THE ESTLANDER FLAP FOR LIP RECONSTRUCTION

7. *Which one of the following statements is correct regarding an Estlander flap?*

   D. **Blood supply is from the contralateral labial artery of the opposite lip.**

   Estlander[1] originally described this flap in 1872 (**Fig. 44.3**). It is a good choice for reconstruction of defects of the oral commissure. The flap receives blood supply from the contralateral labial artery of the opposite lip and reconstruction is accomplished in a single stage, unlike the Abbe flap. The flap can be used for defects of up to two-thirds the lip width but does distort the lip and blunts the oral commissure.

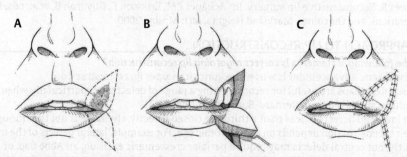

Fig. 44.3 Estlander flap for upper lip reconstruction. *A,* The lower lip flap is designed to be no more than half the size of the upper lip defect. *B,* The flap is rotated about the vermilion, which harbors its blood supply from the contralateral labial artery. *C,* Three-layer closure of the inset flap and donor site. (From Jackson IT. Local Flaps in Head and Neck Reconstruction. St Louis: Quality Medical Publishing, 2007.)

REFERENCE

1. Estlander JA. Eine methode, aus der ienen lippe substanzverluste der anderen zu ersetzen. Langenbecks Arch Klin Chir 1872;14:622

THE KARAPANDZIC FLAP FOR LIP RECONSTRUCTION

8. **Which one of the following statements is correct regarding the Karapandzic flap?**
   D. The flap is only full thickness medially.

The Karapandzic[1] flap may be used to reconstruct large central defects of either the upper or lower lips. A Karapandzic flap usually involves full-thickness dissection a short distance lateral to the defect. The remaining dissection is partial thickness with preservation of the neurovascular pedicle and oral mucosa. Hence, all branches of the facial nerve should be preserved. This is achieved with gentle scissor dissection of the orbicularis oris fibers in the direction in which the nerves and vessels course. Oral competence is usually well maintained but microstomia is likely with larger defects following reconstruction with a Karapandzic flap (**Fig. 44.4**). This may be particularly troublesome for patients who normally wear dentures as they may be unable to use them.[1]

REFERENCE

1. Karapandzic M. Reconstruction of lip defects by local arterial flaps. Br J Plast Surg 1974;27(1):93–97

LOCAL FLAP RECONSTRUCTION OF LARGER LIP DEFECTS

9. **Which one of the following is the key advantage of the Karapandzic flap over the Bernard-Burow flap for lip reconstruction?**
   E. Oral sphincter competence is better preserved.

The Karapanzic flap is a single-stage advancement flap that is useful for reconstruction of one-third to two-thirds of the central upper or lower lip defects. The main advantage of this flap over the Bernard-Burow flap is that muscular continuity of the orbicularis oris is maintained so sphincter continence is superior with this flap. It also preserves the philtrum and modeolus. In contrast, the Bernard-Burow technique can be used to reconstruct central lower lip defects greater than one-third of the lower lip; however, this is at the cost of oral sphincter competence with little or no muscle function afterwards. Furthermore, this flap is insensate. Both flaps can result in microstomia and this has important consequences especially in edentulous patients where mouth opening may be too little to allow them to use their dentures.

The Karapandzic flap is drawn as circumoral flaps passing into the nasolabial folds. Dissection is full thickness on either side of the defect and then partial thickness thereafter in order to preserve muscle, mucosa, and muscle innervation. The Bernard-Burow flap and the Webster modification of this use lateral cheek flaps to advance into the defect and require Burow's triangle excisions in the cheek and chin to facilitate this. These techniques will also need involve reconstruction of the vermilion with buccal mucosal flaps (see **Figs. 44.4** and **44.5**).[1–5]

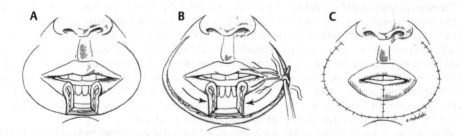

Fig. 44.4 Lower lip reconstruction with a Karapandzic flap. *A,* The width of the circumoral incision must be equal to the height of the defect at all points of the flap. *B,* The labial arteries and buccal nerve branches are identified and preserved bilaterally. *C,* Three-layer closure following medial advancement of the flaps.

REFERENCES

1. Karapandzic M. Reconstruction of lip defects by local arterial flaps. Br J Plast Surg 1974;27(1):93–97
2. Jabaley ME, Clement RL, Orcutt TW. Myocutaneous flaps in lip reconstruction. Applications of the Karapandzic principle. Plast Reconstr Surg 1977;59(5):680–688
3. Freeman BS. Myoplastic modification of the Bernard cheiloplasty. Plast Reconstr Surg Transplant Bull 1958;21(6):453–460
4. Madden JJ Jr, Erhardt WL Jr, Franklin JD, Withers EH, Lynch JB. Reconstruction of the upper and lower lip using a modified Bernard-Burow technique. Ann Plast Surg 1980;5(2):100–107
5. Seo HJ, Bae SH, Nam SB, et al. Lower lip reconstruction after wide excision of a malignancy with barrel-shaped excision or the webster modification of the Bernard operation. Arch Plast Surg 2013;40(1):36–43

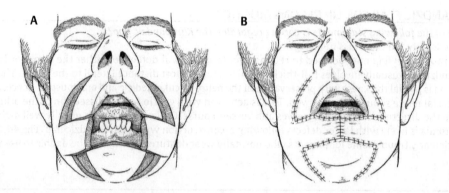

Fig. 44.5 Modified Bernard-Burow procedure. **A,** Excision of the lesion does not violate the labiomental fold, but improved resection of the lesion is achieved by widening the base of the resected area. Burow's triangles are resected more laterally along the nasolabial fold and only involve the resection of skin and some subcutaneous tissue. Along the labiomental fold, skin and subcutaneous Burow's triangles are excised to allow medial rotation of the lower cheek flaps. **B,** Medial advancement of the lower cheek flaps is followed by three-layer closure at the midline and vermilion reconstruction with buccal mucosa. Nasolabial fold defects are closed in a single layer.

TOTAL LIP RECONSTRUCTION

10. *When considering the radial forearm free flap for lower lip reconstruction, which one of the following is true?*

C. Sensory innervation can be achieved by coaptation of the antebrachial cutaneous nerve.

Total lower lip reconstruction can be achieved with a free radial forearm flap and a palmaris longus graft to support lip height. Unfortunately, although the radial forearm remains the best reconstructive option for total lower lip reconstruction overall, the aesthetics and function remain less than ideal; the color match tends to be poor and it can be difficult to achieve aesthetically good reconstruction of specific lip landmarks.

Sensory innervation can be provided with branches of the lateral or medial antebrachial cutaneous nerves, providing a suitable recipient nerve can be identified in the face. Because the radial forearm flap is a fasciocutaneous flap, and does not involve harvesting of the flexor carpi radialis muscle, the reconstruction represents a static sling arrangement (albeit that upper lip movement may be intact) rather than a functional muscle transfer, so poor oral competence is generally observed.

The clinical relevance of the flexor carpi radialis muscle is that it guides elevation of the flap from the forearm as the vascular pedicle lies between this and brachioradialis. The gracilis muscle has been used as an alternative to the radial forearm flap in order to provide functional muscle for the lip, but the aesthetic outcomes when using this flap still tend to be inferior to other reconstructive options such as the radial forearm and it is less commonly used because of this and its short vascular pedicle. One more alternative option to the radial flap is to utilize the soft tissues of the chin and advance this in a hinge fashion to the lower lip. The soft tissues of the submental region will however then need reconstruction due to the defect which is created by this transfer. The advantage here is that the skin match and hair growth (if in a male patient) for the lip is good, but there will still be functional impairment and the vermilion will still need separate reconstruction.

When planning a radial forearm flap, a preoperative Allen's test is required to assess the integrity of the radial and ulnar arterial supply to the hand. Flap elevation should only proceed where there is clear evidence of good ulnar artery flow. The benefit of importing new tissue into the lip with a radial forearm or other free flap is particularly apparent in irradiated fields.[1-7]

REFERENCES

1. Freedman AM, Hidalgo DA. Full-thickness cheek and lip reconstruction with the radial forearm free flap. Ann Plast Surg 1990;25(4):287–294
2. Furuta S, Sakaguchi Y, Iwasawa M, Kurita H, Minemura T. Reconstruction of the lips, oral commissure, and full-thickness cheek with a composite radial forearm palmaris longus free flap. Ann Plast Surg 1994;33(5):544–547
3. Sadove RC, Luce EA, McGrath PC. Reconstruction of the lower lip and chin with the composite radial forearm-palmaris longus free flap. Plast Reconstr Surg 1991;88(2):209–214
4. Godefroy WP, Klop WM, Smeele LE, Lohuis PJ. Free-flap reconstruction of large full-thickness lip and chin defects. Ann Otol Rhinol Laryngol 2012;121(9):594–603
5. Sasidaran R, Zain MA, Basiron NH. Lip and oral commissure reconstruction with the radial forearm flap. Natl J Maxillofac Surg 2012;3(1):21–24

6. Fernandes R, Clemow J. Outcomes of total or near-total lip reconstruction with microvascular tissue transfer. J Oral Maxillofac Surg 2012;70(12):2899–2906
7. Sacak B, Gurunluoglu R. The innervated gracilis muscle for microsurgical functional lip reconstruction: review of the literature. Ann Plast Surg 2015;74(2):204–209

RECONSTRUCTIVE OPTIONS FOR LOWER LIP DEFECTS

11. A 70-year-old man presents with a 3.5-cm wide defect in his lower lip following an excision of a moderately differentiated squamous cell carcinoma. *Which one can best reconstruct this defect?*

   C. Karapandzic flap

   This defect is approximately 70% of the lower lip and of the options listed, it is best reconstructed with a Karapandzic flap. This flap will allow reconstruction of defect this size with rotation/advancement of the residual lower and upper lip components in a single stage. The flap may cause microstomia in cases such as this and should be discussed with patients preoperatively. Due to the design of the flap, sensation and motor innervation are retained (see **Fig. 44.4**).[1]

   The Abbe flap could be used to reconstruct a smaller defect of the lower lip but in general, it is preferable to avoid using the Abbe flap from the upper lip for lower lip reconstruction to avoid tissue distortion.[2] The Estlander flap would be better suited to lateral/commissure defects than the scenario described (see **Fig. 44.3**). The Bernard-Burow flap is a complex flap reserved for reconstruction of larger defects than described in this scenario and is best avoided due to the poor functional outcome. Direct closure in this case would not be a suitable option and even if it is technically possible to close the defect there would be significant tissue distortion as a result (see **Fig. 44.5**).

REFERENCES

1. Karapandzic M. Reconstruction of lip defects by local arterial flaps. Br J Plast Surg 1974;27(1):93–97
2. Abbé RA. A new plastic operation for the relief of deformity due to double harelip. Med Rec 1898;53:477

RECONSTRUCTIVE OPTIONS FOR UPPER LIP DEFECTS

12. A 19-year-old woman is seen after a formal debridement of a facial dog bite. She has a full-thickness, centrally placed upper lip defect that measures 50% of the width. The commissure is preserved. *How best would this defect be managed once the risk of infection has been addressed?*

   D. Reconstruction with an Abbe flap and perialar crescenteric excision

   The Abbe flap is well suited for reconstruction of the upper lip in two stages. In general, this works best for central or lateral defects that do not involve the commissure as in this case. The Abbe flap alone can be used to reconstruct defects of around one-third of lip width. By incorporating a perialar crescenteric excision, additional soft tissue advancement is possible, without compromising function or aesthetics. The scars around the alar base are well disguised and this flap lends itself well to reconstruction of the midline upper lip. In contrast, allowing large facial defects like this to heal by secondary intention will lead to significant tissue distortion and poor functional and aesthetic results. The nasolabial flap can be used for lip reconstruction and in large defects bilateral flaps may be used in unison. These flaps are versatile and can be used for internal lining or skin reconstruction. However, they do not provide any muscle for functional support. The Estlander flap is a single-stage flap indicated for lateral defects involving the commissure rather than central defects as in this case.[1–3]

REFERENCES

1. Zenn MR, Jones G, eds. Reconstructive Surgery: Anatomy, Technique, and Clinical Applications. St Louis: Quality Medical Publishing; 2012
2. Cutting CB, Warren SM. Extended Abbe flap for secondary correction of the bilateral cleft lip. J Craniofac Surg 2013;24(1):75–78
3. Behmand RA, Rees R. Reconstructive lip surgery. In: Achauer BM, Eriksson E, Guyuron B, et al, eds. Plastic Surgery: Indications, Operations, and Outcomes. Maryland Heights, MO: Mosby; 2000

45. Mandibular Reconstruction

See *Essentials of Plastic Surgery*, third edition, pp. 605–614

PRINCIPLES OF MANDIBULAR RECONSTRUCTION

1. *What is the key reason why vascularized bone flaps are preferred for reconstruction of mandibular defects following resection of malignant tumors?*
   A. They are more resistant to the effects of radiotherapy.
   B. They encourage more radical excision margins.
   C. They facilitate re-excision where close margins are obtained.
   D. They are more cost effective than nonvascularized options.
   E. They cause much lower donor site morbidity.

COLLAPSING A MANDIBULAR DEFECT

2. A patient requires partial resection of the ascending ramus of the mandible, including the condylar head. *What is the main disadvantage of collapsing this defect rather than performing a bony reconstruction?*
   A. Technical difficulty
   B. Poor speech outcomes
   C. Long-term temporomandibular joint (TMJ) pain
   D. Difficulty swallowing
   E. Failure to reestablish a normal bite

MANDIBULAR RECONSTRUCTION PLATES

3. *Which one of the following is true of mandibular reconstruction plates as a single modality for mandibular reconstruction?*
   A. They are a reliable choice for most patients.
   B. They are ideal for reconstruction of central mandibular defects.
   C. They must be secured with nonlocking screws.
   D. They have relatively low rates of extrusion.
   E. They usually fail within 18 months following implantation.

SOFT TISSUE FLAPS FOR MANDIBULAR RECONSTRUCTION

4. *Which one of the following represents a disadvantage to using a pectoralis major flap to reconstruct a defect in the mandibular region?*
   A. The blood supply is unreliable.
   B. The vascular pedicle is too short.
   C. The flap is technically difficult to raise.
   D. The flap creates a bulge at the pivot point.
   E. A portion of the clavicle must be removed.

DECISION-MAKING IN MANDIBULAR RECONSTRUCTION

5. *Which one of the following is least relevant when determining the suitability for use of a nonvascularized bone graft in mandibular reconstruction?*
   A. Defect size
   B. Underlying pathology
   C. Subsequent treatment required
   D. Defect location
   E. Method of fixation

BONY RECONSTRUCTION OF THE MANDIBLE

6. You are considering the merits of using vascularized versus nonvascularized bone to reconstruct an edentulous mandible. There is a 4-cm segmental defect in the mandibular body following primary tumor resection. No radiotherapy has been undertaken nor is anticipated and the patient is a nonsmoker. *What is the main indication to use a vascularized bone in this case?*
   A. The size of defect
   B. The location of the defect
   C. The patient's prior medical history
   D. A better chance of bony union
   E. A reduction in donor site morbidity

FIBULA FREE FLAP FOR MANDIBULAR RECONSTRUCTION

7. You are planning to use a free fibular osseocutaneous flap to reconstruct a composite mandibular body and floor of mouth defect. A 7 cm length of bone is required in conjunction with a 3 by 8 cm soft tissue skin paddle. *Which one of the following is correct?*
   A. A separate soft tissue flap is likely to be required as the skin paddle is unreliable.
   B. The bone will need to be double barreled to safely accept dental implants.
   C. Pedicle length will be limited to 5 cm when skin is being harvested.
   D. Osteotomies are safe but bone lengths greater than 2–3 cm should be preserved.
   E. Weight-bearing exercise should not be started before 2 weeks.

THE ILIAC CREST FLAP FOR MANDIBULAR RECONSTRUCTION

8. *Which one of the following is correct regarding the iliac crest free flap?*
   A. Blood supply is from the deep circumflex iliac artery, which arises from the internal iliac artery.
   B. A short pedicle length is a major disadvantage because it rarely exceeds 3–4 cm.
   C. Patients must be counseled regarding the risk of postoperative abdominal pain and hernia formation.
   D. Intraoral soft tissue cover is achieved by harvesting external oblique muscle with the flap.
   E. This flap provides excellent bone stock for implants and has thin pliable skin which is useful for external cover.

FLAP OPTIONS FOR MANDIBULAR RECONSTRUCTION

9. *Which one of the following is considered an advantage of using a deep circumflex iliac artery (DCIA) flap over a fibula flap for reconstruction of a hemimandible?*
   A. Bone height
   B. Intraoral soft tissue cover
   C. Flap harvesting time
   D. Bone length
   E. Vessel diameter

THE SCAPULA FLAP FOR MANDIBULAR RECONSTRUCTION

10. *Which one of the following is correct regarding the scapular osseocutaneous flap?*
   A. The dominant blood supply is the suprascapular artery.
   B. Pedicle length is usually around 20 cm.
   C. Up to 8 cm of bone can be harvested in adult male patients.
   D. Soft tissue availability is less than that of a DCIA flap.
   E. Patient positioning can present a logistical disadvantage.

ANATOMY OF THE SCAPULA FLAP

11. When raising an osseocutaneous scapula free flap, the triangular space must be located to identify the vascular pedicle. *What muscle forms the lateral border of this space?*
   A. Teres major
   B. Teres minor
   C. Rhomboid
   D. Long head of triceps
   E. Latissimus dorsi

COMPUTER AIDED DESIGN IN MANDIBULAR RECONSTRUCTION

12. *What is the major proven benefit of using computer-aided design for mandibular reconstruction?*
   A. Improved functional outcomes
   B. Decreased procedural costs
   C. Reduced duration of preoperative planning
   D. Improved accuracy of reconstruction
   E. Avoidance of multiple osteotomies

Answers

PRINCIPLES OF MANDIBULAR RECONSTRUCTION

1. *What is the key reason why vascularized bone flaps are preferred for reconstruction of mandibular defects following resection of malignant tumors?*

    A. **They are more resistant to the effects of radiotherapy.**

    In general, patients who are likely to undergo postoperative radiotherapy should have autologous reconstruction, preferably using vascularized bone flaps. The principles of malignant tumor resection are that adequate margins are used to achieve complete resection irrespective of the chosen reconstruction method. Margins should not be compromised or tailored to a specific reconstruction type. The cost effectiveness of a reconstructive method is complex to assess and vascularized tissue transfer is expensive and time consuming and is unlikely to be more cost effective in the short term than other techniques. Donor site morbidity is a major consideration in any vascularized or nonvascularized transfer although taking the fibula as an example, most patients would be expected to return to normal or near-normal function after harvest of either vascularized or nonvascularized bone, so it may not make a difference to morbidity which is taken. Perhaps the inclusion of a skin paddle with subsequent need for skin grafting would be a greater concern thereby causing increased, not decreased, morbidity following vascularized bone harvest.[1,2]

REFERENCES

1. Foster RD, Anthony JP, Sharma A, Pogrel MA. Vascularized bone flaps versus nonvascularized bone grafts for mandibular reconstruction: an outcome analysis of primary bony union and endosseous implant success. Head Neck 1999;21(1):66–71
2. Cordeiro PG, Disa JJ, Hidalgo DA, Hu QY. Reconstruction of the mandible with osseous free flaps: a 10-year experience with 150 consecutive patients. Plast Reconstr Surg 1999;104(5):1314–1320

COLLAPSING A MANDIBULAR DEFECT

2. A patient requires partial resection of the ascending ramus of the mandible, including the condylar head. *What is the main disadvantage of collapsing this defect rather than performing a bony reconstruction?*

    E. **Failure to reestablish a normal bite**

    Allowing the mandible to collapse without reconstruction may be acceptable for some ascending ramus or lateral defects, but will lead to deviation of the chin with malocclusion in dentate patients. The outcomes for speech and swallowing are generally good when using this technique. Temporomandibular joint (TMJ) pain is not usually a problem following resection of the joint. Collapse of the mandible is a relatively straightforward procedure so it maintains a role in current practice.[1-6]

REFERENCES

1. Boyd JB, Mulholland RS, Davidson J, et al. The free flap and plate in oromandibular reconstruction: long-term review and indications. Plast Reconstr Surg 1995;95(6):1018–1028
2. Ueyama Y, Naitoh R, Yamagata A, Matsumura T. Analysis of reconstruction of mandibular defects using single stainless steel A-O reconstruction plates. J Oral Maxillofac Surg 1996;54(7):858–862, discussion 862–863
3. Kellman RM, Gullane PJ. Use of the AO mandibular reconstruction plate for bridging of mandibular defects. Otolaryngol Clin North Am 1987;20(3):519–533
4. Schusterman MA, Reece GP, Kroll SS, Weldon ME. Use of the AO plate for immediate mandibular reconstruction in cancer patients. Plast Reconstr Surg 1991;88(4):588–593
5. Kim MR, Donoff RB. Critical analysis of mandibular reconstruction using AO reconstruction plates. J Oral Maxillofac Surg 1992;50(11):1152–1157
6. Papazian MR, Castillo MH, Campbell JH, Dalrymple D. Analysis of reconstruction for anterior mandibular defects using AO plates. J Oral Maxillofac Surg 1991;49(10):1055–1059, discussion 1059–1060

MANDIBULAR RECONSTRUCTION PLATES

3. *Which one of the following is true of mandibular reconstruction plates as a single modality for mandibular reconstruction?*

    E. **They usually fail within 18 months following implantation.**

    The advantages of using mandibular reconstruction plates alone are shorter operating times and avoidance of donor site morbidity. However, extrusion rates are high, especially when used in the anterior mandible. General consensus is that these techniques should be reserved for lateral defects in patients unable to tolerate longer procedures, those with no dentition and display mandibular atrophy, or those with short expected lifespans. Where they are used, they are typically 1.5- to 2.4-mm thick and can use either locking or nonlocking screws into the mandible. Traditional or nonlocking screws simply hold the plate against the bone to create a load-sharing reconstruction. The addition of locking screws that have threaded screw heads that lock into the plate help create a more rigid load-bearing reconstruction. Mandibular reconstruction plates will all fail if the patient survives long enough. Most fail within 18 months, and the mean time is close to 6 months.[1-6]

REFERENCES

1. Boyd JB, Mulholland RS, Davidson J, et al. The free flap and plate in oromandibular reconstruction: long-term review and indications. Plast Reconstr Surg 1995;95(6):1018–1028
2. Ueyama Y, Naitoh R, Yamagata A, Matsumura T. Analysis of reconstruction of mandibular defects using single stainless steel A-O reconstruction plates. J Oral Maxillofac Surg 1996;54(7):858–862, discussion 862–863
3. Kellman RM, Gullane PJ. Use of the AO mandibular reconstruction plate for bridging of mandibular defects. Otolaryngol Clin North Am 1987;20(3):519–533
4. Schusterman MA, Reece GP, Kroll SS, Weldon ME. Use of the AO plate for immediate mandibular reconstruction in cancer patients. Plast Reconstr Surg 1991;88(4):588–593
5. Kim MR, Donoff RB. Critical analysis of mandibular reconstruction using AO reconstruction plates. J Oral Maxillofac Surg 1992;50(11):1152–1157
6. Papazian MR, Castillo MH, Campbell JH, Dalrymple D. Analysis of reconstruction for anterior mandibular defects using AO plates. J Oral Maxillofac Surg 1991;49(10):1055–1059, discussion 1059–1060

SOFT TISSUE FLAPS FOR MANDIBULAR RECONSTRUCTION

4. *Which one of the following represents a disadvantage to using a pectoralis major flap to reconstruct a defect in the mandibular region?*

D. The flap creates a bulge at the pivot point.

The pectoralis major is a workhorse flap for head and neck reconstruction, even with the increased popularity of free tissue transfer. It has many advantages such as the relative ease and speed with which it can be raised, the vascular supply is very reliable (thoracoacromial artery and vein), the reach is adequate for upper neck, and the mandibular region and the donor site are normally closed directly. It allows either muscle only or muscle and skin to be harvested and can be used to reconstruct mandibular, intraoral, or skin defects. The bulge created over the clavicle may be minimized by dissecting the pedicle and reducing muscle bulk at the pivot point. Alternatively, the clavicle can be sectioned but this is not necessary and is rarely performed.[1-5]

REFERENCES

1. Ariyan S. The pectoralis major myocutaneous flap. A versatile flap for reconstruction in the head and neck. Plast Reconstr Surg 1979;63(1):73–81
2. Schneider DS, Wu V, Wax MK. Indications for pedicled pectoralis major flap in a free tissue transfer practice. Head Neck 2012;34(8):1106–1110
3. Rudes M, Bilić M, Jurlina M, Prgomet D. Pectoralis major myocutaneous flap in the reconstructive surgery of the head and neck—our experience. Coll Antropol 2012;36(Suppl 2):137–142
4. Kekatpure VD, Trivedi NP, Manjula BV, Mathan Mohan A, Shetkar G, Kuriakose MA. Pectoralis major flap for head and neck reconstruction in era of free flaps. Int J Oral Maxillofac Surg 2012;41(4):453–457
5. Liu M, Liu W, Yang X, Guo H, Peng H. Pectoralis major myocutaneous flap for head and neck defects in the era of free flaps: harvesting technique and indications. Sci Rep 2017;7:46256

DECISION-MAKING IN MANDIBULAR RECONSTRUCTION

5. *Which one of the following is least relevant when determining the suitability for use of a nonvascularized bone graft in mandibular reconstruction?*

E. Method of fixation

The method of fixation is not a key consideration for determining the suitability of use in nonvascularized bone grafts as a standard approach is taken in all cases. Nonvascular bone grafts may, in principle, be considered for reconstruction of mandibular defects of up to 6 cm after trauma or benign tumor resection. The site of defect is also important and their use in lateral defects is acceptable but use in anterior mandibular defects should be avoided. Even in short defects, they demonstrate lower rates of bony union than vascularized bone. Failure rates of nonvascularized bone grafts vary from more than 50 to 100%, according to site and length. Furthermore, they are less well suited to allow implant-based dental rehabilitation and are also contraindicated in cancer patients and those undergoing subsequent radiotherapy.[1,2]

REFERENCES

1. Adamo AK, Szal RL. Timing, results, and complications of mandibular reconstructive surgery: report of 32 cases. J Oral Surg 1979;37(10):755–763
2. Foster RD, Anthony JP, Sharma A, Pogrel MA. Vascularized bone flaps versus nonvascularized bone grafts for mandibular reconstruction: an outcome analysis of primary bony union and endosseous implant success. Head Neck 1999;21(1):66–71

BONY RECONSTRUCTION OF THE MANDIBLE

6. You are considering the merits of using vascularized versus nonvascularized bone to reconstruct an edentulous mandible. There is a 4-cm segmental defect in the mandibular body following primary tumor resection. No radiotherapy has been undertaken nor is anticipated and the patient is a nonsmoker. *What is the main indication to use a vascularized bone in this case?*

D. A better chance of bony union

Nonvascularized bone can be used to reconstruct short mandibular body segmental defects (<6 cm long) resulting from trauma or benign tumor resection when preoperative or postoperative radiotherapy is not given. Therefore, in this patient, it would be reasonable to consider a bone graft as there are no specific contraindications to its use. However, even in short defects such as in this case, nonvascularized bone grafts still demonstrate lower rates of bony union (55% in all defects, 80% in defects <5 cm) than vascularized bone flaps (100% in all defects).[1]

There are many advantages to using vascularized bone in mandibular reconstruction and this is why it remains the benchmark. In addition to better union rates, vascularized bone flaps provide greater strength, stiffness, and superior functional outcomes.[1] They are also the preferred choice for dental rehabilitation with implants and those in whom aesthetic reconstruction is important. A downside to vascularized bone grafts is the increased duration of surgery and increased technical skill set required. They are generally considered to have less donor site morbidity compared with vascularized flaps.[1–3]

REFERENCES

1. Goldberg VM, Shaffer JW, Field G, Davy DT. Biology of vascularized bone grafts. Orthop Clin North Am 1987;18(2):197–205
2. Foster RD, Anthony JP, Sharma A, Pogrel MA. Vascularized bone flaps versus nonvascularized bone grafts for mandibular reconstruction: an outcome analysis of primary bony union and endosseous implant success. Head Neck 1999;21(1):66–71
3. Cordeiro PG, Disa JJ, Hidalgo DA, Hu QY. Reconstruction of the mandible with osseous free flaps: a 10-year experience with 150 consecutive patients. Plast Reconstr Surg 1999;104(5):1314–1320

FIBULA FREE FLAP FOR MANDIBULAR RECONSTRUCTION

7. *You are planning to use a free fibular osseocutaneous flap to reconstruct a composite mandibular body and floor of mouth defect. A 7 cm length of bone is required in conjunction with a 3 by 8 cm soft tissue skin paddle. Which one of the following is correct?*

D. Osteotomies are safe but bone lengths greater than 2–3 cm should be preserved.

The fibula flap is a workhorse flap for mandibular reconstruction and can provide good volumes of soft tissue and bone. Because of the segmental vascular supply, it is safe to perform osteotomies when contouring to match the resected mandible, but it is advisable to maintain lengths of 3 cm and ensure the periosteum is intact in order to avoid vascular compromise. A separate soft tissue flap, such as a radial forearm, is not required in this case as the skin paddle for a fibula can provide the required skin paddle size. Although the skin island was originally thought to be unreliable, this is no longer considered to be the case, with survival rates close to 100%.

The fibula is suitable for using osseointegrated dental implants, even though it does lack vertical height compared with the native mandible. It does not need to be double barreled in most instances, but some surgeons prefer to do so when reconstructing anterior midline defects. Pedicle length is a real advantage of this flap and varies from 6 to 10 cm and sometimes even more, meaning that there is usually comfortable reach to the facial artery and tributaries of the internal jugular vein for anastomosis. The skin paddle is based on perforators at the junction of the mid to distal thirds of the leg and this helps to extend pedicle length when distal bone is harvested. The skin paddle is based on perforators from the peroneal vessels, which pass in the posterior crural septum arising from the posterior aspect of the fibula. Preoperatively, they may be identified using handheld Doppler and intraoperatively, they can usually be seen running through the septum from the bone and pedicle to the skin.

Weight bearing can be commenced early in the postoperative period (between 2 and 5 days, according to surgeon and patient preference) following fibula flap harvest and most patients can walk normally following this surgery. There are risks of causing damage to other leg nerves and vessels in the anterior, lateral, and posterior compartments. For example, the tibial nerve and vessels as well as the deep peroneal nerve are encountered intraoperatively and may receive traction injuries. Also, the sural and superficial peroneal nerves may be inadvertently damaged during flap harvest leading to altered sensation distally (see **Fig. 45.1**, *Essentials of Plastic Surgery*, third edition).[1–6]

REFERENCES

1. Cordeiro PG, Disa JJ, Hidalgo DA, Hu QY. Reconstruction of the mandible with osseous free flaps: a 10-year experience with 150 consecutive patients. Plast Reconstr Surg 1999;104(5):1314–1320
2. Hidalgo DA. Fibula free flap: a new method of mandible reconstruction. Plast Reconstr Surg 1989;84(1):71–79
3. Garvey PB, Chang EI, Selber JC, et al. A prospective study of preoperative computed tomographic angiographic mapping of free fibula osteocutaneous flaps for head and neck reconstruction. Plast Reconstr Surg 2012;130(4):541e–549e
4. Chang EI, Clemens MW, Garvey PB, Skoracki RJ, Hanasono MM. Cephalometric analysis for microvascular head and neck reconstruction. Head Neck 2012;34(11):1607–1614
5. Momoh AO, Yu P, Skoracki RJ, Liu S, Feng L, Hanasono MM. A prospective cohort study of fibula free flap donor-site morbidity in 157 consecutive patients. Plast Reconstr Surg 2011;128(3):714–720
6. Yu P, Chang EI, Hanasono MM. Design of a reliable skin paddle for the fibula osteocutaneous flap: perforator anatomy revisited. Plast Reconstr Surg 2011;128(2):440–446

THE ILIAC CREST FLAP FOR MANDIBULAR RECONSTRUCTION

8. *Which one of the following is correct regarding the iliac crest free flap?*

   C. Patients must be counseled regarding the risk of postoperative abdominal pain and hernia formation.
   Free vascularized iliac crest bone flaps have a role in mandibular reconstruction and some surgeons prefer to use them instead of the fibula flap. However, this flap carries some additional donor site complications compared with the fibula flap, including risk of postoperative hernia and lower abdominal/hip pain. This can be reduced to some extent by careful reinforced closure of the abdomen during donor site closure. Blood supply is from the deep circumflex iliac artery (DCIA) which arises from the external iliac (not the internal) close to the deep inferior epigastric artery, which is used in a deep inferior epigastric perforator (DIEP) flap. A disadvantage of this flap is its short pedicle (up to 7 cm is typically quoted). This can be improved by moving the site of bone harvest more posteriorly. The skin paddle tends to be bulky and perforating vessels are not consistently present, but muscle can be harvested with the flap to provide intraoral cover. This muscle is the internal oblique (not the external oblique) and mucosalizes rapidly when placed intraorally. The DCIA bone flap provides an excellent foundation for the use of dental implants (see **Fig. 45.2**, *Essentials of Plastic Surgery*, third edition).[1–4]

REFERENCES

1. Urken ML, Vickery C, Weinberg H, Buchbinder D, Lawson W, Biller HF. The internal oblique-iliac crest osseomyocutaneous free flap in oromandibular reconstruction. Report of 20 cases. Arch Otolaryngol Head Neck Surg 1989;115(3):339–349
2. Schardt C, Schmid A, Bodem J, Krisam J, Hoffmann J, Mertens C. Donor site morbidity and quality of life after microvascular head and neck reconstruction with free fibula and deep-circumflex iliac artery flaps. J Craniomaxillofac Surg 2017;45(2):304–311
3. Iqbal M, Lloyd CJ, Paley MD, Penfold CN. Repair of the deep circumflex iliac artery free flap donor site with Protack (titanium spiral tacks) and Prolene (polypropylene) mesh. Br J Oral Maxillofac Surg 2007;45(7):596–597
4. Möhlhenrich SC, Kniha K, Elvers D, et al. Intraosseous stability of dental implants in free revascularized fibula and iliac crest bone flaps. J Craniomaxillofac Surg 2016;44(12):1935–1939

FLAP OPTIONS FOR MANDIBULAR RECONSTRUCTION

9. *Which one of the following is considered an advantage of using a deep circumflex iliac artery (DCIA) flap over a fibula flap for reconstruction of a hemimandible?*

   A. Bone height
   Deep circumflex iliac artery (DCIA) flaps provide superior bone height when compared with fibula flaps. This may be helpful for placing dental implants, although some surgeons feel that positioning a fibula flap more superiorly at the expense of the inferior mandibular contour or double barreling it anteriorly will address this problem. Although a fibula flap can give more bone length (up to 25 cm in adult males), a DCIA gives adequate length for a hemimandible. Both flaps can provide intraoral soft tissue cover. The fibula flap achieves this with a pliable skin paddle, while the DCIA does so with muscle cover from the internal oblique. Harvest time is probably similar and depends on surgeon's experience and patient's body habitus. Both flaps have similar vessel diameter, typically 2–3 mm, so there would not normally be a significant difference in anastomotic difficulty between the two flaps.[1–3]

REFERENCES

1. Urken ML, Vickery C, Weinberg H, Buchbinder D, Lawson W, Biller HF. The internal oblique-iliac crest osseomyocutaneous free flap in oromandibular reconstruction. Report of 20 cases. Arch Otolaryngol Head Neck Surg 1989;115(3):339–349
2. Schardt C, Schmid A, Bodem J, Krisam J, Hoffmann J, Mertens C. Donor site morbidity and quality of life after micro-vascular head and neck reconstruction with free fibula and deep-circumflex iliac artery flaps. J Craniomaxillofac Surg 2017;45(2):304–311
3. Lonie S, Herle P, Paddle A, Pradhan N, Birch T, Shayan R. Mandibular reconstruction: meta-analysis of iliac- versus fibula-free flaps. ANZ J Surg 2016;86(5):337–342

THE SCAPULA FLAP FOR MANDIBULAR RECONSTRUCTION

10. *Which one of the following is correct regarding the scapular osseocutaneous flap?*

    E. Patient positioning can present a logistical disadvantage.

       The dominant blood supply to the osseocutaneous scapula flap is the circumflex scapular artery arising from the subscapular vessels. The skin islands are termed scapular and parascapular and receive blood supply through the transverse or descending branches of the circumflex scapular artery, respectively. Bone is usually harvested from the lateral border of the scapula commencing 2 cm below the glenohumeral joint toward the scapular tip. In addition to the circumflex scapular artery, the scapula also receives blood supply through the thoracodorsal artery, which normally provides the angular branch to the scapula tip. When raised on the thoracodorsal axis, the flap may include the latissimus dorsi muscle and the overlying skin. It is possible to raise a chimeric flap using both thoracodorsal and circumflex scapular vessels. For this reason, the scapular osseocutaneous flap offers a large amount of soft tissue cover in addition to length of bone, up to 14 cm in adult males. Two main disadvantages of this flap are that patients typically require turning intraoperatively, which may limit a two-team simultaneous approach, and that the bone harvested is thin compared with DCIA or fibula. This means that dental rehabilitation is more challenging and the bone is less easy to sculpt especially as it lacks a segmental blood supply and so cannot withstand osteotomies.[1-4]

REFERENCES

1. Swartz WM, Banis JC, Newton ED, Ramasastry SS, Jones NF, Acland R. The osteocutaneous scapular flap for mandibular and maxillary reconstruction. Plast Reconstr Surg 1986;77(4):530–545
2. Dowthwaite SA, Theurer J, Belzile M, et al. Comparison of fibular and scapular osseous free flaps for oromandibular reconstruction: a patient-centered approach to flap selection. JAMA Otolaryngol Head Neck Surg 2013;139(3):285–292
3. Robb GL. Free scapular flap reconstruction of the head and neck. Clin Plast Surg 1994;21(1):45–58
4. Sultan MR. Mandible reconstruction with the scapula osteocutaneous flap. Operative Techniques in Plastic and Reconstructive Surgery 1996;3(4):248–256

ANATOMY OF THE SCAPULA FLAP

11. When raising an osseocutaneous scapula free flap, the triangular space must be located to identify the vascular pedicle. *What muscle forms the lateral border of this space?*

    D. Long head of triceps

       The circumflex scapular pedicle supplies the scapula flaps and passes through the triangular space. This space is formed from the following structures: superiorly, teres minor; inferiorly, teres major; and laterally, long head of triceps (**Fig. 45.1**).[1,2]

REFERENCES

1. Sultan MR. Mandible reconstruction with the scapula osteocutaneous flap. Operative Techniques in Plastic and Reconstructive Surgery 1996;3(4):248–256
2. Swartz WM, Banis JC, Newton ED, Ramasastry SS, Jones NF, Acland R. The osteocutaneous scapular flap for mandibular and maxillary reconstruction. Plast Reconstr Surg 1986;77(4):530–545

COMPUTER AIDED DESIGN IN MANDIBULAR RECONSTRUCTION

12. *What is the major proven benefit of using computer-aided design for mandibular reconstruction?*

    D. Improved accuracy of reconstruction

       Computer-aided design is becoming popular as a tool to help plan and execute reconstruction of complex bony defects such as the mandible and maxilla. Three-dimensional computer images of the mandible and fibula are generated and a virtual mandibular defect is created. Cutting jigs are manufactured preoperatively to assist in bony resection and fibula harvest. A major advantage in using models and computer-designed jigs for fibular reconstruction is that the ischemia time can be minimized. This is because the bone flap can be fully prepared

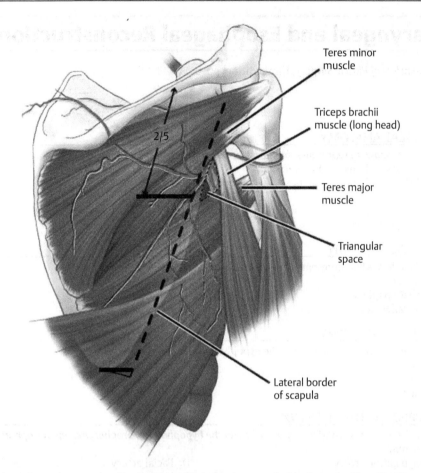

Fig. 45.1   The triangular space contains the vascular pedicle for the scapula flap. It can be identified by palpation approximately two-fifths the distance from the midportion of the scapula spine to its inferior border.

while still attached to the leg, with osteotomies performed and the reconstruction plate fitted. Once the flap is disconnected, it needs to be quickly screwed into place and the anastomoses can be started within a few minutes of transfer.

The other advantage is the accuracy with which the reconstruction is performed. Even with practice and skill, hand sculpting bony flaps cannot match the accuracy and efficiency of using preplanned jigs. As a result, time in the OR is reduced and quality of reconstruction is improved. The other outcomes such as contour aesthetics, correct occlusion, bony union, and temporomandibular joint (TMJ) dynamic function should all be improved by accurate planning. However, this approach is costly and requires additional time for preplanning. Whether this translates into improved functional outcomes is unknown although intuitively it should do so (see **Fig. 45.4**, *Essentials of Plastic Surgery*, third edition).[1-4]

REFERENCES

1. Foley BD, Thayer WP, Honeybrook A, McKenna S, Press S. Mandibular reconstruction using computer-aided design and computer-aided manufacturing: an analysis of surgical results. J Oral Maxillofac Surg 2013;71(2):e111–e119
2. Wilde F, Cornelius CP, Schramm A. Computer-assisted mandibular reconstruction using a patient-specific reconstruction plate fabricated with computer-aided design and manufacturing techniques. Craniomaxillofac Trauma Reconstr 2014;7(2):158–166
3. Tarsitano A, Del Corso G, Ciocca L, Scotti R, Marchetti C. Mandibular reconstructions using computer-aided design/computer-aided manufacturing: a systematic review of a defect-based reconstructive algorithm. J Craniomaxillofac Surg 2015;43(9):1785–1791
4. Deek NFAL, Wei FC. Computer-assisted surgery for segmental mandibular reconstruction with the osteoseptocutaneous fibula flap: can we instigate ideological and technological reforms? Plast Reconstr Surg 2016;137(3):963–970

46. Pharyngeal and Esophageal Reconstruction

See *Essentials of Plastic Surgery*, third edition, pp. 615–633

NASOPHARYNGEAL ANATOMY

1. *Which one of the following represents the posterior boundary of the nasopharynx?*
   A. Lower skull base (clivus) and C1 vertebra
   B. Sphenoid sinus and upper skull base
   C. Soft palate
   D. Choanae
   E. Retropharyngeal space

OROPHARYNGEAL ANATOMY

2. *Which one of the following represents the inferior boundary of the oropharynx?*
   A. Base of tongue
   B. Circumvallate papillae
   C. Hyoid and valleculae
   D. Pharyngeal wall
   E. Tonsillar fossa

HYPOPHARYNGEAL ANATOMY

3. *Which one of the following is a subsite of the hypopharynx?*
   A. Soft palate
   B. Tonsillar fossa
   C. Tongue base
   D. Palatoglossal folds
   E. Piriform sinus

VASCULAR SUPPLY TO THE PHARYNX

4. *Which one of the external carotid artery branches do the hypopharynx, oropharynx, and nasopharynx all receive blood supply from?*
   A. Ascending palatine artery
   B. Ascending pharyngeal artery
   C. Superior thyroid artery
   D. Facial artery
   E. Lingual artery

REFERRED OTALGIA IN HEAD AND NECK CANCER

5. *Which one of the following cranial nerves accounts for a patient presenting with otalgia as the only symptom of a head and neck cancer?*
   A. Trigeminal nerve
   B. Vagus nerve
   C. Vestibulocochlear nerve
   D. Cervical plexus
   E. Accessory nerve

NASOPHARYNGEAL CARCINOMA

6. *Which one of the following is not a risk factor for the development of nasopharyngeal carcinoma?*
   A. A diet high in preservatives and nitrosamines
   B. Wood dust
   C. Epstein-Barr virus
   D. Genetic predisposition
   E. Tobacco smoking

CLINICAL ASSESSMENT OF NASOPHARYNGEAL CARCINOMA

7. A 50-year-old patient presents with nasal obstruction, epistaxis, and conductive hearing loss secondary to otitis media. You obtain a full history and perform a basic examination with fiberoptic nasoendoscopy, which reveals a suspicious area in the nasopharynx. *What is the next most appropriate step in management?*
   A. PET-CT scan
   B. Examination under anesthesia and biopsy
   C. Ultrasound-guided fine-needle aspiration cytology
   D. Multislice CT of the head, neck, and thorax
   E. MRI of the skull base

HUMAN PAPILLOMAVIRUS IN HEAD AND NECK CANCER

8. *Which one of the following tumor sites is strongly associated with human papillomavirus (HPV) 16 and 18 in younger patient groups?*
   A. Cervical esophagus
   B. Larynx
   C. Fossa of Rosenmüller
   D. Tonsils
   E. Nasopharynx

TYPES OF HEAD AND NECK TUMORS

9. *Which one of the following cancers has a much greater incidence in patients with Plummer-Vinson syndrome?*
   A. Oropharyngeal
   B. Medullary thyroid
   C. Unknown primary
   D. Nasopharyngeal
   E. Hypopharyngeal

CLINICAL PRESENTATION IN HEAD AND NECK CANCER

10. *Which one of the following findings is particularly suspicious for nasopharyngeal carcinoma?*
    A. Unilateral otitis media and bilateral level V nodes
    B. Sore throat and gastroesophageal reflux
    C. A single enlarged neck mass
    D. Unilateral otalgia
    E. Dysphagia and jaw pain

PHASES OF SWALLOWING

11. The process of swallowing has multiple phases. *Which one of the following represents the most important phase?*
    A. Oral preparatory
    B. Oral
    C. Pharyngeal
    D. Esophageal
    E. Preparatory

EVALUATION OF SWALLOWING

12. Assessment of swallowing is vital in patients with pharyngeal carcinoma. *Which one of the following modalities provides the most comprehensive noninvasive assessment of all stages of swallowing?*
    A. Bedside assessment with colored fluids
    B. Videofluoroscopy
    C. MRI
    D. Endoscopy
    E. Contrast CT

MANAGEMENT OF HEAD AND NECK TUMORS

13. *Which one of the following is most likely to be avoided by performing robotic surgery in patients with pharyngeal carcinoma?*
    A. Radiotherapy
    B. Neck dissection
    C. Soft tissue reconstruction
    D. Mandibulotomy
    E. Dental extraction

CHEMOTHERAPY AND RADIATION IN HEAD AND NECK CANCER

14. *Which one of the following tumor sites is most likely to receive chemo/radiation therapy as its primary treatment modality?*
    A. Nasopharynx
    B. Oropharynx
    C. Hypopharynx
    D. Oral cavity
    E. Thyroid

OUTCOMES IN HEAD AND NECK CANCER

15. *In general, which site has the worst oncologic outcome of all the head and neck cancers?*
    A. Oral cavity
    B. Thyroid
    C. Oropharynx
    D. Hypopharynx
    E. Nasopharynx

RECONSTRUCTION OF THE HYPOPHARYNX

16. A patient has a circumferential defect after resection of a hypopharyngeal tumor. *According to the classification of Disa et al, what type of defect is this?*
    A. Type I
    B. Type II
    C. Type III
    D. Type IV
    E. Type V

RECONSTRUCTION FOLLOWING TOTAL LARYNGOPHARYNGECTOMY

17. You see a patient in clinic following a total laryngopharyngectomy with reconstruction and insertion of a speech valve for treatment of a T4 tumor. The patient's speech is now reasonably clear, but the patient has a wet, coarse quality to the voice. *Which one of the following is the most likely reconstruction method used?*
    A. Pedicled pectoralis major flap
    B. Free radial forearm flap
    C. Free anterolateral thigh flap
    D. Laryngeal transplantation
    E. Free jejunum flap

RECONSTRUCTION FOLLOWING TOTAL LARYNGOPHARYNGECTOMY

18. *When reconstructing a circumferential defect of the hypopharynx with a free anterolateral thigh (ALT) flap, which one of the following should be undertaken to reduce the risk of early salivary fistula formation?*
    A. Early use of total parenteral nutrition (TPN)
    B. Use of nonabsorbable sutures at the esophageal anastomosis
    C. Delaying postoperative radiotherapy
    D. Use of a salivary pharyngeal bypass tube
    E. Use of a proton pump inhibitor

RECONSTRUCTION OF OROPHARYNGEAL DEFECTS

19. *Which one of the following is correct when managing patients with post-tumor resection defects of the oropharynx?*
    A. Most soft palate defects are well managed with prosthetic devices.
    B. Larger tongue base defects are more safely treated with laryngectomy.
    C. Pharyngeal wall defects usually require free tissue reconstruction.
    D. Local flaps for tongue base reconstruction are associated with low complication rates.
    E. Large tongue defects benefit from free muscle transfer with motor reinnervation.

Answers

NASOPHARYNGEAL ANATOMY

1. *Which one of the following represents the posterior boundary of the nasopharynx?*

A. Lower skull base (clivus) and C1 vertebra

The nasopharynx is a narrow space posterior to the nasal cavity and above the soft palate (**Fig. 46.1**). It is located immediately below the central skull base and has the following boundaries:

- **Superior:** Sphenoid sinus and upper skull base (clivus)
- **Inferior:** Soft palate
- **Anterior:** Choanae
- **Posterior:** Lower skull base (clivus) and first cervical vertebra

The retropharyngeal space is located at the level of the hypopharynx, which forms its posterior boundary.[1-4]

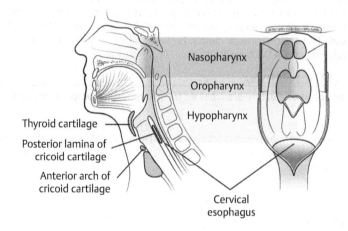

Fig. 46.1   Subdivisions of the pharynx.

REFERENCES

1. Chepeha DB. Reconstruction of the hypopharynx and esophagus. In: Flint PW, Haughey BH, Lund VJ, et al, eds. Cummings Otolaryngology: Head & Neck Surgery. 5th ed. Philadelphia: Elsevier; 2010
2. Gherardini G, Evans RD. Reconstruction of the oral cavity, pharynx, and esophagus. In: Thorne CH, Beasley RW, Aston SJ, et al, eds. Grabb and Smith's Plastic Surgery. 6th ed. Philadelphia: Lippincott Williams & Wilkins; 2007
3. Harreus U. Malignant neoplasms of the oropharynx. In: Flint PW, Haughey BH, Lund VJ, et al, eds. Cummings Otolaryngology: Head & Neck Surgery. 5th ed. Philadelphia: Elsevier; 2010
4. Schecter GL, Wadsworth TT. Hypopharyngeal cancer. In: Bailey BJ, ed. Head & Neck Surgery: Otolaryngology. 2nd ed. Philadelphia: Lippincott Williams & Wilkins; 1998

OROPHARYNGEAL ANATOMY

2. *Which one of the following represents the inferior boundary of the oropharynx?*

C. Hyoid and valleculae

The oropharynx extends from the junction of the hard and soft palates to the aryepiglottic folds, with the hyoid and valleculae representing the inferior boundary. The base of tongue and the circumvallate papillae represent the ventral boundary, whereas the dorsal pharyngeal wall is the dorsal boundary. The lateral boundary is formed by the tonsillar fossa (see **Fig. 46.1**).[1-4]

REFERENCES

1. Chepeha DB. Reconstruction of the hypopharynx and esophagus. In: Flint PW, Haughey BH, Lund VJ, et al, eds. Cummings Otolaryngology: Head & Neck Surgery. 5th ed. Philadelphia: Elsevier; 2010
2. Gherardini G, Evans RD. Reconstruction of the oral cavity, pharynx, and esophagus. In: Thorne CH, Beasley RW, Aston SJ, et al, eds. Grabb and Smith's Plastic Surgery. 6th ed. Philadelphia: Lippincott Williams & Wilkins; 2007

3. Harreus U. Malignant neoplasms of the oropharynx. In: Flint PW, Haughey BH, Lund VJ, et al, eds. Cummings Otolaryngology: Head & Neck Surgery. 5th ed. Philadelphia: Elsevier; 2010
4. Schecter GL, Wadsworth TT. Hypopharyngeal cancer. In: Bailey BJ, ed. Head & Neck Surgery: Otolaryngology. 2nd ed. Philadelphia: Lippincott Williams & Wilkins; 1998

HYPOPHARYNGEAL ANATOMY

3. *Which one of the following is a subsite of the hypopharynx?*

    E. Piriform sinus

        The bilateral piriform sinuses represent subsites of the hypopharynx. The other subsites of the hypopharynx are the postcricoid area and the posterior hypopharyngeal wall. The soft palate, tonsils, tongue base, and oropharyngeal walls are subsites of the oropharynx.[1-3]

REFERENCES

1. Chepeha DB. Reconstruction of the hypopharynx and esophagus. In: Flint PW, Haughey BH, Lund VJ, et al, eds. Cummings Otolaryngology: Head & Neck Surgery. 5th ed. Philadelphia: Elsevier; 2010
2. Gherardini G, Evans RD. Reconstruction of the oral cavity, pharynx, and esophagus. In: Thorne CH, Beasley RW, Aston SJ, et al, eds. Grabb and Smith's Plastic Surgery. 6th ed. Philadelphia: Lippincott Williams & Wilkins; 2007
3. Schecter GL, Wadsworth TT. Hypopharyngeal cancer. In: Bailey BJ, ed. Head & Neck Surgery: Otolaryngology. 2nd ed. Philadelphia: Lippincott Williams & Wilkins; 1998

VASCULAR SUPPLY TO THE PHARYNX

4. *Which one of the external carotid artery branches do the hypopharynx, oropharynx, and nasopharynx all receive blood supply from?*

    B. Ascending pharyngeal artery

        All three of the pharyngeal subdivisions receive blood from the external carotid artery and the vessel supply they each have in common is the ascending pharyngeal artery.[1,2] The branches of the external carotid artery are:

- Ascending pharyngeal
- Facial
- Lingual
- Maxillary
- Posterior auricular
- Superficial temporal
- Superior thyroid
- Occipital

The blood supplies to the three areas of the pharynx are:

- Nasopharynx
  - Ascending pharyngeal
  - Ascending palatine (from facial)
  - Greater palatine (from maxillary)
- Oropharynx
  - Ascending pharyngeal
  - Palatine
  - Lingual
  - Facial
  - Maxillary
- Hypopharynx
  - Ascending pharyngeal
  - Superior thyroid
  - Lingual

REFERENCES

1. Williams PL, Warwick R, eds. Gray's Anatomy. 36th British ed. Philadelphia: WB Saunders; 1980
2. Gherardini G, Evans RD. Reconstruction of the oral cavity, pharynx, and esophagus. In: Thorne CH, Beasley RW, Aston SJ, et al, eds. Grabb and Smith's Plastic Surgery. 6nd ed. Philadelphia: Lippincott Williams & Wilkins; 2007

REFERRED OTALGIA IN HEAD AND NECK CANCER

5. *Which one of the following cranial nerves accounts for a patient presenting with otalgia as the only symptom of a head and neck cancer?*

B. **Vagus nerve**

A patient may present with referred otalgia in the presence of a pharyngeal tumor. This occurs because sensory fibers from the pharyngeal plexus synapse in the jugular ganglion with Arnold's nerve, which supplies the external auditory meatus. Arnold's nerve is primarily formed from the vagus, with contributions from the facial and glossopharyngeal nerves. Such patients generally require a full workup including nasopharyngoscopy and imaging.[1-3]

REFERENCES

1. Williams PL, Warwick R, eds. Gray's Anatomy. 36th British ed. Philadelphia: WB Saunders; 1980
2. Chen RC, Khorsandi AS, Shatzkes DR, Holliday RA. The radiology of referred otalgia. AJNR Am J Neuroradiol 2009;30(10):1817–1823
3. Roland NJ, Palleri V, eds. Head and Neck Cancer: Multidisciplinary Management Guidelines. 4th ed. London: ENTUK; 2011

NASOPHARYNGEAL CARCINOMA

6. *Which one of the following is not a risk factor for the development of nasopharyngeal carcinoma?*

E. **Tobacco smoking**

Although smoking is a risk factor for most head and neck cancers, this is not the case for nasopharyngeal tumors. The key risk factors are ethnicity, genetic alterations with chromosomal deletions, dietary nitrosamines, chemical fumes, wood dust, and Epstein-Barr virus. Incidence is highest in Southeast Asia where it is >30 per 100,000 population compared with 1 per 100,000 population in the US and European Caucasians. Other ethnic groups with a high incidence of nasopharyngeal carcinoma include Eskimos, Polynesian, and indigenous Mediterranean populations.[1-3]

REFERENCES

1. Tan L, Loh T. Benign and malignant tumors of the nasopharynx. In: Flint PW, Haughey BH, Lund VJ, et al, eds. Cummings Otolaryngology: Head & Neck Surgery. 5th ed. Philadelphia: Elsevier; 2010
2. Ong YK, Solares CA, Lee S, Snyderman CH, Fernandez-Miranda J, Gardner PA. Endoscopic nasopharyngectomy and its role in managing locally recurrent nasopharyngeal carcinoma. Otolaryngol Clin North Am 2011;44(5):1141–1154
3. Glastonbury CM, Salzman KL. Pitfalls in the staging of cancer of nasopharyngeal carcinoma. Neuroimaging Clin N Am 2013;23(1):9–25

CLINICAL ASSESSMENT OF NASOPHARYNGEAL CARCINOMA

7. A 50-year-old patient presents with nasal obstruction, epistaxis, and conductive hearing loss secondary to otitis media. You obtain a full history and perform a basic examination with fiberoptic nasoendoscopy, which reveals a suspicious area in the nasopharynx. *What is the next most appropriate step in management?*

B. **Examination under anesthesia and biopsy**

Patients who have visible evidence of tumor during nasoendoscopy in clinic should undergo examination under anesthesia for biopsy and formal assessment of the upper aerodigestive tract. Blind biopsies of the fossa of Rosenmüller should be performed at the same time. Once pathology is diagnosed, it should be staged using a multislice CT of the head, neck, and thorax. An MRI of the skull base is useful if the tumor is advanced. If an occult primary tumor of the nasopharynx is suspected, then a positron emission tomography-computed tomography (PET-CT) scan before biopsy is indicated. If nodal neck disease is evident (which is not the case in this patient), the enlarged node or nodes can be investigated with ultrasound-guided fine-needle aspiration cytology.[1,2]

REFERENCES

1. Roland NJ, Palleri V, eds. Head and Neck Cancer: Multidisciplinary Management Guidelines. 4th ed. London: ENTUK; 2011
2. Tan L, Loh T. Benign and malignant tumors of the nasopharynx. In: Flint PW, Haughey BH, Lund VJ, et al, eds. Cummings Otolaryngology: Head & Neck Surgery. 5th ed. Philadelphia: Elsevier; 2010

HUMAN PAPILLOMAVIRUS IN HEAD AND NECK CANCER

8. *Which one of the following tumor sites is strongly associated with human papillomavirus (HPV) 16 and 18 in younger patient groups?*
   D. Tonsils

   Oropharyngeal cancer has become increasingly common in recent years. Its incidence has doubled in the United States and the United Kingdom over the past decade. More than half of all new oropharyngeal cases are HPV-positive, and the tonsils and tongue base particularly are common subsites. Human papillomavirus (HPV) is also recognized in some oral cavity tumors such as the tongue, lip, and floor of the mouth. It also carries a better prognosis and treatment may be deescalated. HPV-associated squamous cell carcinoma disease typically presents in younger people in whom the usual risk factors for head and neck cancer (that is, high alcohol intake and smoking) are absent.[1,2]

REFERENCES

1. Roland NJ, Palleri V, eds. Head and Neck Cancer: Multidisciplinary Management Guidelines. 4th ed. London: ENTUK; 2011
2. Syrjänen S. HPV infections and tonsillar carcinoma. J Clin Pathol 2004;57(5):449–455

TYPES OF HEAD AND NECK TUMORS

9. *Which one of the following cancers has a much greater incidence in patients with Plummer-Vinson syndrome?*
   E. Hypopharyngeal

   Plummer-Vinson syndrome is a rare condition of unknown cause that is typically seen in postmenopausal, Caucasian women presenting with dysphagia, glossitis, splenomegaly, esophageal stenosis, and iron deficiency anemia. It is also associated with postcricoid cancer and esophageal cancer, which both have a much higher incidence in this population. There is no specific association with the other cancer subtypes listed. This syndrome can usually be effectively treated with iron supplementation and mechanical dilation of the esophagus where there is no evidence of malignancy. However, regular surveillance is often advised because of the risk of malignant transformation.[1]

REFERENCE

1. Novacek G. Plummer-Vinson syndrome. Orphanet J Rare Dis 2006, September 15;1:36

CLINICAL PRESENTATION IN HEAD AND NECK CANCER

10. *Which one of the following findings is particularly suspicious for nasopharyngeal carcinoma?*
    A. Unilateral otitis media and bilateral level V nodes

    Nasopharyngeal cancer most commonly presents in males between 30 and 50 years of age. More than half will present with nodal metastases. The other common presenting symptoms are neck lumps, blood in saliva, deafness, nasal obstruction, tinnitus, and cranial nerve palsy. Particular concern should be raised when any patient presents with unilateral otitis media, bilateral level V nodes, and skull base symptoms.

    Sore throat and gastroesophageal reflux tend to be associated with early stage hypopharyngeal cancer and this may too be associated with referred otalgia. Tonsillar fossa tumors of the oropharynx may present with dysphagia and jaw pain as well as otalgia. A single enlarged neck mass or referred otalgia need urgent assessment and workup. Overall, many of the pharyngeal tumors share presenting symptoms and this highlights the need for accurate and swift assessment in clinic with fine-needle aspiration of neck lumps or core biopsies followed by examination under anesthesia and targeted biopsies in conjunction with appropriate imaging.[1–4]

REFERENCES

1. Tan IB, Chang ET, Chen CJ, et al. Proceedings of the 7th Biannual International Symposium on Nasopharyngeal Carcinoma 2015: Yogyakarta, Indonesia. June 4–6, 2015. BMC Proc. 2016, April 13;10(Suppl 1):1
2. Roland NJ, Palleri V, eds. Head and Neck Cancer: Multidisciplinary Management Guidelines. 4th ed. London: ENTUK; 2011
3. Ho FC, Tham IW, Earnest A, Lee KM, Lu JJ. Patterns of regional lymph node metastasis of nasopharyngeal carcinoma: a meta-analysis of clinical evidence. BMC Cancer 2012;12(1):98
4. Lv J, Wang R, Qing Y, Du Q, Zhang T. [Magnetic resonance imaging analysis of regional lymph node metastasis in 1 298 cases of nasopharyngeal carcinoma]. Lin Chung Er Bi Yan Hou Tou Jing Wai Ke Za Zhi 2012;26(18):769–772

PHASES OF SWALLOWING

11. The process of swallowing has multiple phases. *Which one of the following represents the most important phase?*

C. **Pharyngeal**

Swallowing is the coordinated act that propels a bolus of food from the oral cavity to the esophagus while protecting the airway. It has four key phases which are the oral preparatory, oral, pharyngeal, and esophageal. There is no preparatory phase. Of these, the most important is the pharyngeal phase, as it involves the transit of food into the esophagus while providing airway protection. This key phase may be impaired in patients with pharyngeal tumors, either by the tumor mass itself or secondary to surgical or radiotherapy treatment. The pharyngeal phase is programmed and involves coordination between the medullary inputs of swallow and respiration. Respiration ceases for a fraction of a second during swallow. This requires some cortical input from tongue motion. Triggering of this phase programs five activities: closure of the velopharynx to prevent food reflux, retraction of the tongue base to propel food, contraction of the pharynx to clear residue, elevation and closure of the larynx, and opening of the cricoesophageal and upper esophageal sphincters to allow the food bolus to pass through.[1,2]

REFERENCES

1. Shaw SM, Martino R. The normal swallow: muscular and neurophysiological control. Otolaryngol Clin North Am 2013;46(6):937–956
2. Matsuo K, Palmer JB. Anatomy and physiology of feeding and swallowing: normal and abnormal. Phys Med Rehabil Clin N Am 2008;19(4):691–707, vii

EVALUATION OF SWALLOWING

12. Assessment of swallowing is vital in patients with pharyngeal carcinoma. *Which one of the following modalities provides the most comprehensive noninvasive assessment of all stages of swallowing?*

B. **Videofluoroscopy**

Swallowing may be assessed in a number of different ways. Clinically, it may be assessed at the bedside using small volumes of fluid. During the assessment, the facial, lip, tongue, laryngeal, and respiratory control can each be observed. When checking for postoperative fistula formation, the use of colored fluids can be helpful. The best modality for noninvasive assessment of all phases of the swallow is with videofluoroscopy using a contrast agent such as barium. This is because it is the only procedure that allows observation of the upper aerodigestive tract in all four stages of swallowing. Endoscopic assessment of swallow can be performed such as with the FEEST test. This is a "functional endoscopic evaluation of swallowing with sensory testing" where a trained observer uses an endoscope to watch the swallow process in real time. Sensation can be assessed with puffs of air.[1–3]

REFERENCES

1. Matsuo K, Palmer JB. Anatomy and physiology of feeding and swallowing: normal and abnormal. Phys Med Rehabil Clin N Am 2008;19(4):691–707, vii
2. Nacci A, Ursino F, La Vela R, Matteucci F, Mallardi V, Fattori B. Fiberoptic endoscopic evaluation of swallowing (FEES): proposal for informed consent. Acta Otorhinolaryngol Ital 2008;28(4):206–211
3. Aviv JE, Kaplan ST, Thomson JE, Spitzer J, Diamond B, Close LG. The safety of flexible endoscopic evaluation of swallowing with sensory testing (FEESST): an analysis of 500 consecutive evaluations. Dysphagia 2000;15(1):39–44

MANAGEMENT OF HEAD AND NECK TUMORS

13. *Which one of the following is most likely to be avoided by performing robotic surgery in patients with pharyngeal carcinoma?*

D. **Mandibulotomy**

Mandibulotomy is a technique where the mandible is split in order to obtain access to the pharynx or oral cavity in major tumor resection. It generally involves an extended neck incision (as a continuation of a neck dissection wound) passing over the chin in the midline and through the full thickness of the lower lip. The mandible is then opened like a book (mandibular swing) for access. Minimally invasive surgery with robotic assistance can avoid the need for traditional transcervical access with a mandibulotomy and mandibular swing, thereby reducing postoperative morbidity and scarring.

Transoral Robotic Surgery (TORRS) is one of a number of recent advances in the management of head and neck cancer patients. It has been performed for both tumor extirpation and reconstruction where required. Other developmental advances include free tissue transfer which has allowed more complex defects to be functionally reconstructed, selective neck dissection which has allowed preservation of unaffected lymph node basins and other key structures such as the internal jugular vein (IJV), spinal accessory, and sternocleidomastoid, and Laser surgery which has added another dimension to surgical tumor resection as an alternative to traditional blade dissection. Advances in radiotherapy with intensity modulated radiotherapy (IMRT) have meant that radiotherapy doses are more directed to the malignant tissues, resulting in less dosing to adjacent healthy tissues.

In spite of the benefits of minimally invasive robotic surgery, patients may still require soft tissue reconstruction with local or free tissue transfer, neck dissection, and postoperative radiotherapy depending on tumor type. Dental extractions are not generally performed to help access but are indicated in patients expected to undergo postoperative radiotherapy or those with poor dentition.[1,2]

REFERENCES

1. Selber JC. Transoral robotic reconstruction of oropharyngeal defects: a case series. Plast Reconstr Surg 2010;126(6):1978–1987
2. Selber JC, Robb G, Serletti JM, Weinstein G, Weber R, Holsinger FC. Transoral robotic free flap reconstruction of oropharyngeal defects: a preclinical investigation. Plast Reconstr Surg 2010;125(3):896–900

CHEMOTHERAPY AND RADIATION IN HEAD AND NECK CANCER

14. *Which one of the following tumor sites is most likely to receive chemo/radiation therapy as its primary treatment modality?*

   A. Nasopharynx

Radiation therapy is the main treatment modality for nasopharyngeal carcinoma. Surgery is usually used only in the following selected circumstances:

   • In salvage or recurrent cases
   • To obtain tissue for diagnostic purposes
   • To obtain tissue from clinically involved neck nodes
   • To treat otitis media secondary to effusion

In contrast, surgery is more commonly the first-line treatment for many of the other head and neck tumor subsites, although this will depend on the tumor type and site, as radiotherapy is also used for many patients, often in conjunction with chemotherapy.[1-3]

REFERENCES

1. Tan IB, Chang ET, Chen CJ, et al. Proceedings of the 7th Biannual International Symposium on Nasopharyngeal Carcinoma 2015: Yogyakarta, Indonesia. June 4–6, 2015. BMC Proc. 2016, April 13;10(Suppl 1):1
2. Roland NJ, Palleri V, eds. Head and Neck Cancer: Multidisciplinary Management Guidelines. 4th ed. London: ENTUK; 2011
3. Ho FC, Tham IW, Earnest A, Lee KM, Lu JJ. Patterns of regional lymph node metastasis of nasopharyngeal carcinoma: a meta-analysis of clinical evidence. BMC Cancer 2012;12(1):98

OUTCOMES IN HEAD AND NECK CANCER

15. *In general, which site has the worst oncologic outcome of all the head and neck cancers?*

   D. Hypopharynx

In general, hypopharyngeal tumors have the worst outcomes. At least three quarters of patients with hypopharyngeal tumors present late with stage III or IV disease. Patients with early disease (that is, stage I or II) are often asymptomatic at presentation but may present with gastroesophageal reflux and sore throat. Patients with advanced disease most commonly present with a neck mass. Other symptoms include dysphagia, referred otalgia, and respiratory difficulties. The 5-year survival for patients with locally invasive cancer is less than 35%.[1-4]

REFERENCES

1. Kajanti M, Mäntylä M. Carcinoma of the hypopharynx. A retrospective analysis of the treatment results over a 25-year period. Acta Oncol 1990;29(7):903–907
2. Edge SB, Compton CC. The American Joint Committee on Cancer: the 7th edition of the AJCC cancer staging manual and the future of TNM. Ann Surg Oncol 2010;17(6):1471–1474
3. Uppaluri R, Sunwoo JB. Neoplasms of the hypopharynx and cervical esophagus. In: Flint PW, Haughey BH, Lund VJ, et al, eds. Cummings Otolaryngology: Head & Neck Surgery. 5th ed. Philadelphia: Elsevier; 2010
4. Schecter GL, Wadsworth TT. Hypopharyngeal cancer. In: Bailey BJ, ed. Head & Neck Surgery: Otolaryngology. 2nd ed. Philadelphia: Lippincott Williams & Wilkins; 1998

RECONSTRUCTION OF THE HYPOPHARYNX

16. A patient has a circumferential defect after resection of a hypopharyngeal tumor. *According to the classification of Disa et al, what type of defect is this?*

B. Type II

Disa et al[1] described a classification system for defects of the hypopharynx that require reconstruction. Type I defects involve less than 50% of the circumference, type II involve more than 50% of the circumference, and type III are extensive noncircumferential defects that involve multiple anatomic levels. This is clinically relevant as reconstruction options are based on the extent of the defect created by resection. Local flaps such as pectoralis major are more often used for partial defects, while free tissue transfer flaps are used for larger and circumferential defects.

REFERENCE

1. Disa JJ, Pusic AL, Hidalgo DA, Cordeiro PG. Microvascular reconstruction of the hypopharynx: defect classification, treatment algorithm, and functional outcome based on 165 consecutive cases. Plast Reconstr Surg 2003;111(2):652–660, discussion 661–663

RECONSTRUCTION FOLLOWING TOTAL LARYNGOPHARYNGECTOMY

17. You see a patient in clinic following a total laryngopharyngectomy with reconstruction and insertion of a speech valve for treatment of a T4 tumor. The patient's speech is now reasonably clear, but the patient has a wet, coarse quality to the voice. *Which one of the following is the most likely reconstruction method used?*

E. Free jejunum flap

There are a number of reconstructive procedures used following total laryngopharyngectomy and they include free and pedicled tissue transfers. The primary purpose is to provide a conduit for food and saliva, a safe airway, and the potential for voice rehabilitation. A typical combination is to use a free flap, such as a tubed anterolateral thigh flap (ALT) or free jejunum, and then insert a prosthetic device containing a one-way valve between the posterior trachea and the anterior esophagus. This allows the creation of sound as the air is diverted into the esophagus during speech. There remains debate as to the best flap for circumferential reconstruction of the pharynx, with ALT and jejunum remaining the most popular, each having different advantages. The ALT is useful in thinner patients and is particularly versatile where complex defects are present. Speech outcomes tend to be good and surgery avoids an intraabdominal approach. The free jejunum is a good size match and the moist mucosal tube with retained peristalsis may improve swallowing function. However, the mucus production can impair speech intelligibility and may result in a wet, coarse voice. Also, the jejunum flap is thought to have a long-term reliance on the vascular pedicle and anastomosis, whereas the ALT and other fasciocutaneous flaps will generate blood supply from surrounding tissues fairly soon after reconstruction.[1-5]

REFERENCES

1. Nakatsuka T, Harii K, Asato H, Ebihara S, Yoshizumi T, Saikawa M. Comparative evaluation in pharyngo-oesophageal reconstruction: radial forearm flap compared with jejunal flap. A 10-year experience. Scand J Plast Reconstr Surg Hand Surg 1998;32(3):307–310
2. Reece GP, Schusterman MA, Miller MJ, et al. Morbidity and functional outcome of free jejunal transfer reconstruction for circumferential defects of the pharynx and cervical esophagus. Plast Reconstr Surg 1995;96(6):1307–1316
3. Robb GL, Lewin JS, Deschler DG, et al. Speech and swallowing outcomes in reconstructions of the pharynx and cervical esophagus. Head Neck 2003;25(3):232–244
4. Schusterman MA, Shestak K, de Vries EJ, et al. Reconstruction of the cervical esophagus: free jejunal transfer versus gastric pull-up. Plast Reconstr Surg 1990;85(1):16–21
5. Spyropoulou GC, Lin PY, Chien CY, Kuo YR, Jeng SF. Reconstruction of the hypopharynx with the anterolateral thigh flap: defect classification, method, tips, and outcomes. Plast Reconstr Surg 2011;127(1):161–172

RECONSTRUCTION FOLLOWING TOTAL LARYNGOPHARYNGECTOMY

18. When reconstructing a circumferential defect of the hypopharynx with a free anterolateral thigh (ALT) flap, which one of the following should be undertaken to reduce the risk of early salivary fistula formation?

D. Use of a salivary pharyngeal bypass tube

When reconstructing the pharynx with a free ALT flap, the risk of salivary fistula formation can be reduced by inserting a salivary pharyngeal bypass tube within the neopharynx, bridging both proximal and distal anastomoses. Salivary bypass tubes are clear silicone tubes, also called Montgomery[1] tubes that come in different sizes. The benefits of a bypass tube are to protect the anastomoses from saliva and stent open the neopharynx, thereby potentially also reducing the risk of stricture formation. The anastomoses are usually sutured with absorbable sutures such as Vicryl, as their presence is only required until healing has occurred, which should be 1–2 weeks during which time the patient is given nothing by mouth. Early feeding and hydration can begin with either a nasogastric or gastrostomy tube. There is no role for total parenteral nutrition (TPN) where enteral feeding is possible. Use of a proton pump inhibitor has no direct effect on fistula formation. Many patients will require postoperative radiotherapy, and this typically begins 4–6 weeks after surgery. Therefore, delaying postoperative radiotherapy is not required and of no routine benefit with regard to early fistula formation. Keeping to safe oncologic principles, radiotherapy should be started early once healing is complete. Long-term complications of radiotherapy include both stricture and fistula formation.

REFERENCE

1. Montgomery WW. Plastic esophageal tube. Ann Otol Rhinol Laryngol 1955;64(2):418–421

RECONSTRUCTION OF OROPHARYNGEAL DEFECTS

19. **Which one of the following is correct when managing patients with post-tumor resection defects of the oropharynx?**

   B. **Larger tongue base defects are more safely treated with laryngectomy.**

   The tongue base is critical for airway protection and swallowing. As such, when much of the tongue base will be sacrificed during tumor resection, a laryngectomy should be considered to decrease the risk of aspiration after treatment. Although prosthetic devices are useful for isolated hard palate defects, soft palate defects are usually best reconstructed with local or imported soft tissue. Soft palate defects larger than 50% lead to velopharyngeal insufficiency. Small pharyngeal defects can be left to heal by secondary intention or closed directly. Large defects are often best reconstructed with free tissue flaps such as the radial forearm or ALT. Local flaps may be used for oropharyngeal reconstruction but are not usually recommended for the tongue, as they can cause deformation and tethering. Furthermore, they often lack the bulk required for adequate reconstruction, and flaps such as the platysma myocutaneous flap have high complication rates. Following total or subtotal glossectomy, outcomes for speech and swallowing are typically poor and there is no proven benefit in using muscle flaps with motor reinnervation.[1-3]

REFERENCES

1. Sabri A. Oropharyngeal reconstruction: current state of the art. Curr Opin Otolaryngol Head Neck Surg 2003;11(4):251–254
2. Harreus U. Malignant neoplasms of the oropharynx. In: Flint PW, Haughey BH, Lund VJ, et al, eds. Cummings Otolaryngology: Head & Neck Surgery. 5th ed. Philadelphia: Elsevier; 2010
3. Gherardini G, Evans RD. Reconstruction of the oral cavity, pharynx, and esophagus. In: Thorne CH, Beasley RW, Aston SJ, et al, eds. Grabb and Smith's Plastic Surgery. 6th ed. Philadelphia: Lippincott Williams & Wilkins; 2007

47. Facial Reanimation

See *Essentials of Plastic Surgery*, third edition, pp. 634–655

FACIAL NERVE CLINICAL ANATOMY

1. A patient presents with a progressive left-sided facial nerve palsy. Clinical examination reveals a complete unilateral paralysis of facial mimetic muscles and loss of taste in the anterior two-thirds of the tongue. Hearing is bilaterally normal and sensation of the palate is preserved. *At which anatomic location is the causal lesion likely to be present?*
   A. Intracranially at the facial nerve nucleus
   B. Within the labyrinthine segment
   C. Within the tympanic segment
   D. Within the mastoid segment
   E. Within the parotid gland

FACIAL NERVE CLINICAL ANATOMY

2. You receive a referral letter for a patient with a diagnosis of acoustic neuroma. The letter states the patient has evidence of Hitselberger's sign. *What specifically would you expect to find when examining this patient?*
   A. Decreased taste sensation in the tongue
   B. Pain during facial movement
   C. Reduced sensation in the external auditory canal
   D. The inability to tolerate loud sounds
   E. A dry, gritty, inflamed eye

FACIAL NERVE ANATOMY

3. *Which one of the following is correct regarding the anatomy of the facial nerve?*
   A. The facial nerve nucleus originates in the medulla with the geniculate ganglion.
   B. The first part of the extratemporal nerve lies deeper in children.
   C. There are nine different branching patterns of the extratemporal nerve.
   D. The frontal nerve usually passes 0.5 cm lateral to the lateral end of the brow.
   E. Risk of traumatic shearing is greatest at the junction of labyrinthine and tympanic segments.

FACIAL MUSCULATURE

4 *Which are the three deepest facial mimetic muscles that receive innervation from their superficial surfaces?*
   A. Depressor anguli oris, zygomaticus major, and orbicularis oculi
   B. Depressor labii inferioris, risorius, and platysma
   C. Orbicularis oris, levator labii superioris, and levator labii superioris alaeque nasi
   D. Mentalis, levator anguli oris, and buccinator
   E. Mentalis, levator labii superioris, and buccinator

MUSCLES INVOVED IN SMILING

5. *Which muscle is considered to be the major contributor to production of a perceived smile?*
   A. Levator labii superioris alaeque nasi
   B. Risorius
   C. Levator anguli oris
   D. Zygomaticus major
   E. Levator labii superioris

FACIAL MIMETIC MUSCLES

6. *When treating a patient with botulinum toxin injection, which muscle should be targeted to alleviate obliquely oriented glabellar frown lines?*
   A. Corrugator
   B. Frontalis
   C. Orbicularis oculi
   D. Nasalis
   E. Risorius

IATROGENIC FACIAL NERVE INJURY

7. *Patients undergoing neck dissection need to be counseled about dysfunction of this muscle, which leads to weakness of the lower lip.*
   A. Depressor labii inferioris
   B. Platysma
   C. Mentalis
   D. Levator anguli oris
   E. Orbicularis oris

DIFFERENTIAL DIAGNOSIS OF FACIAL PARALYSIS

8. *An 80-year-old farmer presents with a progressive global unilateral facial paralysis. On examination, he has a firm palpable preauricular swelling and scarring from a partial pinnectomy. What is the most likely diagnosis?*
   A. Primary parotid malignancy
   B. Acoustic neuroma
   C. Metastatic skin cancer
   D. Pleomorphic adenoma
   E. Cholesteatoma

DIFFERENTIAL DIAGNOSIS OF FACIAL PARALYSIS

9. *A 19-year-old pregnant woman presents to her general practitioner with new-onset complete unilateral facial paralysis. She first noticed the problem on waking one morning. On examination, she has no other physical findings of note. Further investigations reveal no obvious abnormality. What is the most likely diagnosis?*
   A. Ramsay Hunt syndrome
   B. Bell's palsy
   C. Möbius syndrome
   D. Acoustic neuroma
   E. Facial myokymia

RECURRENT FACIAL PALSY

10. A 51-year-old woman presents with her third episode of unilateral facial paralysis, which has affected both sides on separate occasions. On examination, she has evidence of facial swelling and tongue fissures. *What is the most likely diagnosis?*
    A. Bell's palsy
    B. Essential blepharospasm
    C. Meige's syndrome
    D. Melkersson-Rosenthal syndrome
    E. Lyme disease

PEDIATRIC FACIAL PALSY

11. *Which one of the following statements is correct regarding pediatric facial palsy and dyskinesia?*
    A. Facial paralysis is a common finding in association with hemifacial microsomia.
    B. In congenital unilateral lower lip palsy (CULLP), the abnormality becomes apparent on crying.
    C. Hemifacial spasm is more commonly observed in children than in adults.
    D. Bell's palsy is not generally found to occur in children.
    E. Cholesteatoma is an infective process leading to dyskinesia in children.

MÖBIUS SYNDROME

12. *Which one of the following would not be expected in a patient with Möbius syndrome?*
    A. Hyperacusis
    B. Limb abnormalities
    C. Inability to abduct the eye
    D. Strabismus
    E. Small jaw

GRADING FACIAL NERVE FUNCTION

13. A patient is seen in the facial palsy clinic after being diagnosed with Bell's palsy. Examination shows complete eye closure with some effort, moderate weakness of the forehead, and the ability to achieve oral competence with maximum effort. *What is the most likely facial palsy grading according to the House-Brackmann scale?*
    A. II
    B. III
    C. IV
    D. V
    E. VI

SURGICAL MANAGEMENT OF FACIAL PALSY

14. A 40-year-old man presents with incompletely resolved Bell's palsy of 5 years' duration that affects his left brow, resulting in ptosis on this side only. This is now starting to affect vision and cosmesis. He has a full head of hair. *How might this be best managed from an aesthetic perspective?*
    A. Upper eyelid blepharoplasty
    B. Tarsorrhaphy
    C. Corneal neurotization
    D. Canthoplasty or an eyelid-shortening procedure
    E. Endoscopic brow lift

EYE SURGERY IN FACIAL PALSY

15. A 53-year-old woman is unable to fully close her right eye 16 months after facial nerve injury. The eye is mildly inflamed, with evidence of epiphora. *How might this be best managed in the longer term?*
    A. Conservatively with regular lubrication
    B. Chemodenervation with botulinum toxin
    C. Tarsorrhaphy
    D. Insertion of gold weight
    E. Upper blepharoplasty

SURGICAL MANAGEMENT OF FACIAL PALSY

16. A patient has lower eyelid ectropion 1 month after a left-sided facial nerve palsy. Examination shows laxity of the lower eyelid soft tissues, corneal irritation, and epiphora. There is no obvious anterior lamella deficiency. *Which one of the following is indicated for this patient?*
    A. Lower eyelid blepharoplasty
    B. Lateral tarsal strip and canthopexy
    C. Tripier flap
    D. Tarsorrhaphy
    E. Frost stitch

SURGICAL APPROACHES TO FACIAL REANIMATION

17. A young adult presents 3 years after iatrogenic damage of the facial nerve and wishes to have facial reanimation surgery to improve resting symmetry and recreate a dynamic smile. *Which one of the following muscle transfer procedures would be most indicated for this patient?*
    A. Temporalis
    B. Masseter
    C. Digastric muscle
    D. Gracilis muscle
    E. Partial rectus abdominis

SURGICAL APPROACHES TO FACIAL REANIMATION

18. A patient presents with partial facial nerve paralysis after a recent wound to the preauricular region. *What surgical intervention is recommended in this case?*
    A. Direct nerve repair
    B. Ipsilateral nerve graft
    C. Cross-face nerve graft
    D. Muscle transfer
    E. Fascial sling

SURGICAL MANAGEMENT OF FACIAL PALSY

19. In a 45-year-old patient with segmental extratemporal facial nerve loss following radical parotidectomy, which one of the following is the most suitable immediate reconstruction method if spontaneous facial movement is desired?
    A. Direct nerve repair
    B. Cross-face nerve graft
    C. Ipsilateral facial nerve graft
    D. Hypoglossal nerve transfer
    E. Spinal accessory nerve transfer

SURGERY IN FACIAL PALSY

20. Which one of the following techniques may be most useful in patients who have sustained marginal mandibular nerve injury?
    A. Temporalis transfer
    B. Masseter transfer
    C. Gracilis transfer
    D. Digastric transfer
    E. Fascia lata slings

Answers

FACIAL NERVE CLINICAL ANATOMY

1. A patient presents with a progressive left-sided facial nerve palsy. Clinical examination reveals a complete unilateral paralysis of facial mimetic muscles and loss of taste in the anterior two-thirds of the tongue. Hearing is bilaterally normal and sensation of the palate is preserved. *At which anatomic location is the causal lesion likely to be present?*

D. Within the mastoid segment

The path of the facial nerve can be divided into three main segments: intracranial, intratemporal, and extratemporal. This is clinically relevant as knowledge of the anatomy can help identify the site of damage or compression of the nerve. There are no branches within the intracranial segment, so a lesion at this site would cause complete loss of facial nerve function with no sparing of individual branches. The intratemporal segment has three subdivisions: labyrinthine, tympanic, and mastoid (**Fig. 47.1**). Four nerve branches are given off within this region in the following order: the greater petrosal nerve (within the labyrinthine section), the nerve to stapedius, the sensory branch to the external auditory canal, and the branch to chorda tympani (within the mastoid section). The patient described has a lesion affecting the chorda tympani and the extratemporal nerve, with sparing of the greater petrosal nerve, the nerve to stapedius, and the nerve to external auditory meatus. Therefore, the lesion is located within the distal mastoid segment. A lesion within the parotid would spare all four of the intratemporal branches.[1-4]

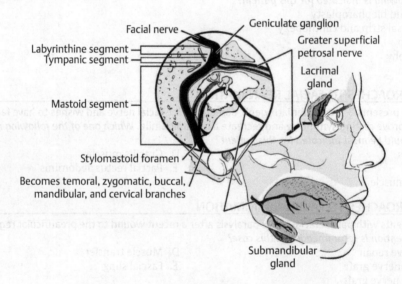

Fig. 47.1 Anatomy and relations of the facial nerve.

REFERENCES

1. Lysek M. Anatomy of the facial nerve. In: Nerves and Nerve Injuries, Vol. 1. April 23, 2015
2. Chu EA, Byrne PJ. Treatment considerations in facial paralysis. Facial Plast Surg 2008;24(2):164–169
3. Gosain AK. Surgical anatomy of the facial nerve. Clin Plast Surg 1995;22(2):241–251
4. Alford BR, Jerger JF, Coats AC, Peterson CR, Weber SC. Neurophysiology of facial nerve testing. Arch Otolaryngol 1973;97(2):214–219

FACIAL NERVE CLINICAL ANATOMY

2. You receive a referral letter for a patient with a diagnosis of acoustic neuroma. The letter states the patient has evidence of Hitselberger's sign. *What specifically would you expect to find when examining this patient?*

C. Reduced sensation in the external auditory canal

Hitselberger's sign refers to hypesthesia of the external auditory canal, secondary to compression or damage to the sensory branch of the facial nerve within the mastoid segment of the intratemporal nerve pathway.[1] Hitselberger and House[1] described this in 1966 as an early diagnostic indicator of acoustic neuroma formation. Decreased taste sensation in the tongue would occur secondary to compression of the chorda tympani, which joins the lingual nerve to supply parasympathetic innervations to the submandibular and sublingual glands, as well as taste to the anterior two-thirds of the tongue. Pain during facial movement is more likely to be associated with trigeminal or dental pain rather than facial nerve compression. Sound dampening is controlled by the nerve to stapedius which originates in the mastoid segment. A dry, gritty eye may well be present in association with a facial nerve palsy as a result of the incomplete eye closure and loss of the corneal reflex but is not specific to Hitselberger's sign.[1,2]

REFERENCES

1. Hitselberger WE, House WF. Acoustic neuroma diagnosis. External auditory canal hypesthesia as an early sign. Arch Otolaryngol 1966;83(3):218–221
2. Alford BR, Jerger JF, Coats AC, Peterson CR, Weber SC. Neurophysiology of facial nerve testing. Arch Otolaryngol 1973;97(2):214–219

FACIAL NERVE ANATOMY

3. Which one of the following is correct regarding the anatomy of the facial nerve?

E. Risk of traumatic shearing is greatest at the junction of labyrinthine and tympanic segments.

The junction between the labyrinthine and tympanic segments is formed by an acute angle, and shearing commonly occurs at this site. In addition, the labyrinthine segment is also the narrowest part so the nerve is at greatest risk of compression, secondary to edema at this site. The facial nerve nucleus is located in the dorsolateral pons, not the medulla; and the geniculate ganglion is present within the intratemporal segment. The first part of the extratemporal facial nerve lies more superficially in children under the age of 2 and is therefore more prone to injury at this site.

Davis et al[1] described six (not nine) different extratemporal facial nerve branching patterns. Of these, type III is the most common, representing 28%. The common theme is that after exiting the stylomastoid foramen, branches are given off to supply the posterior belly of digastric and occipitalis muscles. Then the main nerve trunk divides into superior and inferior segments which collectively form the facial nerve branches most commonly recognized: temporal, zygomatic, buccal, marginal mandibular, and cervical. The surface marking for the temporal nerve passes from 0.5 cm below the tragus to 1.5 cm above the lateral brow. This is referred to as *Pitanguy's line* (**Fig. 47.2**).[2,3]

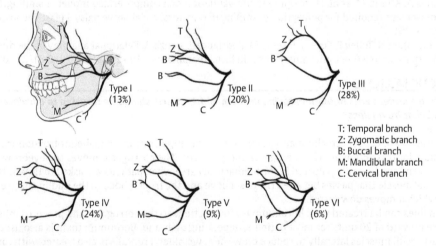

Fig. 47.2 Facial nerve branching patterns. (Adapted from Davis RA, Anson BJ, Budinger JM, et al. Surgical anatomy of the facial nerve and parotid gland based upon a study of 350 cerviofacial halves. Surg Gynecol Obstet 102:385, 1956.)

REFERENCES

1. Davis RA, Anson BJ, Budinger JM, Kurth LR. Surgical anatomy of the facial nerve and parotid gland based upon a study of 350 cervicofacial halves. Surg Gynecol Obstet 1956;102(4):385–412
2. Pitanguy I, Ramos AS. The frontal branch of the facial nerve: the importance of its variations in face lifting. Plast Reconstr Surg 1966;38(4):352–356
3. Gosain AK. Surgical anatomy of the facial nerve. Clin Plast Surg 1995;22(2):241–251

FACIAL MUSCULATURE

4. *Which are the three deepest facial mimetic muscles that receive innervation from their superficial surfaces?*

    D. Mentalis, levator anguli oris, and buccinator

The mentalis, levator anguli oris, and buccinator muscles represent the deepest layer of facial musculature and receive their innervation on their superficial surfaces. All other muscles receive innervation on their deep surface. The facial musculature comprises 23 paired muscles and single orbicularis oris, grouped into four layers. Those described in option A (depressor anguli oris, zygomaticus major, and orbicularis oculi) represent layer one and are the most superficial. Those in option B (depressor labii inferioris, risorius, and platysma) include some of the muscles in layer two. Layer three contains only two muscles: orbicularis oris and levator labii superioris.[1,2]

REFERENCES

1. Moore KL, Dalley AF, eds. Clinically Oriented Anatomy. 4th ed. New York, NY: Lippincott, Williams, and Wilkins; 1999
2. Zabojova J, Thrikutam N, Tolley P, Perez J, Rozen SM, Rodriguez-Lorenzo A. Relational anatomy of the mimetic muscles and its implications on free functional muscle inset in facial reanimation. Ann Plast Surg 2018;81(2):203–207

MUSCLES INVOVED IN SMILING

5. *Which muscle is considered to be the major contributor to production of a perceived smile?*

    D. Zygomaticus major

There are a number of facial mimetic muscles involved in producing a smile, but

the major muscle involved is the zygomaticus major. One particular study has shown that observers perceive a smile when the zygomaticus major functions to achieve 40% of its maximal movement.[1] The zygomaticus minor also has an important contribution to a smile and these two muscles work together to elevate the corner of the mouth and the upper lips as they pass obliquely across the central face between the zygoma to the upper lip. The levator labii superioris alaeque nasi contributes to smile by elevating the medial nasolabial fold and nasal alae. The risorius aids the smile with lateral pull and is more pronounced is some individuals. The levator anguli oris pulls the angle of the mouth upward and medially. The levator labii superioris elevates the upper lip and midportion of the nasolabial fold.[1,2]

REFERENCES

1. Penn JW, James A, Khatib M, et al. Development and validation of a computerized model of smiling: modeling the percentage movement required for perception of smiling in unilateral facial nerve palsy. J Plast Reconstr Aesthet Surg 2013;66(3):345–351
2. Zabojova J, Thrikutam N, Tolley P, Perez J, Rozen SM, Rodriguez-Lorenzo A. Relational anatomy of the mimetic muscles and its implications on free functional muscle inset in facial reanimation. Ann Plast Surg 2018;81(2):203–207

FACIAL MIMETIC MUSCLES

6. *When treating a patient with botulinum toxin injection, which muscle should be targeted to alleviate obliquely oriented glabellar frown lines?*

    A. Corrugator

Some patients are concerned about appearing tired or grumpy because of glabellar frown lines. The muscles responsible for this action are the corrugator and procerus. The corrugator moves the eyebrow medially and downward and can be easily palpated in the medial brow area when patients are asked to frown. The procerus is a pyramidal muscle that passes between the nasal bone and the frontal bone in the midline between the medial brows, which it moves downward.

Frown lines can be treated with botulinum toxin injections to the corrugator and procerus muscles. Starting doses are upward of 20 units for most patients, depending on brand. Botulinum toxin is also used to target the orbicularis oculi muscles laterally to reduce crow's feet wrinkles. Frontalis is also treated with toxin to smooth out wrinkles, particularly in the midline, but care must be taken to avoid lateral and low injection as this can lead to unwanted brow ptosis. The nasalis either flares or dilates the nostrils. The risorius is a muscle that aids lateral pull of the smile. These two muscles would not typically be treated with neurotoxin.[1-4]

REFERENCES

1. Yoelin SG, Aguilera SB, Cohen JL, et al. ABOUT FACE: navigating neuromodulators and injection techniques for optimal results. J Drugs Dermatol 2020;19(4):s5–s15
2. Kordestani R, Small KH, Rohrich RJ. Advancements and refinement in facial neuromodulators. Plast Reconstr Surg 2016;138(4):803–806

3. Nestor MS, Fischer DL, Arnold D. "Masking" our emotions: botulinum toxin, facial expression, and well-being in the age of COVID-19. J Cosmet Dermatol 2020;19(9):2154–2160

4. Freilinger G, Gruber H, Happak W, Pechmann U. Surgical anatomy of the mimic muscle system and the facial nerve: importance for reconstructive and aesthetic surgery. Plast Reconstr Surg 1987;80(5):686–690

IATROGENIC FACIAL NERVE INJURY

7. *Patients undergoing neck dissection need to be counseled about dysfunction of this muscle, which leads to weakness of the lower lip.*

A. **Depressor labii inferioris**

During a neck dissection (particularly level I clearance), the marginal mandibular nerve is at risk of damage because it frequently lies below the lower mandibular border deep to platysma. Damage to this nerve results in elevation of the lower lip on the affected side from paralysis of the depressor labii inferioris. Subsequent treatment can involve injection of botulinum toxin to the depressor labii inferioris on the unaffected side or surgical transfer of the anterior belly of digastric to the lower lip.[1] Platysma receives innervation from the cervical branch of the facial nerve and may be denervated during neck dissection; however, this is not usually of any great clinical concern, so less emphasis is placed on this nerve branch's preservation.

Mentalis is also innervated by the marginal mandibular nerve, but dysfunction tends to be well masked. This muscle pulls the skin of the chin upward. Levator anguli oris pulls the mouth upward, not downward, and is innervated by the buccal branches. Orbicularis oris forms the oral opening and functions to close and compress lips in order to achieve an oral seal. It also receives innervation from the buccal branches.

REFERENCE

1. Tan ST. Anterior belly of digastric muscle transfer: a useful technique in head and neck surgery. Head Neck 2002;24(10):947–954

DIFFERENTIAL DIAGNOSIS OF FACIAL PARALYSIS

8. An 80-year-old farmer presents with a progressive global unilateral facial paralysis. On examination, he has a firm palpable preauricular swelling and scarring from a partial pinnectomy. *What is the most likely diagnosis?*

C. **Metastatic skin cancer**

This man is likely to have a malignancy within the parotid and this must be fully investigated. This clinical presentation can indicate a primary malignancy; however, given his previous partial pinnectomy (presumably for a squamous cell carcinoma of the ear), he is likely to have metastatic disease that has spread to the parotid. This is a common pathway for such disease. In general, presentation with a facial paralysis is a poor prognostic sign and treatment involves parotidectomy at a minimum, often combined with neck dissection, skin resection, and reconstruction. Postoperative radiotherapy may also be indicated. Primary facial reanimation surgery may be incorporated into the surgical plan with static or dynamic midface support, lower eyelid suspension, and brow lifting. Benign parotid tumors such as pleomorphic salivary adenomas typically present in younger patients without facial nerve involvement. Acoustic neuroma would most often present with unilateral hearing loss or tinnitus. Other symptoms typically include vertigo, headache, or ataxia, rather than a parotid swelling. Facial nerve symptoms are observed in a small number of patients at presentation. Cholesteatoma also tends to present with hearing problems as with acoustic neuroma, and facial paralysis is a less common presenting sign. Again parotid swelling would not be expected. Both of these conditions can result in facial nerve paralysis following surgery to remove the primary tumors, and plastic surgeons may only become involved at this stage.[1,2]

REFERENCES

1. O'Brien CJ. The parotid gland as a metastatic basin for cutaneous cancer. Arch Otolaryngol Head Neck Surg 2005;131(7):551–555

2. Haksever M, Akduman D, Demir M, Aslan S, Yanılmaz M, Solmaz F. The treatment of neck and parotid gland in cutaneous squamous cell carcinoma of face and forehead and the review of literature. Ann Med Surg (Lond) 2015;4(1):48–52

DIFFERENTIAL DIAGNOSIS OF FACIAL PARALYSIS

9. A 19-year-old pregnant woman presents to her general practitioner with new-onset complete unilateral facial paralysis. She first noticed the problem on waking one morning. On examination, she has no other physical findings of note. Further investigations reveal no obvious abnormality. *What is the most likely diagnosis?*

B. **Bell's palsy**

The most common cause of facial palsy is Bell's palsy, representing around 85% of cases, and this is a diagnosis of exclusion. It is usually self-limiting and is treated with steroids with or without antiviral medications. The risk of Bell's palsy is significantly increased during pregnancy. Given that this patient has negative findings clinically, on further investigation, Bell's palsy would be the diagnosis given here. The proposed cause of Bell's palsy is viral–vascular insult which causes swelling in the temporal segment and subsequent facial nerve impairment. Ramsay Hunt syndrome is an alternative diagnosis in this patient when otalgia or a facial rash is present. This is caused by varicella zoster virus and is treated accordingly with steroids and acyclovir. Möbius syndrome is a congenital condition associated with bilateral facial nerve absence. Acoustic neuromas present with unilateral hearing loss or vertigo and headaches. Facial myokymia involves continuous undulating, writhing contraction of facial muscles and may be caused by multiple sclerosis, polyradiculopathy, or peripheral nerve injury.[1,2]

REFERENCES

1. de Almeida JR, Guyatt GH, Sud S, et al; Bell Palsy Working Group, Canadian Society of Otolaryngology - Head and Neck Surgery and Canadian Neurological Sciences Federation. Management of Bell palsy: clinical practice guideline. CMAJ 2014;186(12):917–922
2. Somasundara D, Sullivan F. Management of Bell's palsy. Aust Prescr 2017;40(3):94–97

RECURRENT FACIAL PALSY

10. A 51-year-old woman presents with her third episode of unilateral facial paralysis, which has affected both sides on separate occasions. On examination, she has evidence of facial swelling and tongue fissures. *What is the most likely diagnosis?*

   D. Melkersson-Rosenthal syndrome
   Melkersson-Rosenthal syndrome involves recurrent facial paralysis that may alternate sides. The cause is unknown, and treatment is usually conservative. Nerve decompression should be considered in some cases. Bell's palsy is a diagnosis of exclusion and could explain this presentation but would not include the other clinical findings.[1,2] Essential blepharospasm involves an involuntary spastic eyelid closure rather than facial weakness. Meige's syndrome involves blepharospasm, grimacing mouth movements, and tongue protrusion, again without facial nerve paralysis.[3] The most common cause of bilateral facial paralysis is Lyme disease which is itself caused by the spirochete *Borrelia burgdorferi*.[4]

REFERENCES

1. Dhawan SR, Saini AG, Singhi PD. Management strategies of Melkersson-Rosenthal syndrome: a review. Int J Gen Med 2020;13:61–65
2. Cirpaciu D, Goanta CM, Cirpaciu MD. Recurrences of Bell's palsy. J Med Life 2014;7 Spec No. 3(Spec Iss 3):68–77
3. Owecki MK, Bogusz H, Magowska A. Henri Meige (1866–1940). J Neurol 2017;264(11):2348–2350
4. Bamm VV, Ko JT, Mainprize IL, Sanderson VP, Wills MKB. Lyme disease frontiers: reconciling *Borrelia* biology and clinical conundrums. Pathogens 2019;8(4):299

PEDIATRIC FACIAL PALSY

11. *Which one of the following statements is correct regarding pediatric facial palsy and dyskinesia?*

   B. In congenital unilateral lower lip palsy (CULLP), the abnormality becomes apparent on crying.
   Congenital unilateral lower lip palsy (CULLP) affects the marginal mandibular branch on one side only with the remainder of the facial nerve branches intact. There is normal resting tone in the facial muscles and the condition results in an asymmetrical appearance of the lower lip, particularly noticeable when the child cries. Facial paralysis is only present in a small proportion of patients with hemifacial microsomia. Hemifacial spasm is usually seen in middle-aged and elderly adults and reports in children are rare. It is a disorder of the seventh cranial nerve, characterized by irregular, involuntary, and recurrent tonic and clonic contractions of the ipsilateral muscles of facial expression. The cause is usually vascular compression at the brainstem, but can be seen secondary to other tumors.[1] Bell's palsy is a diagnosis of exclusion and is observed in children as well as adults. Cholesteatoma is a localized expanding tumor of the middle ear with keratinizing squamous epithelium that can cause facial nerve palsy in both children and adults. It is not an infective process, but can be associated with or confused with chronic episodes of otitis media.[1]

REFERENCE

1. Masruha MR, Fialho LM, da Nóbrega MV, et al. Hemifacial spasm as a manifestation of pilocytic astrocytoma in a pediatric patient. J Pediatr Neurosci 2011;6(1):72–73

MÖBIUS SYNDROME

12. Which one of the following would not be expected in a patient with Möbius syndrome?

A. Hyperacusis

Möbius syndrome is a congenital condition involving absence of the facial (CN VII) and abducens (CN VI) nerves. This results in facial paralysis, the inability to abduct the eye, and subsequent strabismus. Other cranial nerves may also be affected. Limb abnormalities such as club foot and micrognathia are quite often present. However, hyperacusis is not seen because the cell bodies of the nerve to stapedius are not located in the facial nerve nucleus; therefore, its function is preserved.[1,2]

REFERENCES

1. Morales-Chávez M, Ortiz-Rincones MA, Suárez-Gorrin F. Surgical techniques for smile restoration in patients with Möbius syndrome. J Clin Exp Dent 2013;5(4):e203–e207
2. Parker DL, Mitchell PR, Holmes GL. Poland-Möbius syndrome. J Med Genet 1981;18(4):317–320

GRADING FACIAL NERVE FUNCTION

13. A patient is seen in the facial palsy clinic after being diagnosed with Bell's palsy. Examination shows complete eye closure with some effort, moderate weakness of the forehead, and the ability to achieve oral competence with maximum effort. *What is the most likely facial palsy grading according to the House-Brackmann scale?*

B. III

The House-Brackmann scale categorizes facial nerve function into six grades (I to VI).[1] Grade I is normal facial nerve function, and grade VI is a total paralysis. The remaining grades pass from mild to severe. Each grade is based on gross appearance and motion. Gross appearance assesses muscle power, asymmetry, and tone. Motion assesses forehead, eye, and mouth movement. This patient is classified as having moderate dysfunction according to this scale.

House-Brackman Scale:

- Grade I: Normal facial function
- Grade II: Mild dysfunction
  Gross: Slight weakness on close inspection, normal at rest
  Motion: Forehead, slight to moderate; eye, complete closure with effort; mouth, slightly weak with maximum effort
- Grade III: Moderate dysfunction
  Gross: Obvious but not disfiguring, normal asymmetry and tone at rest
  Motion: Forehead, slight to moderate; eye, complete closure with effort; mouth, slightly weak with maximum effort
- Grade IV: Moderately severe
  Gross: Obvious weakness with disfiguring asymmetry at rest
  Motion: Forehead, none; eye, incomplete closure; mouth, asymmetrical with maximum effort
- Grade V: Severe dysfunction
  Gross: Only barely perceptible motion, asymmetry at rest
  Motion: Forehead, none; eye, incomplete closure; mouth, slight movement
- Grade VI: Total paralysis
  No movement

Other grading systems include the Burres-Fisch and Sunnybrook systems. The latter has become a popular alternative as an objective measuring tool in facial paralysis patients. It has three components: resting symmetry, symmetry of voluntary movement, and synkinesis.[2,3] Comparison is based on the normal side. Assessment of the symmetry of voluntary movement involves five areas: the forehead wrinkle (raising eyebrows), gentle eye closure, open-mouth smile, snarl, and lip pucker. Patients with normal resting symmetry and those with no synkinesis will have a score of zero on this subsection. The composite or final score is calculated by assessing the symmetry of voluntary movement and then subtracting resting symmetry and synkinesis scores. A patient with no evidence of facial palsy should have a score of 100.[1–3]

REFERENCES

1. House JW, Brackmann DE. Facial nerve grading system. Otolaryngol Head Neck Surg 1985;93(2):146–147
2. Ross BG, Fradet G, Nedzelski JM. Development of a sensitive clinical facial grading system. Otolaryngol Head Neck Surg 1996;114(3):380–386
3. Coulson SE, Croxson GR, Adams RD, O'Dwyer NJ. Reliability of the "Sydney," "Sunnybrook," and "House Brackmann" facial grading systems to assess voluntary movement and synkinesis after facial nerve paralysis. Otolaryngol Head Neck Surg 2005;132(4):543–549

SURGICAL MANAGEMENT OF FACIAL PALSY

14. A 40-year-old man presents with incompletely resolved Bell's palsy of 5 years' duration that affects his left brow, resulting in ptosis on this side only. This is now starting to affect vision and cosmesis. He has a full head of hair. *How might this be best managed from an aesthetic perspective?*

E. Endoscopic brow lift

Patients with frontal branch weakness are at high risk of developing brow ptosis, which can be treated with a brow-lift procedure. This candidate is young and probably prefers to minimize visible scarring on the brow. For this reason, an endoscopic approach is probably most favored as the scars are small and well hidden, sensation is retained, alopecia risk is low, and recovery should be fairly quick. Alternative options include open coronal lift, direct mid or lower forehead lift (superciliary), and transpalpebral approaches. The transpalpebral approach can work well with scars hidden in the upper eyelid fold. The other options will leave visible scarring in the forehead. The method of fixation of the brow is probably as important as the approach and once adequate release of the brow soft tissues has been achieved, the brow can be sutured internally from orbicularis to frontalis periosteum or directly to bone with a variety of bone-anchored devices such as Mitek™ or Endotine™, or with screws or drill holes.[1,2] Corneal neurotization can be helpful to protect the globe following facial nerve injury, but will not help brow ptosis. It involves coaptation of the supraorbital and supratrochlear nerves from the contralateral trigeminal to the cornea of the facial palsy eye in order to provide protective sensation on that side.[3]

Tarsorrhaphy is a surgical technique that joins part or all of the upper and lower eyelids to partially or completely close the eye. Temporary tarsorrhaphies are used for protection of the cornea during a short period of exposure or disease. Permanent tarsorraphies are used to protect the cornea from a long-term risk of damage such as where there is facial nerve paralysis, which is unlikely to recover. A permanent tarsorrhaphy usually only closes the lateral (outer) eyelids, so that the patient can still see through the central opening and the eye can still be examined. It tends to round the lateral canthal area and so is not aesthetically pleasing.

REFERENCES

1. Adetayo OA, Wong WW, Motakef S, Frew TG, Campwala I, Gupta SC. Endoscopic brow lift fixation with Mitek suture anchors: a 9-year experience of a new "ideal" technique. Plast Surg (Oakv) 2019;27(2):100–106
2. Karimi N, Kashkouli MB, Sianati H, Khademi B. Techniques of eyebrow lifting: a narrative review. J Ophthalmic Vis Res 2020;15(2):218–235
3. Terzis JK, Dryer MM, Bodner BI. Corneal neurotization: a novel solution to neurotrophic keratopathy. Plast Reconstr Surg 2009;123(1):112–120

EYE SURGERY IN FACIAL PALSY

15. A 53-year-old woman is unable to fully close her right eye 16 months after facial nerve injury. The eye is mildly inflamed, with evidence of epiphora. *How might this be best managed in the longer term?*

D. Insertion of gold weight

Patients with long-standing facial nerve paralysis are at risk of damage of their eyes from incomplete eye closure and loss of blink reflex. Insertion of a gold or platinum weight into the upper eyelid is a technique commonly used to assist with eye closure. The disadvantages are that closure can remain incomplete when a patient is supine, because gravity is not acting to close the eye, the weight may be palpable and visible, and the weight can displace over time. Some patients simply find them uncomfortable and prefer to have them removed after placement. Conservative management with lubrication of the cornea is important but it alone is not the ideal long-term plan.

Chemodenervation with botulinum toxin of levator palpebrae superioris or Muller's muscle is possible, but will risk unwanted or excessive ptosis and inability to open the eyelid adequately. Tarsorrhaphy should not be used as a primary treatment as it is cosmetically disfiguring and reduces the visual field. Upper eyelid blepharoplasty risks making the problem worse as it could leave the eye with insufficient eyelid skin to close (lagophthalmos). For this reason, very careful consideration must be given prior to proceeding with blepharoplasty in facial palsy patients.[1–3]

REFERENCES

1. Neuman AR, Weinberg A, Sela M, Peled IJ, Wexler MR. The correction of seventh nerve palsy lagophthalmos with gold lid load (16 years experience). Ann Plast Surg 1989;22(2):142–145
2. O'Connell JE, Robin PE. Eyelid gold weights in the management of facial palsy. J Laryngol Otol 1991;105(6):471–474
3. Seiff SR, Chang J. Management of ophthalmic complications of facial nerve palsy. Otolaryngol Clin North Am 1992;25(3):669–690

SURGICAL MANAGEMENT OF FACIAL PALSY

16. A patient has lower eyelid ectropion 1 month after a left-sided facial nerve palsy. Examination shows laxity of the lower eyelid soft tissues, corneal irritation, and epiphora. There is no obvious anterior lamella deficiency. *Which one of the following is indicated for this patient?*

 B. Lateral tarsal strip and canthopexy

  Lower eyelid laxity is a common problem in facial palsy patients because of atrophic changes in the orbicularis oculi. Various techniques can be used to tighten or shorten the lower eyelid to reduce ectropion and corneal exposure. Tightening of the canthal tendon with a lateral tarsal strip and canthopexy or canthoplasty can be helpful. In doing this procedure, it is important to ensure that the lateral canthal tendon is lifted deeply and posteriorly into the orbital socket so the eyelid is not pulled away from the globe. This is usually achieved by lifting a periosteal flap from the lateral orbital rim and following this medially into the orbit. The canthal tendon can then be secured to this periosteum for support with a permanent suture. The tarsal strip involves removing the epithelial surface of the canthal tendon (skin/mucosa) so the tendon end can be buried deeply in the orbit as described. A canthopexy involves tightening of the tendon without dividing it, whereas a canthoplasty involves formal division and repositioning of the canthal tendon. A lower eyelid blepharoplasty may include elements of canthal resuspension but this patient is unlikely to have an excess of lower eyelid skin/tissue, but rather flaccid tissue. Therefore, blepharoplasty is not indicated here. If the patient had a cicatricial ectropion with deficiency of the anterior lamella (skin and/or orbicularis muscle) then importation of additional skin such as a full-thickness graft or Tripier transposition flap would be indicated. However, this is not the primary problem in this case. A Frost stitch is part of the surgical procedure in some lower eyelid suspension approaches and it is a temporary suture which holds the eyelids closed. This alone will only help such a problem unless the paralysis is expected to be transient.[1-3]

REFERENCES

1. Custer PL. Ophthalmic management of the facial palsy patient. Semin Plast Surg 2004;18(1):31–38
2. Seiff SR, Chang J. Management of ophthalmic complications of facial nerve palsy. Otolaryngol Clin North Am 1992;25(3):669–690
3. Bergeron CM, Moe KS. The evaluation and treatment of lower eyelid paralysis. Facial Plast Surg 2008;24(2):231–241

SURGICAL APPROACHES TO FACIAL REANIMATION

17. A young adult presents 3 years after iatrogenic damage of the facial nerve and wishes to have facial reanimation surgery to improve resting symmetry and recreate a dynamic smile. *Which one of the following muscle transfer procedures would be most indicated for this patient?*

 D. Gracilis muscle

  The basic principles of facial reanimation surgery are to provide innervation to the mimetic muscles if they are viable, or to supplement them when absent with a muscle transfer. After a period of 3 years, the facial mimetic muscles atrophy and have no potential for useful function even if reinnervated. In this case, a new muscle must be imported to provide dynamic facial movement for "smile surgery." Muscle transfers can be either regional or free tissue subtypes. Regional options include temporalis, masseter, or anterior belly of digastric. Free tissue transfers include gracilis (which is the most favored option), pectoralis minor, partial latissimus dorsi, or partial rectus abdominis. Nerve supply for the free muscle transfers may be provided by the contralateral facial nerve, the hypoglossal nerve, or the nerve to masseter.

  The gracilis is the preferred choice because the excursion suites the requirement to replicate that of zygomaticus major well, it allows a two-team approach, it has a reliable vascular and nerve pedicle, there is no donor site functional loss, harvest is straightforward, and the muscle can be safely thinned to decrease bulk. In general, free tissue transfers are felt to offer the best option for younger patients like in this case to achieve a spontaneous smile.[1,2] Temporalis and masseter are both regional options that can work well but tend to be reserved for older individuals or those who do not want the associated risks of free tissue transfer. They are most often not able to produce a spontaneous smile. Digastric transfer is specific to lower lip dysfunction rather than overall dynamic smile surgery.[3]

REFERENCES

1. Boahene KO, Owusu J, Ishii L, et al. The multivector gracilis free functional muscle flap for facial reanimation. JAMA Facial Plast Surg 2018;20(4):300–306
2. Chuang DC, Lu JC, Chang TN, Laurence VG. Comparison of functional results after cross-face nerve graft-, spinal accessory nerve-, and masseter nerve-innervated gracilis for facial paralysis reconstruction: the Chang Gung experience. Ann Plast Surg 2018;81(6S, Suppl 1):S21–S29
3. Tan ST. Anterior belly of digastric muscle transfer: a useful technique in head and neck surgery. Head Neck 2002;24(10):947–954

SURGICAL APPROACHES TO FACIAL REANIMATION

18. A patient presents with partial facial nerve paralysis after a recent wound to the preauricular region. *What surgical intervention is recommended in this case?*

A. **Direct nerve repair**

In this scenario, direct nerve repair is the best option. It may be worthwhile considering the babysitter procedure as well if an extended denervation time is anticipated in complete transection cases (partial hypoglossal nerve to facial nerve branch). Nerve axons typically regenerate at 1 mm per day so the time to reinnervation depends on the distance of nerve regrowth required. An ipsilateral nerve graft is only indicated where there is nerve loss, that is, repair cannot be made directly or is under tension. A cross-face nerve graft is indicated when the proximal stump of the facial nerve is unavailable for grafting, but a distal stump is present. Neither muscle transfer or fascial slings are indicated in this setting.[1,2]

REFERENCES

1. Humphrey CD, Kriet JD. Nerve repair and cable grafting for facial paralysis. Facial Plast Surg 2008;24(2):170–176
2. Terzis JK, Konofaos P. Nerve transfers in facial palsy. Facial Plast Surg 2008;24(2):177–193

SURGICAL MANAGEMENT OF FACIAL PALSY

19. *In a 45-year-old patient with segmental extratemporal facial nerve loss following radical parotidectomy, which one of the following is the most suitable immediate reconstruction method if spontaneous facial movement is desired?*

C. **Ipsilateral facial nerve graft**

This patient should have both proximal and distal nerve stumps available for grafting and the motor end plates and facial mimetic muscles will be suitable for reinnervation given the immediate reconstruction planned. In this case, interpositional nerve grafting using either sural, great auricular, or antebrachial nerves is indicated. This is most likely to provide spontaneous facial movement in the longer term. Direct repair is clearly not an option given the nerve substance loss. A cross-face nerve graft would only be required if the facial nerve was resected more proximally, thereby leaving no suitable stump for coaptation. The hypoglossal nerve could be used in this setting to coapt directly to the proximal end of the facial nerve as it is easy to access, and provides excellent tone and normal appearance at rest. It also protects the eye and allows intentional facial movement although not spontaneous mimetic function. A major downside is the effect on the tongue which will be partly paralyzed and become atrophic. This can impact speech and swallowing. Furthermore, involuntary grimacing can occur with tongue movement. A compromise is to use a split hypoglossal nerve transfer.[1–3]

REFERENCES

1. Humphrey CD, Kriet JD. Nerve repair and cable grafting for facial paralysis. Facial Plast Surg 2008;24(2):170–176
2. Terzis JK, Konofaos P. Nerve transfers in facial palsy. Facial Plast Surg 2008;24(2):177–193
3. Baker DC, Conley J. Facial nerve grafting: a thirty year retrospective review. Clin Plast Surg 1979;6(3):343–360

SURGERY IN FACIAL PALSY

20. *Which one of the following techniques may be most useful in patients who have sustained marginal mandibular nerve injury?*

D. **Digastric transfer**

Loss of marginal mandibular nerve branch results in functional loss of the depressor anguli oris (DAO) muscle with the inability to pull the corner of the mouth downward. The anterior belly of the digastric muscle can be transferred and inserted into the lower lip, close to the insertion of DAO, just medial to the oral commissure. This provides restoration of lower lip depression. Alternatively, botulinum toxin can be used on the unaffected side to provide better lower lip symmetry, as an alternative to surgery. The other procedures listed target the midface and upper lip in order to reproduce a smile, but do not provide a suitable vector to restore marginal nerve function.[1]

REFERENCE

1. Tan ST. Anterior belly of digastric muscle transfer: a useful technique in head and neck surgery. Head Neck 2002;24(10):947–954

48. Face Transplantation

See *Essentials of Plastic Surgery*, third edition, pp. 656–663

FACE TRANSPLANTATION

1. *Which one of the following statements is correct regarding face transplant surgery?*
   A. Face transplants remain rare, with fewer than 12 performed worldwide since 2000.
   B. Face transplants have yet to be combined with other vascularized composite autograft (VCA).
   C. There have been no reported patient deaths after face transplant surgery.
   D. At least 25% of the facial area should be involved to justify a face transplant.
   E. The recipient will normally assume the appearance of the donor following transplant.

INDICATIONS FOR FACE TRANSPLANTATION

2. *Which one of the following statements is correct regarding face transplant surgery?*
   A. Severe ballistic trauma is considered a poor indication for transplant surgery.
   B. The most common reason for face transplantation is major tumor resection.
   C. Transplants are unsuitable for patients with failed free flap reconstruction.
   D. Primary face transplant following major facial trauma is currently not indicated.
   E. Patients must have a near-total face defect to warrant face transplantation.

CONTRAINDICATIONS TO FACE TRANSPLANT SURGERY

3. *In which one of the following is it reasonable to proceed with face transplantation?*
   A. A patient with systemic lupus
   B. A patient with a large intraoral squamous cell carcinoma (SCC) treated with radiotherapy
   C. A patient who is legally blind
   D. A patient with a known hypercoagulable disorder
   E. A patient with severe depression

PREOPERATIVE EVALUATION IN FACE TRANSPLANT SURGERY

4. You have been asked to use the Cleveland Clinic FACES scoring system when assessing a patient for face transplant surgery. *Which one of the following statements is correct?*
   A. This is a validated scoring system to assess patient suitability before transplant surgery.
   B. Patients receive a score based on a prior surgical history and those having undergone less than five procedures score highest.
   C. Lateral and central defects make up the aesthetic scoring components and are equally weighted.
   D. The patient's functional status assessment is based solely on the Karnofsky score.
   E. Patients receive a composite score of 0–100, which is used postoperatively to monitor successful outcomes.

PREOPERATIVE EVALUATION IN FACE TRANSPLANT SURGERY

5. You are assessing a patient preoperatively for surgery using the Karnovsky performance score as part of the FACES scoring system for which the patient receives a point score of 2. *What does this mean with regards to the patient's current health?*
   A. The patient is fit and well and leads an active life.
   B. The patient is capable of normal activity but this requires additional effort.
   C. The patient is mildly disabled and needs special care and assistance.
   D. The patient is very ill and needs hospital admission.
   E. The patient is a good candidate for face transplant.

SURGICAL PRINCIPLES IN FACE TRANSPLANTION

6. *When undertaking face transplantation surgery, which one of the following statements is correct?*
   A. Motor innervation is usually regained earlier than sensory innervation.
   B. Vascular anastomoses must be undertaken bilaterally of the external carotid and internal jugular vessels.
   C. Procurement of the face takes priority over solid organ retrieval.
   D. Immune suppression therapy is started soon after surgery to minimize rejection risk.
   E. Synkinesis may be minimized by coaptation of nerves close to their target muscle.

SURGICAL PRINCIPLES IN FACE TRANSPLANTION

7. *When undertaking a face transplant, what is the first surgical step performed once the donor face composite has been harvested and the recipient has been prepared?*
   A. Vascular anastomoses
   B. Bony inset
   C. Intraoral and intranasal repairs
   D. Nerve coaptations
   E. Muscle repairs

MAJOR COMPLICATIONS AFTER FACE TRANSPLANT SURGERY

8. *Which one of the following complications is most common after face transplant surgery?*
   A. Microvascular failure with graft loss
   B. Systemic infection
   C. Poor social reintegration
   D. Acute graft rejection
   E. Death

THE PANEL REACTIVE ANTIBODY TEST

9. *A patient awaiting face transplant surgery undergoes a panel reactive antibody test as part of medical clearance. What specific information does this test provide?*
   A. A prediction of hyperacute rejection risk
   B. A prediction of chronic rejection risk
   C. A prediction of whether antithymocyte globulin is required
   D. The blood group type of the patient
   E. The number of maintenance immunosuppressive drugs required

BANFF CLASSIFICATION OF REJECTION

10. A patient who has had face transplant surgery shows some abnormal skin changes in the transplanted area. A biopsy sample shows a dense perivascular infiltrate with mild epidermal and adnexal involvement. *According to the Banff classification, what grade of rejection is present?*
    A. Grade 0 (minimal or no rejection)
    B. Grade I (mild rejection)
    C. Grade II (moderate rejection)
    D. Grade III (severe rejection)
    E. Grade IV (very severe rejection)

MANAGEMENT OF REJECTION FOLLOWING FACE TRANSPLANT

11. *When considering the immunological management for transplant patients, which one of the following is true?*
    A. First-line management of acute rejection is pulsed dose alemtuzumab.
    B. Lifelong therapy includes steroid, tacrolimus, and mycophenolate mofetil.
    C. Both depleting and nondepleting agents act by directly decreasing lymphocyte count.
    D. Steroids such as hydrocortisone have specific targets within immune rejection therapy.
    E. Chronic rejection is not observed in patients following face transplantation.

Answers

FACE TRANSPLANTATION

1. *Which one of the following statements is correct regarding face transplant surgery?*
   D. **At least 25% of the facial area should be involved to justify a face transplant.**
   Face transplantation is used to reconstruct large facial defects that cannot be reconstructed with traditional techniques. The deficit should involve at least 25% of the facial area with loss of at least one central facial feature such as the eyelids, nose, or lips. Although relatively rare, over 40 face transplants have been performed since the first procedure was carried out in France in 2005. Face transplant has been combined with other vascularized composite autograft (VCA) surgery and deaths after face transplant have been reported. Overall, there have been 5 deaths reported of 41 reported face transplants. One patient had a bilateral hand transplant at the same time, but later died from overwhelming postoperative infection. Consequently, combining face transplant with other VCA remains controversial. Another patient died within 2 years of surgery, and this was attributed to compliance issues with immune suppression therapy. The other deaths were documented as secondary to suicide (1) and malignancy (2).[1,2].

   An important point to consider when discussing face transplant surgery is that the recipient does not necessarily take on the facial appearance of the donor. The appearance will be dictated by the nature of the transplant and both donor and recipient features. For example, when the transplant is soft tissue only, the recipients will retain more of their own original appearance. However, where bony reconstruction is also involved, the donor appearance is more likely to be preserved. The site of the facial defect being transplanted is also likely to make a difference, for example, central face versus more peripheral regions.

REFERENCES

1. Siemionow M, Ozturk C. Face transplantation: outcomes, concerns, controversies, and future directions. J Craniofac Surg 2012;23(1):254–259
2. Sosin M, Rodriguez ED. The face transplantation update: 2016. Plast Reconstr Surg 2016;137(6):1841–1850

INDICATIONS FOR FACE TRANSPLANTATION

2. *Which one of the following statements is correct regarding face transplant surgery?*
   D. **Primary face transplant following major facial trauma is currently not indicated.**
   Between 2005 and 2016, 40 patients underwent facial transplantation surgery worldwide. The most common etiology was trauma which had been the presenting injury in more than 30 patients. The major trauma causes were ballistic (17 cases) and burns (10 cases). Other trauma causes included animal bites and blunt injury. In spite of this, facial transplant is **not** currently indicted as a **primary** treatment for major facial trauma, although it could potentially be considered earlier along the treatment pathway rather than subjecting patients to multiple other procedures first. The challenges of undertaking facial transplant surgery in an acute or semi-acute setting are that there are multiple other medical, psychological, and logistical considerations that would need to be addressed and cannot be done without major planning.

   In general, malignant tumor resection is not a recognized indication for face transplantation. Having a failed free flap reconstruction is not a contraindication to transplant surgery. Many of the face transplant patients had undergone previous free tissue reconstruction and many had undergone more than 10 operations previously.[1,2]

   Although the central face is key to face transplantation, the facial deformity does not need to purely involve the central face, nor does it need to involve the full face. However, it would be expected that the defect was complex, not amenable to conventional reconstruction and that one central facial structure is involved.

REFERENCES

1. Siemionow M, Ozturk C. Face transplantation: outcomes, concerns, controversies, and future directions. J Craniofac Surg 2012;23(1):254–259
2. Sosin M, Rodriguez ED. The face transplantation update: 2016. Plast Reconstr Surg 2016;137(6):1841–1850

CONTRAINDICATIONS TO FACE TRANSPLANT SURGERY

3. *In which one of the following is it reasonable to proceed with face transplantation?*
   C. **A patient who is legally blind**
   There has been debate as to whether blindness should be a contraindication to face transplant surgery. This originally stemmed from hand transplant surgery experience that had shown vision to be important in

rehabilitation and not from the concern that a patient would be unable to view the result, although there have been suggestions that the latter is the actual reason. Blind patients have already undergone face transplant and there is no strong reason why a person who is legally blind should not receive a transplant. It would really amount to discrimination if they were unable to have one simply because of blindness. In other areas of plastic surgery, blind patients would not be turned away from procedures considered to be aesthetic such as mastopexy, liposuction, and abdominoplasty.

There are a number of universally accepted contraindications to face transplant surgery. These can be subclassified as psychiatric, medical, or psychosocial. Psychiatric contraindications include an active psychiatric disorder, substance abuse, and cognitive and perceptual inability to understand the procedure. Medical contraindications include an active cancer diagnosis or risk of recurrence, immune deficiency (e.g., human immunodeficiency virus-positive status), active infection (e.g., hepatitis), scleroderma, systemic lupus erythematosus, pregnancy, and hypercoagulable disorders. Psychosocial contraindications include a history of poor compliance with medical therapy and a poor social support network.[1]

REFERENCE

1. Lee J. Face transplantation for the blind: more than being blind in a sighted world. J Med Ethics 2018;44(6):361–365

PREOPERATIVE EVALUATION IN FACE TRANSPLANT SURGERY

4. You have been asked to use the Cleveland Clinic FACES scoring system when assessing a patient for face transplant surgery. *Which one of the following statements is correct?*
    B. Patients receive a score based on prior surgical history and those having undergone less than five procedures score highest.
    The Cleveland Clinic FACES scoring system was developed as a tool to assist in the preoperative evaluation of a patient's suitability for face transplantation. It includes five key areas: functional status, aesthetic deficit, medical comorbidities, depth of tissue involvement, and previous surgical procedures. The system has not been formally validated. The functional status component is based on both the Karnofsky and Strauss-Bacon stability scores. The latter assesses aspects of a patient's social status, including long-term relationships and/or employment. Patients receive a score of 10–60 (not 0–100). A higher score is more favorable for surgery. The analysis tool alone does not represent a complete assessment for the decision-making process. Central defects are weighted more highly than lateral defects (see Table 48.1, *Essentials of Plastic Surgery*, third edition).

PREOPERATIVE EVALUATION IN FACE TRANSPLANT SURGERY

5. You are assessing a patient preoperatively for surgery using the Karnovsky performance score as part of the FACES scoring system for which the patient receives a point score of 2. *What does this mean with regards to the patient's current health?*
    D. The patient is very ill and needs hospital admission.
    The Karnofsky[1] performance score is a commonly used independent assessment tool that grades a patient's health and functional status using a score of 0–100, where 100 is normal health and function without evidence of disease, and where 0 is dead. Scores in between are given in multiples of 10 and lower scores indicate poorer health and functional status. This system is often used in other areas of plastic surgery such as for head and neck cancer patients when assessing their fitness for surgery. It is important to note that the scoring differs as an independent assessment tool, as compared to when it is incorporated into the FACES scoring system.

    When used as part of the FACES system, patients can receive between 2 and 9 points depending on the patient's Karnofsky score/health status. For example, patients will receive 9 points if they have a maximum Karnofsky score of 100 and will receive 2 points if they have a Karnofsky score of 20. This patient scores very badly and a score of this grade suggests that admission to the hospital is indicated (see Table 48.1, *Essentials of Plastic Surgery*, third edition).

REFERENCES

1. Karnofsky DA, Burchenal JH. The clinical evaluation of chemotherapeutic agents in cancer. In: MacLeod CM, ed. Evaluation of Chemotherapeutic Agents. New York: Columbia Univ Press; 1949

SURGICAL PRINCIPLES IN FACE TRANSPLANTION

6. *When undertaking face transplantation surgery, which one of the following statements is correct?*
    E. Synkinesis may be minimized by coaptation of nerves close to their target muscle.
    Synkinesis refers to unwanted involuntary contractions that occur during voluntary muscle activation in another area of the face. It can occur secondary to aberrant regeneration after injury with resultant innervation

of nonnative muscle groups. When undertaking face transplant surgery, coaptation of the motor nerve closer to the target muscle may help reduce subsequent synkinesis. Sensory reinnervation of nerve coaptation occurs earlier than motor reinnervation.

Because of the vascular networks within the head and neck, bilateral vascular anastomoses are not normally required. Unilateral anastomoses of the internal jugular and external carotid (or one of its branches such as the facial artery) are typically used. Immune suppression is started preoperatively to reduce the risk of acute rejection. This may be achieved with a depleting agent such as antithymocyte globulin (a monoclonal antibody) or alemtuzumab (a polyclonal antibody). These are known as depleting agents as they reduce the number of lymphocytes. During harvest from the donor, face procurement may be halted if the donor becomes unstable to allow solid organ procurement. Once facial tissue procurement is complete the donor is fitted with a silicone prosthesis to cover the facial defect created.

SURGICAL PRINCIPLES IN FACE TRANSPLANTION

7. *When undertaking a face transplant, what is the first surgical step performed once the donor face composite has been harvested and the recipient has been prepared?*
    A. Vascular anastomoses
    The priority for face transplantation is to reestablish vascularity in the first instance by performing the arterial anastomosis with the facial artery or other most suitable branch of the external carotid system and performing the venous anastomosis with the internal jugular vein or one of its main tributaries. In many situations with free tissue transfer, obtaining bony stability is considered the primary task such that the vascular anastomoses can be performed with bony stability obtained. For example, in head and neck reconstruction following tumor extirpation where the neomandible is screwed into place, or in lower limb trauma after fracture reduction and application of hardware to long bone fractures. This is traditionally the case for replantation cases too especially those involving the digits. However, minimizing ischemia time is particularly vital for the successful outcome in composite free tissue transfers because tissues such as muscle do not tolerate extended ischemia times well. Once vascularity and bony stability are established, the remaining structures can be repaired from deep to superficial.

MAJOR COMPLICATIONS AFTER FACE TRANSPLANT SURGERY

8. *Which one of the following complications is most common after face transplant surgery?*
    D. Acute graft rejection
    To date, every face transplant patient with follow-up of more than 1 year has recorded at least one episode of acute graft rejection. These episodes were clinically apparent as erythema, edema with nodules, or papules and were treated satisfactorily by adjustment of immune suppression therapy. Microvascular graft failures have been low (4%) which is consistent with expected autologous free tissue transfer failure rates. There have been five deaths reported in the most recent follow-up data set. Significant infection rates have been low. Common localized infections include viral or fungal subtypes such as cytomegalovirus (CMV), herpes, and candida. These are generally well treated with medications such as acyclovir or fluconazole, respectively. One of the benefits of face transplant is improved social reintegration and this has been promising in face transplants undertaken so far.[1-3]

REFERENCES

1. Siemionow M, Ozturk C. Face transplantation: outcomes, concerns, controversies, and future directions. J Craniofac Surg 2012;23(1):254–259
2. Sosin M, Rodriguez ED. The face transplantation update: 2016. Plast Reconstr Surg 2016;137(6):1841–1850
3. Janis JE, MacKenzie KD, Wright SE, et al. Management of steroid-resistant late acute cellular rejection following face transplantation: a case report. Transplant Proc 2015;47(1):223–225

THE PANEL REACTIVE ANTIBODY TEST

9. A patient awaiting face transplant surgery undergoes a panel reactive antibody test as part of medical clearance. *What specific information does this test provide?*
    A. A prediction of hyperacute rejection risk
    Panel reactive antibodies are used to determine whether a patient has specific human leukocyte antigen antibodies.[1] A sample of a patient's blood is tested against the lymphocytes of 100 blood donors. The number of donors to which the patient has a reaction is expressed as a percentage (0–100%). A high percentage indicates that a patient has a high risk of acute rejection and may have to wait an extended time for a suitable donor. It does not reflect chronic rejection status or the blood type of the patient. All patients will require antithymocyte globulin preoperatively as part of the depleting agent process, and all patients will have a typical triple therapy maintenance regimen which will include steroids, tacrolimus, and mycophenolate mofetil.

REFERENCE

1. Bueno EM, Diaz-Siso JR, Pomahac B. A multidisciplinary protocol for face transplantation at Brigham and Women's Hospital. J Plast Reconstr Aesthet Surg 2011;64(12):1572–1579

BANFF CLASSIFICATION OF REJECTION

10. A patient who has had face transplant surgery shows some abnormal skin changes in the transplanted area. A biopsy sample shows a dense perivascular infiltrate with mild epidermal and adnexal involvement. *According to the Banff classification, what grade of rejection is present?*

C. Grade II (moderate rejection)

The Banff classification is used to grade rejection in vascular composite tissue grafts such as face and hand transplants. When evidence of rejection is evident in the skin, small biopsy samples are obtained for analysis.[1,2] The grading system is as follows:

- Grade 0: No rejection
- Grade I: Mild rejection, seen as mild perivascular infiltrate (lymphocytic)
- Grade II: Moderate rejection, seen as moderate to dense perivascular inflammation that can include mild epidermal and adnexal involvement
- Grade III: Severe rejection, seen as dense inflammation with epidermal involvement, epithelial apoptosis/necrosis
- Grade IV: Necrotizing rejection, seen as necrosis of epidermis and/or other skin elements

This patient has evidence of a grade II reaction and may require alterations of the immunosuppressive regimen. Of historic interest, the Banff conference was first held in Banff, Alberta, Canada in 1991. It is an international meeting to discuss transplant pathology. The twelfth meeting was held in Brazil in 2013.

REFERENCES

1. Cendales LC, Kanitakis J, Schneeberger S, et al. The Banff 2007 working classification of skin-containing composite tissue allograft pathology. Am J Transplant 2008;8(7):1396–1400
2. Solez K. History of the Banff classification of allograft pathology as it approaches its 20th year. Curr Opin Organ Transplant 2010;15(1):49–51

MANAGEMENT OF REJECTION FOLLOWING FACE TRANSPLANT

11. When considering the immunological management for transplant patients, which one of the following is true?

B. Lifelong therapy includes steroid, tacrolimus, and mycophenolate mofetil.

Patients undergoing face transplantation will need to take lifelong immunosuppressive therapy. Typical maintenance therapy for patients undergoing face transplant surgery is triple therapy including corticosteroids, tacrolimus, and mycophenolate mofetil. Steroids such as cortisol tend to have generalized immunosuppressant effects with anti-inflammatory properties. Calcineurin inhibitors such as tacrolimus prevent interleukin (IL)-2-dependent activation of lymphocytes. Mycophenolate mofetil is an antiproliferative agent. First-line management of acute rejection is to increase maintenance immunosuppression and ensure close observation of the patient. Second-line management involves steroid boluses, with or without increased doses of maintenance immunosuppressants or topical agents (e.g., clobetasol). Third-line management involves using induction therapy agents.

Agents given as induction therapy can be classified as depleting or nondepleting agents. Depleting agents decrease lymphocyte numbers and include polyclonal antithymocyte globulin and alemtuzumab, which is a monoclonal antibody directed against CD52 (a cell surface marker present on mature lymphocytes). Nondepleting agents do not decrease lymphocyte counts but prevent T-cell activation via the IL-2-dependent pathway (monoclonal anti-IL-2 receptor antibodies). Chronic rejection was initially thought to be less for face transplant and other vascularized composite autograft (VCA) patients than solid organ recipients, but as more data is collected, it appears that chronic rejection is a factor in VCA transfer.

PART IV

Breast

49. Breast Anatomy and Embryology

See *Essentials of Plastic Surgery*, third edition, pp. 667–677

EMBRYOLOGY OF THE BREAST

1. *Which one of the following statements is correct regarding fetal breast tissue development?*
   A. The breasts are primarily formed by mesodermal tissue and the process begins at 6 weeks of gestation.
   B. The milk ridge develops in the 8th week and extends from the fifth rib to the groin.
   C. The lactiferous ducts develop early in fetal development, and are modified sweat glands.
   D. Polymastia can occur anywhere along the milk ridge but most commonly occurs on the right at the level of the inframammary crease.
   E. Polythelia is the second most common congenital breast abnormality, occurring in 0.5–1% of the population.

STAGES OF BREAST DEVELOPMENT

2. An 18-year-old female presents with concern over delayed breast development. Examination of her breasts shows evidence of low-volume glandular tissue in the subareolar region, with the nipple and breast projecting as a single mound. *According to the Tanner classification, which stage does this represent?*
   A. Stage 1   D. Stage 4
   B. Stage 2   E. Stage 5
   C. Stage 3

NORMAL BREAST ANATOMY

3. *Which one of the following is correct regarding the anatomy of adult female breasts?*
   A. The breast footprint extends vertically from the third to the sixth rib in the midclavicular line.
   B. The breast footprint extends horizontally from the midline to the anterior axillary line.
   C. The inframammary fold is a fusion of the pectoralis muscle and the breast.
   D. Cooper's ligaments provide breast support and are implicated in development of breast ptosis.
   E. The tail of Spence is anatomically discrete from the breast as the tissue subtype is different.

BREAST ANATOMY

4. *Which one of the following statements is correct regarding the anatomy of adult female breasts?*
   A. The lobule is the functional unit of the breast and each comprises of 16–24 acini.
   B. Montgomery's glands are small apocrine glands incapable of milk secretion.
   C. Fat represents about two-fifths of the total volume in most breasts.
   D. Morgagni's tubercles are found in the central areola and have no functional role.
   E. The central nipple has orifices to drain the lactiferous ducts which may act as conduits for bacteria.

ARTERIAL SUPPLY OF THE BREAST

5. *Which one of the following provides a significant arterial supply to the breast parenchyma, and is also the dominant blood pedicle supply to the pectoralis major?*
   A. Lateral thoracic artery
   B. Intercostal perforators
   C. Thoracoacromial artery
   D. Internal mammary artery perforators
   E. Circumflex scapular artery

SENSORY INNERVATION TO THE BREAST

6. *When considering the sensory innervation to the breast, which one of the following is true?*
   A. The dermatomal distribution of the breast is T1–T5.
   B. Nipple-areolar sensation is most commonly provided by the sixth intercostal nerve.
   C. The cervical plexus contributes sensory innervation to the medial breast.
   D. Sensory innervation is mainly provided by the anterolateral and anteromedial intercostal nerves.
   E. Breast sensitivity is unrelated to breast size or volume.

LYMPHATIC LEVELS IN THE AXILLA

7. *When performing an axillary dissection for a patient with breast malignancy, which one of the following muscles serves as landmark between the superficial and deep nodes?*
   A. Latissimus dorsi
   B. Long head of triceps
   C. Serratus anterior
   D. Pectoralis minor
   E. Pectoralis major

WÜRINGER'S SEPTUM

8. *Which one of the following statements is correct regarding Würinger's septum?*
   A. The septum carries the motor nerve supply to the pectoralis major muscle.
   B. The septum carries the main arterial supply to the nipple.
   C. The septum makes no structural contribution to the breast.
   D. The septum originates from the third rib and inserts into the NAC.
   E. The septum divides the breast arterial supply into four overlapping zones.

MUSCULATURE OF THE ANTERIOR CHEST WALL

9. *Which one of the following is true regarding muscles of the anterior chest and abdominal wall?*
   A. The pectoralis minor is innervated by the lateral pectoral nerve and inserts on the coronoid process.
   B. The pectoralis major has two heads which insert on the medial side of the intertubercular sulcus.
   C. The serratus anterior originates from the anterior aspects of the first eight ribs and inserts on the medial aspect of the scapula.
   D. The rectus abdominis originates at the seventh to the twelfth costal cartilages and inserts at the pubic line.
   E. The external oblique is innervated by the fourth to tenth intercostal nerves and its key function is to flex the vertebral column.

LYMPHATIC DRAINAGE OF THE BREAST

10. *Which one of the following is true regarding lymphatic drainage of the breast?*
   A. The breast has purely deep lymphatic drainage networks.
   B. All of the breast drains directly into the axillary nodes.
   C. There are four levels of axillary nodes, each relating to pectoralis major.
   D. Lymphatic efferents from the outer quadrants drain directly to the supraclavicular nodes.
   E. Rotter's nodes are found between pectoralis major and minor.

BREAST SHAPE AND AESTHETICS

11. *When considering normal breast aesthetics, which one of the following is true?*
   A. Close side-to-side symmetry is common in younger patients.
   B. Most breast fullness should normally be found within the upper pole.
   C. A normal notch-to-nipple distance is 28 cm.
   D. A description of ptosis is unrelated to nipple position.
   E. The nipple should ideally be at level with the inframammary fold.

POLAND'S SYNDROME

12. *Which one of the following muscles is consistently deficient in patients with Poland's syndrome?*
   A. Pectoralis minor
   B. Sternal head of the pectoralis major
   C. Latissimus dorsi
   D. Serratus anterior
   E. Clavicular head of the pectoralis major

COMPLICATIONS AFTER BREAST SURGERY

13. A patient has axillary dissection for carcinoma of the breast and later develops paresthesia in the upper inner arm. *What is the most likely mechanism underlying the pathology of this symptom?*
   A. Transection of the medial brachial nerve
   B. Transection of the medial antebrachial nerve
   C. Transection of the intercostobrachial nerve
   D. Development of a compressive seroma
   E. Development of a compressive hematoma

Answers

EMBRYOLOGY OF THE BREAST

1. *Which one of the following statements is correct regarding fetal breast tissue development?*
   C. The lactiferous ducts develop early in fetal development, and are modified sweat glands.
   The breast begins to develop in the 4th week of gestation and has an ectodermal origin. Most tissue usually involutes with the exception of a small thoracic portion which penetrates into the underlying mesoderm. The lactiferous ducts are essentially modified sweat glands of ectodermal origin. They develop early in fetal development and toward the end of the gestational period, and acini develop around the tips of the ducts creating the mammary pit. The milk ridge extends from the axilla to the groin (not the fifth rib) and develops in the 6th week (not 8th week). The areolae are usually formed by the 5th month. Polymastia is the term used to describe supernumerary breasts, and can occur anywhere along the milk ridge but is most common on *the left* below the inframammary crease. Polythelia refers to a condition with supernumerary nipples, and is the most common congenital breast abnormality occurring in 2% of the population.[1-3]

REFERENCES

1. Bostwick J III. Anatomy and physiology. In: Bostwick J III, ed. Plastic and Reconstructive Breast Surgery, Vol. 1. 3rd ed. St Louis: Quality Medical Publishing; 2010
2. Moore KL, Persaud TV, Torchia MD, eds. The Developing Human: Clinically Oriented Embryology. 10th ed. Philadelphia: Elsevier; 2016
3. Sadler TW, ed. Langman's Medical Embryology. 13th ed. Philadelphia: Wolters Kluwer Health; 2014

STAGES OF BREAST DEVELOPMENT

2. An 18-year-old female presents with concern over delayed breast development. Examination of her breasts shows evidence of low-volume glandular tissue in the subareolar region, with the nipple and breast projecting as a single mound. *According to the Tanner classification, which stage does this represent?*
   B. Stage 2
   Tanner described five stages of breast development. The case described represents stage 2, which normally occurs at approximately 10–12 years of age. Tanner's stages of breast development are as follows:
   Stage 1: Preadolescent elevation of the nipple is present with no palpable glandular tissue or areolar pigmentation.
   Stage 2: Glandular tissue is present in the subareolar region, and the nipple and breast project as a single mound.
   Stage 3: Glandular tissue is increased and the breast and nipple are enlarged, but the nipple and breast contour remains in a single plane.
   Stage 4: The areolae are enlarged and areolar pigmentation increased, and the nipple and areola form a secondary mound above the level of the breast.
   Stage 5: Adolescent development is complete, with smooth contour and no projection of areola and nipple.[1,2]

REFERENCES

1. Tanner JM, ed. Growth at Adolescence. Oxford: Blackwell Scientific; 1962
2. Bostwick J III. Anatomy and physiology. In: Bostwick J III, ed. Plastic and Reconstructive Breast Surgery, Vol. 1. 3rd ed. St Louis: Quality Medical Publishing; 2010

NORMAL BREAST ANATOMY

3. *Which one of the following is correct regarding the anatomy of adult female breasts?*
   D. Cooper's ligaments provide breast support and are implicated in development of breast ptosis.
   The adult breast extends vertically from the second to the seventh rib (not sixth) in the midclavicular line. Its horizontal extension is from the sternocostal junction to the midaxillary line. The position and dimensions of the breast footprint are key to many aspects of breast surgery including augmentation, reduction, and reconstruction. Internally, the breast is supported by layers of fascia, one near to the dermis and another just superficial to the pectoralis muscle fascia. Cooper's ligaments penetrate the fascial system and the dermis, and ptosis of the breast is said to result from attenuation of these support structures. The inframammary fold (IMF) is a key anatomic

structure of the breast and is formed at the intersection of the lower breast pole and the chest wall. It represents fusion of the deep and superficial fascia with the dermis rather than the pectoralis major muscle and breast tissue. There are distinct criss-crossing fibers which hold the skin in place. In most cases, it is important to respect and preserve the IMF when undertaking breast surgery. Inadvertent damage of the IMF can be difficult to correct. There are, however, some instances when the fold will need to be altered or recreated. For example, in tuberous breasts the IMF is typically abnormally elevated and requires lowering as part of the surgical procedure. Elevating the fold is often more challenging than lowering it, even with suture techniques to the chest wall to support/resuspend/reconstruct it. The tail of Spence is the lateral most extension of the breast into the axilla. This gives the breast a teardrop shape. Appreciation of the relevance of the tail of Spence is key to optimizing aesthetic outcomes after mastectomy and reconstruction. It can be challenging to recreate this area of the breast well, particularly with implant-based approaches.[1,2]

REFERENCES

1. Bostwick J III. Anatomy and physiology. In: Bostwick J III, ed. Plastic and Reconstructive Breast Surgery, Vol. 1. 3rd ed. St Louis: Quality Medical Publishing; 2010
2. Hanna MK, Nahai F. Applied anatomy of the breast. In: Nahai F, ed. Art of Aesthetic Surgery: Principles and Techniques. Vol. 3. 2nd ed. St Louis: Quality Medical Publishing; 2011

BREAST ANATOMY

4. *Which one of the following statements is correct regarding the anatomy of adult female breasts?*

    E. The central nipple has orifices to drain the lactiferous ducts which may act as conduits for bacteria.

The nipple contains orifices which drain each main lactiferous duct and these can act as conduits for infection. This has implications for surgery of the breast, in particular when using breast implants. It is common practice to cover the nipple areola with a dressing when performing augmentation via an inframammary fold approach in order to minimize contamination of bacteria from the nipple to the implant pocket.

The functional unit of the breast is the lobule, and each one is comprised of hundreds of acini, not just 16–24. Each acinus itself has secretory potential and is connected to lactiferous ducts with interlobular ducts. There are 16–24 main lactiferous ducts and these dilate as they approach the nipple, forming a sinus that functions as a reservoir for milk storage. Montgomery's glands are large sebaceous glands capable of milk secretion and also serve to lubricate the areola during lactation. They represent an intermediate stage between sweat and mammary glands. Morgagni's tubercles represent the openings of the Montgomery's glands and are located at the periphery of the areola. Fat is the major component of breast tissue and provides most of the bulk, shape, consistency, and contour of the breast.[1,2]

REFERENCES

1. Moore KL, Dailey AF, Agur AMR. Clinically Oriented Anatomy. 7th ed. Philadelphia: Lippincott Williams & Wilkins; 2013
2. Williams PL, Warwick R, eds. Gray's Anatomy. 36th British ed. Philadelphia: WB Saunders; 1980

ARTERIAL SUPPLY OF THE BREAST

5. *Which one of the following provides a significant arterial supply to the breast parenchyma, and is also the dominant blood pedicle supply to the pectoralis major?*

    C. Thoracoacromial artery

The breast parenchyma is supplied by the internal mammary and intercostal perforators medially and by the lateral thoracic, thoracoacromial, thoracodorsal, and intercostal perforators laterally (**Fig. 49.1**).

Its rich blood supply and arterial collateralization are responsible for maintaining tissue viability during reconstruction or recontouring surgery and allow for invasive resection, dismantling, and rebuilding to be performed safely and consistently with low risk of tissue necrosis, providing the tissues are respected intraoperatively. Venous drainage mirrors the arterial supply and drains to the axilla.

In general, the underlying musculature of the chest wall shares the arterial supply to the breast. The pectoralis major muscle generates blood supply from the internal mammary perforators, thoracoacromial artery, intercostal perforators, and the lateral thoracic artery; however, its main pedicle is the thoracoacromial artery.

Knowledge of the vascular anatomy of this region is particularly important in reconstructive surgery, where a range of flaps are available. Not only is the thoracoacromial pedicle important for transferring the pectoralis major to the head and neck region, it can also be a useful recipient vessel site for free tissue transfer such as clavicular reconstruction with a fibula flap or in a vessel depleted neck for salvage head and neck reconstruction.[1-4]

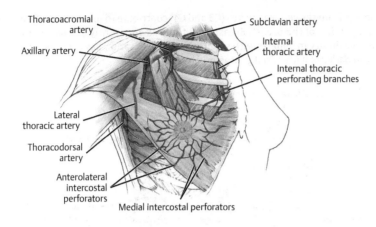

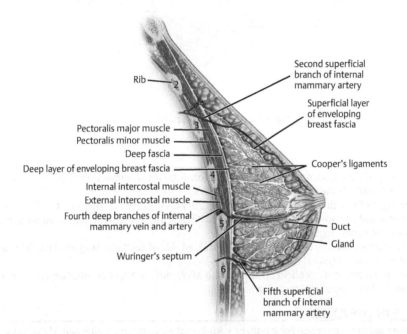

Fig. 49.1 Vascular supply to the breast. (From Hall-Findlay EJ. Aesthetic Breast Surgery: Concepts & Techniques. St Louis: Quality Medical Publishing, 2011.)

REFERENCES

1. van Deventer PV, Graewe FR. The blood supply of the breast revisited. Plast Reconstr Surg 2016;137(5):1388–1397
2. Palmer JH, Taylor GI. The vascular territories of the anterior chest wall. Br J Plast Surg 1986;39(3):287–299
3. Ciudad P, Agko M, Date S, et al. The radial forearm free flap as a "vascular bridge" for secondary microsurgical head and neck reconstruction in a vessel-depleted neck. Microsurgery 2018;38(6):651–658
4. Ye L, Taylor GI. A 10-year follow-up of a free vascularized fibula flap clavicle reconstruction in an adult. Plast Reconstr Surg Glob Open 2017;5(4):e1317

SENSORY INNERVATION TO THE BREAST

6. *When considering the sensory innervation to the breast, which one of the following is true?*

D. Sensory innervation is mainly provided by the anterolateral and anteromedial intercostal nerves.
The dermatomal distribution of the breast is T3–T6 (not T1–T5) and is mainly from the anteromedial and anterolateral branches of the thoracic intercostal nerves. Nipple-areolar sensation is most commonly provided by the fourth anterolateral intercostal nerve, although it is supplied by the third or fifth nerves in some cases.

Supraclavicular nerves from the cervical plexus (C3 and C4) contribute to innervation of the upper lateral portion, but not the medial portion of the breast. Breast sensitivity is apparently related to breast size, with studies showing increased sensitivity in females with smaller breasts. Sensation has been shown to improve after breast reduction surgery in patients with initially large breasts (**Fig. 49.2**).[1-5]

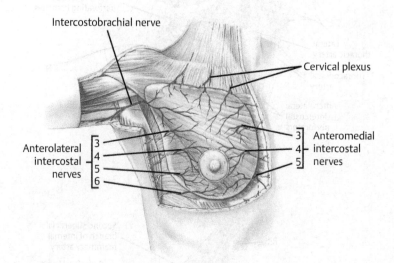

Fig. 49.2   Innervation to the breast.

REFERENCES

1. DelVecchyo C, Caloca J Jr, Caloca J, Gómez-Jauregui J. Evaluation of breast sensibility using dermatomal somatosensory evoked potentials. Plast Reconstr Surg 2004;113(7):1975–1983
2. Moore KL, Dailey AF, Agur AMR. Clinically Oriented Anatomy. 7th ed. Philadelphia: Lippincott Williams & Wilkins; 2013
3. Bostwick J III. Anatomy and physiology. In: Bostwick J III, ed. Plastic and Reconstructive Breast Surgery, Vol. 1. 3rd ed. St Louis: Quality Medical Publishing; 2010
4. Hanna MK, Nahai F. Applied anatomy of the breast. In: Nahai F, ed. Art of Aesthetic Surgery: Principles and Techniques, Vol. 3. 2nd ed. St Louis: Quality Medical Publishing; 2011
5. August DA, Sondak VK. Breast. In: Greenfield LJ, Mulholland MW, Oldham KT, et al, eds. Surgery: Scientific Principles and Practice. 2nd ed. Philadelphia: Lippincott-Raven; 1997

LYMPHATIC LEVELS IN THE AXILLA

7. **When performing an axillary dissection for a patient with breast malignancy, which one of the following muscles serves as landmark between the superficial and deep nodes?**

D. Pectoralis minor

The pectoralis minor is an important landmark during axillary dissection and brachial plexus exploration. The lateral margin divides the superficial from the deep axillary nodes. This muscle may be divided during axillary dissection to access the deep nodes in the apex of the axilla. The axillary nodes are numbered I–III according to pectoralis minor. Level I is the inferior, lateral level, below the lower edge of the pectoralis minor muscle. Level II is located deep to the pectoralis minor and level III is located superior and medial to pectoralis minor.

The pectoralis minor originates from the anterolateral surfaces of third to sixth ribs and inserts into the coracoid process of the scapula. It serves to draw the scapula downward and forward. Its main blood supply is the pectoral branch of thoracoacromial artery, with contribution from the lateral thoracic artery, and a direct branch of the axillary artery. In breast cancer, all three levels are not always removed and there remains some debate about this as there may be no advantage in removing all three levels. In contrast, most surgeons performing a dissection for skin cancer would remove all three levels.[1-3]

REFERENCES

1. Tominaga T, Takashima S, Danno M. Randomized clinical trial comparing level II and level III axillary node dissection in addition to mastectomy for breast cancer. Br J Surg 2004;91(1):38–43

2. Joshi S, Noronha J, Hawaldar R, et al. Merits of level III axillary dissection in node-positive breast cancer: a prospective, single-institution study from India. J Glob Oncol 2019;5:1–8
3. Tsutsumida A, Takahashi A, Namikawa K, et al. Frequency of level II and III axillary nodes metastases in patients with positive sentinel lymph nodes in melanoma: a multi-institutional study in Japan. Int J Clin Oncol 2016;21(4):796–800

WÜRINGER'S SEPTUM

8. *Which one of the following statements is correct regarding Würinger's septum?*

  B. **The septum carries the main arterial supply to the nipple.**

  Würinger et al[1] undertook anatomic dissections and arterial injection studies on female breasts. They found that there is a connective tissue suspensory system of the breast which acts as an internal brassiere. Within the horizontal part of the suspensory system, they identified a septum passing from the pectoral fascia along the fifth rib which is now referred to as Würinger's septum. Within this septum is the neurovascular supply to the nipple-areola complex (NAC). The anatomic nature of the septum means that laterally based breast pedicles are reliable and have a high chance of maintaining sensation following breast surgery. The septum does not carry the motor nerve supply to pectoralis major, nor does it divide the arterial supply of the breast into four zones. It was O'Dey et al[2] who performed an injection study of the breast to map the arterial distribution. They identified four distinct arterial zones, the largest of which were the internal mammary (zone 1) and lateral thoracic (zone 2). This work assessed the vascularity of different breast pedicles in terms of the NAC blood supply and concluded that lateral or medial based pedicles should provide the optimal blood supply to the NAC.

REFERENCES

1. Würinger E, Mader N, Posch E, Holle J. Nerve and vessel supplying ligamentous suspension of the mammary gland. Plast Reconstr Surg 1998;101(6):1486–1493
2. O'Dey DM, Prescher A, Pallua N. Vascular reliability of nipple-areola complex-bearing pedicles: an anatomical micro-dissection study. Plast Reconstr Surg 2007;119(4):1167–1177

MUSCULATURE OF THE ANTERIOR CHEST WALL

9. *Which one of the following is true regarding muscles of the anterior chest and abdominal wall?*

  C. **Serratus anterior originates from the anterior aspects of the first eight ribs and inserts on the medial aspect of the scapula.**

  Serratus anterior plays an important role in stabilization of the scapula against the chest wall. It receives blood supply through the lateral thoracic artery and branches of the thoracodorsal artery. It is innervated by the long thoracic nerve C6–C7, and when this nerve is damaged a winged scapula will occur.

  The pectoralis minor is innervated by the medial (not the lateral) pectoral nerve and is so named because it originates from the medial cord of the brachial plexus (C8 and T1). It originates from the third to sixth ribs and inserts onto the coronoid process. Its function is to draw the scapula downward and forward. Blood supply to the pectoralis minor is from the pectoral branch of thoracoacromial, lateral thoracic, and a direct branch from the axillary artery.

  The pectoralis major originates from the medial clavicle, sternum, second to sixth ribs, external oblique, and rectus abdominis fascia. It inserts on the intertubercular groove of the humerus laterally (not medially). The latissimus dorsi inserts between the pectoralis and teres major muscles. (It is sometimes described as the "lady between two majors.") The functions of pectoralis major are to adduct and medially rotate the arm. Innervation is from the medial and lateral pectoral nerves.

  The rectus abdominis flexes the vertebral column and tenses the abdominal wall. Innervation is from the seventh to twelfth intercostals. It originates from the pubic line and inserts on the third to seventh (not the seventh to twelfth) costal cartilages. External oblique originates from the lower anterior and lateral ribs, inserting at the iliac crest and medial abdominal fascial aponeurosis. Although it may assist in flexion of the vertebral column, a key role is compression of abdominal contents. It receives innervation from the seventh to twelfth intercostal nerves (not the fourth to tenth).[1–3]

REFERENCES

1. Jones G, ed. Bostwick's Plastic and Reconstructive Breast Surgery. 3rd ed. St Louis: Quality Medical Publishing; 2010
2. Zenn M, Jones G, eds. Reconstructive Surgery: Anatomy, Technique and Clinical Applications. New York, NY: Thieme; 2012
3. Moore KL, Dailey AF, Agur AMR. Clinically Oriented Anatomy. 7th ed. Philadelphia: Lippincott Williams & Wilkins; 2013

LYMPHATIC DRAINAGE OF THE BREAST

10. *Which one of the following is true regarding lymphatic drainage of the breast?*

E. **Rotter's nodes are found between pectoralis major and minor.**

The axillary lymph nodes are named according to their relationship with the pectoralis minor. Level 1 is lateral to, level 2 is behind, and level 3 is medial to the pectoralis minor, respectively. The breast has an extensive network of superficial and deep lymphatic drainage. Although most of the breast drains into the axillary nodes, not all areas do so. For example, medial drainage follows the internal mammary perforators and drains to the parasternal nodes. Lymphatic drainage from the outer upper quadrant may pass directly to the subscapular nodes.[1,2] Rotter's nodes are found between the pectoralis major and minor. They are named after the German surgeon, Josef Rotter[1] (1857–1924), who described them in the late nineteenth century, and they may be involved in the metastatic spread of breast cancer.

REFERENCES

1. Vrdoljak DV, Ramljak V, Muzina D, Sarceviç B, Knezević F, Juzbasić S. Analysis of metastatic involvement of interpectoral (Rotter's) lymph nodes related to tumor location, size, grade and hormone receptor status in breast cancer. Tumori 2005;91(2):177–181
2. Haagensen CD, ed. Diseases of the Breast. 3rd ed. Philadelphia: WB Saunders; 1986

BREAST SHAPE AND AESTHETICS

11. *When considering normal breast aesthetics, which one of the following is true?*

E. **The nipple should ideally be at level with the inframammary fold.**

Although there are a number of "typical" measurements for the "normal" breast, there is actually significant variation between individuals. Some of the "typical" measurements are in keeping with the "ideal" or most aesthetic breast appearance. For example, the height of the nipple should ideally be at level with the inframammary fold (IMF), or just above it. This also usually matches with the level of the midhumeral point and a distance of around 19–21 cm from the sternal notch (although this does also depend on the patient's height and breast size). This information is useful when planning breast reduction and mastopexy techniques, as it provides a guide as to where to resite the nipple-areola complex. The normal breast should have a teardrop shape when viewed from the lateral aspect and this is due to greater fullness in the lower pole. The breast is tethered at the IMF so naturally a degree of glandular ptosis occurs where the breast soft tissues fall to sit just below this line. The nipple should still remain above the IMF level in the ideal breast. Therefore, although a minimal amount of glandular ptosis is normal and aesthetically pleasing, more significant amounts are not. Degrees of true ptosis are described by the relationship of the nipple to the IMF and breast parenchyma. Few women have symmetrical breasts at any age and it is important to identify this before performing breast surgery, as the asymmetry may remain or even be exaggerated after surgery. For example, when the nipple is lateralized on the breast mound, augmentation will make this more obvious. Furthermore, surgery tends to increase patients' awareness and focus on detailed specifics of their anatomy, and irregularities and asymmetries are more likely to be noticed.[1-3]

REFERENCES

1. Jones G, ed. Bostwick's Plastic and Reconstructive Breast Surgery. 3rd ed. St Louis: Quality Medical Publishing; 2010
2. Hall-Findlay EJ, ed. Aesthetic Breast Surgery: Concepts & Techniques. St Louis: Quality Medical Publishing; 2011
3. Hanna MK, Nahai F. Applied anatomy of the breast. In: Nahai F, ed. Art of Aesthetic Surgery: Principles and Techniques, Vol. 3. 2nd ed. St Louis: Quality Medical Publishing; 2011

POLAND'S SYNDROME

12. *Which one of the following muscles is consistently deficient in patients with Poland's syndrome?*

B. **Sternal head of the pectoralis major**

Poland's syndrome is a disorder where affected individuals are born with missing or incompletely formed elements of the upper limb and chest on one side. It occurs in 1:30,000 births with no specific gender preference. The right side is affected twice as often as the left. The current theory is that there is in utero compression of the subclavian artery which causes ischemia and hypoplastic development of key chest and limb structures. The main findings include absence of the sternal head of pectoralis major muscle, absence of the costal cartilages, hypoplasia of the breast and nipple-areola complex, deficiency of subcutaneous fat and axillary hair, and syndactyly or hypoplasia of the upper limb. Although it can cause a variety of muscle abnormalities such as those listed, a consistent feature is absence of the sternal portion of the pectoralis major.[1,2]

REFERENCES

1. Urschel HC Jr. Poland's syndrome. Chest Surg Clin N Am 2000;10(2):393–403, viii
2. David TJ. The Poland anomaly and allied disorders. Pediatr Res 1981;15:1184

COMPLICATIONS AFTER BREAST SURGERY

13. A patient has axillary dissection for carcinoma of the breast and later develops paresthesia in the upper inner arm. *What is the most likely mechanism underlying the pathology of this symptom?*

   C. Transection of the intercostobrachial nerve

The medial arm is supplied by the medial brachial and intercostobrachial nerves from T1–T2. The intercostobrachial nerve usually joins with the medial brachial nerve. The medial antebrachial nerve supplies the anterior surfaces of the arm and anteromedial forearm. Transection of any of these can result in paresthesia of the arm; however, the most likely cause is transection of the intercostobrachial nerve. Although a postoperative seroma or hematoma can cause paresthesia in the upper limb, it can also directly irritate the brachial plexus and lead to a combined motor and sensory pathology. Other causes of postoperative upper limb dysfunction include nerve stretch or compression from patient positioning.[1,2]

REFERENCES

1. Sharp E, Roberts M, Żurada-Zielińska A, et al. The most commonly injured nerves at surgery: a comprehensive review. Clin Anat 2021;34(2):244-262
2. Chirappapha P, Arunnart M, Lertsithichai P, Supsamutchai C, Sukarayothin T, Leesombatpaiboon M. Evaluation the effect of preserving intercostobrachial nerve in axillary dissection for breast cancer patient. Gland Surg 2019;8(6):599–608

50. Congenital Breast Deformities

See *Essentials of Plastic Surgery*, third edition, pp. 678–685

CONGENITAL BREAST DEFORMITIES

1. *In which one of the following conditions will nipple reconstruction not be indicated?*
   A. Amastia
   B. Athelia
   C. Amazia
   D. Poland's syndrome
   E. Scalp-ear-nipple syndrome

CONGENITAL BREAST ABNORMALITIES

2. A patient is seen in clinic regarding the management of a congenital hypoplastic breast condition. Examination also shows a unilateral upper limb abnormality with short digits and chest wall asymmetry. *What is the most likely diagnosis?*
   A. Poland's syndrome
   B. Pectus excavatum
   C. Pectus carinatum
   D. Apert's syndrome
   E. Holt-Oram syndrome

POLYTHELIA

3. A 9-year-old girl is seen in clinic with polythelia. She dislikes the appearance of the condition and is embarrassed about it when changing clothes at school for gym and swimming lessons. *What is the most likely intervention required?*
   A. Elliptical excision and direct wound closure
   B. Circular excision and local transposition flap closure
   C. Circular excision and full-thickness skin graft
   D. CO$_2$ Laser therapy
   E. No intervention required

POLYMASTIA

4. *In a patient with polymastia, which one of the following is true?*
   A. The condition only develops after birth.
   B. The cause is genetically linked in most cases.
   C. There may be associated renal abnormalities.
   D. It is most commonly a bilateral finding.
   E. Involved tissues behave differently to normal breast tissue.

HYPOMASTIA

5. You receive a referral for management of bilateral hypomastia in a 19-year-old who wishes to consider breast augmentation as she has minimal breast tissue development and no menstrual cycles. *Which one of the following is true in this case?*
   A. She most likely requires reassurance only.
   B. Hormonal tests should be undertaken prior to surgical intervention.
   C. Surgery should be delayed until age 25.
   D. Round-shaped implants will be preferentially indicated.
   E. A referral to clinical psychology is most indicated.

TUBEROUS BREAST DEFORMITY

6. *Which one of the following is an important consideration in the assessment of tuberous breast deformity but does not form part of the Meara classification system?*
   A. The position of the inframammary fold
   B. The degree of nipple areola herniation
   C. The degree of breast ptosis
   D. The adequacy of the breast volume
   E. The adequacy of the skin envelope

TUBEROUS BREAST DEFORMITY

7. *Which one of the following is true in a patient with a tuberous breast deformity?*
   A. Normal breast function and physiology are likely to be impaired.
   B. The condition is most likely to affect the right side only.
   C. It is present in 15–20% of the population and usually requires no intervention.
   D. The mainstay of treatment is single-stage breast implantation.
   E. Optimal surgical treatment is complex and highly individualized.

CONGENITAL ABNORMALITIES OF THE NIPPLE

8. *When surgically managing the inverted nipple, which one of the following is true?*
   A. Microbial swabs should be sent during the procedure.
   B. Tissue biopsies should be sent intraoperatively to exclude malignancy.
   C. The patients should be advised that they will be unable to breast feed in the future.
   D. The consent form should highlight the risk of recurrence of the inversion.
   E. The single best surgical technique involves division of fibrous bands.

SYNMASTIA

9. *When treating a patient with synmastia, which one of the following is true?*
   A. One of the breasts fails to develop fully.
   B. Single-stage treatment with liposuction is preferred.
   C. The cause will be a genetic abnormality from the mother's side.
   D. Iatrogenic cases are almost never observed.
   E. Treatment may involve plication sutures and local flaps.

Answers

CONGENITAL BREAST DEFORMITIES

1. *In which one of the following conditions will nipple reconstruction not be indicated?*

C. Amazia

Amazia is a condition where there is absence of glandular breast tissue with preservation of the normal nipple-areola complex (NAC). Patients with amazia would therefore not require nipple reconstruction, although they may require breast mound reconstruction with implant-based techniques. Amastia is the total absence of both breast tissue and the NAC, while athelia is the complete absence of a nipple. Poland's syndrome may involve absence of the breast and/or NAC. As the name suggests, scalp-ear-nipple syndrome is a condition in which there are abnormalities of the three described body areas. The nipples may be underdeveloped (hypothelia) or absent. Other features include small, cup-shaped ears, and aplasia cutis congenita. Each of these conditions may require nipple reconstruction.[1-6]

REFERENCES

1. Pryor LS, Lehman JA Jr, Workman MC. Disorders of the Female Breast in the Pediatric Age Group. Disorders of the female breast in the pediatric age group. Plast Reconstr Surg 2009;124(1, Suppl):50e–60e
2. Latham K, Fernandez S, Iteld L, Panthaki Z, Armstrong MB, Thaller S. Pediatric breast deformity. J Craniofac Surg 2006;17(3):454–467
3. Lin KY, Nguyen DB, Williams RM. Complete breast absence revisited. Plast Reconstr Surg 2000;106(1):98–101
4. Trier WC. Complete breast absence. Case report and review of the literature. Plast Reconstr Surg 1965;36(4):431–439
5. Taylor GA. Reconstruction of congenital amastia with complication. Ann Plast Surg 1979;2(6):531–534
6. Banikarim C, De Silva NK. Breast Disorders in Children and Adolescents. In: Torchia MM, ed. UpToDate. Retrieved June 13, 2018. From https://www.uptodate.com/contents/breast-disorders-in-children-and-adolescents

CONGENITAL BREAST ABNORMALITIES

2. A patient is seen in clinic regarding the management of a congenital hypoplastic breast condition. Examination also shows a unilateral upper limb abnormality with short digits and chest wall asymmetry. *What is the most likely diagnosis?*

A. Poland's syndrome

Poland's syndrome is a condition with a variable constellation of findings including hypoplasia or absence of the breast, areola, and subcutaneous tissues. There are associated chest wall and upper limb abnormalities, which can include absent ribs, pectoralis major and minor, and brachysyndactyly of the hand and upper limb on the affected side. These patients are often seen by plastic surgery teams to provide input for either the limb abnormalities or the chest wall and breast abnormalities. Pectus excavatum and pectus carinatum are both defects of the chest wall. Pectus excavatum is the most common chest wall deformity and occurs in 1:400 cases. It involves posterior sternal depression. This tends to be an isolated condition without breast or limb abnormalities; however, the chest wall concavity can affect the appearance of the breasts significantly as effectively the base upon which they sit is retruded. Pectus carinatum is where there is anterior protrusion of the sternum and costal cartilages. Again, this can affect the appearance of the breasts but is not associated with breast or limb abnormalities. Apert's syndrome is one of the craniosynostotic syndromes with associated complex syndactyly of the hands and feet. Chest wall and breast abnormalities are not part of this condition. Holt-Oram syndrome involves radial longitudinal deficiency of the upper limb associated with cardiac defects including septal defects, tetralogy of Fallot, mitral valve prolapse, and patent ductus arteriosus. Again, breast abnormalities are not part of this syndrome.[1,2]

REFERENCES

1. Baldelli I, Baccarani A, Barone C, et al. Consensus based recommendations for diagnosis and medical management of Poland syndrome (sequence). Orphanet J Rare Dis 2020;15(1):201
2. Duflos D, Plu-Bureau G, Thibaud E, et al. Breast diseases in adolescents. In: Sultan C, ed. Pediatric and Adolescent Gynecology: Evidence-Based Clinical Practice (Endocrine Development), Vol. 7. Basel, Switzerland: Karger; 2000:186

POLYTHELIA

3. A 9-year-old girl is seen in clinic with polythelia. She dislikes the appearance of the condition and is embarrassed about it when changing clothes at school for gym and swimming lessons. *What is the most likely intervention required?*

A. **Elliptical excision and direct wound closure**

Polythelia is the presence of supernumerary or accessory nipples and is the most common anomaly of the pediatric breast. It is usually unilateral along the milk line and most often is located just inferior to the normal breast. In most cases surgical excision is performed before puberty while the nipple is small. This can be performed with an elliptical excision and direct closure, leaving a small discreet scar. Local flaps are not normally required due to the small size of the excision and skin grafts are best avoided as the cosmetic outcome would likely be worse than the original accessory nipple. Laser therapy is not used for accessory nipple treatment and would lead to poor scarring following healing by secondary intention. Although no intervention can be considered, in this case, the patient is already concerned about the appearance and earlier treatment before puberty is appropriate as the size of the nipple will be relatively smaller at this stage of her life.[1,2]

REFERENCES

1. Kajava Y. The proportions of supernumerary nipples in the Finnish population. Duodecim 1915;1:143–170
2. Brown J, Schwartz RA. Supernumerary nipples: an overview. Cutis 2003;71(5):344–346

POLYMASTIA

4. *In a patient with polymastia, which one of the following is true?*

C. **There may be associated renal abnormalities.**

Polymastia is the presence of accessory breast tissue and occurs in around 1% of the general population. Familial polymastia has been reported, but is not the most common presentation, and can be associated with chromosomal abnormalities and thoracic and renal anomalies. For this reason, renal ultrasound is indicated especially where other congenital anomalies are noted.

The condition is present at the time of birth, although there will be further development of the breast tissue later in life if left *in situ*. Polymastia may be bilateral but is most often unilateral and the tissues will behave in the same way as other breast tissue. For example, the tissues will be affected by menstruation, pregnancy, and lactation. There is also the potential for development of benign tumors such as fibroadenomas and malignant tumors such as breast cancer. Surgical excision is therefore indicated for other medical, psychological, or cosmetic reasons, rather than cosmetic reasons alone.[1–4]

REFERENCES

1. Sadove AM, van Aalst JA. Congenital and acquired pediatric breast anomalies: a review of 20 years' experience. Plast Reconstr Surg 2005;115(4):1039–1050
2. DiVasta AD, Weldon C, Labow BI. The breast: examination and lesions. In: Emans SJ, Laufer MR, eds. Emans, Laufer, Goldstein's Pediatric & Adolescent Gynecology. 6th ed. Philadelphia: Lippincott Williams & Wilkins; 2012:405
3. Caouette-Laberge L, Borsuk D. Congenital anomalies of the breast. Semin Plast Surg 2013;27(1):36–41
4. Bartsich SA, Ofodile FA. Accessory breast tissue in the axilla: classification and treatment. Plast Reconstr Surg 2011;128(1):35e–36e

HYPOMASTIA

5. You receive a referral for management of bilateral hypomastia in a 19-year-old who wishes to consider breast augmentation as she has minimal breast tissue development and no menstrual cycles. *Which one of the following is true in this case?*

B. **Hormonal tests should be undertaken prior to surgical intervention.**

Hypomastia is commonly seen in young slim patients and, as with other breast developmental conditions, needs to be addressed on an individualized basis. One thing that is key is to be sure there is no underlying treatable reason for the hypomastia. For this reason, medical workup should include hormone function tests including thyroid, estrogen, progesterone, follicle-stimulating hormone (FSH), and luteinizing hormone (LH). This is usually performed by the referring medical team. If there are issues with pubertal development more generally, then a specialist endocrinologist is probably already involved. If so, it is worth working with them to determine the need and timing of surgery. Many slim girls may request augmentation even where hormonal function and puberty is normal. In this case, reassurance alone is unlikely to be sufficient for this patient, although it should be part of the consultation process. If she were 14 or 15 years old then reassurance alone and waiting for breast development to occur would be appropriate.

When considering the timing of breast augmentation in young females, most surgeons would agree that deferring treatment until age 18 is advisable, but waiting until age 25 has no justifiable basis as in the absence of abnormal hormone status or other reason, the hypomastia is unlikely to change.

In cases where there is minimal breast tissue development such as in this case, a more natural look is likely to be achieved with submuscular (dual plane) placement of anatomic implants rather than round. However, patient's preference must be taken into account as some patients will prefer a more rounded look even though it may appear more artificial.

There is a role for clinical psychology in patients undergoing or considering plastic and reconstructive surgery. It can be useful to help patients address their concerns and balance their perceptions of the condition in relation to the physical abnormality they have.

However, in this case it would not be absolutely necessary to do so provided that a full discussion had been undertaken with the patient about the aims, objectives, and understanding of the options and outcomes available.[1,2]

REFERENCES

1. DiVasta AD, Weldon C, Labow BI. The breast: examination and lesions. In: Emans SJ, Laufer MR, eds. Emans, Laufer, Goldstein's Pediatric & Adolescent Gynecology. 6th ed. Philadelphia: Lippincott Williams & Wilkins; 2012:405
2. Duflos D, Plu-Bureau G, Thibaud E, et al. Breast diseases in adolescents. In: Sultan C, ed. Pediatric and Adolescent Gynecology: Evidence-Based Clinical Practice (Endocrine Development), Vol. 7. Basel, Switzerland: Karger; 2000:186

TUBEROUS BREAST DEFORMITY

6. Which one of the following is an important consideration in the assessment of tuberous breast deformity but does not form part of the Meara classification system?

B. The degree of nipple areola herniation

The tuberous breast has a number of key characteristics and when it comes to classification with the Meara system, five key components are considered. These are the degree of constriction of the breast base, the position of the inframammary fold, the adequacy of breast and skin volumes, and the degree of ptosis. Protrusion of the nipple-areola complex is a common finding in the tuberous breast secondary to herniation of the breast tissue anteriorly into the areola area. This is thought to occur because there is constriction within the breast and so development occurs in the path of least resistance, which is through the areola rather than the normal radial breast development. Furthermore, the areola tends to be wider in the tuberous breast. In spite of this, neither areola herniation nor diameter is part of the classification system. Knowledge of the classification system is not only useful for examinations, but helps provide a structural basis for forming surgical management plans.[1]

Von Heimburg is also known for a classification system of the tuberous breast, which also can be useful for clinical practice and examinations. There are four grades (I–IV which range from mild to severe). These can help guide treatment selection:

- Type I: Hypoplasia of the lower medial quadrant
- Type II: Hypoplasia of the lower medial and lateral quadrants, sufficient skin in the subareolar region
- Type III: Hypoplasia of the lower medial and lateral quadrants, deficiency of skin in the subareolar region
- Type IV: Severe breast constriction, minimal breast base[2,3]

REFERENCES

1. Meara JG, Kolker A, Bartlett G, Theile R, Mutimer K, Holmes AD. Tuberous breast deformity: principles and practice. Ann Plast Surg 2000;45(6):607–611
2. von Heimburg D, Exner K, Kruft S, Lemperle G. The tuberous breast deformity: classification and treatment. Br J Plast Surg 1996;49(6):339–345
3. von Heimburg D. Refined version of the tuberous breast classification. Plast Reconstr Surg 2000;105(6):2269–2270

TUBEROUS BREAST DEFORMITY

7. Which one of the following is true in a patient with a tuberous breast deformity?

E. Optimal surgical treatment is complex and highly individualized.

Tuberous breast deformity is a relatively rare condition (not 15–20% of the population) with much inter-patient and intra-patient variation in the degree of deformity observed in the breasts and areolae. It can be quite mild in some cases and very severe in others. There are typically a number of abnormalities which coexist in a tuberous breast. These include a relative skin and volume deficiency, an abnormally developed and elevated inframammary fold (IMF), a reduced breast footprint, and a widened and protruded areolae. Almost all patients with tuberous breast will request some form of surgical treatment and this will be highly individualized to the specific deformity in each case. Most cases will require multiple surgeries and a range of techniques and approaches to be used. A common theme for such patients is the deficiency of skin, particularly in the lower pole, with a short nipple to IMF distance and they will normally need tissue expansion to address this. Patients with coexisting volume deficiencies may secondarily require permanent implants following tissue expansion. Others may have sufficient native breast volume such that implants are not required and instead just need mastopexy or even differential breast reduction with areola repositioning and diameter reduction with release of the constricted inferior pole. Very often patients will need different approaches to each breast so the full repertoire of breast surgery approaches must be in the surgeon's toolbox. Other useful adjuncts include fat transfer and soft tissue flaps.

In spite of the visual abnormality in the tuberous breast, most patients retain normal breast function and physiology. Most patients are affected bilaterally although some cases may be unilateral or display minimal deformity on the second side. Some patients may ask for treatment in a single stage for logistical and financial reasons, but single-stage implant techniques with release of the lower pole and repositioning of the IMF are only likely to be successful in select cases where the deformity is mild.[1-5]

REFERENCES

1. Mandrekas AD, Zambacos GJ, Anastasopoulos A, Hapsas D, Lambrinaki N, Ioannidou-Mouzaka L. Aesthetic reconstruction of the tuberous breast deformity. Plast Reconstr Surg 2003;112(4):1099–1108, discussion 1109
2. Costagliola M, Atiyeh B, Rampillon F. Tuberous breast: revised classification and a new hypothesis for its development. Aesthetic Plast Surg 2013;37(5):896–903
3. Grolleau JL, Lanfrey E, Lavigne B, Chavoin JP, Costagliola M. Breast base anomalies: treatment strategy for tuberous breasts, minor deformities, and asymmetry. Plast Reconstr Surg 1999;104(7):2040–2048
4. Meara JG, Kolker A, Bartlett G, Theile R, Mutimer K, Holmes AD. Tuberous breast deformity: principles and practice. Ann Plast Surg 2000;45(6):607–611
5. Kolker AR, Collins MS. Tuberous breast deformity: classification and treatment strategy for improving consistency in aesthetic correction. Plast Reconstr Surg 2015;135(1):73–86

CONGENITAL ABNORMALITIES OF THE NIPPLE

8. *When surgically managing the inverted nipple, which one of the following is true?*
D. The consent form should highlight the risk of recurrence of the inversion.
Congenital nipple inversion is commonly seen in up to 10% of the population. Patients dislike the appearance of the nipples and also find that function can be impaired for breast feeding. Nipple inversion can have other causes including infection and malignancy and these need to be considered and excluded well before, not during, surgery. For this reason, neither swabs nor biopsies would be indicated intraoperatively. As with all procedure, the consent process is vital and must highlight the key risks of such a procedure and set out a basis for realistic expectations. Even with good surgical technique, there is a risk of the inversion returning once the tissues have healed and scarred down. Sometimes there is a partial improvement so the final nipple prominence ends up being somewhere between the preoperative state and the immediate postoperative state. Other risks include altered sensation, nipple necrosis, and injury to the lactiferous ducts. There is a risk that breast feeding may not be possible in future and this may reflect the original anatomy of the nipple or the surgery performed, although it is not exclusive so patients may well still retain breast feeding function. There are a number of different surgical approaches to the inverted nipple including making a small incision at the base of the nipple and releasing the fibrous bands beneath the nipple base before supporting this with sutures. However, there is not one single recognized best technique and other options include circumferential tightening of the areolar edge and dermal flaps.[1-3]

REFERENCES

1. Hernandez Yenty QM, Jurgens WJFM, van Zuijlen PPM, de Vet HC, Verhaegen PD. Treatment of the benign inverted nipple: a systematic review and recommendations for future therapy. Breast 2016;29:82–89
2. Gould DJ, Nadeau MH, Macias LH, Stevens WG. Inverted nipple repair revisited: a 7-year experience. Aesthet Surg J 2015;35(2):156–164
3. Yukun L, Ke G, Jiaming S. Application of nipple retractor for correction of nipple inversion: a 10-year experience. Aesthetic Plast Surg 2016;40(5):707–715

SYNMASTIA

9. *When treating a patient with synmastia, which one of the following is true?*
E. Treatment may involve plication sutures and local flaps.
Synmastia is a condition where the two breasts join in the midline with disruption or absence of the intermammary sulcus. It is an extremely rare finding as a congenital anomaly and, in fact, is far more commonly seen as an iatrogenic cause following breast surgery. This can be following augmentation where the breast pocket is over dissected medially or it can become apparent following mastectomy and reconstruction with scar tethering

and medialization of the native breast. Either way, it is a challenging deformity to correct and techniques include recruiting skin into the space between the breasts with local flaps, and/or trying to recreate the junction between the breast and the chest wall with plication techniques and/or dermal matrices. Synmastia is therefore not a condition where one breast fails to develop. Liposuction may be helpful to thin the intermammary subcutaneous tissues (breast web) and provide better definition, but is not the only approach.[1,2]

REFERENCES

1. Spence RJ, Feldman JJ, Ryan JJ. Symmastia: the problem of medial confluence of the breasts. Plast Reconstr Surg 1984;73(2):261-269
2. Salgado CJ, Mardini S. Periareolar approach for the correction of congenital symmastia. Plast Reconstr Surg 2004;113(3):992-994

51. Breast Augmentation

See *Essentials of Plastic Surgery*, third edition, pp. 686–709

BACKGROUND TO BREAST AUGMENTATION

1. *Which one of the following statements is correct regarding breast augmentation?*
   A. The Food and Drug Administration (FDA) placed a moratorium on the use of silicone breast implants in 2001.
   B. There is a proven link between silicone implants and systemic autoimmune disease.
   C. There are five generations of silicone implant, if texturing, gel type, and shape are considered.
   D. Saline-filled implants remain the gold standard because they require a smaller incision and more closely maintain body temperature.
   E. In the United States, textured silicone implants do not currently have FDA approval for primary breast augmentation.

PATIENT EVALUATION FOR BREAST AUGMENTATION

2. *Which one of the following is not routinely required during the assessment of patients requesting breast augmentation?*
   A. Assessment of psychological stability and personal motivation for implants
   B. Evidence of recent negative mammograms
   C. Identification of chest wall and vertebral deformities
   D. Measurement of breast base width, notch-to-nipple, and nipple-to-inframammary fold (IMF) distances
   E. Assessment of skin elasticity and upper/lower pole soft tissue cover

SELECTION OF BREAST IMPLANTS FOR COSMETIC AUGMENTATION

3. A slim 30-year-old woman is seen in the outpatient department; she is considering breast augmentation. Examination shows she has good breast symmetry and mild (grade I) ptosis, with nipple-to-notch distances of 26 cm. There are no chest wall deformities evident, and tissue quality is good. *Which one of the following is most useful to guide decision-making for plane of implant placement?*
   A. Placing trial breast sizers within the bra
   B. Measuring the nipple-to-fold distances
   C. Creating computer-generated images
   D. Assessing the superior pole tissue thickness
   E. Measuring breast base width and height

EXPECTED OUTCOMES FOLLOWING BREAST AUGMENTATION

4. A patient is seen in clinic prior to undergoing subglandular breast augmentation. She has grade 1 ptosis and a body mass index (BMI) of 24. She has a number of questions relating to likely outcomes after surgery which is planned with 375-cc smooth round implants. *Which one of the following is true in her case?*
   A. She can reliably expect to have an increase of two bra cup sizes after surgery.
   B. Her ptosis would only be corrected by placement of a much larger implant.
   C. Her future cancer screening and risk of breast cancer will be significantly affected by having implants.
   D. Her lifetime risk of developing BIA-ALCL will be increased to 1:10,0000 following this surgery.
   E. She should expect to be able to feel the implant edges and may see rippling, particularly in the lower pole.

INCISION CHOICE FOR BREAST AUGMENTATION

5. *When choosing the incision site for breast augmentation, which one of the following statements is correct?*
   A. The IMF approach involves scar placement within the fold, centered on the NAC.
   B. The transumbilical approach is well suited to most modern implant types.
   C. The periareolar approach is best achieved with direct parenchymal dissection.
   D. The transaxillary approach avoids a breast scar but risks sensory nerve damage to the arm.
   E. Endoscopic assisted approaches limit implant choice to round saline implants.

PLACEMENT OF BREAST IMPLANTS

6. You are deciding whether to place breast implants in a subglandular or submuscular plane in a young, slim fitness coach. *Which one of the following is correct regarding implant placement relevant to this patient?*
   A. Nipple sensation is equally likely to be preserved with submuscular or subglandular implant placement.
   B. Mammography and breast cancer diagnosis are similarly affected, irrespective of the chosen site.
   C. A submuscular site can result in animation deformities that may be unacceptable for this patient.
   D. Capsular contracture rates are unaffected by the choice of implant site.
   E. A subglandular implant will provide a better contour, which is less prone to palpable implant edges.

DUAL PLANE BREAST IMPLANT PLACEMENT

7. *Which one of the following statements is correct regarding dual plane augmentation?*
   A. By definition, dual plane involves creation of two separate, complete, subglandular and submuscular pockets.
   B. Dual plane I is indicated for breasts in which all of the breast parenchyma is above the IMF.
   C. Dual plane II refers to a modified version of the first published dual plane technique.
   D. Dual plane III involves dissection of the breast from the pectoralis fascia up to the upper pole limit.
   E. Dual plane techniques tend to limit breast parenchymal expansion in the lower pole.

INTRAOPERATIVE APPROACH TO BREAST AUGMENTATION

8. *When undertaking breast augmentation which one of the following is recommended?*
   A. Administration of intravenous (IV) antibiotics (cephalosporin) at the time of implant placement
   B. Delivery of a triple antibiotic solution to the implant pocket created (gentamicin, cefazolin, and bacitracin)
   C. Avoidance of povidone-iodine products contacting the implant and pocket
   D. Avoidance of hypochlorous acid (HOCl) within the implant pocket
   E. Maintaining short incisions when using form-stable implants

THE BAKER CLASSIFICATION

9. A patient has capsular contracture on both sides. On the left, the implant is painful. On the right, the patient is unaware of any changes. *What classification of contraction does she have?*
   A. Baker IV left, Baker III right
   B. Baker II left, Baker III right
   C. Baker II left, Baker IV right
   D. Baker IV left, Baker II right
   E. Baker IV left, Baker I right

CAPSULAR CONTRACTURE

10. *Which one of the following has traditionally been linked to an increased rate of capsular contraction following primary breast augmentation?*
    A. Use of a polyurethane implant
    B. Implant placement in a submuscular plane
    C. Use of a textured implant
    D. Use of a silicone-filled implant
    E. Use of a saline-filled implant

CAPSULAR CONTRACTURE

11. You have a patient with a capsular contracture after revision augmentation and are explaining to her the biofilm theory relating to capsular contracture. *Which one of the following organisms is most likely to be implicated in this theory?*
    A. *Staphylococcus aureus*   D. *Staphylococcus epidermidis*
    B. *Streptococcus pyogenes*   E. *Streptococcus viridans*
    C. *Staphylococcus saprophyticus*

BREAST DEFORMITY FOLLOWING IMPLANT SURGERY

12. *What anatomic structure is primarily responsible for development of a classic or type B double-bubble breast deformity post implant surgery?*
    A. The nipple-areola complex (NAC)   D. The natural inframammary fold (IMF)
    B. The pectoralis major muscle   E. The breast parenchyma
    C. The breast implant capsule

IMAGING AFTER BREAST IMPLANTATION

13. *Which one of the following findings on ultrasound suggest there is extracapsular rupture of a silicone implant?*
    A. Stepladder sign
    B. Linguine sign
    C. Snowstorm sign
    D. Eklund sign
    E. Window shading sign

COUNSELING PATIENTS FOR BREAST AUGMENTATION

14. *Which one of the following represents the greatest risk to a patient undergoing primary subglandular breast augmentation with a silicone, form-stable implant?*
    A. Implant rupture
    B. Altered nipple sensation
    C. Postoperative infection
    D. Capsular contracture
    E. Postoperative hematoma

MANAGEMENT OF PROBLEMATIC BREAST CAPSULES (NEW)

15. You see a 30-year-old patient in clinic who has grade III capsules of the breasts 2 years out following primary augmentation with 450-cc subglandular smooth implants. She is keen to have implants that are smaller and more natural shape. There is no evidence of implant rupture but there is a waterfall deformity. *Which one of the following represents her best option for short- and long-term management of this problem?*
    A. Anterior capsulectomy and subglandular implant
    B. Posterior capsulectomy and submuscular implant
    C. Total capsulectomy and subglandular implant
    D. Total capsulectomy and submuscular implant
    E. Open capsulotomy and submuscular implant

IMPLANT RUPTURE (NEW)

16. *When meeting a patient who is considering breast augmentation, what rupture rate per annum would be most appropriate to quote to her based on current evidence on a latest generation implant?*
    A. 1%
    B. 3%
    C. 5%
    D. 7%
    E. 10%

BREAST IMPLANT–ASSOCIATED ANAPLASTIC LARGE CELL LYMPHOMA (BIA-ALCL)

17. *When discussing the risks of BIA-ALCL with patients preoperatively, which one of the following is true?*
    A. More than 3000 cases have been recorded worldwide at present.
    B. The condition is treatable but normally requires implant removal and chemotherapy.
    C. It is equally likely to occur irrespective of implant brand and texturing technique.
    D. First presentation of BIA-ALCL tends to occur in the second decade after initial implantation.
    E. The baseline risk of developing BIA-ALCL following primary augmentation is around 1:5000.

BREAST IMPLANT–ASSOCIATED ANAPLASTIC LARGE CELL LYMPHOMA (BIA-ALCL)

18. Where a patient presents with a chronic seroma to the breast following breast augmentation and BIA-ALCL is suspected, what is the advised initial management?
    A. Aspiration of peri-implant fluid and cytologic analysis
    B. Capsule tissue biopsy for histologic analysis
    C. Open axillary lymph node biopsy for histologic analysis
    D. Baseline blood tests to include complete blood count (CBC), lactate dehydrogenase (LDH), and electrolytes
    E. MRI of the breast and chest wall

Answers

BACKGROUND TO BREAST AUGMENTATION

1. *Which one of the following statements is correct regarding breast augmentation?*

   C. **There are five generations of silicone implant, if texturing, gel type, and shape are considered.**

   There are five generations of breast implants. The first generation, which appeared in the 1960s, had a thick shell and thick filler with a Dacron patch to help secure it. The second generation appeared in the 1970s and had a thin shell and a less viscous filler. In the 1980s, the third-generation implants were released, and these reverted back to a thicker silicone shell with the addition of a barrier coating. Fourth- and fifth-generation implants represent refined third-generation implants with textured shells and cohesive or form-stable gel fillers. They are available in anatomic or round shapes. Cohesive gel implants rather than saline-filled implants represent the current gold standard because they are more natural in feel, ripple less, and retain their integrity following rupture.

   Breast augmentation is one of the most common cosmetic procedures, and in 1992 (not 2001) a moratorium was placed on its use by the FDA over safety concerns with silicone implants.[1] This was subsequently retracted in 2006, and a number of silicone prostheses are currently approved for use in the United States, both for primary augmentation and reconstruction. Such implants currently include smooth and textured subtypes, although there was debate in 2019 with regards to whether textured subtype should be banned due to an association with breast implant–associated anaplastic large cell lymphoma (BIA-ALCL). However, there is not conclusive evidence to support this action at present. Furthermore, there is no proven link between silicone implant use and breast cancer or systemic autoimmune disease.[1,2]

REFERENCES

1. US Food and Drug Administration. Medical devices: breast implants. Available at https://www.fda.gov/medical-devices/breast-implants/update-safety-silicone-gel-filled-breast-implants-2011-executive-summary
2. Spear SL, Parikh PM, Goldstein JA. History of breast implants and the food and drug administration. Clin Plast Surg 2009;36(1):15–21, v

PATIENT EVALUATION FOR BREAST AUGMENTATION

2. *Which one of the following is not routinely required during the assessment of patients requesting breast augmentation?*

   B. **Evidence of recent negative mammograms**

   Although assessment of a patient's status for breast cancer is important, mammograms are not routinely required prior to undertaking breast augmentation. A general rule of thumb is to arrange a mammogram in patients over the age of 40 or those with a personal or family history of breast cancer. Assessment of the other parameters is absolutely necessary to optimize patient outcomes for implant selection and placement. First, the psychosocial elements must be explored and the patient must be given in-depth information to help understand what the long-term implications are for breast implant placement. Examination must include assessment not only of the breast but also the chest wall shape to identify any asymmetries or irregularities which may affect outcome. Assessment of the breasts themselves will include evaluation of the skin and soft tissues of the breast as well as specific measurements of breast base width, notch-to-nipple, and nipple-to-IMF distances.[1-4]

REFERENCES

1. Selber JC, Nelson JA, Ashana AO, et al. Breast cancer screening prior to cosmetic breast surgery: ASPS members' Adherence to American Cancer Society Guidelines. Plast Reconstr Surg 2009;124(5):1375–1385
2. Smith RA, Cokkinides V, Eyre HJ; American Cancer Society. American Cancer Society guidelines for the early detection of cancer, 2003. CA Cancer J Clin 2003;53(1):27–43
3. Tebbetts JB, Adams WP. Five critical decisions in breast augmentation using five measurements in 5 minutes: the high five decision support process. Plast Reconstr Surg 2006;118(7, Suppl):35S–45S
4. Alpert BS, Lalonde DH. MOC-PS(SM) CME article: breast augmentation. Plast Reconstr Surg 2008;121(4, Suppl):1–7

SELECTION OF BREAST IMPLANTS FOR COSMETIC AUGMENTATION

3. A slim 30-year-old woman is seen in the outpatient department; she is considering breast augmentation. Examination shows she has good breast symmetry and mild (grade I) ptosis, with nipple-to-notch distances of

26 cm. There are no chest wall deformities evident, and tissue quality is good. *Which one of the following is most useful to guide decision-making for plane of implant placement?*

D. **Assessing the superior pole tissue thickness**

There are a number of key decisions to be made when assessing a patient for breast augmentation. These include implant volume, implant shape, and implant pocket selection. In addition, decisions need to be made on textured versus smooth shell devices and saline versus silicone fill.

Assessment of the superior pole fullness is considered to be a key step in helping to decide on the implant pocket selection as where there is minimal upper pole soft tissue cover, submuscular implant placement is generally advocated. Where there is greater volume present, subglandular placement may be preferred.[1]

There are a number of key steps used to help decide what implant size should be used. The first is to measure breast base width and height; this will enable the surgeon to select an appropriate size implant for this patient's current breast and frame size. The next step is to confirm what appearance the patient wishes to achieve and how much bigger she wishes her breasts to be. To achieve this, implant sizers placed in a bra may be helpful to establish a visual image for the patient and surgeon. Alternatively, the use of computer-generated images may be helpful and many surgeons are using this approach for their patients. The risk of using computer-generated imagery is that expectations may be unrealistically set. Once this information is available, the appropriate implant sizes can be selected. Intraoperative decisions on final precise volume can be supported by the use of temporary sizer placement; however, this may increase the risk of complications such as infection as there is more tissue manipulation and passing of the implant multiple times. This can also increase the costs because of increased theater time and equipment. The distance from nipple-areola complex (NAC) to inframammary fold is important when considering the implant base dimensions and the volume of breast implant with respect to the final NAC position. It can also be a factor in decision-making for the need for mastopexy.[2–5]

REFERENCES

1. Tebbetts JB, Adams WP. Five critical decisions in breast augmentation using five measurements in 5 minutes: the high five decision support process. Plast Reconstr Surg 2006;118(7, Suppl):35S–45S
2. Alpert BS, Lalonde DH. MOC-PS(SM) CME article: breast augmentation. Plast Reconstr Surg 2008;121(4, Suppl):1–7
3. Young VL, Watson ME. Breast implant research: where we have been, where we are, where we need to go. Clin Plast Surg 2001;28(3):451–483, vi
4. Tepper OM, Small KH, Unger JG, et al. 3D analysis of breast augmentation defines operative changes and their relationship to implant dimensions. Ann Plast Surg 2009;62(5):570–575
5. Khoo LS, Radwanski HN, Senna-Fernandes V, Antônio NN, Fellet LLF, Pitanguy I. Does the use of intraoperative breast sizers increase complication rates in primary breast augmentation? A retrospective analysis of 416 consecutive cases in a single institution. Plast Surg Int 2016;2016:6584810

EXPECTED OUTCOMES FOLLOWING BREAST AUGMENTATION

4. A patient is seen in clinic prior to undergoing subglandular breast augmentation. She has grade 1 ptosis and a body mass index (BMI) of 24. She has a number of questions relating to likely outcomes after surgery which is planned with 375-cc smooth round implants. *Which one of the following is true in her case?*

E. **She should expect to be able to feel the implant edges and may see rippling, particularly in the lower pole.**

It is vital that patients undergoing breast augmentation understand the implications it will have in the future for them. First, they must understand that implants look, feel, and behave differently to natural breast tissue. Slim patients are most likely to feel and see their implants so must expect rippling and palpability of implants, particularly where soft tissue cover is thinner. This most often affects the lower pole but in subglandular placement such as in this case, upper pole irregularities may also be evident.[1]

Patients frequently inquire how many bra cup sizes they will increase following augmentation, and it is important to explain that no guarantee of specific size can be given. However, a rule of thumb is that for each 125–150 cc of volume added, there will be increase of one cup size. This is just a guide and will be affected by overall breast volume and patient size. In this case an implant of 375 cc would probably increase cup size by two to three sizes.[2] A further key area for discussion is the effect of an implant on ptosis. In cases such as this where there is mild ptosis, and a relatively empty skin envelope, implants can correct the ptosis. However, in moderate or severe ptosis or those patients with thin, stretched tissues such as after massive weight loss, they will almost certainly need a mastopexy in addition to the increased volume provided by an implant. Again, discussing this preoperatively is vital to set out expectations. Patients will often inquire about the risks of breast cancer after implants and as things stand, there is no evidence to suggest that either detection of cancer nor overall risks are affected by implant surgery.[3,4] Risks of breast implant–associated anaplastic large cell lymphoma (BIA-ALCL) must be discussed in relation to breast augmentation; however, as this patient is having smooth implants, there is no quantifiable risk of developing anaplastic large cell lymphoma (ALCL). In spite of this, it is still prudent to have the discussion in clinic.[5]

REFERENCES

1. Laurence GN. Breast implant rippling and palpability. In: Mugea TT, Shiffman MA, eds. Aesthetic Surgery of the Breast. Berlin, Heidelberg: Springer; 2015
2. King NM, Lovric V, Parr WCH, Walsh WR, Moradi P. What is the standard volume to increase a cup size for breast augmentation surgery? A novel three-dimensional computed tomographic approach. Plast Reconstr Surg 2017;139(5):1084–1089
3. Deapen DM, Hirsch EM, Brody GS. Cancer risk among Los Angeles women with cosmetic breast implants. Plast Reconstr Surg 2007;119(7):1987–1992
4. Hoshaw SJ, Klein PJ, Clark BD, Cook RR, Perkins LL. Breast implants and cancer: causation, delayed detection, and survival. Plast Reconstr Surg 2001;107(6):1393–1407
5. de Jong D, Vasmel WLE, de Boer JP, et al. Anaplastic large-cell lymphoma in women with breast implants. JAMA 2008;300(17):2030–2035

INCISION CHOICE FOR BREAST AUGMENTATION

5. *When choosing the incision site for breast augmentation, which one of the following statements is correct?*

   D. The transaxillary approach avoids a breast scar but risks sensory nerve damage to the arm.

   There are four approaches to breast augmentation: inframammary, transaxillary, periareolar, and transumbilical. The pocket dissection may be performed under direct vision where the incision is on the breast as in the IMF or periareolar approaches. Where more distant incisions are used such as the transaxillary or periumbilical approaches, then endoscopic pocket dissection is required.

   The transaxillary approach is less commonly used than the IMF approach but does offer some potential advantages. In experienced hands, it can be a useful technique where avoidance of a breast scar is important to the patient. It begins with an open approach in the axilla with subcutaneous dissection to the lateral border of pectoralis major. Dissection then continues under pectoralis and using the endoscope, the implant pocket is created. The implant, which may be saline or silicone gel filled, can then be passed using an introducer such as a Keller funnel with a no skin touch technique. A disadvantage of this technique (aside from the endoscope skill set required) is the potential risk of injury to sensory nerves including the intercostobrachial and medial brachial cutaneous nerves.[1-3] The IMF approach is commonly used and allows good access to the breast pocket with a scar usually hidden by natural ptosis within a well-defined IMF. The scar should be slightly lateral to the NAC, not in line with it, to minimize visibility medially (1 cm medial and 4 cm lateral). Tissue recruitment from the chest wall may occur during breast augmentation, and this must be considered when choosing the incision height to avoid placing the scar too high or too low on the final augmented breast or chest wall. The periareolar approach can be performed with either direct parenchymal dissection or using a stair-step approach that involves dissection in a subcutaneous plane to the inferior breast before undermining the gland to create the implant pocket. The stair-step approach is considered preferable since it avoids the need to breach the parenchyma, which could lead to potential damage to the ducts and may impact on infection risk. The transumbilical approach is only suitable for saline implants and involves difficult and blind dissection. It is also more challenging to make adjustments or corrections with this approach and can lead to high or asymmetrical implant placement. Because of these limitations, it is the least commonly used approach.[4-6]

REFERENCES

1. Strock LL. Transaxillary endoscopic silicone gel breast augmentation. Aesthet Surg J. 2010 Sep;30(5):745–55.
2. Price CI, Eaves FF, Nahai F. Endoscopic transaxillary subpectoral breast augmentation. Plast Reconstr Surg 1994;94:612–619
3. Tebbetts JB. Axillary endoscopic breast augmentation: processes derived from a 28-year experience to optimize outcomes. Plast Reconstr Surg 2006; 118(7, Suppl):53S–80S
4. Hidalgo DA. Breast augmentation: choosing the optimal incision, implant, and pocket plane. Plast Reconstr Surg 2000;105(6):2202–2216, discussion 2217–2218
5. Alpert BS, Lalonde DH. MOC-PS(SM) CME article: breast augmentation. Plast Reconstr Surg 2008;121(4, Suppl):1–7
6. Mofid MM, Klatsky SA, Singh NK, Nahabedian MY. Nipple-areola complex sensitivity after primary breast augmentation: a comparison of periareolar and inframammary incision approaches. Plast Reconstr Surg 2006;117(6):1694–1698

PLACEMENT OF BREAST IMPLANTS

6. You are deciding whether to place breast implants in a subglandular or submuscular plane in a young, slim fitness coach. *Which one of the following is correct regarding implant placement relevant to this patient?*

   C. A submuscular site can result in animation deformities that may be unacceptable for this patient.

   Placement of the implant under the pectoralis major can result in movement of the implant during activity. This is called an "animation deformity" and may be a major problem for patients involved in athletic activities, such as this patient.[1,2] Various techniques have been described to minimize this including splitting pectoralis major.[2,3]

Nipple sensation is usually preserved following breast augmentation but it is more likely to be preserved with submuscular placement because the fourth intercostal nerve runs within the pectoralis fascia. Standard mammography may be affected by placement of subglandular breast implants, so it is important for patients to inform the radiographer in advance so that screening views may be adapted. Despite this, there is no evidence to suggest breast cancer diagnosis is delayed following breast implant placement in either plane.[4]

Capsular contracture rates are traditionally lower with submuscular implant placement and textured implants.[5,6] Given that she is thin, this patient may benefit from the increased soft tissue coverage that a submuscular site offers. This usually depends on the upper pole soft tissue cover, with more than 2 cm usually required on a pinch test to proceed with subglandular implants.

REFERENCES

1. Dyrberg DL, Bille C, Gunnarsson GL, et al. Breast animation deformity. Arch Plast Surg 2019;46(1):7–15
2. Pelle-Ceravolo M, Del Vescovo A, Bertozzi E, Molinari P. A technique to decrease breast shape deformity during muscle contraction in submuscular augmentation mammaplasty. Aesthetic Plast Surg 2004;28(5):288–294
3. Bracaglia R, Tambasco D, Gentileschi S, D'Ettorre M. Triple-plane technique for breast augmentation: solving animation deformities. Aesthetic Plast Surg 2013;37(4):715–718
4. Jakubietz MG, Janis JE, Jakubietz RG, Rohrich RJ. Breast augmentation: cancer concerns and mammography—a literature review. Plast Reconstr Surg 2004;113(7):117e–122e
5. Wong CH, Samuel M, Tan BK, Song C. Capsular contracture in subglandular breast augmentation with textured versus smooth breast implants: a systematic review. Plast Reconstr Surg 2006;118(5):1224–1236
6. Barnsley GP, Sigurdson LJ, Barnsley SE. Textured surface breast implants in the prevention of capsular contracture among breast augmentation patients: a meta-analysis of randomized controlled trials. Plast Reconstr Surg 2006;117(7):2182–2190

DUAL PLANE BREAST IMPLANT PLACEMENT

7. *Which one of the following statements is correct regarding dual plane augmentation?*

B. Dual plane I is used for breasts in which all of the breast is above the IMF.

The use of the term "dual plane" can sometimes seem confusing in its terminology, but in simple terms it is development of the submuscular approach to breast augmentation that may help reduce some of the problems with either a total submuscular or subglandular implant placement.

The dual plane refers to the fact that the upper part of the implant is submuscular and the lower part is subglandular. However, the implant only lies in one plane, but this plane starts under one tissue type and continues under another. The perceived benefits of using a dual plane approach include a greater soft tissue cover in the upper pole, accurate implant placement at the IMF, and better expansion of the breast parenchyma in the lower pole, thereby helping to reduce a waterfall deformity where the breast tissue slides over the implant.

The dual plane I technique releases the lower border of the pectoralis major at the IMF and continues with a subpectoral dissection. This is used for most typical breasts. The criteria include the following: all of the breast is above the IMF, there is a tight attachment of parenchyma to the pectoralis, and the lower pole is minimally stretched.

Dual planes II and III are used for more ptotic breasts, where there is breast tissue below the IMF and the lower pole is therefore stretched. Dual plane III is also advocated for a constricted breast. The difference between dual planes II and III is the extent of dissection of the subglandular pocket. In dual plane II this is continued to the lower border of the areola, and in dual plane III this is continued to the top of the areola (not the full extent of the superior pole).[1,2]

REFERENCES

1. Tebbetts JB. Dual plane breast augmentation: optimizing implant-soft-tissue relationships in a wide range of breast types. Plast Reconstr Surg 2001;107(5):1255–1272
2. Swanson E. Dual plane versus subpectoral breast augmentation: is there a difference? Plast Reconstr Surg Glob Open 2016;4(12):e1173

INTRAOPERATIVE APPROACH TO BREAST AUGMENTATION

8. *When undertaking breast augmentation which one of the following is recommended?*

B. Delivery of a triple antibiotic solution to the implant pocket created (Gentamicin, cefazolin, and bacitracin)

There are a number of steps which can be undertaken intraoperatively when performing breast augmentation in order to reduce the risk of implant infection. These begin with ensuring meticulous skin preparation with an agent such as alcohol-based chlorhexidine 2%, covering the nipple-areola complex with a temporary dressing, minimizing implant handling, maintaining meticulous prospective hemostasis, and performing irrigation of the newly created pocket. In terms of pocket washout, use of a triple antibiotic is generally advocated. This will include 80 mg of gentamicin, 50,000 units of bacitracin, and 1 g of cefazolin. It is used to soak the pocket for 5 minutes. Alternative pocket irrigation substances include 50 mL of povidone iodine with 1 g of cefazolin and 80 mg of gentamicin in 500 mL of sterile saline. In vitro, this has been shown to eliminate all organisms commonly identified in breast implant pockets. There was a previous FDA warning on directions for use (DFU) disallowing povidone iodine around implants as it was thought to damage the implant shell. This is no longer thought to be the case. A further alternative for pocket washout is hypochlorous acid (HOCl) which can provide antimicrobial activity without risk of cytotoxicity to fibroblasts. Intravenous antibiotics are given 30–60 minutes before surgery rather than at the time of implant placement. Form-stable implants generally require slightly longer, not shorter, incisions due to their construction. Minimizing skin contact with the implants when placing them is key as otherwise bacteria may be dragged in from the skin edges. For this reason, many surgeons will use a device that acts as a funnel (Keller funnel) somewhat like a cake icing bag that transfers the implant through the incision into the pocket with no skin contact at all. They will also change to fresh gloves at the time of implant placement.[1-7]

REFERENCES

1. Jewell ML, Adams WP Jr. Betadine and breast implants. Aesthet Surg J 2018;38(6):623–626
2. Adams WP Jr. Commentary on: surgical site irrigation in plastic surgery: what is essential? Aesthet Surg J 2018;38(3):276–278
3. Adams WP Jr, Conner WC, Barton FE Jr, Rohrich RJ. Optimizing breast pocket irrigation: an in vitro study and clinical implications. Plast Reconstr Surg 2000;105(1):334–338, discussion 339–343
4. Adams WP Jr, Conner WC, Barton FE Jr, Rohrich RJ. Optimizing breast-pocket irrigation: the post-betadine era. Plast Reconstr Surg 2001;107(6):1596–1601
5. Haws MJ, Gingrass MK, Porter RS, Brindle CT. Surgical breast pocket irrigation with hypochlorous acid (HOCl): an in vivo evaluation of pocket protein content and potential HOCl antimicrobial capacity. Aesthet Surg J 2018;38(11):1178–1184
6. Adams WP Jr, Rios JL, Smith SJ. Enhancing patient outcomes in aesthetic and reconstructive breast surgery using triple antibiotic breast irrigation: six-year prospective clinical study. Plast Reconstr Surg 2006;117(1):30–36
7. Moyer HR, Ghazi B, Saunders N, Losken A. Contamination in smooth gel breast implant placement: testing a funnel versus digital insertion technique in a cadaver model. Aesthet Surg J 2012;32(2):194–199

THE BAKER CLASSIFICATION

9. A patient has capsular contracture on both sides. On the left, the implant is painful. On the right, the patient is unaware of any changes. *What classification of contraction does she have?*

   D. Baker IV left, Baker II right

   The Baker classification has four grades, I through IV. A grade I is a soft breast with no evidence of capsule contraction. A grade II breast has a palpable, firm capsule that is not visible; usually only the clinician would notice and diagnose a grade II. A patient is likely to notice grades III and IV. In both grades the breast will have an altered appearance and feel firm. The key difference between grades III and IV is the presence or absence of pain, with IV being painful.[1-3]

REFERENCES

1. Spear SL, Baker JL Jr. Classification of capsular contracture after prosthetic breast reconstruction. Plast Reconstr Surg 1995;96(5):1119–1123, discussion 1124
2. Wan D, Rohrich RJ. Revisiting the management of capsular contracture in breast augmentation: a systematic review. Plast Reconstr Surg 2016;137(3):826–841
3. Zahavi A, Sklair ML, Ad-El DD. Capsular contracture of the breast: working towards a better classification using clinical and radiologic assessment. Ann Plast Surg 2006;57(3):248–251

CAPSULAR CONTRACTURE

10. *Which one of the following has traditionally been linked to an increased rate of capsular contraction following primary breast augmentation?*

    D. Use of a silicone-filled implant

    Traditional rates of capsular contracture before the 1992 FDA ban ranged from around 10% to almost 60%, depending on the type of implant used and its anatomic placement. Silicone implants were associated with much higher contracture rates than either saline or polyurethane. Smooth implants were associated with particularly high rates of capsular contracture and this was the reason for implants being subsequently textured. Placement of the implant in the subpectoral plane was also shown to reduce capsular contracture rates. Most recently collected data show less variation between the factors described above, and the most important factor appears to be the setting in which the implant is used. The rates of capsular contracture are lowest in primary breast augmentation, but are higher in both revision augmentation and reconstruction settings.[1-7]

REFERENCES

1. Calobrace MB, Stevens WG, Capizzi PJ, Cohen R, Godinez T, Beckstrand M. Risk factor analysis for capsular contracture: a 10-year Sientra study using round, smooth, and textured implants for breast augmentation. Plast Reconstr Surg 2018;141(4S Sientra Shaped and Round Cohesive Gel Implants, 4S):20S–28S
2. Gylbert L, Asplund O, Jurell G. Capsular contracture after breast reconstruction with silicone-gel and saline-filled implants: a 6-year follow-up. Plast Reconstr Surg 1990;85(3):373–377
3. Marotta JS, Widenhouse CW, Habal MB, Goldberg EP. Silicone gel breast implant failure and frequency of additional surgeries: analysis of 35 studies reporting examination of more than 8,000 explants. J Biomed Mater Res 1999;48(3):354–364
4. U.S Food and Drug Administration. Center for Devices and Radiological Health. FDA Update on the Safety of Silicone Gel-Filled Breast Implants. 2011
5. Mentor MC. Saline implant premarket approval information. http://www.fda.gov/downloads/medicaldevices/productsandmedicalprocedures/implantsandprosthetics/ breastimpiants/ucm232436.pdf. Published 2001
6. Allergan C. Saline implant premarket approval information. www.fda.gov//downioads/medicaidevices/productsandmedicaiprocedures/impiantsandprosthetics/breastimpiants/ucm064457.pdf. Published 2001
7. FDA. Mentor, Allergan, and Sientra Corporations: Silicone breast implant premarket approval information. www.fda.gov/medicaidevices/productsandmedicaiprocedures/impiantsandprosthetics/breastimpiants/ucm063871.htm. Published 2003

CAPSULAR CONTRACTURE

11. You have a patient with a capsular contracture after revision augmentation and are explaining to her the biofilm theory relating to capsular contracture. *Which one of the following organisms is most likely to be implicated in this theory?*

    D. Staphylococcus epidermidis

    The biofilm theory is currently the single most well-accepted theory for development of capsular contracture. There is a proposed correlation between subclinical infection and subsequent development of a biofilm, although the precise causal relationship has not been shown. As a single organism, *Staphylococcus epidermidis* is the most commonly implicated organism, but other types of bacteria may also be implicated and a polymicrobial cause is also likely.

    Streptococcus pyogenes is a gram-positive bacterium that is the cause of severe group A streptococcal infections. *Staphylococcus saprophyticus* is a gram-positive, coagulase-negative facultative species that is a common cause of urinary tract infections. *Streptococcus viridans* is a commensal of the gastrointestinal and genitourinary tracts that can cause severe infections in immune-compromised patients. *Staphylococcus aureus* is a bacterium that commonly colonizes human skin and mucosa without causing any problems. It can be implicated in severe soft tissue infections and also have a role in capsular contracture formation.[1-8]

REFERENCES

1. Adams WP Jr. Capsular contracture: what is it? What causes it? How can it be prevented and managed? Clin Plast Surg 2009;36(1):119–126, vii
2. Rieger UM, Mesina J, Kalbermatten DF, et al. Bacterial biofilms and capsular contracture in patients with breast implants. Br J Surg 2013;100(6):768–774
3. Wixtrom RN, Stutman RL, Burke RM, Mahoney AK, Codner MA. Risk of breast implant bacterial contamination from endogenous breast flora, prevention with nipple shields, and implications for biofilm formation. Aesthet Surg J 2012;32(8):956–963
4. Burkhardt BRSM, Dempsey PD, Schnur PL, Tofield JJ. Capsular contracture: a prospective study of the effect of local antibacterial agents. Plast Reconstr Surg 1986;77(6):919–932
5. Virden CPSP, Dobke MK, Stein P, Parsons CL, Frank DH. Subclinical infection of the silicone breast implant surface as a possible cause of capsular contracture. Aesthetic Plast Surg 1992;16(2):173–179
6. Dobke MK, Svahn JK, Vastine VL, Landon BN, Stein PC, Parsons CL. Characterization of microbial presence at the surface of silicone mammary implants. Ann Plast Surg 1995;34(6):563–569, 570–571
7. Ajdic D, Zoghbi Y, Gerth D, Panthaki ZJ, Thaller S. The relationship of bacterial biofilms and capsular contracture in breast implants. Aesthet Surg J 2016;36(3):297–309
8. Costerton JW, DeMeo P. Discussion. The role of biofilms: are we hitting the right target? Plast Reconstr Surg 2011;127(Suppl 1):36S–37S

BREAST DEFORMITY FOLLOWING IMPLANT SURGERY

12. *What anatomic structure is primarily responsible for development of a classic or type B double-bubble breast deformity post implant surgery?*

D. **The natural inframammary fold (IMF)**

The double-bubble deformity occurs when the native breast and silicone implant separate to give the appearance of two distinct overlapping mounds. A double-bubble deformity can occur either from the implant displacing inferiorly, leaving breast tissue superiorly, or it can occur with the implant remaining superior and the breast tissue sliding off the implant inferiorly.

These deformities are classified as A if the implant is "Above" the breast or B if the implant is "Below" the breast. A type A double-bubble deformity can occur when a total submuscular plane is used because the implant is then held abnormally high on the chest wall, leaving the loose parenchyma to slide inferiorly. This is called a *waterfall deformity*. Type B can occur with over-dissection of the IMF, which allows the implant to slide into a lower pocket, resulting in the appearance of two separate IMFs. The native IMF will remain as a constricting band of soft tissue to create the classic double bubble.[1,2]

REFERENCES

1. Handel N. The double-bubble deformity: cause, prevention, and treatment. Plast Reconstr Surg 2013;132(6):1434–1443
2. Bresnick SD. Management of a common breast augmentation complication: treatment of the double-bubble deformity with fat grafting. Ann Plast Surg 2016;76(1):18–22

IMAGING AFTER BREAST IMPLANTATION

13. *Which one of the following findings on ultrasound suggest there is extracapsular rupture of a silicone implant?*

C. **Snowstorm sign**

Ultrasonography can demonstrate implant rupture with two commonly described phenomena: the snowstorm and stepladder signs. The snowstorm sign is seen most commonly in conjunction with an extracapsular rupture from small amounts of free silicone mixing with the surrounding breast tissue. The stepladder sign is seen in association with an intracapsular rupture. It is observed as multiple curvilinear low signal intensity lines within a high signal intensity silicone gel. The lines represent the collapsed implant shell floating in the silicone gel. Magnetic resonance imaging (MRI) is the gold standard for assessment of implant rupture. The linguine sign is seen on MRI when intracapsular rupture is present; it is analogous to the stepladder sign on ultrasound. Achieving adequate mammographic views is more challenging when there are breast implants in place, and the Eklund view is a technique used to displace the implant from the breast. Posterosuperior displacement of the implants is performed with simultaneous anterior traction on the implant. Window shading occurs where there is release of the sternal attachments of pectoralis major during breast implantation. This can be avoided by limiting release of the pectoralis to the inferior border medially.[1-4]

REFERENCES

1. Everson LI, Parantainen H, Detlie T, et al. Diagnosis of breast implant rupture: imaging findings and relative efficacies of imaging techniques. AJR Am J Roentgenol 1994;163(1):57–60
2. Gorczyca DP. MR imaging of breast implants. Magn Reson Imaging Clin N Am 1994;2(4):659–672
3. Gorczyca DP, Gorczyca SM, Gorczyca KL. The diagnosis of silicone breast implant rupture. Plast Reconstr Surg 2007;120(7, Suppl 1):49S–61S
4. U.S. Food and Drug Administration. Silicone Gel-Filled Breast Implants. Available online: http://www.fda.gov/Medical-Devices/ProductsandMedicalProcedures/ImplantsandProsthetics/BreastImplants/ucm063871.htm

COUNSELING PATIENTS FOR BREAST AUGMENTATION

14. *Which one of the following represents the greatest risk to a patient undergoing primary subglandular breast augmentation with a silicone, form-stable implant?*

B. **Altered nipple sensation**

The greatest risk of those listed above for a patient undergoing primary breast augmentation as in this case is alteration of nipple sensation. Permanent sensory change occurs in approximately 15% of patients. However, the highest overall risk is actually breast asymmetry as this will be an almost universal finding. The risk of implant rupture is low (probably around 1% per year based on most recent studies with overall rates below 10% at 10 years). Both postoperative infection and hematoma should be discussed with the patient but are also low risks (each less than 1%). The risk of developing capsular contracture is probably about 10% following primary augmentation based on current evidence. This has been traditionally higher for subglandular placement than submuscular placement but things seem to have evened out over time. These numbers highlight the importance of preoperative discussions about risk with patients and putting each into perspective. Often patients are most concerned about the risk of infection as they understand this can have serious negative effects on outcomes with the implant needing to be removed. Overall, each of the risks must be acknowledged and all steps taken to minimize each one from occurring.[1-4]

REFERENCES

1. Pitanguy I, Vaena M, Radwanski HN, Nunes D, Vargas AF. Relative implant volume and sensibility alterations after breast augmentation. Aesthetic Plast Surg 2007;31(3):238–243
2. Mofid MM, Klatsky SA, Singh NK, Nahabedian MY. Nipple-areola complex sensitivity after primary breast augmentation: a comparison of periareolar and inframammary incision approaches. Plast Reconstr Surg 2006;117(6):1694–1698
3. Stevens WG, Calobrace MB, Alizadeh K, Zeidler KR, Harrington JL, d'Incelli RC. Ten-year core study data for Sientra's Food and Drug Administration-approved round and shaped breast implants with cohesive silicone gel. Plast Reconstr Surg 2018;141(4S Sientra Shaped and Round Cohesive Gel Implants, 4S):7S–19S
4. Nava MB, Rancati A, Angrigiani C, Catanuto G, Rocco N. How to prevent complications in breast augmentation. Gland Surg 2017;6(2):210–217

MANAGEMENT OF PROBLEMATIC BREAST CAPSULES (NEW)

15. You see a 30-year-old patient in clinic who has grade III capsules of the breasts 2 years out following primary augmentation with 450-cc subglandular smooth implants. She is keen to have implants that are smaller and more natural shape. There is no evidence of implant rupture but there is a waterfall deformity. *Which one of the following represents her best option for short- and long-term management of this problem?*

C. Total capsulectomy and subglandular implant

The main indications for capsulectomy are Baker III or IV capsules, evidence of a ruptured implant, silicone granulomas, a requirement for an upsized implant, and ALCL. There are different types of capsulectomy characterized by how much of the capsule is to be removed.

When a patient generates a capsule early in the subglandular plane there is a strong indication for complete capsule removal and a change of implant pocket from subglandular to submuscular (dual plane). It would be reasonable to remain with the same plane if the capsular contracture was a much later finding or if the implant size was to be increased.

Anterior-only capsulectomy is often considered in submuscular capsulectomy because removal of the posterior capsule can risk damage to the rib cage and cause a pneumothorax. Patients should be advised of this preoperatively. For this reason, the posterior capsule may be left in situ. Posterior-only capsulectomy may be indicated in cases where the skin is thin and the implant is subglandular as it provides an additional layer of implant cover and avoids the risk of skin damage. In general, capsulotomy is only indicated in cases where the capsule is healthy and soft, i.e., without significant contracture, and the breast needs to be reshaped perhaps with a larger implant. A good example of a setting for capsulotomy is where an expander is being replaced with a permanent implant after breast reconstruction.[1]

An alternative to capsulectomy, where a change of implant pocket is planned, is to leave it in situ and close it down with sutures. A new subpectoral pocket can then be created.[2,3]

REFERENCES

1. Young VL. Guidelines and indications for breast implant capsulectomy. Plast Reconstr Surg 1998;102(3):884–891, discussion 892–894
2. Spear SL, Dayan JH, Bogue D, et al. The "neosubpectoral" pocket for the correction of symmastia. Plast Reconstr Surg 2009;124(3):695–703
3. Maxwell GP, Gabriel A. The neopectoral pocket in revisionary breast surgery. Aesthet Surg J 2008;28(4):463–467

IMPLANT RUPTURE (NEW)

16. *When meeting a patient who is considering breast augmentation, what rupture rate per annum would be most appropriate to quote to her based on current evidence on a latest generation implant?*

A. 1%

Current implant rupture rates with fourth- and fifth-generation silicone or saline implants are estimated to be around 1% per year for both silicone and saline implants, so these are reasonable figures to quote to patients during their consultation. This is much lower than the historical rates which were as follows:
- Mentor MemoryGel implant rupture rates through 8 years
  - 13.6% for primary augmentation
  - 15.5% for revision augmentation

- Allergan Naturelle implant rupture rates through 10 years
  - 9.3% for primary augmentation
  - 5.4% for revision augmentation
- Sientra cohesive gel implants through 8 years
  - 6.4% for primary augmentation
  - 5.2% for revision augmentation

Factors implicated in rupture include manufacturing flaws, underfilling, fold flaws, and surgical technical errors such as passing a needle through the shell.[1-5]

REFERENCES

1. U.S Food and Drug Administration. Center for Devices and Radiological Health. FDA Update on the Safety of Silicone Gel-Filled Breast Implants.; 2011
2. Mentor MC. Saline implant premarket approval information. http://www.fda.gov/downloads/medicaldevices/prod-uctsandmedicalprocedures/implantsandprosthetics/ breastimpiants/ucm232436.pdf. Published 2001
3. Allergan C. Saline implant premarket approval information. www.fda.gov//downioads/medicaidevices/productsand-medicaiprocedures/impiantsandprosthetics/breastimpiants/ucm064457.pdf. Published 2001
4. FDA. Mentor, Allergan, and Sientra Corporations: Silicone breast implant premarket approval information. www.fda.gov/medicaidevices/productsandmedicaiprocedures/impiantsandprosthetics/breastimpiants/ucm063871.htm. Published 2003
5. Spear SL, Murphy DK; Allergan Silicone Breast Implant U.S. Core Clinical Study Group. Natrelle round silicone breast implants: Core Study results at 10 years. Plast Reconstr Surg 2014;133(6):1354–1361

BREAST IMPLANT–ASSOCIATED ANAPLASTIC LARGE CELL LYMPHOMA (BIA-ALCL)

17. When discussing the risks of BIA-ALCL with patients preoperatively, which one of the following is true?

B. The condition is treatable but normally requires implant removal and chemotherapy.

When patients do develop BIA-ALCL, their prognosis is actually excellent and treatment is effective in most cases with complete capsulectomy, implant removal plus/minus chemotherapy, or radiation. Regardless of all the debate and media attention that BIA-ALCL has generated, the numbers remain relatively small overall (less than 600 cases worldwide).[1,2] Contrast this with breast cancer risk at 1:8, which shows the relative risk is still low. That said, minimizing risk of developing BIA-ALCL is paramount and implant type and manufacturing process all seem to play a part. BIA-ALCL is associated with textured implants only (not smooth) and most, but not all, cases are associated with a salt loss texturing process. Mentor use negative imprinting or stamping of the surface, Sientra use ammonium carbonate and heat, while Allergan use sodium chloride crystals which are then washed off. Therefore, risks are affected by different implant types and makes. They are also likely affected by bacterial contamination and genetic predisposition. First presentation of BIA-ALCL is 9 years (median time) but can occur within the first year. The baseline risk is somewhere between 1:1000 and 1:30,000 depending on factors described above.[1-5]

REFERENCES

1. K Groth A, Graf R. Breast implant-associated anaplastic large cell lymphoma (BIA-ALCL) and the textured breast implant crisis. Aesthetic Plast Surg 2020;44(1):1–12
2. de Jong D, Vasmel WLE, de Boer JP, et al. Anaplastic large-cell lymphoma in women with breast implants. JAMA 2008;300(17):2030–2035
3. Health C for D and R. Medical Device Reports of Breast Implant-Associated Anaplastic Large Cell Lymphoma. FDA. April 2019. http://www.fda.gov/medical-devices/breast-implants/medical-device-reports-breast-implant-associated-ana-plastic-large-cell-lymphoma. Accessed July 17, 2019.
4. Gidengil CA, Predmore Z, Mattke S, van Busum K, Kim B. Breast implant-associated anaplastic large cell lymphoma: a systematic review. Plast Reconstr Surg 2015;135(3): 713–720
5. Miranda RN, Aladily TN, Prince HM, et al. Breast implant-associated anaplastic large-cell lymphoma: long-term follow-up of 60 patients. J Clin Oncol 2014;32(2):114–120

BREAST IMPLANT–ASSOCIATED ANAPLASTIC LARGE CELL LYMPHOMA (BIA-ALCL)

18. Where a patient presents with a chronic seroma to the breast following breast augmentation and BIA-ALCL is suspected, what is the advised initial management?

A. Aspiration of peri-implant fluid and cytologic analysis

Clinical suspicion should be raised for BIA-ALCL in patients who present with a late seroma around a breast implant. In this circumstance, fluid should be submitted for cytological evaluation with Wright-Giemsa-stained smears and cell block immunochemistry testing for cluster of differentiation (CD30) and anaplastic lymphoma kinase (ALK) markers. Once the information has been obtained further management may be planned. The surgical management will involve total capsulectomy and implant removal. The capsule tissue can at this stage be sent for histologic analysis. Imaging is useful in the form of ultrasound which can be used to visualize the seroma and sample the fluid. MRI can also be useful for the same reasons. Once a diagnosis has been made, liaison with the hematology team must be made and the case discussed at the appropriate multidisciplinary team meetings. All diagnoses must be recorded and in the US the FDA should be informed.[1-5]

REFERENCES

1. Vu K, Ai W. Update on the treatment of anaplastic large cell lymphoma. Curr Hematol Malig Rep 2018;13(2):135–141
2. K Groth A, Graf R. Breast implant-associated anaplastic large cell lymphoma (BIA-ALCL) and the textured breast implant crisis. Aesthetic Plast Surg 2020;44(1):1–12
3. Health C for D and R. Medical Device Reports of Breast Implant-Associated Anaplastic Large Cell Lymphoma. FDA. April 2019. http://www.fda.gov/medical-devices/breast-implants/medical-device-reports-breast-implant-associated-ana-plastic-large-cell-lymphoma. Accessed July 17, 2019
4. Gidengil CA, Predmore Z, Mattke S, van Busum K, Kim B. Breast implant-associated anaplastic large cell lymphoma: a systematic review. Plast Reconstr Surg 2015;135(3): 713–720
5. Miranda RN, Aladily TN, Prince HM, et al. Breast implant-associated anaplastic large-cell lymphoma: long-term follow-up of 60 patients. J Clin Oncol 2014;32(2):114–120

52. Mastopexy

See *Essentials of Plastic Surgery*, third edition, pp. 710–727

CAUSES OF BREAST PTOSIS

1. A 45-year-old mother of two is seen in the office concerning her breast ptosis. *Which one of the following is not a factor in the development of this condition?*
   A. Loss of skin elasticity with increasing age
   B. Decreased breast parenchyma volume
   C. Effects of pregnancy on breast tissue
   D. Attenuation of fibrous attachments between superficial and deep breast fascia
   E. Alterations in the structural integrity of the inframammary fold

ASSESSMENT OF BREAST PTOSIS

2. You are in clinic and see a woman with concerns about her breast appearance which she feels has changed since losing 26 pounds in weight. Examination shows she has a nipple-areola complex (NAC) positioned at the level of the inframammary fold (IMF), with the majority of the breast below this. *How best is this appearance described?*
   A. Normal
   B. Grade I ptosis
   C. Grade II ptosis
   D. Grade III ptosis
   E. Pseudoptosis

CLINICAL EXAMINATION OF THE BREAST

3. A 50-year-old patient presents with concerns about her breast shape. She feels her breasts have become more droopy over the past 10 years and that there is very little upper pole fullness. Examination shows the breasts to be a reasonable volume with the nipple-areola complex (NAC) and most of the glandular breast tissue being located above the inframammary fold (IMF). There is a degree of upper pole emptiness. *How would this appearance be correctly described?*
   A. Normal
   B. Grade I ptosis
   C. Grade II ptosis
   D. Tuberous breast
   E. Pseudoptosis

MANAGEMENT OF BREAST PSEUDOPTOSIS

4. A 35-year-old patient has bilateral pseudoptosis after removal of 200-cc implants. She still has adequate breast volume and satisfactory nipple positions. *How best might this be managed surgically?*
   A. Wise-pattern mastopexy
   B. Vertical scar mastopexy
   C. Inframammary fold wedge excision
   D. Periareolar resection
   E. Vertical skin wedge resection

IMPROVING BREAST SHAPE FOLLOWING WEIGHT LOSS

5. After significant weight loss, a 50-year-old patient has bilateral grade III ptosis with a nipple-to-notch distance of 32 cm, a large skin excess, and deficient breast volume. She is a nonsmoker, wears an A-cup bra, and wishes to improve both the shape and volume of her breasts. *How best might this be managed?*
   A. Single-stage, vertical scar augmentation-mastopexy
   B. Single-stage, Wise-pattern augmentation-mastopexy
   C. Two-stage, periareolar augmentation-mastopexy
   D. Two-stage, Wise-pattern augmentation-mastopexy
   E. Two-stage, vertical scar augmentation-mastopexy

MANAGEMENT OF BREAST PTOSIS

6. A 30-year-old patient requests unilateral breast surgery to improve the symmetry of her breasts. Examination shows she has breast asymmetry with a notch-to-nipple distance of 28 cm (left) and 24 cm (right). She has adequate breast volume and good quality skin and soft tissues on both sides and prefers the smaller breast. *How might this best be treated?*
   A. Unilateral vertical scar mastopexy
   B. Bilateral vertical scar mastopexy
   C. Unilateral Wise-pattern mastopexy
   D. Bilateral Wise-pattern mastopexy with differential reduction
   E. Unilateral vertical scar mastopexy with low volume reduction

SURGICAL PLANNING IN BREAST SURGERY

7. A patient is scheduled for surgery to have breast implants placed in the submuscular plane and wishes to have a subtle uplift at the same time. Examination shows that the nipple position only needs to be elevated 2 cm and that the overall breast shape is pleasing. *Which one of the following mastopexy skin patterns would be indicated for use in this case?*
   A. Crescent
   B. Periareolar
   C. Circumvertical
   D. Inverted T
   E. J shape

CLINICAL ASSESSMENT IN AESTHETIC BREAST SURGERY

8. *When assessing a patient in clinic, prior to planning for a mastopexy, which one of the following measurements best assesses the skin redundancy in the lower pole?*
   A. The intermammary distance
   B. The notch-to-nipple distance
   C. The nipple-to-inframammary fold (IMF) distance
   D. The clavicle-to-IMF distance
   E. The breast base width

POSTOPERATIVE COMPLICATIONS FOLLOWING MASTOPEXY

9. *Which one of the following is the most common complication after inverted-T (Wise pattern) mastopexy?*
   A. Hematoma
   B. Infection
   C. Wound healing problems
   D. High-riding nipple
   E. Nipple necrosis

VERTICAL SCAR MASTOPEXY

10. *When undergoing mastopexy with a vertical scar approach, which one of the following must be discussed with the patient preoperatively that most specifically relates to this technique?*
   A. The risk of skin pleating around the nipple-areola complex (NAC)
   B. Flattening of the breast and NAC
   C. Risk of T junction breakdown
   D. Risk of inferior skin redundancy
   E. Lack of upper pole fullness early post surgery

MANAGEMENT OF THE BREAST AFTER IMPLANT REMOVAL

11. *When discussing capsulectomy and implant removal in a 55-year-old patient with moderate ptosis and a waterfall deformity, which one of the following is correct?*
   A. She must understand that her ptosis is unlikely to be improved following capsulectomy and explantation alone.
   B. It would not be possible to combine the implant removal and an uplift safely within a single stage.
   C. She would be better to have the implants replaced at the same time as the capsulectomy.
   D. Smoking in the perioperative period would probably have little impact on her outcome of surgery.
   E. Her residual breast volume is likely to be greater than before her implants were placed.

TUBEROUS BREAST DEFORMITY

12. *Which one of the following is a typical feature of the tuberous breast?*
    A. A small areola
    B. Absence of the inframammary fold
    C. Increased breast volume
    D. Herniation of parenchymal tissue
    E. Broad breast base

SURGICAL MANAGEMENT OF THE TUBEROUS BREAST

13. A 17-year-old girl presents with a unilateral tuberous breast deformity. There is severe lower pole skin deficiency and a two-cup size volume difference compared with the contralateral side. The nipple-areola complex is oversized and the nipple height is slightly lower than on the contralateral side. She prefers the volume and shape of her normal, larger breast. *What is the best initial surgical management for this patient's tuberous breast?*
    A. Periareolar mastopexy with immediate permanent implant
    B. Periareolar mastopexy and fat transfer to the lower pole
    C. Vertical scar mastopexy with contralateral reduction
    D. Inferior pole scoring and insertion of a tissue expander
    E. Periareolar mastopexy with second-stage implant insertion

MASTOPEXY TECHNIQUES

14. *When considering different techniques used for mastopexy, which one of the following is correct?*
    A. Lejour, Lassus, and Hall-Findlay techniques all require approximation of the breast parenchymal pillars inferiorly.
    B. Benelli described the periareolar round block technique with polydiaxone periareolar sutures.
    C. Lassus described a vertical mastopexy with undermining.
    D. Hammond is associated with a short scar technique using a lateral pedicle.
    E. Lejour and Hall-Findlay techniques use the same pedicle.

OUTCOMES FOLLOWING MASTOPEXY

15. *Which one of the following is correct regarding outcomes after mastopexy?*
    A. If a vertical scar technique is used, nipple-areolar elevation is not well maintained over time.
    B. In the long term, breast projection and superior pole fullness are significantly improved, especially when fascial sutures are used.
    C. The inverted-T technique has not demonstrated increased rates of "bottoming out" despite historical concerns.
    D. Periareolar techniques have shown the highest rates of surgeon dissatisfaction among board-certified plastic surgeons.
    E. Overelevation of the nipple is an uncommon finding at long-term follow-up.

MASTOPEXY FOLLOWING MASSIVE WEIGHT LOSS

16. You see a massive-weight-loss patient in clinic requesting breast reshaping surgery. On examination, the patient has severe ptosis with notch-to-nipple distance of 38 cm. She also has underfilled breasts with loss of central breast volume. Severe lateral rolls pass to the posterior axillary line on both sides. In the clinical notes, you record the breast appearance as grade III, according to the Rubin scale. *Which one of the following would be the most appropriate technique to improve breast shape and appearance in this case?*
    A. Vertical scar mastopexy alone
    B. Vertical scar augmentation-mastopexy
    C. Wise-pattern mastopexy alone
    D. Wise-pattern augmentation-mastopexy
    E. Wise-pattern autoaugmentation-mastopexy

Answers

CAUSES OF BREAST PTOSIS

1. A 45-year-old mother of two is seen in the office concerning her breast ptosis. *Which one of the following is not a factor in the development of this condition?*
   E. Alterations in the structural integrity of the inframammary fold

   A number of factors are likely to be responsible for the development of breast ptosis. Changes in breast volume or composition following pregnancy, weight fluctuations, and menopause are all implicated. Changes in skin elasticity with age will affect the development of ptosis, and smoking is likely to exacerbate these changes.

   The breast parenchyma is covered by fascia split into two layers. The superficial component passes between the breast and the dermis; the deep component passes between breast and pectoralis major fascia. Cooper's ligaments are fibrous attachments that pass between these two fascial layers to provide support to the breast. Attenuation of Cooper's ligaments is also thought to be responsible for breast ptosis, although some authorities disagree with this theory.

   The appearance of breast ptosis is influenced by the adherence of the lower border of the breast tissue at the inframammary fold (IMF) that secures the lower pole in place and allows the breasts to "fall" or sag over it. Changes at the IMF itself are not responsible for ptosis.[1-5]

REFERENCES

1. Regnault P. Breast ptosis. Definition and treatment. Clin Plast Surg 1976;3(2):193–203
2. Hall-Findlay EJ. Mastopexy. In: Hall-Findlay EJ, ed. Aesthetic Breast Surgery: Concepts & Techniques. St Louis: Quality Medical Publishing; 2011
3. Jones GE. Mastopexy. In: Jones GE, ed. Bostwick's Plastic & Reconstructive Breast Surgery. 3rd ed. St Louis: Quality Medical Publishing; 2010
4. Kirwan L. Augmentation of the ptotic breast: simultaneous periareolar mastopexy/breast augmentation. Aesthet Surg J 1999;19(1):34–39
5. Pang JH, Coombs DM, James I, Fishman J, Rubin JP, Gusenoff JA. Characterizing breast deformities after massive weight loss: utilizing the Pittsburgh rating scale to examine factors affecting severity score and surgical decision making in a retrospective series. Ann Plast Surg 2018;80(3):207–211

ASSESSMENT OF BREAST PTOSIS

2. You are in clinic and see a woman with concerns about her breast appearance which she feels has changed since losing 26 pounds in weight. Examination shows she has a nipple-areola complex (NAC) positioned at the level of the inframammary fold (IMF), with the majority of the breast below this. *How best is this appearance described?*
   E. Pseudoptosis

   Ptosis derives from the Greek, meaning "falling." The term is used to describe the descent of the breast parenchyma that traditionally occurs with advancing age and various physiologic changes. Regnault classified breast ptosis in 1976:[1]

   Grade I: Mild ptosis; the NAC lies at the level of the IMF.

   Grade II: Moderate ptosis; the NAC lies below the IMF but remains above the most dependent part of the breast parenchyma.

   Grade III: Severe ptosis; the NAC lies well below the IMF and is the most dependent part of the breast on the inferior aspect.

   Pseudoptosis is also called *glandular ptosis* and is present when the NAC is above or at the level of the IMF, but the bulk of the breast parenchyma has descended below the level of the fold. This can occur following breast reduction surgery, particularly with inferior pedicle Wise-pattern techniques, and is sometimes described as "bottoming out." In a normal breast, the NAC and the majority of breast tissue should lie above the IMF (**Fig. 52.1**).

REFERENCE

1. Regnault P. Breast ptosis. Definition and treatment. Clin Plast Surg 1976;3(2):193–203

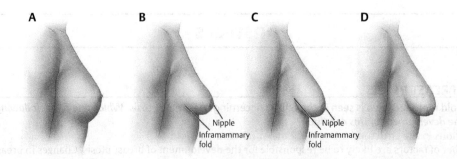

Fig. 52.1   Regnault classification of breast ptosis. *A,* Pseudoptosis. *B,* Grade I ptosis. *C,* Grade II ptosis. *D,* Grade III ptosis. (Adapted from Kirwan L. Augmentation of the ptotic breast: simultaneous periareolar mastopexy/breast augmentation. Aesthet Surg J 19:34–39, 1999.)

CLINICAL EXAMINATION OF THE BREAST

3. A 50-year-old patient presents with concerns about her breast shape. She feels her breasts have become more droopy over the past 10 years and that there is very little upper pole fullness. Examination shows the breasts to be a reasonable volume with the nipple-areola complex (NAC) and most of the glandular breast tissue being located above the inframammary fold (IMF). There is a degree of upper pole emptiness. *How would this appearance be correctly described?*

   A. Normal

   A normal and well-shaped breast should ideally have the nipple-areola complex (NAC) located above the inframammary fold (IMF) with most of the breast volume also situated above the fold. The ideal breast will have a mildly concave upper pole with a convex lower pole and the nipple pointed 20 degrees superiorly from a horizontal plane. There should be a 45:55 upper pole to lower pole ratio.

   When patients present to clinic requesting changes to their breast shape, it is important to understand what they do not like about their breasts and how they should wish to change them. There is much media focus on breast shape that can leave patients confused about what shape normal breasts should really be. This case highlights a normal breast and this lady would not require a mastopexy. However, if she dislikes the lack of upper pole fullness and wishes to accept an overall increase in volume, then she may be a candidate for implant surgery.

   Ptosis refers to breasts becoming droopy, often with increasing age or after weight loss or child birth and breast-feeding. In cases of ptosis, mastopexy may be warranted to uplift and reshape the breast. However, this is not the case in this scenario.[1,2]

REFERENCES

1. Regnault P. Breast ptosis. Definition and treatment. Clin Plast Surg 1976;3(2):193–203
2. Grotting JC, Chen SM. Control and precision in mastopexy. In: Nahai F, ed. The Art of Aesthetic Surgery: Principles & Techniques. 2nd ed. St Louis: Quality Medical Publishing; 2011

MANAGEMENT OF BREAST PSEUDOPTOSIS

4. A 35-year-old patient has bilateral pseudoptosis after removal of 200-cc implants. She still has adequate breast volume and satisfactory nipple positions. *How best might this be managed surgically?*

   C. Inframammary fold wedge excision

   In this case, the nipple height is acceptable, so a standard mastopexy technique is not indicated. The pseudoptosis is caused by bottoming out of the breast with glandular tissue ptosing below the IMF. This may be corrected by performing a transverse wedge excision in the IMF. Rohrich et al[1] have described technique selection for breast contouring at the time of breast implant removal that is based on the degree of ptosis and NAC size and location. This can provide a useful guide in managing this patient group. The IMF wedge excision is also effective at managing the high-riding nipple after Wise-pattern breast reduction although it will not physically change the shortened sternal notch-to-nipple distance if the nipple is genuinely high. It is most effective where there is a degree of pseudoptosis as in this case. The other mastopexy options listed are indicated where the nipple position requires elevation. A vertical skin resection may be helpful following inadequate resection within a previous reduction of mastopexy or may be part of a vertical scar uplift.

REFERENCE

1. Rohrich RJ, Beran SJ, Restifo RJ, Copit SE. Aesthetic management of the breast following explantation: evaluation and mastopexy options. Plast Reconstr Surg 1998;101(3):827–837

IMPROVING BREAST SHAPE FOLLOWING WEIGHT LOSS

5. After significant weight loss, a 50-year-old patient has bilateral grade III ptosis with a nipple-to-notch distance of 32 cm, a large skin excess, and deficient breast volume. She is a nonsmoker, wears an A-cup bra, and wishes to improve both the shape and volume of her breasts. *How best might this be managed?*

  D. **Two-stage, Wise-pattern augmentation-mastopexy**

   After significant weight loss, patients commonly have empty, ptotic breasts that require volume replacement with a prosthesis and mastopexy to reduce skin volume and to raise the NAC. There is debate whether to do this as a single or a multistaged technique because augmentation and mastopexy techniques work against one another. Achieving satisfactory results in a single stage is challenging. Therefore, in this case, a safe, sensible, and reliable approach will be to stage her procedure and uplift the breasts in the first stage, then plan for a second stage 6–12 months later when implants can be inserted. The volume of skin excess in this patient indicates that she would require an inverted-T skin pattern rather than either a periareolar or vertical scar approach.[1-3]

REFERENCES

1. Rubin JP, Toy J. Mastopexy and breast reduction in massive-weight-loss patients. In: Nahai F, ed. The Art of Aesthetic Surgery: Principles & Techniques. 2nd ed. St Louis: Quality Medical Publishing; 2011
2. Rohrich RJ, Gosman AA, Brown SA, Tonadapu P, Foster B. Current preferences for breast reduction techniques: a survey of board-certified plastic surgeons 2002. Plast Reconstr Surg 2004;114(7):1724–1733, discussion 1734–1736
3. Jones GE. Mastopexy. In: Jones GE, ed. Bostwick's Plastic & Reconstructive Breast Surgery. 3rd ed. St Louis: Quality Medical Publishing; 2010

MANAGEMENT OF BREAST PTOSIS

6. A 30-year-old patient requests unilateral breast surgery to improve the symmetry of her breasts. Examination shows she has breast asymmetry with a notch-to-nipple distance of 28 cm (left) and 24 cm (right). She has adequate breast volume and good quality skin and soft tissues on both sides and prefers the smaller breast. *How might this best be treated?*

  E. **Unilateral vertical scar mastopexy with low volume reduction**

   This woman has mild to moderate ptosis, and this may be treated with a vertical scar technique. She also has a volume difference between the breasts and will therefore need some volume to be removed from the larger breast. In this case a vertical scar approach with low volume reduction is probably her best option to achieve symmetry. She could have a small uplift on the contralateral side as well but the additional scars are probably not worth the benefit she would obtain. A Benelli periareolar technique could potentially be used, but a simple periareolar technique is usually useful only in patients with mild ptosis. A Wise-pattern approach could hopefully be avoided in order to minimize her scar length.[1-5]

REFERENCES

1. Lassus C. A 30-year experience with vertical mammaplasty. Plast Reconstr Surg 1996;97(2):373–380
2. Rohrich RJ, Thornton JF, Jakubietz RG, Jakubietz MG, Grünert JG. The limited scar mastopexy: current concepts and approaches to correct breast ptosis. Plast Reconstr Surg 2004;114(6):1622–1630
3. Lejour M. Vertical mammaplasty and liposuction of the breast. Plast Reconstr Surg 1994;94(1):100–114
4. Hammond DC. Short scar periareolar inferior pedicle reduction (SPAIR) mammaplasty. Plast Reconstr Surg 1999;103(3):890–901, discussion 902
5. Hall-Findlay EJ. A simplified vertical reduction mammaplasty: shortening the learning curve. Plast Reconstr Surg 1999;104(3):748–759, discussion 760–763

SURGICAL PLANNING IN BREAST SURGERY

7. A patient is scheduled for surgery to have breast implants placed in the submuscular plane and wishes to have a subtle uplift at the same time. Examination shows that the nipple position only needs to be elevated 2 cm and that the overall breast shape is pleasing. *Which one of the following mastopexy skin patterns would be indicated for use in this case?*

  A. **Crescent**

   Mastopexy can be described by either the skin pattern design, the pedicle design, or a combination of the two. The skin pattern design is selected based on the amount of skin resection that is required. There will be a trade-off between minimizing scar length and achieving improved breast shape.

The crescentic approach to re-siting and uplifting the NAC is ideal in cases where the travel only needs to be small, and where undermining of the breast tissue is ideally avoided. The crescentic approach involves deciding and marking where the NAC should ideally sit and then drawing a crescent in the direction of the travel. The space between the NAC and new position is de-epithelialized and without undermining or with minimal undermining, the NAC is advanced and inset. This approach can work particularly well in combination with an augmentation in patients who have nicely shaped breasts with little ptosis and is safe to perform at the same time as the implant. The addition of an implant begins to take up some of the slack in the soft tissues and this is then further enhanced by the subtle uplift and repositioning. A further benefit is the scars are extremely short and well hidden such that they are unlikely to be noticeable in the longer term. The other skin patterns described are more useful in cases where more involved reshaping and uplifting is required.[1–3]

REFERENCES

1. Puckett CL, Meyer VH, Reinisch JF. Crescent mastopexy and augmentation. Plast Reconstr Surg 1985;75(4):533–543
2. Davison SP, Spear SL. Simultaneous breast augmentation with periareolar mastopexy. Semin Plast Surg 2004;18(3):189–201
3. Grotting JC, Chen SM. Control and precision in mastopexy. In: Nahai F, ed. The Art of Aesthetic Surgery: Principles & Techniques. 2nd ed. St Louis: Quality Medical Publishing; 2011

CLINICAL ASSESSMENT IN AESTHETIC BREAST SURGERY

8. *When assessing a patient in clinic, prior to planning for a mastopexy, which one of the following measurements best assesses the skin redundancy in the lower pole?*
   C. The nipple-to-IMF distance
   Nipple-to-IMF distance is a useful measurement to assess redundancy of the lower pole skin envelope prior to mastopexy. In cases where there is a large excess in a vertical direction, an inverted-T shape scar is indicated. Other key measurements are the notch-to-nipple distances as these provide information on breast ptosis and the need for uplifting and repositioning of the NAC. They also provide information on side-to-side symmetry. The intermammary distance and the breast base width form part of the standard breast measurement series. The base width is worth knowing in cases of reduction, reconstruction, and augmentation. The distance from the clavicle to the IMF is probably most relevant to breast reconstruction cases where a mastectomy has been performed and a soft tissue flap is being designed. This will allow the surgeon to gauge what skin deficiency there is between the mastectomy and contralateral side.[1–3]

REFERENCES

1. Jones GE. Mastopexy. In: Jones GE, ed. Bostwick's Plastic & Reconstructive Breast Surgery. 3rd ed. St Louis: Quality Medical Publishing; 2010
2. Kirwan L. Augmentation of the ptotic breast: simultaneous periareolar mastopexy/breast augmentation. Aesthet Surg J 1999;19(1):34–39
3. Grotting JC, Chen SM. Control and precision in mastopexy. In: Nahai F, ed. The Art of Aesthetic Surgery: Principles & Techniques. 2nd ed. St Louis: Quality Medical Publishing; 2011

POSTOPERATIVE COMPLICATIONS FOLLOWING MASTOPEXY

9. *Which one of the following is the most common complication after inverted-T (Wise pattern) mastopexy?*
   C. Wound healing problems
   The risks of mastopexy are relatively low in most patients and the main risks are issues relating to wound healing and subsequent poor scarring. Delayed wound healing can occur secondary to fat necrosis where breast parenchyma loses its blood supply during surgery. It can also occur at the T junction part of the scar in a Wise-pattern mastopexy as the blood supply to the skin edges corners may be compromised. Providing good wound care is given and patients do not smoke, wounds generally settle well with time. It is vital to warn patients preoperatively that they may have some slowed or delayed healing and that they must not worry about this self-limiting problem.
   The other risks such as hematoma and infection are very low providing strict surgical technique is applied and asepsis is maintained. The addition of breast implants changes the dynamic and increase risk of infection in such cases. All patients must be warned about nipple necrosis when undergoing breast reduction or mastopexy; however, this is extremely rare. A high-riding nipple is a surgical planning error and must be avoided. If there is any doubt it is safer to set the NAC slightly too low than too high as it can always be moved up further if required, but moving a nipple lower may necessitate additional visible scars in the upper pole that are prone to poor scar quality and difficult to camouflage.[1–3]

REFERENCES

1. Swanson E. A retrospective photometric study of 82 published reports of mastopexy and breast reduction. Plast Reconstr Surg 2011;128(6):1282–1301
2. Hall-Findlay EJ. Mastopexy. In: Hall-Findlay EJ, ed. Aesthetic Breast Surgery: Concepts & Techniques. St Louis: Quality Medical Publishing; 2011
3. Jones GE. Mastopexy. In: Jones GE, ed. Bostwick's Plastic & Reconstructive Breast Surgery. 3rd ed. St Louis: Quality Medical Publishing; 2010

VERTICAL SCAR MASTOPEXY

10. When undergoing mastopexy with a vertical scar approach, which one of the following must be discussed with the patient preoperatively that most specifically relates to this technique?

    D. Risk of inferior skin redundancy

There are many advantages of using a vertical scar approach to mastopexy. These include avoidance of the horizontal IMF scar and inferior parenchymal pillar closure which provides internal support and reshaping. The technique is therefore quite effective at improving upper pole fullness. However, it does risk skin excess being present at the lower part of the vertical scar leaving a fullness or standing cone there. In many cases it will settle over time, but patients must be warned about it and understand that if it does not settle a short transverse scar will be required in order to remove the excess. The risk of skin pleating around the NAC is most associated with a periareolar approach (because the wider circular resection incision is being forced to tie in with the smaller new nipple diameter) as is flattening of the breast and NAC (although this can occur to some degree in any technique). The risk of T junction breakdown is associated with an inverted-T approach. There is a risk of having an excess of upper pole fullness (not inadequacy) early postoperatively with a vertical scar mastopexy or reduction. In some cases, the breast will look odd at this early stage and again patients should be warned about this. Often at the time of surgery, inverted-T procedures will look better shaped than vertical scar approaches but with time things even out.[1–5]

REFERENCES

1. Lassus C. A 30-year experience with vertical mammaplasty. Plast Reconstr Surg 1996;97(2):373–380
2. Rohrich RJ, Thornton JF, Jakubietz RG, Jakubietz MG, Grünert JG. The limited scar mastopexy: current concepts and approaches to correct breast ptosis. Plast Reconstr Surg 2004;114(6):1622–1630
3. Lejour M. Vertical mammaplasty and liposuction of the breast. Plast Reconstr Surg 1994;94(1):100–114
4. Hammond DC. Short scar periareolar inferior pedicle reduction (SPAIR) mammaplasty. Plast Reconstr Surg 1999;103(3):890–901, discussion 902
5. Hall-Findlay EJ. A simplified vertical reduction mammaplasty: shortening the learning curve. Plast Reconstr Surg 1999;104(3):748–759, discussion 760–763

MANAGEMENT OF THE BREAST AFTER IMPLANT REMOVAL

11. When discussing capsulectomy and implant removal in a 55-year-old patient with moderate ptosis and a waterfall deformity, which one of the following is correct?

    A. She must understand that her ptosis is unlikely to be improved following capsulectomy and explantation alone.

It is really important that patients are fully on board with likely outcomes following planned aesthetic surgery such that their expectations match the outcome closely. Patients will come requesting to have implants removed many years after having them implanted. Their reasons may include concerns over distortion of the breast shape, pain or firmness, worries about silicone leak or anaplastic large cell lymphoma (ALCL), or they may just wish to be implant free. Unfortunately, capsulectomy and explantation are procedures that are almost certainly going to result in a poorer cosmetic appearance than before surgery unless the preoperative appearance is especially bad. Therefore, helping patients to understand this is a priority. Removing the volume of the implant as well as reducing the thickness of the soft tissue cover provided by the capsule will only serve to make ptosis worse.

It would be absolutely possible to combine the implant removal and mastopexy safely within a single stage and this often works very well for many patients. However, it is still a very reasonable approach to do this in two stages having allowed time for some skin shrinkage. In terms of aesthetics, having the implants replaced would certainly help her volume, but in cases where patients wish to be implant free this is not an option. Her residual breast volume is likely to be less than before her implants were placed as the tissues will have atrophied over time, so it is best for her to expect low volume breasts after this surgery.[1]

REFERENCE

1. Rohrich RJ, Beran SJ, Restifo RJ, Copit SE. Aesthetic management of the breast following explantation: evaluation and mastopexy options. Plast Reconstr Surg 1998;101(3):827–837

TUBEROUS BREAST DEFORMITY

12. *Which one of the following is a typical feature of the tuberous breast?*

D. Herniation of parenchymal tissue

Tuberous breast deformity represents a spectrum of deformity, but typically includes the following features[1]:

- Constricted or narrowed breast base
- High inframammary fold (as opposed to absence of a fold)
- Breast herniation through the areola, leading to large areolae
- Deficiency of breast volume

Tuberous breast may also be classified using the von Heimburg system which was described in 1996 and has four subtypes based on the degree of hypoplasia and the size of the skin envelope:[2]

Type I: Hypoplasia of the lower medial quadrant

Type II: Hypoplasia of the lower medial and lateral quadrants with adequate subareolar skin

Type III: Hypoplasia of the lower medial and lateral quadrants with deficient subareolar skin

Type IV: Severe breast constriction; minimal breast base

Grolleau et al proposed another classification system in 1999 reducing the number of subtypes to three based on the degree of hypoplasia of the breast[3]:

Type I: Hypoplasia of the medial quadrant

Type II: Hypoplasia of the medial and lateral quadrants

Type III: Hypoplasia of all four quadrants

These classification systems can be useful to describe the tuberous breast in medical documentation and also to help guide the most suitable treatment option when planning surgery.

REFERENCES

1. Rees TD, Aston SJ. The tuberous breast. Clin Plast Surg 1976;3(2):339–347
2. von Heimburg D, Exner K, Kruft S, Lemperle G. The tuberous breast deformity: classification and treatment. Br J Plast Surg 1996;49(6):339–345
3. Grolleau JL, Lanfrey E, Lavigne B, Chavoin JP, Costagliola M. Breast base anomalies: treatment strategy for tuberous breasts, minor deformities, and asymmetry. Plast Reconstr Surg 1999;104(7):2040–2048

SURGICAL MANAGEMENT OF THE TUBEROUS BREAST

13. A 17-year-old girl presents with a unilateral tuberous breast deformity. There is severe lower pole skin deficiency and a two-cup size volume difference compared with the contralateral side. The nipple-areola complex is oversized and the nipple height is slightly lower than on the contralateral side. She prefers the volume and shape of her normal, larger breast. *What is the best initial surgical management for this patient's tuberous breast?*

D. Inferior pole scoring and insertion of a tissue expander

Patients with tuberous breast, as in this case, commonly have significant breast asymmetry. Treatment should address both the lower pole skin deficiency and the volume deficiency. It should also lower the IMF, resite the NAC, and reduce the areola diameter as required. This is usually achieved with a combination of techniques including periareolar or vertical scar mastopexy, inferior pole scoring, and tissue expansion followed by augmentation procedures.

Given the number of issues that need to be addressed, a staged approach is justified in this case. In the first stage, the lower pole can be expanded by radial release of the constricted tissues, lowering of the IMF, and placement of a breast expander. Once the expansion and volume have been corrected, either a periareolar or vertical scar approach can be used to reduce the size of the NAC and reposition it on the breast mound. Some surgeons may prefer to incorporate the mastopexy into the first procedure; however, options A, B, and E would still be incorrect because neither a permanent implant nor a fat transfer would be adequate without tissue expansion. In some cases, a contralateral reduction is warranted, but in this case the patient is happy with the larger breast so this should be left alone.[1-3]

REFERENCES

1. Rees TD, Aston SJ. The tuberous breast. Clin Plast Surg 1976;3(2):339–347
2. von Heimburg D, Exner K, Kruft S, Lemperle G. The tuberous breast deformity: classification and treatment. Br J Plast Surg 1996;49(6):339–345
3. Grolleau JL, Lanfrey E, Lavigne B, Chavoin JP, Costagliola M. Breast base anomalies: treatment strategy for tuberous breasts, minor deformities, and asymmetry. Plast Reconstr Surg 1999;104(7):2040–2048

MASTOPEXY TECHNIQUES

14. When considering different techniques used for mastopexy, which one of the following is correct?

A. Lejour, Lassus, and Hall-Findlay techniques all require approximation of the breast parenchymal pillars inferiorly.

The choice of mastopexy technique depends on the degree of ptosis, surgeon's preference, and patient factors. The Lejour, Lassus, and Hall-Findlay techniques use a vertical scar and approximation of the medial and lateral breast pillars to cone the breast, thereby increasing projection. Differences in the techniques are that wide undermining is performed in both the Lejour and Hall-Findlay techniques, whereas no undermining is performed in the Lassus technique. Lejour and Hall-Findlay may also combine liposuction. Lejour uses a superior pedicle, whereas Hall-Findlay uses a medial pedicle. Hammond's technique is a short-scar, periareolar, inferior pedicle procedure (rather than lateral pedicle). Benelli described the purse-string suture using a permanent suture and not a long-acting resorbable suture like polydiaxone.[1-7]

REFERENCES

1. Lejour M. Vertical mammaplasty and liposuction of the breast. Plast Reconstr Surg 1994;94(1):100–114
2. Lassus C. A 30-year experience with vertical mammaplasty. Plast Reconstr Surg 1996;97(2):373–380
3. Hall-Findlay EJ. Mastopexy. In: Hall-Findlay EJ, ed. Aesthetic Breast Surgery: Concepts & Techniques. St Louis: Quality Medical Publishing; 2011
4. Jones GE. Mastopexy. In: Jones GE, ed. Bostwick's Plastic & Reconstructive Breast Surgery. 3rd ed. St Louis: Quality Medical Publishing; 2010
5. Hammond DC. Short scar periareolar inferior pedicle reduction (SPAIR) mammaplasty. Plast Reconstr Surg 1999;103(3):890–901, discussion 902
6. Hall-Findlay EJ. A simplified vertical reduction mammaplasty: shortening the learning curve. Plast Reconstr Surg 1999;104(3):748–759, discussion 760–763
7. Benelli L. A new periareolar mammaplasty: the "round block" technique. Aesthetic Plast Surg 1990;14(2):93–100

OUTCOMES FOLLOWING MASTOPEXY

15. Which one of the following is correct regarding outcomes after mastopexy?

D. Periareolar techniques have shown the highest rates of surgeon dissatisfaction among board-certified plastic surgeons.

A survey of board-certified plastic surgeons found that periareolar techniques had the highest rate of surgeon dissatisfaction and the highest rate of revision.[1] Although most popular, the inverted-T group reported a significantly greater frequency of bottoming out ($p = 0.043$) and excess scarring along the inframammary fold ($p = 0.001$) compared with the short scar and periareolar groups.

A review of 1700 vertical scar procedures showed that the NAC was 1.3 cm higher at day 5 after surgery and remained 1 cm higher 4 years after surgery compared with preoperative measurements, suggesting that elevation of the nipple is well maintained over time.[2]

A review of 82 publications on mastopexy and reduction, including the most popular techniques, showed that neither breast projection or upper pole projection were increased significantly.[3] Methods to increase upper pole fullness or projection, such as fascial sutures and autoaugmentation, generally did not maintain shape in the long term. Nipple over-elevation was observed in around 40% of patients.

REFERENCES

1. Rohrich RJ, Gosman AA, Brown SA, Reisch J. Mastopexy preferences: a survey of board-certified plastic surgeons. Plast Reconstr Surg 2006;118(7):1631–1638
2. Ahmad J, Lista F. Vertical scar reduction mammaplasty: the fate of nipple-areola complex position and inferior pole length. Plast Reconstr Surg 2008;121(4):1084–1091
3. Swanson E. A retrospective photometric study of 82 published reports of mastopexy and breast reduction. Plast Reconstr Surg 2011;128(6):1282–1301

MASTOPEXY FOLLOWING MASSIVE WEIGHT LOSS

16. You see a massive-weight-loss patient in clinic requesting breast reshaping surgery. On examination, the patient has severe ptosis with notch-to-nipple distance of 38 cm. She also has underfilled breasts with loss of central breast volume. Severe lateral rolls pass to the posterior axillary line on both sides. In the clinical notes, you record the breast appearance as grade III, according to the Rubin scale. *Which one of the following would be the most appropriate technique to improve breast shape and appearance in this case?*

E. **Wise-pattern autoaugmentation-mastopexy**

Rubin has classified the severity of the breast deformity following massive weight loss into three grades:

Grade I: Ptosis grade I or II or severe macromastia
Grade II: Ptosis grade III, moderate volume loss or constricted breast
Grade III: Severe lateral roll and/or severe volume loss with loose skin

The grading has clinical relevance as it can guide surgical management of these patients.

In this grade III case, a Wise-pattern approach with long scars is required to address the skin excess. Implant augmentation is best avoided providing the existing volume can create a reasonable result. In such cases a dermal suspension autoaugmentation procedure can be undertaken. This is based on a Wise-pattern technique and uses de-epithelialized tissue from the lateral roll and inferomedial breast to autoaugment the breast volume by anchoring the flaps to the anterior chest wall around a degloved breast mound. Less severe grades I and II may be effectively managed with either vertical scar or Wise-pattern skin approaches and will often need additional volume from prosthetic implant placement either as single- or two-stage procedures.[1,2]

REFERENCES

1. Rubin JP. Mastopexy after massive weight loss: dermal suspension and total parenchymal reshaping. Aesthet Surg J 2006;26(2):214–222
2. Pang JH, Coombs DM, James I, Fishman J, Rubin JP, Gusenoff JA. Characterizing breast deformities after massive weight loss: Utilizing the Pittsburgh rating scale to examine factors affecting severity score and surgical decision making in a retrospective series. Ann Plast Surg 2018;80(3):207–211

53. Augmentation-Mastopexy

See *Essentials of Plastic Surgery*, third edition, pp. 728–734

GENERAL PRINCIPLES IN AUGMENTATION-MASTOPEXY

1. *Which one of the following statements is correct regarding augmentation-mastopexy?*
   A. Most patients with breast skin excess and volume deficiency require augmentation-mastopexy.
   B. It is safer and more cost effective to perform augmentation-mastopexy in a single stage.
   C. Results using two-stage augmentation-mastopexy are usually more predictable.
   D. In spite of high revision rates, levels of malpractice claims following surgery are low.
   E. When staging augmentation-mastopexy, the augmentation should be performed first.

CLASSIFICATION OF BREAST PTOSIS

2. When examining a woman in clinic prior to undergoing an augmentation mastopexy, you record that she has sternal notch-to-nipple distance of 30 cm bilaterally and that the nipples represent the most inferior point of the breasts. *How would this be described using the Regnault classification?*
   A. Grade I ptosis
   B. Grade II ptosis
   C. Grade III ptosis
   D. Pseudoptosis
   E. Glandular ptosis

SELECTION OF BREAST REJUVENATION PROCEDURES

3. A patient presents after two pregnancies because she is considering augmentation-mastopexy. On examination, she has ptotic, underfilled symmetrical breasts. The distance from her sternal notch-to-nipple–areola complex (NAC) measures 30 cm on both sides. Her anterior skin stretch measurement is 5 cm at the nipple-areola complex (NAC), with an inframammary fold (IMF)-to-NAC distance of 12 cm on stretch. You anticipate an excision of 7 cm of skin to adequately uplift her breasts. *Which one of the following is the best option for this patient?*
   A. Breast augmentation alone
   B. Two-stage augmentation-mastopexy
   C. Mastopexy alone
   D. Single-stage augmentation-mastopexy
   E. Staged autoaugmentation-mastopexy

SINGLE-STAGE AUGMENTATION-MASTOPEXY

4. *When a patient is seen in clinic requesting augmentation-mastopexy, which one of the following represents the best scenario for a single-stage approach?*
   A. Tuberous breast deformity
   B. Obvious breast asymmetry
   C. A modest anterior skin excess
   D. A modest vertical skin excess
   E. A modest amount of breast tissue below the IMF

SELECTION OF A SKIN INCISION FOR AUGMENTATION-MASTOPEXY

5. You assess a patient with moderate ptosis for augmentation-mastopexy. Her nipples are sited 4 cm below her IMF, and there is moderate horizontal, but minimal vertical, skin excess. *Which one of the following skin markings is best suited to this patient?*
   A. Short inverted-T scar
   B. Full Wise-pattern scar
   C. Vertical scar
   D. Horizontal scar
   E. Periareolar scar

INTRAOPERATIVE SEQUENCE FOR AUGMENTATION-MASTOPEXY

6. *In which clinical setting is it advisable to perform the augmentation before the mastopexy?*
   A. Where the vertical skin excess is more than 6 cm
   B. When performing a single-stage procedure
   C. Where the notch-to-nipple distances are greater than 30 cm
   D. When a two-stage procedure is planned
   E. Where there is significant breast asymmetry

REOPERATION RATES AFTER AUGMENTATION-MASTOPEXY

7. You plan a single-stage augmentation-mastopexy for a 40-year-old woman. *What is the approximate risk of revision surgery?*
   A. Less than 1%
   B. 5%
   C. 10%
   D. 20%
   E. 33%

Answers

GENERAL PRINCIPLES IN AUGMENTATION-MASTOPEXY

1. *Which one of the following statements is correct regarding augmentation-mastopexy?*

   C. **Results using two-stage augmentation-mastopexy are usually more predictable.**

   Augmentation-mastopexy can be undertaken as a single-stage procedure, but a two-stage approach is generally thought to be more predictable. Many patients with combined breast volume deficiency and skin excess can be managed successfully with either augmentation or mastopexy alone. Augmentation-mastopexy is only required for patients who require additional breast volume and have skin excess that cannot be compensated for by augmentation or mastopexy alone. It may be more cost effective in the short term to undertake augmentation-mastopexy in a single stage, but the long-term costs as a result of high revision rates can offset this.

   It is not necessarily safer to undertake a single- rather than a two-stage procedure, although the number of general anesthetic procedures will be reduced. Augmentation-mastopexy techniques are associated with high revision rates of up to one in five, although this may be reduced to less than 1 in 10 by staging the procedure.

   Augmentation-mastopexy is one of the most common causes for malpractice claims. It represents a real challenge for the surgeon who has to balance the two opposing factors, namely, skin excess and volume deficiency, with augmentation and mastopexy techniques, essentially working against one another.

   The order of augmentation-mastopexy will be guided by the clinical situation and either stage may be undertaken first. In general, if the primary goal is ptosis correction, then the mastopexy should be performed first. If the primary goal is to improve projection or upper pole fullness, then the implant should be placed first.[1]

REFERENCE

1. Lee MR, Unger JG, Adams WP Jr. The tissue-based triad: a process approach to augmentation mastopexy. Plast Reconstr Surg 2014;134(2):215–225

CLASSIFICATION OF BREAST PTOSIS

2. When examining a woman in clinic prior to undergoing an augmentation mastopexy, you record that she has sternal notch-to-nipple distance of 30 cm bilaterally and that the nipples represent the most inferior point of the breasts. *How would this be described using the Regnault classification?*

   C. **Grade III ptosis**

   Ptosis derives from the Greek, meaning "falling." The term is used to describe the descent of the breast parenchyma that traditionally occurs with advancing age and various physiologic changes. Ptosis is essentially the main indication for mastopexy, and ptosis combined with more significant volume deficiency represents an indication for augmentation-mastopexy. Regnault classified breast ptosis in 1976[1]:

   Grade I: Mild ptosis; the NAC lies at the level of the IMF.
   Grade II: Moderate ptosis; the NAC lies below the IMF but remains above the most dependent part of the breast parenchyma.
   Grade III: Severe ptosis; the NAC lies well below the IMF and is the most dependent part of the breast on the inferior aspect.

   Pseudoptosis is also called *glandular ptosis* and is present when the NAC is above or at the level of the IMF, but the bulk of the breast parenchyma has descended below the level of the fold. In a normal breast, the NAC and the majority of breast tissue should lie above the IMF.

REFERENCE

1. Regnault P. Breast ptosis. Definition and treatment. Clin Plast Surg 1976;3(2):193–203

SELECTION OF BREAST REJUVENATION PROCEDURES

3. A patient presents after two pregnancies because she is considering augmentation-mastopexy. On examination, she has ptotic, underfilled symmetrical breasts. The distance from her sternal notch-to-nipple–areola complex (NAC) measures 30 cm on both sides. Her anterior skin stretch measurement is 5 cm at the nipple-areola complex (NAC), with an inframammary fold (IMF)-to-NAC distance of 12 cm on stretch. You anticipate an excision of 7 cm of skin to adequately uplift her breasts. *Which one of the following is the best option for this patient?*

B. **Two-stage augmentation-mastopexy**

Lee et al[1] have developed an algorithm to guide selection of augmentation-mastopexy procedures (**Fig. 53.1**). The following three key measurements need to be considered:

1. NAC anterior skin stretch
2. NAC-to-IMF vertical skin stretch
3. Vertical skin and parenchymal excess

Skin stretch refers to nipple excursion on light anterior traction and provides information on the laxity in the anteroposterior (AP) plane. Nipple-to-IMF distance on maximal stretch provides information on the laxity in the vertical dimension. *Vertical excess* is the anticipated excess skin/parenchyma to be resected. A two-stage augmentation-mastopexy procedure is advocated for this patient because of her large skin excess. Furthermore, she is likely to need an inverted-T or Wise-pattern approach to adequately deal with this excess.

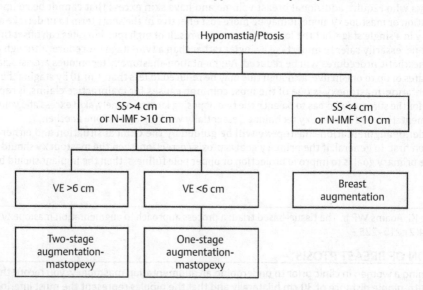

Fig. 53.1   Algorithm for selecting mastopexy, one-stage augmentation-mastopexy, or two-stage mastopexy. *(N-IMF,* Nipple-to-IMF distance; *SS,* skin stretch; *VE,* vertical excess.) (Adapted from Lee MR, Unger JG, Adams WP. The tissue triad: a process approach to augmentation mastopexy. Plast Reconstr Surg 134(2):215–225, 2014.)

REFERENCE

1. Lee MR, Unger JG, Adams WP Jr. The tissue-based triad: a process approach to augmentation mastopexy. Plast Reconstr Surg 2014;134(2):215–225

SINGLE-STAGE AUGMENTATION-MASTOPEXY

4. ***When a patient is seen in clinic requesting augmentation-mastopexy, which one of the following represents the best scenario for a single-stage approach?***

   D. **A modest vertical skin excess**

   The best indication for a single-stage augmentation-mastopexy is the patient in whom augmentation alone will not quite correct the deformity and yet the vertical skin excess remains modest. To place figures on this, patients with anterior skin stretch of >4 cm *or* NAC-to-IMF distance on stretch of >10 cm typically benefit from both augmentation and mastopexy. Once this is established, assessment of the vertical skin excess is made. To do this, the required NAC-to-IMF distance is calculated based on the new planned NAC position and the implant size selected. The difference between the vertical skin present and what is required is the vertical skin excess. In patients with mild/modest vertical excess, a single-stage approach should work well. Such patients typically have less than 6 cm of vertical excess.[1]

   Other contraindications to single-stage augmentation-mastopexy are a tuberous breast deformity (which is usually challenging to treat and has high variability of breast shape and size characteristics), significant side-to-side asymmetry, and in patients where a subglandular implant is preferred. In patients with poorly shaped breasts and asymmetry, performing mastopexy first can be very helpful as this allows a fairly aggressive approach to mastopexy without the need to worry about the effects of the implant on vascularity and tissue healing. It allows shape, volume, and NAC alterations to be made. In some cases, patients will be sufficiently pleased with the outcome that they will choose to avoid the second augmentation stage.

Beyond this tissue triad approach as described by Lee et al,[1] consideration needs to be given to the patient's aims. If a patient has a ptotic breast, then mastopexy will help. However, if they are unhappy about the upper pole volume, then it is likely they will need to consider augmentation to address it. Therefore, if both elements are important to them, augmentation-mastopexy may be indicated.

The presence of less than 2 cm of breast tissue below the IMF suggests minimal ptosis or pseudoptosis. In this case, where the breasts are underfilled, the patient will probably do well without mastopexy and by having the empty soft tissue envelope filled with a suitable size implant.

REFERENCE

1. Lee MR, Unger JG, Adams WP Jr. The tissue-based triad: a process approach to augmentation mastopexy. Plast Reconstr Surg 2014;134(2):215–225

SELECTION OF A SKIN INCISION FOR AUGMENTATION-MASTOPEXY

5. You assess a patient with moderate ptosis for augmentation-mastopexy. Her nipples are sited 4 cm below her IMF, and there is moderate horizontal, but minimal vertical, skin excess. *Which one of the following skin markings is best suited to this patient?*

C. Vertical scar

Selection of a skin pattern for an augmentation-mastopexy depends on the anticipated amount of skin excess after augmentation. The guidelines for selection are as follows:

A periareolar pattern is recommended for patients with minimal ptosis.
- The nipple is less than 2 cm below the IMF.
- The NAC is at or above the breast border (and does not point inferiorly).
- No more than 3 or 4 cm of associated breast ptosis is present.

A vertical pattern is recommended for patients with moderate ptosis.
- The nipple is greater than 2 cm below the IMF.
- Horizontal skin excess and minimal vertical skin excess are present.

A Wise pattern is recommended for patients with severe ptosis.
- The nipple is greater than 2 cm below the IMF.
- Both vertical and horizontal skin excess are present.

As this patient has horizontal skin excess without vertical skin excess in the presence of moderate ptosis, she could be managed with a vertical scar approach, according to these guidelines. The use of a short T-scar can be useful when undertaking a vertical scar technique if it is found that there remains an excess of skin which is difficult to absorb in the vertical scar alone.[1–3]

REFERENCES

1. Lee MR, Unger JG, Adams WP Jr. The tissue-based triad: a process approach to augmentation mastopexy. Plast Reconstr Surg 2014;134(2):215–225
2. Davison SP, Spear SL. Simultaneous breast augmentation with periareolar mastopexy. Semin Plast Surg 2004;18(3):189–201
3. Kirwan L. A classification and algorithm for treatment of breast ptosis. Aesthet Surg J 2002;22(4):355–363

INTRAOPERATIVE SEQUENCE FOR AUGMENTATION-MASTOPEXY

6. *In which clinical setting is it advisable to perform the augmentation before the mastopexy?*

B. When performing a single-stage procedure

Often, there has been debate about the order of performing augmentation-mastopexy as well as whether to do it as a single- or two-stage procedure. It is wise to plan things defensively such that you have not committed to any step until you are sure about this and that it is needed. For this reason, it is best to place the implant first during a single-stage augmentation-mastopexy before committing to the final skin resection. This will avoid over-resection of skin and having to compromise on implant volume or incur overly tight wound closure. All planned markings should be made preoperatively with the patient upright. This allows the correct NAC position to be determined. However, there may be some alterations required on table which can be assessed with tailor tacking once the implant is in place.

It is also important to obtain the best outcome at each stage for the patient who will have to live with things following surgery and this is particularly relevant when a two-stage procedure is selected. In general, it is best to perform the mastopexy first in any staged procedure and this is particularly true where asymmetry correction is planned. A vertical skin excess of more than 6 cm is also an indication for a two-stage procedure as is a notch-to-nipple distance greater than 30 cm. Performing the mastopexy first in these cases allows the best shape and symmetry to be obtained and facilitates the best interim outcome for the patient. Once the shape has been optimized, if further volume is still desired, it is straightforward to subsequently augment the reshaped breasts in the second procedure.[1-3]

REFERENCES

1. Spear SL, Giese SY. Simultaneous breast augmentation and mastopexy. Aesthet Surg J 2000;20:155–164
2. Kirwan L. A classification and algorithm for treatment of breast ptosis. Aesthet Surg J 2002;22(4):355–363
3. Jones GE, ed. Bostwick's Plastic and Reconstructive Breast Surgery. 3rd ed. St Louis: Quality Medical Publishing; 2010

REOPERATION RATES AFTER AUGMENTATION-MASTOPEXY

7. You plan a single-stage augmentation-mastopexy for a 40-year-old woman. *What is the approximate risk of revision surgery?*

D. 20%

Two large series have published reoperation rates of 15–20% for single-stage augmentation-mastopexy procedures. Therefore, it is prudent to counsel patients to expect this level of risk from a conservative standpoint. Data from Lee et al show lower revision rates than this with similarly low rates of approximately 7% for either the single-stage or the two-stage procedure. The authors applied their algorithm to determine the appropriate augmentation-mastopexy procedure for each patient. This highlights that careful patient selection and preoperative planning can help reduce risk and optimize outcomes in augmentation-mastopexy, but it doesn't change the fact that a one-stage procedure can be challenging to get just right.[1-3]

REFERENCES

1. Lee MR, Unger JG, Adams WP Jr. The tissue-based triad: a process approach to augmentation mastopexy. Plast Reconstr Surg 2014;134(2):215–225
2. Stevens WG, Freeman ME, Stoker DA, Quardt SM, Cohen R, Hirsch EM. One-stage mastopexy with breast augmentation: a review of 321 patients. Plast Reconstr Surg 2007;120(6):1674–1679
3. Calobrace MB, Herdt DR, Cothron KJ. Simultaneous augmentation/mastopexy: a retrospective 5-year review of 332 consecutive cases. Plast Reconstr Surg 2013;131(1):145–156

54. Breast Reduction

See *Essentials of Plastic Surgery*, third edition, pp. 735–752

IDEAL BREAST AESTHETIC MEASUREMENTS

1. *Which one of the following is a characteristic of an ideal breast, as described by Penn in his 1955 study?*
   A. The notch-to-nipple distance is equivalent to the internipple distance.
   B. The base width is 11–12 cm.
   C. The notch-to-nipple distance is 24 cm.
   D. The nipple-to-inframammary fold (IMF) distance is 4 cm.
   E. The areolar diameter is 5 cm.

AESTHETICS OF THE NORMAL BREAST

2. *In general, when marking the new nipple position for a bilateral breast reduction, where should the nipple be vertically positioned?*
   A. A distance of 26 cm from the sternal notch
   B. A distance of 8 cm from the inframammary fold
   C. At level with the humerus proximal one-third to two-third junction
   D. At Pitanguy's point transposed to the anterior breast
   E. At a distance of 20 cm from the midclavicular point

PATHOPHYSIOLOGY OF HYPERMASTIA

3. *Which one of the following statements is thought to occur in patients with hypermastia?*
   A. An increase in the level of circulating estrogens
   B. An increase in the number of estrogen receptors
   C. Volume increases that predominate in glandular tissue
   D. An imbalance between estrogen and progesterone production
   E. An altered response to circulating estrogens

JUVENILE VIRGINAL HYPERTROPHY OF THE BREAST

4. *You see a 12-year-old girl in clinic who has developed excessively large breasts over the past 12 months. Examination shows her to be of slim build with symmetrical breasts that have an estimated volume in excess of 2000 g per side. Which one of the following is correct?*
   A. The condition is likely to regress once puberty stops.
   B. Medical management is the first-line therapy.
   C. Following surgical resection, recurrence does not occur.
   D. Blood tests are likely to show an abnormal sex hormone profile.
   E. Symptoms are likely to have developed just after her first menstrual period.

SUCTION LIPECTOMY FOR BREAST REDUCTION

5. *In which one of the following settings might suction lipectomy represent a reasonable alternative to standard breast reduction techniques in the management of hypermastia?*
   A. In young patients with large, dense nonptotic breasts
   B. In young, slim patients with mild ptosis wanting to breast-feed
   C. In older patients with soft, heavy breasts and less concern for cosmesis
   D. In patients of any age where only small volumes (<250 cc) need to be removed
   E. None of the above, as it should only be used in conjunction with an excisional technique

PEDICLE DESIGNS IN BREAST REDUCTION

6. All young patients undergoing breast reduction must be warned of the potential risks associated with breast-feeding and loss of nipple sensation following surgery. The effects of these are related to pedicle design. *Which one of the following pedicles should be particularly avoided in young patients who hope to breast-feed and maintain nipple sensation following their breast reduction?*
   A. Central pedicle
   B. Inferior pedicle
   C. Superior pedicle
   D. Superomedial pedicle
   E. Lateral pedicle

PEDICLE SELECTION IN BREAST REDUCTION

7. *Which one of the following pedicle designs best allows for preservation of Würinger's septum and may subsequently lead to improved vascular supply and sensory innervation to the nipple?*
   A. Medial pedicle
   B. Inferior pedicle
   C. Superior pedicle
   D. Superomedial pedicle
   E. Lateral pedicle

SKIN PATTERN EXCISION IN BREAST REDUCTION

8. *Which one of the following statements is correct regarding breast reduction techniques?*
   A. A Wise pattern relies on parenchyma to shape and hold the skin.
   B. Inverted-T and vertical scar techniques invariably require subsequent dog-ear excision.
   C. Free nipple grafts do not preserve nipple sensation, but lactation is usually possible.
   D. Vertical scar techniques rely on skin to shape and hold the breast.
   E. Periareolar patterns are not usually useful for breast reduction cases and can stretch the NAC.

MARKINGS FOR INVERTED-T BREAST REDUCTION

9. *Which one of the following statements is correct when marking a patient for an inverted-T breast reduction?*
   A. The breast meridian will determine the vertical nipple position.
   B. The vertical limbs should be 5 cm long to minimize bottoming out.
   C. The NAC cut-out should be designed slightly larger than the areolar diameter.
   D. In heavy pendulous breasts the nipple should be marked slightly lower.
   E. The horizontal lines joining the vertical limbs and IMF should be straight.

INFILTRATION FOR BREAST REDUCTION

10. You are planning a bilateral breast reduction procedure and have decided to inject the breast tissue with an infiltration of a solution that contains dilute epinephrine and local anesthetic. *Based on evidence from multiple studies, which one of the following has consistently been demonstrated to be significantly reduced by this strategy?*
    A. Operating duration
    B. Hospital stay
    C. Postoperative pain at 9 hours
    D. Intraoperative blood loss
    E. Skin flap viability

PROBLEMS WITH PERFUSION OF THE NIPPLE-AREOLA COMPLEX (NAC)

11. You are using an inverted-T pattern with an inferior pedicle to perform a bilateral breast reduction in a 37-year-old woman. You have satisfactorily reduced the first side and are in the process of elevating the pedicle on the second side when you notice that the nipple appears severely compromised. *What is your next step in the management of this patient?*
    A. Continue with the procedure as planned
    B. Temporarily stop the procedure, assess temperature, urine output, and blood pressure
    C. Apply topical nitroglycerin
    D. Convert to a free nipple graft on that side
    E. Confirm that the pedicle is not kinked, then resect more tissue from the pedicle to decrease bulk and oxygen requirements

EVIDENCE IN BREAST REDUCTION

12. You are trying to evaluate evidence to guide your practice in breast reduction surgery. *Which one of the following is correct?*
    A. A correlation exists between increasing excision volume and greater symptom relief.
    B. The use of drains in breast reduction surgery is not proven to decrease hematomas.
    C. Most patients with hypermastia seek treatment for purely cosmetic reasons.
    D. The symptoms of hypermastia are much less severe than with chronic medical conditions.
    E. Patients with a BMI greater than 25 have more severe functional symptoms.

Answers

IDEAL BREAST AESTHETIC MEASUREMENTS

1. *Which one of the following is a characteristic of an ideal breast, as described by Penn in his 1955 study?*

    A. The notch-to-nipple distance is equivalent to internipple distance.

        Penn[1] studied breast aesthetics in the 1950s. He reviewed a number of females and concluded that certain measurements provided an aesthetically pleasing breast. In Penn's ideal breast measurements, the sternal notch-to-nipple distance was 21 cm and was equivalent to the internipple distance. The vertical nipple-to-inframammary fold (IMF) distance was 7 cm. Breast base width was not described. A normal nipple-areola complex is between 3.8 and 4.5 cm but there is significant variation beyond this. A clear understanding of normal breast aesthetics is vital for performing corrective breast surgery (**Fig. 54.1**).

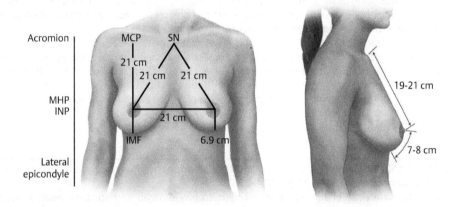

Fig. 54.1 Ideal breast measurements. *(IMF,* Inframammary fold; *INP,* ideal nipple plane; *MCP,* midclavicular point; *MHP,* midhumeral plane; *SN,* sternal notch.) (B, From Hall-Findlay EJ. Aesthetic Breast Surgery: Concepts & Techniques. St Louis: Quality Medical Publishing, 2011.)

REFERENCE

1. Penn J. Breast reduction. Br J Plast Surg 1955;7(4):357–371

AESTHETICS OF THE NORMAL BREAST

2. *In general, when marking the new nipple position for a bilateral breast reduction, where should the nipple be vertically positioned?*

    D. At Pitanguy's point transposed to the anterior breast

        Classic numbers associated with an aesthetic breast for nipple position are 21 cm from the sternal notch to nipple and a nipple-to-inframammary fold (IMF) distance of approximately 7cm.[1] Of course, these can vary considerably between individuals based on their frame and breast shape/size. When marking up a patient for bilateral breast reduction, there are three useful guides to vertical nipple placement: the IMF, the distance from the sternal notch, and the midhumeral point when arms are placed by the patient's side. The point at which the IMF level is transposed to the anterior breast is known as *Pitanguy's point* and is a reliable guide to ideal nipple position in most patients. A range of distances (21–24 cm) from the sternal notch-to-nipple are generally applicable, but 26 cm would be too low in most cases. Many surgeons will use all three measurements/landmarks to guide their decision-making. The main aim is to ensure the nipple-areola complex (NAC) is placed at an aesthetically pleasing point on the most projected part of the breast, while ensuring it is not placed too high, otherwise this makes it visible above the bra or a low cut dress. Furthermore, it is difficult to correct without additional unwanted scarring.[2]

REFERENCES

1. Penn J. Breast reduction. Br J Plast Surg 1955;7(4):357–371
2. Elsahy NI. Correction of abnormally high nipples after reduction mammaplasty. Aesthetic Plast Surg 1990;14(1):21–26

PATHOPHYSIOLOGY OF HYPERMASTIA

3. *Which one of the following statements is thought to occur in patients with hypermastia?*

    E. An altered response to circulating estrogens

        In most patients with hypermastia, there are both normal estrogen levels and receptor number, which suggests that the abnormal excessive breast growth may be the result of an altered response to normal circulating estrogens. The main increase in breast volume is observed in fibrous and fatty tissue rather than within glandular tissue.[1]

REFERENCE

1. Jabs AD, Frantz AG, Smith-Vaniz A, Hugo NE. Mammary hypertrophy is not associated with increased estrogen receptors. Plast Reconstr Surg 1990;86(1):64–66

JUVENILE VIRGINAL HYPERTROPHY OF THE BREAST

4. You see a 12-year-old girl in clinic who has developed excessively large breasts over the past 12 months. Examination shows her to be of slim build with symmetrical breasts that have an estimated volume in excess of 2000 g per side. *Which one of the following is correct?*

    E. Symptoms are likely to have developed just after her first menstrual period.

        Juvenile virginal hypertrophy of the breast (gigantomastia) has an unknown etiology and patients usually have a normal endocrine profile. Onset occurs shortly after the girl's first menstruation with excessive growth of both breasts. Surgical management with breast reduction is the mainstay of treatment with at least 1800 g typically removed. There is a risk of recurrence following resection and this is particularly high during pregnancy. Regression is rare without intervention.[1,2]

REFERENCES

1. Hoppe IC, Patel PP, Singer-Granick CJ, Granick MS. Virginal mammary hypertrophy: a meta-analysis and treatment algorithm. Plast Reconstr Surg 2011;127(6):2224–2231
2. Menekşe E, Önel S, Karateke F, et al. Virginal breast hypertrophy and symptomatic treatment: a case report. J Breast Health 2014;10(2):122–124

SUCTION LIPECTOMY FOR BREAST REDUCTION

5. *In which one of the following settings might suction lipectomy represent a reasonable alternative to standard breast reduction techniques in the management of hypermastia?*

    C. In older patients with soft, heavy breasts and less concern for cosmesis

        Suction lipectomy has limited indications for use as a stand-alone technique in breast reduction. It is more commonly used in conjunction with an excisional technique to shape specific areas of the breast. When used independently as a reduction technique it is best reserved for older patients with large, heavy breasts as they tend to have a higher proportion of fat within the breast that can be removed with liposuction. Suction lipectomy is less effective in younger patients as they have more parenchyma and less fatty tissue. This is particularly true in slimmer patients. Advantages of lipectomy over excisional techniques include reduced scarring and preservation of nipple innervations and lactation. However, it is less effective at correcting ptosis and can lead to a flatter breast shape. Suction lipectomy has been used successfully to treat macromastia in certain patient groups and this was not limited to small volume reduction. For example, in a series published by Courtiss[1] volumes of up to 835 cc was removed from each breast, and in a study by Gray[2] up to 2250 cc was removed with good outcomes and no reported complications.

REFERENCES

1. Courtiss EH. Reduction mammaplasty by suction alone. Plast Reconstr Surg 1993;92(7):1276–1284, discussion 1285–1289
2. Gray LN. Liposuction breast reduction. Aesthetic Plast Surg 1998;22(3):159–162

PEDICLE DESIGNS IN BREAST REDUCTION

6. All young patients undergoing breast reduction must be warned of the potential risks associated with breast-feeding and loss of nipple sensation following surgery. The effects of these are related to pedicle design. *Which one of the following pedicles should be particularly avoided in young patients who hope to breast-feed and maintain nipple sensation following their breast reduction?*

    C. Superior pedicle

        With all pedicle designs there is a risk of poor breast-feeding potential and altered sensation, but the superior pedicle is particularly poor because the nipple-areola complex (NAC) is based on dermal rather than dermoglandular tissue. The perceived benefit of this technique is that ptosis may be reduced and projection improved because of inferior tissue excision. The inferior pedicle and central mound are reasonable choices for maintenance of sensation and breastfeeding potential. Around three-quarters of patients with inferior pedicle reductions will secrete postpartum milk.[1]

REFERENCE

1. Schlenz I, Rigel S, Schemper M, Kuzbari R. Alteration of nipple and areola sensitivity by reduction mammaplasty: a prospective comparison of five techniques. Plast Reconstr Surg 2005;115(3):743–751, discussion 752–754

PEDICLE SELECTION IN BREAST REDUCTION

7. *Which one of the following pedicle designs best allows for preservation of Würinger's septum and may subsequently lead to improved vascular supply and sensory innervation to the nipple?*

    E. Lateral pedicle

        Würinger's septum is part of a brassiere-like connective tissue suspensory system of the breast. It is a horizontal septum originating from the pectoral fascia along the fifth rib and merges with lateral and medial vertical ligaments. Within it are branches of the thoracoacromial, lateral thoracic, and fourth to sixth intercostal arteries. It also carries the main contributory nerve to the nipple (fourth intercostal). The lateral pedicle is most likely to maintain this septum although the central mound should also do so with careful dissection. In spite of this potential advantage, the lateral pedicle is less popular than the inferior, central, or superomedial pedicles because many patients need tissue removal from the lateral breast area and the pedicle design precludes this.[1-3]

REFERENCES

1. Würinger E, Mader N, Posch E, Holle J. Nerve and vessel supplying ligamentous suspension of the mammary gland. Plast Reconstr Surg 1998;101(6):1486–1493
2. Würinger E. Secondary reduction mammaplasty. Plast Reconstr Surg 2002;109(2): 812–814
3. Nahai F, ed. The Art of Aesthetic Surgery. 2nd ed. St Louis: Quality Medical Publishing; 2011

SKIN PATTERN EXCISION IN BREAST REDUCTION

8. *Which one of the following statements is correct regarding breast reduction techniques?*

    E. Periareolar patterns are not usually useful for breast reduction cases and can stretch the NAC.

        Although periareolar approaches can be used for small mastopexy cases, their use for reduction mammaplasty is limited to very small reductions. Instead, their main role remains within mastopexy surgery or for gynecomastia resection.

        An inverted-T or Wise pattern relies on the skin to act as an external brassiere and support the breast. This can lead to bottoming out in the long term. For this reason, it receives criticism from proponents of the vertical scar techniques, which aim to reshape the breast and provide support from within using parenchymal pillar sutures. Skin is then redraped over the top. The ability to lactate after breast reduction is highly variable and seems to be affected by pedicle selection. Two issues require consideration: Is any amount of lactation possible, and is the volume adequate to successfully breast-feed? In theory, the ducts can recannulate after free nipple grafts, but the likelihood of successful lactation is negligible.[1-3]

REFERENCES

1. Nahai F, ed. The Art of Aesthetic Surgery. 2nd ed. St Louis: Quality Medical Publishing; 2011
2. Hall-Findlay EJ, ed. Aesthetic Breast Surgery: Concepts & Techniques. St Louis: Quality Medical Publishing; 2011
3. Jones G, ed. Bostwick's Plastic and Reconstructive Breast Surgery. 3rd ed. St Louis: Quality Medical Publishing; 2010

MARKINGS FOR INVERTED-T BREAST REDUCTION

9. *Which one of the following statements is correct when marking a patient for an inverted-T breast reduction?*

D. In heavy pendulous breasts the nipple should be marked slightly lower.

When marking a breast for an inverted-T scar technique in breast reduction, the nipple is usually placed at the level of the IMF, which equates to Pitanguy's line. However, in heavy pendulous breasts it is prudent to lower the nipple slightly to avoid overcorrection with the nipple ending up too high postoperatively. This is because once the weight of the breast parenchyma has been reduced, the elastic recoil of the skin will tend to lift the NAC above the estimated level. Correction of the high-riding nipple is difficult following uplift procedures and will create scars above the NAC. The breast meridian will provide a guide for the horizontal rather than vertical placement of the nipple. The vertical limbs should be 7–8 cm and are left this short to minimize bottoming out of the breast postoperatively. If they are too short however, there will be excessive skin tension during closure that can lead to wound dehiscence. The cut-out for the NAC should be slightly smaller than the NAC to minimize postoperative stretch. The vertical limbs of a breast reduction are straight but the horizontal limbs should be curvilinear with a lazy S-pattern, as this helps to reduce the medial and lateral dog-ears, while maintaining adequate skin at the T-junction. The use of curvilinear limbs on the lateral skin flaps increases the wound edge length on this side which can help any length discrepancy which exists compared with the IMF wound edge.[1,2]

REFERENCES

1. Nahai F, ed. The Art of Aesthetic Surgery. 2nd ed. St Louis: Quality Medical Publishing; 2011
2. Jones G, ed. Bostwick's Plastic and Reconstructive Breast Surgery. 3rd ed. St Louis: Quality Medical Publishing; 2010

INFILTRATION FOR BREAST REDUCTION

10. You are planning a bilateral breast reduction procedure and have decided to inject the breast tissue with an infiltration of a solution that contains dilute epinephrine and local anesthetic. *Based on evidence from multiple studies, which one of the following has consistently been demonstrated to be significantly reduced by this strategy?*

D. Intraoperative blood loss

Multiple studies have shown that infiltration with a solution of dilute epinephrine for breast reduction can significantly decrease intraoperative blood loss.[1-5] This seems to be a fairly consistent finding across multiple studies and represents the major reproducible benefit of performing such a technique.

Solutions that contain a local anesthetic have been shown to decrease postoperative pain in some studies. However, this was true only during the very early postoperative period. This is expected because the effects of local anesthetic agents are short-lived. Some studies have shown decreased operating time, presumably attributable to a blood-free operating field, whereas others have shown reduced postoperative drainage, but these results have not been consistent across the studies. Hospital stays at times trended toward shorter time periods, but they were not significantly different. Many surgeons will use intraoperative pectoralis blocks with infiltration of local anesthetic between pectoralis major and minor and further injections into serratus anterior. This can help reduce the opiate requirement post breast reduction.

REFERENCES

1. Soueid A, Nawinne M, Khan H. Randomized clinical trial on the effects of the use of diluted adrenaline solution in reduction mammaplasty: same patient, same technique, same surgeon. Plast Reconstr Surg 2008;121(3):30e–33e
2. Thomas SS, Srivastava S, Nancarrow JD, Mohmand MH. Dilute adrenaline infiltration and reduced blood loss in reduction mammaplasty. Ann Plast Surg 1999;43(2):127–131
3. Rosaeg OP, Bell M, Cicutti NJ, Dennehy KC, Lui AC, Krepski B. Pre-incision infiltration with lidocaine reduces pain and opioid consumption after reduction mammaplasty. Reg Anesth Pain Med 1998;23(6):575–579
4. Wilmink H, Spauwen PH, Hartman EH, Hendriks JC, Koeijers VF. Preoperative injection using a diluted anesthetic/adrenaline solution significantly reduces blood loss in reduction mammaplasty. Plast Reconstr Surg 1998;102(2):373–376
5. Samdal F, Serra M, Skolleborg KC. The effects of infiltration with adrenaline on blood loss during reduction mammaplasty. Scand J Plast Reconstr Surg Hand Surg 1992;26(2): 211–215

PROBLEMS WITH PERFUSION OF THE NIPPLE-AREOLA COMPLEX (NAC)

11. You are using an inverted-T pattern with an inferior pedicle to perform a bilateral breast reduction in a 37-year-old woman. You have satisfactorily reduced the first side and are in the process of elevating the pedicle on the second side when you notice that the nipple appears severely compromised. *What is your next step in the management of this patient?*

B. Temporarily stop the procedure, assess temperature, urine output, and blood pressure

The NAC can become compromised during or after a breast reduction procedure. This can result from poor arterial inflow leading to a pale nipple with no red bleeding evident or from venous congestion leading to a purple-colored nipple. Management of a compromised nipple is dependent on the likely cause and timing of the problem. Several key factors need to be confirmed. Patients should be warm and well perfused, with adequate blood pressure and urine output. The pedicle should be examined for signs of damage or kinking. Cessation of the procedure for a short time is advocated to assess these parameters and to allow the pedicle vasculature to recover from possible spasm. Local anesthetic infiltration with epinephrine may be contributing to an arterial inflow problem. If a patient is cardiovascularly optimized and the nipple continues to appear nonviable, then conversion to a free nipple graft may be sensible providing that all other factors have been addressed. If the compromise occurs during closure, or begins postoperatively, then it may be due to localized swelling causing vessel compression. Intraoperatively, the sutures can be removed to see if the nipple appearance improves. If so, loose closure may be indicated. If the compromise occurs postoperatively, it may be necessary to return to surgery, for example, to evacuate a hematoma (and reduce compression), to check for pedicle compression, or to convert to a free nipple graft.

Nitroglycerine is a potent topical vasodilator that increases local blood flow by dilating arteries and veins. Although application of a topical nitroglycerine patch or ointment to the compromised nipple might be tempting, if the cause of inadequate perfusion is compromise of the pedicle for which the nipple is an indicator, then this will not be helped because the vascularity of the deeper tissues will not be affected.[1,2]

REFERENCES

1. Hall-Findlay EJ, ed. Aesthetic Breast Surgery: Concepts & Techniques. St Louis: Quality Medical Publishing; 2011
2. Hallock GG, Cusenz BJ. Salvage of the congested nipple during reduction mammoplasty. Aesthetic Plast Surg 1986;10(3):143–145

EVIDENCE IN BREAST REDUCTION

12. You are trying to evaluate evidence to guide your practice in breast reduction surgery. *Which one of the following is correct?*

    B. The use of drains in breast reduction surgery is not proven to decrease hematomas.

        A number of studies have confirmed that there is no benefit in using drains in breast reduction patients with regard to hematoma rates.[1-3] A randomized controlled study by Collis et al[4] compared the use of drains in reduction mammaplasty with no drains in 150 patients and showed no difference in hematoma rates when a drain was or was not used. The incidence of wound healing or other complication was also unaffected by drain use.

        The American Society of Plastic Surgeons (ASPS) have published evidence-based guidelines[5,6] on breast reduction and concluded that there is no correlation between volume excision and symptom relief. Most patients seek breast reduction surgery for functional reasons, although cosmesis is also often identified as a secondary concern.[7] The functional symptoms of hypermastia are reported to be of comparable severity to those of a patient with a chronic medical condition, but there is no evidence to show that patients with a higher body mass index (BMI) (>25) have more severe symptoms. Reduction weights of greater than 800 g are associated with higher rates of complications including fat necrosis, wound dehiscence, delayed wound healing, seroma, and hematoma.

REFERENCES

1. Wrye SW, Banducci DR, Mackay D, Graham WP, Hall WW. Routine drainage is not required in reduction mammaplasty. Plast Reconstr Surg 2003;111(1):113–117
2. Corion LU, Smeulders MJ, van Zuijlen PP, van der Horst CM. Draining after breast reduction: a randomised controlled inter-patient study. J Plast Reconstr Aesthet Surg 2009;62(7):865–868
3. Matarasso A, Wallach SG, Rankin M. Reevaluating the need for routine drainage in reduction mammaplasty. Plast Reconstr Surg 1998;102(6):1917–1921
4. Collis N, McGuiness CM, Batchelor AG. Drainage in breast reduction surgery: a prospective randomised intra-patient trial. Br J Plast Surg 2005;58(3):286–289
5. American Society of Plastic Surgeons. Evidence-based clinical practice guideline: reduction mammaplasty. Available at https://journals.lww.com/plasreconsurg/Abstract/9900/American_Society_of_Plastic_Surgeons.590.aspx
6. American Society of Plastic Surgeons. Reduction mammaplasty: ASPS recommended insurance coverage criteria for third-party payers. Available at www.plasticsurgery.org/Documents/medical-professionals/health-policy/insurance/Reduction_Mammaplasty_Coverage_Criteria.pdf
7. Schnur PL, Hoehn JG, Ilstrup DM, Cahoy MJ, Chu CP. Reduction mammaplasty: cosmetic or reconstructive procedure? Ann Plast Surg 1991;27(3):232–237

55. Gynecomastia

See *Essentials of Plastic Surgery*, third edition, pp. 753–762

GENERAL ASPECTS OF GYNECOMASTIA

1. **Which one of the following is correct regarding gynecomastia?**
   A. Causes of gynecomastia are either physiologic or pathologic.
   B. Fewer than 1 in 10 males experience it during their lifetime.
   C. More than half of cases are bilateral.
   D. Adolescent males are very commonly affected.
   E. It is associated with an increased risk of breast cancer.

GENERAL CAUSES OF GYNECOMASTIA

2. **What is the most common cause of gynecomastia?**
   A. Pubertal circulating hormone excess
   B. Use of anabolic steroids
   C. Testicular tumors
   D. Liver cirrhosis
   E. Idiopathic cause

PHARMACOLOGIC CAUSES OF GYNECOMASTIA

3. It is vital to review prescription and nonprescription drugs of patients with gynecomastia. **Which one of the following is not usually expected to cause gynecomastia?**
   A. Marijuana
   B. Spironolactone
   C. Cimetidine
   D. Simvastatin
   E. Anabolic steroids

EXAMINATION OF THE MALE CHEST

4. **Which one of the following is true when examining a normal male chest?**
   A. The nipple areola diameter is usually 3.5 cm in diameter.
   B. The sternal notch-to-nipple distance is usually less than 14 cm.
   C. The inframammary fold is elevated compared with the female breast.
   D. Mild fullness is observed around the nipple-areola complex (NAC).
   E. The breast base width is normally 10–12 cm.

PREOPERATIVE WORKUP

5. **When assessing a patient in clinic with gynecomastia, which one of the following is correct?**
   A. There is no strong need to differentiate between excess glandular and adipose tissue.
   B. Testicular examination and an ultrasound scan should be performed in every case.
   C. Blood tests for beta human chorionic gonadotropin (HCG), follicle-stimulating hormone (FSH), luteinizing hormone (LH), and testosterone are rarely required.
   D. A tall, lanky patient with an abnormal testicular examination may require genetic testing.
   E. The neck and abdomen do not routinely need to be examined.

BREAST CANCER IN MALES

6. A 55-year-old man presents with a 3-month history of unilateral gynecomastia. Examination reveals mild glandular gynecomastia, with no evidence of testicular abnormality or axillary lymphadenopathy. He takes nifedipine and aspirin and no other medications. His older sister had a mastectomy for right-sided breast cancer at age 70 and continues to do well. **Which one of the following statements is correct regarding the patient?**
   A. His risk of developing breast cancer is typically one-twentieth that of his sister.
   B. None of his medications are likely to account for gynecomastia.
   C. His age is the most common age for a diagnosis of male breast cancer.
   D. Mammography is the best clinical investigation to exclude malignancy.
   E. His risk of malignancy is unaffected by his sister's previous disease.

CLASSIFICATION AND STAGING

7. *What is the most clinically relevant aspect of the various staging systems for gynecomastia?*
   A. They allow data collection for comparative research.
   B. They enable doctors to communicate about the nature of the patient's disease.
   C. They inform the patients of their likely long-term outcome.
   D. They guide the surgical decision-making process.
   E. They provide information on the likely risk of recurrence.

MANAGEMENT OF GYNECOMASTIA

8. *Which one of the following statements is correct regarding management of gynecomastia?*
   A. Idiopathic gynecomastia consistently regresses spontaneously within 3 months of enlargement.
   B. Tamoxifen or testosterone may be useful for managing lumpy gynecomastia.
   C. Idiopathic gynecomastia that presents for longer than 1 year is unlikely to fully regress.
   D. Liposuction and excision are combined as a single procedure for most patients.
   E. Excisional techniques generally have better outcomes than liposuction techniques.

MANAGEMENT OF GYNECOMASTIA

9. A 20-year-old man presents with unilateral idiopathic gynecomastia. On examination he has moderate breast enlargement with palpable soft glandular and fatty breast tissue. Skin quality is good with modest excess. *Which one of the following is correct?*
   A. His condition would be best suited to ultrasound-assisted liposuction.
   B. He would be very likely to require concurrent surgical resection.
   C. Postoperative bruising is worse when using ultrasound-assisted liposuction compared with suction-assisted liposuction.
   D. Incision sites for liposuction should be placed symmetrically at the inframammary fold.
   E. Postoperative use of compression garments is not normally required.

LIPOSUCTION TECHNIQUE IN GYNECOMASTIA

10. *What is the key difference in technique for liposuction of the male breast versus the female breast?*
    A. That ultrasound assisted liposuction should be used
    B. That larger bore cannulas should be used
    C. That tumescent infiltration should be used
    D. That the inframammary fold (IMF) should be purposefully disrupted
    E. That the deeper layers of fatty tissue are predominantly targeted

SURGICAL MANAGEMENT OF GYNECOMASTIA

11. You consult a 40-year-old patient with a 1-year history of idiopathic bilateral gynecomastia. Examination reveals large symmetrical breasts with more than 500 g of excess fibrofatty tissue and significant skin excess on each side. The nipple-to-IMF distance is 30 cm and the nipple is situated below the inframammary fold. *Which one of the following surgical options is most likely to provide the best aesthetic result?*
    A. Single-stage liposuction only
    B. Single-stage surgical excision only
    C. Single-stage liposuction with surgical excision
    D. Staged liposuction, then surgical excision
    E. Staged surgical excision, then liposuction

COMPLICATIONS FOLLOWING EXCISIONAL SURGERY FOR GYNECOMASTIA

12. *What is the most common perioperative complication following surgical management of gynecomastia?*
    A. Hematoma
    B. Seroma
    C. Infection
    D. Inadequate resection
    E. Poor wound healing

Answers

GENERAL ASPECTS OF GYNECOMASTIA

1. *Which one of the following is correct regarding gynecomastia?*
   D. Adolescent males are very commonly affected.

   Two-thirds of males have gynecomastia during puberty and most often this is self-limiting, requiring no intervention. Gynecomastia may be classified as idiopathic, physiologic, pathologic, or pharmacologic, and most males have it to some degree during their lives. Approximately half of cases are bilateral. No evidence suggests an increased risk of breast cancer in association with gynecomastia in the general population.[1,2]

REFERENCES

1. Wise GJ, Roorda AK, Kalter R. Male breast disease. J Am Coll Surg 2005;200(2):255–269
2. Braunstein GD. Clinical practice. Gynecomastia. N Engl J Med 2007;357(12):1229–1237

GENERAL CAUSES OF GYNECOMASTIA

2. *What is the most common cause of gynecomastia?*
   E. Idiopathic cause

   All the options presented are potential causes of gynecomastia, but most cases have no obvious precipitating cause. A thorough history should be obtained and an examination performed to exclude a potentially treatable cause before surgical management begins. Once this has been established, decisions can be made regarding the choice of surgical intervention for each individual patient. Many obese patients will display gynecomastia which tends to be bilateral and of fatty origin. In these circumstances, weight reduction can be beneficial.[1,2]

REFERENCES

1. Wise GJ, Roorda AK, Kalter R. Male breast disease. J Am Coll Surg 2005;200(2):255–269
2. Braunstein GD. Clinical practice. Gynecomastia. N Engl J Med 2007;357(12):1229–1237

PHARMACOLOGIC CAUSES OF GYNECOMASTIA

3. It is vital to review prescription and nonprescription drugs of patients with gynecomastia. *Which one of the following is not usually expected to cause gynecomastia?*
   D. Simvastatin

   Numerous medications are known to cause gynecomastia (see **Box 55.1**).

   This highlights the importance of obtaining a thorough medical history during assessment of these patients. Reversible causes can be established and managed accordingly. Whether or not statins can cause gynecomastia has been debated. This was discussed in the *New England Journal of Medicine* in 2007.[1,2] The available evidence linking statins to gynecomastia was based on case reports only and involved pravastatin and atorvastatin rather than simvastatin. Overall, the evidence was weak. Simvastatin is unlikely to be a significant factor in gynecomastia.

BOX 55.1 *PATHOLOGIC CLASSIFICATION OF GYNECOMASTIA*

Increased Serum Estrogen	**Decreased Testosterone Synthesis**
Increased Endogenous Production	*Primary Gonadal Failure*
Leydig or Sertoli cell tumors	Trauma
Eutopic or ectopic human chorionic	Radiation
gonadotropin–secreting tumors	Drugs
Adrenocortical tumors	Klinefelter's syndrome
Higher Aromatization	**Congenital anorchia**
Aging	*Secondary Hypogonadism*
Obesity	Hypothalamic diseases
Hyperthyroidism	Pituitary failure
Liver disease	Kallmann's syndrome
Familial or sporadic aromatase excess syndrome	*Decreased Androgen Action*
Klinefelter's syndrome	Androgen receptor defect
Testicular tumors	Antiandrogen drugs
Adrenal tumors	**MISCELLANEOUS**
Refeeding after starvation	*Chronic Renal Failure*
Exogenous Sources	*Liver Disease*
Topical estrogen creams	*Human immunodeficiency virus (HIV)*
Oral estrogen ingestion	*Chronic Illness*
Displacement of Estrogen from Sex Hormone-	*Enhanced Breast Tissue Sensitivity*
Binding Globulin	*Environmental Agents*
Medications such as spironolactone and	Embalming agents
ketoconazole	Lavender and tea tree oils
Decreased Estrogen Metabolism	Phenothrin in delousing agents
Cirrhosis	

REFERENCES

1. Braunstein GD. Clinical practice. Gynecomastia. N Engl J Med 2007;357(12):1229–1237
2. Westenend PJ, Storm R, Oostenbroek RJ. Gynecomastia. N Engl J Med 2007;357(25): 2636–2637, author reply 2636–2637

EXAMINATION OF THE MALE CHEST

4. *Which one of the following is true when examining a normal male chest?*
    D. Mild fullness is observed around the nipple-areola complex (NAC).
        There are a number of key differences in the male and female breast and understanding these is important when managing patients with gynecomastia. The male breast has a far smaller volume of glandular tissue that tends to be located close to and beneath the nipple-areola complex (NAC). In gynecomastia, the excess glandular tissue is also centered around the nipple with a predominantly fibrous component. The breast base width and NAC are smaller than in the female breast. The NAC diameter is usually around 2.8 cm and ranges from 2 to 4 cm. It is located approximately 20 cm from the sternal notch most commonly. The inframammary fold is less well defined in males but sits at the same level in both sexes.[1–3]

REFERENCES

1. Wise GJ, Roorda AK, Kalter R. Male breast disease. J Am Coll Surg 2005;200(2):255–269
2. Johnson RE, Murad MH. Gynecomastia: pathophysiology, evaluation, and management. Mayo Clin Proc 2009;84(11):1010–1015
3. Blau M, Hazani R, Hekmat D. Anatomy of the gynecomastia tissue and its clinical significance. Plast Reconstr Surg Glob Open 2016;4(8):e854

PREOPERATIVE WORKUP

5. When assessing a patient in clinic with gynecomastia, which one of the following is correct?

D. A tall, lanky patient with an abnormal testicular examination may require genetic testing.

Young, lanky patients with gynecomastia and abnormal testicular development may have the chromosomal abnormality 47,XXY. This condition is known as Klinefelter's syndrome[1] following its description in 1942. It is also associated with other feminizing features such as a lack of male hair distribution. Patients are likely to be infertile and have an increased risk of developing breast cancer (greater than 60 times). Further confirmation of the diagnosis is required.

A thorough breast examination can help to differentiate between glandular and adipose tissue and is important as it can affect the surgical options available for treatment. It also helps to identify or exclude the presence of potential breast malignancy. A routine assessment should also continue with examination of the neck and abdomen to identify thyroid, liver, or other abdominal masses. Examination of the testes is routine but further imaging, such as ultrasound, is only required if pathology is suspected. It is standard practice to obtain a set of baseline blood tests to assess the hormone profile in cases of gynecomastia, if this has not already been completed by the referring physician.[2,3]

REFERENCES

1. Klinefelter HF Jr, Reifenstein EC Jr, Albright F. Syndrome characterized by gynecomastia, aspermatogenesis without a-Leydigism, and increased excretion of follicle-stimulating hormone. J Clin Endocrinol Metab 1942;2(11):615–627
2. Swerdlow AJ, Schoemaker MJ, Higgins CD, Wright AF, Jacobs PA; UK Clinical Cytogenetics Group. Cancer incidence and mortality in men with Klinefelter syndrome: a cohort study. J Natl Cancer Inst 2005;97(16):1204–1210
3. Brinton LA. Breast cancer risk among patients with Klinefelter syndrome. Acta Paediatr 2011;100(6):814–818

BREAST CANCER IN MALES

6. A 55-year-old man presents with a 3-month history of unilateral gynecomastia. Examination reveals mild glandular gynecomastia, with no evidence of testicular abnormality or axillary lymphadenopathy. He takes nifedipine and aspirin and no other medications. His older sister had a mastectomy for right-sided breast cancer at age 70 and continues to do well. Which one of the following statements is correct regarding the patient?

D. Mammography is the best clinical investigation to exclude malignancy.

Male breast cancer accounts for only 1% of all breast cancer (not 5%). Therefore, the risk for a male is usually only one-hundredth that of a female patient. The risk increases if a female family member is diagnosed with breast cancer. The most common age at diagnosis in males is around 65 years of age. Although nifedipine may be a cause of gynecomastia, new-onset unilateral disease requires exclusion of malignancy. Mammography is the best modality, with a 94% sensitivity and specificity for distinguishing between benign and malignant lesions. It has a negative predictive value very near to 100 in this setting because of the low overall prevalence of male breast cancer.[1-3]

REFERENCES

1. Wise GJ, Roorda AK, Kalter R. Male breast disease. J Am Coll Surg 2005;200(2):255–269
2. Yalaza M, İnan A, Bozer M. Male breast cancer. J Breast Health 2016;12(1):1–8
3. Chau A, Jafarian N, Rosa M. Male breast: clinical and imaging evaluations of benign and malignant entities with histologic correlation. Am J Med 2016;129(8):776–791

CLASSIFICATION AND STAGING

7. What is the most clinically relevant aspect of the various staging systems for gynecomastia?

D. They guide the surgical decision-making process.

The key purpose of each of the classification systems for gynecomastia is that they help to guide the surgical decision-making process. This is true for the UTSW, Simon, and McMaster classifications as they focus on the composition and volume of the glandular/fatty breast constituents and the quality and volume of the skin. Of the three systems, the McMaster example includes a proposed treatment within it. Higher grades in all classifications correlate to more severe gynecomastia which often involves skin excess. Where there is an isolated volume excess or where the skin excess is mild, no skin resection is required. Conversely where there is a significant excess of skin and breast tissue then both will have to be removed. In general, having classification systems also helps clinicians communicate with one another and can be useful for research and forecasting outcomes, but these are less important in clinical practice within gynecomastia.[1-4]

REFERENCES

1. Waltho D, Hatchell A, Thoma A. Gynecomastia classification for surgical management: a systematic review and novel classification system. Plast Reconstr Surg 2017;139(3):638e–648e
2. Simon BE, Hoffman S, Kahn S. Classification and surgical correction of gynecomastia. Plast Reconstr Surg 1973;51(1):48–52
3. Rohrich RJ, Ha RY, Kenkel JM, Adams WP Jr. Classification and management of gynecomastia: defining the role of ultrasound-assisted liposuction. Plast Reconstr Surg 2003;111(2):909–923, discussion 924–925
4. Waltho D, Hatchell A, Thoma A. Gynecomastia classi fi cation for surgical management: a systematic review and novel classi fi cation system. Plast Reconstr Surg 2017;139(3): 638e–648e

MANAGEMENT OF GYNECOMASTIA

8. Which one of the following statements is correct regarding management of gynecomastia?

C. Idiopathic gynecomastia that presents for longer than 1 year is unlikely to fully regress.

Idiopathic gynecomastia often regresses between 3 and 18 months. Once it has been present for longer than a year, it is unlikely to completely regress because of tissue fibrosis, so progression along a surgical pathway would be indicated at this stage. Although tamoxifen is useful for lump-type gynecomastia, testosterone appears to have a limited benefit. Aromatase inhibitors have also been shown to help regression in pubertal gynecomastia without side effects. Danazol and clomiphene citrate have had only limited success and are not currently recommended for gynecomastia treatment.[1,2] Surgical treatments may involve liposuction or gland/skin resection and may be combined in a single procedure. However, most patients tend to be treated with one or the other modality. In general, liposuction is the best treatment for mild to moderate glandular hypertrophy with no skin excess, whereas more dense glandular tissue, or those with skin excess, may need resectional techniques involving either gland only or skin and gland. The key benefit of liposuction is reduced scarring and shorter down times, but if the density of the glandular tissue is firm then it alone will not be successful.[3-5]

REFERENCES

1. Lawrence SE, Faught KA, Vethamuthu J, Lawson ML. Beneficial effects of raloxifene and tamoxifen in the treatment of pubertal gynecomastia. J Pediatr 2004;145(1):71–76
2. Viani GA, Bernardes da Silva LG, Stefano EJ. Prevention of gynecomastia and breast pain caused by androgen deprivation therapy in prostate cancer: tamoxifen or radiotherapy? Int J Radiat Oncol Biol Phys 2012;83(4):e519–e524
3. Johnson RE, Murad MH. Gynecomastia: pathophysiology, evaluation, and management. Mayo Clin Proc 2009;84(11):1010–1015
4. Petty PM, Solomon M, Buchel EW, Tran NV. Gynecomastia: evolving paradigm of management and comparison of techniques. Plast Reconstr Surg 2010;125(5):1301–1308
5. Waltho D, Hatchell A, Thoma A. Gynecomastia classification for surgical management: a systematic review and novel classification system. Plast Reconstr Surg 2017;139(3):638e–648e

MANAGEMENT OF GYNECOMASTIA

9. A 20-year-old man presents with unilateral idiopathic gynecomastia. On examination he has moderate breast enlargement with palpable soft glandular and fatty breast tissue. Skin quality is good with modest excess. Which one of the following is correct?

A. His condition would be best suited to ultrasound-assisted liposuction.

This patient has a moderate excess of both fatty and glandular tissue in the breast with a mild skin excess. His condition is ideally suited to ultrasound-assisted liposuction (UAL), rather than suction-assisted liposuction, as this has shown good results in treating gynecomastia. Given his age, skin and gland quality, he should not require skin excision or concurrent glandular tissue excision. UAL is associated with reduced bleeding and bruising, and radiographic dye studies have shown significantly less vascular disruption with UAL than with traditional techniques. The incision sites should be placed away from the inframammary fold in order to achieve adequate cross-hatching across the fold and into the glandular tissue. Compression garments are uniformly recommended following this procedure. Duration for compression is usually 4–6 weeks.[1,2]

REFERENCES

1. Gingrass MK, Shermak MA. The treatment of gynecomastia with ultrasound-assisted lipoplasty. Semin Plast Surg 1999;12(2):101–112
2. Rohrich RJ, Ha RY, Kenkel JM, Adams WP Jr. Classification and management of gynecomastia: defining the role of ultrasound-assisted liposuction. Plast Reconstr Surg 2003;111(2):909–923, discussion 924–925

LIPOSUCTION TECHNIQUE IN GYNECOMASTIA

10. *What is the key difference in technique for liposuction of the male breast versus the female breast?*

    D. That the inframammary fold (IMF) should be purposefully disrupted

       Liposuction for gynecomastia can be highly effective in certain cases where there is good quality skin and no or mild excess, combined with fatty tissue present. The process has many similarities to liposuction in the female breast and other body areas; however, the key difference is that the IMF would be preserved in the female whereas in the male, it is should be intentionally disrupted with multiple passes across it. This is because the IMF gives female characteristics to the breast and its disruption can help masculinize the chest appearance. In all cases tumescent liposuction is generally preferred in order to reduce bleeding, improve pain control, and help to separate the fat. The choice of cannula will be personal preference and relate to the tissues being targeted rather than a difference due to male or female gender. Ultrasound-assisted liposuction can be particularly useful in cases where a degree of skin tightening is required. However, this technique is equally applicable to the male or female breast. In traditional liposuction techniques the deeper layers are targeted with the aim of preserving the superficial fat layer beneath the dermis. In gynecomastia, this approach is different because the intermediate and immediate subdermal adipose layers are also targeted. When using ultrasound-assisted liposuction it is important to keep the probe tip moving constantly to avoid thermal injury.[1-3]

REFERENCES

1. Rohrich RJ, Ha RY, Kenkel JM, Adams WP Jr. Classification and management of gynecomastia: defining the role of ultrasound-assisted liposuction. Plast Reconstr Surg 2003;111(2):909–923, discussion 924–925
2. Fagerlund A, Lewin R, Rufolo G, Elander A, Santanelli di Pompeo F, Selvaggi G. Gynecomastia: a systematic review. J Plast Surg Hand Surg 2015;49(6):311–318
3. Brown RH, Chang DK, Siy R, Friedman J. Trends in the surgical correction of gynecomastia. Semin Plast Surg 2015;29(2):122–130

SURGICAL MANAGEMENT OF GYNECOMASTIA

11. You consult a 40-year-old patient with a 1-year history of idiopathic bilateral gynecomastia. Examination reveals large symmetrical breasts with more than 500 g of excess fibrofatty tissue and significant skin excess on each side. The nipple-to-IMF distance is 30 cm and the nipple is situated below the inframammary fold. *Which one of the following surgical options is most likely to provide the best aesthetic result?*

    D. Staged liposuction, then surgical excision

       This man has a combination of significant skin and glandular excess giving a feminine appearance to the breasts. This condition cannot be treated adequately with liposuction alone as this will leave a significant skin excess and ongoing ptosis. Proceeding with liposuction first as part of a two-stage process is beneficial because it can reduce the breast volume significantly and allow for skin shrinkage prior to surgical excision. The subsequent scarring incurred during the second stage should be reduced by adopting this approach. In a large study by Rohrich et al,[1] most patients with a similar degree of gynecomastia to the patient described were initially treated with ultrasound-assisted liposuction and went on to have a second-stage excision at 6–9 months, once skin retraction had taken place.

REFERENCE

1. Rohrich RJ, Ha RY, Kenkel JM, Adams WP Jr. Classification and management of gynecomastia: defining the role of ultrasound-assisted liposuction. Plast Reconstr Surg 2003;111(2):909–923, discussion 924–925

COMPLICATIONS FOLLOWING EXCISIONAL SURGERY FOR GYNECOMASTIA

12. *What is the most common perioperative complication following surgical management of gynecomastia?*

    A. Hematoma

       There are a number of key risks involved with surgery for gynecomastia and these can be classified as early (perioperative) or late (long term). The most common early complication is hematoma and this is most prevalent following open resection techniques (approximately 10–15%). The combination of highly vascular tissue being resected via small access incisions probably explains this. Hematoma risks can be minimized during open surgery by careful and meticulous hemostasis throughout and checking again at the end of the procedure, ensuring the anesthetized patient has a normal systolic blood pressure. Hematoma rates tend to be far lower in liposuction-only cases (approximately 1%). Infection and poor wound healing are low risk early complications. Inadequate resection needing revision surgery is the most common long-term complication.[1-3]

REFERENCES

1. Petty PM, Solomon M, Buchel EW, Tran NV. Gynecomastia: evolving paradigm of management and comparison of techniques. Plast Reconstr Surg 2010;125(5):1301–1308
2. Colombo-Benkmann M, Buse B, Stern J, Herfarth C. Indications for and results of surgical therapy for male gynecomastia. Am J Surg 1999;178(1):60–63
3. Li CC, Fu JP, Chang SC, Chen TM, Chen SG. Surgical treatment of gynecomastia: complications and outcomes. Ann Plast Surg 2012;69(5):510–515

56. Breast Cancer

See *Essentials of Plastic Surgery*, third edition, pp. 763–776

BREAST CANCER STATISTICS

1. *What is the approximate lifetime risk for a woman to develop breast cancer?*
   A. 5%
   B. 12%
   C. 20%
   D. 28%
   E. 42%

RISK FACTORS FOR BREAST CANCER

2. A woman is seen in clinic wishing to assess her risk for development of breast cancer. She had an early menarche at age 11, but has never had any children. She drinks more the recommended daily amount of alcohol. Her mother and sister have both developed breast cancer within the past 5 years. *Which one of the following factors is most significant with respect to elevation of her risk status?*
   A. Social status
   B. Alcohol consumption
   C. Nulliparity
   D. Early menarche
   E. Family history

TRIPLE ASSESSMENT IN BREAST CANCER

3. *What does triple assessment involve when a patient presents to clinic with a palpable breast mass?*
   A. Physical examination, MRI, and fine-needle aspiration cytology (FNAC) sampling
   B. Physical examination, genetic screening, and multidisciplinary team meeting (MDT) discussion
   C. Physical examination, breast imaging, and pathologic evaluation
   D. Physical examination, pathologic evaluation, and genetic screening
   E. Formal history, physical examination, and breast imaging

IMAGING IN BREAST CANCER

4. *When considering imaging of the breast in relation to breast cancer, which one of the following is true?*
   A. Screening and diagnostic mammography utilize the same protocols and breast views.
   B. Effectiveness of mammographic screening is dependent on breast density.
   C. Breast imaging must be performed with the patient supine and standing.
   D. Ultrasound imaging is reserved for patients unable to tolerate mammography.
   E. Magnetic resonance imaging (MRI) is reserved for use in recurrent tumor cases.

DIFFERENT SUBTYPES OF BREAST CANCER

5. *Which one of the following represents the most common type of malignant breast tumor?*
   A. Ductal carcinoma in situ (DCIS)
   B. Paget's disease
   C. Lobular carcinoma in situ (LCIS)
   D. Invasive ductal carcinoma
   E. Invasive lobular carcinoma

MOLECULAR SUBTYPES AND PROGNOSTIC FACTORS IN BREAST TUMORS

6. *Why do triple negative breast tumors tend to have a particularly poor short-term prognosis?*
   A. Because they are detected later
   B. Because there are no targeted therapies for them
   C. Because they are unresponsive to radiotherapy
   D. Because they are always T4 lesions
   E. Because they always involve metastatic disease

TNM STAGING OF BREAST TUMORS

7. A patient is discussed in the setting of the breast multidisciplinary team meeting (MDT) with a 2.5-cm breast tumor, six positive axillary nodes, and no evidence of distant spread. *What would the staging be based on the current American Joint Committee on Cancer (AJCC) guidelines?*
   A. T1N1M0
   B. T2N3M0
   C. T2N2M0
   D. T3N2M0
   E. T4N2M0

BREAST CONSERVATION THERAPY

8. *Which one of the following represents an absolute contraindication to breast conservation therapy?*
   A. Previous breast irradiation
   B. Tumors larger than 3 cm diameter
   C. Unifocal disease
   D. Ductal carcinoma in situ
   E. Tumors in large fatty breasts

TYPES OF MASTECTOMY

9. A patient is referred to clinic for delayed reconstruction following a modified radical mastectomy for breast cancer. *Which one of the following anatomic structures will certainly have been completely preserved?*
   A. Nipple-areola complex
   B. Breast skin
   C. Axillary nodes
   D. Pectoralis major
   E. Breast parenchyma

MANAGEMENT OF THE AXILLA IN BREAST CANCER

10. *Which one of the following is true in respect of a patient with breast cancer?*
   A. A positive axillary sentinel lymph node biopsy will mean a completion lymphadenectomy is required.
   B. Combining blue dye and isotope in sentinel lymph node biopsy increases procedural effectiveness.
   C. The disease status of the axilla has only modest clinical importance in breast cancer cases.
   D. When formal axillary dissection is required, levels I–III should all be cleared.
   E. Axillary clearance is best avoided where possible, as it has rates of chronic lymphedema in 70–80% of cases.

SYSTEMIC TREATMENT IN BREAST CANCER

11. *Which one of the following is true in relation to systemic management of breast cancer?*
   A. Chemotherapy is most often used in the adjuvant setting for high-risk breast cancer patients.
   B. Newer chemotherapy regimens combine anthracyclines and taxanes with anti-HER2 directed agents such as trastuzumab.
   C. Tamoxifen treatment is used for estrogen receptor (ER)-negative tumors and should not be administered for more than 5 years.
   D. Aromatase inhibitors are routinely prescribed to all premenopausal patients with breast cancers.
   E. Adjuvant capecitabine therapy can be used to prolong disease-free and overall survival among all patients with ER-negative breast cancer.

TREATMENT AND PROGNOSIS IN BREAST CANCER

12. *In a female patient with a primary T2N0M0 breast cancer, which one of the following is correct?*
   A. Her overall survival is unaffected whether breast conservation surgery or mastectomy is performed.
   B. Her risk of local recurrence is significantly increased if the nipple-areola complex (NAC) is preserved compared with a skin-sparing, nipple-sacrificing approach.
   C. Postoperative radiotherapy is required irrespective of whether breast conservation surgery or mastectomy is performed.
   D. Immediate breast reconstruction should be avoided in this patient.
   E. A requirement for postoperative radiotherapy would have little impact if immediate reconstruction were performed.

Answers

BREAST CANCER STATISTICS

1. *What is the approximate lifetime risk for a woman to develop breast cancer?*

B. 12%

Breast cancer is the most common cancer in females (not including nonmelanoma skin cancers), with a lifetime risk of 1 in 8, or 12%. It is the second most common cause of cancer deaths in females (after lung cancer) and is most commonly sporadic (80% of cases). Approximately, 15% of cases are familial. Patients who are *BRCA* positive represent only a small proportion (5%) of all breast cancer patients. However, this patient group has a significantly increased risk of developing breast cancer (estimated at 70%). Male breast cancer is much less common and represents approximately 1% of all breast cancer cases with a lifetime risk of 1 in 1000.[1,2]

REFERENCES

1. American Cancer Society. Breast cancer facts & figures. The Society: Atlanta, GA, USA
2. Momenimovahed Z, Salehiniya H. Epidemiological characteristics of and risk factors for breast cancer in the world. Breast Cancer (Dove Med Press) 2019;11:151–164

RISK FACTORS FOR BREAST CANCER

2. *A woman is seen in clinic wishing to assess her risk for development of breast cancer. She had an early menarche at age 11, but has never had any children. She drinks more the recommended daily amount of alcohol. Her mother and sister have both developed breast cancer within the past 5 years.* **Which one of the following factors is most significant with respect to elevation of her risk status?**

E. Family history

This patient has a number of risk factors for development of breast cancer. The most significant of these is her family history, having two first-degree relatives affected. Risk of developing breast cancer is generally stratified into three groups: strong, moderate, and low.

Strong risk factors (RR >4) include age over 65, BRCA positive status, biopsy-confirmed atypical hyperplasia, and a personal history of breast cancer, none of which this patient has. Moderate risk factors (RR 2.1–4) include two first-degree relatives with breast cancer, high endogenous estrogen, high dose radiation to the chest, and high postmenopausal bone density, one of which this patient has. Low-risk factors (RR 1.1–2.0) include high alcohol consumption, early menarche (<age 12), late menopause (>age 55), nulliparity, late age at first pregnancy (>30), hormone replacement therapy (HRT), personal history of endometrial, ovarian, or colon cancer, obesity, and high socioeconomic status, a number of which this lady has.[1,2]

REFERENCES

1. American Cancer Society. Breast cancer facts & figures. The Society: Atlanta, GA, USA
2. Momenimovahed Z, Salehiniya H. Epidemiological characteristics of and risk factors for breast cancer in the world. Breast Cancer (Dove Med Press) 2019;11:151–164

TRIPLE ASSESSMENT IN BREAST CANCER

3. *What does triple assessment involve when a patient presents to clinic with a palpable breast mass?*

C. Physical examination, breast imaging, and pathologic evaluation

Patients seen in breast clinic with new-onset breast symptoms such as a mass, skin changes, or bloody discharge undergo formal assessment which begins with a complete medical history detailing specific information about the onset and duration of symptoms. It then progresses to include family and personal history of breast cancer and nonmalignant breast disease, information on menstrual status, pregnancies, lactation, hormone use, and previous breast surgery. In addition, all other aspects of a standard medical history such as long-term medical conditions, medications, allergies, and smoking status must be reviewed.

This marks the beginning of the consultation but does not form part of the so-called "triple assessment" which starts with the physical examination and continues with imaging using mammography and ultrasound, and then pathologic assessment using image-guided core biopsy.

Fine-needle aspiration cytology (FNAC) may be useful in some situations but is less preferable because it provides less information than a biopsy and in particular cannot distinguish between in situ and invasive disease. The triple assessment is, of course, undertaken as part of the multidisciplinary team meeting (MDT) process but the MDT *per se* is not one of the triple assessment parameters, nor is genetic screening which is only indicated in specific cases anyway.

The aim of the triple assessment process is to be able to diagnose or exclude breast cancers in a "one-stop shop" setting so delay in diagnosis is minimized and patient attendances to clinic are also reduced.[1-6]

REFERENCES

1. Bland KI, Beenken S, Copeland EM. Schwartz's Principles of Surgery. New York: McGraw-Hill Education. Breast 2005:454–459
2. Iglehart JD, Kaelin CM. SabistonText Book of Surgery, Vol. 1. Amsterdam, Netherlands: Elsevier Health Sciences. Diseases of the breast; 2004:877
3. Ahmed I, Nazir R, Chaudhary MY, Kundi S. Triple assessment of breast lump. J Coll Physicians Surg Pak 2007;17(9):535–538
4. NICE. Early and locally advanced breast cancer: diagnosis and treatment. Available at https://www.nice.org.uk/guidance/cg80; 2009
5. Khoda L, Kapa B, Singh GK, Gojendra T, Singh LR, Sharma KL. Evaluation of modified triple test (clinical breast examination, ultrasonography, and fine-needle aspiration cytology) in the diagnosis of palpable breast lumps. J Med Soc 2015;29:26–30
6. Jan M, Mattoo JA, Salroo NA, Ahangar S. Triple assessment in the diagnosis of breast cancer in Kashmir. Indian J Surg 2010;72(2):97–103

IMAGING IN BREAST CANCER

4. *When considering imaging of the breast in relation to breast cancer, which one of the following is true?*

B. Effectiveness of mammographic screening is dependent on breast density.

Breast screening has been shown to reduce mortality from breast cancer. However, the effectiveness of screening is dependent on the density of the breast, with lower sensitivity in higher density breast tissue. Screening mammography and diagnostic mammography differ in their protocols and views. Screening mammography consists of a mediolateral oblique view and a craniocaudal view of each breast. Diagnostic mammography involves additional views such as compression or magnification views used to further evaluate abnormalities found on screening or supplement clinical findings. Clinical examination, rather than imaging, must be performed with the patient supine and upright so as to avoid missing subtle changes in the skin and nipple not evident in only one position. In addition, the axillae must be examined. Ultrasound imaging is part of the standard assessment of the breast and can help to differentiate between solid and cystic lesions. It is also useful to guide biopsy sampling in clinic. MRI has a number of roles in breast imaging, not only recurrent tumor cases. For example, it may be useful in assessing tumor multifocality in patients wishing to pursue breast conservation treatment, and can be useful for assessing response to treatment with neoadjuvant chemotherapy and investigating occult primary tumors where patients present with axillary nodal metastases.[1-3]

REFERENCES

1. Vourtsis A, Berg WA. Breast density implications and supplemental screening. Eur Radiol 2019;29(4):1762–1777
2. Bartella L, Smith CS, Dershaw DD, Liberman L. Imaging breast cancer. Radiol Clin North Am 2007;45(1):45–67
3. Menezes GL, Knuttel FM, Stehouwer BL, Pijnappel RM, van den Bosch MA. Magnetic resonance imaging in breast cancer: a literature review and future perspectives. World J Clin Oncol 2014;5(2):61–70

DIFFERENT SUBTYPES OF BREAST CANCER

5. *Which one of the following represents the most common type of malignant breast tumor?*

D. Invasive ductal carcinoma

Invasive ductal carcinoma is the most common histological subtype of malignant mammary tumors representing between 65 and 80% of all mammary carcinomas. Subtypes of ductal carcinoma include tubular, medullary, metaplastic, mucinous (colloid) papillary, and adenoid cystic carcinoma.

Ductal carcinoma in situ (DCIS) represents an abnormal proliferation of malignant epithelial cells within the mammary ductal-lobular system without invasion into the surrounding stroma. Increased use of screening mammography during the past two decades has led to a marked increase in the number of patients with a diagnosis of DCIS and currently about 85% of all DCIS cases are detected solely based on mammography. The natural history of DCIS is only partially understood and its potential to progress to invasive breast cancer is uncertain.

Paget's disease of the nipple is a rare type of breast cancer involving the skin of the nipple. It starts in the breast ducts and spreads to the skin of the nipple and then to the areola. Paget's disease can be associated with an underlying in situ or invasive component.

Lobular carcinoma in situ (LCIS) is characterized by a solid proliferation of small cells with round to oval nuclei that distort the involved spaces in the terminal duct-lobular units. Although it is a marker for breast cancer risk, it is not a malignant finding. Invasive lobular carcinoma constitutes approximately 10–14% of invasive mammary carcinomas.[1-3]

REFERENCES

1. American Cancer Society. Breast cancer facts & figures. The Society: Atlanta, GA, USA
2. Yersal O, Barutca S. Biological subtypes of breast cancer: prognostic and therapeutic implications. World J Clin Oncol 2014;5(3):412–424
3. Sotiriou C, Neo SY, McShane LM, et al. Breast cancer classification and prognosis based on gene expression profiles from a population-based study. Proc Natl Acad Sci U S A 2003;100(18):10393–10398

MOLECULAR SUBTYPES AND PROGNOSTIC FACTORS IN BREAST TUMORS

6. *Why do triple negative breast tumors tend to have a particularly poor short-term prognosis?*

B. Because there are no targeted therapies for them

Breast tumors can be assessed in response to their molecular profiling. Estrogen (ER), progesterone (PR), and HER2 receptors can be measured by immunohistochemical (IHC) studies. Positivity generally correlates with response to endocrine therapy and better prognosis. Therefore, triple negative tumors tend to have a poorer short-term prognosis in part because there are currently no targeted therapies for these tumors.

Molecular profiling techniques have allowed better understanding of the molecular subtypes of breast cancers, and four main molecular subtypes have been identified:

1. **Luminal A:** This is ER/PR positive and HER2 negative. It constitutes approximately 70% of invasive mammary carcinomas. It is associated with the most favorable prognosis and it is responsive to antihormone therapy.

2. **Luminal B:** This is ER+ and/or PR+ and is further defined by being highly positive for Ki67 or HER2. It tends to be a higher grade and is associated with poorer survival than a Luminal A cancer.

3. **HER2-enriched:** This is both ER/PR− and HER2+ and represents about 5% of invasive breast cancers. It tends to behave more aggressively than other subtypes and is associated with poorer short-term prognosis compared to HR+ breast cancers. Widespread use of targeted anti-HER2 therapies and use of dual anti-HER2 therapies have improved outcomes for these patients.

4. **Triple negative:** This is ER−, PR−, and HER2−. As discussed, triple negative breast cancers have a poorer short-term prognosis than other subtypes, in part because there are currently no targeted therapies for these tumors.[1-3]

REFERENCES

1. Aysola K, Desai A, Welch C, et al. Triple negative breast cancer—an overview. Hereditary Genet 2013;2013(2, Suppl 2):1
2. Yersal O, Barutca S. Biological subtypes of breast cancer: prognostic and therapeutic implications. World J Clin Oncol 2014;5(3):412–424
3. Sotiriou C, Neo SY, McShane LM, et al. Breast cancer classification and prognosis based on gene expression profiles from a population-based study. Proc Natl Acad Sci U S A 2003;100(18):10393–10398

TNM STAGING OF BREAST TUMORS

7. A patient is discussed in the setting of the breast MDT with a 2.5-cm breast tumor, six positive axillary nodes, and no evidence of distant spread. *What would the staging be based on the current American Joint Committee on Cancer (AJCC) guidelines?*

C. T2N2M0

This patient has T2N2M0 disease and this is calculated based on the American Joint Committee on Cancer system[1,2] as follows:

Primary Tumor (T)

- TX: Cannot be assessed
- T0: No evidence of tumor
- Tis: Carcinoma in situ
- T1: Smaller than 2 cm
- T2: 2–5 cm
- T3: Larger than 5 cm
- T4: Any size and invades chest wall or skin (includes inflammatory breast cancer)

Lymph Nodes (N)

- NX: Cannot be assessed

- N0: No evidence of spread
- N1: 1–3 axillary nodes
- N2: 4–9 axillary nodes or enlarged internal mammary node
- N3: 10 or more axillary plus mammary or supraclavicular nodes
Metastasis (M)
- MX: Cannot be assessed
- M0: No distant disease
- M1: Metastatic (most commonly bone, lung, brain, and liver)

REFERENCES

1. Edge SB; American Joint Committee on Cancer. AJCC Cancer Staging Manual. 7th ed. New York: Springer; 2010:xiv, 648
2. Amin MB; American Joint Committee on Cancer and American Cancer Society. AJCC Cancer Staging Manual. 8th ed. Editor-in-chief, Mahul B. Amin, MD, FCAP; editors, Stephen B. Edge, MD, FACS and 16 others; Donna M. Gress, RHIT, CTR - Technical editor; Laura R. Meyer, CAPM - Managing editor. Chicago IL: American Joint Committee on Cancer, Springer; 2017:xvii, 1024

BREAST CONSERVATION THERAPY

8. *Which one of the following represents an absolute contraindication to breast conservation therapy?*

   A. **Previous breast irradiation**

   Breast conservation therapy may be considered in patients with small primary tumors including nipple-areola complex (NAC), particularly in moderate to large breasts. Often the ratio of tumor to breast size is a major factor in the decision-making process and having large fatty breasts can lend itself well to wide local excision with a therapeutic mammoplasty, combined with a symmetrizing reduction performed on the opposite side. This approach relies on the principles of reduction mammoplasty, adapted to allow tumor resection with a more cosmetic approach. These are so-called "oncoplastic techniques." The key contraindications to breast-conserving therapy are previous breast irradiation (as it cannot be given twice and will be required in breast-conserving treatment), recurrent or multifocal disease, tumors greater than 5 cm in diameter, inflammatory breast disease, and a high tumor size to breast size ratio. The need for clear margins is paramount in breast-conserving surgery as otherwise there is a two-fold risk of recurrence compared with negative margin results.[1–4]

REFERENCES

1. Buchholz TA, Somerfield MR, Griggs JJ, et al. Margins for breast-conserving surgery with whole-breast irradiation in stage I and II invasive breast cancer: American Society of Clinical Oncology endorsement of the Society of Surgical Oncology/American Society for Radiation Oncology consensus guideline. J Clin Oncol 2014;32(14):1502–1506
2. Morrow M, Van Zee KJ, Solin LJ, et al. Society of Surgical Oncology-American Society for Radiation Oncology-American Society of Clinical Oncology consensus guideline on margins for breast-conserving surgery with whole-breast irradiation in ductal carcinoma in situ. J Clin Oncol 2016;34(33):4040–4046
3. Darby S, McGale P, Correa C, et al; Early Breast Cancer Trialists' Collaborative Group (EBCTCG). Effect of radiotherapy after breast-conserving surgery on 10-year recurrence and 15-year breast cancer death: meta-analysis of individual patient data for 10,801 women in 17 randomised trials. Lancet 2011;378(9804):1707–1716
4. Kronowitz SJ, Kuerer HM, Buchholz TA, Valero V, Hunt KK. A management algorithm and practical oncoplastic surgical techniques for repairing partial mastectomy defects. Plast Reconstr Surg 2008;122(6):1631–1647

TYPES OF MASTECTOMY

9. A patient is referred to clinic for delayed reconstruction following a modified radical mastectomy for breast cancer. *Which one of the following anatomic structures will certainly have been completely preserved?*

   D. **Pectoralis major**

   This patient would have the pectoralis major muscle preserved. A simple mastectomy involves removal of the nipple-areola complex, breast parenchyma, and some of the breast skin (usually in a horizontal ellipse around the nipple), but the axilla is spared. A radical mastectomy as was originally described by Halsted, combined a simple mastectomy with axillary clearance and removal of pectoralis major. A modified radical mastectomy, as described in this case, involves a simple mastectomy and an axillary clearance with preservation of the chest wall musculature. Other, less-invasive mastectomy procedures include nipple-areola-sparing or skin-sparing techniques, which are regularly performed as prophylactic risk-reducing procedures in the absence of proven disease. These are also becoming more popular when breast disease is present and probably have similar overall survival and local recurrence rates to simple mastectomy for many patients.[1,2]

REFERENCES

1. Zurrida S, Bassi F, Arnone P, et al. The changing face of mastectomy (from mutilation to aid to breast reconstruction). Int J Surg Oncol 2011;2011:980158
2. De La Cruz L, Moody AM, Tappy EE, Blankenship SA, Hecht EM. Overall survival, disease-free survival, local recurrence, and nipple-areolar recurrence in the setting of nipple-sparing mastectomy: a meta-analysis and systematic review. Ann Surg Oncol 2015;22(10):3241–3249

MANAGEMENT OF THE AXILLA IN BREAST CANCER

10. *Which one of the following is true in respect of a patient with breast cancer?*
    B. Combining blue dye and isotope in sentinel lymph node biopsy increases procedural effectiveness.
        Sentinel lymph node biopsy (SNLB) has evolved out of efforts to minimize the morbidity associated with axillary lymph node clearance yet provide clinical information about the disease status of the axilla. It is a standard practice to combine blue dye and isotope as this better identifies the sentinel lymph node and when used in combination, the positive predictive value of the technique approaches 100%, with a negative predictive value close to 95%. Although sentinel lymph node metastases usually prompt axillary lymph node dissection, it is not always necessary because patients with a lower tumor burden (such as one to two positive nodes) undergoing whole breast irradiation will not need to have this performed. The disease status of the axilla is highly important in breast cancer as it represents one of the most significant prognostic factors. When formal axillary clearance is required, level II dissection is the extent of dissection preferred unlike in melanoma cases where all three levels are taken. Lymphedema is one of the key complications following axillary clearance but only a quarter of patients will normally develop lymphedema. Other potential complications include seroma, hematoma, infection, delayed wound heling, and potential nerve damage to the pectoral, long thoracic, and intercostobrachial nerves.[1-7]

REFERENCES

1. Bromham N, Schmidt-Hansen M, Astin M, Hasler E, Reed MW. Axillary treatment for operable primary breast cancer. Cochrane Database Syst Rev 2017;1(1):CD004561
2. Chatterjee A, Serniak N, Czerniecki BJ. Sentinel lymph node biopsy in breast cancer: a work in progress. Cancer J 2015;21(1):7–10
3. Mansel RE, Fallowfield L, Kissin M, et al. Randomized multicenter trial of sentinel node biopsy versus standard axillary treatment in operable breast cancer: the ALMANAC Trial. J Natl Cancer Inst 2006;98(9):599–609
4. Krag DN, Anderson SJ, Julian TB, et al. Sentinel-lymph-node resection compared with conventional axillary-lymph-node dissection in clinically node-negative patients with breast cancer: overall survival findings from the NSABP B-32 randomised phase 3 trial. Lancet Oncol 2010;11(10):927–933
5. Kuehn T, Bauerfeind I, Fehm T, et al. Sentinel-lymph-node biopsy in patients with breast cancer before and after neoadjuvant chemotherapy (SENTINA): a prospective, multicentre cohort study. Lancet Oncol 2013;14(7):609–618
6. Boughey JC, Suman VJ, Mittendorf EA, et al; Alliance for Clinical Trials in Oncology. Sentinel lymph node surgery after neoadjuvant chemotherapy in patients with node-positive breast cancer: the ACOSOG Z1071 (Alliance) clinical trial. JAMA 2013;310(14):1455–1461
7. Giuliano AE, Hunt KK, Ballman KV, et al. Axillary dissection vs no axillary dissection in women with invasive breast cancer and sentinel node metastasis: a randomized clinical trial. JAMA 2011;305(6):569–575

SYSTEMIC TREATMENT IN BREAST CANCER

11. *Which one of the following is true in relation to systemic management of breast cancer?*
    B. Newer chemotherapy regimens combine anthracyclines and taxanes with anti-HER2 directed agents such as trastuzumab.
        Chemotherapy is commonly used for breast cancer patients and has been shown to improve overall survival. It may be used in the adjuvant or neoadjuvant setting. Decisions on its use include size of the primary tumor, lack of expression of estrogen or progesterone receptors, axillary involvement, HER2 status, and metastatic disease.
        One of the key indications for neoadjuvant chemotherapy is high-risk breast cancers, with the intention to downstage the primary breast and axillary nodal disease, thereby minimizing the extent of surgery. Furthermore, neoadjuvant chemotherapy allows for assessment of tumor response to treatment, which can be a vital information that would not otherwise be gleaned. Anthracycline-based regimens have become the basis for the adjuvant treatment of high-risk patients with breast cancer, often incorporating taxanes and targeted agents (anti-HER2 directed agents, e.g., trastuzumab and pertuzumab). Four major adjuvant trials, Herceptin Adjuvant (HERA), National Surgical Adjuvant Breast and Bowel Project (NSABP) B-31, North Central Cancer Treatment Group (NCCTG) N9831, and Breast Cancer International Research Group (BCIRG) 006, have confirmed the effectiveness of trastuzumab in the adjuvant setting. These trials have shown that trastuzumab reduces the 3-year risk of recurrence by about 50% in this population.[1-5] The addition of pertuzumab to trastuzumab and neoadjuvant chemotherapy has demonstrated increased frequency of complete pathological response rates.[6]

Tamoxifen has been shown to reduce the risk of relapse and mortality in randomized trials of women with estrogen receptor (ER)-positive (not negative) breast cancer. The standard treatment is for 5 years, but recent evidence from the Adjuvant Tamoxifen: Longer Against Shorter (ATLAS) trial showed that extending to 10 years reduced the recurrence and mortality for patients.[7] A 10-year treatment plan is now currently recommended.

Aromatase inhibitors such as Exesmestane are used to treat estrogen receptor–positive breast tumors in postmenopausal patients. Three double-blind, randomized, prospective studies—ATAC, the Intergroup Exesmestane Study (EIS), and the BIG 1-98 trial—have confirmed the superiority of aromatase inhibitors over tamoxifen in early stage cancers in postmenopausal women. All three studies have demonstrated an increase in disease-free survival.[8,9,10] The American Society of Clinical Oncology now recommends aromatase inhibitors be used to lower the risk of recurrence in receptor-positive postmenopausal breast cancers as initial therapy or after treatment with tamoxifen.[11]

REFERENCES

1. Perez EA, Romond EH, Suman VJ, et al. Four-year follow-up of trastuzumab plus adjuvant chemotherapy for operable human epidermal growth factor receptor 2-positive breast cancer: joint analysis of data from NCCTG N9831 and NSABP B-31. J Clin Oncol 2011;29(25):3366–3373
2. Perez EA, Romond EH, Suman VJ, et al. Trastuzumab plus adjuvant chemotherapy for human epidermal growth factor receptor 2-positive breast cancer: planned joint analysis of overall survival from NSABP B-31 and NCCTG N9831. J Clin Oncol 2014;32(33):3744–3752
3. Cameron D, Piccart-Gebhart MJ, Gelber RD, et al; Herceptin Adjuvant (HERA) Trial Study Team. 11 years' follow-up of trastuzumab after adjuvant chemotherapy in HER2-positive early breast cancer: final analysis of the HERceptin Adjuvant (HERA) trial. Lancet 2017;389(10075):1195–1205
4. Piccart-Gebhart MJ, Procter M, Leyland-Jones B, et al; Herceptin Adjuvant (HERA) Trial Study Team. Trastuzumab after adjuvant chemotherapy in HER2-positive breast cancer. N Engl J Med 2005;353(16):1659–1672
5. Slamon D, Eiermann W, Robert N, et al; Breast Cancer International Research Group. Adjuvant trastuzumab in HER2-positive breast cancer. N Engl J Med 2011;365(14):1273–1283
6. Gianni L, Pienkowski T, Im YH, et al. Efficacy and safety of neoadjuvant pertuzumab and trastuzumab in women with locally advanced, inflammatory, or early HER2-positive breast cancer (NeoSphere): a randomised multicentre, open-label, phase 2 trial. Lancet Oncol 2012;13(1):25–32
7. Davies C, Pan H, Godwin J, et al; Adjuvant Tamoxifen: Longer Against Shorter (ATLAS) Collaborative Group. Long-term effects of continuing adjuvant tamoxifen to 10 years versus stopping at 5 years after diagnosis of oestrogen receptor-positive breast cancer: ATLAS, a randomised trial. Lancet 2013;381(9869):805–816
8. Coates AS, Keshaviah A, Thürlimann B, et al. Five years of letrozole compared with tamoxifen as initial adjuvant therapy for postmenopausal women with endocrine-responsive early breast cancer: update of study BIG 1-98. J Clin Oncol 2007;25(5):486–492
9. Morden JP, Alvarez I, Bertelli G, et al. Long-term follow-up of the intergroup Exemestane study. J Clin Oncol 2017;35(22):2507–2514
10. Cuzick J, Sestak I, Baum M, et al; ATAC/LATTE investigators. Effect of anastrozole and tamoxifen as adjuvant treatment for early-stage breast cancer: 10-year analysis of the ATAC trial. Lancet Oncol 2010;11(12):1135–1141
11. Winer EP, Hudis C, Burstein HJ, et al. American Society of Clinical Oncology technology assessment on the use of aromatase inhibitors as adjuvant therapy for postmenopausal women with hormone receptor-positive breast cancer: status report 2004. J Clin Oncol 2005;23(3):619–629

TREATMENT AND PROGNOSIS IN BREAST CANCER

12. In a female patient with a primary T2N0M0 breast cancer, which one of the following is correct?

A. Her overall survival is unaffected whether breast conservation surgery or mastectomy is performed.

For most small to medium breast cancers, the survival rates are equivalent for breast conservation surgery or mastectomy.[1] Breast conservation surgery is sometimes described as a lumpectomy or partial mastectomy and involves removal of the tumor with the surrounding portion of the breast. In almost all cases, postoperative radiotherapy is given. In contrast, patients who opt for a mastectomy do not usually require radiotherapy unless the tumor is particularly aggressive. Most patients have to weigh the risks and benefits involved with respect to either complete mastectomy or breast conservation surgery and radiotherapy.

Her risk of local recurrence, overall survival, and disease-free survival is unlikely to be different whether the nipple is preserved or sacrificed, unless of course the nipple is involved with the disease. This evidence is based on a recent meta-analysis.[2]

There remains debate regarding immediate reconstruction, and two main issues need to be considered. First, should radiotherapy be required, will this treatment be compromised by the presence of a breast reconstruction in place. Second, will the reconstruction itself be compromised by the radiotherapy if required. Ideally, if radiotherapy is planned then reconstruction should wait until treatment is complete. If radiotherapy is unlikely to be required then immediate reconstruction is more safely indicated. As it stands there is evidence in both directions with some studies showing that radiotherapy did compromise delivery of radiotherapy,[3,4] whereas other reports suggest that postoperative outcomes did not differ where reconstruction was or was not performed.[5] In general, autologous reconstruction fairs better in response to radiotherapy than implant-based modalities. Overall decisions must be taken with the patients on an individual case-by-case basis to determine the best option for them bearing in mind the likely cancer treatment and the available reconstructive options for them.

REFERENCES

1. Darby S, McGale P, Correa C, et al; Early Breast Cancer Trialists' Collaborative Group (EBCTCG). Effect of radiotherapy after breast-conserving surgery on 10-year recurrence and 15-year breast cancer death: meta-analysis of individual patient data for 10,801 women in 17 randomised trials. Lancet 2011;378(9804):1707–1716
2. De La Cruz L, Moody AM, Tappy EE, Blankenship SA, Hecht EM. Overall survival, disease-free survival, local recurrence, and nipple-areolar recurrence in the setting of nipple-sparing mastectomy: a meta-analysis and systematic review. Ann Surg Oncol 2015;22(10):3241–3249
3. Motwani SB, Strom EA, Schechter NR, et al. The impact of immediate breast reconstruction on the technical delivery of postmastectomy radiotherapy. Int J Radiat Oncol Biol Phys 2006;66(1):76–82
4. Koutcher L, Ballangrud A, Cordeiro PG, et al. Postmastectomy intensity modulated radiation therapy following immediate expander-implant reconstruction. Radiother Oncol 2010;94(3):319–323
5. Barry M, Kell MR. Radiotherapy and breast reconstruction: a meta-analysis. Breast Cancer Res Treat 2011;127(1):15–22

57. Autologous Breast Reconstruction

See *Essentials of Plastic Surgery*, third edition, pp. 777–793

OPTIMAL APPROACH TO RECONSTRUCTION OF THE BREAST POST MASTECTOMY

1. *Which one of the following types of free tissue reconstruction is considered to be the "gold standard" for breast reconstruction?*
   A. Back flap
   B. Medial thigh flap
   C. Abdominal flap
   D. Buttock flap
   E. Lateral thigh flap

TIMING OF BREAST RECONSTRUCTION

2. *Which one of the following adjuvant therapies is most important to consider when deciding whether to proceed with immediate or delayed breast reconstruction?*
   A. Chemotherapy
   B. Radiotherapy
   C. Hormone therapy
   D. Immunotherapy
   E. Axillary surgery

PEDICLED LATISSIMUS DORSI FLAP FOR BREAST RECONSTRUCTION

3. *Which one of the following statements is correct regarding breast reconstruction with the latissimus dorsi (LD) flap?*
   A. The vascular supply is robust and arises from the thoracoacromial vessels and intercostal perforators.
   B. Its main clinical indication is for breast reconstruction salvage cases following failed free tissue transfer.
   C. The main advantage of this flap is the avoidance of a permanent prosthetic implant.
   D. Assessing normal arm and shoulder adduction preoperatively helps guide whether there has been previous damage to the vascular pedicle.
   E. Many patients incur significant permanent functional loss on the ipsilateral shoulder following surgery.

ELEVATION OF THE LATISSIMUS DORSI FLAP FOR BREAST RECONSTRUCTION

4. *When elevating a latissimus dorsi flap for breast reconstruction, which of the following is advised?*
   A. Positioning the patient prone for the flap elevation to improve access and ease of pedicle dissection.
   B. Having a rigid standardized approach to muscle elevation, always starting at the anterior muscle border.
   C. Placement of quilting sutures and fibrin glue when closing back the donor site.
   D. Preservation of the serratus vascular branch to optimize flap tissue viability and reduce necrosis.
   E. Preservation of the thoracodorsal nerve to help preserve long-term maintenance of tissue bulk.

PEDICLED TRAM FLAP FOR BREAST RECONSTRUCTION

5. *Which one of the following characteristics is shared between the pedicled and free transverse rectus abdominis myocutaneous (TRAM) approaches to breast reconstruction?*
   A. The blood supply
   B. The complication rate
   C. The number of surgical procedures required
   D. The donor site morbidity
   E. The skin and fat transferred

CONTRAINDICATIONS TO ABDOMINAL FREE TISSUE TRANSFER IN BREAST RECONSTRUCTION

6. A patient is seen in clinic requesting breast reconstruction using an abdominal free flap. *Which one of the following prior surgical procedures would represent an absolute contraindication to proceeding with free abdominal breast reconstruction?*
   A. Abdominal laparoscopic surgery
   B. Open appendectomy
   C. Abdominal liposuction
   D. Midline laparotomy
   E. Abdominoplasty

ABDOMINAL FREE TISSUE TRANSFER FOR BREAST RECONSTRUCTION

7. *What is the main advantage of a superficial inferior epigastric artery (SIEA) flap over a deep inferior epigastric artery (DIEA) flap for abdominal based breast reconstruction?*
   A. Reach of the vascular pedicle
   B. Decreased donor site morbidity
   C. Avoidance of rib harvest
   D. Increased vessel diameter
   E. More reliable contralateral flap vascularity

FREE FLAP ABDOMINAL RECONSTRUCTION OF THE BREAST

8. *When discussing abdominal free flap breast reconstruction with patients, which one of the following should you advise them of?*
   A. Their hospital stay will normally be 10 nights.
   B. They will likely need to be off work for 1 year.
   C. The flap may completely fail in 15% of cases.
   D. They may benefit from preoperative imaging with CT or MRI.
   E. Their abdominal function will be retained irrespective of the flap type used.

AUTOLOGOUS FREE TISSUE BREAST RECONSTRUCTION

9. While performing free tissue transfer for breast reconstruction, you have been trying for an extended period of time to achieve a satisfactory venous anastomosis with the internal mammary vein but are unsuccessful. The arterial anastomosis is running well and you do not wish to redo it. *Which one of the following vessels can be used as an alternative venous outflow source in this situation without preparing a vessel graft or re-siting the artery?*
   A. The lateral thoracic vein
   B. The axillary vein
   C. The thoracodorsal vein
   D. The cephalic vein
   E. The internal jugular vein

FREE ABDOMINAL FLAP RECONSTRUCTION

10. You are supervising a senior resident as he or she raises a free TRAM flap. *What is the main reason to encourage to dissect the superficial epigastric vein during this procedure?*
    A. To perform the primary venous anastomosis of the flap
    B. As backup in case a vein graft is subsequently required
    C. To develop their skills in vessel dissection in a relaxed setting
    D. In case the flap turns out to have a dominant superficial drainage
    E. To minimize the risk of hematoma in the groin

FREE THIGH BASED FLAPS FOR BREAST RECONSTRUCTION

11. *Which one of the following is true of thigh based free flaps for breast reconstruction?*
    A. They should be reserved for patients planning further pregnancies.
    B. They are well suited to reconstructing all shapes and sizes of breast.
    C. They require longer hospital stay than equivalent abdominal flaps.
    D. They are associated with low donor site morbidity and discreet scars.
    E. They provide long pedicles for relatively easy vascular anastomosis.

THIGH BASED FREE FLAPS FOR BREAST RECONSTRUCTION

12. *Which one of the following characteristics do the transverse upper gracilis (TUG) flap and profunda artery perforator (PAP) flap have in common?*
    A. They share the same vascular supply.
    B. They share the same skin paddle design.
    C. They are both harvested in the lithotomy position.
    D. They both involve perforator dissection.
    E. They both involve muscle sacrifice/harvest.

FREE GLUTEAL FLAPS FOR BREAST RECONSTRUCTION

13. *When raising free gluteal flaps for breast reconstruction, which one of the following is true?*
- A. Where laterally based perforators are identified, effective pedicle length can be increased.
- B. Such flaps frequently require vein grafts to provide sufficient pedicle length.
- C. Pedicle length is similar for both inferior gluteal artery perforator (IGAP) and superior gluteal artery perforator (SGAP) flaps.
- D. Gluteal flaps are challenging for venous anastomoses due to small diameter of flap vessels.
- E. Proximal intramuscular pedicle dissection is rapid due to the paucity of side branches.

RECIPIENT VESSELS IN FREE FLAP BREAST RECONSTRUCTION

14. *Which one of the following represents a disadvantage of using the internal mammary vessels when performing breast reconstruction with a free TRAM flap?*
- A. There is a high risk of pneumothorax.
- B. There is commonly a vessel size mismatch.
- C. The internal mammary vein is often absent.
- D. The operating field is mobile during the anastomosis.
- E. The flap pedicle often has insufficient length.

Answers

OPTIMAL APPROACH TO RECONSTRUCTION OF THE BREAST POST MASTECTOMY

1. *Which one of the following types of free tissue reconstruction is considered to be the "gold standard" for breast reconstruction?*

    C. Abdominal flap

    Abdominal flap breast reconstruction, including the free muscle-sparing transverse rectus abdominis myocutaneous (MS-TRAM) and deep inferior epigastric artery perforator (DIEAP) flaps, is considered the gold standard in suitable patients, and is ideal for those in whom a cosmetic abdominoplasty is seen as an advantage. Shared decision-making in carefully selected patients, and close communication between the oncological and reconstructive teams achieves excellent outcomes for the majority of patients with a high level of patient satisfaction.[1–3]

    Breast reconstruction plays a significant role in the woman's physical, emotional, and psychological recovery from breast cancer. Autologous breast reconstruction allows creation of a breast whose texture and appearance closely match that which has been lost, with the breast appearance improving or remaining stable rather than deteriorating with time.

    Flaps taken from the back, buttock, or thigh are each able to provide high-quality breast reconstructions but, in general, there is less soft tissue volume available from these flaps and the donor site scars are less well hidden and consequently they remain less commonly popular.[4,5]

REFERENCES

1. Macadam SA, Zhong T, Weichman K, et al. Quality of life and patient-reported outcomes in breast cancer survivors: a multicenter comparison of four abdominally based autologous reconstruction methods. Plast Reconstr Surg 2016;137(3):758–771
2. Panchal H, Matros E. Current trends in postmastectomy breast reconstruction. Plast Reconstr Surg 2017;140(5S Advances in Breast Reconstruction):7S–13S
3. Hamdi M, Rebecca A. The deep inferior epigastric artery perforator flap (DIEAP) in breast reconstruction. Semin Plast Surg 2006;20(2):95–102
4. LoTempio MM, Allen RJ. Breast reconstruction with SGAP and IGAP flaps. Plast Reconstr Surg 2010;126(2):393–401
5. Fattah A, Figus A, Mathur B, Ramakrishnan VV. The transverse myocutaneous gracilis flap: technical refinements. J Plast Reconstr Aesthet Surg 2010;63(2):305–313

TIMING OF BREAST RECONSTRUCTION

2. *Which one of the following adjuvant therapies is most important to consider when deciding whether to proceed with immediate or delayed breast reconstruction?*

    B. Radiotherapy

    When considering the timing of reconstructive surgery after mastectomy, there are a number of points to consider. These relate to both medical and psychological elements individual to each patient and include the adjuvant therapy anticipated for the patient.

    Where there is a possibility of needing adjuvant radiotherapy, serious consideration should be given to delaying reconstruction because the reconstruction may affect the delivery of radiotherapy secondary to delay in commencing this (if delayed wound healing occurs) or due to the increased tissue bulk. Furthermore, the reconstruction may itself be compromised by the radiotherapy treatment leading to skin changes, distortion, or implant extrusion.[1]

    There are studies supporting each approach and any decisions must be taken jointly with the patient and breast surgeon. If reconstruction is to be delayed, then waiting for 6 months following radiotherapy is probably reasonable to allow the soft tissues to settle.[2–4] The main consideration when dealing with any cancer is whether an intervention not required to cure the cancer may potentially delay cancer treatment. In any situation that this may potentially occur, nonurgent treatment should in principle be deferred.

    Many patients will need chemotherapy as part of their treatment, but the delivery of this should not be affected by reconstruction nor the reconstruction affected by the treatment. Likewise, patients may require subsequent axillary surgery, immunotherapy, or hormone therapy as part of their breast cancer treatment, but these normally have far less impact, if any, on decisions regarding timing of surgery than radiotherapy.

REFERENCES

1. Yoon AP, Qi J, Brown DL, et al. Outcomes of immediate versus delayed breast reconstruction: results of a multicenter prospective study. Breast 2018;37:72–79
2. Motwani SB, Strom EA, Schechter NR, et al. The impact of immediate breast reconstruction on the technical delivery of postmastectomy radiotherapy. Int J Radiat Oncol Biol Phys 2006;66(1):76–82
3. Koutcher L, Ballangrud A, Cordeiro PG, et al. Postmastectomy intensity modulated radiation therapy following immediate expander-implant reconstruction. Radiother Oncol 2010;94(3):319–323
4. Barry M, Kell MR. Radiotherapy and breast reconstruction: a meta-analysis. Breast Cancer Res Treat 2011;127(1):15–22

PEDICLED LATISSIMUS DORSI FLAP FOR BREAST RECONSTRUCTION

3. *Which one of the following statements is correct regarding breast reconstruction with the latissimus dorsi (LD) flap?*

D. **Assessing normal arm and shoulder adduction preoperatively helps guide whether there has been previous damage to the vascular pedicle.**

Prior to undertaking breast reconstruction with the latissimus dorsi muscle flap, it is prudent to assess normal muscle function with arm and shoulder adduction, extension, and internal rotation. The preservation of function is a good indicator that both the vascular pedicle and nerve supply are intact and is relevant in patients who have previously undergone axillary or thoracic surgery. Where iatrogenic damage has occurred previously there would likely be muscle atrophy and dysfunction evident.

The vascular supply to the latissimus dorsi is robust, but it is from the thoracodorsal artery (not the thoracoacromial) as well as the posterior intercostal and lumbar perforators. This makes it a type V flap according to the Mathes and Nahai classification.[1]

There are many indications for using the latissimus dorsi for breast reconstruction and its use is certainly not limited to salvage cases following free tissue transfer failure, although this is one useful scenario in which to use it. It is particularly useful in patients who require bilateral reconstruction and have had radiotherapy but don't have enough soft tissue for free tissue transfer.

Most patients still require a breast prosthesis when using this flap to provide adequate projection and volume. The extended or volume-added latissimus dorsi can be useful for obtaining more soft tissue cover in breast reconstruction, as this includes adipose tissue above and below the muscle, but even this can usually only be used without an implant in small to medium or partial reconstructions. Larger breasts will almost always require a supplementary implant.[2]

Few patients experience long-term significant problems with shoulder function after using this flap, which is surprising given its functional importance. Patients with more specific physical requirements such as those involved in physical activities such as climbing or swimming may be more affected. Even so it is important to discuss this as a potential problem with patients and ensure that physical therapy is considered.

REFERENCES

1. Mathes SJ, Nahai F. Classification of the vascular anatomy of muscles: experimental and clinical correlation. Plast Reconstr Surg 1981;67(2):177–187
2. Hammond DC. Latissimus dorsi flap breast reconstruction. Plast Reconstr Surg 2009;124(4):1055–1063

ELEVATION OF THE LATISSIMUS DORSI FLAP FOR BREAST RECONSTRUCTION

4. *When elevating a latissimus dorsi flap for breast reconstruction, which of the following is advised?*

C. **Placement of quilting sutures and fibrin glue when closing back the donor site.**

When elevating a latissimus dorsi flap for breast reconstruction it is important to minimize the risk of postoperative seroma as this procedure carries a high risk of this complication at the donor site. Seroma formation is estimated to be as high as 80% in some series.[1] The use of progressive tension sutures has been shown to significantly reduce seroma formation, as this reduces the effective size of the dissected subcutaneous pocket with quilting.[2]

Combining quilting sutures with fibrin glue has also been shown to be effective in reducing seroma rates. Where seroma does occur, drainage followed by intracavity steroid injections can be helpful.[3]

In terms of patient positioning, the lateral decubitus position is preferred as this allows for good access and facilitates passage of the flap to the anterior breast pocket. It also allows the arm to be abducted, thereby creating space to safely dissect out the pedicle proximally. To elevate the flap in the prone position is also possible but it is usually reserved for bilateral cases and two surgeons working simultaneously. Although a "set piece" or standardized approach to the elevation may seem ideal, in reality it is often best to be adaptable in the approach as there may be times when dissection is slowed or landmarks are more difficult to visualize. The key landmarks include the spinous processes, trapezius, scapula, teres major, serratus anterior, and the boundaries of the latissimus itself.

Preservation of the serratus muscle vascular branch of the thoracodorsal pedicle (which itself is another useful landmark) is not usually possible as this will likely limit the flap movement and reach. The elevated flap will not be reliant on this branch for vascularity so there is no need to preserve it for that reason.

Innervation of the latissimus dorsi is from the thoracodorsal nerve, which originates from the posterior cord of the brachial plexus and many surgeons divide this segmentally during flap harvest to stop unwanted postoperative contractions. It can usually be identified close to the pedicle in the axilla and its identification confirmed with gentle compression using forceps. This elicits a contraction in the muscle. The muscle is likely to atrophy anyway following its transfer so there is no strong indication to preserve this nerve for maintenance of bulk alone.

REFERENCES

1. Delay E, Gounot N, Bouillot A, Zlatoff P, Rivoire M. Autologous latissimus breast reconstruction: a 3-year clinical experience with 100 patients. Plast Reconstr Surg 1998;102(5):1461–1478
2. Rios JL, Pollock T, Adams WP Jr. Progressive tension sutures to prevent seroma formation after latissimus dorsi harvest. Plast Reconstr Surg 2003;112(7):1779–1783
3. Hart AM, Duggal C, Pinell-White X, Losken A. A prospective randomized trial of the efficacy of fibrin glue, triamcinolone acetonide, and quilting sutures in seroma prevention after latissimus dorsi breast reconstruction. Plast Reconstr Surg 2017;139(4):854e–863e

PEDICLED TRAM FLAP FOR BREAST RECONSTRUCTION

5. *Which one of the following characteristics is shared between the pedicled and free transverse rectus abdominis myocutaneous (TRAM) approaches to breast reconstruction?*

E. The skin and fat transferred

The pedicled and free TRAM flaps are very different to one another. For a start they have different blood supplies, with the free TRAM being based on the deep inferior epigastric vessels and the pedicled TRAM being based on the superior epigastric vessels, which are the continuation of the internal mammary vessels. The complication rates are higher for the pedicled flap including fat necrosis and wound healing problems. Again, this relates to the blood supply which is usually predominantly from the inferior vessels. Because the full width and length of the rectus muscle, as well as the overlying fascia, is harvested in the pedicled TRAM, there is far more donor site morbidity and mesh is required to reconstruct this deficit. The risk of hernia and abdominal wall weakness are thereby markedly increased. The number of surgical procedures may be the same for each flap, but ideally the pedicled flap will involve delay by ligation of the ipsilateral deep inferior epigastric vessels a couple of weeks prior to surgery, so this will add a further operative step. Therefore, the only real similarity is that the same piece of skin and fat is transferred, i.e., the transverse part of the anterior lower abdomen between the umbilicus and the mons pubis.

Given the negative points associated with the pedicled TRAM it is no longer commonly used where microsurgically trained surgeons are available and has been superseded by its free tissue alternatives.[1-3]

REFERENCES

1. Serletti JM. Breast reconstruction with the TRAM flap: pedicled and free. J Surg Oncol 2006;94(6):532–537
2. Golpanian S, Gerth DJ, Tashiro J, Thaller SR. Free versus pedicled TRAM flaps: cost utilization and complications. Aesthetic Plast Surg 2016;40(6):869–876
3. Moran SL, Serletti JM. Outcome comparison between free and pedicled TRAM flap breast reconstruction in the obese patient. Plast Reconstr Surg 2001;108(7):1954–1960, discussion 1961–1962

CONTRAINDICATIONS TO ABDOMINAL FREE TISSUE TRANSFER IN BREAST RECONSTRUCTION

6. A patient is seen in clinic requesting breast reconstruction using an abdominal free flap. *Which one of the following prior surgical procedures would represent an absolute contraindication to proceeding with free abdominal breast reconstruction?*

E. Abdominoplasty

There are a number of contraindications to breast reconstruction with abdominal tissue relating to previous surgery. They can be absolute or relative. Absolute contraindications include previous planned or inadvertent deep inferior epigastric artery (DIEA) pedicle ligation (during abdominal or gynecologic surgery) or previous abdominoplasty because the perforating vessels from the DIEA pedicle will have already been sacrificed at the suprafascial level during this procedure. Other relative contraindications include previous abdominal liposuction, which also risks damage to multiple perforators between the abdominal wall and the skin, and multiple previous abdominal surgeries leaving complex scars such as midline laparotomies and open cholecystectomy. In the latter scenario it may be necessary to use a hemi flap, if it provides sufficient volume, or a bipedicled flap harvesting both DIEA, if it does not. These can then be anastomosed to the internal mammary artery (IMA) and internal mammary vein (IMV) antegrade and retrograde or by joining the pedicles directly. Other contraindications not specifically related to previous surgery include smoking, metastatic disease, coagulopathies, and chronic medical conditions. Interestingly, a recent case report has described successful use of a deep inferior epigastric perforator (DIEP) flap for breast reconstruction flap 10 years post abdominoplasty, suggesting that there can be recanalization of perforators after this surgery. However, this is a rarely described finding and there should always be preoperative imaging in this setting as well as an alternative flap plan made for the reconstruction should it not work out. Successful use of free abdominal flaps has also been described after liposuction, but this is less surprising as one might expect the majority of perforators to remain intact after this surgery. Again, in these circumstances, preoperative imaging would be strongly recommended to assess the vasculature of the abdominal wall.[1-3]

REFERENCES

1. Zeltzer AA, De Baerdemaeker RA, Hendrickx B, Seidenstücker K, Brussaard C, Hamdi M. Deep inferior epigastric artery perforator flap harvest after full abdominoplasty. Acta Chir Belg 2019;119(5):322–327
2. De Frene B, Van Landuyt K, Hamdi M, et al. Free DIEAP and SGAP flap breast reconstruction after abdominal/gluteal liposuction. J Plast Reconstr Aesthet Surg 2006;59(10):1031–1036
3. Rozen WM, Garcia-Tutor E, Alonso-Burgos A, Corlett RJ, Taylor GI, Ashton MW. The effect of anterior abdominal wall scars on the vascular anatomy of the abdominal wall: a cadaveric and clinical study with clinical implications. Clin Anat 2009;22(7):815–822

ABDOMINAL FREE TISSUE TRANSFER FOR BREAST RECONSTRUCTION

7. *What is the main advantage of a superficial inferior epigastric artery (SIEA) flap over a deep inferior epigastric artery (DIEA) flap for abdominal based breast reconstruction?*

B. Decreased donor site morbidity

The superficial inferior epigastric vessels, which supply the superficial inferior epigastric artery (SIEA) flap, arise from the common femoral artery and saphenous bulb. The use of this flap is limited by the variability of vessel caliber and quality, a short vascular pedicle, and unreliable perfusion to the contralateral flap. The main advantage of this flap is that donor site morbidity is minimal as there is no violation of the rectus sheath. Furthermore, operative time should be shortened as a result of the reduced dissection and lack of abdominal wall closure. An issue with the short pedicle arises when trying to anastomose to the internal mammary vessels in that reach may be inadequate and finding suitable perforators from this vessel may be necessary. In these circumstances rib harvest may be avoided, but this does not represent the key advantage of this flap.[1-3]

REFERENCES

1. Grünherz L, Wolter A, Andree C, et al. Autologous breast reconstruction with SIEA flaps: an alternative in selected cases. Aesthetic Plast Surg 2020;44(2):299–306
2. Selber JC, Samra F, Bristol M, et al. A head-to-head comparison between the muscle-sparing free TRAM and the SIEA flaps: is the rate of flap loss worth the gain in abdominal wall function? Plast Reconstr Surg 2008;122(2):348–355
3. Macadam SA, Zhong T, Weichman K, et al. Quality of life and patient-reported outcomes in breast cancer survivors: a multicenter comparison of four abdominally based autologous reconstruction methods. Plast Reconstr Surg 2016;137(3):758–771

FREE FLAP ABDOMINAL RECONSTRUCTION OF THE BREAST

8. *When discussing abdominal free flap breast reconstruction with patients, which one of the following should you advise them of?*

D. They may benefit from preoperative imaging with CT or MRI.

Preoperative imaging using computed tomographic angiography (CTA) or magnetic resonance angiography (MRA) is generally advocated for patients undergoing free tissue transfer from the abdomen to the breast. This helps to confirm that the deep inferior epigastric vessels are intact and helps to map out their pathway in relation to the rectus muscle and identify the number, location, and caliber of perforating vessels.

This can help preoperative planning and speed up intraoperative decision-making in terms of perforator selection and deciding whether to undertake a muscle-sparing TRAM or a DIEP.[1-3] There are other modalities that can be useful; for example, handheld Doppler to assess for perforators is highly recommended for all such patients. However, this alone does not fully predict the anatomic pathway of the vessels in relation to the abdominal wall and rectus abdominis. Despite this not all surgeons agree that preoperative imaging is helpful or needed and there is a potential cost implication as well as an increased radiation dose when CT is chosen.

Patients do need to understand that autologous breast reconstruction is a major undertaking and they are likely to have both an extended stay in hospital (2–6 nights typically with Enhanced Recovery After Surgery (ERAS) protocols, not 10 nights) and 3–6 months overall recovery time. Depending on their occupation, patients will normally be back to work 6–10 weeks following surgery. Flap failure rates are fairly low and most surgeons would quote rates of around 5% for failure. However, this may be even lower in many units. Donor site morbidity is proportional to the amount of muscle included with the flap so patients need to understand that if a muscle-sparing TRAM is required rather than a DIEP, their abdominal wall function may be more significantly affected. However, once the procedure has been started, the major focus should be on maintaining a well-vascularized flap to reconstruct the breast and muscle sacrifice must be accepted if necessary.[4]

REFERENCES

1. Teunis T, Heerma van Voss MR, Kon M, van Maurik JF. CT-angiography prior to DIEP flap breast reconstruction: a systematic review and meta-analysis. Microsurgery 2013;33(6):496–502
2. Chhaya N, Sarbeng P, Stuart S, Angullia F, Mosahebi A, Malhotra A. Benefits of CT-angiography localisation in the surgical planning of deep inferior epigastric perforator flap breast reconstruction. Breast Cancer Res 2010;12:48
3. Aubry S, Pauchot J, Kastler A, Laurent O, Tropet Y, Runge M. Preoperative imaging in the planning of deep inferior epigastric artery perforator flap surgery. Skeletal Radiol 2013;42(3):319–327
4. Macadam SA, Zhong T, Weichman K, et al. Quality of life and patient-reported outcomes in breast cancer survivors: a multicenter comparison of four abdominally based autologous reconstruction methods. Plast Reconstr Surg 2016;137(3):758–771

AUTOLOGOUS FREE TISSUE BREAST RECONSTRUCTION

9. While performing free tissue transfer for breast reconstruction, you have been trying for an extended period of time to achieve a satisfactory venous anastomosis with the internal mammary vein but are unsuccessful. The arterial anastomosis is running well and you do not wish to redo it. *Which one of the following vessels can be used as an alternative venous outflow source in this situation without preparing a vessel graft or re-siting the artery?*

D. The cephalic vein

There are two main options available in this situation that will avoid both re-anastomosing the artery and utilizing a vein graft. The first of these is a cephalic turndown, where the cephalic vein is elevated from distal to proximal in the upper arm into the deltopectoral groove. It is then transposed medially to allow direct venous anastomosis. The second option (not listed) is to dissect the external jugular vein (not the internal) in the neck from cranial to caudal and pass the vessel from the neck into the zone where the arterial anastomosis is sited. The other options would each require a vein graft to adequately reach the TRAM flap pedicle. Where there is a long pedicle as may be the case in a DIEP flap, it may be possible to separate the artery from the vein and reach laterally but this still may present problems with adequate vessel length.[1,2]

REFERENCES

1. Shankhdhar VK, Yadav PS, Dushyant J, Seetharaman SS, Chinmay W. Cephalic vein: saviour in the microsurgical reconstruction of breast and head and neck cancers. Indian J Plast Surg 2012;45(3):485–493
2. Chang EI, Fearmonti RM, Chang DW, Butler CE. Cephalic vein transposition versus vein grafts for venous outflow in free-flap breast reconstruction. Plast Reconstr Surg Glob Open 2014;2(5):e141

FREE ABDOMINAL FLAP RECONSTRUCTION

10. You are supervising a senior resident as he or she raises a free TRAM flap. *What is the main reason to encourage to dissect the superficial epigastric vein during this procedure?*

D. In case the flap turns out to have a dominant superficial drainage

The reason for dissecting and preserving length of the superficial inferior epigastric vessels is that some abdominal flaps are heavily reliant on this system for venous outflow. In some cases, the superficial system is the dominant system. This may display as a grossly congested flap following completion of satisfactory anastomoses at the recipient site. In such cases, it can be helpful to perform a second venous anastomosis to one of the lateral chest wall or axillary vessels in order to generate satisfactory venous outflow and maintain flap viability. The primary anastomosis for a typical TRAM flap is the deep inferior epigastric vein. If the vein graft is required, then this can be harvested at the necessary time. Practicing dissection skills on vessels not primarily used in a reconstruction can be a useful training exercise but it should not compromise patient's safety or unnecessarily extend the operating duration.[1-6]

REFERENCES

1. Ochoa O, Pisano S, Chrysopoulo M, Ledoux P, Arishita G, Nastala C. Salvage of intraoperative deep inferior epigastric perforator flap venous congestion with augmentation of venous outflow: flap morbidity and review of the literature. Plast Reconstr Surg Glob Open 2013;1(7):e52
2. Schaverien M, Saint-Cyr M, Arbique G, Brown SA. Arterial and venous anatomies of the deep inferior epigastric perforator and superficial inferior epigastric artery flaps. Plast Reconstr Surg 2008;121(6):1909–1919
3. Carramenha e Costa MA, Carriquiry C, Vasconez LO, Grotting JC, Herrera RH, Windle BH. An anatomic study of the venous drainage of the transverse rectus abdominis musculocutaneous flap. Plast Reconstr Surg 1987;79(2):208–217
4. Rozen WM, Pan WR, Le Roux CM, Taylor GI, Ashton MW. The venous anatomy of the anterior abdominal wall: an anatomical and clinical study. Plast Reconstr Surg 2009;124(3):848–853
5. Sbitany H, Mirzabeigi MN, Kovach SJ, Wu LC, Serletti JM. Strategies for recognizing and managing intraoperative venous congestion in abdominally based autologous breast reconstruction. Plast Reconstr Surg 2012;129(4):809–815
6. Eom JS, Sun SH, Lee TJ. Selection of the recipient veins for additional anastomosis of the superficial inferior epigastric vein in breast reconstruction with free transverse rectus abdominis musculocutaneous or deep inferior epigastric artery perforator flaps. Ann Plast Surg 2011;67(5):505–509

FREE THIGH BASED FLAPS FOR BREAST RECONSTRUCTION

11.Which one of the following is true of thigh based free flaps for breast reconstruction?

   D. They are associated with low donor site morbidity and discreet scars.

   Free thigh flaps utilize thigh tissue that is typically discarded during a medial thigh lift. A significant advantage of their use is the discreet placement of scars and low donor site morbidity. Although they are good secondary choices for free autologous breast reconstruction in patients unsuitable for an abdominal flap, they may also be primary options in women with significant soft tissue excess of the medial/posterior thigh, in younger patients with a known genetic mutation with insufficient abdominal tissue for bilateral reconstruction, and those who wish to become pregnant in the future.[1] Tissue quality is similar to breast tissue and is indicated for reconstruction of small or moderate-sized breasts only.

   The hospital stay is similar to other free tissue transfer techniques but may if anything be slightly shorter and overall recovery is generally shorter than free abdominal flaps at 6–8 weeks. One challenge is the relatively short vascular pedicles for anastomosis, meaning that internal mammary perforators may need to be used rather than the main source vessels.[2,3]

REFERENCES

1. Allen RJ Jr, Lee ZH, Mayo JL, Levine J, Ahn C, Allen RJ Sr. The profunda artery perforator flap experience for breast reconstruction. Plast Reconstr Surg 2016;138(5):968–975
2. Haddock NT, Gassman A, Cho MJ, Teotia SS. 101 consecutive profunda artery perforator flaps in breast reconstruction: lessons learned with our early experience. Plast Reconstr Surg 2017;140(2):229–239
3. Fattah A, Figus A, Mathur B, Ramakrishnan VV. The transverse myocutaneous gracilis flap: technical refinements. J Plast Reconstr Aesthet Surg 2010;63(2):305–313

THIGH BASED FREE FLAPS FOR BREAST RECONSTRUCTION

12.Which one of the following characteristics do the transverse upper gracilis (TUG) flap and profunda artery perforator (PAP) flap have in common?

   C. They are both harvested in the lithotomy position.

   The transverse upper gracilis (TUG) flap and profunda artery perforator (PAP) flap are both free tissue flaps used for breast reconstruction. They are both harvested in the lithotomy position and use thigh skin flaps. The vascular supply differs between the two flaps; the TUG flap is based on the medial circumflex femoral artery, while the PAP flap, as the name suggests, is based on the profunda femoris artery. The skin paddles used are similar, but not identical because of placement of the perforators from the PAP which can display variation in their location. The TUG flap is designed as a transverse skin ellipse with the scar positioned in the groin crease anteriorly and the gluteal crease posteriorly. The PAP flap can be designed with a transverse, vertical, oblique, L-shaped, or fleur-de-lis skin paddle design and can facilitate recruitment of more abundant soft tissue volume lateral to the midline of the posterior thigh region. The PAP flap is a perforator flap with no harvest of muscle, whereas the TUG flap is a muscle based flap. The profunda artery may be septocutaneous or musculocutaneous through the adductor magnus. Therefore, some muscle dissection may be necessary. Two advantages of the PAP flap over the TUG flap are that the pedicle length is greater, and the vessel diameter is wider. The mean arterial diameter is 1.6 mm for the TUG versus 2.2 mm for the PAP. The mean pedicle length is 5.4 cm for the TUG versus 10 cm for the PAP. A shared approach can be undertaken intraoperatively to first identify the PAP perforator. If this is present, then continuation of the PAP can be continued, otherwise the TUG flap can be elevated instead.[1-3]

REFERENCES

1. Allen RJ Jr, Lee ZH, Mayo JL, Levine J, Ahn C, Allen RJ Sr. The profunda artery perforator flap experience for breast reconstruction. Plast Reconstr Surg 2016;138(5):968–975
2. Haddock NT, Gassman A, Cho MJ, Teotia SS. 101 consecutive profunda artery perforator flaps in breast reconstruction: lessons learned with our early experience. Plast Reconstr Surg 2017;140(2):229–239
3. Fattah A, Figus A, Mathur B, Ramakrishnan VV. The transverse myocutaneous gracilis flap: technical refinements. J Plast Reconstr Aesthet Surg 2010;63(2):305–313

FREE GLUTEAL FLAPS FOR BREAST RECONSTRUCTION

13. *When raising free gluteal flaps for breast reconstruction, which one of the following is true?*

A. Where laterally based perforators are identified, effective pedicle length can be increased.

Superior and inferior gluteal artery perforator (S/IGAP) flaps are based on the superior and inferior gluteal artery perforators, respectively. One of the main challenges of using free gluteal flaps for breast reconstruction is that the pedicle length is fairly short. This differs between the IGAP and SGAP flaps, with pedicle length being longer in the IGAP (typically 7–10 cm) versus SGAP (typically 5–8 cm). Where there are laterally based perforators, they tend to run obliquely in the gluteal muscle so dissecting them out can increase the effective pedicle length. Although the pedicles are relatively short, they do not normally require vein grafts. The vessel caliber in gluteal flaps is usually a reasonable match for the internal mammary vessels although the artery tends to be smaller than the internal mammary artery (IMA) (1.8–2.0 mm) and the vein tends to be larger (3.5 mm). Proximal pedicle dissection into the muscle can be slow and tedious because there are a high number of deep branches present.[1-3]

REFERENCES

1. LoTempio MM, Allen RJ. Breast reconstruction with SGAP and IGAP flaps. Plast Reconstr Surg 2010;126(2):393–401
2. Allen RJ, Levine JL, Granzow JW. The in-the-crease inferior gluteal artery perforator flap for breast reconstruction. Plast Reconstr Surg 2006;118(2):333–339
3. Ahmadzadeh R, Bergeron L, Tang M, Morris SF. The superior and inferior gluteal artery perforator flaps. Plast Reconstr Surg 2007;120(6):1551–1556

RECIPIENT VESSELS IN FREE FLAP BREAST RECONSTRUCTION

14. *Which one of the following represents a disadvantage of using the internal mammary vessels when performing breast reconstruction with a free TRAM flap?*

D. The operating field is mobile during the anastomosis.

One particular challenge of performing a free flap anastomosis to the internal mammary vessels is that respiration causes the operating field to move. This can interfere with the focus of the microscope and make the process significantly more difficult. It is important to communicate with the anesthesiologist so that the effects of ventilation on the operative field can be minimized. This may be achieved by using high-volume, low-rate settings on the ventilator. The other challenges of using the internal mammary vessels are that access can be difficult, especially in patients after radiation. Access generally requires removal of a section of rib cartilage and careful dissection of the vessels just superficial to pleura. Although the risk is only small, it is possible to cause a pneumothorax while doing this part of the procedure. The vessels are usually well matched for size to the deep inferior epigastric pedicle and are consistently present in most patients. However, the vessels may be thin walled and friable, especially following radiotherapy. They are rarely absent but may be smaller on the left than the right. The inferior epigastric pedicle does have sufficient length to comfortably reach this area for anastomosis.[1-4]

REFERENCES

1. Hamdi M, Blondeel P, Van Landuyt K, Monstrey S. Algorithm in choosing recipient vessels for perforator free flap in breast reconstruction: the role of the internal mammary perforators. Br J Plast Surg 2004;57(3):258–265
2. Saint-Cyr M, Chang DW, Robb GL, Chevray PM. Internal mammary perforator recipient vessels for breast reconstruction using free TRAM, DIEP, and SIEA flaps. Plast Reconstr Surg 2007;120(7):1769–1773
3. Santanelli Di Pompeo F, Longo B, Sorotos M, Pagnoni M, Laporta R. The axillary versus internal mammary recipient vessel sites for breast reconstruction with diep flaps: a retrospective study of 256 consecutive cases. Microsurgery 2015;35(1):34–38
4. Lhuaire M, Hivelin M, Dramé M, et al. Determining the best recipient vessel site for autologous microsurgical breast reconstruction with DIEP flaps: An anatomical study. J Plast Reconstr Aesthet Surg 2017;70(6):781–791

58. Implant-Based Breast Reconstruction

See *Essentials of Plastic Surgery*, third edition, pp. 794–804

IMPLANT-BASED BREAST RECONSTRUCTION

1. You are discussing breast reconstruction with a patient. *Which one of the following statements is correct to tell her regarding implant-based versus autologous reconstruction techniques?*
   A. They are less commonly performed.
   B. They provide long-term cost benefits.
   C. They result in fewer long-term complications.
   D. They are harder to match with a natural breast.
   E. They are less likely to require revision surgery.

ACELLULAR DERMAL MATRIX IN BREAST RECONSTRUCTION

2. *Which one of the following is true regarding acellular dermal matrix (ADM) in breast reconstruction?*
   A. Its use is considered "off-label" by the FDA at present.
   B. The sole indication for use is in immediate subpectoral reconstruction.
   C. The matrix should always be tightly adherent to the prosthesis without obvious laxity.
   D. It has a proven role in reducing capsular contracture and radiation effects.
   E. It has been shown to be cost effective for immediate and delayed procedures.

PREPECTORAL BREAST IMPLANT RECONSTRUCTION

3. *What is currently the main reason for avoiding prepectoral breast implant reconstruction?*
   A. The lack of long-term evidence to support its use
   B. The technical difficulty of the procedure
   C. The resultant breast animation that occurs
   D. The need to stage the procedure
   E. The requirement for incorporating acellular dermal matrix (ADM)

SURGICAL PLANNING IN BREAST RECONSTRUCTION

4. Following mastectomy and radiotherapy, a patient requests implant-based reconstruction. *Which type of reconstruction would be preferable in her case with respect to minimizing complications?*
   A. Single-stage submuscular implant and ADM
   B. Two-stage submuscular expander/implant
   C. Single-stage latissimus dorsi and implant
   D. Single-stage prepectoral implant and ADM
   E. Two-stage prepectoral expander/implant

TWO-STAGE RECONSTRUCTION

5. You have decided to perform a two-stage implant breast reconstruction for a patient. *Which one of the following statements is correct regarding this procedure?*
   A. The tissue expander should routinely be placed in the subcutaneous plane.
   B. The expander should remain empty at the end of the first surgical procedure.
   C. The expansion process normally begins 6 weeks after the initial surgery.
   D. The patient's response can be helpful in gauging optimal expansion volumes in clinic.
   E. The expander should never be overfilled beyond the required final volume.

EVALUATING MASTECTOMY FLAP VIABILITY

6. *Which one of the following is true regarding mastectomy skin flaps?*
   A. Their vascularity can only be accurately evaluated by clinical assessment.
   B. Flap thickness and vascularity is fairly uniform across different patient groups.
   C. Reconstruction should be delayed if flap vascularity is in question.
   D. Viability of mastectomy flaps bears little relation to surgical skills or technique.
   E. Poor flap perfusion does not consistently correlate with increased complication rates.

SELECTION OF BREAST RECONSTRUCTION TECHNIQUE

7. A 40-year-old woman is to have bilateral prophylactic mastectomies as she is BRCA positive. A skin-sparing approach is planned with preservation of the nipple-areola complex. She is otherwise fit and well and is a nonsmoker. On examination, she has small breasts; estimated volume is 300 cc with good skin quality. Her body mass index (BMI) is 21 and she wishes to moderately increase her breast size. *Which one of the following is the most suitable reconstructive option for this patient?*
   A. Implants only
   B. Implants and de-epithelialized inferiorly based skin flaps
   C. Implants and acellular dermal matrix
   D. Pedicled transverse rectus abdominis myocutaneous (TRAM) flaps
   E. Pedicled musculocutaneous latissimus dorsi (LD) flaps with implants

EFFECTS OF RADIATION ON BREAST RECONSTRUCTION

8. *When considering implant-based breast reconstruction, which one of the following elements is unaffected by radiotherapy?*
   A. Infection rate
   B. Seroma rate
   C. Implant rupture rate
   D. Skin flap necrosis
   E. Capsular contraction

COMPLICATIONS FOLLOWING IMPLANT-BASED BREAST RECONSTRUCTION

9. *Within the first year following two-stage, implant-based breast reconstruction, what is the most common complication?*
   A. Implant extrusion
   B. Implant infection
   C. Total reconstruction failure
   D. Seroma
   E. Capsular contracture

Answers

IMPLANT-BASED BREAST RECONSTRUCTION

1. You are discussing breast reconstruction with a patient. *Which one of the following statements is correct to tell her regarding implant-based versus autologous reconstruction techniques?*

   D. They are harder to match with a natural breast.

   Implant-based reconstruction is the most common form of breast reconstruction in the US and it carries with it a number of advantages over autologous techniques. These include a lower initial cost, reduced operating room (OR) time, reduced hospital stay, avoidance of a donor scar, and in most cases, the technique is technically simpler and microvascular skills are not required. In the longer term, many of the advantages may be lost because the need for subsequent revision is increased as a result of complications such as capsular contracture, implant malposition, or implant rupture. In addition, it is difficult to achieve satisfactory symmetry in unilateral reconstruction as the soft tissue characteristics of a natural breast cannot be recreated and natural ptosis does not develop over time in the implant reconstructed breast. This is a key point to highlight to patients undergoing unilateral reconstruction to ensure they are well informed preoperatively and have realistic expectations from surgery.[1-4] A technique that may help both the appearance and feel of an implant reconstruction is fat transfer, as this alters the ratio of autologous to implant volume, although this will add further procedures and costs to the process.[5]

REFERENCES

1. Kroll SS, Evans GR, Reece GP, et al. Comparison of resource costs between implant-based and TRAM flap breast reconstruction. Plast Reconstr Surg 1996;97(2):364–372
2. Spear SL, Mardini S, Ganz JC. Resource cost comparison of implant-based breast reconstruction versus TRAM flap breast reconstruction. Plast Reconstr Surg 2003;112(1): 101–105
3. Cordeiro PG, McCarthy CM. A single surgeon's 12-year experience with tissue expander/implant breast reconstruction: part I. A prospective analysis of early complications. Plast Reconstr Surg 2006;118(4):825–831
4. Cordeiro PG, McCarthy CM. A single surgeon's 12-year experience with tissue expander/implant breast reconstruction: part II. An analysis of long-term complications, aesthetic outcomes, and patient satisfaction. Plast Reconstr Surg 2006;118(4):832–839
5. Salgarello M, Visconti G, Barone-Adesi L. Fat grafting and breast reconstruction with implant: another option for irradiated breast cancer patients. Plast Reconstr Surg 2012;129(2):317–329

ACELLULAR DERMAL MATRIX IN BREAST RECONSTRUCTION

2. *Which one of the following is true regarding acellular dermal matrix (ADM) in breast reconstruction?*

   A. Its use is considered "off-label" by the FDA at present.

   The use of ADM has dramatically increased for breast reconstruction during the past decade with a number of different sources providing the matrices (bovine, porcine, human) and many manufacturers producing it. However, its use remains "off-label" from the FDA perspective in breast reconstruction. There are many indications and it is certainly not limited only to immediate subpectoral reconstruction. It is useful for both immediate and delayed reconstruction and prepectoral and submuscular reconstructions. The matrix should be tightly adherent to a permanent implant; however, some laxity should be left in the setting of planned tissue expansion. The matrix acts as an internal bra to support the implant in the correct place and also provide more soft tissue cover for the prosthesis. A further proposed advantage is that single-stage immediate reconstruction can be performed with the ADM providing inferior and lateral cover for the implant where the pectoralis muscle fails to provide cover. This may be the case, but overlying tissue vascularity in the inferior pole will be reduced given the thickness of the postmastectomy skin flap and wound healing problems can occur. Care must be taken to carefully suture the ADM to the pectoralis muscle superiorly and to the inframammary fold (IMF) inferiorly. Postreconstruction animation can still occur with this technique and also there is unlikely to be much development of natural breast ptosis due to the rigid fixity of the reconstruction. ADM does not have a proven role in reducing capsular contracture rates nor the effects of radiation therapy. One major concern with ADM is the cost effectiveness of its use as it is expensive and generally costs more than the implants themselves.[1-4]

   In patients with larger breasts, it is preferable to utilize a de-epithelialized inferior dermal pedicle to cover the implant caudal to pectoralis major as this often provides thicker soft tissue cover than a matrix, is vascularized, and saves the cost of the ADM. The procedure is performed in the same way as an inferior pedicle breast reconstruction is undertaken but is only really applicable to immediate reconstruction (ideally prophylactic skin-sparing mastectomies) in patients with large ptotic breasts.

REFERENCES

1. Spear SL, Seruya M, Clemens MW, Teitelbaum S, Nahabedian MY. Acellular dermal matrix for the treatment and prevention of implant-associated breast deformities. Plast Reconstr Surg 2011;127(3):1047–1058
2. Nguyen KT, Mioton LM, Smetona JT, Seth AK, Kim JY. Esthetic outcomes of ADM-assisted expander-implant breast reconstruction. Eplasty 2012;12:e58
3. Nahabedian MY. AlloDerm performance in the setting of prosthetic breast surgery, infection, and irradiation. Plast Reconstr Surg 2009;124(6):1743–1753
4. de Blacam C, Momoh AO, Colakoglu S, Slavin SA, Tobias AM, Lee BT. Cost analysis of implant-based breast reconstruction with acellular dermal matrix. Ann Plast Surg 2012;69(5):516–520

PREPECTORAL BREAST IMPLANT RECONSTRUCTION

3. *What is currently the main reason for avoiding prepectoral breast implant reconstruction?*

   A. The lack of long-term evidence to support its use

     Prepectoral breast implant reconstruction has grown in popularity over the past decade. Historically, implant reconstruction had been performed in the subcutaneous plane but poor implant support and high complication rates led to the change in favor toward submuscular implant placement. Due to the problems with animation and disruption of the pectoralis muscle, prepectoral placement has seen a resurgence in use. However, while there is some evidence to show that early results are reasonable, there is no long-term evidence to support its use and it may be that with time the procedure falls out of favor once more.[1–3] The procedure itself is not especially difficult and breast animation is avoided. The procedure may be staged but can also be performed in a single stage. The requirement for any procedure to need ADM needs careful consideration as there are cost implications and the risk of seroma development may be increased. Prepectoral breast implant reconstruction most often involves completely wrapping the implant in ADM and then suturing this to the chest wall. The concern some plastic and reconstructive surgeons have with this approach is the use of nonvascularized tissue being placed in a poorly vascularized pocket in combination with an implant. The long-term outcome reports of these techniques will be useful to guide practice preferences in the future.

REFERENCES

1. Sigalove S, Maxwell GP, Sigalove NM, et al. Prepectoral implant-based breast reconstruction: rationale, indications, and preliminary results. Plast Reconstr Surg 2017;139(2): 287–294
2. Ter Louw RP, Nahabedian MY. Prepectoral breast reconstruction. Plast Reconstr Surg 2017;140(5S Advances in Breast Reconstruction):51S–59S
3. Sbitany H, Piper M, Lentz R. Prepectoral breast reconstruction: a safe alternative to submuscular prosthetic reconstruction following nipple-sparing mastectomy. Plast Reconstr Surg 2017;140(3):432–443

SURGICAL PLANNING IN BREAST RECONSTRUCTION

4. Following mastectomy and radiotherapy, a patient requests implant-based reconstruction. *Which type of reconstruction would be preferable in her case with respect to minimizing complications?*

   C. Single-stage latissimus dorsi and implant

     The challenge for this patient in terms of breast reconstruction is twofold. First, she is missing both breast volume and an adequate soft tissue envelope. Second, she has had radiotherapy to the chest wall and will therefore be at an increased risk of developing wound healing problems post surgery. In this setting most surgeons would prefer to import fresh soft tissue into the area for reconstruction and perform an autologous tissue. However, in the situation where implant-based reconstruction is desired, or when autologous reconstruction is not possible, reconstruction in this setting is best undertaken in combination with the latissimus dorsi transfer. This has been shown to reduce implant-based complication rates by 66–72%.[1,2] The other options would all be likely to result in postoperative complications including wound healing issues, infection, and implant extrusion. A single-stage, submuscular or prepectoral implant and ADM would not work for this patient given her skin deficiency. In principle, two-stage reconstruction with tissue expansion may work but the effects of radiotherapy on chest wall skin makes it respond poorly to this process.

REFERENCES

1. Lee K-T, Mun G-H. Prosthetic breast reconstruction in previously irradiated breasts: a meta-analysis. J Surg Oncol 2015;112(5):468–475
2. Fischer JP, Basta MN, Shubinets V, Serletti JM, Fosnot J. A systematic meta-analysis of prosthetic-based breast reconstruction in irradiated fields with or without autologous muscle flap coverage. Ann Plast Surg 2016;77(1):129–134

TWO-STAGE RECONSTRUCTION

5. You have decided to perform a two-stage implant breast reconstruction for a patient. *Which one of the following statements is correct regarding this procedure?*

   D. **The patient's response can be helpful in gauging optimal expansion volumes in clinic.**
      When undertaking tissue expansion in the breast there are a number of key principles that should be adhered to. First, the expander is most often, but not always, placed in the submuscular (subpectoral) plane and not the subcutaneous plane. The advantage of doing so is the additional soft tissue cover provided by this. The expander should have all of the air removed from it intraoperatively to completely empty it, and then a small volume of fluid should be injected (50–100 cc). Many surgeons will use a tiny amount of methylene blue to slightly color the fluid blue for confirmation of the needle being correctly placed in the implant port, which can subsequently be made by withdrawing and visualizing colored fluid prior to injection. Leaving a small volume at the end of the procedure is often helpful, but too much may risk vascular compromise to the mastectomy skin flaps and negate the benefit of choosing a two-stage expansion method. The expansion process can be commenced a few weeks after surgery and does not need to be delayed to 6 weeks unless there have been problems with wound healing. In clinic most surgeons will inject between 30 and 120 cc of fluid per session. However, the patient's response to injection is often one of the most helpful guides. Patients are able to guide the procedure by advising when the injection starts to feel too tight and discomfort is experienced. On reaching this point, the volume can be reduced slightly. Patients' input is also important at the end of the expansion process as they can guide the surgeon how large they wish the reconstructed breasts to be. The other factor to observe during expansion is the skin flap perfusion as this provides useful information via capillary refill and blanching to avoid causing vascular compromise. Once the desired volume has been reached it is prudent to overinflate the implant slightly to allow for skin recoil with removal of the expander for implant placement.[1–3]

REFERENCES

1. Bertozzi N, Pesce M, Santi P, Raposio E. Tissue expansion for breast reconstruction: methods and techniques. Ann Med Surg (Lond) 2017;21:34–44
2. McCue JD, Migliori M, Cunningham BL. Expanders and breast reconstruction with gel and saline implants. In: Hall-Findlay EJ, Evans GRD, eds. Aesthetic and Reconstructive Surgery of the Breast. 1st ed. New York: Elsevier Ltd.; 2010:29–50
3. Cordeiro PG, Jazayeri L. Two-stage implant-based breast reconstruction: an evolution of the conceptual and technical approach over a two-decade period. Plast Reconstr Surg 2016;138(1):1–11

EVALUATING MASTECTOMY FLAP VIABILITY

6. *Which one of the following is true regarding mastectomy skin flaps?*

   C. **Reconstruction should be delayed if flap vascularity is in question.**
      The adequacy of mastectomy flap vascularity is absolutely vital to successful breast reconstruction as the flaps provide the final soft tissue cover for the reconstructed breast. Mastectomy flaps by their very nature have compromised vascularity by the fact that they have been separated from the breast and thinned, sometimes close to the subdermal level. Flap vascularity is best assessed clinically with consideration given to tissue thickness, amount of exposed dermis, skin color, and capillary refill. Dark, congested flaps are likely to incur necrosis or wound dehiscence particularly if placed under additional stress and tension over an implant. In such circumstances, reconstruction is better delayed to allow for recovery or demarcation of the mastectomy flaps. Months down the line, the flaps may be progressively expanded safely and reconstruction still completed. Flap thickness following mastectomy varies considerably according to the patient and the surgeon performing the procedure. Clinical assessment is not the only way to assess the flaps and there are adjuncts including indocyanine green (ICG) fluorescence imaging and ICG laser angiography which may help to evaluate perfusion intraoperatively if uncertainty remains.[1,2]

REFERENCES

1. Moyer HR, Losken A. Predicting mastectomy skin flap necrosis with indocyanine green angiography: the gray area defined. Plast Reconstr Surg 2012;129(5):1043–1048
2. Newman MI, Jack MC, Samson MC. SPY-Q analysis toolkit values potentially predict mastectomy flap necrosis. Ann Plast Surg 2013;70(5):595–598

SELECTION OF BREAST RECONSTRUCTION TECHNIQUE

7. A 40-year-old woman is to have bilateral prophylactic mastectomies as she is BRCA positive. A skin-sparing approach is planned with preservation of the nipple-areola complex. She is otherwise fit and well and is a nonsmoker. On examination, she has small breasts; estimated volume is 300 cc with good skin quality. Her body

mass index (BMI) is 21 and she wishes to moderately increase her breast size. *Which one of the following is the most suitable reconstructive option for this patient?*

C. Implants and acellular dermal matrix

The simplest approach to reconstruction for this patient is to utilize an implant-based technique. As she is disease free, her skin envelope is maintained and no postoperative radiotherapy will be needed. These factors support the use of a prosthetic device. It is important to provide complete soft tissue cover for the implants as the skin flaps will be thin in this patient. For such cases, the use of dermal matrix has become popular.

Superiorly the implant/expander can be covered by the pectoralis major muscle and serratus anterior. Inferiorly the dermal matrix can cover the implant from the inframammary fold to the pectoralis muscle. In larger breasted patients, the use of a de-epithelialized inferior skin flap is favored to provide additional implant cover without a dermal matrix. This patient does not have sufficient breast tissue for this approach. To use bilateral pedicled TRAM flaps in this patient would be a poor choice, particularly given her age, because of the morbidity associated with sacrifice of both rectus muscles. In addition, given her BMI it is unlikely she will have sufficient tissue for autologous reconstruction. Bilateral LD flaps could be used to provide additional implant cover but there is no need for harvesting skin as the native breast skin is preserved. Use of LD muscle flaps would also involve significant back scarring, which can be avoided by using an implant and matrix combination.[1-4]

REFERENCES

1. Salzberg CA. Nonexpansive immediate breast reconstruction using human acellular tissue matrix graft (AlloDerm). Ann Plast Surg 2006;57(1):1–5
2. Stevens LA, McGrath MH, Druss RG, Kister SJ, Gump FE, Forde KA. The psychological impact of immediate breast reconstruction for women with early breast cancer. Plast Reconstr Surg 1984;73(4):619–628
3. Colwell AS, Christensen JM. Nipple-sparing mastectomy and direct-to-implant breast reconstruction. Plast Reconstr Surg 2017;140(5S Advances in Breast Reconstruction):44S–50S
4. Colwell AS, Damjanovic B, Zahedi B, Medford-Davis L, Hertl C, Austen WG Jr. Retrospective review of 331 consecutive immediate single-stage implant reconstructions with acellular dermal matrix: indications, complications, trends, and costs. Plast Reconstr Surg 2011;128(6):1170–1178

EFFECTS OF RADIATION ON BREAST RECONSTRUCTION

8. *When considering implant-based reconstruction, which one of the following elements is unaffected by radiotherapy?*

C. Implant rupture rate

Radiation therapy is often utilized as a component of breast cancer treatment, particularly in patients with larger or more aggressive tumors or those with axillary lymph node involvement. Radiation has known detrimental effects on the skin and subcutaneous tissues, including altered vascularity, radiation dermatitis, atrophy, dryness, discoloration, and chronic fibrosis. Lee and Mun[1] analyzed 20 different studies looking at complication rates with implant reconstruction in patients who had previously undergone radiation therapy. Pooled analysis showed a significant increase in complications after radiation therapy, including reconstructive failure, infection, seroma formation, and mastectomy flap necrosis. Complication rates were higher regardless of reconstructive method used, including use of ADM, one versus two stage reconstruction, immediate versus delayed reconstruction, or nipple-sparing mastectomy. Although radiation does therefore affect the cosmetic outcome in terms of the soft tissues, there is no evidence to show that it will reduce the longevity of the implant itself nor increase the risk of implant failure/rupture. The reason therefore for early revision being necessary in implant-based reconstruction after radiation is soft tissue related rather than device related. It may be that the negative effects of radiation on an implant-based reconstruction are more severe when an expander is in place as opposed to a permanent implant.[2,3]

REFERENCES

1. Lee K-T, Mun G-H. Prosthetic breast reconstruction in previously irradiated breasts: a meta-analysis. J Surg Oncol 2015;112(5):468–475
2. El-Sabawi B, Sosin M, Carey JN, Nahabedian MY, Patel KM. Breast reconstruction and adjuvant therapy: a systematic review of surgical outcomes. J Surg Oncol 2015;112(5):458–464
3. El-Sabawi B, Carey JN, Hagopian TM, Sbitany H, Patel KM. Radiation and breast reconstruction: algorithmic approach and evidence-based outcomes. J Surg Oncol 2016;113(8): 906–912

COMPLICATIONS FOLLOWING IMPLANT-BASED BREAST RECONSTRUCTION

9. *Within the first year following two-stage, implant-based breast reconstruction, what is the most common complication?*

B. Implant infection

The most common complication within the first year after implant-based breast reconstruction is infection[1] and the rates are markedly higher following radiation therapy. This highlights the importance of meticulous surgical technique including adequate skin preparation with 2% alcohol-based chlorhexidine, use of systemic and pocket irrigation with antibiotics, and minimizing hematoma risk. Ensuring adequacy of mastectomy skin flaps and thereby minimizing risk of wound healing complications should also be a high priority as should swift management of seromas which could themselves become infected. The other options all represent risks in the first year with the exception of capsular contracture, which is a later complication and is estimated to be around 10% risk. In the long term, 88% of patients have good aesthetic outcomes[1] and most are satisfied with the outcomes of their surgery.[2]

REFERENCES

1. Cordeiro PG, McCarthy CM. A single surgeon's 12-year experience with tissue expander/implant breast reconstruction: part I. A prospective analysis of early complications. Plast Reconstr Surg 2006;118(4):825–831
2. Cordeiro PG, McCarthy CM. A single surgeon's 12-year experience with tissue expander/implant breast reconstruction: part II. An analysis of long-term complications, aesthetic outcomes, and patient satisfaction. Plast Reconstr Surg 2006;118(4):832–839

59. Secondary Breast Reconstruction

See *Essentials of Plastic Surgery*, third edition, pp. 805–811

BREAST RECONSTRUCTION

1. *When discussing implant-based breast reconstruction with a patient preoperatively, which one of the following should you advise her based on current available evidence?*
   A. Their reconstructive surgery should be limited to a maximum of two surgical procedures.
   B. They should expect to need some form of revision surgery after the primary procedure.
   C. They are more likely to be satisfied with their reconstruction than if autologous tissue was used.
   D. Obvious rippling is almost certainly going to be evident with this type of reconstruction.
   E. Their long-term risk of capsular contracture will be more than 40%.

BREAST RECONSTRUCTION

2. In 2009, Blondeel published a paper describing a three-point approach to breast surgery that is applicable to both aesthetic breast surgery and breast reconstruction. *What three concepts did he highlight as key to guide surgical thought processes, planning, and achieving successful outcomes?*
   A. Breast footprint, soft tissue shape/volume, and skin envelope
   B. Breast footprint, nipple-areola complex, and breast cone
   C. Nipple-areola complex, breast cone, and skin envelope
   D. Chest wall, breast footprint, and breast soft tissue volume
   E. Chest wall, breast volume, and skin envelope

BREAST RECONSTRUCTION

3. A patient attends clinic 6 months after delayed breast reconstruction with a deep inferior epigastric perforator (DIEP) flap. Examination shows the reconstructed breast to have an elliptical skin paddle with more volume than the contralateral breast centrally and laterally. As yet, the nipple has not been reconstructed. The breast footprints are well matched as are the inframammary fold (IMF) positions, but there is a vertical skin excess on the DIEP flap side (3 cm). The contralateral breast is well shaped with adequate volume. *What would be the most appropriate management for this patient?*
   A. Liposuction of the reconstructed breast
   B. Skin and fat resection with or without liposuction of the reconstructed breast
   C. Formal mastopexy/low volume reduction of the reconstructed breast
   D. Fat transfer to the contralateral breast
   E. Prosthetic augmentation of the contralateral breast

FAT GRAFTING FOLLOWING BREAST RECONSTRUCTION

4. *When considering fat grafting to the reconstructed breast following abdominal based reconstruction, which one of the following is true?*
   A. This is only indicated for small volume contour deformities.
   B. Injection volumes should be kept to less than 75 cc per procedure.
   C. Patients should be warned that more than one treatment session may be required.
   D. Placement of a prosthesis is probably preferable for most patients.
   E. Donor site harvest from the abdomen must be avoided.

ACHIEVING SYMMETRY FOLLOWING BREAST RECONSTRUCTION

5. A patient is seen 6 months following unilateral breast reconstruction with a free muscle-sparing transverse rectus abdominis myocutaneous (MS-TRAM) flap. Examination shows a good result of the reconstructed breast but marked asymmetry between the breasts with grade III ptosis on the contralateral side and 30% more volume within it. The patient would be happy with either breast volume but just wishes to have optimal symmetry. Nipple reconstruction has not yet been performed. *Which one of the following procedures would be most indicated in this case to achieve optimal symmetry?*
   A. Breast reduction
   B. Liposuction
   C. Mastopexy
   D. Breast augmentation
   E. Fat transfer

INFRAMAMMARY FOLD RECONSTRUCTION

6. During mastectomy it is noted there has been effacement of the inframammary fold. *Which one of the following is true in this case?*

   A. It is probably best repaired at the time of surgery with sutures.
   B. Reconstructive approaches are categorized as either flap or template subtypes.
   C. Delayed reconstruction is the most successful technique.
   D. External devices have been designed specifically for use in inframammary fold (IMF) reconstruction.
   E. The Ryan procedure is the preferred option for immediate reconstruction in this case.

Answers

BREAST RECONSTRUCTION

1. *When discussing implant-based breast reconstruction with a patient preoperatively, which one of the following should you advise her based on current available evidence?*

   B. **They should expect to need some form of revision surgery after the primary procedure.**

   There is significant variation in the number of revision surgeries required following primary breast reconstruction and this varies according to reconstruction type, number of breasts reconstructed, previous treatment such as radiotherapy, and patient factors such as diabetes, smoking, and obesity.

   For example, Losken et al reviewed nearly 900 patients after breast reconstruction, with an average of 4 revision procedures for unilateral reconstruction, and 5.5 for bilateral reconstruction being required,[1] whereas Enajat et al reviewed more than 300 patients following free tissue breast reconstruction, with an average of 1.06 revision procedures per patient.[2] Revision of the reconstructed breast can be undertaken for a variety of reasons including aesthetic appearance, implant problems, and soft tissue changes after adjuvant radiotherapy.

   What is important to stress to all breast reconstruction patients preoperatively is that they should expect to need more than one procedure in total for the initial reconstruction to be completed, and those undergoing implant-based reconstruction should expect further surgery to be needed in the longer term for management of capsular problems or implant replacement.

   In terms of unilateral autologous reconstruction, patients will often need two or three procedures to achieve optimal symmetry. Typically, the primary procedure involves transfer of tissue to the breast to provide a skin envelope and volume filler. The second procedure typically involves revision to the contralateral breast with perhaps a mastopexy or reduction with or without subtle ipsilateral alterations such as fat transfer or scar/shape alteration and perhaps donor site revision. The third stage would normally involve recreation of the nipple-areola complex under local anesthetic.

   In terms of patient satisfaction, autologous reconstruction patients tend to have higher satisfaction rates than implant reconstruction.[3] It is important to discuss rippling and palpability of the implant post reconstruction and while this is a common problem it is not uniformly seen as it depends on other factors such as the thickness and quality of the overlying soft tissue envelope. The medium- to long-term risk of capsular contracture is likely to be between 10 and 15% rather than 35% in implant-based reconstruction.

REFERENCES

1. Losken A, Carlson GW, Schoemann MB, Jones GE, Culbertson JH, Hester TR. Factors that influence the completion of breast reconstruction. Ann Plast Surg 2004;52(3):258–261, discussion 262
2. Enajat M, Smit JM, Rozen WM, et al. Aesthetic refinements and reoperative procedures following 370 consecutive DIEP and SIEA flap breast reconstructions: important considerations for patient consent. Aesthetic Plast Surg 2010;34(3):306–312
3. Yueh JH, Slavin SA, Adesiyun T, et al. Patient satisfaction in postmastectomy breast reconstruction: a comparative evaluation of DIEP, TRAM, latissimus flap, and implant techniques. Plast Reconstr Surg 2010;125(6):1585–1595

BREAST RECONSTRUCTION

2. In 2009, Blondeel published a paper describing a three-point approach to breast surgery that is applicable to both aesthetic breast surgery and breast reconstruction. *What three concepts did he highlight as key to guide surgical thought processes, planning, and achieving successful outcomes?*

   A. **Breast footprint, soft tissue shape/volume, and skin envelope**

   Blondeel et al wrote a seminal paper describing the breast footprint, soft tissue shape and volume (conus), and skin envelope.[1] These principles can be applied to secondary breast reconstruction to guide decision-making and surgical planning. It is helpful to think about the breast in this way so that reconstructive tools can be tailored to specific problems. For example, in patients who have undergone a standard mastectomy, there will be both a skin envelope and soft tissue deficiency. There may also be distortion or changes to the breast footprint secondary to surgery, scarring, or radiation changes. In a patient who has chronic problems after implant-based reconstruction, where a significant capsular contracture has occurred, there is likely to be a reduction in the breast footprint, which will need to be addressed. There may also be an apparent volume deficiency, or it may be that the volume is simply located in the wrong place. For example, if there is a double-bubble deformity. Like with any building structure, there must be a solid foundation to build upon, and in the breast, this refers to both the chest wall on which the breast sits and the breast footprint. Although the chest wall is not part of Blondeel's three, it is vital to consider this and discuss things preoperatively with the patient. For example, where there is pectus excavatum or chest wall asymmetry, the result will be affected. In most secondary breast reconstruction, the breast base will need adjustment, to reset the footprint at the correct place on the chest and with the correct dimensions. Then the appropriate volume can be found and the skin envelope created accordingly. The nipple-areola complex is not one of the three components in Blondeel's description although it does, of course, form part of the skin envelope and would ideally be located on the most prominent point of the breast mound. The key parts of Blondeel's description are as follows (**Figs. 59.1** and **59.2**)[2]:

1. **Footprint (Outline of breast on the chest wall)**
   - Lateral: 1–2 cm behind anterior axillary line
   - Inferior: Inframammary fold
   - Medial: Within 1–2 cm of sternal midline
   - Superior: Cranially curved line connecting medial and lateral, most superior at midclavicular line
2. **Soft Tissue (Conus)**
   - Three-dimensional shape and volume of breast
   - More fullness inferiorly
   - Most projection at nipple-areola complex
3. **Skin Envelope**
   - Functions to hold the breast parenchyma in place
   - Excess skin results in breast ptosis
   - Skin shortage results in flattening of the breast
   - Skin quality also critical to maintaining shape and position

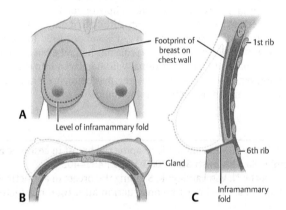

Fig. 59.1 Frontal (**A**), axial (**B**), and sagittal (**C**) views of the breast footprint on the chest wall as described by Blondeel et al.

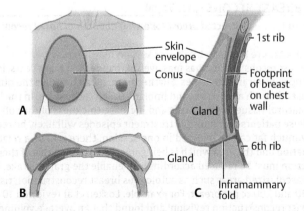

Fig. 59.2 Frontal (**A**), axial (**B**), and sagittal (**C**) views of the breast footprint, conus, and skin envelope as described by Blondeel et al.

REFERENCES

1. Blondeel PN, Hijjawi J, Depypere H, Roche N, Van Landuyt K. Shaping the breast in aesthetic and reconstructive breast surgery: an easy three-step principle. Plast Reconstr Surg 2009;123(2):455–462
2. Blondeel PN, Hijjawi J, Depypere H, Roche N, Van Landuyt K. Shaping the breast in aesthetic and reconstructive breast surgery: an easy three-step principle. Part II—Breast reconstruction after total mastectomy. Plast Reconstr Surg 2009;123(3):794–805

BREAST RECONSTRUCTION

3. A patient attends clinic 6 months after delayed breast reconstruction with a deep inferior epigastric perforator (DIEP) flap. Examination shows the reconstructed breast to have an elliptical skin paddle with more volume than the contralateral breast centrally and laterally. As yet, the nipple has not been reconstructed. The breast footprints are well matched as are the inframammary fold (IMF) positions, but there is a vertical skin excess on the DIEP flap side (3 cm). The contralateral breast is well shaped with adequate volume. *What would be the most appropriate management for this patient?*

   B. Skin and fat resection with or without liposuction of the reconstructed breast

   There may often be some subtle volume differences between the breasts after unilateral autologous tissue reconstruction. Sometimes there is more volume on the reconstructed side and sometimes on the contralateral side. This can be affected by wound healing and if, for example, there has been some flap loss due to fat necrosis laterally then volume would be reduced. Decision-making for symmetrizing surgery will therefore depend on the patient's preferred volume and shape characteristics of each breast.

   In cases such as this, an incision at the end of the previous skin paddle may be used to allow reduction of both skin and fat volume directly without creation of additional scars. Use of tailor tacking is useful to gauge resections required. Sometimes it is also necessary to perform liposuction to further refine symmetry. If there is no skin excess this can be performed as the only intervention. Although it may be reasonable to perform a formal mastopexy or low volume reduction to improve symmetry, it is not required for this deep inferior epigastric perforator (DIEP) reconstruction especially as the nipple areola has not yet even been reconstructed.

   In some situations, patients may prefer to have additional volume placed into the contralateral breast and fat transfer may be considered. However, this will result in fat necrosis being present in the breast and will need to be taken into account in subsequent mammography examinations.[1-3]

REFERENCES

1. Blondeel PN, Hijjawi J, Depypere H, Roche N, Van Landuyt K. Shaping the breast in aesthetic and reconstructive breast surgery: an easy three-step principle. Plast Reconstr Surg 2009;123(2):455–462
2. Blondeel PN, Hijjawi J, Depypere H, Roche N, Van Landuyt K. Shaping the breast in aesthetic and reconstructive breast surgery: an easy three-step principle. Part II—Breast reconstruction after total mastectomy. Plast Reconstr Surg 2009;123(3):794–805
3. Beahm EK, Walton RL. Revision in autologous breast reconstruction: principles and approach. Clin Plast Surg 2007;34(1):139–162, abstract vii–viii

FAT GRAFTING FOLLOWING BREAST RECONSTRUCTION

4. *When considering fat grafting to the reconstructed breast following abdominal based reconstruction, which one of the following is true?*

   C. Patients should be warned that more than one treatment session may be required.

   The use of fat transfer in breast reconstruction has massively expanded in recent years. It can be very useful for adding volume or correcting contour irregularities. Furthermore, it can improve the quality of tissues treated with prior radiation. It is used in both autologous and implant-based techniques. In the latter, the primary aim is to increase the ratio of natural tissue to prosthesis and increase thickness of the soft tissue envelope. In all cases, it is important to advise patients that multiple treatment episodes will likely be required. Although there is no specific limit to how much fat can be injected in one session, there will be a relative limit according to each patient's specific situation and the area which is being injected. For example, if there is only a thin pocket for injection, then fat injection must be reduced accordingly to enable the grafts to take. Larger volumes can be injected into larger, well-vascularized areas such as autologous breast reconstruction tissue. Injection volumes can often range between 40 and 200 cc per breast. For example, Losken et al reviewed 107 patients receiving fat grafting for secondary breast reconstruction revision[1] and found that an average volume of 40 cc was injected. Weichman et al reviewed 228 patients with free flap reconstruction with fat grafting and found that the average volume was 148 cc per breast.[2] A proportion of injected fat is likely to resorb leaving somewhere between 50 and 100% of the injected fat within the breast in the longer term. Therefore, fat transfer is indicated in small to medium volume deficiencies and can be used in larger ones if there is adequate donor site availability and multiple procedures are acceptable to the surgeon and patient. Popular donor sites include the abdomen, flanks, thighs, and buttocks and are patient specific. After abdominal based breast reconstruction, it may be wise to harvest fat with caution centrally and keep the more lateral and the flanks, but there is no absolute contraindication to using the abdomen as a donor site.[1–3]

REFERENCES

1. Losken A, Pinell XA, Sikoro K, Yezhelyev MV, Anderson E, Carlson GW. Autologous fat grafting in secondary breast reconstruction. Ann Plast Surg 2011;66(5):518–522
2. Weichman, KE, Peter NB, Neil T, Stelios CW, Anna A, Jamie PL, Christina A, Mihye C, Nolan SK, and Robert A. The role of autologous fat grafting in secondary microsurgical breast reconstruction. Annals of plastic surgery 71, no. 1 (2013): 24-30
3. Spear SL, Wilson HB, Lockwood MD. Fat injection to correct contour deformities in the reconstructed breast. Plast Reconstr Surg 2005;116(5):1300–1305

ACHIEVING SYMMETRY FOLLOWING BREAST RECONSTRUCTION

5. A patient is seen 6 months following unilateral breast reconstruction with a free muscle-sparing transverse rectus abdominis myocutaneous (MS-TRAM) flap. Examination shows a good result of the reconstructed breast but marked asymmetry between the breasts with grade III ptosis on the contralateral side and 30% more volume within it. The patient would be happy with either breast volume but just wishes to have optimal symmetry. Nipple reconstruction has not yet been performed. *Which one of the following procedures would be most indicated in this case to achieve optimal symmetry?*

A. Breast reduction

In this case, the patient would almost certainly have had bilateral breast ptosis and macromastia prior to mastectomy and reconstruction, and this is now displayed as a unilateral ptosis and oversized breast on the unoperated side. The reconstructive process provides the opportunity to address these preexisting features of the breast and provide breast cancer patients with uplifted and better shaped breasts than perhaps they began with. The first question to consider is what the patients' preferences are for their breasts. Sometimes patients will prefer to try to match their existing breast, other times they will prefer to match the newly reconstructed one. In this case, the patient has expressed a desire for volume and shape symmetry. A contralateral breast reduction would be the preferred choice as this will address the volume difference and the ptosis the patient displays. This should be performed prior to nipple reconstruction on the transverse rectus abdominis myocutaneous (TRAM) side so that nipple position can be optimized to match the native breast. Breast reduction is the most commonly performed symmetry procedure for autologous reconstruction.[1,2]

Liposuction may be useful where there is a volume difference between the breasts without a skin difference or ptosis. It is also useful for making subtle adjustments to breast shape. Mastopexy is commonly performed to the contralateral side following autologous or implant-based breast reconstruction and is indicated where there is ptosis without volume differences.

Breast augmentation is sometimes used to balance breast asymmetry post reconstruction and perhaps is useful in select small autologous breast reconstruction cases. However, adding a prosthetic to an autologous reconstruction does go against the main principles of autologous reconstruction in that it is intended to create a permanent and natural breast that is unlikely to require long-term alteration. If there is a significant size difference between the breasts and the shape is otherwise good, then an implant may be considered. When implant-based techniques are used, a differential implant on the nonoperated side may be helpful to improve shape and symmetry for some patients. Fat transfer in this case would help address the volume difference but would not address the ptosis. This can be effective for use in TRAM flaps to increase volume or correct specific contour or volume irregularities such as can occur in the upper pole.

REFERENCES

1. Losken A, Carlson GW, Bostwick J III, Jones GE, Culbertson JH, Schoemann M. Trends in unilateral breast reconstruction and management of the contralateral breast: the Emory experience. Plast Reconstr Surg 2002;110(1):89–97
2. Nahabedian MY. Managing the opposite breast: contralateral symmetry procedures. Cancer J 2008;14(4):258–263

INFRAMAMMARY FOLD RECONSTRUCTION

6. During mastectomy it is noted there has been effacement of the inframammary fold. *Which one of the following is true in this case?*

A. It is probably best repaired at the time of surgery with sutures.

The inframammary fold (IMF) is the inferior defining border of the breast footprint and is generally described as being at the level of the fifth or sixth rib, extending from midline to the anterior axillary line.[1] The IMF can become effaced during mastectomy or during breast reconstruction, particularly delayed reconstruction. If it is damaged during mastectomy, it is probably best repaired at the time with a suture-based technique as delayed reconstruction can be more difficult to achieve satisfactorily.

Reconstruction of the IMF can generally be grouped into three categories:
1. Flap-based reconstruction
2. Suture-based reconstruction
3. Template-based reconstruction

Many of these methods are reported either without patient data or only have data reported in the index publication, and there is no single most successful procedure. The Ryan procedure is a local tissue arrangement/flap approach that involves utilization of a lower thoracic advancement flap to create a neo-IMF.[2] A number of external devices have been described for use in the IMF repair but none are specifically designed devices. They include bending an endotracheal tube stylet to the shape of the contralateral IMF and creating a paper template of the hemi-abdomen and IMF and transposing this to the opposite side.[3-6]

REFERENCES

1. Nava M, Quattrone P, Riggio E. Focus on the breast fascial system: a new approach for inframammary fold reconstruction. Plast Reconstr Surg 1998;102(4):1034–1045
2. Ryan JJ. A lower thoracic advancement flap in breast reconstruction after mastectomy. Plast Reconstr Surg 1982;70(2):153–160
3. Chun YS, Pribaz JJ. A simple guide to inframammary-fold reconstruction. Ann Plast Surg 2005;55(1):8–11, discussion 11
4. Ching JA, Dayicioglu D. The stylet technique for inframammary fold definition in breast reconstruction. J Plast Reconstr Aesthet Surg 2014;67(2):273–275
5. Pozzi M, Zoccali G, Buccheri EM, de Vita R. Technique to achieve the symmetry of the new inframammary fold. Can J Surg 2014;57(4):278–279
6. Akhavani M, Sadri A, Ovens L, Floyd D. The use of a template to accurately position the inframammary fold in breast reconstruction. J Plast Reconstr Aesthet Surg 2011;64(10):e259–e261

60. Nipple-Areolar Reconstruction

See *Essentials of Plastic Surgery*, third edition, pp. 812–826

NIPPLE RECONSTRUCTION

1. *Which one of the following statements is correct regarding nipple reconstruction?*
   A. It is ideally performed at the same time as breast mound reconstruction.
   B. There is a single gold standard technique that has been uniformly adopted by surgeons.
   C. It is usually performed as an inpatient procedure under general anesthesia.
   D. Patient downtime is usually 2–3 weeks following nipple reconstruction.
   E. It correlates highly with enhanced patient satisfaction following breast reconstruction.

NIPPLE POSITIONING

2. *Which one of the following statements is correct regarding markings for a C-V flap nipple reconstruction?*
   A. The patient should be marked when lying supine on the operating room (OR) table.
   B. The surgeon should independently select the new nipple position.
   C. The nipple must overlie the point of maximal breast projection.
   D. Accurate anatomic placement is less important than optimizing symmetry.
   E. The V flaps must be oriented transversely, with the base of the C flap inferior.

NIPPLE RECONSTRUCTION TECHNIQUES

3. *Which one of the following nipple reconstruction techniques traditionally uses a central dermal/fat flap with bilateral partial- or full-thickness wings and a full-thickness skin graft for closure?*
   A. Skate flap
   B. Bell flap
   C. Star flap
   D. Fishtail flap
   E. S flap

LONG-TERM PROBLEMS WITH NIPPLE RECONSTRUCTION

4. *Which one of the following is the most significant long-term challenge of nipple reconstruction with local flap techniques?*
   A. Minimizing fading of the areola
   B. Avoiding scar stretch
   C. Maintaining projection
   D. Achieving patient satisfaction
   E. Eliminating hypertrophic scarring

LOSS OF PROJECTION AFTER NIPPLE RECONSTRUCTION

5. You are consenting a patient for nipple reconstruction using a local skin flap technique. *What is the expected approximate projection loss 2 years after nipple reconstruction?*
   A. 5%
   B. 15%
   C. 25%
   D. 35%
   E. 50%

FLAP DESIGN FOR NIPPLE RECONSTRUCTION

6. *When designing a C-V flap for nipple reconstruction, which one of the following dimensions will dictate the initial nipple projection?*
   A. Width of the C component
   B. Length of the C component
   C. Width of the V component
   D. Length of the V component
   E. Depth of the V component

INVERTED NIPPLES

7. **What is the most common cause of nipple inversion?**
   A. Acute mastitis
   B. Chronic mastitis
   C. Breast carcinoma
   D. Paget's disease
   E. Congenital

NIPPLE INVERSION

8. **What is the key feature to consider when grading nipple inversion?**
   A. The underlying cause
   B. The chronicity
   C. The ability to successfully breast-feed
   D. The ability to manually correct the inversion
   E. The projection compared with the opposite side

Answers

NIPPLE RECONSTRUCTION

1. *Which one of the following statements is correct regarding nipple reconstruction?*

E. It correlates highly with enhanced patient satisfaction following breast reconstruction.

Nipple-areolar reconstruction is undertaken to complete a breast reconstruction such that it looks more natural-looking breast. Retrospective analyses have shown that patient satisfaction with their breast reconstruction highly correlates with the presence of a nipple and areola.[1] It is best to wait a few months following breast mound reconstruction before reconstructing the nipple, irrespective of the original breast mound reconstructive technique, as this allows the breast tissue to stabilize and develop a more natural ptosis. Performing the nipple reconstruction early increases the risk of incorrect placement.

Unfortunately, there is no gold standard technique for consistently producing the ideal nipple and many different techniques are, therefore, in use. Such techniques include local flaps and nipple sharing, each of which is simple and can be undertaken with local anesthetic as an outpatient procedure.[2] The downtime is very short, and most patients can return to normal activities the following day.

REFERENCES

1. Wellisch DK, Schain WS, Noone RB, Little JW III. The psychological contribution of nipple addition in breast reconstruction. Plast Reconstr Surg 1987;80(5):699–704
2. Farhadi J, Maksvytyte GK, Schaefer DJ, Pierer G, Scheufler O. Reconstruction of the nipple-areola complex: an update. J Plast Reconstr Aesthet Surg 2006;59(1):40–53

NIPPLE POSITIONING

2. *Which one of the following statements is correct regarding markings for a C-V flap nipple reconstruction?*

D. Accurate anatomic placement is less important than optimizing symmetry.

A key goal of nipple reconstruction is to achieve symmetry between the two breasts and for this reason the new nipple may need to be placed in a nonanatomic position. Ideally the nipple will be sited at the point of maximal projection (or convexity), but this is not always possible when considering symmetry.

Nipple position is an important contributor to the final result of breast reconstruction and the patient should be involved in the decision-making process because this improves patient satisfaction. Patients should be marked standing straight with the shoulders relaxed, in the presence of a chaperone. The orientation of the C-V flap will depend on the orientation of scars on the breast mound rather than be limited to a set transverse design.[1,2]

REFERENCES

1. Bostwick J. Nipple areolar reconstruction. In: Jones G, ed. Bostwick's Plastic & Reconstructive Breast Surgery. 3rd ed. St Louis: Quality Medical Publishing; 2010
2. Spear SL, Little JW, Bogue DP. Nipple areola reconstruction. In: Spear SL, ed. Surgery of the Breast: Principles and Art. 3rd ed. Philadelphia: Lippincott Williams & Wilkins; 2011

NIPPLE RECONSTRUCTION TECHNIQUES

3. *Which one of the following nipple reconstruction techniques traditionally uses a central dermal/fat flap with bilateral partial- or full-thickness wings and a full-thickness skin graft for closure?*

A. Skate flap

There are a range of different local flap techniques used in nipple reconstruction. The skate flap remains a popular traditional flap that uses local flaps and a skin graft to provide predictable, versatile nipple reconstruction (**Fig. 60.1**). A central dermal fat pedicle is elevated from the breast mound with lateral wings that may be either partial or full thickness. The wings are wrapped around the central dermal fat pedicle and the donor site is closed with a skin graft. The modified skate flap avoids skin grafting by using local flaps to achieve direct closure. The Bell flap is useful for reconstructing a nipple that requires little projection and involves a local flap without skin grafting (**Fig. 60.2**). It involves a pull-out flap that is folded on itself and the donor site is closed primarily with a purse-string suture. Maximal projection of the flap is half the flap length because it is folded on itself. The star flap is a derivative of the skate flap that avoids the use of a skin graft. It is simple to create but tends not to provide much projection (**Fig. 60.3**). The fishtail flap is a modification of the C-V flap where the V flaps are angulated to be less than 180 degrees from one another. The S flap uses two adjacent flaps in conjunction with a full-thickness skin graft and is useful in areas where a scar crosses the proposed location for the nipple. For further reading, see also the review article by Farhadi et al.[1]

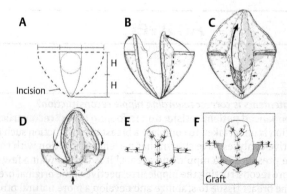

Fig. 60.1   ***A–C***, Skate flap with primary closure of donor site. ***D–F***, With skin graft. (Adapted from Spear SL, Little JW, Bogue DP. Nipple areola reconstruction. In: Spear SL, Willey SW, Robb GL, et al, eds. Surgery of the Breast: Principles and Art, 2nd ed. Philadelphia: Lippincott Williams & Wilkins, 2006.)

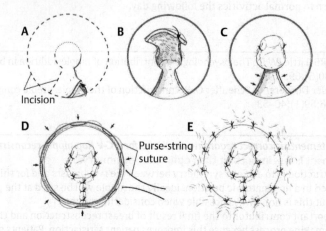

Fig. 60.2   Bell flap. (Adapted from Spear SL, Little JW, Bogue DP. Nipple areola reconstruction. In: Spear SL, Willey SW, Robb GL, et al, eds. Surgery of the Breast: Principles and Art, 2nd ed. Philadelphia: Lippincott Williams & Wilkins, 2006.)

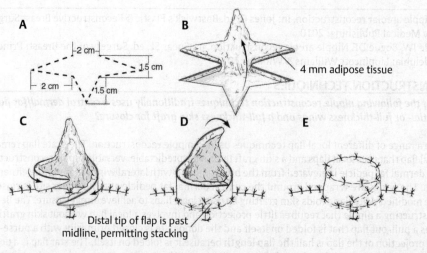

Fig. 60.3   Star flap. (Adapted from Hartrampf CR, Culbertson JH. A dermal-fat flap for nipple reconstruction. Plast Reconstr Surg 73:982, 1984.)

REFERENCE

1. Farhadi J, Maksvytyte GK, Schaefer DJ, Pierer G, Scheufler O. Reconstruction of the nipple-areola complex: an update. J Plast Reconstr Aesthet Surg 2006;59(1):40–53

LONG-TERM PROBLEMS WITH NIPPLE RECONSTRUCTION

4. *Which one of the following is the most significant long-term challenge of nipple reconstruction with local flap techniques?*

C. Maintaining projection

The main problem with local flap nipple reconstruction techniques is a lack of long-term projection. Areolar fading occurs after tattooing but can easily be touched up in clinic. In fact, patients may need to do so multiple times. Patient satisfaction is a very important goal of nipple reconstruction, and patients are generally very satisfied after this procedure. Some studies suggest that the principal determinant of patient dissatisfaction with nipple reconstruction is excessive flattening.[1] However, this is not uniformly the case, and patients have been shown to have high levels of satisfaction even where nipple projection is not well maintained.[2] Scar stretch can be a problem as scars do not reliably accept tattoo pigments, but hypertrophic scarring is uncommon and may be treated with conservative measures such as massage, silicone therapy, and steroid injection.

REFERENCES

1. Jabor MA, Shayani P, Collins DR Jr, Karas T, Cohen BE. Nipple-areola reconstruction: satisfaction and clinical determinants. Plast Reconstr Surg 2002;110(2):457–463, discussion 464–465
2. Jones AP, Erdmann M. Projection and patient satisfaction using the "Hamburger" nipple reconstruction technique. J Plast Reconstr Aesthet Surg 2012;65(2):207–212

LOSS OF PROJECTION AFTER NIPPLE RECONSTRUCTION

5. You are consenting a patient for nipple reconstruction using a local skin flap technique. *What is the expected approximate projection loss 2 years after nipple reconstruction?*

E. 50%

Loss of nipple projection will depend on several factors such as flap design and tissue quality. Reports of projection loss vary within the literature and range from 43 to 71% when C-V–type skin flaps are used.[1] Banducci et al[2] reported a decrease of 71% at 3 years using a modified star flap. Shestak et al[3] observed a 50–70% reduction at 2 years with local flaps (including star, skate, and bell flaps). Attempts to improve projection include placing auricular cartilage or AlloDerm within the nipple construct and these have reported varied results. Jones and Erdmann[4] found a 67% reduction at 2 years even when cartilage grafts were placed inside the construct.

The dressings placed around the nipple reconstruction may affect the reconstruction, and compression should be avoided. This is usually achieved by placing a donut-shaped dressing around the nipple and avoiding direct pressure from garments.

REFERENCES

1. Farhadi J, Maksvytyte GK, Schaefer DJ, Pierer G, Scheufler O. Reconstruction of the nipple-areola complex: an update. J Plast Reconstr Aesthet Surg 2006;59(1):40–53
2. Banducci DR, Le TK, Hughes KC. Long-term follow-up of a modified Anton-Hartrampf nipple reconstruction. Ann Plast Surg 1999;43(5):467–469, discussion 469–470
3. Shestak KC, Gabriel A, Landecker A, Peters S, Shestak A, Kim J. Assessment of long-term nipple projection: a comparison of three techniques. Plast Reconstr Surg 2002;110(3): 780–786
4. Jones AP, Erdmann M. Projection and patient satisfaction using the "Hamburger" nipple reconstruction technique. J Plast Reconstr Aesthet Surg 2012;65(2):207–212

FLAP DESIGN FOR NIPPLE RECONSTRUCTION

6. *When designing a C-V flap for nipple reconstruction, which one of the following dimensions will dictate the initial nipple projection?*

C. Width of the V component

The C-V flap has evolved from the skate flap and preoperative markings are shown in **Fig. 60.4**.
It comprises a central C flap with bilateral V flaps. The V flaps wrap around to form a cylinder-shaped construct which creates the walls of the nipple papule and the C component then forms the construct lid. The main factor that will dictate the initial nipple projection will therefore be the width of the V flaps. The length and depth of the V flaps will dictate how wide or bulky the papule is. It is advisable to oversize the flaps to allow for subsequent shrinkage. A rule of thumb is to create a nipple that starts off twice the desired final height.[1,2]

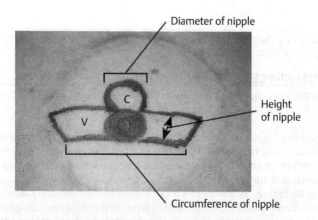

Diameter of nipple

Height
of nipple

Circumference of nipple

Fig. 60.4 C-V flap. The width of the V flap determines nipple projection, and the diameter of the C flap determines nipple diameter. (From Bostwick J III. Nipple-areolar reconstruction. In: Bostwick J III, ed. Plastic and Reconstructive Breast Surgery, 2nd ed. St Louis: Quality Medical Publishing, 2000.)

REFERENCES

1. Bostwick J. Nipple areolar reconstruction. In: Jones G, ed. Bostwick's Plastic & Reconstructive Breast Surgery. 3rd ed. St Louis: Quality Medical Publishing; 2010
2. Losken A, Mackay GJ, Bostwick J III. Nipple reconstruction using the C-V flap technique: a long-term evaluation. Plast Reconstr Surg 2001;108(2):361–369

INVERTED NIPPLES

7. What is the most common cause of nipple inversion?

   E. Congenital

   Nipple inversion is relatively common and affects 1 in 10 women of child-bearing age. It is usually bilateral and many cases are as a result of chronic mastitis, but the most common cause is congenital. Other important causes include breast cancer and Paget's disease of the nipple and these must be diagnosed and treated early. Inversion results from relative shortness of the lactiferous ducts that tether the nipple and prevent normal projection, and a paucity of normal dense collagenous tissue surrounding the ducts.[1]

REFERENCE

1. Schwager RG, Smith JW, Gray GF, Goulian D Jr. Inversion of the human female nipple, with a simple method of treatment. Plast Reconstr Surg 1974;54(5):564–569

NIPPLE INVERSION

8. What is the key feature to consider when grading nipple inversion?

   D. The ability to manually correct the inversion

   Evaluation of patients with inverted nipples involves an assessment of whether the inversion can be manually corrected and whether it maintains correction following release of traction. This is important as it provides information on the severity and guides surgical management. The classification system by Han and Hong[1] formally grades the severity of nipple inversion based on the findings of this assessment:

   Grade I: Nipple can be easily pulled out manually and maintains projection without traction.

   Grade II: Nipple can be pulled out manually but with less ease than grade I and tends to retract.

   Grade III: Nipple is inverted, difficult to pull out manually, and promptly retracts.

   Surgical management involves release of the pathologic bands with or without release of the lactiferous ducts and creation of tightness at the neck of the inverted nipple using a purse-string suture. Additional bulk may also be added beneath the nipple using cartilage or adjacent dermal fat flaps providing that full release has been undertaken.

REFERENCE

1. Han S, Hong YG. The inverted nipple: its grading and surgical correction. Plast Reconstr Surg 1999;104(2):389–395, discussion 396–397

PART V

Trunk and Lower Extremity

61. Chest Wall Reconstruction

See *Essentials of Plastic Surgery*, third edition, pp. 829–844

ANATOMY OF THE CHEST WALL

1. *Which one of the following statements is correct regarding the anatomy of the chest wall?*
   A. The visceral and parietal pleura have identical embryologic origins.
   B. Of the 12 paired ribs, up to 8 directly articulate with the sternum.
   C. The sternum has three distinct components in all patient groups.
   D. Neurovascular bundles lie at the inferior margin of the ribs, between the external and internal intercostal muscles.
   E. The internal mammary vessels usually bifurcate at the level of the fifth interspace.

MUSCLES OF RESPIRATION

2. *Which one of the following is a primary muscle of respiration?*
   A. Serratus posterior
   B. Middle scalene
   C. Sternocleidomastoid
   D. Internal intercostal
   E. Pectoralis major

RECONSTRUCTION OF CHEST WALL DEFECTS

3. *Which one of the following statements is correct regarding the causes and management of chest wall defects?*
   A. Sternal defects are usually classified according to the site and size of the soft tissue defect.
   B. The thoracic skeleton should usually be reconstructed if more than two ribs are resected.
   C. Omentum may be used to reconstruct the chest wall and is supplied by the superior epigastric vessels.
   D. Some large skeletal defects may not need reconstruction if they are posterior or at sites of previous radiotherapy.
   E. The Eloesser flap is used to treat bronchopleural fistula in preference to thoracoplasty.

CLASSIFICATION OF STERNOTOMY DEFECTS

4. *Which one of the following is a key component of the Pairolero classification for sternal defects?*
   A. Defect location
   B. Defect size
   C. Chronicity of wound
   D. Underlying cause of defect
   E. Volume of bone loss

SOFT TISSUE RECONSTRUCTION OF THE CHEST WALL

5. A 68-year-old man with right-sided Poland's syndrome is referred 4 weeks after coronary bypass surgery. He has a 10 cm by 5 cm dehisced midline sternotomy wound passing from the inferior xiphisternum to the fifth intercostal space. His left internal mammary artery was harvested as a graft. The wound is clean, with negative results of bone biopsy and swab analyses. *How best should this patient be managed surgically?*
   A. Left pectoralis major turnover
   B. Right pectoralis major turnover
   C. Right pectoralis major advancement
   D. Left vertical rectus abdominis myocutaneous flap
   E. Right vertical rectus abdominis myocutaneous flap

SOFT TISSUE RECONSTRUCTION OF THE CHEST WALL

6. A 65-year-old patient presents with a history of left-sided thoracotomy for excision of a lung tumor. He is referred by the cardiothoracic team following an infection after open cardiac valve replacement. He has an 8 cm by 4 cm defect over the left upper third of his sternum, with sternal loss and exposed mediastinum. The right internal mammary vessels are preserved on arteriography. *How best should this defect be managed surgically?*
   A. Right free anterolateral thigh flap
   B. Right pectoralis major flap
   C. Left vertical rectus abdominis flap
   D. Left pedicled latissimus dorsi flap
   E. Left serratus anterior flap.

SOFT TISSUE RECONSTRUCTION OF THE CHEST WALL

7. A slim, 47-year-old woman has a 20 cm by 15 cm defect of her anterior chest wall after resection of a recurrent sarcoma. Her left pectoralis major and minor were resected, along with large portions of ribs three through seven. Her first reconstruction involved a pedicled latissimus dorsi flap from the left side. Her past surgical history also includes an open cholecystectomy. *Which one of the following represents the best reconstruction procedure in her case?*
   A. Right vertical rectus abdominis myocutaneous flap
   B. Free right-sided deep inferior epigastric perforator (DIEP) flap
   C. Free right-sided latissimus dorsi flap
   D. Right pectoralis major advancement flap and split graft
   E. Pedicled omental flap

POLAND'S SYNDROME

8. *Which one of the following statements is correct regarding Poland's syndrome?*
   A. The incidence is 1:500,000 live births.
   B. The left side is most commonly affected.
   C. It can occur after subclavian artery compression during the second trimester.
   D. Facial weakness and a squint are occasionally also evident.
   E. The clavicular head of the pectoralis major is normally absent.

KEY FINDINGS IN POLAND'S SYNDROME

9. *Which one of the following is a less common finding in patients with Poland's syndrome?*
   A. Absence of the sternal head of pectoralis major
   B. Breast hypoplasia that may affect the nipple-areola complex
   C. Absence of pectoralis minor muscle
   D. Deficiency of subcutaneous fat and axillary hair
   E. Hypoplasia of ipsilateral extremity with syndactyly

PECTUS EXCAVATUM

10. A 4-year-old boy is brought to your clinic with a moderate pectus excavatum. *Which one of the following statements is correct regarding this diagnosis?*
   A. This is also called *pigeon chest* and results from excessive growth of the lower costal cartilages.
   B. This is less common than pectus carinatum and has an equal sex distribution.
   C. His sternum will have a tendency to rotate if costal growth is mismatched and untreated.
   D. His abnormality should improve with increasing age but will never fully resolve.
   E. Surgery should be delayed until growth is complete.

PECTUS CARINATUM

11. A teenage girl presents with concerns about her overly prominent sternum, which she would like to have altered. *Which one of the following statements is correct regarding pectus carinatum?*
   A. It is characterized by an anterior protrusion of the sternum and costal cartilages, commonly causing respiratory difficulties.
   B. Females are most commonly affected and most have a positive family history.
   C. Surgical correction specifically relies on the Ravitch technique.
   D. The most common site of protrusion is the manubrium, with depression of the sternal body.
   E. One defect subtype is commonly seen in conjunction with Poland's syndrome.

Answers

ANATOMY OF THE CHEST WALL

1. *Which one of the following statements is correct regarding the anatomy of the chest wall?*

   B. Of the 12 paired ribs, up to 8 directly articulate with the sternum.

   There are 12 paired ribs, 7 or 8 of which are true ribs and articulate directly with the sternum. The first rib articulates with the T1 vertebra only and does not contact C7. The remaining true ribs articulate with their corresponding vertebra and the one above. False ribs articulate with the costal cartilages and the vertebra. The two floating ribs articulate only with their vertebral bodies.

   The parietal and visceral pleura have separate embryologic origins, including vascular, lymphatic, and neural supply.

   The sternum has three separate but connected divisions, the manubrium, body, and xiphoid. By the start of the fifth decade, the xiphoid has usually ossified and united with the body of the sternum so it is no longer a three-part construct. The neurovascular bundles are found between the internal and innermost intercostals (not the external and internal). They are arranged as vein, artery, and nerve in descending order and are generally well protected at the inferior aspect of each rib.[1]

   The internal mammary artery arises from the first part of the subclavian artery passing 1 cm lateral to the sternum. The internal mammary vessels are highly relevant to chest wall reconstruction because they supply commonly used flaps such as the rectus abdominus and pectoralis major muscles. Furthermore, they may be sacrificed during cardiac procedures such as coronary bypass grafting or major chest wall resections. The internal mammary vessels are also relevant to free tissue transfer to the chest wall such as for anastomoses in breast reconstruction. Knowledge of their anatomy is therefore important. When using these vessels for free tissue transfer, the third intercostal space or higher is often used for access, because the veins get progressively smaller distally and usually bifurcate at or distal to this point. The veins and artery are usually a good caliber at this level.[2]

REFERENCES

1. Moore KL, Dalley AF, Agur AMR, eds. Clinically Oriented Anatomy. 7th ed. Philadelphia: Wolters Kluwer/Lippincott Williams & Wilkins; 2013
2. Clark CP III, Rohrich RJ, Copit S, Pittman CE, Robinson J. An anatomic study of the internal mammary veins: clinical implications for free-tissue-transfer breast reconstruction. Plast Reconstr Surg 1997;99(2):400–404

MUSCLES OF RESPIRATION

2. *Which one of the following is a primary muscle of respiration?*

   D. Internal intercostal

   Muscles involved in respiration can be classified in three groups, primary, secondary, and accessory (used in times of respiratory distress).[1] Primary muscles are the diaphragm and intercostals (external, internal, and innermost), which are supplied by the phrenic nerve and intercostal nerves, respectively. The intercostal nerves are formed by the anterior divisions of the T1–T11 thoracic nerves.

   Secondary muscles of respiration are the sternocleidomastoid, serratus posterior, scalenes (anterior, middle, and posterior) and levatores costarum. The innervations of these muscles are the spinal accessory for the sternocleidomastoid, T9–T12 intercostal nerves for the serratus posterior, C4–C6 for the scalenes, and the lateral divisions of the posterior primary rami of the corresponding spinal nerves for the levatores costarum.

   Accessory muscles of respiration include the serratus anterior, supplied by the long thoracic nerve (C5–C7), and the pectoralis major, supplied by medial and lateral pectoral nerves (C5–C7 and C8, T1, respectively).[1,2]

REFERENCES

1. Standring S, ed. Gray's Anatomy: The Anatomical Basis of Clinical Practice, Expert Consult. 40th ed. Philadelphia: Churchill Livingstone Elsevier; 2008. Available at https://www.elsevier.com/books/grays-anatomy/standring/978-0-7020-7705-0
2. Moore KL, Dalley AF, Agur AMR, eds. Clinically Oriented Anatomy. 7th ed. Philadelphia: Wolters Kluwer/Lippincott Williams & Wilkins; 2013

RECONSTRUCTION OF CHEST WALL DEFECTS

3. *Which one of the following statements is correct regarding the causes and management of chest wall defects?*

   D. **Some large skeletal defects may not need reconstruction if they are posterior or at sites of previous radiotherapy.**

   Decisions regarding reconstruction of the thoracic skeleton will be made on an individual patient basis depending on baseline respiratory function and the impact of the defect on respiratory function; however, the usual guidelines for reconstruction of the thoracic skeleton are:

   1. Defects where four contiguous ribs have been removed
   2. Defects larger than 5 cm in diameter

   But these indications will differ as follows:

   1. Previous radiation treatment stiffens the chest wall so larger defects may be tolerated without reconstruction.
   2. Posterior defects are better tolerated without reconstruction given the support of the bony scapula and musculature.
   3. Patients with poor respiratory reserve such as chronic obstructive pulmonary disease (COPD) will tolerate defects less well and may benefit from reconstruction of smaller defects.

   Sternal defects can be classified by using either the Pairolero and Arnold[1] or Starzynski et al[2] classifications. These are significantly different to one another, although each has the same number of grades/types. The Starzynski classification is based on the anatomic structures missing, as well as the physiological deficit incurred. The Pairolero classification is based on chronicity and the presence or absence of infection.

   The omental flap is a useful option for chest wall reconstruction and receives blood supply from the gastroepiploic vessels, not the superior epigastric vessels. The Eloesser flap is an inferiorly based U-shaped flap from the posterior chest wall that is turned into the thoracic cavity to facilitate passive drainage of empyema. It does not address bronchopleural fistula. Thoracoplasty treats both bronchopleural fistula and empyema in a single surgery, but results in rib cage deformity and interferes with upper limb function.

REFERENCES

1. Pairolero PC, Arnold PG. Management of infected median sternotomy wounds. Ann Thorac Surg 1986;42(1):1–2
2. Starzynski TE, Snyderman RK, Beattie EJ Jr. Problems of major chest wall reconstruction. Plast Reconstr Surg 1969;44(6):525–535

CLASSIFICATION OF STERNOTOMY DEFECTS

4. *Which one of the following is a key component of the Pairolero classification for sternal defects?*

   C. **Chronicity of wound**

   Pairolero and Arnold[1] described a classification for sternotomy wounds in 1986. The classification is based on the timing of the defect relative to surgery (early, intermediate, or late) and the presence or absence of active infection as evidenced by cellulitis, positive swabs, or osteomyelitis. They described treatment according to the subtype as follows:

   - **Type 1:**
     - Serosanguineous drainage within the first 3 days of surgery
     - No active infection
     - Treatment: Re-exploration, debridement, and closure of the defect directly
   - **Type 2:**
     - Purulent discharge within the first 3 weeks of surgery
     - Active infection evident
     - Treatment: Exploration, debridement, and coverage of the defect with a soft tissue flap
   - **Type 3:**
     - Chronically infected wound months or years after surgery

   The other factors listed do not form part of the Pairolero description. This classification system is often discussed in the setting of clinical viva scenarios in plastic surgery.

REFERENCE

1. Pairolero PC, Arnold PG. Management of infected median sternotomy wounds. Ann Thorac Surg 1986;42(1):1–2

SOFT TISSUE RECONSTRUCTION OF THE CHEST WALL

5. A 68-year-old man with right-sided Poland's syndrome is referred 4 weeks after coronary bypass surgery. He has a 10 cm by 5 cm dehisced midline sternotomy wound passing from the inferior xiphisternum to the fifth intercostal space. His left internal mammary artery was harvested as a graft. The wound is clean, with negative results of bone biopsy and swab analyses. *How best should this patient be managed surgically?*

E. Right vertical rectus abdominis myocutaneous flap

This patient probably requires reconstruction with a right vertical rectus abdominis myocutaneous flap. This is the most appropriate option because it provides good soft tissue cover, is able to fill the dead space, and provides robust skin to close the wound directly. Although infection is no longer present, importation of well-vascularized muscle into such defects is preferable. The internal mammary vessels supplying the flap are intact, whereas they are not on the other side. The defect is probably too low for a left pectoralis major advancement and a turnover flap should be avoided anyway due to harvest of the internal mammary artery on this side. Given the diagnosis of Poland's syndrome the sternal head of the muscle is not available for harvest on the right-hand side. Alternative options not listed may include an omental pedicled flap but would require a skin graft and the abdominal cavity would have to be opened. A left latissimus dorsi myocutaneous flap could be used. A disadvantage would be a need to turn the patient intraoperatively. Achieving adequate reach is possible in these scenarios, but normally requires detachment at the humeral insertion and division of the thoracodorsal nerve to stop muscle contractions.[1-3] The rectus abdominis is normally reserved for patients with an intact superior vascular supply. However, rectus muscle advancement for sternal wound reconstruction has been described using the deep inferior epigastric system and releasing the other fascial and tendinous attachments to provide a 12 cm advancement.[4]

REFERENCES

1. Levy AS, Ascherman JA. Sternal wound reconstruction made simple. Plast Reconstr Surg Glob Open 2019;7(11): e2488
2. Clarkson JH, Probst F, Niranjan NS, et al. Our experience using the vertical rectus abdominis muscle flap for reconstruction in 12 patients with dehiscence of a median sternotomy wound and mediastinitis. Scand J Plast Reconstr Surg Hand Surg 2003;37(5):266-271
3. Davison SP, Clemens MW, Armstrong D, Newton ED, Swartz W. Sternotomy wounds: rectus flap versus modified pectoral reconstruction. Plast Reconstr Surg 2007;120(4):929-934
4. Pantelides NM, Young SS, Iyer S. The rectus abdominis muscle advancement flap as a salvage option for chest wall reconstruction. Ann R Coll Surg Engl 2017;99(5):e142-e144

SOFT TISSUE RECONSTRUCTION OF THE CHEST WALL

6. A 65-year-old patient presents with a history of left-sided thoracotomy for excision of a lung tumor. He is referred by the cardiothoracic team following an infection after open cardiac valve replacement. He has an 8 cm by 4 cm defect over the left upper third of his sternum, with sternal loss and exposed mediastinum. The right internal mammary vessels are preserved on arteriography. *How best should this defect be managed surgically?*

B. Right pectoralis major flap

This patient has a proximal left-sided defect that is relatively small, and the contralateral internal mammary is preserved. Therefore, a right pectoralis major turnover flap combined with a split-skin graft is a suitable option. A pedicled ipsilateral latissimus dorsi is usually an option if reach is sufficient. However, neither this nor the serratus flap will be available on the ipsilateral side in this patient because of the previous thoracotomy. A free flap could be used with anastomoses into the right internal mammary vessels, but this would be unnecessary in a complex patient where the simpler and reliable alternative of a pectoralis major flap was an option. The vertical rectus flap is more usually reserved for long and inferior sternal defects and, in this case, we have no information to suggest the left internal mammary vessels are intact, so it is best avoided.[1,2]

REFERENCES

1. Levy AS, Ascherman JA. Sternal wound reconstruction made simple. Plast Reconstr Surg Glob Open 2019;7(11):e2488
2. Davison SP, Clemens MW, Armstrong D, Newton ED, Swartz W. Sternotomy wounds: rectus flap versus modified pectoral reconstruction. Plast Reconstr Surg 2007;120(4):929-934

SOFT TISSUE RECONSTRUCTION OF THE CHEST WALL

7. A slim, 47-year-old woman has a 20 cm by 15 cm defect of her anterior chest wall after resection of a recurrent sarcoma. Her left pectoralis major and minor were resected, along with large portions of ribs three through seven. Her first reconstruction involved a pedicled latissimus dorsi flap from the left side. Her past surgical history also includes an open cholecystectomy. *Which one of the following represents the best reconstruction procedure in her case?*

E. Pedicled omental flap

This patient has no remaining local muscle flap options to reconstruct a defect of this size. In this case, an omental flap would represent the best choice from the options listed. Omental flaps are traditionally used more often than free tissue transfers to reconstruct extensive chest wall defects. If a free muscle transfer was used in this case, a free contralateral latissimus dorsi, or a free anterolateral thigh (ALT) or deep inferior epigastric perforator (DIEP) would also be reasonable choices. She is not a good candidate for reconstruction with a right vertical rectus flap because of the previous cholecystectomy incision.[1-3]

REFERENCES

1. Vaziri M, Jesmi F, Pishgahroudsari M. Omentoplasty in deep sternal wound infection. Surg Infect (Larchmt) 2015;16(1):72–76
2. Chittithavorn V, Rergkliang C, Chetpaophan A, Simapattanapong T. Single-stage omental flap transposition: modality of an effective treatment for deep sternal wound infection. Interact Cardiovasc Thorac Surg 2011;12(6):982–986
3. van Wingerden JJ, Lapid O, Boonstra PW, de Mol BA. Muscle flaps or omental flap in the management of deep sternal wound infection. Interact Cardiovasc Thorac Surg 2011;13(2):179–187

POLAND'S SYNDROME

8. *Which one of the following statements is correct regarding Poland's syndrome?*

   D. Facial weakness and a squint are occasionally also evident.

   Poland's syndrome is a congenital condition in which there are a number of upper limb and chest wall abnormalities. It occurs in approximately 1:30,000 births and affects males and females equally. The right side is affected more often than the left side by a ratio of 2:1. It is postulated that the subclavian vessels are compressed in the first (not second) trimester. A consistent finding is the absence of the sternal head (not the clavicular head) of the pectoralis major. Although rare, Poland's syndrome can be associated with Möbius syndrome and therefore with the absence of cranial nerves VI and VII. Patients with Poland's syndrome are often seen by plastic surgeons with regard to reconstruction of both the upper limb and chest/breast deformities. Sometimes the latissimus dorsi muscle is transferred to the anterior chest wall to reconstruct the pectoralis deficiency. This is particularly useful in female patients to provide a foundation for future breast reconstruction using implant-based techniques.[1-4]

REFERENCES

1. Freire-Maia N, Chautard EA, Opitz JM, Freire-Maia A, Quelce-Salgado A. The Poland syndrome-clinical and genealogical data, dermatoglyphic analysis, and incidence. Hum Hered 1973;23(2):97–104
2. Hester TR Jr, Bostwick J III. Poland's syndrome: correction with latissimus muscle transposition. Plast Reconstr Surg 1982;69(2):226–233
3. Ohmori K, Takada H. Correction of Poland's pectoralis major muscle anomaly with latissimus dorsi musculocutaneous flaps. Plast Reconstr Surg 1980;65(4):400–404
4. Ravitch MM. Poland's syndrome—a study of an eponym. Plast Reconstr Surg 1977;59(4):508–512

KEY FINDINGS IN POLAND'S SYNDROME

9. *Which one of the following is a less common finding in patients with Poland's syndrome?*

   C. Absence of pectoralis minor muscle

   Poland's syndrome represents a spectrum of abnormalities affecting the ipsilateral chest wall and upper limb. Common key findings include the following:

   - Absence of the sternal head of the pectoralis major
   - Absence of costal cartilages
   - Hypoplasia of breast tissue, including the nipple-areola complex
   - Deficiency of subcutaneous fat and axillary hair
   - Syndactyly or hypoplasia of the ipsilateral extremity

   Additional features that occur less commonly include the following:

   - Absence of the pectoralis minor
   - Shortening of the forearm
   - Deformity of chest wall muscles, including the serratus, latissimus dorsi, and external oblique
   - Total absence of anterolateral ribs with herniation of the lung
   - Associations with Möbius syndrome
   - Symphalangism

   Common surgical procedures for the chest in Poland's patients include latissimus dorsi transfer to reconstruct the pectoralis major deficiency, and breast reconstruction with a variety of implant of autologous techniques. Surgery for the limb may include syndactyly release and, occasionally, free toe-to-hand transfer.[1-4]

REFERENCES

1. Freire-Maia N, Chautard EA, Opitz JM, Freire-Maia A, Quelce-Salgado A. The Poland syndrome-clinical and genealogical data, dermatoglyphic analysis, and incidence. Hum Hered 1973;23(2):97–104
2. Hester TR Jr, Bostwick J III. Poland's syndrome: correction with latissimus muscle transposition. Plast Reconstr Surg 1982;69(2):226–233
3. Ohmori K, Takada H. Correction of Poland's pectoralis major muscle anomaly with latissimus dorsi musculocutaneous flaps. Plast Reconstr Surg 1980;65(4):400–404
4. Ravitch MM. Poland's syndrome—a study of an eponym. Plast Reconstr Surg 1977;59(4):508–512

PECTUS EXCAVATUM

10. A 4-year-old boy is brought to your clinic with a moderate pectus excavatum. *Which one of the following statements is correct regarding this diagnosis?*

    C. **His sternum will have a tendency to rotate if costal growth is mismatched and untreated.**

Pectus excavatum is the most common chest wall deformity affecting 1 in 400 children and affects males more than females with a ratio of 4:1. It occurs 10 times more frequently than pectus carinatum and is called *funnel chest*, not pigeon chest. (Pigeon chest refers to *pectus carinatum*.) Funnel chest occurs secondary to excess growth of the lower costal cartilages resulting in a sternal depression. The sternum will rotate if growth is greater on one side. The condition becomes progressively worse with time and continued growth, leaving a cosmetic and sometimes functional deformity. It is treated surgically relatively early (2–5 years of age is recommended) using Nuss procedure, sternal turnover, or sternal osteotomies. A key motivation for patients to consider surgery is the aesthetics of the deformity. Surgery with the Nuss procedure involves a minimally invasive approach that slips concave steel bars behind the sternum through two small incisions. The bar is flipped to a convex position to anteriorly displace the sternum and correct the deformity.[1-4]

REFERENCES

1. Shamberger RC, Welch KJ. Surgical repair of pectus excavatum. J Pediatr Surg 1988;23(7):615–622
2. Shamberger RC, Welch KJ, Castaneda AR, Keane JF, Fyler DC. Anterior chest wall deformities and congenital heart disease. J Thorac Cardiovasc Surg 1988;96(3):427–432
3. Shamberger RC, Welch KJ. Chest wall deformities. In: Ashcraft KW, Holder TM, eds. Pediatric Surgery. 2nd ed. Philadelphia: WB Saunders; 1993
4. Ravitch MM. Congenital Deformities of the Chest Wall and Their Operative Correction. 5th ed. Philadelphia: Saunders-Elsevier; 2010

PECTUS CARINATUM

11. A teenage girl presents with concerns about her overly prominent sternum, which she would like to have altered. *Which one of the following statements is correct regarding pectus carinatum?*

    E. **One defect subtype is commonly seen in conjunction with Poland's syndrome.**

Pectus carinatum (pigeon chest) is characterized by anterior protrusion of the sternum but rarely causes physiologic symptoms. It affects males more than females (4:1 ratio), and a positive family history is present in a third of cases. Three subtypes are recognized: chondrogladiolar (most common), pouter pigeon chest, and lateral depression of the ribs. The latter is commonly associated with Poland's syndrome. Pouter pigeon chest is least common and involves protrusion of the manubrium and depression of the sternal body. Chondrogladiolar is most common and involves anterior displacement of the sternal body and symmetrical concavity of costal cartilages. Several surgical options are available, including repositioning of the sternum, excision of costal cartilages, and the use of strut techniques such as the Ravitch procedure. This technique is, however, not absolutely required and is not totally specific to pectus carinatum.[1-3]

REFERENCES

1. Crump HW. Pectus excavatum. Am Fam Physician 1992;46(1):173–179
2. Shamberger RC, Welch KJ. Surgical correction of pectus carinatum. J Pediatr Surg 1987;22(1):48–53
3. Ravitch MM. Congenital Deformities of the Chest Wall and Their Operative Correction. 5th ed. Philadelphia: Saunders-Elsevier; 2010

62. Abdominal Wall Reconstruction

See *Essentials of Plastic Surgery*, third edition, pp. 845–862

ANATOMY OF THE ANTERIOR ABDOMINAL WALL

1. *Which one of the following statements is correct regarding the myofascial structure of the anterior abdominal wall?*
   A. The anterior axillary line represents the lateral border of the anterior abdominal wall.
   B. The linea semilunaris delineates the midline decussation of abdominal wall muscle fascia.
   C. The anterior rectus sheath composition is consistent throughout its course.
   D. Below the arcuate line, the posterior rectus sheath is devoid of thick, strong fascia.
   E. The pyramidalis is a functionally important triangular muscle that tenses the linea alba.

VASCULAR ANATOMY OF THE ANTERIOR ABDOMINAL WALL

2. *When considering the vascular anatomy of the anterior abdominal wall, which one of the following is true?*
   A. The central area of the abdominal wall is considered zone I and the dominant blood supply is received from the superior epigastric vessels.
   B. The inferolateral anterior abdominal wall is termed zone II and its blood supply is largely limited to the deep and superficial epigastric vessels.
   C. The superolateral aspect of the anterior abdominal wall is considered zone III and has particularly precarious blood supply reliant solely on the external pudendal arteries.
   D. The deep inferior epigastric vessels normally have medial and lateral perforator rows, of which the lateral ones are usually dominant.
   E. Most perforators in the midline anterior abdominal wall arise within close proximity to the umbilicus.

GRADING OF VENTRAL ABDOMINAL WALL HERNIA DEFECTS

3. In 2010 the Ventral Hernia Working Group (VHWG) published guidelines for the management of ventral abdominal wall hernias. *Which one of the following is a key component of this system?*
   A. Hernia size
   B. Hernia site
   C. Method of repair
   D. Functional impairment
   E. Infection

GRADING OF VENTRAL ABDOMINAL WALL HERNIA DEFECTS

4. The Ventral Hernia Working Group (VHWG) classification system was revised by Kanters et al. *What was the main improvement compared to the previous grading system?*
   A. It was formally validated.
   B. The number of grades were increased.
   C. The grades were determined based on method of repair.
   D. The grades were based on hernia size.
   E. Repair material choice affected the grading system.

PRINCIPLES OF ABDOMINAL WALL RECONSTRUCTION

5. *Which one of the following statements is true when reconstructing abdominal wall defects?*
   A. Blood sugar levels should ideally be less than 110 mg/dL.
   B. Smoking must be stopped 4 months before reconstruction.
   C. Repairs should always be reinforced using acellular dermal matrix.
   D. Debridement and repair must be performed in separate stages.
   E. Reinforcing materials should be avoided in previous fistulation sites.

ADJUNCTS TO CLOSURE OF ABDOMINAL WALL DEFECTS

6. *Which one of the following statements is correct regarding techniques for abdominal wall reconstruction?*
   A. Heavyweight, small-pore polypropylene is an absorbable mesh with poor resistance to bacterial contamination and demonstrates low extrusion rates.
   B. Gore-Tex sheet is manufactured from expanded polytetrafluoroethylene (ePTFE) and can facilitate fluid egress and fibrous ingrowth in abdominal wounds.
   C. Tissue expanders in the abdominal region should always be placed in the subcutaneous plane.
   D. Polyglycolic acid is useful as temporary support in abdominal wall defects but may lead to hernia formation in the longer term.
   E. AlloDerm (LifeCell, Branchburg, NJ) is a freeze-dried porcine acellular dermis that is stronger than fascia lata.

ALLOPLASTIC COMPOSITE MATERIALS

7. *What is the main proposed benefit of using newer composite or barrier-coated prosthetic materials for abdominal wall repair as compared to traditional alloplastic materials?*
   A. They provide financial cost savings.
   B. They resorb completely, leaving less foreign body material.
   C. They provide far better tissue integration.
   D. They may reduce formation of tissue adhesions.
   E. They negate the need for omental bowel cover.

BIOPROSTHETIC MATERIALS

8. *Which one of the following statements is correct regarding biologic materials in abdominal wall reconstruction?*
   A. They are recommended for use in all wound types.
   B. They are all crosslinked to control enzymatic degradation.
   C. Hernia recurrence rates are uniformly low following their use.
   D. They are ideal for use in bridging interpositional repairs.
   E. They may be placed directly on the bowel with low adhesion rates.

MESH POSITION IN VENTRAL WALL ABDOMINAL REPAIR

9. *Which one of the following represents the ideal plane for mesh placement when performing abdominal wall hernia repair?*
   A. Onto peritoneum beneath deep fascia
   B. Onto omentum beneath deep fascia
   C. Beneath rectus muscle on posterior rectus sheath
   D. Above rectus muscle under anterior rectus sheath
   E. Above rectus fascia beneath skin flap and Scarpa's fascia

COMPONENT SEPARATION

10. You are planning a component separation on a patient with an anterior abdominal wall defect. *Which one of the following statements is correct regarding this procedure?*
   A. Abdominal wall closure is significantly enhanced when the rectus abdominis is advanced with the external oblique.
   B. The key plane of dissection is between the internal oblique and transversus abdominis.
   C. The main neurovascular structures supplying the abdominal wall are found between the internal and external oblique muscles.
   D. The original component separation technique takes a perforator-sparing approach.
   E. Release of the rectus from its posterior sheath can increase advancement by an additional 2 cm at all levels.

COMPONENT SEPARATION

11. *According to the original study by Ramirez et al, how much advancement can be achieved at the waist after a bilateral component separation?*
   A. 6 cm
   B. 10 cm
   C. 20 cm
   D. 24 cm
   E. 30 cm

APPROACHES TO ABDOMINAL WALL REPAIR

12. You have just completed a free tissue transfer for breast reconstruction using a muscle-sparing transverse rectus abdominis myocutaneous (TRAM) flap instead of the planned deep inferior epigastric perforator (DIEP) flap. A 5 by 8 cm fascial defect of the anterior rectus sheath is present. *How should this defect be reconstructed?*
    A. Direct fascial repair alone
    B. Onlay graft with acellular dermal matrix
    C. Inlay repair with polyglactin mesh
    D. Inlay repair with polypropylene mesh
    E. Component separation

MANAGEMENT OF ABDOMINAL WALL HERNIAS

13. A 50-year-old woman has a large, chronic rectus sheath hernia following emergency paramedian laparotomy for bowel perforation. The initial abdominal wall repair took months to heal after partial dehiscence occurred. She has a 5 by 10 cm abdominal wall hernia to the left of the midline and is concerned about function, cosmesis, and discomfort. *Which one of the following is the most appropriate option for management of this patient?*
    A. Lifestyle modification
    B. Direct repair of the hernia with permanent mesh
    C. Direct repair of the hernia with acellular dermal matrix
    D. Component separation with synthetic permanent mesh
    E. Component separation with direct repair

Answers

ANATOMY OF THE ANTERIOR ABDOMINAL WALL

1. **Which one of the following statements is correct regarding the myofascial structure of the anterior abdominal wall?**

   D. **Below the arcuate line, the posterior rectus sheath is devoid of thick, strong fascia.**

   The anterior abdominal wall comprises a myofascial complex consisting of five paired muscles and a number of key fascial layers and interfaces enveloping them. The five key muscles are the rectus abdominus, external and internal oblique, transversus abdominis, and pyramidalis. Each has an important functional role with the exception of the pyramidalis. The two rectus abdominis or "six pack" muscles are para-midline paired muscles that run from the pubic ramus to the xiphisternum and ribs five through seven. They are enclosed by fascia anteriorly and posteriorly that joins in the midline as the linea alba or "white line" (not the linea semilunaris which represents the lateral fascial adherence of these muscles). The composition of this fascial arrangement, which includes anterior and posterior components, differs above and below the arcuate line, which is a transverse line passing across the lower abdomen at the level of the anterior superior iliac spines. The anterior sheath comprises the external oblique aponeurosis and the anterior leaf of the internal oblique aponeurosis throughout its length. Above the arcuate line, the posterior leaf of the internal oblique aponeurosis forms the posterior sheath, along with the transversus abdominis and transversalis fascia. Below the arcuate line, the posterior sheath consists of only transversalis fascia, and everything else is anterior to the rectus abdominis and contained within the anterior sheath. This is why patients are at increased risk of developing iatrogenic hernias of the lower abdomen following laparotomy or free transverse rectus abdominis myocutaneous (TRAM) harvest when the anterior fascia is deficient.[1]

   The lateral border of the anterior abdominal wall is the midaxillary line (not the anterior axillary line). The superior border is the xiphisternum and the seventh to twelfth costal cartilages. The inferior border is the pubic tubercle and inguinal ligament. The paired pyramidalis muscles are small triangular structures sited between the rectus abdominis and the posterior surface of the rectus sheath. They are functionally unimportant and often absent. It has been postulated that they serve to tense the linea alba.[1–3]

REFERENCES

1. Moore KL, Dalley AF, Agur AMR, eds. Clinically Oriented Anatomy. 7th ed. Philadelphia: Wolters Kluwer/Lippincott Williams & Wilkins; 2013
2. Lovering RM, Anderson LD. Architecture and fiber type of the pyramidalis muscle. Anat Sci Int 2008;83(4):294–297
3. Khansa I, Janis JE. Modern reconstructive techniques for abdominal wall defects after oncologic resection. J Surg Oncol 2015;111(5):587–598

VASCULAR ANATOMY OF THE ANTERIOR ABDOMINAL WALL

2. **When considering the vascular anatomy of the anterior abdominal wall, which one of the following is true?**

   E. **Most perforators in the midline anterior abdominal wall arise within close proximity to the umbilicus.**

   Knowledge of the blood supply to the anterior lower abdomen is vital to free tissue harvest from the abdomen and abdominal wall reconstruction. The vasculature has been classified by Huger into three zones: a central midline zone (zone I) which overlies the rectus muscles, an inferolateral zone (zone II) which overlaps zone I and continues laterally toward the anterior superior iliac crests and paired groin creases, and a superolateral zone (zone III) which lies above zone II and lateral to zone I.

   Zone I is supplied by the superior and inferior epigastric vessels (not just superior), which collateralize in the middle third of the rectus muscle near the umbilicus. It is in this area that most perforators are found. The deep inferior epigastric vessels provide the dominant blood supply and usually have medial and lateral perforator rows, of which the medial (not lateral) is usually dominant and allows perfusion of a greater amount of the contralateral hemiabdomen. These perforators are utilized in free tissue harvest of the anterior abdominal wall and are preserved in minimally invasive component separation procedures.

   Zone II does share blood supply from zone I with input from the deep inferior epigastric vessels, but also receives blood from other branches of the common femoral artery, namely, the superficial circumflex femoral artery, superficial inferior epigastric artery, and external pudendal artery.

   Zone III has a robust blood supply which is why the entire abdominal wall remains viable after abdominoplasty, component separation, or double deep inferior epigastric perforator (DIEP) harvest as thoracic intercostal and lumbar perforators contribute to its vascularity (**Fig. 62.1**).[1,2]

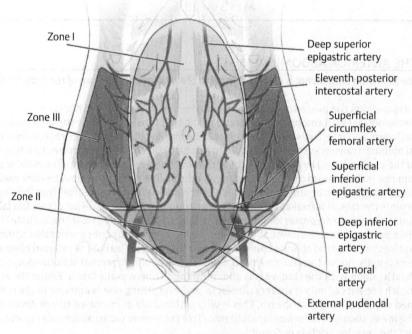

Fig. 62.1   Huger zones.

REFERENCES

1. Huger WE Jr. The anatomic rationale for abdominal lipectomy. Am Surg 1979;45(9):612–617
2. Schaverien M, Saint-Cyr M, Arbique G, Brown SA. Arterial and venous anatomies of the deep inferior epigastric perforator and superficial inferior epigastric artery flaps. Plast Reconstr Surg 2008;121(6):1909–1919

GRADING OF VENTRAL ABDOMINAL WALL HERNIA DEFECTS

3. In 2010 the Ventral Hernia Working Group (VHWG) published guidelines for the management of ventral abdominal wall hernias. *Which one of the following is a key component of this system?*

   E. Infection

   The Ventral Hernia Working Group[1] (VHWG) has described a four-grade system for classifying hernias. The intention of this system was to improve risk stratification for patients with ventral wall hernia. The key factor within this system is either the presence or absence of infection or the risk of its subsequent development. *Grade 1* represents a low-risk hernia without infection or wound contamination. *Grade 2* represents a hernia without active infection but with an increased systemic risk of infection such as smoking, diabetes, or obesity. *Grade 3* refers to a potentially contaminated hernia, as seen in patients with a stoma or previous infection. *Grade 4* is an actively infected hernia. This classification system does not refer to hernia size, specific location, method of repair, or functional impairment.

REFERENCE

1. Breuing K, Butler CE, Ferzoco S, et al; Ventral Hernia Working Group. Incisional ventral hernias: review of the literature and recommendations regarding the grading and technique of repair. Surgery 2010;148(3):544–558

GRADING OF VENTRAL ABDOMINAL WALL HERNIA DEFECTS

4. The Ventral Hernia Working Group (VHWG) classification system was revised by Kanters et al. *What was the main improvement compared to the previous grading system?*

   A. It was formally validated.

   The revised ventral hernia classification system proposed by Kanters et al[1] followed a review of a group of 299 patients who had undergone ventral wall hernia repair. The study was undertaken to evaluate the accuracy of the original classification by the Ventral Hernia Working Group (VHWG)[2] in predicting surgical site occurrence after open ventral hernia repair. Following the study, the authors concluded that modification of the original

VHWG classification system to three grades, instead of four, with redistribution of patients from the original grades, significantly improves the accuracy of predicting surgical site occurrence.[1] Using the revised system, patients are stratified according to their comorbidities, their prior history of wound infection, and their Centers for Disease Control and Prevention (CDC) wound contamination status. The Kanters classification is currently the only formally validated system for ventral hernia repair. The grade of abdominal wall hernia using this system helps guide the nature of the surgical repair.[1,2]

REFERENCES

1. Kanters AE, Krpata DM, Blatnik JA, Novitsky YM, Rosen MJ. Modified hernia grading scale to stratify surgical site occurrence after open ventral hernia repairs. J Am Coll Surg 2012;215(6):787–793
2. Breuing K, Butler CE, Ferzoco S, et al; Ventral Hernia Working Group. Incisional ventral hernias: review of the literature and recommendations regarding the grading and technique of repair. Surgery 2010;148(3):544–558

PRINCIPLES OF ABDOMINAL WALL RECONSTRUCTION

5. Which one of the following statements is true when reconstructing abdominal wall defects?

A. Blood sugar levels should ideally be less than 110 mg/dL.

Principles in repair of abdominal wall hernias include patient optimization, preparation of the wound, and appropriate surgical techniques. Blood sugar levels should be less than 110 mg/dL and elective surgery should be postponed if HBA1C is greater than 7.5. Smoking cessation must be complete at least 4 weeks before surgery (not 4 months) to optimize postoperative healing. Furthermore, patients must be able to maintain cessation through the postoperative healing phase as smoking has been shown to affect many elements of patient outcomes including wound healing and chest complications, not just only in abdominal wall reconstruction.[1-4]

The wound must be adequately debrided and may require serial procedures before reconstruction. However, the two procedures do not always need to be staged. Repairs should always be reinforced and this fact is supported by level A evidence. The repair material will differ according to the grade of ventral wall hernia. Nonabsorbable mesh is preferred in low-risk repairs. Fistulas must be adequately addressed prior to reconstruction, but these sites still need reinforcement.[4,5]

REFERENCES

1. Duncan AE. Hyperglycemia and perioperative glucose management. Curr Pharm Des 2012;18(38):6195–6203
2. Trang K, Spain DA. Smoking cessation in elective surgery. Am Surg 2019;85(4):e193–e194
3. Møller AM, Pedersen T, Villebro N, Munksgaard A. Effect of smoking on early complications after elective orthopaedic surgery. J Bone Joint Surg Br 2003;85(2):178–181
4. Khansa I, Janis JE. The 4 principles of complex abdominal wall reconstruction. Plast Reconstr Surg Glob Open 2019;7(12):e2549
5. Breuing K, Butler CE, Ferzoco S, et al; Ventral Hernia Working Group. Incisional ventral hernias: review of the literature and recommendations regarding the grading and technique of repair. Surgery 2010;148(3):544–558

ADJUNCTS TO CLOSURE OF ABDOMINAL WALL DEFECTS

6. Which one of the following statements is correct regarding techniques for abdominal wall reconstruction?

D. Polyglycolic acid is useful as temporary support in abdominal wall defects but may lead to hernia formation in the longer term.

Polyglycolic acid and polyglactin 910 are both absorbable materials that can be used as temporary mesh supports in abdominal wall reconstruction. They are not suitable for repairs of areas deficient in fascia, because their lack of permanence can result in hernia formation in the long term. Nonabsorbable polypropylene mesh, such as Marlex, is durable and strong with good resistance to bacterial contamination. Gore-Tex sheet is produced with ePTFE, but its use is limited because it does not allow fluid egress or fibrous ingrowth. Tissue expanders can be placed between the internal and external oblique muscles and in the subcutaneous plane. AlloDerm is acellular human cadaver dermis and is not available in the United Kingdom. Furthermore, it tends to stretch over time and may be insufficient to prevent bulging and herniation. Instead, a porcine acellular dermal matrix, which is less prone to stretching and has comparable strength to fascia lata, can be used in many countries.[1-6]

REFERENCES

1. Brown GL, Richardson JD, Malangoni MA, Tobin GR, Ackerman D, Polk HC Jr. Comparison of prosthetic materials for abdominal wall reconstruction in the presence of contamination and infection. Ann Surg 1985;201(6):705–711

2. Mathes SJ, Steinwald PM, Foster RD, Hoffman WY, Anthony JP. Complex abdominal wall reconstruction: a comparison of flap and mesh closure. Ann Surg 2000;232(4):586–596

3. Khansa I, Janis JE. Abdominal wall reconstruction using retrorectus self-adhering mesh: a novel approach. Plast Reconstr Surg Glob Open 2016;4(11):e1145

4. Butler CE. The role of bioprosthetics in abdominal wall reconstruction. Clin Plast Surg 2006;33(2):199–211, v–vi

5. Turza KC, Butler CE. Adhesions and meshes: synthetic versus bioprosthetic. Plast Reconstr Surg 2012;130(5, Suppl 2):206S–213S

6. Janis JE, O'Neill AC, Ahmad J, Zhong T, Hofer SOP. Acellular dermal matrices in abdominal wall reconstruction: a systematic review of the current evidence. Plast Reconstr Surg 2012;130(5, Suppl 2):183S–193S

ALLOPLASTIC COMPOSITE MATERIALS

7. *What is the main proposed benefit of using newer composite or barrier-coated prosthetic materials for abdominal wall repair as compared to traditional alloplastic materials?*

  D. They may reduce formation of tissue adhesions.

  There are a number of newer composite prosthetics that combine both absorbable and nonabsorbable materials such as polypropylene and polyglactin, or nonabsorbable and tissue-separating barrier materials such as polypropylene and cellulose. Proceed and Supramesh are examples of the latter type and should help maintain tissue separation and adhesion formation. The benefits of materials such as Vypro and Ultrapro, which contain a combination of absorbable and nonabsorbable alloplastic materials, are that handling and initial strength may be improved while reducing the amount of foreign body present in the longer term. None of these materials contain purely absorbable material and will not resorb completely, and tissue integration differs between materials, but will never match that of normal tissue. A caveat with these materials is that they tend to be more expensive than traditional prosthetics. Although these newer materials should reduce bowel adhesions, it is still advisable to cover the bowel with omentum to separate the bowel from the mesh.[1–3]

REFERENCES

1. Turza KC, Butler CE. Adhesions and meshes: synthetic versus bioprosthetic. Plast Reconstr Surg 2012;130(5, Suppl 2):206S–213S

2. Janis JE, O'Neill AC, Ahmad J, Zhong T, Hofer SOP. Acellular dermal matrices in abdominal wall reconstruction: a systematic review of the current evidence. Plast Reconstr Surg 2012;130(5, Suppl 2):183S–193S

3. Butler CE. The role of bioprosthetics in abdominal wall reconstruction. Clin Plast Surg 2006;33(2):199–211, v–vi

BIOPROSTHETIC MATERIALS

8. *Which one of the following statements is correct regarding biologic materials in abdominal wall reconstruction?*

  E. They may be placed directly on the bowel with low adhesion rates.

  There are a variety of acellular dermal matrices (ADMs) in use. They are either bovine, porcine, or human in origin. They are expensive compared with alloplastic materials and their use should be targeted to contaminated wounds in which prosthetic mesh must be avoided. Permacol is an example of a crosslinked porcine ADM. Cross-linking will help to control enzymatic degradation of the graft, but it tends to make the product behave more like a synthetic with less tissue integration. A vast majority of ADMs such as Surgimend, AlloDerm, XenMatrix, and Strattice are not crosslinked. Hernia recurrence rates are highly variable when using ADMs[1] and the highest rates are when used as a bridging technique. A major benefit of their use is that they produce few visceral adhesions compared with prosthetics and may be placed directly onto the bowel. Their use is however off-label from an Food and Drug Administration (FDA) perspective.

REFERENCE

1. Janis JE, O'Neill AC, Ahmad J, Zhong T, Hofer SOP. Acellular dermal matrices in abdominal wall reconstruction: a systematic review of the current evidence. Plast Reconstr Surg 2012;130(5, Suppl 2):183S–193S

MESH POSITION IN VENTRAL WALL ABDOMINAL REPAIR

9. *Which one of the following represents the ideal plane for mesh placement when performing abdominal wall hernia repair?*

  C. Beneath rectus muscle on posterior rectus sheath

  The placement of mesh in the abdominal wall is generally required for abdominal wall hernia reconstruction. The position of this mesh will depend on a number of factors according to the defect and associated soft tissues. In principle, the best place for the mesh is away from the intra-abdominal contents and yet with sufficient vascularized soft tissue cover to protect it from the external environment. Accordingly, the ideal position is probably retrorectus as there is no contact with either the external environment nor the intra-abdominal contents. Furthermore, the rectus muscle should be well vascularized to help with healing and tissue integration. From a biomechanical perspective, mesh placed internally to a fascial layer, that is, an inlay mesh, will be preferable as when intra-abdominal pressure increases the mesh will be forced close to the native fascial layer and close the repair gap. This will apply to deeper placement beneath any one of the deep fascial layers. In contrast, an onlay mesh placed suprafascially will tend to be forced away from the fascial attachment with increased abdominal pressure. Interpositional bridges represent the weakest repair biomechanically as their strength has no additional fascial support. For this reason, they are associated with the highest rate of recurrence and bulge. Where meshes must be placed intraperitoneally, it is best if they can be placed flat without bulges and on top of omentum to reduce adhesion and its subsequent complications. In all cases, where mesh is used, 3–5 cm of overlap between the material and fascia is advised.[1-3]

REFERENCES

1. Khansa I, Janis JE. Abdominal wall reconstruction using retrorectus self-adhering mesh: a novel approach. Plast Reconstr Surg Glob Open 2016;4(11):e1145
2. Sosin M, Nahabedian MY, Bhanot P. The perfect plane: a systematic review of mesh location and outcomes, update 2018. Plast Reconstr Surg 2018;142(3, Suppl):107S–116S
3. Holihan JL, Bondre I, Askenasy EP, et al; Ventral Hernia Outcomes Collaborative (VHOC) Writing Group. Sublay versus underlay in open ventral hernia repair. J Surg Res 2016;202(1):26–32

COMPONENT SEPARATION

10. You are planning a component separation on a patient with an anterior abdominal wall defect. *Which one of the following statements is correct regarding this procedure?*

E. Release of the rectus from its posterior sheath can increase advancement by an additional 2 cm at all levels.

In 1990, Ramirez et al[1] published results of a clinical and anatomic study to determine whether separation of the components of the abdominal wall musculature allows increased mobilization of each to close large abdominal wall defects. They dissected 10 cadavers and found that the external and internal oblique muscles could be separated in a relatively avascular plane. This allowed medial advancement of the rectus (once elevated from the posterior sheath) as a composite with the internal oblique (not external oblique) and transversus abdominis muscles. The advancement was far greater than with direct closure of all components as a single composite. The neurovascular structures were identified between the internal oblique and transversus abdominis, and these two structures were tightly adherent to one another.

To perform the procedure, the external oblique aponeurosis is split longitudinally at the linea alba. This plane is developed laterally between the external and internal oblique muscles to the midaxillary line. The posterior rectus sheath is also separated from the rectus via a midline incision to facilitate advancement.

After their anatomic study, Ramirez et al performed the procedure in 11 clinical cases, which were also presented in the paper. Good clinical outcomes were observed in all cases. In four of the patients who had preoperative back pain, the problem resolved after surgery.

Although Ramirez et al are quoted as having originally described the technique, the first description of this concept actually dates back to a paper by Young[2] in 1961 for repair of epigastric hernias.

The original description did not take a perforator-sparing approach. This has been subsequently described by a number of authors to decrease risk of dehiscence and seroma. This is achieved by using access tunnels or endoscopic approaches.[3-5]

REFERENCES

1. Ramirez OM, Ruas E, Dellon AL. "Components separation" method for closure of abdominal-wall defects: an anatomic and clinical study. Plast Reconstr Surg 1990;86(3):519–526
2. Young D. Repair of epigastric incisional hernia. Br J Surg 1961;48:514–516
3. Saulis AS, Dumanian GA. Periumbilical rectus abdominis perforator preservation significantly reduces superficial wound complications in "separation of parts" hernia repairs. Plast Reconstr Surg 2002;109(7):2275–2280, discussion 2281–2282
4. Butler CE, Campbell KT. Minimally invasive component separation with inlay bioprosthetic mesh (MICSIB) for complex abdominal wall reconstruction. Plast Reconstr Surg 2011;128(3):698–709
5. Lowe JB, Garza JR, Bowman JL, Rohrich RJ, Strodel WE. Endoscopically assisted "components separation" for closure of abdominal wall defects. Plast Reconstr Surg 2000;105(2):720–729, quiz 730

COMPONENT SEPARATION

11. *According to the original study by Ramirez et al, how much advancement can be achieved at the waist after a bilateral component separation?*

    C. 20 cm

    Ramirez et al[1] quoted the following figures for unilateral advancement: 5 cm at the epigastrium, 10 cm at the middle third, and 3 cm in the suprapubic region. These figures are doubled for the bilateral advancement. Although some surgeons report much greater advancement at the midabdomen, they also indicate that advancement of the upper and lower third are difficult to achieve without posterior sheath release or extension over the costal margins.

REFERENCE

1. Ramirez OM, Ruas E, Dellon AL. "Components separation" method for closure of abdominal-wall defects: an anatomic and clinical study. Plast Reconstr Surg 1990;86(3):519–526

APPROACHES TO ABDOMINAL WALL REPAIR

12. You have just completed a free tissue transfer for breast reconstruction using a muscle-sparing transverse rectus abdominis myocutaneous (TRAM) flap instead of the planned deep inferior epigastric perforator (DIEP) flap. A 5 by 8 cm fascial defect of the anterior rectus sheath is present. *How should this defect be reconstructed?*

    D. Inlay repair with polypropylene mesh

    When a planned DIEP flap requires conversion to a muscle-sparing TRAM flap, a residual fascial defect in the anterior rectus sheath warrants repair. If the defect is small (less than 2 cm wide), direct closure may be possible; otherwise, reinforced closure is required. Although the benefits of mesh over direct repair are debated, Luijendijk et al[1] conducted a large study that showed significantly lower rates of incisional hernia recurrence where mesh repairs were used compared with direct suture repair only. Wan et al[2] showed similar rates of hernia in patients after a TRAM flap with mesh repair compared with those who had a DIEP procedure. Without a mesh repair, the rates were higher in the TRAM group.

    Permanent mesh such as polypropylene is probably the best option for this clean, elective surgery. These products are inert, readily available, inexpensive, and provide good long-term strength and support. Inlay mesh repair is in theory biomechanically superior because the forces acting on it by intra-abdominal pressure will push the interface between mesh and abdominal wall firmly together at the areas of overlap. Debate exists over the benefits of underlay versus overlay techniques. However, the VHWG[3] suggested the use of an underlay rather than an overlay in open procedures for abdominal wall repair. Polyglactin 910 is less appropriate, given that it is absorbable and cannot provide long-term support. Acellular dermal matrix has a role in abdominal wound closure, but the benefits in this situation do not support the increased cost. Component separation would not be required for a defect of this nature.

REFERENCES

1. Luijendijk RW, Hop WC, van den Tol MP, et al. A comparison of suture repair with mesh repair for incisional hernia. N Engl J Med 2000;343(6):392–398
2. Wan DC, Tseng CY, Anderson-Dam J, Dalio AL, Crisera CA, Festekjian JH. Inclusion of mesh in donor-site repair of free TRAM and muscle-sparing free TRAM flaps yields rates of abdominal complications comparable to those of DIEP flap reconstruction. Plast Reconstr Surg 2010;126(2):367–374
3. Breuing K, Butler CE, Ferzoco S, et al; Ventral Hernia Working Group. Incisional ventral hernias: review of the literature and recommendations regarding the grading and technique of repair. Surgery 2010;148(3):544–558

MANAGEMENT OF ABDOMINAL WALL HERNIAS

13. A 50-year-old woman has a large, chronic rectus sheath hernia following emergency paramedian laparotomy for bowel perforation. The initial abdominal wall repair took months to heal after partial dehiscence occurred. She has a 5 by 10 cm abdominal wall hernia to the left of the midline and is concerned about function, cosmesis, and discomfort. *Which one of the following is the most appropriate option for management of this patient?*

    D. Component separation with synthetic permanent mesh

    This patient has a number of options, including lifestyle modification or revision surgery. The former is unlikely to be acceptable to this patient given her age and lifestyle demands. A key principle in repair of this hernia is to reapproximate and centralize the rectus muscles and for this, a component separation should be used. The repair will also need reinforcement with a mesh. In this case a permanent mesh such as polypropylene would be a good choice, although there are other options too, as there is no ongoing infection and the bowel is not likely to be involved. A further option not listed is a Rives-Stoppa procedure. The Rives-Stoppa technique can be useful in patients with a large ventral hernia. It employs a reinforcing mesh sublay in the retromuscular space between the rectus muscle and the posterior rectus sheath, but it can be limited by the lateral edge of the posterior rectus sheath. Therefore, for larger defects, a larger inlay mesh is sometimes placed behind the rectus sheath but outside of the peritoneum.[1-7]

REFERENCES

1. Janis JE, Khansa I. Evidence-based abdominal wall reconstruction: the maxi-mini approach. Plast Reconstr Surg 2015;136(6):1312–1323
2. Khansa I, Janis JE. Complex open abdominal wall reconstruction: management of the skin and subcutaneous tissue. Plast Reconstr Surg 2018;142(3, Suppl):125S–132S
3. Ramirez OM, Ruas E, Dellon AL. "Components separation" method for closure of abdominal-wall defects: an anatomic and clinical study. Plast Reconstr Surg 1990;86(3):519–526
4. Yaghoobi Notash A, Yaghoobi Notash A Jr, Seied Farshi J, Ahmadi Amoli H, Salimi J, Mamarabadi M. Outcomes of the Rives-Stoppa technique in incisional hernia repair: ten years of experience. Hernia 2007;11(1):25–29
5. Shestak KC, Edington HJD, Johnson RR. The separation of anatomic components technique for the reconstruction of massive midline abdominal wall defects: anatomy, surgical technique, applications, and limitations revisited. Plast Reconstr Surg 2000;105(2):731–738, quiz 739
6. Girotto JA, Ko MJ, Redett R, Muehlberger T, Talamini M, Chang B. Closure of chronic abdominal wall defects: a long-term evaluation of the components separation method. Ann Plast Surg 1999;42(4):385–394, discussion 394–395
7. Butler CE, Campbell KT. Minimally invasive component separation with inlay bioprosthetic mesh (MICSIB) for complex abdominal wall reconstruction. Plast Reconstr Surg 2011;128(3):698–709

63. Posterior Trunk Reconstruction

See *Essentials of Plastic Surgery*, third edition, pp. 863–871

MUSCULAR ANATOMY OF THE POSTERIOR TRUNK

1. *When operating on the posterior trunk, which muscle is found just deep to the latissimus dorsi in the midline at the level of T10?*
   - A. Trapezius
   - B. Serratus posterior
   - C. Paraspinal
   - D. Intercostals
   - E. Rhomboid

FREE TISSUE TRANSFER FOR THE LATERAL POSTERIOR TRUNK

2. *When faced with reconstruction of a lateral posterior thoracic wall defect, what would be the greatest potential challenge of undertaking free tissue transfer to reconstruct the defect?*
   - A. Finding a suitable donor site to obtain a good soft tissue match
   - B. Positioning the patient safely during the procedure
   - C. Finding suitable recipient vessels for vascular anastomoses
   - D. Ensuring a comfortable reach for the microscope
   - E. Facilitating a dual team approach to surgery

PRINCIPLES OF MANAGING MIDLINE WOUNDS OF THE POSTERIOR TRUNK

3. *In what way do the principles of managing infected midline back wounds post spinal surgery differ from those principles generally applied elsewhere?*
   - A. That debridement and reconstruction must be performed in a single stage
   - B. That metalwork is preferably not removed
   - C. That unincorporated bone graft should be left in situ
   - D. That intraoperative placement of drains should be avoided
   - E. That negative pressure dressings should be avoided

MANAGEMENT OF POSTERIOR CERVICAL WOUNDS FOLLOWING SPINAL SURGERY

4. A patient has undergone cervical spine fusion via a posterior approach and has since had problems with postoperative wound healing. There is now a deep wound overlying the spinous processes of C6/7 with exposed bone. There is no visible metalwork although imaging shows this to be in place. The defect size is 8 cm. The local surrounding tissues are firm and woody. There is some granulation evident. A debridement is performed with bone and soft tissue removal. *Once clean, which one of the following would be the preferred choice for defect reconstruction?*
   - A. Latissimus dorsi flap
   - B. Trapezius flap
   - C. Keystone island flap
   - D. Lumbar perforator flap
   - E. Pectoralis major flap

RECONSTRUCTION OF THE MIDLINE THORACIC AND LUMBAR REGION

5. *Which one of the following is generally considered to be the first-line reconstructive option for smaller midline thoracolumbar soft tissue defects?*
   - A. Paraspinal muscles
   - B. Reverse latissimus dorsi
   - C. Vertical rectus abdominis (VRAM)
   - D. Pedicled latissimus dorsi
   - E. Lumbar perforator

SECONDARY RECOSTRUCTION OF THE POSTERIOR TRUNK

6. A patient is seen in clinic following reconstructive surgery to the posterior cervical spine with a trapezius myocutaneous flap 6 months before. The vast majority of the flap has healed well but there is a small defect measuring 2 × 2 cm at the leading edge of the flap, where necrosis had occurred. The surrounding soft tissues are soft. *Which one of the following may be best to reconstruct this defect?*
   - A. Healing by secondary intention
   - B. Direct closure
   - C. Split-skin graft
   - D. Local fasciocutaneous flap
   - E. Paraspinal flap

Answers

MUSCULAR ANATOMY OF THE POSTERIOR TRUNK

1. **When operating on the posterior trunk, which muscle is found just deep to the latissimus dorsi in the midline at the level of T10?**

   B. Serratus posterior

   The main muscles of the back when considering posterior trunk reconstruction are the paired latissimus dorsi, the trapezius, the paired paraspinal muscles (erector spinae), and the paired serratus anterior and posterior. The latissimus dorsi muscles are the largest muscles in the body and span the lower and mid back from their origin on the posterior iliac crest and thoracolumbar fascia, passing cranially from T12 to T7 vertebrae just over the scapula tip and inserting on the anterior humerus. The latissimus is a real workhorse flap for reconstruction and this is the case for both anterior and posterior trunk defect reconstruction.[1]

   In the midline, cranially the trapezius is the most superficial muscle of the posterior trunk commencing at the nuchal fold of the occiput and passing inferiorly to T12 spinous process and inserting along the scapulae. Caudally, it overlaps the latissimus dorsi medially between T7 and T12. When raising a latissimus muscle flap, one should carefully identify the inferior tip and lower border as it passes over the latissimus to avoid damage to this muscle.

   The erector spinae run parallel to the spine and function to stabilize and extend the vertebrae.

   They are made up of three distinct muscle bellies—spinalis, longissimus, and iliocostalis—travelling the length of the spine. Along the medial posterior trunk, the paraspinous muscles are immediately deep to the latissimus dorsi, except in the T10–L1 location, where the serratus posterior inferior muscle fibers may be found sandwiched between them and latissimus dorsi.[1,2]

   There are anterior and posterior serratus muscles. The serratus posterior has two components (superior and inferior) and is located in the thoracolumbar region at the level of C7–L2 where it passes from the spinous processes of the vertebrae to the ribs. It helps to stabilize the vertebral column and to elevate and depress the ribs. The serratus anterior originates from the 1st to 9th or 10th ribs on the lateral chest wall and inserts on the medial border of the scapula. It acts to pull the scapula onto the thorax. The lower part of this muscle can be used for reconstruction in its own right, either free or pedicled, or used as part of a composite muscle flap with latissimus (**Fig. 63.1**).[3]

REFERENCES

1. Bakri K, Mardini S, Evans KK, Carlsen BT, Arnold PG. Workhorse flaps in chest wall reconstruction: the pectoralis major, latissimus dorsi, and rectus abdominis flaps. Semin Plast Surg 2011;25(1):43–54
2. Moore KL, Dalley AF, Agur AMR, eds. Clinically Oriented Anatomy. 7th ed. Philadelphia: Wolters Kluwer/Lippincott Williams & Wilkins; 2013
3. Godat DM, Sanger JR, Lifchez SD, et al. Detailed neurovascular anatomy of the serratus anterior muscle: implications for a functional muscle flap with multiple independent force vectors. Plast Reconstr Surg 2004;114(1):21–29, discussion 30–31

FREE TISSUE TRANSFER FOR THE LATERAL POSTERIOR TRUNK

2. **When faced with reconstruction of a lateral posterior thoracic wall defect, what would be the greatest potential challenge of undertaking free tissue transfer to reconstruct the defect?**

   C. Finding suitable recipient vessels for vascular anastomoses

   Reconstruction of the lateral posterior trunk is most commonly required after wide local excision of cutaneous or soft tissue malignancies. Defects can range from small to large and lateral posterior trunk reconstruction adheres to the standard reconstructive principles of plastic surgery in terms of replacing tissue in a like for like fashion. Where primary closure is not possible and there is a well-vascularized bed, which is often the case, the wound can be closed with a skin graft. Alternatively, the lateral posterior trunk is well suited to local flap or regional flap options of which there are many where there are larger defects. As a result, the need for free tissue transfer is rarely necessary compared with other sites such as the limbs or head and neck. The major challenge of undertaking free tissue transfer in this anatomic area, when needed, is the relative paucity of recipient vessels. If a free flap is required, a vein graft or arteriovenous loop is often needed to achieve sufficient reach to appropriate vessels. Finding a suitable donor site should not be a problem as the usual free flap choices may be used. Likewise, positioning the patient is standard operating practice as either a lateral or prone position may be used. The position of the microscope should be just as simple to set up as with any

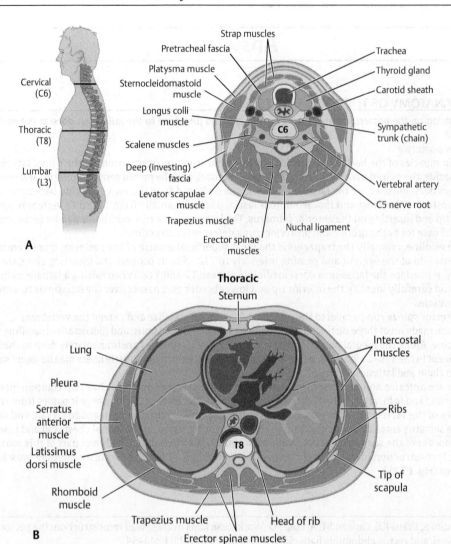

A

Cervical (C6)

Thoracic (T8)

Lumbar (L3)

Strap muscles

Pretracheal fascia

Platysma muscle

Sternocleidomastoid muscle

Longus colli muscle

Scalene muscles

Deep (investing) fascia

Levator scapulae muscle

Trapezius muscle

Erector spinae muscles

Trachea

Thyroid gland

Carotid sheath

Sympathetic trunk (chain)

Vertebral artery

C5 nerve root

Nuchal ligament

C6

Thoracic

Sternum

Lung

Pleura

Serratus anterior muscle

Latissimus dorsi muscle

Rhomboid muscle

Trapezius muscle

Erector spinae muscles

Intercostal muscles

Ribs

Tip of scapula

Head of rib

T8

B

Lumbar

Inferior vena cava   Aorta

Rectus abdominus muscle

External oblique muscle

Internal oblique muscle

Transversus abdominus muscle

Peritoneum

Latissimus dorsi muscle

Quadratus lumborum muscle

Psoas major muscle

Erector spinae muscles

Ureter

Lumbodorsal fascia

L3

C

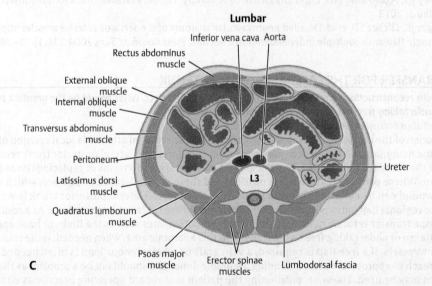

Fig. 63.1 Cross-sectional musculoskeletal anatomy at the cervical, thoracic, and lumbar levels.

other case, and a dual team approach should still be possible with most donor site flaps, especially those from the contralateral side.[1-6]

REFERENCES

1. Clemens MW, Chang EI, Selber JC, Lewis VO, Oates SD, Chang DW. Composite extremity and trunk reconstruction with vascularized fibula flap in postoncologic bone defects: a 10-year experience. Plast Reconstr Surg 2012;129(1): 170–178
2. Houdek MT, Rose PS, Bakri K, et al. Outcomes and complications of reconstruction with use of free vascularized fibular graft for spinal and pelvic defects following resection of a malignant tumor. J Bone Joint Surg Am 2017;99(13):e69
3. Lee YJ, Baek SE, Lee J, Oh DY, Rhie JW, Moon SH. Perforating vessel as an alternative option of a recipient selection for posterior trunk-free flap reconstruction. Microsurgery 2018;38(7):763–771
4. Mathes DW, Thornton JF, Rohrich RJ. Management of posterior trunk defects. Plast Reconstr Surg 2006;118(3): 73e–83e
5. Harry BL, Deleyiannis FW. Posterior trunk reconstruction using an anteromedial thigh free flap and arteriovenous loop. Microsurgery 2013;33(5):416–417
6. Arkudas A, Horch RE, Regus S, et al. Retrospective cohort study of combined approach for trunk reconstruction using arteriovenous loops and free flaps. J Plast Reconstr Aesthet Surg 2018;71(3):394–401

PRINCIPLES OF MANAGING MIDLINE WOUNDS OF THE POSTERIOR TRUNK

3. *In what way do the principles of managing infected midline back wounds post spinal surgery differ from those principles generally applied elsewhere?*

B. That metalwork is preferably not removed

Patients will occasionally be referred for plastic surgery following spinal surgery with dehisced or infected wounds overlying hardware. The usual principles of performing thorough debridement and reconstructing tissue apply. For this debridement a dual specialty approach is generally advised. During the debridement it is important to remove all nonviable soft tissue and unincorporated bone graft. In this scenario, however, the usual principles of removing metalwork cannot be followed as this may leave patients with an unstable spine. Only if the hardware is broken, loose, or chronically infected, should it be removed and replaced. If hardware is removed, it should be replaced at the same sitting by the spinal team. The debridement should ideally be performed in a single stage, but where necessary, wounds can and should be temporized. Use of drains and/or negative pressure dressings is normal practice in posterior trunk reconstruction. However, care should be taken when there may be a dural leak as negative pressure would be contraindicated in this case.[1-5]

REFERENCES

1. Anghel EL, DeFazio MV, Barker JC, Janis JE, Attinger CE. Current concepts in debridement: science and strategies. Plast Reconstr Surg 2016;138(3, Suppl)82S–93S
2. Chang DW, Friel MT, Youssef AA. Reconstructive strategies in soft tissue reconstruction after resection of spinal neo-plasms. Spine 2007;32(10):1101–1106
3. Mericli AF, Tarola NA, Moore JH Jr, Copit SE, Fox JW IV, Tuma GA. Paraspinous muscle flap reconstruction of complex midline back wounds: risk factors and postreconstruction complications. Ann Plast Surg 2010;65(2):219–224
4. Hultman CS, Jones GE, Losken A, et al. Salvage of infected spinal hardware with paraspinous muscle flaps: anatomic considerations with clinical correlation. Ann Plast Surg 2006;57(5):521–528
5. Chun JK, Lynch MJ, Poultsides GA. Distal trapezius musculocutaneous flap for upper thoracic back wounds associated with spinal instrumentation and radiation. Ann Plast Surg 2003;51(1):17–22

MANAGEMENT OF POSTERIOR CERVICAL WOUNDS FOLLOWING SPINAL SURGERY

4. A patient has undergone cervical spine fusion via a posterior approach and has since had problems with postoperative wound healing. There is now a deep wound overlying the spinous processes of C6/7 with exposed bone. There is no visible metalwork although imaging shows this to be in place. The defect size is 8 cm. The local surrounding tissues are firm and woody. There is some granulation evident. A debridement is performed with bone and soft tissue removal. *Once clean, which one of the following would be the preferred choice for defect reconstruction?*

B. Trapezius flap

This scenario is not uncommon in clinical practice. A key component of the debridement is to remove all necrotic tissue and the prominent bone before reconstruction as the bony prominences with thin soft tissue coverage are often a contributory factor in the wound healing problem. In this scenario, a robust local muscle flap option is preferred and the trapezius works well for such defects due to its close proximity to the defect and reliable blood supply. The trapezius flap is supplied by the descending branch of the transverse cervical artery. The midline part of the trapezius can be harvested with a skin paddle to close defect of this size with the donor site closing directly and the flap tunneling to the defect or with elevation of skin flaps to join the two wounds together. Because the donor is away from the wound, the woody nature of the wound edge tissue has less relevance in this scenario. The muscle is ideal for filling the defect, especially in the presence of previous infection and the skin will provide a robust cover. The latissimus dorsi flap as an alternative may reach but would be a second choice. The keystone island flap can work well on the back but in this instance, it would probably fail to move sufficiently due to the woody nature of the tissues, nor would it fill the defect depth adequately. The lumbar perforator flap would not reach this defect, nor would a pectoralis major flap. The pectoralis major flap would also involve turning the patient half way through the procedure. The lumbar perforator flap is indicated for more distal wounds and the pectoralis major for anterior trunk or head and neck wounds.[1-3]

REFERENCES

1. Chun JK, Lynch MJ, Poultsides GA. Distal trapezius musculocutaneous flap for upper thoracic back wounds associated with spinal instrumentation and radiation. Ann Plast Surg 2003;51(1):17–22
2. Disa JJ, Smith AW, Bilsky MH. Management of radiated reoperative wounds of the cervicothoracic spine: the role of the trapezius turnover flap. Ann Plast Surg 2001;47(4):394–397
3. Oh TS, Hallock G, Hong JP. Freestyle propeller flaps to reconstruct defects of the posterior trunk: a simple approach to a difficult problem. Ann Plast Surg 2012;68(1):79–82

RECONSTRUCTION OF THE MIDLINE THORACIC AND LUMBAR REGION

5. *Which one of the following is generally considered to be the first-line reconstructive option for smaller midline thoracolumbar soft tissue defects?*

A. Paraspinal muscles

The paraspinal muscle flaps are considered the first-line option for reconstruction of smaller thoracic or lumbar midline regions. When used in this setting, the paraspinous muscle flaps should be released from their lateral fascial attachments to allow for medial advancement. The muscle bellies can be imbricated into the wound and obliterate dead space with the use of a Lembert suture technique.[1-3]

The latissimus dorsi can be used as either an advancement flap on the main pedicle or as a reverse flap on its segmental vessel supply. Alternative options also include the omentum or a lumbar perforator fasciocutaneous flap. The omentum can be isolated on the right or left gastroepiploic vessels and tunneled through the diaphragm or retroperitoneum to fill dead space and protect hardware along the thoracic spine. A transpelvic vertical rectus abdominis myocutaneous (VRAM) flap is an option for lower defects involving the sacrum where anterior and posterior approaches are combined. Gluteal flaps, either V-Y or rotational, can also be useful for lower lumbar or sacral defect coverage.

REFERENCES

1. Garvey PB, Rhines LD, Dong W, Chang DW. Immediate soft-tissue reconstruction for complex defects of the spine following surgery for spinal neoplasms. Plast Reconstr Surg 2010;125(5):1460–1466
2. Mericli AF, Tarola NA, Moore JH Jr, Copit SE, Fox JW IV, Tuma GA. Paraspinous muscle flap reconstruction of complex midline back wounds: risk factors and postreconstruction complications. Ann Plast Surg 2010;65(2):219–224
3. Hultman CS, Jones GE, Losken A, et al. Salvage of infected spinal hardware with paraspinous muscle flaps: anatomic considerations with clinical correlation. Ann Plast Surg 2006;57(5):521–528

SECONDARY RECOSTRUCTION OF THE POSTERIOR TRUNK

6. A patient is seen in clinic following reconstructive surgery to the posterior cervical spine with a trapezius myocutaneous flap 6 months before. The vast majority of the flap has healed well but there is a small defect measuring 2 × 2 cm at the leading edge of the flap, where necrosis had occurred. The surrounding soft tissues are soft. *Which one of the following may be best to reconstruct this defect?*

D. Local fasciocutaneous flap

In this instance there is justification for secondary reconstruction of this defect with a small local fasciocutaneous flap such as a rhomboid. This will advance adjacent tissue into the defect, which is relatively superficial. Leaving this to heal by secondary intention is unlikely to work given the duration since surgery. Direct closure may be possible, but in general, the local tissues tend not to move well in chronic wounds. A split-skin graft may be an option if there is a granulating bed, but really, importation of new vascularized tissue is required. A paraspinal flap would be indicated for a deeper wound with exposed metalwork, but not a more superficial defect as in this case (**Table 63.1**).[1-2]

Table 63.1 *Common Local and Regional Flaps for Posterior Trunk Reconstruction*

Flap	Included Tissues	Vascular Supply	Lateral Posterior Trunk	Cervical	Thoracic	Lumbosacral
Paraspinous	Muscle	Thoracic and lumbar perforators		×	×	×
Trapezius	Muscle or myocutaneous	Transverse cervical; dorsal scapular		×	×	
Latissimus dorsi	Muscle or myocutaneous	Thoracodorsal	×		×	
Reverse latissimus dorsi	Muscle or myocutaneous	Thoracic and lumbar perforators	×		×	×
Omentum	Visceral adipose	Right or left gastroepiploic			×	×
Gluteal	Muscle, myocutaneous, or fasciocutaneous	Superior gluteal; inferior gluteal				×
Lumbar perforator	Fasciocutaneous	Lumbar perforator	×			×
Intercostal artery perforator	Fasciocutaneous	Intercostal perforator	×		×	
Keystone flap	Fasciocutaneous	Random	×	×	×	×
Rotation-advancement flap	Fasciocutaneous	Random	×	×	×	×

REFERENCES

1. Hallock GG. Reconstruction of posterior trunk defects. Semin Plast Surg 2011;25(1):78–85
2. Janis JE, Kwon RK, Attinger CE. The new reconstructive ladder: modifications to the traditional model. Plast Reconstr Surg 2011(127):205S–212S

64. Perineal Reconstruction

See *Essentials of Plastic Surgery*, third edition, pp. 872–879

CAUSES OF PERINEAL DEFECTS

1. *What is the most common reason for a patient to require perineal reconstruction?*
   A. Radiotherapy
   B. Tumor extirpation
   C. Trauma
   D. Infection
   E. Vascular event

ANATOMY OF THE PERINEUM

2. *Which one of the following represents the anterior border of the perineum?*
   A. Pubic arch and the arcuate ligament of the pubis
   B. Tip of the coccyx
   C. Inferior rami of the pubis
   D. Ischial tuberosity
   E. Pelvic floor

SKIN GRAFTS IN PERINEAL DEFECTS

3. *What is the main limitation to using skin grafts in the perineal region?*
   A. They are difficult to bolster or stent.
   B. Recipient vascularity is suboptimal.
   C. They provide poor long-term aesthetics.
   D. Intraoperative patient positioning is a challenge.
   E. Negative pressure dressings cannot be used.

FLAP SELECTION IN PERINEAL RECONSTRUCTION

4. *What is generally considered to be the main workhorse flap for perineal reconstruction?*
   A. Rectus abdominis
   B. Gracilis
   C. Anterolateral thigh
   D. Singapore
   E. Posterior thigh

VASCULAR SUPPLY OF FLAPS USED IN PERINEAL RECONSTRUCTION

5. *Which one of the following represents the arterial blood supply to the gracilis flap when used for perineal reconstruction?*
   A. Deep inferior epigastric artery
   B. Profunda femoris artery
   C. Pudendal arteries
   D. Medial circumflex femoral artery
   E. Lateral circumflex femoral artery

RECONSTRUCTION OF VAGINAL WALL DEFECTS

6. A patient is seen in clinic who is planned for wide resection of a vaginal wall tumor. It is expected that a 6 × 2 cm lateral wall defect will be created and will require reconstruction. *Which one of the following would be best suited to reconstructing this defect?*
   A. Singapore flap (pudendal thigh flap)
   B. Posterior thigh flap
   C. Anterolateral thigh flap
   D. Gracilis flap
   E. Groin flap

RECONSTRUCTION OF THE PENIS

7. *When performing a phalloplasty which one of the following is true?*
   A. The free fibula flap is the gold standard for functional penile reconstruction.
   B. Sensation is normally provided by coapting the superficial radial nerve to the pudendal nerve.
   C. Regional flaps are generally preferred as they can be completed in a single stage.
   D. The risk of reconstructive failure is much higher than in other reconstructions.
   E. If the radial forearm flap is used, the antebrachial cutaneous nerves are used to provide sensation.

DEFECT CLASSIFICATION IN VAGINAL DEFECTS

8. *Which one of the following is true of the Cordeiro classification for vaginal defects?*

    A. It categorizes the defect by physical size in cm.

    B. It categorizes the defect by cause.

    C. It categorizes the defect by chronicity.

    D. It considers external tissue loss to the labia, perineum, and anus.

    E. It provides an algorithm for reconstructive approaches.

Answers

CAUSES OF PERINEAL DEFECTS

1. What is the most common reason for a patient to require perineal reconstruction?

B. Tumor extirpation

Perineal reconstruction is most commonly performed after tumor extirpation. Common cancers affecting the perineum include colorectal, vulvar, vaginal, uterine, and bladder subtypes.

The unique anatomy of the perineum often requires many considerations for maintaining function, cosmesis, obliteration of dead space, and achieving a healed wound. Often reconstruction following tumor extirpation is further complicated by prior radiotherapy for the same cancer. This makes reconstruction more challenging and highlights the importance of importing healthy vascularized tissue into the area. Radiotherapy alone can, of course, be a requirement for needing perineal reconstruction but this is less likely. Trauma is an occasional cause for a need to undertake perineal reconstruction and serious burns are one of the more likely examples. Infection is a cause for patients to require perineal reconstruction, particularly in cases such as necrotizing fasciitis and Fournier's gangrene, once debridement has been undertaken and the infection is controlled. A need for reconstruction for an isolated vascular event would be rare other than in the context of a necrotizing infection.[1,2]

REFERENCES

1. Weichman KE, Matros E, Disa JJ. Reconstruction of peripelvic oncologic defects. Plast Reconstr Surg 2017;140(4): 601e–612e
2. Mericli AF, Martin JP, Campbell CA. An algorithmic anatomical subunit approach to pelvic wound reconstruction. Plast Reconstr Surg 2016;137(3):1004–1017

ANATOMY OF THE PERINEUM

2. Which one of the following represents the anterior border of the perineum?

A. Pubic arch and the arcuate ligament of the pubis

The perineal area can be divided into two triangular zones, the anterior urogenital triangle and the posterior anal triangle (**Fig. 64.1**).

The perineum represents the area between the scrotum or vagina and the anus. The anatomic boundaries are as follows:

- Anterior: Pubic arch and the arcuate ligament of the pubis
- Posteriorly: Tip of the coccyx
- Lateral and medial: Inferior rami of the pubis and the ischial tuberosity
- Superior: Pelvic floor
- Inferiorly: Skin and fascia

In the female the external genitalia comprise of the mons pubis, labia majora, labia minora, clitoris, and vestibule. The vagina is a tubular structure that extends from the vaginal opening to the uterus. In the male, the external genitalia comprises the penis, which has a root (radix), a body (corpus), and epithelium (glans penis). In addition, there is the scrotum which is a sack of skin and smooth muscle that houses the external spermatic fascia,

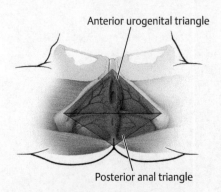

Anterior urogenital triangle

Posterior anal triangle

Fig. 64.1   Perianal triangle.

testes, epididymis, and ductus deferens. Knowledge of the anatomy of the perineum is key to understanding the principles of reconstruction and the flaps available for doing so.[1-3]

REFERENCES

1. Weichman KE, Matros E, Disa JJ. Reconstruction of peripelvic oncologic defects. Plast Reconstr Surg 2017;140(4): 601e–612e
2. Mericli AF, Martin JP, Campbell CA. An algorithmic anatomical subunit approach to pelvic wound reconstruction. Plast Reconstr Surg 2016;137(3):1004–1017
3. Moore KL, Dalley AF, Agur AMR, eds. Clinically Oriented Anatomy. 7th ed. Philadelphia: Wolters Kluwer/Lippincott Williams & Wilkins; 2013

SKIN GRAFTS IN PERINEAL DEFECTS

3. *What is the main limitation to using skin grafts in the perineal region?*

A. **They are difficult to bolster or stent.**

Skin grafts certainly have a role in perineal defects, both in split- and full-thickness forms. One of the main challenges is ensuring they remain secure on the recipient bed without movement due to friction or shear in the early days post surgery. This affects the perineum because of a number of factors including the anatomic contour as well as external compression forces that act upon them. One option that is sometimes employed to help grafts remain secure is to use a negative pressure dressing. This approach can be taken in the perineum, but the same limitation applies in that the contours, movement, local hair growth, and moisture make this a relative challenge. Recipient vascularity is suboptimal after radiation, but not uniformly so in perineal reconstruction cases. The aesthetic outcome is generally adequate and patient positioning is unaffected as this will normally be the same irrespective of whether flaps or grafts are used.[1-3]

REFERENCES

1. Hollenbeck ST, Toranto JD, Taylor BJ, et al. Perineal and lower extremity reconstruction. Plast Reconstr Surg 2011;128(5):551e–563e
2. Mughal M, Baker RJ, Muneer A, Mosahebi A. Reconstruction of perineal defects. Ann R Coll Surg Engl 2013;95(8):539–544
3. Orhan E, Şenen D. Using negative pressure therapy for improving skin graft taking on genital area defects following Fournier gangrene. Turk J Urol 2017;43(3):366–370

FLAP SELECTION IN PERINEAL RECONSTRUCTION

4. *What is generally considered to be the main workhorse flap for perineal reconstruction?*

A. **Rectus abdominis**

The rectus abdominis flap is considered to be the workhorse flap for perineal reconstruction.

It is used for large perineal defects and, in particular, following abdominoperineal resection. It also is useful for vaginal reconstruction. One of the key benefits of using this flap is that it obliterates pelvic dead space with the muscle component and also provides skin cover where necessary in the form of a vertical rectus myocutaneous (VRAM) flap or transverse rectus abdominis myocutaneous (TRAM) flap. Traditionally, when anteroposterior (AP) resection was performed as an open procedure, the harvest of this muscle was particularly favorable. With moves toward laparoscopic AP resection, other flaps such as a gluteal advancement have gained popularity and provide a fair alternative.[1,2]

REFERENCES

1. Butler CE, Gündeslioglu AO, Rodriguez-Bigas MA. Outcomes of immediate vertical rectus abdominis myocutaneous flap reconstruction for irradiated abdominoperineal resection defects. J Am Coll Surg 2008;206(4):694–703
2. McAllister E, Wells K, Chaet M, Norman J, Cruse W. Perineal reconstruction after surgical extirpation of pelvic malignancies using the transpelvic transverse rectus abdominal myocutaneous flap. Ann Surg Oncol 1994;1(2):164–168

VASCULAR SUPPLY OF FLAPS USED IN PERINEAL RECONSTRUCTION

5. *Which one of the following represents the arterial blood supply to the gracilis flap when used for perineal reconstruction?*

D. **Medial circumflex femoral artery**

There are a number of locoregional flaps commonly used for perineal reconstruction. These include the gracilis, the rectus abdominis, the posterior thigh, the Singapore, and anterolateral thigh flaps. The blood supplies to these flaps are as follows:

- Rectus flap = Deep inferior epigastric artery

- Posterior thigh flap = Profunda femoris artery perforators
- Singapore flap = Pudendal arteries (giving rise to labial arteries)
- Gracilis flap = Medial circumflex femoral artery
- Anterolateral thigh flap = Lateral circumflex femoral artery (most commonly the descending branch)[1-5]

REFERENCES

1. McCraw JB, Massey FM, Shanklin KD, Horton CE. Vaginal reconstruction with gracilis myocutaneous flaps. Plast Reconstr Surg 1976;58(2):176–183
2. Shibata D, Hyland W, Busse P, et al. Immediate reconstruction of the perineal wound with gracilis muscle flaps following abdominoperineal resection and intraoperative radiation therapy for recurrent carcinoma of the rectum. Ann Surg Oncol 1999;6(1):33–37
3. Westbom CM, Talbot SG. An algorithmic approach to perineal reconstruction. Plast Reconstr Surg Glob Open 2019;7(12):e2572
4. Coelho JAJ, McDermott FD, Cameron O, Smart NJ, Watts AM, Daniels IR. Single centre experience of bilateral gracilis flap perineal reconstruction following extra-levator abdominoperineal excision. Colorectal Dis 2019;21(8):910–916
5. Stein MJ, Karir A, Ramji M, et al. Surgical outcomes of VRAM versus gracilis flaps for the reconstruction of pelvic defects following oncologic resection*. J Plast Reconstr Aesthet Surg 2019;72(4):565–571

RECONSTRUCTION OF VAGINAL WALL DEFECTS

6. A patient is seen in clinic who is planned for wide resection of a vaginal wall tumor. It is expected that a 6 × 2 cm lateral wall defect will be created and will require reconstruction. *Which one of the following would be best suited to reconstructing this defect?*

   A. Singapore flap (pudendal thigh flap)

   The Singapore flap is a neurovascular island flap that is very useful for reconstructing vaginal wall defects where there is no significant dead space to fill (i.e., more superficial defects requiring relining and no dead space to fill). This flap receives its arterial supply from the labial arteries which, in turn, derive their supply from the pudendal arteries. Advantages of using this flap are that it is reliable, uses thin pliable tissue from adjacent to the defect (medial thigh/groin crease), has good reach to the vaginal area, and is sensate, and the donor can be closed directly leading to high levels of cosmesis and function. A limitation may be the inability to fill a large dead space, and in this scenario, a bulkier flap containing muscle would be indicated such as a rectus or gracilis. Where the defect dictates a larger thin pliable flap, bilateral Singapore flaps can be reliably used.[1,2]

   The posterior thigh flap receives its blood supply from the inferior gluteal artery, or profunda femoris perforators. This flap can be useful for pressure sore management or in perineal reconstruction where other flaps are not available.[3] The anterolateral thigh flap is a reliable flap to use for both regional reconstruction and as a free tissue transfer. It is supplied by the descending branch of the lateral circumflex femoral vessels but tends to be used as a second-line choice for perineal reconstruction. It is used as a pedicle flap for abdominal wall reconstruction and groin defects, for example, following complications of groin dissection. The gracilis flap is based on the medial circumflex femoral vessels. It could be used for this scenario but would be better reserved for defects which require dead space filling such as a rectovaginal fistula. Groin flaps are supplied by the superficial circumflex iliac vessels and can be used for many defects as free tissue transfers or some local defects. They tend not to be used for vaginal reconstruction.[4]

REFERENCES

1. Pope RJ, Brown RH, Chipungu E, Hollier LH Jr, Wilkinson JP. The use of Singapore flaps for vaginal reconstruction in women with vaginal stenosis with obstetric fistula: a surgical technique. BJOG 2018;125(6):751–756
2. Woods JE, Alter G, Meland B, Podratz K. Experience with vaginal reconstruction utilizing the modified Singapore flap. Plast Reconstr Surg 1992;90(2):270–274
3. Djedovic G, Morandi EM, Metzler J, et al. The posterior thigh flap for defect coverage of ischial pressure sores—a critical single-centre analysis. Int Wound J 2017;14(6):1154–1159
4. Hollenbeck ST, Toranto JD, Taylor BJ, et al. Perineal and lower extremity reconstruction. Plast Reconstr Surg 2011;128(5):551e–563e

RECONSTRUCTION OF THE PENIS

7. *When performing a phalloplasty which one of the following is true?*

   E. If the radial forearm flap is used, the antebrachial cutaneous nerves are used to provide sensation.

   Phalloplasty techniques are sometimes required after trauma, gender reassignment surgery, or resectional surgery for penile carcinoma. The tubed free radial forearm free flap is considered to be the gold standard. When this flap is used, sensation is provided by coapting the antebrachial cutaneous nerves in the flap to the pudendal nerve. Other options and considerations include the fibula flap. One advantage of this is that the bony construct eliminates the need for a secondary procedure to place a prosthesis. However, it does mean the phallus is permanently rigid. In addition to these free tissue options, pedicled rectus or lateral thigh flaps may be considered, although these flaps will add additional stages to the reconstruction.[1-3]

REFERENCES

1. Morrison SD, Shakir A, Vyas KS, Kirby J, Crane CN, Lee GK. Phalloplasty: a review of techniques and outcomes. Plast Reconstr Surg 2016;138(3):594–615
2. Schechter LS, Safa B. Introduction to phalloplasty. Clin Plast Surg 2018;45(3):387–389
3. Zaheer U, Granger A, Ortiz A, Terrell M, Loukas M, Schober J. The anatomy of free fibula osteoseptocutaneous flap in neophalloplasty in transgender surgery. Clin Anat 2018;31(2):169–174

DEFECT CLASSIFICATION IN VAGINAL DEFECTS

8. ***Which one of the following is true of the Cordeiro classification for vaginal defects?***

    E. It provides an algorithm for reconstructive approaches.

The Cordeiro classification is used for vaginal defects ad their reconstruction.

It categorizes defects according to whether they are partial or circumferential into types I or II, respectively. These subtypes are then further split into either A or B groupings. Type IA defect involves the anterior or lateral wall, whereas type IB involves the posterior wall.[1] Type IIA defects involve the upper two-thirds of the vagina whereas type IIB defects are total circumferential defects (**Fig. 64.2**):

- Type I: Partial
- Type IA: Partial defect of the anterior or lateral wall
- Type IB: Partial defect of the posterior wall
- Type 2: Circumferential
- Type IIA: Circumferential defects of the upper two-thirds of the vagina
- Type IIB: Circumferential total vaginal defects

The classification does not therefore consider the measured size, the cause, nor the chronicity of the defect. Furthermore, it does not consider the labia, perineum, or anus. The classification includes an algorithm which guides reconstruction as follows:

- Type IA defects: Singapore flaps or other perforator based fasciocutaneous flap
- Types IB and IIA: Pedicled rectus abdominis, can be rolled or tubed
- Type IIB: Bilateral pedicle gracilis or rectus abdominis flap
- Free jejunum has also been used for circumferential vaginal defects

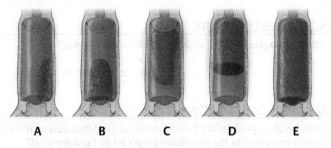

   A   **B**   **C**   **D**   **E**

Fig. 64.2 Vaginal defect classification.

REFERENCE

1. Cordeiro PG, Pusic AL, Disa JJ. A classification system and reconstructive algorithm for acquired vaginal defects. Plast Reconstr Surg 2002;110(4):1058–1065

65. Genitourinary Reconstruction

See *Essentials of Plastic Surgery*, third edition, pp. 880–889

EMBRYOLOGY OF THE GENITOURINARY (GU) SYSTEM

1. *When considering the embryology of the genitourinary (GU) tract, from which germinal layer does the external genitalia originate?*
   - A. Endoderm
   - B. Mesoderm
   - C. Ectoderm
   - D. Exoderm
   - E. Lameladerm

EMBRYOLOGY OF THE GENITOURINARY SYSTEM

2. *During embryonic development of the GU system, which one of the following is true?*
   - A. Male and female differentiation begins at the beginning of the second trimester.
   - B. The default process for fetal differentiation is development of male external genitalia.
   - C. The external genitalia for both sexes develop from the mesonephric ducts.
   - D. The interstitial cells of Leydig produce a testosterone analog that directs male development.
   - E. Müllerian inhibiting substance (MIS) activates the Sertoli cells to direct female differentiation.

VAGINAL DEFECTS

3. A young patient is seen in clinic with congenital absence of the vagina. *Which one of the following statements is correct?*
   - A. Her condition is caused by the congenital absence of the mesonephric ducts.
   - B. She will almost certainly have associated urinary abnormalities.
   - C. She will have a nonfunctional uterus, even if it is present.
   - D. Her diagnosis is synonymous with Mayer-Rokitansky-Küster-Hauser syndrome.
   - E. Her condition is relatively common, affecting 1 in 1000 live births.

MANAGEMENT OF VAGINAL AGENESIS

4. *Which one of the following techniques for vaginal reconstruction involves vulvoperineal fasciocutaneous flaps?*
   - A. McIndoe procedure
   - B. Málaga technique
   - C. Davydov procedure
   - D. Vecchietti procedure
   - E. Frank's technique

CLASSIFICATION OF VAGINAL WALL DEFECTS

5. *In the Cordeiro classification for vaginal defects, defects are classified by what?*
   - A. Size
   - B. Chronicity
   - C. Cause
   - D. Location
   - E. Infection risk

CLINICAL CASES OF VAGINAL RECONSTRUCTION

6. A patient has a partial lateral wall vaginal defect that requires surgical management. *What would be the most appropriate treatment option according to the algorithm proposed by Cordeiro et al?*
   - A. Split-thickness skin graft and prosthetic
   - B. Bilateral gracilis myocutaneous flaps
   - C. Lotus petal flap
   - D. Singapore flap
   - E. Rolled rectus abdominis flap

HYPOSPADIAS

7. A young baby with hypospadias is referred to you by the pediatric team. *Which one of the following statements is correct regarding this condition?*
   - A. The male urethral meatus is abnormally located dorsally between the corona and perineum.
   - B. The incidence ranges from 1:4000 to 1:6000 live births.
   - C. Surgical treatment usually begins after the fifth birthday.
   - D. The presence of chordee can cause a ventral penile curvature.
   - E. It least commonly involves the middle third of the penile shaft.

SURGICAL CORRECTION OF HYPOSPADIAS

8. *Which one of the following represents a single-stage technique used in hypospadias that involves a longitudinal incision through the midline epithelium of the urethral plate, which is subsequently tubularized?*
   A. Meatal advancement and glanuloplasty (MAGPI) technique
   B. Urethral advancement
   C. Snodgrass (tubular incised plate [TIP]) technique
   D. Flip-flap technique
   E. Bracka technique (full-thickness graft urethroplasty)

EPISPADIAS

9. A new patient with a diagnosis of epispadias is referred to you. *Which one of the following is a key feature occurring with this condition?*
   A. Bladder exstrophy
   B. Absent testes
   C. Undescended testes
   D. Duplication of the urethra
   E. A short, straight penis

PEYRONIE'S DISEASE

10. *Which one of the following statements is correct regarding Peyronie's disease?*
   A. 1 in 500 men aged 40–60 years are affected.
   B. Painful erections are the only presenting symptom.
   C. Almost all patients also have Dupuytren's disease.
   D. Surgical treatment involves plication or dermal grafting.
   E. Plication techniques are ideal if the penis is short.

TREATMENT OF PEYRONIE'S DISEASE

11. You are planning surgical correction of a penile curvature caused by Peyronie's disease. *Which one of the following is the abnormal tissue layer?*
   A. Skin
   B. Dartos fascia
   C. Buck's fascia
   D. Tunica albuginea
   E. Corpus cavernosa

FOURNIER'S GANGRENE

12. You are called to the operating room (OR) by a general surgical colleague to assist with a case of Fournier's gangrene. You jointly debride the perineal and scrotal region until healthy viable tissue remains. *What is the next step in management of this patient?*
   A. Local wound care with topical antibiotics and early reassessment
   B. Split-thickness skin graft reconstruction
   C. Direct closure if possible, with or without undermining
   D. Application of a negative-pressure dressing and early reassessment
   E. Local tissue flap wound closure over drains and minimal dressings to facilitate observation

Answers

EMBRYOLOGY OF THE GENITOURINARY (GU) SYSTEM

1. *When considering the embryology of the genitourinary (GU) tract, from which germinal layer does the external genitalia originate?*

   C. **Ectoderm**

There are three germinal components in the embryo, the endoderm, ectoderm, and mesoderm. Most structures within the GU system arise from the mesoderm. These include the nephric system, the Müllerian and Wolffian ducts, and the gonads. However, the external genitalia is formed from the ectodermal layer.

The endoderm forms the cloaca and membrane. In general terms, the ectoderm gives rise to the nervous system and skin, the mesoderm gives rise to muscle and other connective tissues, while the endoderm gives rise to the digestive system and other internal organs. Embryological knowledge helps to explain and understand congenital abnormalities of the GU system.[1,2]

REFERENCES

1. Moore KL, Persaud TV, Torchia MD, eds. The Developing Human: Clinically Oriented Embryology. 10th ed. Philadelphia: Elsevier; 2016
2. Sadler TW, ed. Langman's Medical Embryology. 13th ed. Philadelphia: Wolters Kluwer Health; 2014

EMBRYOLOGY OF THE GENITOURINARY SYSTEM

2. *During embryonic development of the GU system, which one of the following is true?*

   D. **The interstitial cells of Leydig produce a testosterone analog that directs male development.**

A developing fetus has the ability to develop into male or female and the default differentiation is female (not male) unless this process is interrupted. Male and female differentiation begins at week 6 in the first (not second) trimester. At this point, all fetuses have the precursors for both male and female differentiation. These are the mesonephric (Wolffian) and paramesonephric (Müllerian) ducts that develop into male and female reproductive structures, respectively. The differentiation into a male is influenced by Müllerian inhibiting substance (MIS) which is produced by (and not acts on) Sertoli cells. This substance causes paramesonephric duct regression. A testosterone analog is produced by the interstitial cells of Leydig, which serves to stimulate masculine development of the mesonephric ducts which then form the epididymis, vas deferens, and seminal vesicles. In the absence of MIS, the paramesonephric ducts develop into the upper vagina, fallopian tubes, and uterus.[1,2]

REFERENCES

1. Moore KL, Persaud TV, Torchia MD, eds. The Developing Human: Clinically Oriented Embryology. 10th ed. Philadelphia: Elsevier; 2016
2. Sadler TW, ed. Langman's Medical Embryology. 13th ed. Philadelphia: Wolters Kluwer Health; 2014

VAGINAL DEFECTS

3. A young patient is seen in clinic with congenital absence of the vagina. *Which one of the following statements is correct?*

   D. **Her diagnosis is synonymous with Mayer-Rokitanksy-Küster-Hauser syndrome.**

Mayer-Rokitansky-Küster-Hauser syndrome is a condition of vaginal agenesis, with or without an absent uterus. Although it is a rare condition, incidence varies from 1:4000 to 1:80,000. It is not caused by a congenital absence of the mesonephric duct. It may be caused by either a defect in the paramesonephric duct or fusion of the urogenital sinus with the paramesonephric duct. Associated urinary abnormalities such as ectopy, duplication, and agenesis occur in 25–50%, but not all patients. The clinical findings are of two types: a genetic female with or without a functioning uterus and absent vagina, who is otherwise normal; or a genetic female with or without a functioning uterus and absent vagina, who also has associated skeletal, urinary, or digestive system anomalies.[1–3]

REFERENCES

1. Chmel R Jr, Pastor Z, Mužík M, Brtnický T, Nováčková M. Syndrome Mayer-Rokitansky-Küster-Hauser-uterine and vaginal agenesis: current knowledge and therapeutic options. Ceska Gynekol 2019;84(5):386–392
2. Avino A, Răducu L, Tulin A, et al. Vaginal reconstruction in patients with Mayer-Rokitansky-Küster-Hauser syndrome—one centre experience. Medicina (Kaunas) 2020;56(7):327

3. Committee on Adolescent Health Care. ACOG Committee Opinion No. 728: Müllerian agenesis: diagnosis, management, and treatment. Obstet Gynecol 2018;131(1):e35–e42

MANAGEMENT OF VAGINAL AGENESIS

4. Which one of the following techniques for vaginal reconstruction involves vulvoperineal fasciocutaneous flaps?

   B. Málaga technique

   Several reconstructive options are available for vaginal agenesis.

   Málaga technique uses vulvoperineal fasciocutaneous flaps, whereas a McIndoe procedure involves a skin graft after dissection of a tunnel in the perineum, between the rectum and the bladder. This is associated with subsequent stricture and fistula formation. Vascularized bowel can be used to reconstruct the vagina but is associated with excessive mucus secretion and bleeding during intercourse. Other flaps have been described, including rectus abdominis, gracilis, and pudendal thigh flaps.[1-3] The Vecchietti procedure is performed laparoscopically and uses traction sutures to help form a neovagina.[4] The Davydov procedure combines transabdominal and transperineal approaches to dissect space between the bladder and rectum which is lined with peritoneal flaps to avoid skin grafts.[5] Vaginal agenesis can be associated with other anomalies, including imperforate hymen, double vagina, and an introitus obstruction. These can be treated surgically. An imperforate hymen can be treated with perforation and oversewing of the edges. A double vagina can be treated with a transverse incision of the septum. An obstructed introitus can be treated with a vaginoplasty. Frank's technique is a nonsurgical serial dilation procedure.[1-5]

REFERENCES

1. Gürlek A, Evans GR. The Málaga flap for vaginoplasty in the Mayer-Rokitansky-Kuster-Hauser syndrome: experience and early-term results. Plast Reconstr Surg 1997;100(3):806–809
2. Eldor L, Friedman JD. Reconstruction of congenital defects of the vagina. Semin Plast Surg 2011;25(2):142–147
3. Giraldo F. Cutaneous neovaginoplasty using the Málaga flap (vulvoperineal fasciocutaneous flap): a 12-year follow-up. Plast Reconstr Surg 2003;111(3):1249–1256
4. Nahas S, Yi J, Magrina J. Mayo Clinic experience with modified Vecchietti procedure for vaginal agenesis: it is easy, safe, and effective. J Minim Invasive Gynecol 2013;20(5):553
5. Takahashi K, Nakamura E, Suzuki S, et al. Laparoscopic Davydov procedure for the creation of a neovagina in patients with Mayer-Rokitansky-Kuster-Hauser syndrome: analysis of 7 cases. Tokai J Exp Clin Med 2016;41(2):81–87

CLASSIFICATION OF VAGINAL WALL DEFECTS

5. In the Cordeiro classification for vaginal defects, defects are classified by what?

   D. Location

   The Cordeiro classification[1] considers two main features of the vaginal defect: the location (e.g., anterior, posterior, or lateral wall) and the extent of the defect (for example, partial or circumferential defect). The actual size, cause, infection risk, and chronicity are not considered. The classification is as follows (**Fig. 65.1**):

   Type IA: Partial defect involving the anterior or lateral wall
   Type IIA: Circumferential defect involving the upper two-thirds
   Type IB: Partial defect involving the posterior wall
   Type IIB: Circumferential total defect

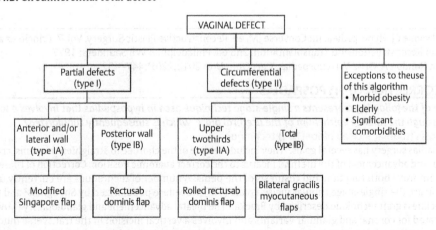

Fig. 65.1 Classification system and algorithm proposed by Cordeiro based on anatomic location.

REFERENCE

1. Cordeiro PG, Pusic AL, Disa JJ. A classification system and reconstructive algorithm for acquired vaginal defects. Plast Reconstr Surg 2002;110(4):1058–1065

CLINICAL CASES OF VAGINAL RECONSTRUCTION

6. A patient has a partial lateral wall vaginal defect that requires surgical management. *What would be the most appropriate treatment option according to the algorithm proposed by Cordeiro et al?*

   D. Singarore flap

   Vaginal and vulvar defects most commonly occur following oncologic resection, but may also be secondary to radiation therapy, infection, and trauma. Cordeiro has proposed a treatment algorithm in keeping with the classification system for vaginal wall defects. Partial defects (Type I) as in this case are either reconstructed with a modified Singapore flap, if they are anterior or lateral, or a rectus abdominis flap, if they are posterior.[1] The Singapore flap is a really useful and reliable flap for reconstruction of partial defects of the vagina. It is a fasciocutaneous flap based on the posterior labial arteries. The flap is designed running parallel to the medial thigh crease and raised deep-to-deep fascia from anterior to posterior. The flap can then be tunneled subcutaneously under the labia to be inset into the vaginal vault. The donor defect can be closed directly within the thigh crease with minimal cosmetic consequence. Although not part of the Cordeiro algorithm for partial posterior defects, the modified Singapore flap can be reliably used for these defects too. In larger defects, bilateral Singapore flaps may be combined.[2,3] Circumferential defects can be reconstructed using a rolled rectus abdominis flap, if the upper two-thirds are involved, or bilateral gracilis flaps if the defect is total (see **Fig. 65.1**).[4]

REFERENCES

1. Cordeiro PG, Pusic AL, Disa JJ. A classification system and reconstructive algorithm for acquired vaginal defects. Plast Reconstr Surg 2002;110(4):1058–1065
2. Pope RJ, Brown RH, Chipungu E, Hollier LH Jr, Wilkinson JP. The use of Singapore flaps for vaginal reconstruction in women with vaginal stenosis with obstetric fistula: a surgical technique. BJOG 2018;125(6):751–756
3. Woods JE, Alter G, Meland B, Podratz K. Experience with vaginal reconstruction utilizing the modified Singapore flap. Plast Reconstr Surg 1992;90(2):270–274
4. Cortinovis U, Sala L, Bonomi S, et al. Rectus abdominis myofascial flap for vaginal reconstruction after pelvic exenteration. Ann Plast Surg 2018;81(5):576–583

HYPOSPADIAS

7. A young baby with hypospadias is referred to you by the pediatric team. *Which one of the following statements is correct regarding this condition?*

   D. The presence of chordee can cause a ventral penile curvature.

   Hypospadias is a congenital abnormality of the male urogenital tract that occurs in 1:150 to 1:300 males. It involves a proximally based ventral meatus (occurring anywhere between the glans and perineum), a hooded prepuce, and chordee, which may cause a ventral curvature of the penis. Hypospadias can be subdivided based on the meatal position into proximal, middle, or distal third subtypes. Distal are most common (50%), and proximal are least common (20%). Treatment is surgical and is usually performed between 6 and 9 months of age.[1,2]

REFERENCES

1. Horton CE, Devine CJ. Hypospadiea. In: Converse JM, ed. Reconstructive Plastic Surgery, Vol. 7. Principles and Procedures in Correction Reconstruction and Transplantation. 2nd ed. Philadelphia: WB Saunders; 1977
2. Macedo A Jr, Rondon A, Ortiz V. Hypospadias. Curr Opin Urol 2012;22(6):447–452

SURGICAL CORRECTION OF HYPOSPADIAS

8. *Which one of the following represents a single-stage technique used in hypospadias that involves a longitudinal incision through the midline epithelium of the urethral plate, which is subsequently tubularized?*

   C. Snodgrass (tubular incised plate [TIP]) technique

   Hypospadias surgery has several goals.[1] They include release of the chordee to straighten the penis, creation of a new urethra, and advancement of the urethral meatus to the correct anatomic position. Correction of these abnormalities should improve both function and cosmesis of the penis. A number of techniques are currently used. The most common are the single-stage tubular incised plate (TIP) procedure popularized by Snodgrass[2] and the two-stage, full-thickness graft technique described by Bracka.[3] The meatal advancement and glanuloplasty (MAGPI) technique is indicated for coronal and glanular variants and involves a vertical incision in the transverse mucosal bar distal to the meatal opening, which is closed transversely. A glanuloplasty is achieved by midline approximation of the lateral glans wings. This technique does not treat chordee.

In the TIP procedure a longitudinal incision is made through the midline epithelium of the urethral plate, extending from the hypospadias meatus to the end of the glans. The plate is then tubularized on itself, and the dorsal prepuce is mobilized and used to cover the urethroplasty.

Mathieu[4] described the flip-flap technique, which transposes the proximal soft tissues over the urethral defect. Duckett[5] described the preputial flap. This involves an island flap from the prepuce to the ventral surface of the penis that is used as a tube for the urethra. The Cantwell-Ramsey, Young, and W-flap techniques are used for the correction of epispadias rather than hypospadias.

REFERENCES

1. Baskin LS, Ebbers MB. Hypospadias: anatomy, etiology, and technique. J Pediatr Surg 2006;41(3):463–472
2. Snodgrass W. Tubularized, incised plate urethroplasty for distal hypospadias. J Urol 1994;151(2):464–465
3. Bracka A. The role of two-stage repair in modern hypospadiology. Indian J Urol 2008;24(2):210–218
4. Mathieu P. Treatment in a time of the balanic and juxta-balanic hypospadias. J Chir (Paris) 1932;39:481–484
5. Duckett JW Jr. Transverse preputial island flap technique for repair of severe hypospadias. Urol Clin North Am 1980;7(2):423–430

EPISPADIAS

9. A new patient with a diagnosis of epispadias is referred to you. *Which one of the following is a key feature occurring with this condition?*

A. Bladder exstrophy

Epispadias is a severe congenital anomaly involving the penis, which is typically short, wide, and stubby with clefting and flattening of the glans and a dorsally placed urethral meatus. The penis usually has a dorsal curvature. It usually occurs in conjunction with bladder exstrophy, but the other abnormalities listed are not specifically associated with this condition. Epispadias occurs in 1 in 30,000 males (compared with 1 in 350 for hypospadias). Principles of reconstruction are similar in each condition but with specific techniques described for epispadias.[1,2]

REFERENCES

1. Dunn EA, Kasprenski M, Facciola J, et al. Anatomy of classic bladder exstrophy: MRI findings and surgical correlation. Curr Urol Rep 2019;20(9):48
2. Frimberger D. Diagnosis and management of epispadias. Semin Pediatr Surg 2011;20(2):85–90

PEYRONIE'S DISEASE

10. *Which one of the following statements is correct regarding Peyronie's disease?*

D. Surgical treatment involves plication or dermal grafting.

Peyronie's disease is a fibroproliferative condition of unknown cause that affects the penile shaft. It results in abnormal curvature and painful erections and affects approximately 1 in 100 men between 40 and 60 years of age. Although plication techniques are regularly used, they tend to leave a 20% reduction in erect length, which can be unacceptable to men whose penis was short preoperatively.[1–3]

REFERENCES

1. Levine LA, Burnett AL. Standard operating procedures for Peyronie's disease. J Sex Med 2013;10(1):230–244
2. Ostrowski KA, Gannon JR, Walsh TJ. A review of the epidemiology and treatment of Peyronie's disease. Res Rep Urol 2016;8:61–70
3. Miner MM, Seftel AD. Peyronie's disease: epidemiology, diagnosis, and management. Curr Med Res Opin 2014;30(1): 113–120

TREATMENT OF PEYRONIE'S DISEASE

11. You are planning surgical correction of a penile curvature caused by Peyronie's disease. *Which one of the following is the abnormal tissue layer?*

D. Tunica albuginea

Peyronie's disease is a localized penile disorder of collagen primarily involving the tunica albuginea. The penis has a number of key layers. From superficial to deep, these are the skin, Dartos fascia, and then Buck's fascia. The tunica albuginea lies deeper still and surrounds each corpus cavernosa which are the erectile components of the penile shaft. The deep arteries lie within this tissue. There are two dorsal veins, one deep to skin and the other deep to the deep fascia (Buck's). The dorsal arteries and nerves are also found in this layer. The urethra is located in the midline and is covered by the corpus spongiosum which is also covered by deep fascia (Buck's). Knowledge of these layers is important in penile surgery and understanding techniques for hypospadias, epispadias, and Peyronie's disease. About 10% of patients also have Dupuytren's contracture of the palmar fascia, and trials of collagenase therapy have been undertaken as an alternative to surgery in this condition.[1–4]

REFERENCES

1. Levine LA, Burnett AL. Standard operating procedures for Peyronie's disease. J Sex Med 2013;10(1):230–244

2. Ostrowski KA, Gannon JR, Walsh TJ. A review of the epidemiology and treatment of Peyronie's disease. Res Rep Urol 2016;8:61–70

3. Gelbard M, Goldstein I, Hellstrom WJ, et al. Clinical efficacy, safety and tolerability of collagenase Clostridium histolyticum for the treatment of Peyronie disease in 2 large double-blind, randomized, placebo controlled phase 3 studies. J Urol 2013;190(1):199–207

4. Gholami SS, Gonzalez-Cadavid NF, Lin CS, Rajfer J, Lue TF. Peyronie's disease: a review. J Urol 2003;169(4):1234–1241

FOURNIER'S GANGRENE

12. You are called to the operating room (OR) by a general surgical colleague to assist with a case of Fournier's gangrene. You jointly debride the perineal and scrotal region until healthy viable tissue remains. *What is the next step in management of this patient?*

A. Local wound care with topical antibiotics and early reassessment
Fournier's gangrene is a potentially life-threatening, rapidly progressing, soft tissue infection within the spectrum of necrotizing fasciitis. Patients need urgent resuscitation, intravenous antibiotics, and early debridement in the OR, as in this case. Following initial debridement, the wounds should be temporized with simple dressings with or without topical antibiotics. Sometimes it is necessary to place the testes in temporary thigh pouches or suture them together to stop retraction. The wounds should then be revisited in the OR within 24 hours, or sooner if the patient remains unwell or has visible spread of continued infection/necrosis. There is no justification for attempting to close the wounds at this stage or apply a negative-pressure dressing. A negative-pressure dressing can, however, be very useful beyond the second assessment to manage wound exudate and reduce the defect size, providing that infection is controlled and a satisfactory seal can be achieved. Reconstruction should only be initiated once the infection has completely resolved. Skin grafts are usually preferred for the lower abdomen and groin rather than attempts at direct closure, with or without local tissue flaps or undermining.[1–3]

REFERENCES

1. Hagedorn JC, Wessells H. A contemporary update on Fournier's gangrene. Nat Rev Urol 2017;14(4):205–214

2. Singh A, Ahmed K, Aydin A, Khan MS, Dasgupta P. Fournier's gangrene. A clinical review. Arch Ital Urol Androl 2016;88(3):157–164

3. Eke N. Fournier's gangrene: a review of 1726 cases. Br J Surg 2000;87(6):718–728

66. Pressure Sores

See *Essentials of Plastic Surgery*, third edition, pp. 890–901

SITES OF PRESSURE SORE DEVELOPMENT

1. **What is the most common anatomic site for development of a pressure sore?**
   A. Ischial tuberosity
   B. Greater trochanter
   C. Scalp
   D. Sacrum
   E. Heel

ETIOLOGIC FACTORS IN PRESSURE SORES

2. **Which one of the following is an extrinsic factor in development of pressure sores?**
   A. Ischemia
   B. Infection
   C. Malnutrition
   D. Smoking
   E. Moisture

THE BRADEN SCALE

3. **When considering a patient's risk of pressure sore development, which one of the following scores indicates the highest risk on the Braden scale?**
   A. 0
   B. 3
   C. 6
   D. 9
   E. 12

PRESSURE SORE STAGING

4. A patient has a pressure sore on the left heel measuring 5 cm. It involves full-thickness tissue loss to, but not through, fascia or bone. **What stage is this sore?**
   A. Stage I
   B. Stage II
   C. Stage III
   D. Stage IV
   E. Unstageable

PRESSURE VALUES RECORDED IN PRESSURE SORE STUDIES

5. **What is the external pressure measured at the ischial tuberosity of a patient who is sitting with feet supported according to the scientific literature?**
   A. 12 mm Hg
   B. 32 mm Hg
   C. 45 mm Hg
   D. 80 mm Hg
   E. 100 mm Hg

PREVENTION OF PRESSURE SORES

6. **Which one of the following is aimed at treating pressure sores on the basis of Kosiak's principle?**
   A. Meticulous skin care
   B. Care with transfers
   C. Minimization of spasticity
   D. Regular turning
   E. Smoking cessation

ASSESSMENT OF PRESSURE SORES

7. A patient is referred to you with a grade IV pressure sore in the sacral region. The patient has multiple comorbidities and sepsis. Osteomyelitis is suspected. **Which one of the following tests is the benchmark for diagnosis?**
   A. Culture swab
   B. Contrast CT
   C. MRI
   D. Bone biopsy
   E. Plain radiographs

ASSESSMENT OF OSTEOMYELITIS IN PRESSURE SORES

8. A patient requires imaging for suspected osteomyelitis from a trochanteric pressure sore. *What is the sensitivity of MRI in detecting osteomyelitis?*
   A. 25%
   B. 56%
   C. 68%
   D. 80%
   E. 97%

DAKIN'S SOLUTION

9. You are reviewing a patient who has a trochanteric pressure sore, and the nurse suggests cleaning the wound with Dakin's solution. You have not used this before and decide to research the product before you proceed. *Which one of the following statements is correct regarding Dakin's solution?*
   A. It contains silver sulfadiazine.
   B. It is nontoxic to healthy tissue.
   C. It should be used in undiluted form.
   D. Treatment duration should be limited to 14 days.
   E. It is useful where *Pseudomonas* is suspected.

PRESSURE SORE SURGERY

10. *When performing surgical debridement and reconstruction of grade IV pressure sores, which one of the following should generally be avoided?*
    A. Methylene blue application
    B. Tumescent infiltration
    C. Excision of unaffected bony prominences
    D. Obliteration of dead space
    E. Flap design to allow re-advancement

RECURRENCE RATES AFTER PRESSURE SORE RECONSTRUCTION

11. *Which one of the following statements is correct regarding recurrence rates after pressure sore reconstruction?*
    A. Myocutaneous flaps have a higher ulcer recurrence rate than fasciocutaneous flaps.
    B. Paraplegic patients have a 30% risk of recurrence at the same site over 18 months.
    C. Nonparaplegic patients have a higher rate of recurrence than paraplegic patients.
    D. Myocutaneous and fasciocutaneous reconstructions have comparable ulcer recurrence rates in many series.
    E. Young posttraumatic paraplegic patients generally heal better than other subgroups.

Answers

SITES OF PRESSURE SORE DEVELOPMENT

1. What is the most common anatomic site for development of a pressure sore?

D. Sacrum

The site of pressure sore development will depend on several factors such as patient's mobility, body mass index, positioning, and local anatomy. However, the most common overall site is the sacrum (28–36%). This occurs most frequently in bed-bound patients, particularly those with spinal cord injuries and other individuals such as frail, elderly patients with decreased mobility who spend long periods of time in a lying position. Other common anatomic sites are the ischial tuberosity (17–20%) in seated patients who spend long periods in wheelchairs, for example. The heels are also quite commonly affected (9%) in bed-bound patients lying supine. The greater trochanter is at risk in individuals lying in a lateral position for extended periods. The posterior scalp (occiput) is at risk for patients in intensive care for extended periods due to immobility.[1]

REFERENCE

1. Ricci JA, Bayer LR, Orgill DP. Evidence-based medicine: the evaluation and treatment of pressure injuries. Plast Reconstr Surg 2017;139(1):275e–286e

ETIOLOGIC FACTORS IN PRESSURE SORES

2. Which one of the following is an extrinsic factor in development of pressure sores?

E. Moisture

Causal factors in the development of pressure sores can be classified as intrinsic or extrinsic. Key extrinsic factors are the forces of shear, friction, and pressure (compression). However, moisture is also an extrinsic factor, and this increases the risk of pressure sore development in incontinent patients. Intrinsic factors include ischemia, infection, sensory loss, vascular disease, altered consciousness, decreased autonomic control, anemia, and malnutrition. Management of pressure sores is based on addressing both intrinsic and extrinsic factors.[1–4]

REFERENCES

1. Janis JE, Kenkel JM. Pressure sores. Sel Read Plast Surg 2003;9(39):1–42
2. VanGilder C, Amlung S, Harrison P, Meyer S. Results of the 2008–2009 International Pressure Ulcer Prevalence Survey and a 3-year, acute care, unit-specific analysis. Ostomy Wound Manage 2009;55(11):39–45
3. O'Sullivan KL, Engrav LH, Maier RV, Pilcher SL, Isik FF, Copass MK. Pressure sores in the acute trauma patient: incidence and causes. J Trauma 1997;42(2):276–278
4. Enis JE, Sarmiento A. The pathophysiology and management of pressure sores. Orthop Rev 1973;2:25–34

THE BRADEN SCALE

3. When considering a patient's risk of pressure sore development, which one of the following scores indicates the highest risk on the Braden scale?

C. 6

A number of scoring systems have been created to assess the risk of developing a pressure sore. The Braden scale is one example. It has subscales, including sensory perception, skin moisture, activity, mobility, nutrition, and local mechanical forces that act on wounds. Composite scores range from 6 to 23, with lower scores indicating an increased risk for pressure sore development.[1,2] Other systems include the Waterlow score, which places patients in different risk categories (low, medium, and high) based on factors such as body mass index (BMI), skin type, sex, malnutrition, continence, mobility, and age.[3]

Although the assessment and scoring of a pressure sore are typically undertaken by the nursing team, understanding the workings of these systems is highly relevant to the surgical team both for delivery of high-quality, safe patient care and for the preparation for clinical exams. Assessment of pressure areas now forms part of the surgical check listing process before starting and after completing surgery. This is particularly important in longer procedures and in high-risk patients.

REFERENCES

1. Chen HL, Cao YJ, Zhang W, Wang J, Huai BS. Braden scale (ALB) for assessing pressure ulcer risk in hospital patients: a validity and reliability study. Appl Nurs Res 2017;33:169–174

2. Bergstrom N, Braden BJ. Predictive validity of the Braden Scale among Black and White subjects. Nurs Res 2002;51(6):398–403
3. Waterlow J. Pressure sores: a risk assessment card. Nurs Times 1985;81(48):49–55

PRESSURE SORE STAGING

4. A patient has a pressure sore on the left heel measuring 5 cm. It involves full-thickness tissue loss to, but not through, fascia or bone. *What stage is this sore?*

   C. Stage III

      Pressure sores are graded into one of four stages according to the National Pressure Ulcer Advisory Panel. Stage I involves nonblanching erythema of intact skin. Stage II is a partial-thickness defect presenting as a blister. Stage III is a full-thickness skin defect, as in this case, that does not go through fascia. Stage IV includes underlying bone, muscle, tendon, or joint capsule. In cases in which full assessment is not possible clinically (e.g., soft tissue cover obscures deeper structures) two alternative grades can be used: unstageable and suspected deep.[1] Pressure sores evolve over time, so they should be repeatedly inspected during the early stages to prevent under-staging because of overlooked deep tissue damage (**Fig. 66.1**). Assessment of pressure areas is now part of the World Health Organization (WHO) checklist during surgery, so all surgeons should be regularly involved in this assessment. Being able to reliably assess grade of the pressure sore in the context of a patient's overall health is important with respect to selecting the best management plan for them.[1–3]

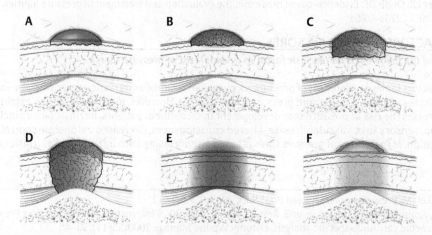

Fig. 66.1 National Pressure Ulcer Advisory Panel stages. *A,* Stage I. *B,* Stage II. *C,* Stage III. *D,* Stage IV. *E,* Unstageable. *F,* Suspected deep tissue injury. (Adapted from National Pressure Ulcer Advisory Panel (NPUAP). Pressure ulcer stages/categories 2007. Available at http://www.npuap.org/resources/educational-and-clinical-resources/.)

REFERENCES

1. National Pressure Ulcer Advisory Panel (NPUAP). Pressure Ulcer Stages/Categories 2007. Available at http://www.npuap.org/resources/educational-and-clinical-resources/npuap-pressure-ulcer-stagescat-egories/
2. Edsberg LE, Black JM, Goldberg M, McNichol L, Moore L, Sieggreen M. Revised National Pressure Ulcer Advisory Panel pressure injury staging system: revised pressure injury staging system. J Wound Ostomy Continence Nurs 2016;43(6):585–597
3. Spear M. Pressure ulcer staging-revisited. Plast Surg Nurs 2013;33(4):192–194

PRESSURE VALUES RECORDED IN PRESSURE SORE STUDIES

5. *What is the external pressure measured at the ischial tuberosity of a patient who is sitting with feet supported according to the scientific literature?*

   E. 100 mm Hg

      Capillary blood pressure ranges from 12 mm Hg at the venous end to 32 mm Hg at the arterial end. If external pressure exceeds the capillary opening pressure, then perfusion is reduced. For short time periods, this will have no detrimental effect. However, if it is continued for an extended time, ischemia and tissue damage will occur. An inverse relationship exists between the amount of pressure and the duration required to cause pressure necrosis.

      Animal studies have shown that a pressure of 70 mm Hg applied over 2 hours was sufficient to cause pathologic changes in dogs. In a porcine model, pressure of 100 mm Hg for only 10 minutes caused muscle necrosis. Changes in the skin occur later than those in muscle, suggesting that pressure sores begin deep and the skin changes are late signs. Lindan et al[1] performed a landmark study in 1965. They observed pressures of up to 60 mm Hg in the sacral area of humans who were in a supine position (**Fig. 66.2**). Pressure in the heels, occiput, and buttocks was approximately 40 mm Hg. Measurements of patients in the seated position were greatest at the ischial tuberosities and were in the order of 100 mm Hg. This helps explain the high incidence of ischial pressure sores.

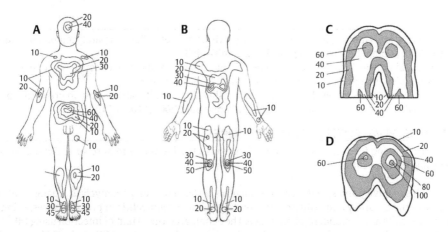

Fig. 66.2 Pressure-distribution maps (in mm Hg) of a male figure. *A,* Supine. *B,* Prone. *C,* Sitting with feet hanging freely. *D,* Sitting with feet supported. (Adapted from Lindan O, Greenway RM, Piazza JM. Pressure distribution on the surface of the human body. I. Evaluation in lying and sitting positions using a bed of springs and nails. Arch Phys Med Rehabil 46:378, 1965.)

REFERENCE

1. Lindan O, Greenway RM, Piazza JM. Pressure distribution on the surface of the human body. I. Evaluation in lying and sitting positions using a "bed of springs and nails." Arch Phys Med Rehabil 1965;46:378–385

PREVENTION OF PRESSURE SORES

6. *Which one of the following is aimed at treating pressure sores on the basis of Kosiak's principle?*

   D. Regular turning

     All of the choices are vital components of prevention and nonsurgical management of pressure sores. However, according to the Kosiak's principle, tissues tolerate increased pressure if it is interspersed with pressure-free periods.[1] Seated patients should therefore be lifted every 10 minutes for 10 seconds, and supine patients should be turned every 2 hours.

     Kosiak[2] first demonstrated the principle in 1959 by applying varying loads to the trochanters and ischial tuberosities of dogs. He found that high loads for short periods or low loads for long periods caused pressure ulcers. He later used a rat model to show that removal of pressure for short periods of time provided relief and resulted in less tissue damage.[3] Tissues are more susceptible to a constant load as opposed to an intermittent load.

     Similarly, Dinsdale[4] showed prevention of injury when pressure was relieved for short durations, for example, 5 minutes of relief from a pressure of more than 400 mm Hg.

REFERENCES

1. Kosiak M, Kubicek WG, Olson M, Danz JN, Kottke FJ. Evaluation of pressure as a factor in the production of ischial ulcers. Arch Phys Med Rehabil 1958;39(10):623–629
2. Kosiak M. Etiology and pathology of ischemic ulcers. Arch Phys Med Rehabil 1959;40(2):62–69
3. Kosiak M. Etiology of decubitus ulcers. Arch Phys Med Rehabil 1961;42:19–29
4. Dinsdale SM. Decubitus ulcers: role of pressure and friction in causation. Arch Phys Med Rehabil 1974;55(4):147–152

ASSESSMENT OF PRESSURE SORES

7. A patient is referred to you with a grade IV pressure sore in the sacral region. The patient has multiple comorbidities and sepsis. Osteomyelitis is suspected. *Which one of the following tests is the benchmark for diagnosis?*

   D. Bone biopsy

     The benchmark test for diagnosis of osteomyelitis within a deep pressure area is a positive bone biopsy. However, this is not always technically possible unless the patient is in the OR. Routine microbiology swabs from pressure sores will show growth of multiple organisms and interpretation of these results needs to be combined with a clinical evaluation to assess for evidence of local infection. The best noninvasive option for patients with suspected osteomyelitis would be an MRI. Plain radiographs and CT may be useful but are less accurate. The clinical importance of osteomyelitis is that if the extent is unknown or underappreciated, then any reconstruction is destined to fail.[1-3]

REFERENCES

1. Huang AB, Schweitzer ME, Hume E, Batte WG. Osteomyelitis of the pelvis/hips in paralyzed patients: accuracy and clinical utility of MRI. J Comput Assist Tomogr 1998;22(3):437–443
2. Larson DL, Gilstrap J, Simonelic K, Carrera GF. Is there a simple, definitive, and cost-effective way to diagnose osteomyelitis in the pressure ulcer patient? Plast Reconstr Surg 2011;127(2):670–676
3. Han H, Lewis VL Jr, Wiedrich TA, Patel PK. The value of Jamshidi core needle bone biopsy in predicting postoperative osteomyelitis in grade IV pressure ulcer patients. Plast Reconstr Surg 2002;110(1):118–122

ASSESSMENT OF OSTEOMYELITIS IN PRESSURE SORES

8. A patient requires imaging for suspected osteomyelitis from a trochanteric pressure sore. *What is the sensitivity of MRI in detecting osteomyelitis?*

E. 97%

MRI has a high sensitivity and specificity for evaluation of the extent of osteomyelitis. Huang et al[1] conducted a study to assess the accuracy and utility of MRI for diagnosing osteomyelitis in pressure sores, using histologic/microbiologic results as the standard of reference. They compared the extent of infection using MRI and surgical margins. The overall accuracy of MRI was high with only one false-negative MRI study. MRI for the diagnosis of osteomyelitis yielded a sensitivity of 97% and a specificity of 89%.

A total of 21 patients underwent limited surgical resection guided by MRI findings in which only the enhancing area was resected. Osteomyelitis recurred only once, at the surgical margins. The authors concluded that MRI is accurate in the diagnosis of osteomyelitis and associated soft tissue abnormalities in spinal cord–injured patients. It can delineate the extent of infection and help to guide limited surgical resection and preserve viable tissue.

REFERENCE

1. Huang AB, Schweitzer ME, Hume E, Batte WG. Osteomyelitis of the pelvis/hips in paralyzed patients: accuracy and clinical utility of MRI. J Comput Assist Tomogr 1998;22(3):437–443

DAKIN'S SOLUTION

9. You are reviewing a patient who has a trochanteric pressure sore, and the nurse suggests cleaning the wound with Dakin's solution. You have not used this before and decide to research the product before you proceed. *Which one of the following statements is correct regarding Dakin's solution?*

E. It is useful where Pseudomonas is suspected.

Dakin's solution can be useful for cleaning wounds such as pressure sores that have *Pseudomonas* growth, but should be used cautiously and for limited periods because of its toxicity to healthy tissue. It contains sodium hypochlorite and boric acid, not silver sulfadiazine. It should be diluted to quarter strength and used for a few days only (not 14 days). Wounds with *Pseudomonas* typically appear green and have a characteristic malodor. Other popular dressings for pressure sores include hydrogels if there is black eschar, hydrocolloids if there is granulation tissue, and an alginate and absorbent foam in wounds with high exudate. Manuka honey has also become popular for chemical debridement of pressure sores and this works in a number of ways which include antibacterial as well as debriding. The use of a dressing containing silver is particularly useful in cases of *Pseudomonas* infection. Irrespective of dressing used, the propensity for a pressure sore to heal will be dependent on the vascularity of the wound itself and removal of the instigating cause.[1-3]

REFERENCES

1. Ueno CM, Mullens CL, Luh JH, Wooden WA. Historical review of Dakin's solution applications. J Plast Reconstr Aesthet Surg 2018;71(9):e49–e55
2. Norman G, Dumville JC, Moore ZE, Tanner J, Christie J, Goto S. Antibiotics and antiseptics for pressure ulcers. Cochrane Database Syst Rev 2016;4(4):CD011586
3. Chuangsuwanich A, Chortrakarnkij P, Kangwanpoom J. Cost-effectiveness analysis in comparing alginate silver dressing with silver zinc sulfadiazine cream in the treatment of pressure ulcers. Arch Plast Surg 2013;40(5):589–596

PRESSURE SORE SURGERY

10. When performing surgical debridement and reconstruction of grade IV pressure sores, which one of the following should generally be avoided?

    C. Excision of unaffected bony prominences

        Although any nonviable or infected bone should be fully debrided, healthy bony prominences should not be routinely excised. If healthy bony prominences are excised to relieve pressure at the site of the sore, this can have unintended consequences from pressure transfer to other sites. An example is perineal ulceration following over-resection of the ischial tuberosity.

        Coating the bursa with methylene blue dye before excision can help verify that all bursal tissue has been completely excised. Infiltration of the peribursal area with a liposuction solution can help reduce/control bleeding during debridement. During reconstruction, any dead space must be obliterated with the chosen flap. Flaps should always be designed to allow for further revision surgery. For this reason, advancement and rotation flaps are generally preferred.[1-3]

REFERENCES

1. Cushing CA, Phillips LG. Evidence-based medicine: pressure sores. Plast Reconstr Surg 2013;132(6):1720–1732
2. Conway H, Griffith BH. Plastic surgery for closure of decubitus ulcers in patients with paraplegia; based on experience with 1,000 cases. Am J Surg 1956;91(6):946–975
3. Larson DL, Hudak KA, Waring WP, Orr MR, Simonelic K. Protocol management of late-stage pressure ulcers: a 5-year retrospective study of 101 consecutive patients with 179 ulcers. Plast Reconstr Surg 2012;129(4):897–904

RECURRENCE RATES AFTER PRESSURE SORE RECONSTRUCTION

11. Which one of the following statements is correct regarding recurrence rates after pressure sore reconstruction?

    D. Myocutaneous and fasciocutaneous reconstructions have comparable ulcer recurrence rates in many series.

        Several authors have assessed recurrence rates after reconstruction of pressure sores. The overall rates range from 19% at 3.7 years (Kierney et al[1]) to 69% at 9.3 months (Disa et al[2]). Disa et al indicated that young posttraumatic paraplegics had a particularly high recurrence rate of 79% at 11 months.

        In a meta-analysis of pressure sore recurrence rates from 55 studies, Sameem et al[3] identified similar recurrence rates with myocutaneous (8.9%) and fasciocutaneous (11.2%) flaps. Perforator flaps appeared to fare best overall with a 5.6% recurrence rate, but the differences between the three flap types were not statistically significant.

REFERENCES

1. Kierney PC, Engrav LH, Isik FF, Esselman PC, Cardenas DD, Rand RP. Results of 268 pressure sores in 158 patients managed jointly by plastic surgery and rehabilitation medicine. Plast Reconstr Surg 1998;102(3):765–772
2. Disa JJ, Carlton JM, Goldberg NH. Efficacy of operative cure in pressure sore patients. Plast Reconstr Surg 1992;89(2): 272–278
3. Sameem M, Au M, Wood T, Farrokhyar F, Mahoney J. A systematic review of complication and recurrence rates of musculocutaneous, fasciocutaneous, and perforator-based flaps for treatment of pressure sores. Plast Reconstr Surg 2012;130(1):67e–77e

67. Lower Extremity Reconstruction

See *Essentials of Plastic Surgery*, third edition, pp. 902–921

GUSTILO CLASSIFICATION IN LOWER LIMB TRAUMA

1. *A patient presents with an open tibial fracture after a motor vehicle accident. Surgery reveals extensive soft tissue damage involving skin and muscle with associated periosteal stripping of bone. How should this injury be correctly described using the Gustilo-Anderson classification system?*
   A. Gustilo I
   B. Gustilo IIa
   C. Gustilo IIb
   D. Gustilo IIIb
   E. Gustilo IIIc

CLASSIFICATION OF OPEN TIBIAL FRACTURES

2. *What is the key difference between a Gustilo type I and type II open lower limb injury?*
   A. The degree of wound contamination
   B. The presence or absence of a vascular injury
   C. The degree of fracture comminution
   D. The measured wound size
   E. The location of soft tissue injury

BYRD CLASSIFICATION OF OPEN TIBIAL FRACTURES

3. *Which one of the following is considered in the Byrd classification system but not in the Gustilo classification?*
   A. The degree of force involved to sustain the injury
   B. The size of the soft tissue defect
   C. The presence of a vascular injury
   D. The chronicity of the injury
   E. The degree of skin and soft tissue loss

PROGNOSTIC FACTORS IN OPEN TIBIAL FRACTURES

4. *Which one of the following has no prognostic significance following an open tibial shaft fracture?*
   A. Comminution
   B. Infection
   C. Concomitant fibula fracture
   D. Bone loss
   E. Soft tissue injury

ORDER OF ACUTE TREATMENT IN LOWER LIMB OPEN FRACTURES

5. *After initial resuscitation measures, which one of the following should generally be performed first when managing an open tibial fracture?*
   A. Fasciotomies
   B. Soft tissue wound debridement
   C. Arterial repair
   D. Fracture reduction and stabilization
   E. Nerve repair

TIMING OF SOFT TISSUE RECONSTRUCTION IN OPEN FRACTURES OF THE LOWER LIMB

6. *Following adequate debridement and external fixator stabilization of a grade IIIb open tibial fracture, when should definitive free flap reconstruction be performed based on current evidence?*
   A. At the same time
   B. Within 24 hours
   C. Within the first week
   D. After 2 weeks
   E. Once bone healing is complete

BLOOD SUPPLY TO THE TIBIA

7. *Which one of the following statements is correct regarding tibial blood supply?*
   A. The periosteal circulation derives from the metaphyseal artery.
   B. The inner third of the cortex is supplied by the endosteal circulation.
   C. The outer two-thirds of the cortex are supplied by the periosteal vessels.
   D. Endosteal circulation derives from the nutrient artery on the posterior tibia.
   E. When a long bone is fractured, the nutrient artery is disrupted and the entire distal fragment becomes avascular.

BONY RECONSTRUCTION OF THE LOWER LIMB

8. A 60-year-old man sustains an open midshaft tibial fracture with extensive soft tissue loss after being hit by a car. Exploration in the operating room (OR) shows a segment of nonviable tibia measuring 8 cm, which is removed. Following debridement, a soft tissue defect measuring 16 by 8 cm is planned for reconstruction using an anterolateral thigh flap with vastus lateralis. A spanning external fixation device is used to temporarily stabilize the fracture and a longer term plan is made for bone transport with distraction osteogenesis. *Which one of the following is true of the distraction process?*
   A. After the device is applied, distraction is postponed for 1 month.
   B. Distraction is commonly performed at a rate of 3 mm per day.
   C. Blood transfusions are commonly required intraoperatively.
   D. A corticotomy is performed outside the zone of injury before distraction.
   E. Distraction is usually reserved for bone defects larger than 20 cm.

LOCAL FLAP OPTIONS IN LOWER LIMB RECONSTRUCTION

9. *Which one of the following statements is correct regarding reconstruction of lower limb soft tissue defects in physically active patients?*
   A. An extensor digitorum longus flap is supplied by the peroneal vessels, and the use of this flap can result in permanent loss of toe extension.
   B. A flexor digitorum longus flap can be used for small to medium size midshaft defects but leads to a significant functional loss.
   C. A flexor hallucis longus flap should not be used in athletes for middle third defects because of its important role in running.
   D. Sacrifice of the medial head of gastrocnemius to reconstruct anterior knee defects is preferred to the lateral head because the functional deficit is less.
   E. A proximally based soleus flap can be used to cover the tibial tuberosity but leaves a functional deficit.

RECONSTRUCTIVE OPTIONS FOR THE LOWER LIMB

10. A patient has a 10 cm long by 15 cm wide wound in the anterolateral thigh with exposed muscle belly and an underlying femoral fracture. No nerve, bone, or vessel exposure is noted. *How best should this be managed surgically?*
   A. Split-thickness skin graft (STSG)
   B. Direct closure
   C. Anterolateral thigh flap
   D. Free gracilis and STSG
   E. Free latissimus dorsi and STSG

RECONSTRUCTIVE OPTIONS FOR THE LOWER LIMB

11. A patient has a 5 by 8 cm anterior knee wound with an exposed total knee replacement prosthesis. *How best should this be managed surgically?*
   A. Split-thickness skin graft (STSG)
   B. Medial gastrocnemius and STSG
   C. Lateral gastrocnemius and STSG
   D. Free gracilis and STSG
   E. Free latissimus dorsi and STSG

RECONSTRUCTIVE OPTIONS FOR THE LOWER LIMB

12. A patient has a 3 by 5 cm distal tibial wound with exposed bone over the medial malleolus and posterior tibial vessels. *How best should this be managed surgically?*
   A. Split-thickness skin graft (STSG)
   B. Medial gastrocnemius and STSG
   C. Proximally based soleus and STSG
   D. Free gracilis and STSG
   E. Free latissimus dorsi and STSG

RECONSTRUCTION OF TIBIAL AND KNEE SOFT TISSUE DEFECTS

13. You have a patient with a full-thickness soft tissue defect over the proximal tibia with exposure of the tibial tuberosity measuring 7 by 4 cm. The wound is clean and ready for definitive reconstruction. *Which one of the following options is best for coverage of this defect?*
   A. Distally based on soleus flap
   B. Medial gastrocnemius flap
   C. Lateral gastrocnemius flap
   D. Bipedicled tibialis anterior flap
   E. Reverse sural artery flap

COMPARTMENT SYNDROME

14. *Which one of the following is true of compartment syndrome in the lower limb?*
    A. It occurs in less than 1% of tibial shaft fractures.
    B. An open tibial fracture usually decompresses the anterior compartment.
    C. Loss of distal pulses is a reliable early sign suggestive of compartment syndrome.
    D. Sensation will be preserved to the medial calf and foot.
    E. Decompression involves release of all three compartments.

OSTEOMYELITIS FOLLOWING OPEN TIBIAL INJURY

15. *Which one of the following statements is correct regarding the prevention and treatment of osteomyelitis in patients with Gustilo type IIIb tibial fracture?*
    A. The most common pathogens leading to osteomyelitis are anaerobic *Streptococcus* spp.
    B. A single dose of prophylactic cephalosporin and aminoglycoside is sufficient in clean wounds.
    C. All small fragments of bone should be removed during surgical debridement.
    D. The expected infection rate is greater than 20% without antibiotic therapy.
    E. Negative-pressure dressings should not be used in cases of osteomyelitis.

CHRONIC WOUNDS OF THE LOWER EXTREMITY

16. You assess a patient with a nonhealing ulcer to the lower limb. Examination shows a 3 by 3 cm ulcer between the malleoli and gastrocnemius myotendinous junction. There is surrounding soft tissue firmness and swelling with pigmentation changes and varicosities. *Which one of the following is the most appropriate management of this ulcer?*
    A. Excision biopsy
    B. Referral for revascularization surgery
    C. Hyperbaric oxygen therapy
    D. Compression bandaging
    E. Negative pressure wound therapy

Answers

GUSTILO CLASSIFICATION IN LOWER LIMB TRAUMA

1. A patient presents with an open tibial fracture after a motor vehicle accident.
   Surgery reveals extensive soft tissue damage involving skin and muscle with associated periosteal stripping of bone. *How should this injury be correctly described using the Gustilo-Anderson classification system?*
   D. Gustilo IIIb

   The Gustilo classification was first published in 1976[1] and was later modified in 1984.[2] It describes three types of open tibial fractures: I, II, and III. The latter is further divided into types a, b, and c, depending on associated soft tissue damage. It is generally accepted that an accurate assessment of the fracture in relation to the Gustilo classification can only be performed intraoperatively. Plastic surgical input is required to reconstruct most IIIb and IIIc fractures as in this case. The usual standard of care for open tibial fractures is early operative debridement with a team comprising a senior orthopaedic surgeon and a senior plastic surgeon. The aim of this early intervention is to debride the limb and make a joint formal assessment of the bony and soft tissue injuries such that a suitable plan for stabilization and soft tissue cover can be made. Where possible this will be performed at the same time, but if more complex intervention is required the wound can be temporized with negative pressure and a temporary external fixation device or external splintage.

REFERENCES

1. Gustilo RB, Anderson JT. Prevention of infection in the treatment of one thousand and twenty-five open fractures of long bones: retrospective and prospective analyses. J Bone Joint Surg Am 1976;58(4):453–458
2. Gustilo RB, Mendoza RM, Williams DN. Problems in the management of type III (severe) open fractures: a new classification of type III open fractures. J Trauma 1984;24(8): 742–746

CLASSIFICATION OF OPEN TIBIAL FRACTURES

2. *What is the key difference between a Gustilo type I and type II open lower limb injury?*
   D. The measured wound size

   Measured wound size is the key discriminator between type I and II injuries. The degree of wound contamination and the presence of a vascular injury are considered in type III injuries. The location of soft tissue injury and the degree of comminution are not specifically considered in this classification. The description of types I through IIIc are as follows:

   Type I: An open fracture with a clean laceration less than 1 cm long

   Type II: An open fracture with a clean laceration greater than 1 cm long without extensive soft tissue injury, flaps, or avulsions

   Type IIIa: Open fractures with extensive soft tissue damage, involving muscle, skin, and neurovascular structures, but with adequate soft tissue coverage

   Type IIIb: As above, except a more extensive injury with periosteal stripping, exposed bone, and/or massive contamination

   Type IIIc: Similar to a type IIIb injury with an additional arterial injury that requires repair

   In-depth knowledge of this classification is useful for everyday practice and for clinical exams as it is often tested in both written and viva examinations.[1–3]

REFERENCES

1. Gustilo RB, Anderson JT. Prevention of infection in the treatment of one thousand and twenty-five open fractures of long bones: retrospective and prospective analyses. J Bone Joint Surg Am 1976;58(4):453–458
2. Gustilo RB, Mendoza RM, Williams DN. Problems in the management of type III (severe) open fractures: a new classification of type III open fractures. J Trauma 1984;24(8): 742–746
3. Byrd HS, Spicer TE, Cierney G III. Management of open tibial fractures. Plast Reconstr Surg 1985;76(5):719–730

BYRD CLASSIFICATION OF OPEN TIBIAL FRACTURES

3. *Which one of the following is considered in the Byrd classification system but not in the Gustilo classification?*
   A. The degree of force involved to sustain the injury

   The Byrd[1] classification is primarily based on the energy level of injury, ranging from low through moderate to high. It also differs from the Gustilo classification[2,3] in that the fracture pattern and mechanism of injury are considered for some of the gradings. For example, whether the fracture is displaced, comminuted, or a simple oblique or spiral pattern is considered. Similarity between the two systems is that the degree of the soft tissue injury, including defect size and vascular injury, is considered in both classifications. Chronicity is not specifically considered in either classification, as it is assumed that all are acute injuries as follows:

Type I: Low-energy forces causing a spiral or oblique fracture pattern with a skin laceration less than 2 cm and a relatively clean wound.

Type II: Moderate-energy forces causing a comminuted or displaced fracture pattern with a skin laceration greater than 2 cm and moderate adjacent skin and muscle contusion, but without devitalized muscle.

Type III: High-energy forces causing a significantly displaced fracture pattern with severe comminution, segmental fracture, or bone defect with extensive associated skin loss and devitalized muscle.

Type IV: Fracture pattern as in type III but with extreme energy forces as in high-velocity gunshot or shotgun wounds, a history of degloving, or associated vascular injury requiring repair.

REFERENCES

1. Byrd HS, Spicer TE, Cierney G III. Management of open tibial fractures. Plast Reconstr Surg 1985;76(5):719–730
2. Gustilo RB, Anderson JT. Prevention of infection in the treatment of one thousand and twenty-five open fractures of long bones: retrospective and prospective analyses. J Bone Joint Surg Am 1976;58(4):453–458
3. Gustilo RB, Mendoza RM, Williams DN. Problems in the management of type III (severe) open fractures: a new classification of type III open fractures. J Trauma 1984;24(8): 742–746

PROGNOSTIC FACTORS IN OPEN TIBIAL FRACTURES

4. Which one of the following has no prognostic significance following an open tibial shaft fracture?

C. Concomitant fibular fracture

In 1983 Keller[1] reviewed 10,000 tibial shaft fractures. In this review, neither fracture location or concomitant fibular fracture showed prognostic significance. Complications did increase in the presence of comminution, displacement, bone loss, distraction, soft tissue injury, infection, and polytrauma. For this reason, management of open tibial fractures has become more formalized in recent years in order to prioritize their early management with an orthoplastic approach. If the bone and soft tissue injury is managed optimally, this should reduce the chances of infection and other complications such as nonunion and chronic wounds. It stands to reason that the greater the energy of the injury involved, the greater the tissue damage and increased risk of complications. Low-energy injuries even when open tend to have reasonable outcomes with only modest intervention unless the host has significant other comorbidities.[1–5]

REFERENCES

1. Keller CS. The principles of the treatment of tibial shaft fractures: a review of 10,146 cases from the literature. Orthopedics 1983;6(8):993–999
2. Yaremchuk MJ, Brumback RJ, Manson PN, Burgess AR, Poka A, Weiland AJ. Acute and definitive management of traumatic osteocutaneous defects of the lower extremity. Plast Reconstr Surg 1987;80(1):1–14
3. Godina M. Early microsurgical reconstruction of complex trauma of the extremities. Orthop Trauma Dir 2006;4(05): 29–35
4. Young K, Aquilina A, Chesser TJS, et al; MTC-22. Open tibial fractures in major trauma centres: a national prospective cohort study of current practice. Injury 2019;50(2): 497–502
5. Wordsworth M, Lawton G, Nathwani D, et al. Improving the care of patients with severe open fractures of the tibia: the effect of the introduction of Major Trauma Networks and national guidelines. Bone Joint J 2016;98-B(3):420–424

ORDER OF ACUTE TREATMENT IN LOWER LIMB OPEN FRACTURES

5. After initial resuscitation measures, which one of the following should generally be performed first when managing an open tibial fracture?

D. Fracture reduction and stabilization

Each of the above factors is highly relevant to the acute management of lower limb open tibial fractures. In general, the wound is washed and fully assessed in the OR with joint orthopaedic and plastic surgical teams present; then bony stabilization is performed in order to provide a stable base for further management. This often entails application of an external fixation device. The bone ends must, of course, be debrided fully before reduction. Vascular inflow must be established early to ensure distal limb perfusion. Thorough debridement of soft tissues must be performed with removal of any devitalized tissue and fasciotomies undertaken as required.

Recent evidence has shown that the most important factor affecting outcome after an open tibial fracture is a thorough debridement of devitalized tissues. This is because it optimizes healing and minimizes infection risk. Recent advances in both civilian and military experience indicate that an aggressive washout protocol, temporary fracture stabilization, and application of a negative pressure dressing can also buy some time before formal reconstruction is performed.[1,2]

REFERENCES

1. Hou Z, Irgit K, Strohecker KA, et al. Delayed flap reconstruction with vacuum-assisted closure management of the open IIIB tibial fracture. J Trauma 2011;71(6):1705–1708
2. Kumar AR, Grewal NS, Chung TL, Bradley JP. Lessons from operation Iraqi freedom: successful subacute reconstruction of complex lower extremity battle injuries. Plast Reconstr Surg 2009;123(1):218–229

TIMING OF SOFT TISSUE RECONSTRUCTION IN OPEN FRACTURES OF THE LOWER LIMB

6. *Following adequate debridement and external fixator stabilization of a grade IIIb open tibial fracture, when should definitive free flap reconstruction be performed based on current evidence?*

    C. Within the first week

    Based on current evidence, definitive free tissue cover for open tibial fractures should ideally be performed within the first week. Many authorities now prefer to achieve a so-called "fix and flap" approach within 48 hours. Timing will, of course, be affected by factors such as the nature of the injury, the presence of infection, degree of contamination, and bone loss. It will also be affected by other injuries and the general condition of the patient. For example, when patients have other life-threatening injuries and are in the intensive care unit (ICU), it will generally be preferable to delay free tissue transfer until they are more stable.

    Evidence presented by Byrd[1] in the 1980s supported early debridement and soft tissue cover within the first 5–6 days. The authors found that this approach resulted in fewest complications and the shortest length of hospital admission. Godina[2] found that patients who had debridement and free flap cover within 3 days had very low flap failure rates (less than 1%) and postoperative infection rates (1.5%). They found that patients who received their flaps between 3 days and 3 months had an increased flap failure rate (12%) and infection rate (17.5%). It should be noted that this is a relatively wide timeframe as it crosses both the acute, subacute, and chronic biologic phases involved in open fracture wounds. Patients who received flaps beyond 3 months had complication rates that fell somewhere between those managed in the early and intermediate phases. Yaremchuk et al[3] had infection rates of 14% in a cohort of patients who received flap coverage at a mean of 17 days. Recent military and civilian experiences suggest that soft tissue cover can be safely delayed for a few days providing that adequate debridement has been performed and the wound temporized with a negative pressure wound therapy (NPWT) device.[4,5] Some of the military data relates to injuries sustained with improvised explosive devices that alter the timeframe because of the requirement for multiple debridement procedures.[5]

    In the UK, guidelines have been published jointly by the British orthopaedic and plastic surgery associations based on current available evidence.[6] They suggest that most open tibial fractures are initially debrided, stabilized, and scheduled for surgery within 24 hours with both senior plastic surgeons and orthopaedic surgeons present. Exceptions are those with vascular compromise or severe contamination, as these need immediate management. The guidelines also suggest that soft tissue free flap cover should ideally be performed within the first week, in part to ensure that the flap recipient vessels are still in a healthy condition.

REFERENCES

1. Byrd HS, Spicer TE, Cierney G III. Management of open tibial fractures. Plast Reconstr Surg 1985;76(5):719–730
2. Godina M. Early microsurgical reconstruction of complex trauma of the extremities. Plast Reconstr Surg 1986;78(3):285–292
3. Yaremchuk MJ, Brumback RJ, Manson PN, Burgess AR, Poka A, Weiland AJ. Acute and definitive management of traumatic osteocutaneous defects of the lower extremity. Plast Reconstr Surg 1987;80(1):1–14
4. Hou Z, Irgit K, Strohecker KA, et al. Delayed flap reconstruction with vacuum-assisted closure management of the open IIIB tibial fracture. J Trauma 2011;71(6):1705–1708
5. Kumar AR, Grewal NS, Chung TL, Bradley JP. Lessons from operation Iraqi freedom: successful subacute reconstruction of complex lower extremity battle injuries. Plast Reconstr Surg 2009;123(1):218–229
6. British Association of Plastic Reconstructive and Aesthetic Surgeons. Standards for the management of open fractures of the lower limb. London: Royal Society of Medicine Press, 2009. Available at http:// www.bapras.org.uk/downloaddoc. asp?id-141

BLOOD SUPPLY TO THE TIBIA

7. *Which one of the following statements is correct regarding tibial blood supply?*

    D. Endosteal circulation derives from the nutrient artery on the posterior tibia.

    The tibia has three types of blood supply: periosteal, metaphyseal, and nutrient artery supply. The periosteal circulation derives from the primary limb vessels (not the metaphyseal artery) to supply the outer third of the cortex. The endosteal circulation derives from the nutrient artery and supplies the inner two-thirds (not one-third) of the cortex. When a long bone is fractured, the distal blood supply is usually preserved because of the structure of the periosteal circulation in which the vessels are oriented transversely.[1,2]

REFERENCES

1. Rhinelander FW. Tibial blood supply in relation to fracture healing. Clin Orthop Relat Res 1974;(105):34–81
2. Macnab I, De Haas WG. The role of periosteal blood supply in the healing of fractures of the tibia. Clin Orthop Relat Res 1974;(105):27–33

BONY RECONSTRUCTION OF THE LOWER LIMB

8. A 60-year-old man sustains an open midshaft tibial fracture with extensive soft tissue loss after being hit by a car. Exploration in the operating room (OR) shows a segment of nonviable tibia measuring 8 cm, which is removed. Following debridement, a soft tissue defect measuring 16 by 8 cm is planned for reconstruction using an anterolateral thigh flap with vastus lateralis. A spanning external fixation device is used to temporarily stabilize the fracture and a longer term plan is made for bone transport with distraction osteogenesis. *Which one of the following is true of the distraction process?*

   D. A corticotomy is performed outside the zone of injury before distraction.

   Distraction osteogenesis was pioneered by Ilizarov and this is typically indicated in segmental long bone gaps of up to 12 cm. It involves placement of an external distraction device with a corticotomy performed outside the zone of injury. Bone distraction is slow (1 mm per day, not 3 mm), so this method does take an extended time to achieve required bone length but probably represents the benchmark for long segmental defects of the tibia. The amount of bone generated is anatomically correct for the size of the defect and soft tissues can be closed by the docking method during the same process. Intraoperative blood loss is low so transfusion is not generally required. Distraction begins a week after device application. In cases like this scenario where there is segmental bone loss and soft tissue loss, it is appropriate to achieve wound closure with a free tissue transfer such as a latissimus dorsi or anterolateral thigh flap in the subacute setting. Temporary fracture stabilization can be achieved with a simple external frame. Once the soft tissues have healed (2–3 weeks), the external frame can be exchanged for a circular frame. The benefit of such fixation is that weight bearing can begin, so general mobility is improved and where bone ends are together, healing is accelerated.

   Nonvascularized bone is traditionally used for reconstructing smaller defects but some authors state that they can be used beneath vascularized muscle flaps for defects of up to 10 cm.[1] Free osseous flaps such as fibula, scapula, and iliac crest may reliably be used to reconstruct segmental bone gaps. Fibula flaps can be harvested at lengths of up to 20 cm in adult patients, if required. The use of free tissue flaps is generally indicated for segmental gaps larger than 6 cm. Free flaps are still less favorable than bone transport for segmental tibial defect reconstruction because of the difference in bone shape and quality compared with the native tibia. Their role in upper limb segmental defect reconstruction (e.g., humerus) is probably more significant.

REFERENCE

1. Kumar AR, Grewal NS, Chung TL, Bradley JP. Lessons from operation Iraqi freedom: successful subacute reconstruction of complex lower extremity battle injuries. Plast Reconstr Surg 2009;123(1):218–229

LOCAL FLAP OPTIONS IN LOWER LIMB RECONSTRUCTION

9. *Which one of the following statements is correct regarding reconstruction of lower limb soft tissue defects in physically active patients?*

   C. A flexor hallucis flap should not be used in athletes for middle third defects because of its important role in running.

   The flexor hallucis longus flap can be used to reconstruct middle third soft tissue defects. However, this muscle is important in push off for the great toe; therefore, it should not be sacrificed in physically active patients. With the current focus on the availability of surgeons skilled in free tissue transfer, local flap reconstruction in the lower limb is less commonly used, particularly for higher energy injuries. However, there remain some robust flaps that are particularly useful such as the gastrocnemius for mid and upper third defects. The extensor digitorum longus flap is supplied by the anterior tibial vessels (not the peroneal vessels) and can be used to close small wounds of the middle third. It is important to preserve the peroneal nerve during dissection of this flap. If the entire muscle is harvested, then permanent loss of toe extension will occur. A flexor digitorum longus flap can be used for small defects of the lower portion of the middle third, without significant functional loss. The medial head of gastrocnemius is preferentially chosen over the lateral head for reconstruction purposes, as it is larger and not because the functional outcome differs between the two. A proximally based soleus flap can be reliably used to cover the middle third anterior leg defects without causing a functional deficit, particularly if it is harvested as a hemisoleus.[1–5]

REFERENCES

1. Ozer H, Ergisi Y, Harput G, Senol MS, Baltaci G. Short-term results of flexor hallucis longus transfer in delayed and neglected Achilles tendon repair. J Foot Ankle Surg 2018;57(5):1042–1047

2. Arnold PG, Hodgkinson DJ. Extensor digitorum turn-down muscle flap. Plast Reconstr Surg 1980;66(4):599–604
3. Durand S, Sita-Alb L, Ang S, Masquelet AC. The flexor digitorum longus muscle flap for the reconstruction of soft-tissue defects in the distal third of the leg: anatomic considerations and clinical applications. Ann Plast Surg 2013;71(5): 595–599
4. Moscona RA, Fodor L, Har-Shai Y. The segmental gastrocnemius muscle flap: anatomical study and clinical applications. Plast Reconstr Surg 2006;118(5):1178–1182
5. Islam MS, Hossain MT, Uddin MN, Chowdhury MR, Hasan MS. Wound coverage of infected open fracture of distal third of tibia by distally based medial hemi-soleus muscle flap. Mymensingh Med J 2018;27(4):798–804

RECONSTRUCTIVE OPTIONS FOR THE LOWER LIMB

10. A patient has a 10 cm long by 15 cm wide wound in the anterolateral thigh with exposed muscle belly and an underlying femoral fracture. No nerve, bone, or vessel exposure is noted. *How best should this be managed surgically?*

   A. **Split-thickness skin graft (STSG)**

   This wound should be amenable to skin grafting with or without partial closure, because the wound bed is healthy and vascularized. Although it might be tempting to try and close the wound directly if tissue laxity appears to be adequate, this can be risky because of the underlying fracture and anticipated swelling. Direct closure would not be an option due to soft tissue loss and free tissue transfer would be unnecessary.[1,2]

REFERENCES

1. Janis JE, Kwon RK, Attinger CE. The new reconstructive ladder: modifications to the traditional model. Plast Reconstr Surg 2011;127(Suppl 1):205S–212S
2. Hollenbeck ST, Toranto JD, Taylor BJ, et al. Perineal and lower extremity reconstruction. Plast Reconstr Surg 2011;128(5):551e–563e

RECONSTRUCTIVE OPTIONS FOR THE LOWER LIMB

11. A patient has a 5 by 8 cm anterior knee wound with an exposed total knee replacement prosthesis. *How best should this be managed surgically?*

   B. **Medial gastrocnemius and STSG**

   This wound is best covered with a medial gastrocnemius local flap and split-thickness skin graft (STSG). This is preferable to a lateral gastrocnemius because of its greater size and reach. The medial gastrocnemius muscle flap has become a real workhorse flap for this sort of case. It has a reliable blood supply based on the medial sural artery and venae comitantes. It is quick to raise and has good reach to the anterior knee over the patella. Raising this flap is often best performed using a separate incision running longitudinally on the medial aspect of the leg relatively close to the midline or just medial to it. This allows a clear view of the muscle and the midline raphe such that it can be separated from the lateral gastrocnemius while causing minimal damage to the Achilles tendon. The muscle can then be passed underneath a skin bridge to the defect site. If more reach is required, additional measures include proximal release or scoring of the under-surface of the muscle. The flap harvest incision can be closed directly and the muscle covered with split-skin graft. Free tissue transfer is not generally required in such cases unless local flap options have failed, where the defect includes the proximal patella or above, or in areas where there has been previous radiotherapy.[1–3]

REFERENCES

1. Kilic A, Denney B, de la Torre J. Reconstruction of knee defects using pedicled gastrocnemius muscle flap with split-thickness skin grafting: a single surgeon's experience with 21 patients. J Knee Surg 2019;32(5):463–467
2. Walton Z, Armstrong M, Traven S, Leddy L. Pedicled rotational medial and lateral gastrocnemius flaps: surgical technique. J Am Acad Orthop Surg 2017;25(11):744–751
3. Lamaris GA, Carlisle MP, Durand P, Couto RA, Hendrickson MF. Maximizing the reach of the pedicled gastrocnemius muscle flap: a comparison of 2 surgical approaches. Ann Plast Surg 2017;78(3):342–346

RECONSTRUCTIVE OPTIONS FOR THE LOWER LIMB

12. A patient has a 3 by 5 cm distal tibial wound with exposed bone over the medial malleolus and posterior tibial vessels. *How best should this be managed surgically?*

   D. **Free gracilis and STSG**

   This defect can be covered with a range of different free flaps or with a local fasciocutaneous propeller flap. However, because of its small size and the logistics of harvesting a gracilis versus a latissimus dorsi flap, a gracilis free flap is a better option in this case. Other popular alternatives include fasciocutaneous flaps such as the anterolateral thigh (ALT), scapula, groin, or lateral arm flaps. The benefit of such flaps is avoidance of a skin graft. There are no local options that will so reliably reconstruct this defect, aside perhaps from a dorsalis pedis or extensor digitorum brevis flap, which are not mentioned as options in this scenario. The medial gastrocnemius is useful as a local flap for proximal third tibial defects or after complications of total knee replacement (TKR). A variant of this vascular supply that may be useful for a defect of this size is a medial sural artery perforator (MSAP) flap which can be harvested on one or two perforators without sacrifice of the gastrocnemius muscle. The proximally based soleus is another potential option for proximal third defects and can also be used in the middle third. However, it would not be able to cover this defect. Split graft alone is only useful in distal third leg injuries where there is healthy muscle at the wound base.[1-3]

REFERENCES

1. Pederson WC, Grome L. Microsurgical reconstruction of the lower extremity. Semin Plast Surg 2019;33(1):54–58
2. Franco MJ, Nicoson MC, Parikh RP, Tung TH. Lower extremity reconstruction with free gracilis flaps. J Reconstr Microsurg 2017;33(3):218–224
3. Sue GR, Kao HK, Borrelli MR, Cheng MH. The versatile free medial sural artery perforator flap: an institutional experience for reconstruction of the head and neck, upper and lower extremities. Microsurgery 2020;40(4):427–433

RECONSTRUCTION OF TIBIAL AND KNEE SOFT TISSUE DEFECTS

13. You have a patient with a full-thickness soft tissue defect over the proximal tibia with exposure of the tibial tuberosity measuring 7 by 4 cm. The wound is clean and ready for definitive reconstruction. **Which one of the following options is best for coverage of this defect?**

B. Medial gastrocnemius flap

A gastrocnemius flap is a very good source for soft tissue coverage in mid to upper anterior tibial defects after trauma or tumor resection. It is particularly useful for reconstruction of anterior knee defects with an exposed knee prosthesis.

The gastrocnemius muscle has two heads (medial and lateral); the medial is the larger and is most commonly employed for reconstructions. It receives its blood supply from the medial sural artery, which arises from the popliteal artery. When a medial gastrocnemius flap is raised, an incision is typically made on the medial aspect of the leg, 2 cm posterior to the tibia at midcalf level, and is continued proximally to the popliteal fossa. During this part of the dissection, care is required to prevent injury to the long saphenous vein and saphenous nerve. The fascia and overlying skin are then elevated off the medial gastrocnemius to the midline, where the medial and lateral heads meet. During this part of the dissection, the sural nerve and small saphenous vein are identified and preserved. The medial raphe between the medial and lateral heads should be divided, and the plane is developed down to soleus muscle. Within this plane, the plantaris tendon is identified. Next, the distal tendon is transected so that the flap can be raised from distal to proximal. Visualization of the sural artery pedicle is not usually required for coverage of a lower defect, as in this case. Where the arc of rotation is greater than 100 degrees, it can be useful to continue the dissection proximally and identify the medial sural artery pedicle and medial sural motor nerve supplying the flap. The nerve can also be transected to stop subsequent muscle contractions. The proximal gastrocnemius attachment or hamstring tendons can also be divided to improve flap reach, although this is not usually required in most cases.[1]

The proximally based (not distally based) soleus flap is a reasonable alternative and can be carried to a point 5 cm above its tendinous insertion. The bipedicled tibialis anterior flap is more suitable for middle third coverage. The reverse sural artery flap is used for the distal third.

REFERENCE

1. Masquelet AC, Sassu P. Gastrocnemius flap. In: Wei FC, Mardini S, eds. Flaps and Reconstructive Surgery. Philadelphia: Saunders Elsevier; 2009

COMPARTMENT SYNDROME

14. Which one of the following is true of compartment syndrome in the lower limb?

D. Sensation will be preserved to the medial calf and foot.

Sensation to the medial calf is preserved in compartment syndrome because this area is supplied by the saphenous nerve that is located outside the compartments of the lower leg. Compartment syndrome is a condition where the intracompartmental pressure exceeds perfusion pressure, leading to ischemia and subsequent necrosis of the muscle compartments. It occurs in approximately 1 in 10 tibial fractures and must be recognized and treated early in order to avoid irreversible tissue damage. It can occur with both open and closed injuries and the fact that a fracture can breach a given compartment does not mean that the compartment is adequately decompressed. The main signs of compartment syndrome are the six p's: pain (out of proportion to the injury and with passive stretch), pressure from swollen compartments, paresthesia of the involved compartment, paralysis or decreased strength of the involved compartment, pallor, and pulselessness as a result of vascular compromise. Loss of distal pulses is a late sign of compartment syndrome and is more likely because of vascular injury. To supplement clinical examination, intracompartmental pressures can be measured using devices specifically made for this purpose. A difference of 30 mm Hg or less between the measured pressure and diastolic pressure is considered a justification for decompression. When decompression is performed, a number of approaches are available. One example is to use combined medial and lateral approaches where longitudinal incisions are made 1–2 cm medial and 1–2 cm lateral to the tibial borders overlying the soft tissue compartments. This facilitates decompression of all four (not three) compartments: anterior, lateral, superficial posterior, and deep posterior. This also preserves the medial perforating vessels in case a local fasciocutaneous flap is required.[1,2]

REFERENCES

1. Frink M, Hildebrand F, Krettek C, Brand J, Hankemeier S. Compartment syndrome of the lower leg and foot. Clin Orthop Relat Res 2010;468(4):940–950
2. Guo J, Yin Y, Jin L, Zhang R, Hou Z, Zhang Y. Acute compartment syndrome: cause, diagnosis, and new viewpoint. Medicine (Baltimore) 2019;98(27):e16260

OSTEOMYELITIS FOLLOWING OPEN TIBIAL INJURY

15. **Which one of the following statements is correct regarding the prevention and treatment of osteomyelitis in patients with Gustilo type IIIb tibial fracture?**

    D. **The expected infection rate is greater than 20% without antibiotic therapy.**

    The most common pathogen in osteomyelitis is *S. aureus*. Prophylactic use of antibiotics can significantly reduce the infection rate in lower limb trauma wounds, but a single dose is not sufficient. Thorough debridement and removal of all devitalized tissue are required, but small viable bone fragments can remain in situ. Negative pressure dressings are appropriate for patients with debrided osteomyelitic wounds in conjunction with antibiotic therapy.[1]

REFERENCE

1. Patzakis MJ, Wilkins J, Moore TM. Use of antibiotics in open tibial fractures. Clin Orthop Relat Res 1983;(178):31–35

CHRONIC WOUNDS OF THE LOWER EXTREMITY

16. You assess a patient with a nonhealing ulcer to the lower limb. Examination shows a 3 by 3 cm ulcer between the malleoli and gastrocnemius myotendinous junction. There is surrounding soft tissue firmness and swelling with pigmentation changes and varicosities. **Which one of the following is the most appropriate management of this ulcer?**

    D. **Compression bandaging**

    The clinical description above suggests a diagnosis of venous ulcer. These tend to be located in the gaiter region between the malleoli and the gastrocnemius myotendinous junction, sometimes termed "boot strap distribution." The other findings include chronic edema, varicosities, lipodermatosclerosis, and a history of deep vein thrombosis. Either incision or excision biopsy is indicated in suspected skin cancers such as a Marjolin's ulcer arising in a chronic wound. Referral to the vascular team may be warranted in patients with a suspected arterial ulcer. These present as punched-out, painful ulcers with a history of claudication and absent pulses. Hyperbaric oxygen therapy may be indicated in radiation ulcers before surgical resection and soft tissue cover. It is not indicated in venous ulcers and neither is negative pressure wound therapy.[1,2]

REFERENCES

1. Guest JF, Fuller GW, Vowden P. Venous leg ulcer management in clinical practice in the UK: costs and outcomes. Int Wound J 2018;15(1):29–37
2. O'Donnell TF Jr, Passman MA, Marston WA, et al; Society for Vascular Surgery; American Venous Forum. Management of venous leg ulcers: clinical practice guidelines of the Society for Vascular Surgery ® and the American Venous Forum. J Vasc Surg 2014;60(2, Suppl):3S–59S

68. Foot Ulcers

See *Essentials of Plastic Surgery*, third edition, pp. 922–941

EPIDEMIOLOGY OF FOOT ULCERS

1. You see a 50-year-old patient in your clinic who has a chronic foot ulcer. *In Europe and the United States, what is the most likely underlying condition associated with this diagnosis?*
   A. Diabetes mellitus
   B. Malignancy
   C. Infection
   D. Venous insufficiency
   E. Arterial insufficiency

RISKS OF FOOT ULCER COMPLICATIONS IN DIABETIC PATIENTS

2. *What is the approximate risk of a diabetic patient developing a foot ulcer in his or her lifetime?*
   A. 1 in 2
   B. 1 in 4
   C. 1 in 10
   D. 1 in 20
   E. 1 in 50

RISK FACTORS IN DIABETIC FOOT ULCER DEVELOPMENT

3. *What is the classic triad of risk factors for diabetic foot ulcer development?*
   A. Poor footwear, foot deformity, and peripheral neuropathy
   B. Peripheral neuropathy, foot deformity, and minor trauma
   C. Smoking, minor trauma, and peripheral arterial disease
   D. Elevated blood glucose, foot deformity, and poor hygiene
   E. Peripheral neuropathy, previous amputation, and smoking

CLASSIFICATION OF DIABETIC FOOT ULCERS

4. *Which one of the following statements is correct regarding classification systems for diabetic foot ulcers?*
   A. The Meggitt-Wagner system is most commonly used and consistently considers infection status across all grades.
   B. The University of Texas system assesses wound size, depth, and chronicity, but not tissue perfusion.
   C. When using the PEDIS system as described by the International Working Group on the Diabetic Foot (IWGDF), the *P* stands for paresthesia.
   D. The main strength of the Infectious Disease Society of America (IDSA) classification system is that it incorporates wound size, depth, and sensation.
   E. Wound depth, infection, and vascularity are the key predictive factors and should ideally be featured within a classification system.

THE AMERICAN DIABETES ASSOCIATION ALGORITHM FOR DIABETIC FOOT ULCERATION

5. The American Diabetes Association (ADA) algorithm for managing neuropathic foot ulcers in diabetic patients has six essential components. *Which one of these components represents the most important aspect to facilitate healing?*
   A. Off-loading
   B. Early debridement
   C. Management of infection
   D. Correction of ischemia
   E. Early amputation

MANAGEMENT OF THE DIABETIC FOOT

6. While you are on call, the emergency department refers a 64-year-old diabetic man with a provisional diagnosis of cellulitis of his foot. Erythema has developed over the course of a few days and his entire foot is warm with moderate swelling. Further examination shows bounding pulses, reduced sensation, and absent deep tendon reflexes. The patient is systemically well, pain free, and afebrile. Blood glucose control is chronically poor. Recent blood test findings are unremarkable. *Which one of the following statements is correct regarding the management of this patient?*
   A. He should be given high-dose intravenous floxacillin and metronidazole.
   B. Early mobilization, elevation, and nonsteroidal anti-inflammatory drugs (NSAIDs) are beneficial to reduce swelling.
   C. Serial radiographs are unlikely to alter management.
   D. Incision and drainage of the swelling within 24 hours are advisable.
   E. Strict immobilization of the affected foot and ankle is critically important.

FOOT DEFORMITY IN DIABETES

7. *Which one of the following is the most common site for development of a diabetic foot ulcer?*
   A. Heel
   B. Arch
   C. Lateral sole
   D. Region of the great toe
   E. Tips of the toes

TOTAL CONTACT CASTING

8. You are considering the use of total contact casting for a patient with a problematic diabetic foot ulcer. *Which one of the following statements is correct regarding this technique?*
   A. Patient compliance is typically poor.
   B. Infection should be aggressively managed simultaneously.
   C. Healing rates are only 40–50% within the first 6 weeks.
   D. The entire plantar aspect of the foot and lower leg should be in contact with the cast.
   E. Casts can be easily placed by patients or their caregivers.

DEBRIDEMENT OF DIABETIC FOOT ULCERS

9. A patient presents in the diabetic foot clinic with a necrotic, malodorous foot ulcer. *Which one of the following statements is correct regarding selection of a debridement method for such patients?*
   A. Wet-to-dry dressings are nonselective in the tissue removed but provide pain-free dressing changes.
   B. When used for wound debridement, maggots are effective against methicillin-resistant *Staphylococcus aureus* (MRSA) and vancomycin-resistant *Enterococcus* (VRE).
   C. Hydrosurgical debridement will commonly result in excessive removal of healthy granulation tissue.
   D. Where dry gangrene is present, this should be routinely debrided before revascularization is attempted.
   E. *P. sericata* larvae are left in situ for 1 week but nonselectively debride devitalized and healthy tissue.

DIAGNOSIS OF LOWER LIMB ULCERS

10. A patient has a painful, punched-out ulcer with a yellow, fibrinous base. Further examination reveals shiny, hairless skin and dystrophic toe nails. *What is the most likely underlying pathology?*
    A. Arterial insufficiency
    B. Venous insufficiency
    C. Skin malignancy
    D. Diabetes mellitus
    E. Radiotherapy

MANAGEMENT OF LOWER LIMB ULCERS

11. A patient has a rapidly enlarging ulcer in a previous burn site. *What is the most appropriate next step in management?*
    A. Surgical debridement
    B. Diagnostic tissue biopsy
    C. Hyperbaric oxygen
    D. Ankle and toe-brachial indices
    E. Revascularization

Answers

EPIDEMIOLOGY OF FOOT ULCERS

1. You see a 50-year-old patient in your clinic who has a chronic foot ulcer. *In Europe and the United States, what is the most likely underlying condition associated with this diagnosis?*

    A. Diabetes mellitus

    Diabetes is now the leading cause of foot ulcers and their complications, with an incidence of 2.0–6.8% per year in Europe and the United States. Other common causes include venous and arterial ulcers. Skin malignancies represent a fair proportion of foot ulcers and suspicious lesions warrant early biopsy. It is clearly important to be able to recognize the different ulcers in clinical practice as their management differs significantly. Diabetic foot ulcer management should focus on prevention as diabetes continues to affect more people worldwide.[1,2]

REFERENCES

1. Lavery LA, Armstrong DG, Wunderlich RP, Tredwell J, Boulton AJ. Diabetic foot syndrome: evaluating the prevalence and incidence of foot pathology in Mexican Americans and non-Hispanic whites from a diabetes disease management cohort. Diabetes Care 2003;26(5):1435–1438
2. Pecoraro RE, Reiber GE, Burgess EM. Pathways to diabetic limb amputation. Basis for prevention. Diabetes Care 1990;13(5):513–521

RISKS OF FOOT ULCER COMPLICATIONS IN DIABETIC PATIENTS

2. *What is the approximate risk of a diabetic patient developing a foot ulcer in his or her lifetime?*

    B. 1 in 4

    One quarter of patients with diabetes will develop a foot ulcer during their lifetime. Half of these will become infected at some stage. Of the infected ulcers, a fifth will ultimately require amputation. More than half of all nontraumatic limb amputations across all health care are performed because of diabetes. Of the foot ulcers occurring, half are on the plantar surface and the consequences of problematic foot ulcers are the leading cause of hospitalization in the UK and Europe. These figures highlight the importance of preventing and treating ulcers early in this population group with patient education, tight control of blood glucose, and practical steps to avoid foot trauma.[1,2]

REFERENCES

1. Singh N, Armstrong DG, Lipsky BA. Preventing foot ulcers in patients with diabetes. JAMA 2005;293(2):217–228
2. Skrepnek GH, Armstrong DG, Mills JL. Open bypass and endovascular procedures among diabetic foot ulcer cases in the United States from 2001 to 2010. J Vasc Surg 2014;60(5):1255–1265

RISK FACTORS IN DIABETIC FOOT ULCER DEVELOPMENT

3. *What is the classic triad of risk factors for diabetic foot ulcer development?*

    B. Peripheral neuropathy, foot deformity, and minor trauma

    The classic triad of risk factors for development of diabetic foot ulcers is peripheral neuropathy, foot deformity, and minor trauma. Neuropathy is the most significant single factor. Other contributing factors include poor selection of footwear (which can contribute to repeated minor trauma), poor self-care, smoking, peripheral arterial disease, obesity, and hypertension.[1]

REFERENCE

1. Reiber GE, Vileikyte L, Boyko EJ, et al. Causal pathways for incident lower-extremity ulcers in patients with diabetes from two settings. Diabetes Care 1999;22(1):157–162

CLASSIFICATION OF DIABETIC FOOT ULCERS

4. *Which one of the following statements is correct regarding classification systems for diabetic foot ulcers?*

    E. Wound depth, infection, and vascularity are key predictive factors and should ideally be featured within a classification system.

    Numerous classification systems have been developed for diabetic foot ulcers, suggesting that no uniformly accepted ideal exists. Three factors are particularly relevant to healing and these are wound depth, infection status, and vascularity as indicated by the presence or absence of peripheral arterial disease. For this reason, the ideal classification should include these three factors as a minimum. The Meggitt-Wagner system is most commonly used and has six grades as follows:

0: Preulcerative/high-risk foot
1: Superficial ulcer
2: Deep to tendon, bone, or joint
3: Deep with abscess/osteomyelitis
4: Forefoot gangrene
5: Whole foot gangrene

Weaknesses of this system are that the presence or absence of wound infection is not considered in grades 0 to 2, and peripheral arterial disease is considered only in grades 4 and 5.[1] The University of Texas Wound Classification System uses a 4 × 4 matrix and considers wound depth, infection, and peripheral arterial disease, so it contains the three key criteria described above. It is therefore a useful system, but does not take into account wound size or chronicity, which are two additional factors that will influence healing.[2] The International Working Group on the Diabetic Foot (IWGDF) developed the PEDIS (perfusion, extent/size, depth/tissue loss, infection, and sensation) system, which does cover the key criteria. The Infectious Disease Society of America (IDSA) system describes the presence of infection in diabetic foot ulcers and has four grades: not infected, mild, moderate, and severe infection.[3] It is essentially the same as the *infection* component of the PEDIS classification. However, it does not assess other key components such as wound size, depth, and sensation.[3,4]

REFERENCES

1. Wagner FW Jr. The dysvascular foot: a system for diagnosis and treatment. Foot Ankle 1981;2(2):64–122
2. Armstrong DG, Lavery LA, Harkless LB. Validation of a diabetic wound classification system. The contribution of depth, infection, and ischemia to risk of amputation. Diabetes Care 1998;21(5):855–859
3. Lipsky BA, Berendt AR, Cornia PB, et al; Infectious Diseases Society of America. 2012 Infectious Diseases Society of America clinical practice guideline for the diagnosis and treatment of diabetic foot infections. Clin Infect Dis 2012;54(12):e132–e173
4. Lipsky BA, Aragón-Sánchez J, Diggle M, et al; International Working Group on the Diabetic Foot. IWGDF guidance on the diagnosis and management of foot infections in persons with diabetes. Diabetes Metab Res Rev 2016;32(Suppl 1):45–74

THE AMERICAN DIABETES ASSOCIATION ALGORITHM FOR DIABETIC FOOT ULCERATION

5. The American Diabetes Association (ADA) algorithm for managing neuropathic foot ulcers in diabetic patients has six essential components. *Which one of these components represents the most important aspect to facilitate healing?*

A. Off-loading

According to the American Diabetes Society (ADA), the management of neuropathic diabetic foot ulcers requires six essential factors. Of these, off-loading pressure is the most important. The goal is to off-load pressure at the ulcer site while the patient remains ambulatory. The other essential factors are the following:

• Debridement early and often
• Moist wound healing environment
• Treatment of infection
• Correction of ischemia (below-the-knee disease)
• Prevention of amputation

All factors should be addressed in conjunction with optimization of medical therapy to successfully manage diabetic foot ulcers.[1]

REFERENCE

1. Bus SA. The role of pressure offloading on diabetic foot ulcer healing and prevention of recurrence. Plast Reconstr Surg 2016; 138(3, Suppl):179S–187S

MANAGEMENT OF THE DIABETIC FOOT

6. While you are on call, the emergency department refers a 64-year-old diabetic man with a provisional diagnosis of cellulitis of his foot. Erythema has developed over the course of a few days and his entire foot is warm with moderate swelling. Further examination shows bounding pulses, reduced sensation, and absent deep tendon reflexes. The patient is systemically well, pain free, and afebrile. Blood glucose control is chronically poor. Recent blood test findings are unremarkable. *Which one of the following statements is correct regarding the management of this patient?*

E. Strict immobilization of the affected foot and ankle is critically important.

This patient demonstrates Charcot foot, which is a condition of unknown cause that occurs in diabetic patients. It presents as a red, hot, swollen foot and ankle and can be confused with either cellulitis or deep venous thrombosis.[1] If it is not diagnosed, the outcome is poor with irreversible destruction of the bony architecture of the foot. Serial radiographs can be useful for monitoring bony changes. If a wound is present, osteomyelitis should be excluded with an MRI. It may be reasonable to begin antibiotic therapy for this patient. However, he is less likely to have infection because he is well and has normal blood results such as white blood cell count.

REFERENCE

1. American Family Physician. The Charcot foot in diabetes: six key points. Available at http://www.aafp.org/afp/1998/0601/p2705.html

FOOT DEFORMITY IN DIABETES

7. *Which one of the following is the most common site for development of a diabetic foot ulcer?*
   D. Region of the great toe
   Common sites for diabetic foot ulcers are those where pressure and shear are most likely to occur, in conjunction with the poorest areas of blood supply. Overall, the most common site is under the hallux. Other areas include the heel (because pressure is transmitted when lying or standing), the tips of the toes (especially with clawing and pressure when weight bearing), and those that are exposed to high repetitive trauma during walking.[1]

REFERENCE

1. Neville RF, Kayssi A, Buescher T, Stempel MS. The diabetic foot. Curr Probl Surg 2016;53(9):408–437

TOTAL CONTACT CASTING

8. You are considering the use of total contact casting for a patient with a problematic diabetic foot ulcer. *Which one of the following statements is correct regarding this technique?*
   D. The entire plantar aspect of the foot and lower leg should be in contact with the cast.
   The goal of contact casting is to evenly distribute pressure across the foot, rather than to completely relieve the ulcer site of pressure at the expense of other vulnerable areas. Infection and ischemia should be aggressively treated before casting begins. Casts should be applied by a skilled clinician to prevent iatrogenic ulceration. Patient compliance is very good because it is difficult to remove a full cast. Healing rates are 72–100% over 5–7 weeks.[1]

REFERENCE

1. Sinacore DR, Mueller MJ, Diamond JE, Blair VP III, Drury D, Rose SJ. Diabetic plantar ulcers treated by total contact casting. A clinical report. Phys Ther 1987;67(10):1543–1549

DEBRIDEMENT OF DIABETIC FOOT ULCERS

9. A patient presents in the diabetic foot clinic with a necrotic, malodorous foot ulcer. *Which one of the following statements is correct regarding selection of a debridement method for such patients?*
   B. When used for wound debridement, maggots are effective against methicillin-resistant *Staphylococcus aureus* (MRSA) and vancomycin-resistant *Enterococcus* (VRE).
   Debridement of chronic ulcers is important in order to remove devitalized tissue and biofilm in order to reset the acute healing process. Debridement may be achieved mechanically or chemically. Mechanical debridement includes wet-to-dry dressings, surgical debridement, and maggot therapy. Chemical debridement includes enzymatic debridement with collagenases or other active dressings such as honey. Maggots *(Phaenicia sericata)* are the larvae of green blowfly and they selectively consume devitalized tissue in wounds, while preserving healthy tissue. A secondary benefit is that they are resistant to both methicillin-resistant Staphylococcus aureus (MRSA) and vancomycin-resistant Enterococcus (VRE). They are normally left in situ for 3 days (not 1 week) beneath a mesh dressing before being changed. Not only are wet-to-dry dressings nonselective in the tissue removed, they are also painful for patients, can lead to surface cooling, and are labor intensive. Surgical debridement can be with a traditional blade or can be hydrosurgical debridement using systems like the Versajet (Smith & Nephew, Memphis, TN). Such systems are highly effective at debriding wounds accurately using high-velocity streams of saline and a vacuum. This appears to remove necrotic tissue and the biofilm. Wet gangrene should be debrided promptly to minimize systemic illness, but dry gangrene without cellulitis should remain in situ until revascularization is achieved to minimize progressive tissue loss and promote subsequent wound healing.[1–6]

REFERENCES

1. Greer N, Foman N, Dorrian J, et al. Advanced Wound Care Therapies for Non-Healing Diabetic, Venous, and Arterial Ulcers: A Systematic Review. Washington (DC): 2012
2. Falch BM, de Weerd L, Sundsfjord A. [Maggot therapy in wound management]. Tidsskr Nor Laegeforen 2009;129(18):1864–1867
3. Malekian A, Esmaeeli Djavid G, Akbarzadeh K, et al. Efficacy of maggot therapy on Staphylococcus aureus and Pseudomonas aeruginosa in diabetic foot ulcers: a randomized controlled trial. J Wound Ostomy Continence Nurs 2019;46(1):25–29
4. Attinger CE, Janis JE, Steinberg J, Schwartz J, Al-Attar A, Couch K. Clinical approach to wounds: débridement and wound bed preparation including the use of dressings and wound-healing adjuvants. Plast Reconstr Surg 2006;117(7, Suppl):72S–109S
5. Game FL, Jeffcoate WJ. Dressing and diabetic foot ulcers: a current review of the evidence. Plast Reconstr Surg 2016;138(3, Suppl):158S–164S
6. Sumpio BE, Lee T, Blume PA. Vascular evaluation and arterial reconstruction of the diabetic foot. Clin Podiatr Med Surg 2003;20(4):689–708

DIAGNOSIS OF LOWER LIMB ULCERS

10. A patient has a painful, punched-out ulcer with a yellow, fibrinous base. Further examination reveals shiny, hairless skin and dystrophic toe nails. *What is the most likely underlying pathology?*

A. **Arterial insufficiency**

Lower limb ulcers have some distinct features according to the cause. Factors to be considered when assessing an ulcer include location, appearance, symptoms, and risk factors. The hallmark features of an arterial ulcer are a round or punched-out appearance with a well-demarcated border. There may be a fibrinous yellow base or true eschar. Bone and/or tendon may be evident in the wound base. The typical location is over the distal bony prominences. Other features include a shiny appearance in the adjacent skin, loss of hair, dystrophic toenails, and absence of foot pulses.

The hallmark features of a venous lesion are a shallow ulcer with irregular borders located near the medial malleolus. Other features include varicose veins, leg edema, dermatitis, lipodermatosclerosis, and purple pigmentary changes.

Diabetic ulcers arise on pressure points on the feet. There is often callus surrounding the wound with undermined edges, blisters, hemorrhage, or necrosis present. Exposure of deeper structures may be observed. The key indicators of a skin malignancy, such as squamous cell carcinoma (SCC) or melanoma, are rapid growth with bleeding and ulceration. There may well be a keratin scabs itch, an SCC, and the lesion may appear de novo or in the setting of a chronic wound. Wound edges may be poorly defined and such lesions require biopsy to exclude or confirm the suspected diagnosis. Other skin malignancies such as basal cell carcinoma (BCC) or melanoma can also present with nonhealing ulcerated appearances. Melanomas are often, but not always, pigmented. Radiotherapy ulcers arise in previous treatment sites and appear as unstable patches of skin. A high suspicion for malignancy should be maintained until biopsies have been performed.[1,2]

REFERENCES

1. Federman DG, Ladiiznski B, Dardik A, et al. Wound Healing Society 2014 update on guidelines for arterial ulcers. Wound Repair Regen 2016;24(1):127–135
2. Hinchliffe RJ, Brownrigg JR, Andros G, et al; International Working Group on the Diabetic Foot. Effectiveness of revascularization of the ulcerated foot in patients with diabetes and peripheral artery disease: a systematic review. Diabetes Metab Res Rev 2016;32(Suppl 1):136–144

MANAGEMENT OF LOWER LIMB ULCERS

11. A patient has a rapidly enlarging ulcer in a previous burn site. *What is the most appropriate next step in management?*

B. **Diagnostic tissue biopsy**

The presence of a new ulcer in a chronic wound or old injury such as a burn should be investigated with a tissue biopsy under local anesthetic in order to exclude a skin malignancy such as a squamous cell carcinoma. The development of skin cancers in chronic wounds is termed a *Marjolin's ulcer.*[1]

Surgical debridement is warranted in chronic wounds that are not healing in order to help remove dead tissue and biofilm and thereby kick-start the healing process. Hyperbaric oxygen has a potential role in management of diabetic foot ulcers and may contribute to reducing subsequent need for amputation.[2] Ankle and toe-brachial indices are useful markers of arterial insufficiency. An ankle-brachial index less than 0.9 is suggestive of arterial insufficiency, while a toe-brachial index above 0.6 can be predictive of healing. Vascular intervention can be very useful in the management of leg ulcers. Revascularization with angioplasty and/or bypass can help healing in both diabetic foot and arterial ulcers. In this case once a tissue diagnosis has been confirmed, in the absence of malignancy, a vascular referral should be made. [3,4]

REFERENCES

1. Kanth AM, Heiman AJ, Nair L, et al. Current trends in management of Marjolin's ulcer: a systematic review. J Burn Care Res 2021 4;42(2):144–151
2. Liu R, Li L, Yang M, Boden G, Yang G. Systematic review of the effectiveness of hyperbaric oxygenation therapy in the management of chronic diabetic foot ulcers. Mayo Clin Proc 2013;88(2):166–175
3. Hinchliffe RJ, Brownrigg JR, Andros G, et al; International Working Group on the Diabetic Foot. Effectiveness of revascularization of the ulcerated foot in patients with diabetes and peripheral artery disease: a systematic review. Diabetes Metab Res Rev 2016;32(Suppl 1):136–144
4. Greer N, Foman N, Dorrian J, et al. Advanced Wound Care Therapies for Non-Healing Diabetic, Venous, and Arterial Ulcers: A Systematic Review. Washington (DC): 2012

69. Lymphedema

See *Essentials of Plastic Surgery*, third edition, pp. 942–956

DEMOGRAPHICS OF LYMPHEDEMA

1. *Which one of the following statements is correct regarding the demographics of lymphedema?*
   A. It currently affects around one million people worldwide.
   B. It is limited to the limbs and genital areas.
   C. It affects 1 in 10 patients following mastectomy.
   D. Worldwide, 90% of cases affect the lower limb.
   E. Globally, the most common cause is iatrogenic.

PHYSIOLOGY OF THE LYMPHATIC SYSTEM

2. *Which one of the following statements is correct regarding the lymphatic system?*
   A. Derived embryologically from the venous system, it serves to move interstitial proteins and lipids from the vascular system.
   B. It is comprised of a collection of valveless, superficial interconnecting vessels with no deeper component.
   C. Muscle does not contain lymphatic channels but its contraction is vital to lymphatic fluid transport.
   D. The basic functional unit of the lymphatic system is the noncontractile lymphangion.
   E. Lymphatic channels share very similar basement membrane properties to blood vessels.

STAGING OF LYMPHEDEMA

3. *According to the International Society of Lymphology classification system, what disease stage is characterized by resolution of lymphedema with elevation of the limb?*
   A. Stage 0
   B. Stage I
   C. Stage II
   D. Stage III
   E. Stage IV

PRIMARY LYMPHEDEMA

4. *Which one of the following statements is correct regarding primary lymphedema?*
   A. Congenital lymphedema is sometimes known as *Milroy's disease* and usually involves unilateral arm and leg lymphedema.
   B. Most cases of primary lymphedema are inherited in an autosomal recessive fashion.
   C. Most patients with primary lymphedema, irrespective of cause, present with some form of upper limb swelling.
   D. Lymphedema tarda is the least common subtype and occurs in the fourth decade.
   E. The most common form of primary lymphedema presents within the first 2 years of life.

CLINICAL PRESENTATION IN LYMPHEDEMA

5. A 14-year-old girl develops new-onset lymphedema involving the left leg and foot. A thorough review suggests a strong family history of this condition on her mother's side. *Which one of the following findings you might expect to see on clinical examination?*
   A. Absence of her eyebrows
   B. Epicanthic folds
   C. Lower eyelid coloboma
   D. Double row of eyelashes
   E. Blepharoptosis

CONSEQUENCES AND COMPLICATIONS OF LYMPHEDEMA

6. *What does the term pseudosarcoma mean with respect to lymphedema?*
   A. A streptococcal dermal infection
   B. Infection of the lymphatic vessels starting distally
   C. A rare malignant soft tissue tumor
   D. Massive local edema with skin thickening
   E. Infection of the skin presenting with erythema

CLINICAL EXAMINATION IN LYMPHEDEMA

7. *What does a positive "Stemmer sign" refer to with reference to physical examination of a lymphedematous patient?*
   A. That there is a significant size discrepancy between the limbs
   B. That the skin has a "peau de orange" appearance to it
   C. That there is active infection in a lymphedematous limb
   D. That there is a doughy swelling of the extremities
   E. That the skin cannot be pinched over the dorsum of the second toe

IMAGING IN CASES OF LYMPHEDEMA

8. *Which one of the following imaging modalities is considered the "gold standard" and is most commonly used for patients with lymphedema?*
   A. Contrast lymphangiography
   B. Contrast CT scan
   C. Contrast MRI scan
   D. Lymphoscintigraphy
   E. Doppler ultrasound

LYMPHEDEMA IN BREAST CANCER PATIENTS

9. *Which one of the following statements is correct when considering lymphedema in patients treated for breast cancer?*
   A. Breast cancer represents the second most common cause of upper limb lymphedema resulting from malignancy.
   B. There is no strong supporting evidence that the affected limb must not be used for venipuncture.
   C. Breast conservation surgery is associated with a similar risk of lymphedema compared with mastectomy.
   D. The incidence of lymphedema is the same after sentinel lymph node biopsy or axillary clearance.
   E. Obesity and weight gain after breast cancer treatment does not affect development of lymphedema.

NATURAL COURSE OF LYMPHEDEMA

10. You see a patient years after she had a left mastectomy and axillary dissection for breast cancer. She now presents with evidence of blue-red subcutaneous nodules and ecchymosis in the left upper limb. There has been no history of trauma. *What does this most likely suggest?*
    A. The presence of lymphangitis
    B. Metastatic spread of breast cancer
    C. The presence of pseudosarcoma
    D. Development of erysipelas
    E. Development of a new malignancy

MANAGEMENT OF SECONDARY LYMPHEDEMA

11. *What is the usual drug of choice for management of secondary lymphedema as a result of filariasis?*
    A. Suramin
    B. Ivermectin
    C. Mebendazole
    D. Penicillin
    E. Erythromycin

MANAGEMENT OF PATIENTS WITH LYMPHEDEMA

12. A 50-year-old man presents with lymphedema of 6 months after a groin dissection for penile squamous cell carcinoma. No evidence of disease recurrence or infection is present, but he is troubled by the differential volumes present in the lower limb. *What would be the preferred first-line treatment in this case?*
    A. Long-term compression garment
    B. Complete decongestive therapy
    C. Circumferential limb liposuction
    D. The Charles procedure
    E. The modified Charles procedure

MANAGEMENT OF LYMPHEDEMA ACCORDING TO THE BARCELONA ALGORITHM

13. A 45-year-old woman presents with long-standing upper limb lymphedema after treatment for breast cancer, despite compliance with a good compression garment and general conservative measures. Lymphoscintigraphy reveals evidence of lymphatic vessel activity with no axillary tethering. *How might this be best treated surgically according to the Barcelona algorithm?*
    A. Lymphaticovenular bypass anastomoses
    B. Vascularized lymph node transfer (VLNT)
    C. Power assisted liposuction
    D. The Miller procedure
    E. Interposition lymph vessel transplantation

Answers

DEMOGRAPHICS OF LYMPHEDEMA

1. **Which one of the following statements is correct regarding the demographics of lymphedema?**

D. **Worldwide, 90% of cases affect the lower limb.**

Lymphedema is the build-up of proteinaceous fluid within the interstitial compartment secondary to an imbalance of lymphatic fluid production and its clearance by the lymphatic transport system. Although estimates vary in the literature, lymphedema probably affects in excess of 200 million people worldwide. The most common cause by far is the parasite *Wuchereria bancrofti,* which is estimated to affect more than 90 million people worldwide. (Again, this varies in the literature, as it is difficult to accurately record incidence in many developing countries.) This parasitic disease, transmitted by mosquitoes, results in adult filarial worms physically blocking lymphatic channels. The World Health Organization (WHO) has implemented major programs to target the problem of filariasis.[1] The lower limb is affected far more commonly than any other site. The ratio between lower to upper limb involvement is 9:1 across all causes. Lymphedema is not, however, limited to the limbs and genitalia, as it can occur in the head and neck region in patients treated for head and neck cancer.[2]

In the developed world, the most common cause of secondary lymphedema is malignancy.[3] This occasionally occurs secondary to a primary tumor but is far more common after surgical excision or radiotherapy of tumor or lymph node basins. Between 25 and 50% of patients develop lymphedema of the ipsilateral upper limb after mastectomy. Lymph node dissection can lead to lymphedema in up to 70% of cases depending on anatomic site, while even sentinel lymph node biopsy is associated with rates of up to 10%.

REFERENCES

1. World Health Organization. Global programme to eliminate lymphatic filariasis. Available at https://www.who.int/publications/i/item/who-wer9641-497-508
2. Deng J, Ridner SH, Dietrich MS, et al. Prevalence of secondary lymphedema in patients with head and neck cancer. J Pain Symptom Manage 2012;43(2):244–252
3. Warren AG, Brorson H, Borud LJ, Slavin SA. Lymphedema: a comprehensive review. Ann Plast Surg 2007;59(4):464–472

PHYSIOLOGY OF THE LYMPHATIC SYSTEM

2. **Which one of the following statements is correct regarding the lymphatic system?**

C. **Muscle does not contain lymphatic channels but its contraction is vital to lymphatic fluid transport.**

Although muscle itself does not have lymphatic channels, it serves an important role in lymphatic function by moving lymph from areas of low to high pressure. The propulsion of lymph relies on valves within the lymphatic system combined with both smooth muscle in the vessels themselves, and skeletal muscle externally compressing the vessels to propel fluid from the periphery to the trunk. Other modalities of propulsion are arterial and respiratory movements.

The lymphatic system is derived embryologically from the venous system and serves to move fluid, proteins, and lipids from the interstitial space into the venous system (not away from it). The lymphatic system contains both deep and superficial components. Some channels such as those within the dermis contain valves. The superficial components drain into the deep components at three main sites: the cubital fossa, the inguinal fossa, and the popliteal fossa. The cisterna chyli is a sac at the level of L1–L2 that receives lymphatic drainage from the lower limbs and trunk. From the cisterna, lymph travels within the thoracic duct from T12 and drains into the confluence of the left internal jugular and left subclavian veins. Knowledge of this anatomy is clinically relevant when undertaking a neck dissection, as damage to the lymphatic system here can result in a chyle leak. The lymphangion is the functional unit of the lymphatic system but is noncontractile. While blood vessels have a defined basement membrane, lymphatics have several intercellular gaps that allow movement of fat and proteins into the lymphatics.[1-3]

REFERENCES

1. Beahm EK, Walton RL, Lohman RF. Vascular insufficiency of the lower extremity: lymphatic, venous, and arterial. In: Mathes SJ, ed. Plastic Surgery. 2nd ed. Philadelphia: Saunders Elsevier; 2006
2. Witte MH, Hanto D, Witte CL. Clinical and experimental techniques to study the lymphatic system. Vasc Surg 1977;11(3):120–129
3. Executive Committee. The diagnosis and treatment of peripheral lymphedema: 2016 Consensus Document of the International Society of Lymphology. Lymphology 2016;49(4):170–184

STAGING OF LYMPHEDEMA

3. *According to the International Society of Lymphology classification system, what disease stage is characterized by resolution of lymphedema with elevation of the limb?*

B. Stage I

The International Society of Lymphology has developed a four-stage classification for lymphedema.[1] Stage 0 represents a latent or subclinical condition without evidence of edema, even though lymphatic transport is impaired. Stage I involves early accumulation of proteinaceous fluid that can cause pitting or nonpitting edema, which resolves with limb elevation. Stage II involves tissue fibrosis, and limb elevation alone will no longer resolve tissue swelling. Stage III is associated with lymphostatic elephantiasis with absent pitting, acanthosis, and other tropic skin changes.

An alternative way to classify the degree of lymphedema is by assessment of relative volume excess as compared to the contralateral unaffected side. Minimal lymphedema is present where there is less than 20% volume excess, 20–40% volume excess is considered moderate, and >40% is considered severe.[2-4]

REFERENCES

1. International Society of Lymphology. The diagnosis and treatment of peripheral lymphedema. Consensus document of the International Society of Lymphology. Lymphology 2003;36(2):84–91
2. Allen RJ Jr, Cheng MH. Lymphedema surgery: patient selection and an overview of surgical techniques. J Surg Oncol 2016;113(8):923–931
3. Cheng MH, Pappalardo M, Lin C, Kuo CF, Lin CY, Chung KC. Validity of the novel Taiwan lymphoscintigraphy staging and correlation of Cheng lymphedema grading for unilateral extremity lymphedema. Ann Surg 2018;268(3):513–525
4. Douglass J, Kelly-Hope L. Comparison of staging systems to assess lymphedema caused by cancer therapies, lymphatic filariasis, and podoconiosis. Lymphat Res Biol 2019;17(5): 550–556

PRIMARY LYMPHEDEMA

4. *Which one of the following statements is correct regarding primary lymphedema?*

D. Lymphedema tarda is the least common subtype and occurs in the fourth decade.

Primary lymphedema most commonly affects the lower limbs and can be unilateral or bilateral. It is classified by age of onset as congenital (younger than 2 years), praecox (puberty), or tarda (35 years of age).[1,2] Of these, lymphedema tarda is the rarest subtype (<10%) and lymphedema praecox is the most common, representing up to 80% of all primary lymphedema. Milroy's disease refers to lymphedema congenita and affects females more commonly than males with a 2:1 ratio. It usually presents with bilateral lower limb lymphedema in children before their second birthday. The inheritance pattern for primary lymphedema varies depending on subtype and is most commonly autosomal dominant, but can be sporadic in Milroy's disease.

Wolfe and Kinmonth[3] have classified primary lymphedema as anaplastic, hypoplastic, or hyperplastic based on the appearance during lymphangiography. Hypoplastic lymphedema is the most common subtype (67% of cases) and can be obstructive or nonobstructive.

REFERENCES

1. Warren AG, Brorson H, Borud LJ, Slavin SA. Lymphedema: a comprehensive review. Ann Plast Surg 2007;59(4):464–472
2. Richards AM. Key Notes on Plastic Surgery. Oxford, UK: Blackwell Press; 2002
3. Wolfe JH, Kinmonth JB. The prognosis of primary lymphedema of the lower limbs. Arch Surg 1981;116(9):1157–1160

CLINICAL PRESENTATION IN LYMPHEDEMA

5. A 14-year-old girl develops new-onset lymphedema involving the left leg and foot. A thorough review suggests a strong family history of this condition on her mother's side. *Which one of the following findings you might expect to see on clinical examination?*

D. Double row of eyelashes

The history suggests this patient has Meige's syndrome, which is a type of primary lymphedema occurring in puberty that usually presents as new-onset unilateral lymphedema affecting the foot and calf. Associated inflammation is often present, and this can be complicated by cellulitis. Associated abnormalities include vertebral and cerebrovascular malformations, sensorineural (as opposed to conductive) hearing loss, and a double row of eyelashes (distichiasis). The latter can result from abnormal development of the meibomian glands. Meige's disease is also known as familial lymphedema praecox and more typically affects females with a ratio of 4:1. It is the most common form of primary lymphedema representing 65–80% of cases.[1-2]

REFERENCES

1. Wheeler ES, Chan V, Wassman R, Rimoin DL, Lesavoy MA. Familial lymphedema praecox: Meige's disease. Plast Reconstr Surg 1981;67(3):362–364
2. Grisolia ABD, Nelson CC. Lymphedema-distichiasis syndrome in a male patient followed for 16 years. Ophthal Plast Reconstr Surg 2018;34(2):e63–e65

CONSEQUENCES AND COMPLICATIONS OF LYMPHEDEMA

6. *What does the term pseudosarcoma mean with respect to lymphedema?*

D. Massive local edema with skin thickening

The term *pseudosarcoma* relates to a massive local edema in severely obese patients where there are folds of fat that compress the lymphatics and lead to a thickened epidermis with dermal fibrosis. The most common anatomic location is the medial thigh but this process can also occur in the abdomen in the presence of a large panniculus.[1,2]

Erysipelas refers to a streptococcal dermal infection that can be seen in patients with lymphedema. Infection of the lymphatics is often a problem in patients with lymphedema and is termed lymphangitis. This tends to start distally. Lymphangiosarcoma is a rare form of soft tissue cancer that can occur in patients with chronic lymphedema. Cellulitis is also a frequent complication in lymphedema patients and may be seen in association with lymphangitis. Infections are generally managed well with short courses of intravenous targeted antibiotics.[1–3]

REFERENCES

1. Bahrami A, Ronaghan JE, O-Yurvati AH. Pseudosarcoma of the thigh: a rare case of massive localized lymphedema. Int Surg 2015;100(3):461–465
2. Kurt H, Arnold CA, Payne JE, Miller MJ, Skoracki RJ, Iwenofu OH. Massive localized lymphedema: a clinicopathologic study of 46 patients with an enrichment for multiplicity. Mod Pathol 2016;29(1):75–82
3. Petrova TV, Karpanen T, Norrmén C, et al. Defective valves and abnormal mural cell recruitment underlie lymphatic vascular failure in lymphedema distichiasis. Nat Med 2004;10(9):974–981

CLINICAL EXAMINATION IN LYMPHEDEMA

7. *What does a positive "Stemmer sign" refer to with reference to physical examination of a lymphedematous patient?*

E. That the skin cannot be pinched over the dorsum of the second toe

There are a range of signs that should be noted during examination of a patient with suspected lymphedema. The Stemmer sign is elicited by attempting to pinch skin over the dorsum of the second toe. This will not be possible in a patient with significant lymphedema. Other clinical findings are not specific to the lower limb and include doughy swelling, peau de orange skin changes, and circumferential limb measurements with a side-to-side difference greater than 2 cm. Assessing whether the edema is pitting or nonpitting is also important, as well as looking for evidence of active infection such as cellulitis or lymphangitis. The peau de orange sign is due to swelling within the dermis.[1–3]

REFERENCES

1. Maclellan RA, Couto RA, Sullivan JE, Grant FD, Slavin SA, Greene AK. Management of primary and secondary lymphedema: analysis of 225 referrals to a center. Ann Plast Surg 2015;75(2):197–200
2. Stemmer R. [A clinical symptom for the early and differential diagnosis of lymphedema]. Vasa 1976;5(3):261–262
3. Garza R III, Skoracki R, Hock K, Povoski SP. A comprehensive overview on the surgical management of secondary lymphedema of the upper and lower extremities related to prior oncologic therapies. BMC Cancer 2017;17(1):468

IMAGING IN CASES OF LYMPHEDEMA

8. *Which one of the following imaging modalities is considered the "gold standard" and is most commonly used for patients with lymphedema?*

D. Lymphoscintigraphy

Lymphoscintigraphy is currently considered to be the benchmark for diagnosing lymphedema, although other modalities can be very useful in some circumstances.[1] For example, where deep venous thrombosis or chronic vascular disease is suspected, an ultrasound examination is useful. If malignancy is suspected, then CT or MRI may be helpful. Each of these modalities has a high sensitivity and specificity in confirming the diagnosis of lymphedema while facilitating tumor identification. An MRI is particularly good for providing detail of lymphatic architecture and preventing radiation exposure. Because of the success of these less-invasive imaging modalities, contrast lymphangiography is no longer commonly performed.

Lymphoscintigraphy involves injection of nonionizing contrast agent (Tc 99M, Tc 99m-HAS, or Tc 99m dextran) into the interstitial space. It can help to assess the function of the lymphatic channels and drainage of lymph to nodal basins. The downside is that poor resolution prohibits anatomic evaluation and it is unable to quantify changes in the limb. Furthermore, it is generally not useful in planning lymphaticovenular anastomoses, and for this purpose, CT is better. Lastly, it requires injection which can be painful for patients.[1-3]

REFERENCES

1. Warren AG, Brorson H, Borud LJ, Slavin SA. Lymphedema: a comprehensive review. Ann Plast Surg 2007;59(4):464–472
2. Pappalardo M, Cheng MH. Lymphoscintigraphy for the diagnosis of extremity lymphedema: current controversies regarding protocol, interpretation, and clinical application. J Surg Oncol 2020;121(1):37–47
3. Bae JS, Yoo RE, Choi SH, et al. Evaluation of lymphedema in upper extremities by MR lymphangiography: comparison with lymphoscintigraphy. Magn Reson Imaging 2018;49:63–70

LYMPHEDEMA IN BREAST CANCER PATIENTS

9. *Which one of the following statements is correct when considering lymphedema in patients treated for breast cancer?*

   B. There is no strong supporting evidence that the affected limb should not be used for venipuncture.

   It is a myth that venipuncture should not be performed on the affected side after treatment of the axilla (particularly in breast cancer patients), because it will exacerbate lymphedema or result in infection. Green et al[1] reviewed literature from 1966 to 2004 and found no evidence to support this common dictum. They stated that the main theoretical risk for patients with lymphedema having cannulation is the introduction of infection, leading to cellulitis and further lymphatic damage. They found no evidence that aseptic placement of a cannula or needle will regularly cause infection or that such an approach will worsen or exacerbate lymphedema. Injections are required for lymphoscintigraphy, lymphangiography, and liposuction, yet these are not regularly complicated by cellulitis or worsening of lymphedema. In the absence of robust evidence, the alternative limb should probably be used preferentially. However, the affected side can be considered for safe use in venipuncture when required.

   van der Veen et al[2] attempted to identify risk factors for the development of lymphedema after breast surgery with axillary clearance. In a cohort of 245 women, they found that risk increased with body mass index (BMI) over 25, axillary radiotherapy, and pathologic lymph node status. In general, the greatest risk of developing lymphedema is after mastectomy but is still high after a lumpectomy or axillary node surgery. The rates of lymphedema following sentinel lymph node biopsy (SNLB) and axillary clearance differ significantly with rates after SNLB of up to 10% compared with rates of up to 65% after full axillary clearance. This does, however, make the point that patients must be aware of the risk of lymphedema with SNLB particularly as this is only a staging/diagnostic procedure yet carries this risk. In contrast although the risk of lymphedema is far higher with formal lymph node dissection, this is a treatment procedure.

REFERENCES

1. Greene AK, Borud L, Slavin SA. Blood pressure monitoring and venipuncture in the lymphedematous extremity. Plast Reconstr Surg 2005;116(7):2058–2059
2. van der Veen P, De Voogdt N, Lievens P, Duquet W, Lamote J, Sacre R. Lymphedema development following breast cancer surgery with full axillary resection. Lymphology 2004;37(4):206–208

NATURAL COURSE OF LYMPHEDEMA

10. You see a patient years after she had a left mastectomy and axillary dissection for breast cancer. She now presents with evidence of blue-red subcutaneous nodules and ecchymosis in the left upper limb. There has been no history of trauma. *What does this most likely suggest?*

    E. Development of a new malignancy

    The description given is suspicious for development of a new malignancy and this is likely to be Stewart-Treves syndrome. This is a type of lymphangiosarcoma arising within chronic lymphedema, classically described after radical mastectomy. It is difficult to treat and has a very poor prognosis (life expectancy is less than 18 months after diagnosis). Wide local resection of the tumor is the preferred treatment modality.[1] Erysipelas and lymphangitis both present with a red swollen limb and would not be expected to display the above features. Breast cancer more commonly would metastasize to the lungs, bone, or liver, although it may recur locally in the chest wall. The term *pseudosarcoma* refers to massive local edema in severely obese patients where folds of fat compress the lymphatics leading to edema, thickened epidermis, and dermal fibrosis. It most commonly occurs on the thighs.

REFERENCE

1. Sharma A, Schwartz RA. Stewart-Treves syndrome: pathogenesis and management. J Am Acad Dermatol 2012;67(6): 1342–1348

MANAGEMENT OF SECONDARY LYMPHEDEMA

11. *What is the usual drug of choice for management of secondary lymphedema as a result of filariasis?*

B. Ivermectin

Ivermectin is the drug of choice used for treatment of filariasis and is used in the World Health Organization (WHO) program.[1] It is a broad-spectrum antiparasitic agent that may be combined with albendazole in the case of coendemicity with onchocerciasis (another parasitic disease transmitted by black flies that can lead to skin disease and blindness). The other treatment option is to use diethylcarbamazine citrate with albendazole. Suramin is another antiparasitic drug that was developed almost 100 years ago. It is used to treat trypanosomes (sleeping sickness). Mebendazole is a drug used to treat parasitic worm infections such as threadworms (*Enterobius vermicularis*), roundworm (ascariasis), or hook worm (*Ancylostoma*). Penicillin is a broad-spectrum antibiotic derived from penicillium molds, first discovered in 1928 and used for a variety of soft tissue, visceral, and bone infections. Erythromycin is another antibiotic with similar indications to penicillin but for individuals with a penicillin allergy.[1,2]

REFERENCES

1. World Health Organization. Global programme to eliminate lymphatic filariasis. Available at https://www.who.int/publications/i/item/who-wer9641-497-508
2. Taylor MJ, Hoerauf A, Bockarie M. Lymphatic filariasis and onchocerciasis. Lancet 2010;376(9747):1175–1185

MANAGEMENT OF PATIENTS WITH LYMPHEDEMA

12. A 50-year-old man presents with lymphedema of 6 months after a groin dissection for penile squamous cell carcinoma. No evidence of disease recurrence or infection is present, but he is troubled by the differential volumes present in the lower limb. *What would be the preferred first-line treatment in this case?*

B. Complete decongestive therapy

Complete decongestive therapy (CDT) can be very effective for managing lymphedema and reducing volume by 40–60% in patients with pitting edema. It is the benchmark first-line treatment for lymphedema as in this case and is administered by a certified lymphedema therapist. It combines an initial volume reduction phase of 3–8 weeks (involving manual drainage, exercise, skin care, elastic compression, and patient education delivered by therapist) with a maintenance phase of self-administered lymph drainage, exercise, skin care, and compression garments. A compression garment alone is far less effective than these combined measures.

Circumferential liposuction can be extremely effective at reducing volume in lymphedema. It is best indicated where there is a volume excess largely due to fat hypertrophy and there is minimal pitting. The caveat of liposuction is that lifelong compression must be used to maintain the results. It would not be the first-line treatment, however, as CDT would be undertaken first.[1-3]

The Charles procedure is a procedure described by Charles in 1912. It involves radical, circumferential excision of skin and lymphedematous tissue above the deep fascial layer with immediate split-thickness skin grafting, much like the management of deep burn injury. This is clearly a very deforming undertaking and is not commonly used in clinical practice.[4] The modified Charles procedure stages the reconstruction using split-thickness skin grafts with temporization of the wounds with negative pressure therapy. Skin grafts are then applied at 1 week.[5]

REFERENCES

1. Brorson H, Svensson H, Norrgren K, Thorsson O. Liposuction reduces arm lymphedema without significantly altering the already impaired lymph transport. Lymphology 1998;31(4):156–172
2. Brorson H. Liposuction gives complete reduction of chronic large arm lymphedema after breast cancer. Acta Oncol 2000;39(3):407–420
3. Brorson H. Liposuction in lymphedema treatment. J Reconstr Microsurg 2016;32(1):56–65
4. Charles RH. Elephantiasis scroti. In: Latham AC, English TC, eds. A System of Treatment, Vol. 3. London: Churchill; 1912
5. van der Walt JC, Perks TJ, Zeeman BJ, Bruce-Chwatt AJ, Graewe FR. Modified Charles procedure using negative pressure dressings for primary lymphedema: a functional assessment. Ann Plast Surg 2009;62(6):669–675

MANAGEMENT OF LYMPHEDEMA ACCORDING TO THE BARCELONA ALGORITHM

13. A 45-year-old woman presents with long-standing upper limb lymphedema after treatment for breast cancer, despite compliance with a good compression garment and general conservative measures. Lymphoscintigraphy reveals evidence of lymphatic vessel activity with no axillary tethering. *How might this be best treated surgically according to the Barcelona algorithm?*

A. **Lymphaticovenular bypass anastomoses**

The Barcelona algorithm for the management of lymphedema aims to guide clinicians on decision-making for surgery in lymphedema (**Fig. 69.1**).[1]

As can be seen from the figure, clinical assessment and imaging must be performed first. The recommended imaging includes indocyanine green (ICG) lymphography, lymphoscintigraphy, and MRI lymphography. This should provide information on the nature of the cause. If there is a functional lymphatic system, then a decision needs to be made as to whether there is impairment of lymphatic flow through the axilla or not. If there is no impairment then lymphaticovenular anastomoses (LVA) may be indicated. In this technique, super microsurgery is performed to connect distal subdermal lymphatic vessels to the adjacent venues and thereby improve lymphatic drainage. Three or four bypass anastomoses per patient provide good symptomatic and objective improvements in breast cancer patients. VLNT is an alternative technique which is indicated where there is impairment of flow within the axilla. It involves transfer of vascularized tissue such as the superficial circumflex iliac flap (SCIP flap) containing lymph nodes to the lymphedema limb either distally or proximally. It may be combined with LVA. In patients who have undergone mastectomy, autologous breast reconstruction may be offered. The term "total breast anatomy reconstruction" (TBAR) may be used. This entails abdominal free tissue transfer to reconstruct the breast and incorporates lymph nodes within this flap. In addition, LVA would be incorporated into the surgical procedure.[1]

Power assisted liposuction has a place in the Barcelona algorithm where there is a nonfunctional lymphatic system. The Miller procedure is not part of the algorithm and involves an excisional approach with a longitudinal medial excision of skin and subcutaneous tissue from the limb.

Interposition lymph vessel transplantation was first reported by Baumeister et al in 1986 and involves harvesting two or three ventromedial thigh lymph vessels from the thigh and using these as interposition grafts to bypass a lymphatic obstruction and optimize flow. This procedure is not part of the Barcelona algorithm.[2,3]

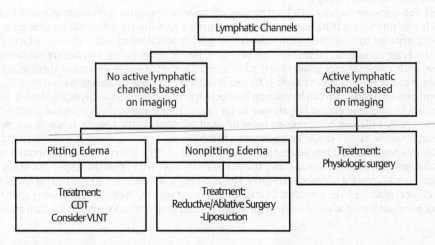

Fig. 69.1 Barcelona lymphedema algorithm for surgical treatment of lymphedema. CDT, complete decongestive therapy; VLNT, vascularized lymph node transfer.

REFERENCES

1. Masià J, Pons G, Rodríguez-Bauzà E. Barcelona lymphedema algorithm for surgical treatment in breast cancer-related lymphedema. J Reconstr Microsurg 2016;32(5):329–335

2. Baumeister RG, Siuda S, Bohmert H, Moser E. A microsurgical method for reconstruction of interrupted lymphatic pathways: autologous lymph-vessel transplantation for treatment of lymphedemas. Scand J Plast Reconstr Surg 1986;20(1): 141–146

3. Baumeister RG, Siuda S. Treatment of lymphedemas by microsurgical lymphatic grafting: what is proved? Plast Reconstr Surg 1990;85(1):64–74, discussion 75–76

PART VI

Hand, Wrist, and Upper Extremity

70. Hand Anatomy and Biomechanics

See *Essentials of Plastic Surgery*, third edition pp. 959–974

JOINTS		
CMC joint: Carpometacarpal joint **DIP joint:** Distal interphalangeal joint	**IP joint:** Interphalangeal joint **MCP joint:** Metacarpophalangeal joint	**PIP joint:** Proximal interphalangeal joint

MUSCLES		
ADM: Acellular dermal matrix **AdP:** Adductor pollicis **APB:** Abductor pollicis brevis **APL:** Abductor pollicis longus **BR:** Brachioradialis **ECRB:** Extensor carpi radialis brevis **ECRL:** Extensor carpi radialis longus **ECU:** Extensor carpi ulnaris	**EDC:** Extensor digiti communis **EDM:** Extensor digiti minimi **EIP:** Extensor indicis proprius **EPL:** Extensor pollicis longus **FCR:** Flexor carpi radialis **FCU:** Flexor carpi ulnaris **FDM:** Flexor digiti minimi **FDP:** Flexor digitorum profundus	**FDS:** Flexor digitorum superficialis **FPB:** Flexor pollicis brevis **FPL:** Flexor pollicis longus **ODM:** Opponens digiti minimi **PL:** Palmaris longus **PT:** Pronator teres

RETINACULAR SYSTEM OF THE DIGITS

1. *Which one of the following structures can prevent bowstringing of the neurovascular bundle during finger flexion?*
   - A. Cleland's ligament
   - B. Ligament of Landsmeer
   - C. Transverse retinacular ligament
   - D. Grayson's ligament
   - E. Superficial volar fascia

DEEP FASCIAL SPACES OF THE HAND

2. *Which one of the following is the location of a collar button abscess?*
   - A. Thenar space
   - B. Midvolar space
   - C. Interdigital space
   - D. Parona's space
   - E. Hypothenar space

DORSAL WRIST COMPARTMENTS

3. *Which one of the following statements is correct regarding the dorsal wrist compartments?*
   - A. There are five dorsal wrist compartments.
   - B. EPL is located within the first compartment.
   - C. ECRL and ECRB are located within the third compartment.
   - D. EDC travels with EIP in the fourth compartment.
   - E. EDM and ECU are located within the fifth compartment.

EXTENSOR TENDONS OF THE HAND AND FOREARM

4. A patient is referred to you with a zone VI extensor tendon injury and who is unable to fully extend the long finger. *Where will the division have occurred?*
   - A. Over the MCP joint
   - B. At the level of the wrist
   - C. Over the proximal phalanx
   - D. In the forearm
   - E. At the level of the metacarpal

EXTENSOR TENDONS OF THE HAND

5. A patient presents with painful flicking of the extensor tendon over the ring finger MCP joint when making a fist. **Which structure is likely to be damaged?**
    A. Central slip
    B. Juncturae tendinum
    C. Lateral slip
    D. Sagittal band
    E. Transverse retinacular ligament

INSERTIONS OF THE EXTENSOR TENDONS

6. **Which one of the following statements is correct regarding extensor tendon insertions in the hand and wrist?**
    A. EPL passes around Lister's tubercle to insert on the thumb proximal phalanx.
    B. The ECRL tendon inserts on the base of the third metacarpal.
    C. The EDC tendons insert directly onto the proximal phalanges.
    D. EIP and EDM insert ulnar to the EDC tendons of their respective digits.
    E. The APL tendon inserts on the base of the proximal phalanx of the thumb.

CONTENTS OF THE CARPAL TUNNEL

7. **Which one of the following statements is correct when exploring the contents of the carpal tunnel?**
    A. It usually contains nine structures, including the median nerve and flexor tendons.
    B. The FDS tendons to the middle and ring fingers lie superficial to those of the index and little fingers.
    C. The median nerve lies deep to the FDP tendons.
    D. The median nerve lies between the FDS and FDP tendons.
    E. The FPL lies superficial to the median nerve.

FLEXOR TENDON INJURIES IN THE HAND

8. Flexor tendon injuries are commonly seen in hand trauma patients. A thorough knowledge of flexor tendon anatomy in the hand is vital to diagnosing and managing these injuries. **Which one of the following statements is correct regarding the anatomy of this area?**
    A. Verdan described six zones of flexor tendon injury that relate to treatment and prognosis.
    B. Even-numbered annular pulleys arise from the volar plates of the MCP, PIP, and DIP joints.
    C. *No-man's land* describes the flexor sheath from the A1 pulley to the FDP insertion.
    D. The C1 cruciate pulley lies between the A1 and A2 annular pulleys.
    E. The A2 and A4 annular pulleys are considered to be the most important to preserve.

FLEXOR TENDON INJURY TO THE HAND

9. You are repairing a complete FPL division from a knife wound over the proximal phalanx. The injury occurred during full flexion of the thumb. **Which one of the following statements is correct regarding the anatomy of this region?**
    A. This represents a zone III injury.
    B. The proximal tendon is unlikely to have retracted proximally.
    C. Preservation of the oblique pulley is most important.
    D. The thumb has both annular and cruciate pulleys.
    E. The neurovascular bundles of the thumb are more protected than in the fingers.

ARTERIAL SUPPLY TO THE HAND

10. **Which one of the following statements is correct regarding the arterial supply to the hand?**
    A. The princeps pollicis arises consistently from the superficial palmar arch.
    B. The ulnar artery lies ulnar to the ulnar nerve and FCU at the wrist.
    C. In the fingers, the digital vessels lie volar to the digital nerves.
    D. The deep volar arch arises from the larger terminal branch of the ulnar artery.
    E. Kaplan's line is a useful marker of the superficial palmar arch.

INNERVATION OF THE HAND AND UPPER LIMB

11. **Which one of the following actions would be lost after an injury to the ulnar nerve at the elbow?**
    A. Flexion of the thumb at the IP joint
    B. Flexion of the ring finger at the DIP joint
    C. Flexion of the wrist
    D. Flexion of the little finger at the PIP joint
    E. Flexion of the index finger at the DIP joint

BRANCHES OF THE MEDIAN NERVE

12. *Which one of the following is usually innervated by a branch of the median nerve?*
    A. FDP to ring finger
    B. Dorsal interossei
    C. APB
    D. Deep portion of FPB
    E. ADM

SENSORY INNERVATION OF THE HAND

13. *Which nerve usually supplies the skin of the dorsal hand overlying the index metacarpal?*
    A. Dorsal branch of the ulnar nerve
    B. Lateral antebrachial cutaneous nerve
    C. Posterior antebrachial cutaneous nerve
    D. Superficial branch of the radial nerve
    E. Medial antebrachial cutaneous nerve

POSTERIOR INTEROSSEOUS NERVE PALSY

14. *Which one of the following is usually spared in a posterior interosseous nerve palsy?*
    A. ECRL
    B. ECU
    C. EDM
    D. EDC
    E. EPL

NERVE ANATOMY IN THE HAND

15. *Which one of the following is correct?*
    A. The Martin-Gruber anastomosis is a sensory fiber connection between the ulnar and median nerves in the forearm.
    B. The superficial radial nerve passes between the tendons of the ECRL and ECRB.
    C. The Riche-Cannieu anastomosis is a motor fiber connection between the ulnar and median nerves in the hand.
    D. The dorsal sensory branch of the ulnar nerve arises 1–3 cm proximal to the ulnar styloid process.
    E. The palmar cutaneous branch of the median nerve arises 3 cm proximal to the wrist crease.

BONES OF THE WRIST

16. *Which one of the following bones links the proximal and distal carpal rows?*
    A. Trapezoid
    B. Scaphoid
    C. Trapezium
    D. Pisiform
    E. Capitate

Answers

RETINACULAR SYSTEM OF THE DIGITS

1. *Which one of the following structures can prevent bowstringing of the neurovascular bundle during finger flexion?*

    D. Grayson's ligament

        The retinacular system is comprised of palmar (volar) fascia and the retaining ligaments of the fingers. Grayson's and Cleland's ligaments flank the neurovascular bundle and can play a role in anchoring the skin envelope to the digital skeleton without impeding movement. Grayson's ligaments pass transversely from the flexor sheath to the skin and lie volar to the neurovascular bundles. They are thought to prevent bowstringing of the neurovascular bundles. Cleland's ligaments lie dorsally, arising from periosteum and inserting into the skin. The transverse retinacular ligaments anchor the lateral bands to the volar aspect of the proximal phalanx, near the PIP joint. Their function is to prevent excessive dorsal displacement of the lateral bands in PIP joint extension (which occurs in a swan-neck deformity). The ligament of Landsmeer originates on the volar aspect of the middle phalanx and inserts on the dorsal aspect of the distal phalanx. It helps coordinate PIP joint and DIP joint motion (**Figs. 70.1** and **70.2**).[1,2]

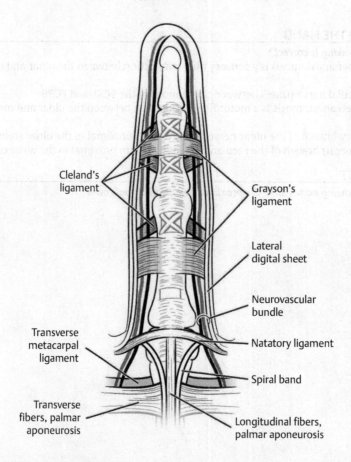

Cleland's ligament

Grayson's ligament

Lateral digital sheet

Neurovascular bundle

Natatory ligament

Transverse metacarpal ligament

Spiral band

Transverse fibers, palmar aponeurosis

Longitudinal fibers, palmar aponeurosis

Fig. 70.1   Distal volar digital fascia. (Adapted from Doyle JR, Botte MJ, eds. Surgical Anatomy of the Upper Extremity. Philadelphia: Lippincott Williams & Wilkins, 2003.)

REFERENCES

1. Doyle JR, Botte MJ, eds. Surgical Anatomy of the Hand & Upper Extremity. Philadelphia: Lippincott Williams & Wilkins; 2003

2. Beasley RW, ed. Beasley's Surgery of the Hand. New York: Thieme; 2003

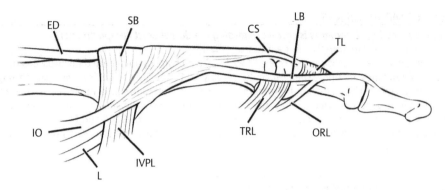

Fig. 70.2   Extensor mechanism. *CS*, Central slip; *ED*, extensor digitorum; *IO*, interosseous; *IVPL*, intervolar plate ligament (deep transverse metacarpal ligament); *L*, lumbrical; *LB*, lateral band; *ORL*, oblique retinacular ligament of Landsmeer; *SB*, sagittal band; *TL*, triangular ligament; *TRL*, transverse retinacular ligament. (Adapted from Lluch AL. Repair of the extensor tendon system. In: Aston SJ, Beasley RW, Thorne CHM, eds. Grabb and Smith's Plastic Surgery, 5th ed. Philadelphia: Lippincott-Raven, 1997.)

DEEP FASCIAL SPACES OF THE HAND

2. *Which one of the following is the location of a collar button abscess?*

    C. Interdigital space

        The fascial spaces of the hand are potential spaces that are clinically relevant with respect to hand infections. The interdigital web space is the site of a collar button abscess. Drainage usually requires both volar and dorsal approaches.

        Parona's space is important with respect to proximal spread of infection from either the midvolar space or from the radial or ulna bursa. It is important to look deep to the digital flexors for pus lying superficial to the pronator quadratus when draining palmar digital infections.[1-4] The palmar spaces are illustrated in **Fig. 70.3**.

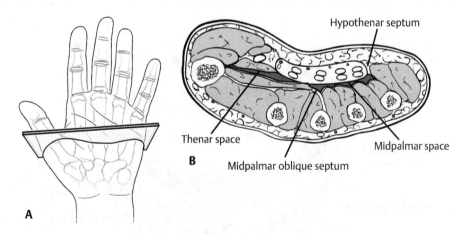

Fig. 70.3   *A* and *B*, Fascial spaces of the hand.

REFERENCES

1. Doyle JR, Botte MJ, eds. Surgical Anatomy of the Hand & Upper Extremity. Philadelphia: Lippincott Williams & Wilkins; 2003
2. Beasley RW, ed. Beasley's Surgery of the Hand. New York: Thieme; 2003
3. Teo WZW, Chung KC. Hand infections. Clin Plast Surg 2019;46(3):371–381
4. Jebson PJ. Deep subfascial space infections. Hand Clin 1998;14(4):557–566, viii

DORSAL WRIST COMPARTMENTS

3. *Which one of the following statements is correct regarding the dorsal wrist compartments?*

D. EDC travels with EIP in the fourth compartment.

The wrist contains six extensor compartments (not five), which are synovial lined fibro-osseus tunnels through which extensor tendons pass under the retinaculum (**Table 70.1**). The EIP and EDC tendons pass through the fourth extensor compartment. The posterior interosseous nerve is also found in this compartment, where it terminates to supply the wrist joint. Knowledge of its anatomic location is useful because it can be intentionally resected to treat wrist pain or can be a potential donor for digital nerve grafts. EDM and ECU are located in different compartments (fifth and sixth, respectively). ECRL and ECRB are located in the second compartment and EPL within the third compartment (**Fig. 70.4**).[1-3]

Table 70.1 *Muscles of the Dorsal Wrist Compartments*

Compartment	Muscle	Insertion	Action
First	APL	Base of first metacarpal	Extensor of first metacarpal and aids in abduction of thumb
	EPB	Base of proximal phalanx of thumb	Combines with EPL to extend thumb IP joint
Second	ECRL	Base of second metacarpal	Primarily radial deviation of wrist and secondarily wrist extension
	ECRB	Base of third metacarpal	Prime wrist extensor
Third	EPL	Passes around Lister's tubercle of radius and inserts on distal phalanx of thumb	Extends thumb IP joint
Fourth	EDC	No direct bony attachment to proximal phalanx (see Extensor mechanism below)	Extends MCP joints and, with intrinsic muscles, extends IP joints
			EDC to small finger absent in 50% of population
	EIP	Tendon lies ulnar to EDC tendon; functionally independent	Extends index finger while others are flexed
Fifth	EDM	Tendon lies ulnar to EDC tendon	Prime extensor of fifth MCP joint, allows independent small finger extension
			Abducts small finger
Sixth	ECU	Inserts on base of fifth metacarpal	Primarily ulnar deviation of wrist Secondarily wrist extension

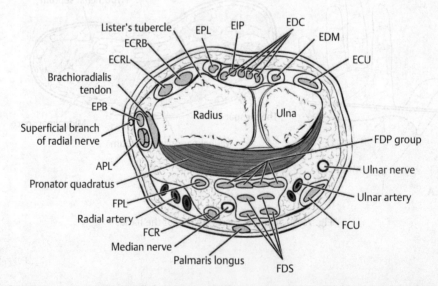

Fig. 70.4 Cross section of the wrist illustrating basic anatomic relations of major structures. Note the configuration of the flexor tendons (flexor digitorum superficialis *[FDS]* and flexor digitorum profundus *[FDP]* groups). *APL,* Abductor pollicis longus; *ECRB,* extensor carpi radialis brevis; *ECRL,* extensor carpi radialis longus; *ECU,* extensor carpi ulnaris; *EDC,* extensor digitorum communis; *EDM,* extensor digiti minimi; *EIP,* extensor indicis proprius; *EPB,* extensor pollicis brevis; *EPL,* extensor pollicis longus; *FCR,* flexor carpi radialis; *FCU,* flexor carpi ulnaris; *FPL,* flexor pollicis longus. (Adapted from Bentz ML, Bauer BS, Zuker RM. Principles & Practice of Pediatric Plastic Surgery. St Louis: Quality Medical Publishing, 2008.)

REFERENCES

1. Doyle JR, Botte MJ, eds. Surgical Anatomy of the Hand & Upper Extremity. Philadelphia: Lippincott Williams & Wilkins; 2003
2. Beasley RW, ed. Beasley's Surgery of the Hand. New York: Thieme; 2003
3. Lluch AL. Repair of the extensor tendon system. In: Aston SJ, Beasley RW, Throne CH, eds. Grabb and Smith's Plastic Surgery. 5th ed. Philadelphia: Lippincott Williams & Wilkins; 1997

EXTENSOR TENDONS OF THE HAND AND FOREARM

4. A patient is referred to you with a zone VI extensor tendon injury and who is unable to fully extend the long finger. *Where will the division have occurred?*

    E. **At the level of the metacarpal**

    There are nine extensor tendon zones. Odd numbers are over the joints, starting with zone I over the DIP joint, and even numbers are between joints (**Fig. 70.5**). The injury described is located over the metacarpal. The presence of juncturae tendinum connecting the extensor digitorum communis tendons means that a patient may still be able to partially, even fully, extend a finger at the MCP joint despite a complete division of the tendon slip to that digit. Note that the zones are different in the thumb, with TI at the IP joint, TII at the proximal phalanx, TIII at the MCP joint, TIV at the first metacarpal, and TV at the wrist.[1-3]

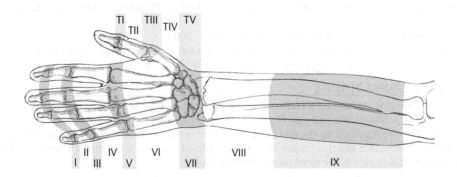

Fig. 70.5   Extensor zones of the hand and forearm. The thumb has only two zones.

REFERENCES

1. Doyle JR, Botte MJ, eds. Surgical Anatomy of the Hand & Upper Extremity. Philadelphia: Lippincott Williams & Wilkins; 2003
2. Beasley RW, ed. Beasley's Surgery of the Hand. New York: Thieme; 2003
3. Lluch AL. Repair of the extensor tendon system. In: Aston SJ, Beasley RW, Throne CH, eds. Grabb and Smith's Plastic Surgery. 5th ed. Philadelphia: Lippincott Williams & Wilkins; 1997

EXTENSOR TENDONS OF THE HAND

5. A patient presents with painful flicking of the extensor tendon over the ring finger MCP joint when making a fist. *Which structure is likely to be damaged?*

    D. **Sagittal band**

    The sagittal bands arise from the volar plate and help to stabilize the extensor tendon over the MCP joint. They may be torn during a punching injury, or sharply divided by a tooth or other sharp object. Although the intact extensor tendon may continue to extend the digit at the MCP joint, there may be painful jumping of the extensor tendon into the gutter between the metacarpal heads in flexion. Initiating extension may also be difficult or painful as the tendon loses some of its mechanical advantage when dropped between the metacarpal heads instead of being held over the dorsum of the metacarpal head by the sagittal bands.

    Central slip is the insertion of the extensor mechanism on the dorsal base of the middle phalanx where it extends the PIP joint. The juncturae tendinum are tendinous interconnections between EDC tendons on the dorsum of the hand which prevent fully independent action of EDC on a single digit. The lateral bands are formed by the intrinsics and the lateral slips. They insert onto the distal phalanx as the terminal extensor tendon. The transverse retinacular ligament prevents dorsal subluxation of the lateral bands during PIP joint extension.[1-3]

REFERENCES

1. Lluch AL. Repair of the extensor tendon system. In: Aston SJ, Beasley RW, Throne CH, eds. Grabb and Smith's Plastic Surgery. 5th ed. Philadelphia: Lippincott Williams & Wilkins; 1997
2. Kleinhenz BP, Adams BD. Closed sagittal band injury of the metacarpophalangeal joint. J Am Acad Orthop Surg 2015;23(7):415–423
3. Watson HK, Weinzweig J, Guidera PM. Sagittal band reconstruction. J Hand Surg Am 1997;22(3):452–456

INSERTIONS OF THE EXTENSOR TENDONS

6. *Which one of the following statements is correct regarding extensor tendon insertions in the hand and wrist?*
   D. EIP and EDM insert ulnar to the EDC tendons of their respective digits.
   All four fingers have an EDC tendon which effects a mass extension action. In addition, the index and little finger each have another tendon (EIP and EDM, respectively), which allows for independent extension. These may be used as tendon transfers and it is important to be able to differentiate them anatomically from EDC (see **Table 70.1**). EPL inserts on the distal phalanx of the thumb. ECRL inserts on the second metacarpal base. The EDC tendons extend over the proximal phalanges as the extensor expansion, including lateral bands and central slip, but do not insert directly into these bones. APL inserts on the base of the thumb metacarpal.[1-3]

REFERENCES

1. Doyle JR, Botte MJ, eds. Surgical Anatomy of the Hand & Upper Extremity. Philadelphia: Lippincott Williams & Wilkins; 2003
2. Beasley RW, ed. Beasley's Surgery of the Hand. New York: Thieme; 2003
3. Lluch AL. Repair of the extensor tendon system. In: Aston SJ, Beasley RW, Throne CH, eds. Grabb and Smith's Plastic Surgery. 5th ed. Philadelphia: Lippincott Williams & Wilkins; 1997

CONTENTS OF THE CARPAL TUNNEL

7. *Which one of the following statements is correct when exploring the contents of the carpal tunnel?*
   B. The FDS tendons to the middle and ring fingers lie superficial to those of the index and little fingers.
   The carpal tunnel usually contains the median nerve and nine flexor tendons (four FDS, four FDP, and FPL). The FDS tendons to the middle and ring fingers lie most superficially alongside the median nerve. FPL lies deep and just ulnar to the FCR tendon at the wrist crease (see **Fig. 70.4**).[1,2]

REFERENCES

1. Doyle JR, Botte MJ, eds. Surgical Anatomy of the Hand & Upper Extremity. Philadelphia: Lippincott Williams & Wilkins; 2003
2. Rotman MB, Donovan JP. Practical anatomy of the carpal tunnel. Hand Clin 2002;18(2):219–230

FLEXOR TENDON INJURIES IN THE HAND

8. Flexor tendon injuries are commonly seen in hand trauma patients. A thorough knowledge of flexor tendon anatomy in the hand is vital to diagnosing and managing these injuries. *Which one of the following statements is correct regarding the anatomy of this area?*
   E. The A2 and A4 annular pulleys are considered to be the most important to preserve.
   Originally Verdan[1] described five zones (not six) of flexor tendon injury, which relate to treatment and prognosis (**Fig. 70.6**). Bunnell[2] had previously described zone II as *no-man's land* because of the poor outcomes of repair in this area. This zone lies between the A1 pulley and the FDS (not the FDP) insertion and represents a tight sheath that contains both flexors. The sheath comprises five annular and three cruciate pulleys (**Fig. 70.7**). These function to prevent bowstringing and improve the mechanical advantage of tendons. The A2 and A4 pulleys are most important in preventing bowstringing and should be preserved during surgery. The odd-numbered annular pulleys are sited at the joints (MCP, PIP, and DIP), whereas the even-numbered pulleys lie over the shafts of the phalanges. All cruciate pulleys lie between the annular pulleys; however, no cruciate pulley exists between A1 and A2. The cruciate pulleys are thinner and more pliable and are thought to distort to accommodate flexion of the digit.

REFERENCES

1. Verdan CE. Primary repair of flexor tendons. J Bone Joint Surg Am 1960;42-A:647–657
2. Bunnell S. Surgery of the Hand. 2nd ed. Philadelphia: JB Lippincott; 1948

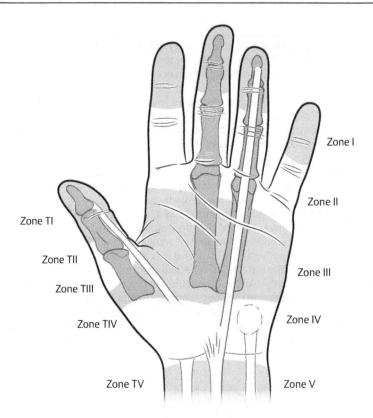

Fig. 70.6 Flexor zones of the hand. (Adapted from Zidel P. Tendon healing and flexor tendon surgery. In: Aston SJ, Beasley RW, Thorne CHM, eds. Grabb and Smith's Plastic Surgery, 5th ed. Philadelphia: Lippincott-Raven, 1997.)

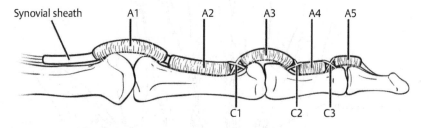

Fig. 70.7 Flexor tendon sheath pulley system. (Adapted from Zidel P. Tendon healing and flexor tendon surgery. In: Aston SJ, Beasley RW, Thorne CHM, eds. Grabb and Smith's Plastic Surgery, 5th ed. Philadelphia: Lippincott-Raven, 1997.)

FLEXOR TENDON INJURY TO THE HAND

9. You are repairing a complete FPL division from a knife wound over the proximal phalanx. The injury occurred during full flexion of the thumb. *Which one of the following statements is correct regarding the anatomy of this region?*

   C. Preservation of the oblique pulley is most important.

   The thumb flexor zones differ from those of the other digits and an injury over the proximal phalanx is located in zone II (see **Fig. 70.6**). The thumb contains only one long flexor and three pulleys (one oblique and two annular) but does not have a cruciate pulley like the fingers. The most important pulley is the oblique pulley and this is at risk of damage in a zone II injury. It is a continuation of the adductor pollicis insertion and lies between the two annular pulleys. These are located at the MCP joint and IP joints. When completely divided, the FPL tendon retracts proximally and is usually found just ulnar/deep to the FCR tendon in the wrist. The neurovascular bundles are less well protected in the thumb as they lie more superficially than in the other digits.[1-5]

REFERENCES

1. Verdan CE. Primary repair of flexor tendons. J Bone Joint Surg Am 1960;42-A:647–657
2. Bunnell S. Surgery of the Hand. 2nd ed. Philadelphia: JB Lippincott; 1948
3. Rigo IZ, Røkkum M. Predictors of outcome after primary flexor tendon repair in zone 1, 2 and 3. J Hand Surg Eur Vol 2016;41(8):793–801
4. Tonkin MA. Primary flexor tendon repair: surgical techniques based on the anatomy and biology of the flexor tendon system. World J Surg 1991;15(4):452–457
5. Zidel P. Tendon healing and flexor tendon surgery. In: Aston SJ, Beasley RW, Thorne CH, eds. Grabb and Smith's Plastic Surgery. 5th ed. Philadelphia: Lippincott Williams & Wilkins; 1997

ARTERIAL SUPPLY TO THE HAND

10. Which one of the following statements is correct regarding the arterial supply to the hand?

E. Kaplan's line is a useful marker of the superficial palmar arch.

Kaplan[1] originally described the *cardinal line* in 1953 as a line "drawn from the apex of the interdigital fold between the thumb and index finger toward the ulnar side of the hand, parallel with the middle crease of the hand." It has also been described as a line drawn across the palm from the first web space to the hook of the hamate (**Fig. 70.8**). Various authors have identified it as a useful landmark in carpal tunnel release because the superficial palmar arch is usually distal to this line, and ensuring dissection stops here should protect it from damage. The princeps pollicis artery usually arises from the deep palmar arch or from the radial artery direct (not the superficial arch) and is the dominant blood supply to the thumb. The ulnar artery lies radial (not ulnar) to the nerve and FCU at the wrist. The digital vessels lie dorsal to the nerves within the fingers, and when patients describe profuse bleeding after sustaining a knife wound to the volar aspect of the digit, they are likely to have also transected the digital nerve. The deep palmar arch is formed by the largest branch of the radial, not ulnar, artery.

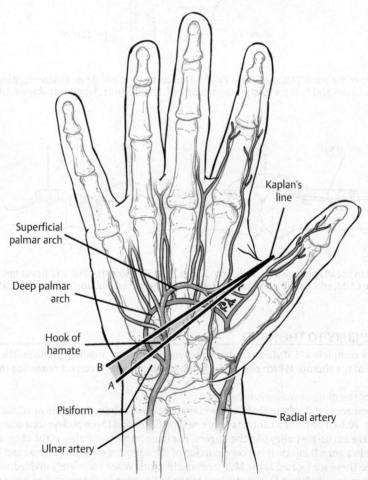

Fig. 70.8 Kaplan's line in relation to vascular anatomy of the hand.

REFERENCE

1. Kaplan EB. Surface anatomy of the hand and wrist. In: Spinner E, ed. Functional and Surgical Anatomy of the Hand. Philadelphia: JB Lippincott; 1953

INNERVATION OF THE HAND AND UPPER LIMB

11. Which one of the following actions would be lost after an injury to the ulnar nerve at the elbow?

B. Flexion of the ring finger at the DIP joint

Most of the extrinsic flexors are innervated by the median nerve, with the exception of the FDP to the little and ring fingers and the FCU. Loss of ulnar nerve function would affect the ability to flex both the little and ring fingers at the DIP joint. Flexion at the PIP joint would be spared because this is controlled by the median nerve innervated FDS. Flexion at the thumb IP joint and index finger DIP joint would also be spared as they are innervated by the anterior interosseous branch of the median nerve. The main wrist flexor is the FCU; however, wrist flexion is still possible with loss of FCU function because of the action of FCR.[1]

REFERENCE

1. Beasley RW, ed. Beasley's Surgery of the Hand. New York: Thieme; 2003

BRANCHES OF THE MEDIAN NERVE

12. Which one of the following is usually innervated by a branch of the median nerve?

C. APB

APB is innervated by the recurrent motor branch of the median nerve. It is a useful guide to median nerve function in the hand in relation to carpal tunnel syndrome. All of the other listed muscles are usually innervated by the ulnar nerve.[1]

REFERENCE

1. Beasley RW, ed. Beasley's Surgery of the Hand. New York: Thieme; 2003

SENSORY INNERVATION OF THE HAND

13. Which nerve usually supplies the skin of the dorsal hand overlying the index metacarpal?

D. Superficial branch of radial nerve

The sensory nerve supply to the hand and wrist arises from branches of the radial, ulnar, median, medial antebrachial cutaneous, and musculocutaneous nerves. The lateral antebrachial cutaneous nerve arises from the musculocutaneous nerve, and the posterior antebrachial cutaneous nerve arises from the radial nerve. The sensory distribution differs on the volar surface compared with the dorsal surface (**Fig. 70.9**).[1]

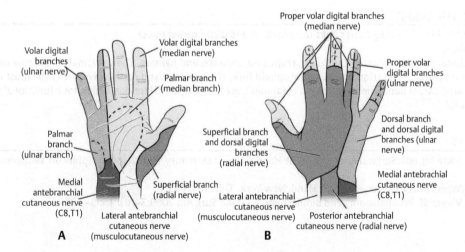

Fig. 70.9 Sensory distribution. *A*, Volar. *B*, Dorsal. (Adapted from Beasley RW, ed. Beasley's Surgery of the Hand. New York: Thieme, 2003.)

REFERENCE

1. Beasley RW, ed. Beasley's Surgery of the Hand. New York: Thieme; 2003

POSTERIOR INTEROSSEOUS NERVE PALSY

14. Which one of the following is usually spared in a posterior interosseous nerve palsy?
   A. ECRL
      BR and ECRL are usually supplied by the radial nerve before it branches into the superficial radial nerve and the posterior interosseous nerve (PIN), although sometimes ECRL is also supplied by the PIN. Therefore, patients with a posterior interosseous nerve palsy may still be able to extend their wrist.[1-3]

REFERENCES

1. Sigamoney KV, Rashid A, Ng CY. Management of atraumatic posterior interosseous nerve palsy. J Hand Surg Am 2017;42(10):826–830
2. Doyle JR, Botte MJ, eds. Surgical Anatomy of the Hand & Upper Extremity. Philadelphia: Lippincott Williams & Wilkins; 2003
3. Beasley RW, ed. Beasley's Surgery of the Hand. New York: Thieme; 2003

NERVE ANATOMY IN THE HAND

15. Which one of the following is correct?
   C. The Riche-Cannieu anastomosis is a motor fiber connection between the ulnar and median nerves in the hand.
      A Riche-Cannieu anastomosis is a motor fiber connection from the ulnar to median nerve in the hand and is thought to be present in as many as 70% of individuals. This can result in preservation of APB function despite a complete division of the median nerve at the wrist. A Martin-Gruber anastomosis is a motor fiber connection from the median to ulnar nerve in the forearm that is present in 10–25% of the United States population.[1] A Berretini sensory anastomosis can arise between the common digital nerves derived from the median and ulnar nerves.[2] A Martin-Gruber anastomosis can result in preserved ulnar nerve motor function in the hand after a high ulnar nerve injury. The presence of these variations can lead to confusion in a clinical examination, particularly in a trauma setting. When exploring wounds, it is important to be aware of the usual anatomical locations of key branches. The dorsal sensory branch of the ulnar nerve usually arises 5–7 cm proximal to the ulnar styloid process and the palmar cutaneous branch of the median nerve usually arises 5 cm proximal to the wrist crease.

REFERENCES

1. Rodriguez-Niedenführ M, Vazquez T, Parkin I, Logan B, Sañudo JR. Martin-Gruber anastomosis revisited. Clin Anat 2002;15(2):129–134
2. Tagil SM, Bozkurt MC, Ozçakar L, Ersoy M, Tekdemir I, Elhan A. Superficial palmar communications between the ulnar and median nerves in Turkish cadavers. Clin Anat 2007;20(7):795–798

BONES OF THE WRIST

16. Which one of the following bones links the proximal and distal carpal rows?
   B. Scaphoid
      The distal row includes the trapezium, trapezoid, capitate, and hamate. The proximal carpal row includes the scaphoid, lunate, and triquetrum. The scaphoid links the proximal and distal rows and is the most commonly fractured carpal bone (the pisiform is a sesamoid bone within the FCU tendon and is not a functional part of the carpus).[1-3]

REFERENCES

1. Doyle JR, Botte MJ, eds. Surgical Anatomy of the Hand & Upper Extremity. Philadelphia: Lippincott Williams & Wilkins; 2003
2. Beasley RW, ed. Beasley's Surgery of the Hand. New York: Thieme; 2003
3. Kijima Y, Viegas SF. Wrist anatomy and biomechanics. J Hand Surg Am 2009;34(8): 1555–1563

71. Basic Hand Examination

See *Essentials of Plastic Surgery*, third edition, pp. 975–987

NORMAL RANGE OF MOVEMENT IN THE HAND AND WRIST

1. A 35-year-old mechanic presents with pain and stiffness in his dominant hand and wrist after a fall 6 weeks earlier. *Which one of the following is most likely to represent a normal active joint range for this individual?*
   A. Index finger metacarpophalangeal (MCP) joint: -15 to +80 degrees
   B. Little finger metacarpophalangeal (MCP) joint: 0 to +70 degrees
   C. Middle finger proximal interphalangeal (PIP) joint: -25 to +55 degrees
   D. Wrist extension/flexion: -30 to +75 degrees
   E. Wrist radial/ulnar deviation: -10 to ±10 degrees

EXAMINING MOTOR FUNCTION OF THE HAND

2. *When examining a patient following a hand injury, which one of the following is correct?*
   A. The flexor digitorum profundus (FDP) tendon is assessed by testing isolated flexion of the proximal interphalangeal (PIP) joint.
   B. Isolated active flexion at the MCP joint specifically tests integrity of the flexor pollicis longus (FPL) tendon.
   C. Assessment of flexor digitorum superficialis (FDS) requires isolation of the adjacent digits in flexion.
   D. Adductor pollicis (AdP) weakness may be masked by thumb interphalangeal (IP) joint flexion.
   E. Abductor pollicis brevis (APB) is assessed with the hand placed flat with the palm down.

EXAMINING THE HAND AFTER INJURY

3. *When examining a patient following lacerations to the dorsum of the hand and wrist, which one of the following is correct?*
   A. Extensor digitorum communis (EDC) function can be confirmed by extending all four MCP joints with IP joints in flexion.
   B. Isolated active extension at the thumb IP joint specifically tests the integrity of the extensor pollicis longus (EPL) tendon.
   C. Extensor carpi radialis longus (ECRL) and extensor carpi radialis brevis (ECRB) cannot normally be independently assessed.
   D. Abductor pollicis longus (APL) and extensor pollicis brevis (EPB) are tested independently with different movements.
   E. Extensor carpi ulnaris (ECU) is best independently assessed by extending the wrist in neutral.

CLINICAL SIGNS OF PATHOLOGY IN THE HAND

4. *When seeing a patient with de Quervain's tenosynovitis, which one of the following movements will most exacerbate their pain?*
   A. Wrist flexion
   B. Finger extension
   C. Thumb extension
   D. Ulnar deviation of the wrist
   E. Radial deviation of the wrist

TINEL'S TEST IN THE UPPER LIMB

5. Tinel's test is a technique used to assess nerve pathology in the upper limb. *Which one of the following is correct?*
   A. An advancing Tinel's sign over time is unreliable as a guide to nerve recovery.
   B. A positive Tinel's sign is tingling along the course of a nerve upon percussion.
   C. A positive Tinel's sign at the carpal tunnel is diagnostic for carpal tunnel syndrome.
   D. The extent of a positive Tinel's sign is proportional to the severity of nerve compression.
   E. Tinel's sign is applicable only to the median nerve and carpal tunnel syndrome.

ASSESSING SPECIFIC NERVES IN THE UPPER LIMB

6. A patient has reduced sensation in the little and ring fingers and hypothenar eminence, with normal sensation on the dorsoulnar aspect of the hand. *Which one of the following is most likely?*
   A. Diabetic neuropathy
   B. T1 nerve root compression
   C. Brachial plexus tumor
   D. Ulnar nerve compression at the elbow
   E. Ulnar nerve compression at the wrist

ASSESSING SPECIFIC NERVES IN THE UPPER LIMB

7. A patient presents for a medicolegal assessment, claiming a nerve injury 6 weeks ago when he cut his finger at work. He reports reduced sensation in the index finger. The skin feels moist and wrinkles on immersion in water. Static two-point discrimination at the tip is 4 mm. *Which one of the following is most likely?*
   A. Complete division of the digital nerve
   B. 50% division of the digital nerve
   C. No significant digital nerve injury
   D. Neuroma in continuity
   E. Compression of the digital nerve by scar tissue

ASSESSING SPECIFIC NERVES IN THE UPPER LIMB

8. A patient has 6/10 sensation in the dorsal first web space following a night in handcuffs. *Which one of the following is most likely?*
   A. Posterior interosseous nerve neurapraxia
   B. Proximal radial nerve injury from prolonged pronation
   C. Superficial radial nerve neuropraxia
   D. Lateral antebrachial cutaneous nerve neurapraxia
   E. Superficial radial nerve neurotmesis

Answers

NORMAL RANGE OF MOVEMENT IN THE HAND AND WRIST

1. A 35-year-old mechanic presents with pain and stiffness in his dominant hand and wrist after a fall 6 weeks earlier. *Which one of the following is most likely to represent a normal active joint range for this individual?*

   A. Index finger metacarpophalangeal (MCP) joint: –15 to +80 degrees

   Joint range of motion does vary widely within the general population because of differences in age, joint laxity, and individual anatomy. Furthermore, active and passive ranges frequently differ with range increased on passive movement. The American Society for Surgery of the Hand (ASSH) offers a guide to normal joint ranges, which is worth reviewing (**Table 71.1**).[1]

   All of the ranges described in the clinical scenario are reduced for a healthy 35-year-old male, with the exception of answer option A. The MCP joints have a large range of motion, both passive and active. This also differs between the digits, with most being present in the little finger which can commonly have 40 degrees of extension and 90 degrees of flexion. Range of motion progressively decreases in the MCP joints moving radially from the little finger to index. This is in contrast to the PIP joint which normally has a range of 0 to 100 degrees only because of the box ligamentous structure and it is more consistent between the digits. It is vital to have a good understanding of normal and abnormal joint ranges when assessing hand patients in clinic. The best approach is to compare left with right in most cases, as this helps ascertain the "normal" or baseline range for each individual. Joint ranges must be documented in the notes, especially in conditions such as Dupuytren's disease or following a hand injury.

Table 71.1   *Normal Range of Motion Reference Values for the Upper Limb*

	Typical Range of Motion (Degrees)	
Elbow	Extension/flexion	0/145
Forearm	Pronation/supination	70/85
Wrist	Extension/flexion	70/75
	Radial/ulnar	20/35
Thumb basal joint	Palmar adduction/abduction	Contact or 45
	Radial adduction/abduction	Contact or 60
Thumb interphalangeal (IP) joint	Hyperextension/flexion	15/80
Thumb metacarpophalangeal (MCP) joint	Hyperextension/flexion	10/55
Finger distal interphalangeal (DIP) joint	Extension/flexion	0/80
Finger proximal interphalangeal (PIP) joint	Extension/flexion	0/100
Finger MCP joint	Hyperextension/flexion	(0–45/90)

REFERENCE

1. American Society for Surgery of the Hand. Normal range of motion reference values. Available at: http://www.assh.org/Public/HandAnatomy/Anatomy/Pages/Normal-Range-Motion.aspx. Accessed June 30, 2021

EXAMINING MOTOR FUNCTION OF THE HAND

2. *When examining a patient following a hand injury, which one of the following is correct?*

   D. Adductor pollicis (AdP) weakness may be masked by thumb IP joint flexion.

   To assess the AdP, a paper sheet is placed between the thumb and index finger, and the patient is asked to forcibly grasp it against resistance (**Fig. 71.1**).

   Flexion at the thumb IP joint can occur to compensate when AdP is weak (positive Froment's test, which is a classic test for ulnar nerve function).

   The flexor digitorum profundus (FDP) is assessed by immobilizing the digit and testing for isolated distal interphalangeal (DIP) joint flexion. Assessment of the flexor digitorum superficialis (FDS) requires that the adjacent digits are held in extension while flexion of the proximal interphalangeal (PIP) joint is attempted (**Figs. 71.2** and **71.3**). Immobilization is required to prevent the FDP from contributing to PIP joint flexion as it also crosses the

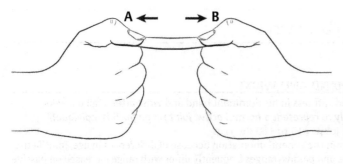

Fig. 71.1 Froment's sign. Test is positive in six (compensatory flexion at interphalangeal [IP] joint). (Adapted from American Society for Surgery of the Hand. The Hand: Examination and Diagnosis, 3rd ed. Philadelphia: Churchill Livingstone, 1990.)

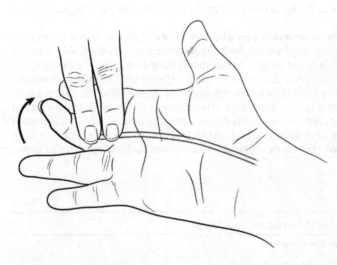

Fig. 71.2 Test for FDP myotendinous function. (Adapted from American Society for Surgery of the Hand. The Hand: Examination and Diagnosis, 3rd ed. Philadelphia: Churchill Livingstone, 1990.)

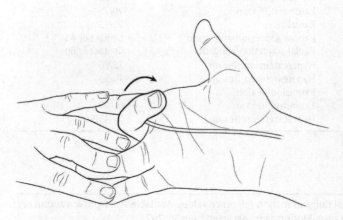

Fig. 71.3 Test for flexor digitorum superficialis (FDS) myotendinous function. (Adapted from American Society for Surgery of the Hand. The Hand: Examination and Diagnosis, 3rd ed. Philadelphia: Churchill Livingstone, 1990.)

joint. The flexor pollicis longus (FPL) is assessed by active flexion of the IP joint, not the MCP joint, which is flexed by the thenar muscles abductor pollicis brevis (APB), opponens pollicis, and flexor pollicis brevis (**Figs. 71.4** and **71.5**). The APB is tested with the hand placed on a table and the palm facing upward not downward (**Fig. 71.6**). The assessment of APB is a classic test for the recurrent motor branch of the median nerve at the wrist.[1-3]

REFERENCES

1. American Society for Surgery of the Hand. The Hand: Examination and Diagnosis. 3rd ed. New York: Churchill Livingstone, 1990
2. Day CS, Wu WK, Smith CC. Examination of the hand and wrist. N Engl J Med 2019;380(12):e15
3. Tubiana R, Thomine J, Mackin E. Examination of the Hand and Wrist. 1st ed. London: CRC Press; 1998

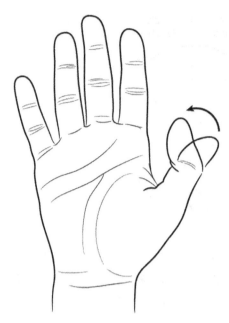

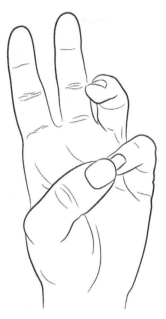

Fig. 71.4 Test for flexor pollicis longus (FPL) myotendinous function. (Adapted from American Society for Surgery of the Hand. The Hand: Examination and Diagnosis, 3rd ed. Philadelphia: Churchill Livingstone, 1990.)

Fig. 71.5 Test for thumb opposition. (Adapted from American Society for Surgery of the Hand. The Hand: Examination and Diagnosis, 3rd ed. Philadelphia: Churchill Livingstone, 1990.)

EXAMINING THE HAND AFTER INJURY

3. *When examining a patient following lacerations to the dorsum of the hand and wrist, which one of the following is correct?*

A. Extensor digitorum communis (EDC) function can be confirmed by extending all four MCP joints with IP joints in flexion.

EDC function is assessed by asking the patient to extend the fingers at the knuckles (MCP joint) with IP joints flexed or asking them to straighten all fingers simultaneously. To independently assess the extensor indicis proprius (EIP) and extensor digiti minimi/extensor digiti quinti (EDM/EDQ), the respective digits should be extended independently (**Fig. 71.7**). Isolated active extension at the thumb IP joint does not specifically test for integrity of the EPL tendon, because the extensor pollicis brevis (EPB) can also cross this joint and be responsible for IP joint extension. The EPB insertion is highly variable: it is absent in around 5% of hands, inserts into the MCP joint extensor hood in around 25%, into the base of the proximal phalanx in around 25%, and continues right up to the distal phalanx in 25%.[1] Therefore, to accurately assess EPL function, the patient should be asked to put their hand flat on a surface and lift their thumb off that surface. The full length of the EPL tendon from the extensor retinaculum to IP joint will usually be seen and be palpable (**Fig. 71.8**).

Extensor carpi radialis longus (ECRL) and extensor carpi radialis brevis (ECRB) share the same action but can be independently assessed by palpation while asking the patient to make a fist and extend the wrist (see **Fig. 71.8**).

Abductor pollicis longus (APL) and EPB are tested with the same movement but may also be differentiated by palpation of the tendons. The patient should be instructed to move their thumb out to the side or do a thumbs-up gesture (see Fig. 71.7).

Extensor carpi ulnaris (ECU) is best tested by having the patient extend the wrist with ulnar deviation while palpating the tendon at the wrist (see Fig. 71.11).[2-4]

REFERENCES

1. Jabir S, Lyall H, Iwuagwu FC. The extensor pollicis brevis: a review of its anatomy and variations. Eplasty 2013;13:e35
2. Doyle J. Extensor tendons: acute injuries. In: Green's Operative Hand Surgery. New York: Churchill Livingstone; 1993
3. Yoon AP, Chung KC. Management of acute extensor tendon injuries. Clin Plast Surg 2019;46(3):383–391
4. Tubiana R, Thomine J, Mackin E. Examination of the Hand and Wrist. 1st ed. London: CRC Press; 1998

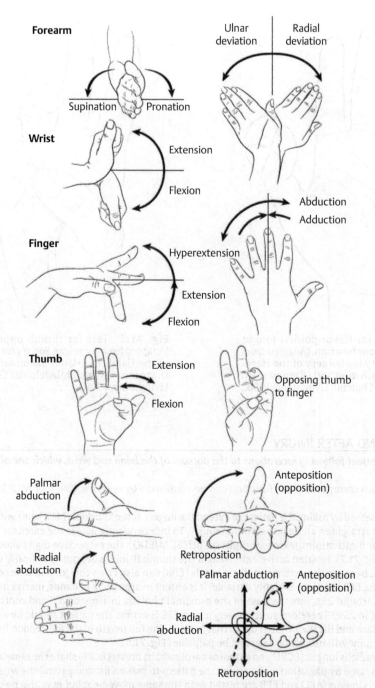

Fig. 71.6   Terminology of the hand and digit motion. (Adapted from American Society for Surgery of the Hand. The Hand: Examination and Diagnosis, 3rd ed. Philadelphia: Churchill Livingstone, 1990.)

CLINICAL SIGNS OF PATHOLOGY IN THE HAND

4. *When seeing a patient with de Quervain's tenosynovitis, which one of the following movements will most exacerbate their pain?*

   D. Ulnar deviation of the wrist

   Patients with de Quervain's tenosynovitis have tenderness and swelling affecting the first extensor compartment. Pain is exacerbated by stretching the tendons passing within this compartment, namely APL and EPB. This can be tested with either Finkelstein's test or Eichhoff's test. Both involve stretching of the tendon by pulling the hand into

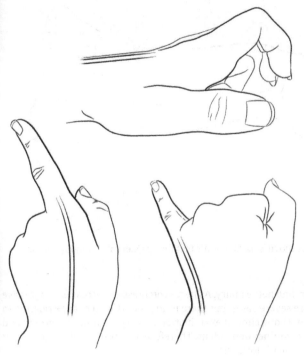

Fig. 71.7 Test for extensor digitorum communis (EDC), extensor indicis proprius (EIP), and extensor digiti minimi (EDM) (extensor digiti quinti [EDQ]) myotendinous function. (Adapted from American Society for Surgery of the Hand. The Hand: Examination and Diagnosis, 3rd ed. Philadelphia: Churchill Livingstone, 1990.)

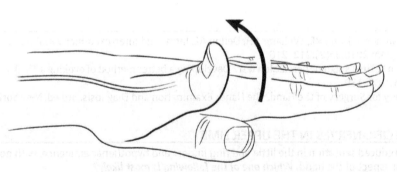

Fig. 71.8 Test for extensor pollicis longus (EPL) myotendinous function. (Adapted from American Society for Surgery of the Hand. The Hand: Examination and Diagnosis, 3rd ed. Philadelphia: Churchill Livingstone, 1990.)

ulnar deviation and applying traction on the thumb. Although the test can be performed with the thumb clasped within the patient's own fingers, it is generally thought to generate more false-positive results than placement of traction on the relaxed thumb (**Fig. 71.9**). There may also be discomfort during other movements, such as thumb extension where APL and EPB may be active, but ulnar deviation of the wrist is usually the most painful.[1-3]

REFERENCES

1. Finkelstein H. Stenosing tenosynovitis at the radial styloid process. J Bone Joint Surg 1930;12:509–540
2. Wu F, Rajpura A, Sandher D. Finkelstein's test is superior to Eichhoff's test in the investigation of de Quervain's disease. J Hand Microsurg 2018;10(2):116–118
3. Nakamura T. De Quervain's tenosynovitis. J Wrist Surg 2019;8(2):89

TINEL'S TEST IN THE UPPER LIMB

5. Tinel's test is a technique used to assess nerve pathology in the upper limb. *Which one of the following is correct?*

    B. A positive Tinel's sign is tingling along the course of a nerve upon percussion.

        A positive Tinel's sign is indicated by a tingling sensation along the course of a nerve when it is tapped at the site of compression or regeneration. It is a useful method to assess nerve regeneration in cases such as two-stage

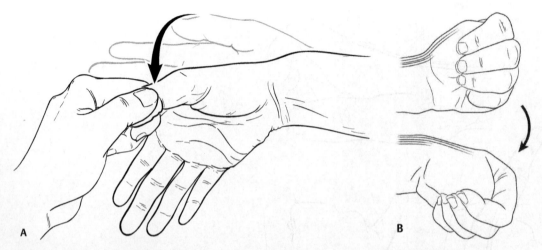

Fig. 71.9 *A,* Finkelstein's test for de Quervain's tenosynovitis. *B,* Eichhoff's test for de Quervain's tenosynovitis.

facial reanimation techniques and following upper limb nerve injury. As nerve compression increases, progressive axonal loss can lead to a loss of Tinel's sign in more severe cases, but there is no proportional change relating to greater damage. Although Tinel's sign is used as part of a clinical examination for carpal tunnel syndrome and nerve regeneration, the results are variable and examiner dependent. Therefore, this test is not diagnostic or reliable in isolation and should be combined with other information.[1–3]

REFERENCES

1. Lifchez SD, Means KR Jr, Dunn RE, Williams EH, Dellon AL. Intra- and inter-examiner variability in performing Tinel's test. J Hand Surg Am 2010;35(2):212–216
2. Monsivais JJ, Sun Y. Tinel's sign or percussion test? Developing a better method of evoking a Tinel's sign. J South Orthop Assoc 1997;6(3):186–189
3. American Society for Surgery of the Hand. The Hand: Examination and Diagnosis. 3rd ed. New York: Churchill Livingstone; 1990

ASSESSING SPECIFIC NERVES IN THE UPPER LIMB

6. A patient has reduced sensation in the little and ring fingers and hypothenar eminence, with normal sensation on the dorsoulnar aspect of the hand. *Which one of the following is most likely?*
   E. Ulnar nerve compression at the wrist
   Sparing of the dorsal sensory branch of the ulnar nerve suggests pathology distal to this branch, which arises 5 to 7 cm proximal to the ulnar styloid. More proximal lesions, or a diffuse neuropathy, would usually affect all the distal functions of the nerve, both motor and sensory.[1–3]

REFERENCES

1. Strohl AB, Zelouf DS. Ulnar tunnel syndrome, radial tunnel syndrome, anterior interosseous nerve syndrome, and pronator syndrome. J Am Acad Orthop Surg 2017;25(1):e1–e10
2. Staples JR, Calfee R. Cubital tunnel syndrome: current concepts. J Am Acad Orthop Surg 2017;25(10):e215–e224
3. Boone S, Gelberman RH, Calfee RP. The management of cubital tunnel syndrome. J Hand Surg Am 2015;40(9):1897–1904, quiz 1904

ASSESSING SPECIFIC NERVES IN THE UPPER LIMB

7. A patient presents for a medicolegal assessment, claiming a nerve injury 6 weeks ago when he cut his finger at work. He reports reduced sensation in the index finger. The skin feels moist and wrinkles on immersion in water. Static two-point discrimination at the tip is 4 mm. *Which one of the following is most likely?*
   C. No significant digital nerve injury
   This patient has objectively normal findings despite his subjective complaints. Although a degree of reduced sensation is reported, a significant digital nerve injury is very unlikely, with the normal two-point discrimination displayed (normal values for two-point discrimination are static, up to 6 mm in the fingertip, and dynamic 2 to 3

mm). Six weeks is too early for normal two-point discrimination to return after a complete or 50% nerve injury. Moist skin suggests preserved sweating and wrinkling on immersion also suggests a largely intact digital nerve. Sweating is very useful to assess when suspecting digital nerve injury, as where a patient describes altered sensation distal to a laceration and the finger also feels smooth over the same distribution, division of the nerve is likely.[1-3]

REFERENCES

1. American Society for Surgery of the Hand. The Hand: Examination and Diagnosis. 3rd ed. New York: Churchill Livingstone; 1990
2. Strauch B, Lang A, Ferder M, Keyes-Ford M, Freeman K, Newstein D. The ten test. Plast Reconstr Surg 1997;99(4): 1074–1078
3. Dunlop RLE, Wormald JCR, Jain A. Outcome of surgical repair of adult digital nerve injury: a systematic review. BMJ Open 2019;9(3):e025443

ASSESSING SPECIFIC NERVES IN THE UPPER LIMB

8. A patient has 6/10 sensation in the dorsal first web space following a night in handcuffs. *Which one of the following is most likely?*

   C. Superficial radial nerve neurapraxia

   This patient has most likely had a compression of the superficial radial nerve at the wrist from the handcuffs, resulting in a neurapraxia rather than a complete nerve division. The lateral antebrachial cutaneous nerve territory does not extend onto the hand. The posterior interosseous nerve has mainly motor function with the exception of sensory supply to the dorsal wrist capsule. A proximal radial nerve injury would involve motor weakness with decreased extension and wrist drop.[1-2]

REFERENCES

1. Tubiana R, Thomine J, Mackin E. Examination of the Hand and Wrist. 1st ed. London: CRC Press; 1998
2. American Society for Surgery of the Hand. The Hand: Examination and Diagnosis. 3rd ed. New York: Churchill Livingstone; 1990

72. Congenital Hand Anomalies

See *Essentials of Plastic Surgery*, third edition, pp. 988–1013

GENERAL PRINCIPLES IN CONGENITAL HAND ANOMALIES

1. *When managing children with congenital hand anomalies, which one of the following is true?*
   A. Parents should be advised that although anomalies are rare, they typically lead to severe functional and psychological disabilities.
   B. Parents should ideally be provided with all the relevant clinical and psychosocial information in the initial consultation.
   C. Assessment of function in clinic is assisted by observing the child using different toys.
   D. The timing of surgery is normally delayed until after 4 years of age to facilitate the child's compliance with rehabilitation.
   E. Following surgery, parents should be encouraged to change dressings on a regular basis to facilitate early mobilization.

EMBRYOLOGY OF THE UPPER LIMB

2. *Which one of the following is the most likely effect of interference with the zone of polarizing activity in the developing limb?*
   A. A truncated limb
   B. An absent limb
   C. A limb with absent fingernails
   D. A limb with abnormal ulnar development
   E. A limb with a hypoplastic thumb

CLASSIFICATION OF CONGENITAL ANOMALIES

3. *According to the International Federation of Societies for Surgery of the Hand classification system, how would a patient with syndactyly be best described?*
   A. Failure of formation
   B. Failure of differentiation
   C. Duplication
   D. Overgrowth
   E. Undergrowth

SYNDACTYLY OF THE UPPER LIMB

4. A 2-month-old baby with complex syndactyly involving all four fingers is referred to you. *Which one of the following statements is correct regarding this condition?*
   A. The term *complex* implies additional hidden phalanges or joint anomalies.
   B. Radiographs will reliably predict the subtype of syndactyly.
   C. Correctional surgery can be performed in a single stage.
   D. A Buck-Gramko stiletto flap would be the only reliable technique for correcting the tip deformities.
   E. This pattern of syndactyly is often associated with a syndrome.

SYNDACTYLY OF THE UPPER LIMB

5. You assess a 1-year-old white girl who has syndactyly of both hands. This is her initial presentation. *Which one of the following statements is correct regarding this condition?*
   A. The optimal time for surgery has passed.
   B. It is most likely to affect the middle and ring fingers.
   C. Her condition is more common than camptodactyly.
   D. The frequency of this condition is much higher in the black population.
   E. Other family members are unlikely to be affected.

CLASSIFICATION SYSTEMS FOR CONGENITAL LIMB ABNORMALITIES

6. *Which one of the following congenital limb anomalies is predominantly classified according to its radiologic features rather than clinical findings?*
   A. Thumb hypoplasia
   B. Constriction ring syndrome
   C. Macrodactyly
   D. Syndactyly
   E. Thumb duplication

CAMPTODACTYLY

7. A 13-year-old girl presents with lifelong mild flexion contractures to both little finger proximal interphalangeal (PIP) joints, which have become worse during puberty. Her range of motion in these joints is now 20 to 75 degrees. *Which one of the following statements is correct regarding her condition?*
   A. It more frequently affects the thumb and index finger.
   B. Presentation in girls of this age is fairly unusual.
   C. It is caused by an abnormal flexor digitorum profundus tendon insertion.
   D. Her condition is easily correctable with modern surgical techniques.
   E. She should be treated nonoperatively with physiotherapy.

CLINODACTYLY

8. A patient with a diagnosis of clinodactyly is referred to you. *Which one of the following statements is correct regarding this condition?*
   A. Patients often present with painful, stiff digits.
   B. The head of the proximal phalanx is often abnormal.
   C. The ring finger is most commonly affected.
   D. K-wires should be used during surgical correction.
   E. Physiotherapy and splinting are sufficient treatments in many cases.

POLYDACTYLY OF THE UPPER LIMB

9. *Which one of the following statements is correct regarding polydactyly?*
   A. The true incidence is accurately recorded at 1:1,000 live births.
   B. Classification systems are the same for preaxial and postaxial subtypes.
   C. Incidence remains fairly consistent across all racial groups.
   D. Treatment is almost always surgery, performed at 1 year of age.
   E. Other syndromes must be excluded in well-developed ulnar polydactyly.

MACRODACTYLY

10. You are referred a young patient with one digit significantly larger than the others. *Which one of the following is correct?*
    A. This condition only affects the soft tissues.
    B. Amputation is rarely indicated as the primary intervention.
    C. The digit will continue to grow disproportionately unless treated.
    D. The condition is usually bilateral and symmetrical.
    E. The patient may have associated soft-tissue nodules and café au lait spots.

RADIAL LONGITUDINAL DEFICIENCY

11. *When seeing an infant in clinic with an absent radius and confirmed cardiac anomalies, what would be the most likely diagnosis?*
    A. Holt-Oram syndrome
    B. VACTERL syndrome
    C. TAR syndrome
    D. Fanconi anemia
    E. Pollex abductus

THUMB HYPOPLASIA

12. *When considering the patient with a hypoplastic thumb, what is the clinical significance of a type 3B or greater deformity?*
    A. That the child will use the thumb normally.
    B. That the child is unlikely to require surgery.
    C. That the child will likely require pollicization.
    D. That the web space will need reconstruction with Z-plasty techniques.
    E. That ulnar collateral ligament (UCL) reconstruction will be required.

CLEFT HAND

13. You receive a referral letter about a child with typical cleft hand. *Which one of the following statements is correct?*
    A. The child is likely to have poor hand function.
    B. Syndactyly is unlikely to be a feature.
    C. Both hands are likely to be involved.
    D. Chest wall deformities are likely to be present.
    E. Metacarpal development is most likely to be normal.

CONSTRICTION BAND SYNDROME

14. You are asked to see a baby in the neonatal unit who has a grossly swollen purple toe distal to a tight band. You notice another constriction band at the ankle in the same limb. *Which one of the following statements is incorrect?*
    A. A hair tourniquet should be promptly excluded before diagnosing constriction ring syndrome in a digit.
    B. The full circumference of the band on the affected toe should be released.
    C. The band at the ankle can cause lymphedema as the child grows.
    D. A distal segment that is blue or purple should receive early surgical intervention.
    E. Plain radiographs can be helpful in planning treatment for the ankle.

PEDIATRIC TRIGGER THUMB

15. You are on call and receive a referral for a toddler whose thumb has spontaneously stuck in flexion at the interphalangeal (IP) joint. Gentle manipulation resolves the situation in clinic, and the thumb now functions normally. *Which one of the following is correct regarding this condition?*
    A. It is associated with Notta's node on the flexor pollicis longus (FPL) tendon.
    B. Treatment is usually the same in children as it is in adults.
    C. Imaging should be requested to exclude bony pathology.
    D. The child should be scheduled for definitive correction on an elective basis.
    E. The chance that the contralateral thumb is affected is 50%.

Answers

GENERAL PRINCIPLES IN CONGENITAL HAND ANOMALIES

1. When managing children with congenital hand anomalies, which one of the following is true?

C. Assessment of function in clinic is assisted by observing the child using different toys.

In contrast to adults, where clinical assessment can be directed by specific commands and copied movements, the examination of young children can be far more challenging. It is often most effective to observe the child in a calm environment with toys and see how they utilize their hand/s and assess what function is possible and what deficiencies are evident.

Congenital hand anomalies are relatively common, with an incidence of up to 1:626 live births[1] and many children with such deformities generally function very well as they adapt to the limbs with which they are born.

When meeting with parents for the first time in clinic, it is important to provide sufficient information without overloading them. Parents often go through a grieving process over the loss of the "perfect baby" that was expected,[2] and many families will not have known about the congenital difference until the baby was born. Therefore, the first visit with a family and their new born will involve careful counseling. Further information can be provided in subsequent consultations and supported with appropriate written and web-based resources.

The timing of surgery is multifactorial and there is no hard and fast rule around age. In general, it is preferable to delay elective surgery in children until they reach 1 year of age from an anesthetic perspective. Surgery may be technically easier if the hand is bigger and on this basis leaving surgery until later may be preferable. Early surgery is sometimes indicated for reasons such as differential growth in border digits in syndactyly, and in general surgery preschool is helpful for psychosocial reasons. Compliance fluctuates with age and temperament and children tend to be quite robust and fair well after surgery at most ages. When surgery has been performed it is vital to protect the limb from interference in the early phases of healing. For this reason, a meticulous, nonconstrictive dressing that is unlikely to spontaneously be removed is imperative. An above-elbow full cast with the elbow flexed at 90 degrees is frequently necessary in order to protect skin grafts or osteotomies. Prolonged postoperative immobilization is tolerated much better by children than adults, and persistent stiffness is rare.[1,2]

REFERENCES

1. Carter P, Ezaki M, Oishi S, et al. Disorders of the upper extremity. In: Herring JA, ed. Tachdjian's Pediatric Orthopedics, Vol. 1, 4th ed. Philadelphia: Saunders Elsevier; 2007
2. Waters PM, Bae DS, eds. Pediatric Hand and Upper Limb Surgery: A Practical Guide. Philadelphia: Lippincott Williams & Wilkins; 2012

EMBRYOLOGY OF THE UPPER LIMB

2. Which one of the following is the most likely effect of interference with the zone of polarizing activity in the developing limb?

D. A limb with abnormal ulnar development

Embryologic development of the limb occurs primarily between weeks 5 and 8. Growth and development occur in three main directions: proximal to distal (axial), radial to ulnar (preaxial and postaxial), and volar to dorsal.

The zone of polarizing activity (ZPA) is a cluster of mesenchymal cells on the postaxial (ulnar) border and plays a role in preaxial/postaxial (radial to ulnar) differentiation. It induces ulnar formation and the four ulnar sided digits in the hand. Consequently, interference with the ZPA results in abnormal ulnar side development such as ulnar longitudinal deficiency. Volar/dorsal development is controlled by the dorsal ectoderm and the wingless-type protein (WNT7) and Lim homeodomain transcription factor (LMX1B). Altered development in this field can result in absence of the fingernails. The apical ectodermal ridge (AER) is an ectodermal thickening at the leading edge of the limb bud, responsible for axial development. Its removal leads to limb truncation. Progressive loss of fibroblast growth factor (FGF) function at the AER leads to a loss of radial structures (e.g., thumb hypoplasia).[1-4]

REFERENCES

1. Moore KL, Persaud TV, Torchia MD, eds. The Developing Human: Clinically Oriented Embryology. 10th ed. Philadelphia: Elsevier; 2016
2. Sadler TW, ed. Langman's Medical Embryology. 13th ed. Philadelphia: Wolters Kluwer Health; 2014
3. Waters PM, Bae DS, eds. Pediatric Hand and Upper Limb Surgery: A Practical Guide. Philadelphia: Lippincott Williams & Wilkins; 2012

4. Oberg KC, Feenstra JM, Manske PR, Tonkin MA. Developmental biology and classification of congenital anomalies of the hand and upper extremity. J Hand Surg Am 2010;35(12):2066–2076

CLASSIFICATION OF CONGENITAL ANOMALIES

3. *According to the International Federation of Societies for Surgery of the Hand classification system, how would a patient with syndactyly be best described?*
   B. **Failure of differentiation**
   Swanson[1] described the uniformly accepted classification system for congenital hand anomalies in 1976. This has been adopted by most hand authorities, including the International Federation of Societies for Surgery of the Hand and the American Society for Surgery of the Hand. It has seven categories and is a popular topic for examination questions (**Table 72.1**). Syndactyly is the congenital fusion of two or more digits and is an example of failure to differentiate. The precise cause is unknown, but the theory is that there may be a failure of digital patterning, failure of apoptosis between the digits, or failure of the apical ectodermal ridge (AER) regression.[2]
   Examples of failure to form would be phocomelia or radial/ulnar longitudinal deformities. Examples of duplication include polydactyly and mirror hand. An example of overgrowth would be macrodactyly, while an example of undergrowth would be brachydactyly. There are two further categories to this classification: constriction band and generalized anomalies and syndromes. Constriction band syndrome (congenital band syndrome or Streeter's syndrome) represents a range of abnormalities where limbs or digits have linear indentations or, when severe, become circumferentially constricted leading to deformity or loss of the distal part. It is also associated with acrosyndactyly and may be confused with symbrachydactyly. It is thought to occur secondary to abnormal amniotic band material settling on the developing embryo in utero. Some conditions such as trigger thumb are not considered to be true congenital deformities and so do not fit within the classification scheme.

Table 72.1 *Classification for Congenital Hand Anomalies*[1]

Type		Examples
I	Failure of formation	Phocomelia, hypoplastic thumb, radial, central, or ulnar longitudinal deficiency
II	Failure of differentiation	Synostosis, syndactyly, radial head dislocation, symphalangism, camptodactyly, clinodactyly, Kirner's deformity
III	Duplication	Polydactyly, mirror hand, duplicate thumb
IV	Overgrowth	Macrodactyly
V	Undergrowth	Brachydactyly
VI	Constriction band	Constriction band
VII	Generalized	

REFERENCES

1. Swanson AB. A classification for congenital limb malformations. J Hand Surg Am 1976;1(1):8–22
2. Choi M, Sharma S, Louie O. Congenital hand abnormalities. In: Thorne C, ed. Grabb & Smith's Plastic Surgery. 6th ed. Philadelphia: Lippincott Williams & Wilkins; 2006

SYNDACTYLY OF THE UPPER LIMB

4. *A 2-month-old baby with complex syndactyly involving all four fingers is referred to you. Which one of the following statements is correct regarding this condition?*
   E. **This pattern of syndactyly is often associated with a syndrome.**
   This pattern of syndactyly can occur as part of Apert's syndrome. The term *complex syndactyly* refers to bony fusion of the distal phalanges. Additional phalanges (polysyndactyly) and abnormal joints (e.g., symphalangism) are classified as *complicated syndactyly*. This term is used inconsistently. It is sometimes used to describe significant neurovascular or tendinous anomalies or syndactyly that occurs as part of a syndrome (**Fig. 72.1**). Upton[1] classified the hand anomalies in Apert's syndrome as follows:
   Type I: Complex syndactyly of all four fingers, the first web space is spared
   Type II: Complex syndactyly of all four fingers, simple first web syndactyly
   Type III: Complex syndactyly of all digits, including the thumb
   Radiographs are critical for evaluating bony involvement but can give false results as a result of incomplete ossification. A rule of thumb is that surgery should be performed only on one side of a digit at a time to minimize risk to the vascular supply; therefore, surgery for this child will require staging. Tip reconstruction can be performed with a Hentz "pulp plasty" or Buck-Gramko (stiletto) flaps.

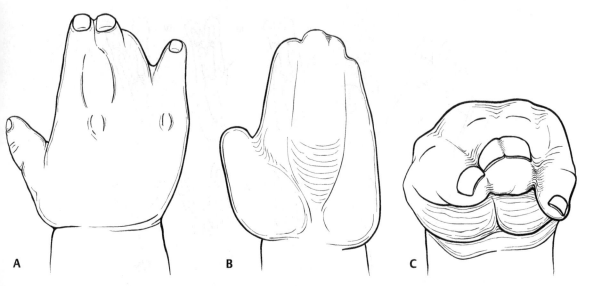

Fig. 72.1 *A*, Typical type I or spade-shaped hand. *B*, Type II or mitten hand. *C*, Type III or rosebud hand.

REFERENCE

1. Upton J. Apert syndrome. Classification and pathologic anatomy of limb anomalies. Clin Plast Surg 1991;18(2):321–355

SYNDACTYLY OF THE UPPER LIMB

5. You assess a 1-year-old white girl who has syndactyly of both hands. This is her initial presentation. *Which one of the following statements is correct regarding this condition?*
   B. It is most likely to affect the middle and ring fingers.

   The most common site for syndactyly is the third web space, with the first web space being seen least often. In the United States, the incidence of syndactyly is 1:2,000 live births. This condition is 10 times more common in white people than in black people and up to 40% of cases have a family history of syndactyly. Syndactyly is much less common than camptodactyly, the incidence of which is probably closer to 1:100. It is difficult to define the optimal time for surgery, but it is commonly performed between 1 and 2 years of age provided it does not affect the border digits. If border digits are involved, correction is usually carried out earlier so that differential growth of the digits is not affected.[1–3]

REFERENCES

1. Lumenta DB, Kitzinger HB, Beck H, Frey M. Long-term outcomes of web creep, scar quality, and function after simple syndactyly surgical treatment. J Hand Surg Am 2010;35(8):1323–1329
2. Goldfarb CA. Congenital hand differences. J Hand Surg Am 2009;34(7):1351–1356
3. Kay SP, McCombe DB, Kozin SH. Deformities of the hand and fingers. In: Wolfe SW, Hotchkiss RN, Pederson WC, et al, eds. Green's Operative Hand Surgery, Vol. 2. 6th ed. Philadelphia: Elsevier; 2011

CLASSIFICATION SYSTEMS FOR CONGENITAL LIMB ABNORMALITIES

6. *Which one of the following congenital limb anomalies is predominantly classified according to its radiologic features rather than clinical findings?*
   E. Thumb duplication

   Wassel[1] classified thumb duplication according to the underlying bony anatomy (**Fig. 72.2**).
   Type I: Least common, occurs in 2%[2]
   Type IV: Most common, occurs in 43%[2]
   Type VII: Most complex, requires at least one triphalangeal thumb.
   Syndactyly is classified into incomplete/complete, simple/complex/complicated, according to both soft-tissue and skeletal features. Classification systems for other abnormalities have also been described and these are largely based on clinical appearance.
   Blauth[3] classified hypoplastic thumb anomalies, and Manske and McCaroll[4] modified them as follows:
   Type 1: Diminution of thenar muscle bulk, smaller thumb elements
   Type 2: Absence of thenar intrinsic muscles, decreased thumb–index web space, metacarpophalangeal (MCP) joint instability from the ulnar collateral ligament

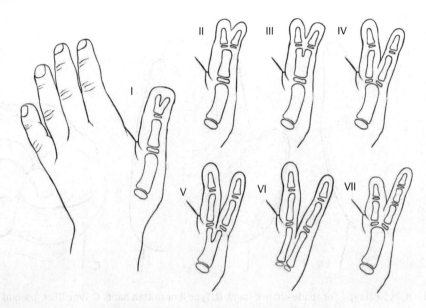

Fig 72.2   Wassel classification of thumb polydactyly.

Type 3A: Type 2 with extrinsic muscle abnormalities, even less bony (metacarpal) element, stable carpometacarpal (CMC) joint

Type 3B: Type 3A with an unstable CMC joint

Type 4: Floating thumb (pouce flottant): Small pedicle holding a floating thumb

Type 5: Completely absent thumb

A key point is that the presence or absence of a stable CMC joint will guide surgical management.

Patterson[5] classified constriction ring syndrome as follows:

Type I: Simple constriction ring

Type II: Constriction ring with deformity of the distal part

Type III: Constriction with variable fusion of distal parts (acrosyndactyly)

Type IV: Complete intrauterine disruption

Upton[6] classified macrodactyly as follows:

Type I: Macrodactyly with lipofibromatosis of the nerve(s)

Type II: Associated with neurofibromatosis (von Recklinghausen's disease)

Type III: Macrodactyly with hyperostosis (very rare)

Type IV: Macrodactyly with hemihypertrophy

REFERENCES

1. Wassel HD. The results of surgery for polydactyly of the thumb. A review. Clin Orthop Relat Res 1969;64:175–193
2. Flatt AE, ed. The Care of Congenital Hand Anomalies. 2 ed. St Louis: Quality Medical Publishing; 1994
3. Blauth W. [The hypoplastic thumb]. Arch Orthop Unfallchir 1967;62(3):225–246
4. Manske PR, McCaroll HR Jr. Index finger pollicization for a congenitally absent or nonfunctioning thumb. J Hand Surg Am 1985;10(5):606–613
5. Patterson TJ. Congenital ring-constrictions. Br J Plast Surg 1961;14:1–31
6. Upton J. Congenital anomalies of the hand and forearm. In: McCarthy JG, ed. Plastic Surgery, Vol. 8. 2nd ed. Philadelphia: WB Saunders; 1990

CAMPTODACTYLY

7. A 13-year-old girl presents with lifelong mild flexion contractures to both little finger proximal interphalangeal (PIP) joints, which have become worse during puberty. Her range of motion in these joints is now 20 to 75 degrees. *Which one of the following statements is correct regarding her condition?*

   E. She should be treated nonoperatively with physiotherapy.

   Camptodactyly is a common condition typically affecting the little finger. It can be present and first noticed at birth or it can worsen with accelerated growth and only become evident around the time of puberty. Females are more commonly affected than males and presentation is common at this age. The underlying cause is not confirmed, but theories include abnormal flexor digitorum superficialis (FDS), tendons (such as additional FDS slips), abnormal extensor tendons, bony deformities of the proximal interphalangeal (PIP) joint, or abnormal lumbrical muscle insertions. Mild contractures should be managed with physiotherapy and extension splinting. More severe contractures may occasionally require surgical release; however, surgery has a high failure rate. Plain radiographs should be obtained to exclude bony abnormalities. The lateral view is particularly important to assess the joint shape and articular surfaces.[1-3]

REFERENCES

1. Carter P, Ezaki M, Oishi S, et al. Disorders of the upper extremity. In: Herring JA, ed. Tachdjian's Pediatric Orthopedics, Vol. 1, 4th ed. Philadelphia: Saunders Elsevier; 2007
2. Goldfarb CA. Congenital hand differences. J Hand Surg Am 2009;34(7):1351–1356
3. Kozin SH, Kay SP, Griffin JR, et al. Congenital contracture. In: Wolfe SW, Hotchkiss RN, Pederson WC, et al, eds. Green's Operative Hand Surgery, Vol. 2. 6th ed. Philadelphia: Elsevier; 2011

CLINODACTYLY

8. A patient with a diagnosis of clinodactyly is referred to you. *Which one of the following statements is correct regarding this condition?*

D. K-wires should be used during surgical correction.

Clinodactyly refers to a curvature of the finger in a radial/ulnar direction and often features an abnormal middle phalanx. The physis may be **C**-shaped (bracketed) around one corner of the phalangeal base (**Fig. 72.3**). The middle phalanx may be triangular or trapezoidal in shape and the former is termed a "delta" phalanx. These features prevent normal growth on one side resulting in uneven growth of the digit. The presence of a deformed head of the proximal phalanx is more typical of camptodactyly. Clinodactyly is usually painless and affects the little finger most frequently. Surgical correction nearly always requires a stabilizing K-wire. A Z-plasty may be required to release the soft tissues. Splinting is not an effective treatment for clinodactyly.[1-4]

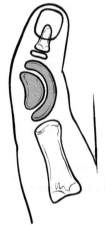

Fig. 72.3 Clinodactyly caused by a longitudinally bracketed physis.

REFERENCES

1. Carter P, Ezaki M, Oishi S, et al. Disorders of the upper extremity. In: Herring JA, ed. Tachdjian's Pediatric Orthopedics, Vol. 1. 4th ed. Philadelphia: Saunders Elsevier; 2007
2. Goldfarb CA. Congenital hand differences. J Hand Surg Am 2009;34(7):1351–1356
3. Kay SP, McCombe DB, Kozin SH. Deformities of the hand and fingers. In: Wolfe SW, Hotchkiss RN, Pederson WC, et al, eds. Green's Operative Hand Surgery, Vol. 2. 6th ed. Philadelphia: Elsevier; 2011
4. Kozin SH. Upper-extremity congenital anomalies. J Bone Joint Surg Am 2003;85(8): 1564–1576

POLYDACTYLY OF THE UPPER LIMB

9. *Which one of the following statements is correct regarding polydactyly?*

E. Other syndromes must be excluded in well-developed ulnar polydactyly.

Polydactyly is a condition where there are more than five digits on one hand. In well-developed ulnar-side polydactyly, there is a 30% risk of syndromic association; therefore, a full workup should be arranged in such cases. In contrast, mild ulnar polydactyly is rarely associated with other conditions and normally represents an isolated finding. Although conditions such as Holt-Oram syndrome and Fanconi anemia are more common with radial longitudinal deficiency, an association also exists between them and radial polydactyly (specifically, triphalangeal thumb or Wassel type VII). Therefore, it is prudent to ensure that the children with radial polydactyly are also fully assessed by a pediatrician.[1,2] Polydactyly is classified as preaxial or postaxial, depending on whether the radial or ulnar digits are duplicated. Postaxial subtypes are classified as A or B, depending on how well the extra digit is formed (A is well formed and B is rudimentary). Preaxial subtypes are classified using the Wassel system.[3] Both classifications are useful to guide management. Incidence is estimated to be between 1:300 and 1:3,000 depending on subtype and race. These may be underestimates because of autoamputation of rudimentary digits at an early age. Complex surgery is not required for the majority of polydactyly cases. Treatment requirements depend on the subtype and extent of the abnormality. For example, mild ulnar polydactyly may autoamputate or be managed with simple ligation, whereas complex radial polydactyly may require complex reconstruction of the thumb with ligamentous, bony, and muscle insertion alteration.

REFERENCES

1. Castilla EE, Lugarinho R, da Graça Dutra M, Salgado LJ. Associated anomalies in individuals with polydactyly. Am J Med Genet 1998;80(5):459–465
2. Wilks DJ, Kay SP, Bourke G. Fanconi's anaemia and unilateral thumb polydactyly–don't miss it. J Plast Reconstr Aesthet Surg 2012;65(8):1083–1086
3. Upton J. Congenital anomalies of the hand and forearm. In: McCarthy JG, ed. Plastic Surgery, Vol 8. 2nd ed. Philadelphia: WB Saunders; 1990

MACRODACTYLY

10. You are referred a young patient with one digit significantly larger than the others. *Which one of the following is correct?*

E. The patient may have associated soft-tissue nodules and café au lait spots.

Macrodactyly is a condition of overgrowth of a digit and is usually an isolated unilateral finding but may be associated with other conditions such as neurofibromatosis. For this reason, a full assessment of the other features associated with neurofibromatosis should be explored. The etiology of macrodactyly is largely unknown, but the most common theory is that the growth is somehow nerve induced. There are different types of macrodactyly (static or progressive) and growth may therefore be proportional or disproportionate to other digits. Both soft tissue and bone are usually affected, and amputation may be the best option for some patients, although debulking is generally performed as a first-line treatment. The psychological effects of this condition can be severe, so a multidisciplinary approach including counseling is advised.[1-3]

REFERENCES

1. Kay SP, McCombe DB, Kozin SH. Deformities of the hand and fingers. In: Wolfe SW, Hotchkiss RN, Pederson WC, et al, eds. Green's Operative Hand Surgery, Vol. 2, 6th ed. Philadelphia: Elsevier; 2011
2. Labow BI, Pike CM, Upton J. Overgrowth of the hand and upper extremity and associated syndromes. J Hand Surg Am 2016;41(3):473–482, quiz 482
3. Upton J. Congenital anomalies of the hand and forearm. In: McCarthy JG, ed. Plastic Surgery, Vol. 8, 2nd ed. Philadelphia: WB Saunders; 1990

RADIAL LONGITUDINAL DEFICIENCY

11. *When seeing an infant in clinic with an absent radius and confirmed cardiac anomalies, what would be the most likely diagnosis?*

A. Holt-Oram syndrome

Radial longitudinal deficiency is a congenital condition affecting the radial structures of the arm and may include either a hypoplastic or absent radius and thumb anomalies. It is essential to evaluate such patients for other associated conditions.

Holt-Oram syndrome is an autosomal dominant condition where patients have a radial longitudinal deformity and a number of cardiac defects including septal defects, tetralogy of Fallot, mitral valve prolapse, and a patent ductus arteriosus.

VACTERL syndrome involves vertebral, anal, cardiac, tracheoesophageal fistula, renal and lower extremity abnormalities, as well as the radial longitudinal deficiency. Blood dyscrasias associated with radial longitudinal deficiency include TAR syndrome (thrombocytopenia and absent radius) and Fanconi anemia which is an autosomal dominant condition with bone marrow failure. Pollex abductus is a situation where the long thumb flexor tendon inserts onto the extensor mechanism, thereby causing abduction on forced thumb flexion. It may be present in radial longitudinal deficiency or polydactyly.

All patients with radial longitudinal deficiency should receive a cardiac workup (auscultation, echocardiography), a renal ultrasound, complete blood count (CBC) with differential and medical genetics referral. However, in most cases, these have already been done by the referring team prior to review in the plastic surgery clinic.[1-4]

REFERENCES

1. Al-Qattan MM, Al-Sahabi A, Al-Arfaj N. Ulnar ray deficiency: a review of the classification systems, the clinical features in 72 cases, and related developmental biology. J Hand Surg Eur Vol 2010;35(9):699–707
2. Goldfarb CA, Wall L, Manske PR. Radial longitudinal deficiency: the incidence of associated medical and musculoskeletal conditions. J Hand Surg Am 2006;31(7):1176–1182
3. James MA, Bedmar MS. Malformations and deformities of the wrist and forearm. In: Wolfe SW, Hotchkiss RN, Pederson WC, et al, eds. Green's Operative Hand Surgery, Vol. 2. 6th ed. Philadelphia: Elsevier; 2011
4. Solomon BD. The etiology of VACTERL association: current knowledge and hypotheses. Am J Med Genet C Semin Med Genet 2018;178(4):440–446

THUMB HYPOPLASIA

12. When considering the patient with a hypoplastic thumb, what is the clinical significance of a type 3B or greater deformity?

C. That the child will likely require pollicization.

Thumb hypoplasia is a type of radial longitudinal deficiency with a spectrum of severity that is classified using the modified Blauth system. This classification is useful clinically, as it directs likely treatment.

Type I is a mild deformity where the thenar intrinsic muscles are hypoplastic and the thumb is generally reduced in size. This rarely requires surgical intervention. Type 2 involves thenar intrinsic hypoplasia with a narrowed first web space, metacarpophalangeal (MCP) joint instability from ulnar collateral ligament (UCL) laxity. Type 3A is similar to type 2 but also involves extrinsic muscle abnormalities, hypoplastic bony elements, and a stable carpometacarpal (CMC) joint. Both 2 and 3a subtypes are treated with web space deepening such as Z-plasties or a jumping man flap. Opponensplasty with ring finger FDS, extensor indicis proprius (EIP), or Huber transfer may be required. UCL stabilization may also be needed.

Type 3B has the same features as type 3A, but the defining difference is the lack of a stable CMC joint. Type 4 is a floating thumb and type 5 is a complete aplasia. Therefore, types 3B and above are typically treated with pollicization.

Routine use of the thumb by the child helps the clinician to distinguish a type 3A from a type 3B deformity, as the child will tend to ignore the thumb, instead preferring a scissor grip with the index and long fingers.[1-4]

REFERENCES

1. Kay SP, McCombe DB, Kozin SH. Deformities of the hand and fingers. In: Wolfe SW, Hotchkiss RN, Pederson WC, et al, eds. Green's Operative Hand Surgery, Vol. 2. 6th ed. Philadelphia: Elsevier; 2011
2. Kozin SH. Deformities of the thumb. In: Wolfe SW, Hotchkiss RN, Pederson WC, et al, eds. Green's Operative Hand Surgery, Vol. 2. 6th ed. Philadelphia: Elsevier; 2011
3. Light TR, Gaffey JL. Reconstruction of the hypoplastic thumb. J Hand Surg Am 2010;35(3):474–479
4. Tay SC, Moran SL, Shin AY, Cooney WP III. The hypoplastic thumb. J Am Acad Orthop Surg 2006;14(6):354–366

CLEFT HAND

13. You receive a referral letter about a child with typical cleft hand. Which one of the following statements is correct?

C. Both hands are likely to be involved.

Typical cleft hand is normally bilateral and familial. Syndactyly is a common finding. Hand function is usually very good, but cosmesis is poor. For this reason, Flatt described it as a "functional triumph, but a social disaster." Metacarpal abnormalities are common, as these bones can be absent, bifid, or duplicated. This condition may be associated with cleft lip or cleft palate; so, the oral cavity should be assessed during examination. Atypical cleft hand differs from typical cleft hand and can occur as part of Poland's syndrome. Therefore, it can be associated with any of the other common features of Poland's syndrome such as chest wall deformity, upper limb abnormality, or breast hypoplasia. Atypical cleft hand is unilateral and spontaneous with syndactyly occurring infrequently. The remaining digits can be markedly hypoplastic.[1,2]

REFERENCES

1. Miura T, Komada T. Simple method for reconstruction of the cleft hand with an adducted thumb. Plast Reconstr Surg 1979;64(1):65–67
2. Upton J, Taghinia AH. Correction of the typical cleft hand. J Hand Surg Am 2010;35(3): 480–485

CONSTRICTION BAND SYNDROME

14. You are asked to see a baby in the neonatal unit who has a grossly swollen purple toe distal to a tight band. You notice another constriction band at the ankle in the same limb. Which one of the following statements is incorrect?

B. The full circumference of the band on the affected toe should be released.

Vascular compromise in the toe warrants prompt surgical release. However, it is advisable to release no more than 50% of the circumference at one time to reduce the risk of exacerbating vascular compromise. If the toe were simply lymphedematous, observation and elevation would be sufficient at this early stage. As a child grows, constriction bands can interfere with deeper structures, and plain radiographs can be helpful to monitor the underlying ankle joint. Hair tourniquets around the toes of infants are commonly referred to plastic surgery for review. The hair is usually very difficult to visualize even with loupe magnification and management may require blade division of the hair down to or through the skin to ensure adequate release.[1-3]

REFERENCES

1. Upton J, Tan C. Correction of constriction rings. J Hand Surg Am 1991;16(5):947–953
2. Patterson TJ. Congenital ring-constrictions. Br J Plast Surg 1961;14:1–31
3. Kay SP, McCombe DB, Kozin SH. Deformities of the hand and fingers. In: Wolfe SW, Hotchkiss RN, Pederson WC, et al, eds. Green's Operative Hand Surgery, Vol. 2. 6th ed. Philadelphia: Elsevier; 2011

PEDIATRIC TRIGGER THUMB

15. You are on call and receive a referral for a toddler whose thumb has spontaneously stuck in flexion at the interphalangeal (IP) joint. Gentle manipulation resolves the situation in clinic, and the thumb now functions normally. *Which one of the following is correct regarding this condition?*

    A. It is associated with Notta's node on the flexor pollicis longus (FPL) tendon.

    Trigger thumb in a child is treated differently from that in adults. Half of all cases of pediatric trigger thumb will settle without surgery within 6 months with conservative measures including stretching. Steroid injections and splinting usually provide no benefit. It is bilateral in only a quarter (not half) of cases, and imaging is rarely indicated unless trauma has occurred. Notta's node is a thickening on the FPL tendon that catches on the A1 pulley. This pulley is surgically released only in persistent cases. The diagnosis should be explained to the parents and follow-up planned for approximately 6 to 8 weeks.[1,2]

REFERENCES

1. Kozin SH. Deformities of the thumb. In: Wolfe SW, Hotchkiss RN, Pederson WC, et al, eds. Green's Operative Hand Surgery, Vol. 2. 6th ed. Philadelphia: Elsevier; 2011
2. Bae DS, Sodha S, Waters PM. Surgical treatment of the pediatric trigger finger. J Hand Surg Am 2007;32(7):1043–1047

73. Carpal Bone Fractures

See *Essentials of Plastic Surgery*, third edition, pp. 1014–1024

THE SCAPHOID BONE

1. *Which one of the following statements is correct regarding the scaphoid bone?*
   A. It is most commonly fractured in children and adolescents.
   B. Its entire surface is covered with articular cartilage.
   C. It is the only bone to bridge the proximal and distal carpal rows.
   D. It is supplied by a single distal vascular pedicle originating from the radial artery.
   E. The volar portion of the scapholunate ligament is stronger than the dorsal component.

DIAGNOSING A SCAPHOID FRACTURE

2. *Which one of the following statements is correct regarding the process of diagnosing a scaphoid fracture?*
   A. Forced hyperextension is the only mechanism causing scaphoid waist fractures.
   B. Tenderness in the anatomical snuffbox is highly specific for a scaphoid fracture.
   C. Comprehensive five-view radiographic imaging can reliably exclude a scaphoid fracture.
   D. An MRI scan of the wrist should normally be obtained in the acute setting.
   E. Bone scans can be a useful aid in fracture diagnosis after a few weeks.

TREATMENT OF SCAPHOID FRACTURES

3. A 20-year-old woman presents with an acute, proximal pole scaphoid fracture. Plain radiographs confirm the fracture is nondisplaced. *Which one of the following statements is correct regarding management of this patient?*
   A. Nonoperative management in a short-arm cast should be undertaken.
   B. She would benefit from internal fixation with a differential pitch screw.
   C. Splinting in a thumb spica cast is required for up to 6 weeks.
   D. Her profession will be the main factor in guiding treatment selection.
   E. If internal fixation is selected, a volar approach must be used.

COMPLICATIONS AFTER SCAPHOID FRACTURES

4. A 30-year-old man is referred to you with a persistent nonunion of a scaphoid fracture after 8 weeks of immobilization. *Which one of the following statements is correct regarding the sequelae of scaphoid fractures?*
   A. Nonunion of a scaphoid fracture typically results in a volar intercalated segment instability (VISI) deformity.
   B. Scaphoid nonunion is the main cause of a scapholunate advanced collapse (SLAC) wrist deformity.
   C. A humpback deformity following scaphoid malunion requires surgical intervention.
   D. Degenerative arthritis of the wrist is very common after proximal scaphoid nonunion.
   E. A delayed union is diagnosed if pain is ongoing and no radiographic evidence of union is seen at 6 weeks of immobilization.

CARPAL BONE FRACTURES

5. *Which one of the following statements is correct regarding carpal bone fractures?*
   A. Fractures of the hook of the hamate are often associated with a median nerve injury.
   B. Hamate fractures have a low rate of nonunion with nonoperative care.
   C. Fractures to the pisiform are easily viewed on anteroposterior (AP) and lateral radiographs.
   D. Hamate body fractures can occur with fourth and fifth CMC joint dislocations and often require fixation.
   E. The triquetrum tends to fracture with forced thumb hyperextension.

CARPAL BONE FRACTURES

6. *Which carpal bone is the least commonly fractured, as a result of the protection of the surrounding bony anatomy and strong carpal ligaments?*
    A. Scaphoid
    B. Triquetrum
    C. Trapezoid
    D. Trapezium
    E. Lunate

KIENBOCK'S DISEASE OF THE WRIST

7. *A patient is referred with a diagnosis of Kienbock's disease. Which one of the following carpal bones is most likely to have been injured preceding this diagnosis?*
    A. Trapezium
    B. Capitate
    C. Lunate
    D. Trapezoid
    E. Pisiform

THE ANVIL MECHANISM IN WRIST INJURY

8. *Which one of the following carpal bones may be fractured during a wrist hyperextension injury through the "anvil mechanism."*
    A. Triquetrum
    B. Hamate
    C. Trapezium
    D. Capitate
    E. Lunate

DELAYED PRESENTATION OF CARPAL BONE FRACTURES

9. A young male patient presents with a spontaneous inability to flex the little finger at the proximal interphalangeal and distal interphalangeal joints. There has been no recent trauma to the little finger itself, but about 3 months ago he sustained a fall onto his outstretched hand while mountain biking. He sought no medical intervention but has continued to have a tender wrist. Plain radiographs confirm evidence of a carpal bone fracture. *Which one of the following is most likely to be involved?*
    A. Hook of hamate
    B. Body of hamate
    C. Body of triquetrum
    D. Volar pole of lunate
    E. Body of capitate

IMAGING OF THE WRIST

10. *Which one of the following radiographic views of the wrist best demonstrates a hook of hamate fracture?*
    A. Anteroposterior (AP) view of wrist
    B. Carpal tunnel view
    C. 45-degree pronated oblique view
    D. AP in ulnar deviation
    E. Reverse oblique view

Answers

THE SCAPHOID BONE

1. Which one of the following statements is correct regarding the scaphoid bone?

C. It is the only bone to bridge the proximal and distal carpal rows.

The scaphoid is a component of the proximal carpal row and is the only bone to bridge both proximal and distal rows. It is an important component in normal wrist function. While it is the most commonly fractured bone of the carpus, fractures are uncommon in children and it remains cartilaginous. Approximately 80% of the surface is covered with articular cartilage, leaving a thin strip around the dorsal waist where most blood supply enters. The scaphoid has two (not one) vascular pedicles, both of which originate from the radial artery: one at the distal tubercle, supplying 20%, and the other along the dorsal ridge which supplies the remaining 80%. There are no vessels entering proximal to the wrist, hence the higher rate of nonunion and avascular necrosis with proximal fractures. During surgery, care should be taken to preserve the dorsal ridge region of vascular supply. The dorsal scapholunate ligament is far stronger than its volar counterpart and this serves to prevent excessive flexion of the scaphoid relative to the lunate.[1-4]

REFERENCES

1. Garcia-Ellis M. Carpal bone fractures. In: Weinzweig J, ed. The Wrist. Philadelphia: Lippincott Williams & Wilkins; 2001
2. Nakamura R, Imaeda T, Horii E, Miura T, Hayakawa N. Analysis of scaphoid fracture displacement by three-dimensional computed tomography. J Hand Surg Am 1991;16(3): 485–492
3. Wolfe S. Fractures of the Carpus: scaphoid fractures. In: RA Berger AW, ed. Hand Surgery. Philadelphia: Lippincott Williams & Wilkins; 2004
4. Gelberman RH, Panagis JS, Taleisnik J, Baumgaertner M. The arterial anatomy of the human carpus. Part I: The extraosseous vascularity. J Hand Surg Am 1983;8(4):367–375

DIAGNOSING A SCAPHOID FRACTURE

2. Which one of the following statements is correct regarding the process of diagnosing a scaphoid fracture?

E. Bone scans can be a useful aid in fracture diagnosis after a few weeks.

The standard approach to imaging for suspected scaphoid fractures is five-view radiographs. There are variations between institutions regarding the series of images acquired. A typical series includes posteroanterior (PA), lateral, oblique, clenched fist, and scaphoid views. Despite this, normal radiographs cannot always exclude a scaphoid fracture, so they may need to be repeated after 2 or 3 weeks or augmented by additional investigations. CT imaging can provide a more detailed examination of the scaphoid. After a few weeks, bone scans can also be useful because they show increased isotope activity along the fracture line. However, they may tend to overdiagnose fractures. While CT is helpful in identifying the scaphoid and its alignment, MRI is preferred by many in the acute phase, as other causes of pain (such as bone contusions) may also be demonstrated. However, the cost of this modality and the difficulties in getting timely access to scans precludes its routine use in most patients. Furthermore, MRI and CT may each still underdiagnose scaphoid fractures. There are two main mechanisms of injury for scaphoid fracture: axial loading from a punch injury and hyperextension injuries, such as occurring during a fall onto the outstretched hand. Axial loading frequently results in fractures of the scaphoid waist. Although tenderness in the anatomic snuffbox is common in scaphoid fractures, it is nonspecific and is seen in some normal people and with many other conditions. When there is an acute scaphoid fracture present, there is normally additional volar or dorsal tenderness identified.[1-5]

REFERENCES

1. Gelberman RH, Menon J. The vascularity of the scaphoid bone. J Hand Surg Am 1980;5(5):508–513
2. Steinmann SP, Adams JE. Scaphoid fractures and nonunions: diagnosis and treatment. J Orthop Sci 2006;11(4):424–431
3. Nakamura R, Imaeda T, Horii E, Miura T, Hayakawa N. Analysis of scaphoid fracture displacement by three-dimensional computed tomography. J Hand Surg Am 1991;16(3): 485–492
4. Carpenter CR, Pines JM, Schuur JD, Muir M, Calfee RP, Raja AS. Adult scaphoid fracture. Acad Emerg Med 2014;21(2): 101–121
5. de Zwart AD, Beeres FJ, Rhemrev SJ, Bartlema K, Schipper IB. Comparison of MRI, CT and bone scintigraphy for suspected scaphoid fractures. Eur J Trauma Emerg Surg 2016;42(6):725–731

TREATMENT OF SCAPHOID FRACTURES

3. A 20-year-old woman presents with an acute, proximal pole scaphoid fracture. Plain radiographs confirm the fracture is nondisplaced. *Which one of the following statements is correct regarding management of this patient?*

B. She would benefit from internal fixation with a differential pitch screw.

Most nondisplaced scaphoid fractures heal well with immobilization. However, internal fixation is recommended for proximal pole fractures because of high rates of nonunion. Otherwise, internal fixation is usually reserved for displaced fractures and those with delayed union. Internal fixation uses a solid or cannulated screw placed across the fracture site. Screws with a differential pitch are preferred to provide compression across the fracture site. Nonoperative management requires an extended duration of immobilization for a total of 6 to 12 weeks depending on the fracture location. There is debate surrounding the type of cast. Some would recommend that the first 6 weeks should be in a long-arm thumb spica cast and the second 6 weeks in a short-arm thumb spica cast, whereas others would recommend leaving the thumb free and splinting in slight dorsal extension for 6 to 12 weeks until clinical union.[1] Consequently, a patient's profession should be taken into account when selecting treatment, as internal fixation may be preferable to reduce the immobilization period. It is not the main factor, however, in guiding treatment for a proximal pole fracture. Either a dorsal or volar approach can be used for internal fixation, but the dorsal approach provides a better exposure of the proximal pole.[1-3]

REFERENCES

1. Rhemrev SJ, Ootes D, Beeres FJ, Meylaerts SA, Schipper IB. Current methods of diagnosis and treatment of scaphoid fractures. Int J Emerg Med 2011;4:4
2. Slade JF III, Jaskwhich D. Percutaneous fixation of scaphoid fractures. Hand Clin 2001;17(4):553–574
3. Krimmer H. Management of acute fractures and nonunions of the proximal pole of the scaphoid. J Hand Surg [Br] 2002;27(3):245–248

COMPLICATIONS AFTER SCAPHOID FRACTURES

4. A 30-year-old man is referred to you with a persistent nonunion of a scaphoid fracture after 8 weeks of immobilization. *Which one of the following statements is correct regarding the sequelae of scaphoid fractures?*

D. Degenerative arthritis of the wrist is very common after proximal scaphoid nonunion.

One of the main problems with inadequately treated scaphoid fractures is chronic wrist pain and development of degenerative osteoarthritis. Scaphoid nonunion can result in instability of the intercalated segment of the wrist (the lunate and associated components of the proximal carpal row). This usually results in extension of or a dorsal angulation of the lunate (i.e., dorsal intercalated segment instability [DISI], not volar intercalated segment instability [VISI]). Over time, the resulting degenerative change in the wrist can lead to a scaphoid nonunion-advanced collapse (SNAC) (not scapholunate advanced collapse [SLAC]) wrist deformity. A SLAC wrist refers to SLAC and is most often secondary to untreated scapholunate ligament injury.[1] A humpback deformity of the scaphoid is the most common example of a nonunion and leaves the distal pole of the scaphoid flexed while the proximal pole is extended. It can be associated with DISI deformity and reduced function, but it is not always symptomatic and does not therefore always require surgical correction.[2] Delayed union is diagnosed if symptoms persist with no radiographic evidence of healing after 4 months (not 6 weeks) of immobilization, although many would conclude this earlier than 4 months. If the fracture lines appear sclerotic, this is nonunion.[1-3]

REFERENCES

1. Taleisnik J, Watson HK. Midcarpal instability caused by malunited fractures of the distal radius. J Hand Surg Am 1995;20:57–62
2. Jiranek WA, Ruby LK, Millender LB, Bankoff MS, Newberg AH. Long-term results after Russe bone-grafting: the effect of malunion of the scaphoid. J Bone Joint Surg Am 1992;74(8):1217–1228
3. Krimmer H. Management of acute fractures and nonunions of the proximal pole of the scaphoid. J Hand Surg [Br] 2002;27(3):245–248

CARPAL BONE FRACTURES

5. *Which one of the following statements is correct regarding carpal bone fractures?*

D. Hamate body fractures can occur with fourth and fifth CMC joint dislocations and often require fixation.

Hamate fractures either involve the body or the hook (hamulus). Fractures of the body most commonly occur because of a high axial load through the wrist, such as occurs during a punch injury. In patients who present with fourth and fifth metacarpal base fractures following an axial loading, careful examination of the carpometacarpal

(CMC) joints and hamate is required during assessment. These injuries may cause a hamate body fracture in the coronal plane with dorsal translation of the fractured segment. A CT scan is usually warranted in this situation and the hamate fracture may require K-wire or screw fixation. Hamulus fractures may directly injure the ulnar nerve and artery, or cause compression due to hematoma in Guyon's canal. Therefore, careful examination of ulnar nerve function must be performed. Hamate fractures are relatively common, and some patterns have around a >50% rate of nonunion with immobilization alone.[1] The scaphoid is most commonly fractured (70%) followed by the triquetrum. The pisiform is a sesamoid bone in the flexor carpi ulnaris (FCU) that can be fractured due to direct trauma. Plain radiographs frequently do not demonstrate these injuries and specific carpal tunnel views or CT scans are required. Trapezium (not triquetrum) fractures are thought to occur with combined hyperextension and abduction forces to the thumb.[1–2]

REFERENCES

1. Scheufler O, Andresen R, Radmer S, Erdmann D, Exner K, Germann G. Hook of hamate fractures: critical evaluation of different therapeutic procedures. Plast Reconstr Surg 2005;115(2):488–497
2. Garcia-Ellis M. Carpal bone fractures. In: Weinzweig J, ed. The Wrist Philadelphia: Lippincott Williams & Wilkins; 2001

CARPAL BONE FRACTURES

6. *Which carpal bone is the least commonly fractured, as a result of the protection of the surrounding bony anatomy and strong carpal ligaments?*

   C. Trapezoid

   The trapezoid is the least commonly fractured carpal bone, as it is well protected by the surrounding osseous anatomy and the strong carpal ligaments surrounding tissues. However, it may be injured during significant trauma to the wrist in conjunction with other associated injuries. Displaced fractures should be treated with anatomic reduction and fixation. Chronic injuries may require second CMC joint arthrodesis. The scaphoid is the most commonly fractured carpal bone, accounting for 70% of all such fractures. It may be injured by either forced hyperextension or severe axial loading of the wrist. The triquetrum is the second most commonly fractured carpal bone and occurs most often as an avulsion fracture secondary to ligamentous injury pulling small bony fragments off the dorsal rim. Trapezium and lunate fractures are both rare fracture types. Trapezium fractures are not usually seen in isolation and tend to be associated with ligamentous injury. They can occur secondary to a crush injury against the radial styloid or with first metacarpal base fractures. Lunate fractures usually occur in association with ligamentous injuries of the wrist or from axial compression between the capitate and lunate fossa on the radius.[1,2]

REFERENCES

1. Nammour M, Desai B, Warren M, Godshaw B, Suri M. Approach to isolated trapezoid fractures. Ochsner J 2019;19(3):271–275
2. Garcia-Ellis M. Carpal bone fractures. In: Weinzweig J, ed. The Wrist. Philadelphia: Lippincott Williams & Wilkins; 2001

KIENBOCK'S DISEASE OF THE WRIST

7. *A patient is referred with a diagnosis of Kienbock's disease. Which one of the following carpal bones is most likely to have been injured preceding this diagnosis?*

   C. Lunate

   Kienbock's disease is a condition of avascular necrosis of the lunate. It may occur spontaneously or following a nonunion of a lunate fracture. Kienbock's disease may first present with a pathologic fracture of the lunate. Prompt management of displaced lunate body fractures is therefore advocated to minimize the risk of nonunion and subsequent development of Kienbock's disease. Overall, lunate fractures are thankfully rare and occur in association with ligamentous wrist injuries.

   Kienbock's disease most commonly occurs in young adult males and the main presenting symptom is dorsal wrist pain which tends to be activity related. Management will depend on severity of the condition. This includes conservative options with nonsteroidal anti-inflammatory drugs and immobilization as well as operative options including radial wedge osteotomy, partial wrist fusion, complete wrist fusion, proximal carpectomy, total wrist arthroplasty, or vascularized bone grafts.[1,2]

REFERENCES

1. Fontaine C. Kienböck's disease. Chir Main 2015;34(1):4–17
2. Schuind F, Eslami S, Ledoux P. Kienbock's disease. J Bone Joint Surg Br 2008;90(2):133–139

THE ANVIL MECHANISM IN WRIST INJURY

8. *Which one of the following carpal bones may be fractured during a wrist hyperextension injury through the "anvil mechanism."*

   D. Capitate

   The capitate is at risk of transverse body fracture during forced hyperextension when it is forced against the distal radius through the anvil mechanism (**Fig. 73.1**). This can result in 180-degree rotation of the proximal fragment which cannot heal without formal reduction and stabilization. Patients remain at risk of avascular necrosis of the proximal fragment.[1]

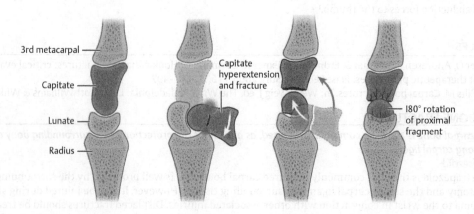

3rd metacarpal

Capitate

Capitate hyperextension and fracture

Lunate

180° rotation of proximal fragment

Radius

Fig. 73.1   Anvil mechanism resulting in capitate body fracture.

REFERENCE

1. Shah MA, Viegas SF. Fractures of the carpal bones excluding the scaphoid. J Am Soc Surg Hand 2002;2:129–140

DELAYED PRESENTATION OF CARPAL BONE FRACTURES

9. A young male patient presents with a spontaneous inability to flex the little finger at the proximal interphalangeal and distal interphalangeal joints. There has been no recent trauma to the little finger itself, but about 3 months ago he sustained a fall onto his outstretched hand while mountain biking. He sought no medical intervention but has continued to have a tender wrist. Plain radiographs confirm evidence of a carpal bone fracture. *Which one of the following is most likely to be involved?*

   A. Hook of hamate

   Hamate fractures may be subdivided as either hamulus fractures (hook of hamate) or hamate body fractures. Hook of hamate fractures occur secondary to direct trauma to the hand while holding an object such as a bat or racket. Alternatively, they may occur during falls onto the outstretched hand. Untreated hook fractures can present with delayed spontaneous rupture of the little finger flexor tendons. Attrition ruptures of the tendon occur secondary to degenerative bony changes at the fracture site where nonunion has occurred. In this case, the hamulus fragment should be excised in addition to addressing the flexor tendon ruptures. Hamate body fractures tend to be associated with fourth and fifth metacarpal base fractures rather than delayed tendon injuries. A careful ulnar nerve examination is needed in hook of hamate fractures as the deep motor branch is particularly at risk of injury.[1-5]

REFERENCES

1. Mandegaran R, Gidwani S, Zavareh A. Concomitant hook of hamate fractures in patients with scaphoid fracture: more common than you might think. Skeletal Radiol 2018;47(4):505–510
2. Wright TW, Moser MW, Sahajpal DT. Hook of hamate pull test. J Hand Surg Am 2010;35(11):1887–1889
3. Neviaser RJ. Fractures of the hook of the hamate. J Hand Surg Am 1986;11(1):146
4. Scheufler O, Andresen R, Radmer S, Erdmann D, Exner K, Germann G. Hook of hamate fractures: critical evaluation of different therapeutic procedures. Plast Reconstr Surg 2005;115(2):488–497
5. Kadar A, Morsy M, Sur YJ, Akdag O, Moran SL. Capitate fractures: a review of 53 patients. J Hand Surg Am 2016;41(10): e359–e366

IMAGING OF THE WRIST

10. Which one of the following radiographic views of the wrist best demonstrates a hook of hamate fracture?

   B. Carpal tunnel view

   Hook of hamate fractures are demonstrated in lateral, oblique, and carpal tunnel views. The AP view of wrist is a core component of a wrist series. The 45-degree pronated oblique view is used to image the triquetrum. AP in ulnar deviation is a component of a scaphoid series. The reverse oblique view is a 45-degree supination view with the wrist extended that demonstrates pisiform fractures.[1,2]

REFERENCES

1. Neviaser RJ. Fractures of the hook of the hamate. J Hand Surg Am 1986;11(1):146
2. Scheufler O, Andresen R, Radmer S, Erdmann D, Exner K, Germann G. Hook of hamate fractures: critical evaluation of different therapeutic procedures. Plast Reconstr Surg 2005;115(2):488–497

74. Carpal Instability and Dislocations

See *Essentials of Plastic Surgery*, third edition, pp. 1025–1051

WRIST ANATOMY

1. *Which one of the following carpal bones forms part of the proximal row in the carpus?*
   - A. Trapezium
   - B. Hamate
   - C. Triquetrum
   - D. Capitate
   - E. Trapezoid

2. *When considering wrist anatomy, which one of the following is true?*
   - A. There are no muscle or tendon attachments to the carpal bones.
   - B. Intrinsic ligaments link the carpal bones to the radius and ulna.
   - C. There are three functional columns in the carpus.
   - D. There are eight bones involved in the combined wrist articulations.
   - E. The pisiform lies within the flexor carpi radialis (FCR) tendon.

WRIST INSTABILITY

3. *What does the term "dissociative instability" refer to when discussing the wrist?*
   - A. Altered biomechanics between the proximal carpal row and the ulna.
   - B. Altered biomechanics between the distal carpal row and the metacarpals.
   - C. Altered biomechanics between carpal bones within the same row.
   - D. Altered biomechanics between the different rows of carpal bones.
   - E. Altered biomechanics between the proximal carpal row and the radius.

CARPAL INSTABILITY CLASSIFICATION

4. *Which one of the following statements is correct when describing carpal instability?*
   - A. Carpal instability dissociative (CID) is instability between the distal radius and the carpus.
   - B. Carpal instability nondissociative (CIND) is instability that does not show on a plain radiograph.
   - C. Carpal instability adaptive (CIA) is caused by a malunion of the scaphoid.
   - D. Malalignment of the carpal bones will be present in plain radiographs in dynamic instability.
   - E. Predynamic instability is usually confirmed only during wrist arthroscopy.

INTERCALATED SEGMENT INSTABILITY OF THE WRIST

5. *The orientation of which one of the following bones on lateral radiograph defines whether there is a dorsal intercalated segment instability (DISI) versus a volar intercalated segment instability (VISI) in a wrist injury?*
   - A. Scaphoid
   - B. Lunate
   - C. Capitate
   - D. Hamate
   - E. Triquetrum

RADIOGRAPHIC SIGNS OF SCAPHOLUNATE LIGAMENT INJURY

6. *Which of the following would be most suggestive of an isolated scapholunate ligament injury on a plain radiograph?*
   - A. Spilled teapot sign
   - B. Cortical ring sign
   - C. A volar intercalated segment instability (VISI) sign
   - D. Piano key sign
   - E. The wedding band sign

EXAMINATION FINDINGS IN CARPAL INSTABILITY

7. *A patient with chronic wrist pain has a positive Watson test on examination. Which one of the following structures is most likely to be injured?*
   - A. Scaphoid bone
   - B. Radial styloid
   - C. Radioscapholunate ligament
   - D. Lunotriquetral ligament
   - E. Scapholunate ligament

WRIST INJURY ASSESSMENT

8. A patient is referred with a stage III perilunate injury after a fall on the outstretched hand. *Which one of the following findings is least likely to be present?*
    A. Median nerve paresthesia
    B. A fracture of the radial styloid
    C. A tear in the space of Poirier
    D. Lunate dislocation into the carpal tunnel
    E. Lunotriquetral ligament rupture

LIGAMENTS OF THE WRIST

9. You are opening a wrist to reduce and repair a perilunate dislocation. *Which one of the following statements is correct?*
    A. A dorsal capsular flap must be used to preserve the ligaments.
    B. A triangular capsular flap is required to preserve the volar ligaments.
    C. The dorsal scapholunate ligament usually requires repair.
    D. The lunate is commonly dislocated into the carpal tunnel.
    E. A volar incision should be avoided to protect the median nerve.

MANAGEMENT OF CARPAL INSTABILITY

10. A young patient presents with persistent wrist pain and instability 6 months after a closed wrist injury. A scapholunate ligament disruption is confirmed. *Which one of the following is the most likely treatment?*
    A. Bone anchor repair of the ligament
    B. Radiolunate fusion
    C. Flexor carpi radialis (FCR) ligament reconstruction
    D. Radioscapholunate fusion
    E. Percutaneous K-wiring

WRIST ARTHROSCOPY

11. You are performing arthroscopy to investigate chronic wrist pain in a 40-year-old woman. *Which one of the following is correct?*
    A. Your first portal is likely to be the 1–2 interval portal.
    B. The extensor pollicis longus (EPL) tendon is at risk of injury at the 4–5 interval portal.
    C. The 4–5 interval portal is the most common viewing portal.
    D. Ligamentous injuries should be graded according to the Geissler system.
    E. A 4-mm wide, 30-degree viewing scope is most appropriate.

RECOGNITION OF A CARPAL INJURY

12. *Which one of the following statements is correct regarding assessment of a plain radiograph of an injured wrist?*
    A. Lesser arc injuries involve ligamentous disruption with a scaphoid fracture.
    B. A scapholunate angle of less than 30 degrees implies a scapholunate ligament disruption.
    C. Volar angulation of the lunate implies disruption of the lunotriquetral ligament.
    D. A proximal pole capitate fracture is most likely to represent an isolated injury.
    E. The Terry Thomas sign represents hyperflexion of the scaphoid.

Answers

WRIST ANATOMY

1. *Which one of the following carpal bones forms part of the proximal row in the carpus?*

C. Triquetrum

The carpal bones are arranged into proximal and distal rows. The proximal row contains three bones: the scaphoid, the lunate, and the triquetrum. These are joined by the scapholunate and lunotriquetral ligaments. The distal row contains the trapezium, trapezoid, capitate, and hamate. There is also a sesamoid bone located in the flexor carpi ulnaris (FCU) tendon called the pisiform.

The two rows must move in synchrony during flexion, extension, and ulnar/radial deviation to allow smooth movement of the wrist. Disruption of the normal biomechanics of the carpus can result in significant functional problems.[1-4]

REFERENCES

1. Moore KL, Dalley AF, eds. Clinically Oriented Anatomy. 4th ed. New York, NY: Lippincott Williams & Wilkins; 1999
2. Idler RS. Anatomy and biomechanics of the digital flexor tendons. Hand Clin 1985;1(1): 3–11
3. Lewis OJ, Hamshere RJ, Bucknill TM. The anatomy of the wrist joint. J Anat 1970;106(Pt 3):539–552
4. Macconaill MA. The mechanical anatomy of the carpus and its bearings on some surgical problems. J Anat 1941; 75(Pt 2):166–175

2. *When considering wrist anatomy, which one of the following is true?*

A. There are no muscle or tendon attachments to the carpal bones.

The carpal bones are unusual in that they have no muscle or tendon attachments. Instead they are joined by a complex set of ligamentous structures.

The ligaments of the carpus may be subdivided as intrinsic and extrinsic. The intrinsic ones link the carpal bones to one another, whereas the extrinsic ones link the carpal bones to the radius and ulna. There are two, not three, functional columns of the carpus.

Although there are 8 carpal bones, there are 14 bones involved in the articulations of the carpus. The proximal row of the carpus articulates with the distal radius and ulna and the distal row articulates with the five metacarpals. The pisiform is a sesamoid bone forming a lever arm for the flexor carpi ulnaris (FCU) (not FCR) tendon and is not a true carpal bone.[1-4]

REFERENCES

1. Moore KL, Dalley AF, eds. Clinically Oriented Anatomy. 4th ed. New York, NY: Lippincott Williams & Wilkins; 1999
2. Idler RS. Anatomy and biomechanics of the digital flexor tendons. Hand Clin 1985;1(1): 3–11
3. Mayfield JK, Johnson RP, Kilcoyne RK. Carpal dislocations: pathomechanics and progressive perilunar instability. J Hand Surg Am 1980;5(3):226–241
4. Macconaill MA. The mechanical anatomy of the carpus and its bearings on some surgical problems. J Anat 1941; 75(Pt 2):166–175

WRIST INSTABILITY

3. *What does the term "dissociative instability" refer to when discussing the wrist?*

C. Altered biomechanics between carpal bones within the same row.

The term "dissociative instability" of the carpus refers to disruption of the normal support structures and biomechanics within a row of the carpus, either proximal or distal, such as when there is a scapholunate or lunotriquetral ligament disruption. The term "nondissociative instability" refers to a situation where there is altered biomechanics of the entire proximal row relative to the radiocarpal or midcarpal joints (**Figs. 74.1** and **74.2**).[1]

REFERENCE

1. Wolfe SW, Garcia-Elias M, Kitay A. Carpal instability nondissociative. J Am Acad Orthop Surg 2012;20(9):575–585

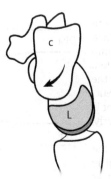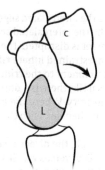

Volar inclination lunate
with volar subluxation of
capitate

Dorsal inclination lunate
with dorsal subluxation of
capitate

Fig. 74.1 Carpal instability dissociative (CID). (Adapted from Wolfe SW, Garcia-Elias M, Kitay A. Carpal instability nondissociative. J Am Acad Orthop Surg 20:575–585, 2012.)

CARPAL INSTABILITY CLASSIFICATION

4. *Which one of the following statements is correct when describing carpal instability?*

E. **Predynamic instability is usually confirmed only during wrist arthroscopy.**

Carpal instability may be described as static, dynamic, or predynamic. In cases of static instability, there is malalignment of the carpus on plain radiographs. In cases of dynamic instability, patients will have normal plain radiographs, but malalignment is seen on stress views. Predynamic instability occurs with mild scapholunate joint instability such as when the ligament is only stretched or partially ruptured. It therefore tends to be diagnosed only during arthroscopy because in this scenario, there are normal plain radiographs and normal stress views.

Carpal instability dissociative (CID) refers to instability between bones of the same carpal row (e.g., scaphoid and lunate or lunate and triquetrum). Carpal instability nondissociative (CIND) refers to instability of the entire proximal row (e.g., scaphoid, lunate, and triquetrum), relative to either the distal carpal row or the radius and triangular fibrocartilaginous complex (TFCC). Carpal instability adaptive (CIA) refers to compensatory changes in the carpus to accommodate an extrinsic problem, the most common of which is an uneven platform following a distal radius fracture malunion.[1]

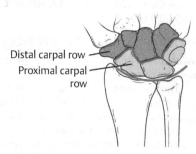

Distal carpal row
Proximal carpal row

Fig. 74.2 Carpal instability nondissociative (CIND) represents radiocarpal and/or midcarpal joint instability with **no** break between bones within either the proximal carpal or distal carpal row. (Adapted from Wolfe SW, Garcia-Elias M, Kitay A. Carpal instability nondissociative. J Am Acad Orthop Surg 20:575–585, 2012.)

REFERENCE

1. Wolfe SW, Garcia-Elias M, Kitay A. Carpal instability nondissociative. J Am Acad Orthop Surg 2012;20(9):575–585

INTERCALATED SEGMENT INSTABILITY OF THE WRIST

5. *The orientation of which one of the following bones on lateral radiograph defines whether there is a dorsal intercalated segment instability (DISI) versus a volar intercalated segment instability (VISI) in a wrist injury?*

B. **Lunate**

The proximal row of the carpus is formed by the scaphoid, lunate, and triquetrum. It is a highly mobile unit, which is held by balanced competing forces between the distal radius and triangular fibrocartilaginous complex (TFCC), and the distal carpal row. These forces tend to push the scaphoid into flexion, and the triquetrum into extension. The lunate is held suspended between these two competing forces of rotation by tough scapholunate and lunotriquetral ligaments. These ligaments normally allow the proximal row to function as one gently twisting unit as the wrist moves. In the normal wrist, as the scaphoid flexes in radial deviation, the lunate and triquetrum follow to a degree due to the ligamentous attachments. When there is ligamentous damage, there is dissociation between the three bones and they no longer move smoothly in relation to one another.

If the proximal row is the intercalated segment of the wrist, one can consider the lunate to be the intercalated segment of this row. When the scapholunate ligament is disrupted, the scaphoid tends to slump into flexion and the unrestrained lunate tilts dorsally in extension, pulled in part by its attachment to the triquetrum. Therefore, as the lunate rotates into dorsal tilt, there is a dorsal intercalated segment instability (DISI) deformity. Where the lunotriquetral ligament is disrupted, the lunate can then flex with the scaphoid and tilt volarly, hence VISI deformity.

So, in a lateral radiograph, the direction of tilt of the lunate is the key factor that defines a DISI versus a VISI and the cause is primarily a ligamentous injury in the proximal row, or a scaphoid fracture, as part of the progressive range of perilunate injuries, mild to severe.

A DISI deformity is characterized by extension of the lunate in the lateral view with flexion of the scaphoid, giving a scapholunate angle greater than 60 degrees (**Fig. 74.3**). A VISI deformity is characterized by a reduced scapholunate angle less than 30 degrees.[1,2]

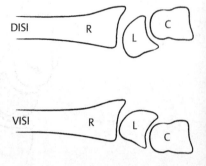

Fig. 74.3 In dorsal intercalated segment instability *(DISI)*, the lunate tilts dorsally. In volar intercalated segment instability *(VISI)*, the lunate tilts volarly. (*C*, capitate; *L*, lunate; *R*, radius.)

REFERENCES

1. Lee DJ, Elfar JC. Carpal ligament injuries, pathomechanics, and classification. Hand Clin 2015;31(3):389–398
2. Larsen CF, Amadio PC, Gilula LA, Hodge JC. Analysis of carpal instability: I. Description of the scheme. J Hand Surg Am 1995;20(5):757–764

RADIOGRAPHIC SIGNS OF SCAPHOLUNATE LIGAMENT INJURY

6. *Which of the following would be most suggestive of an isolated scapholunate ligament injury on a plain radiograph?*
   B. Cortical ring sign

   There are two key radiographic features of scapholunate ligament disruption. They are the Terry Thomas and cortical ring signs. The Terry Thomas sign reflects an increased gap between the scaphoid and the lunate. It refers to a famous English comedian with a large gap between his central upper incisors. The cortical ring sign (also called the "signet ring sign") represents a hyperflexed scaphoid wherein the distal pole is seen on end and appears as a cortical ring within 7 mm of the proximal pole.

   The scapholunate ligament is a b-shaped structure that connects the dorsal, proximal, and volar surfaces of the scaphoid and lunate. When this ligament is injured, it usually pulls away from the scaphoid and remains attached to the lunate. This allows unwanted movement between the scaphoid and lunate leading to chronic wrist problems. A VISI deformity (or VISI sign) refers to volar angulation of the lunate in the lateral view. This occurs with disruption of the lunotriquetral ligament rather than the scapholunate ligament (which would result in dorsal angulation of the lunate, or DISI). The spilled teapot sign indicates volar displacement of the lunate on a lateral radiograph in association with a more severe perilunate injury (stage IV). The cortical ring or signet ring sign is a term also used to describe radiographic signs seen in bronchiectasis when the dilated bronchus and accompanying artery branch are seen in cross-section. Normally the two should be the same diameter, but in this condition the dilated airway appears larger. The Tram track sign also refers to bronchiectasis where the dilated airways are shown in horizontal rather than cross-sectional orientation. There is no wedding band sign described in radiology.[1-4]

REFERENCES

1. Walsh JJ, Berger RA, Cooney WP. Current status of scapholunate interosseous ligament injuries. J Am Acad Orthop Surg 2002;10(1):32–42
2. Butterfield WL, Joshi AB, Lichtman D. Lunotriquetral injuries. J Am Soc Surg Hand 2002;2:195–203
3. Garcia-Elias M, Geissler WB. Carpal instability. In: Green DP, Hotchkiss RN, Pederson WC, et al, eds. Green's Operative Hand Surgery. 5th ed. Philadelphia: Churchill Livingstone; 2005
4. Pasławski M, Złomaniec J. Small bronchiectases and bronchiolectases in high resolution computed tomography (HRCT). Ann Univ Mariae Curie Sklodowska Med 2003;58(2): 402–406

EXAMINATION FINDINGS IN CARPAL INSTABILITY

7. A patient with chronic wrist pain has a positive Watson test on examination. *Which one of the following structures is most likely to be injured?*
   E. Scapholunate ligament

   A positive Watson test corresponds to a "clunk" felt during dynamic wrist loading. The Watson (scaphoid shift) test assesses scaphoid instability (**Fig. 74.4**).

It particularly stresses the scapholunate ligament but may be positive in other problems affecting carpal stability. The test is performed as follows:

The examiner holds the scaphoid in full extension by placing pressure over the tubercle on the volar side, while the wrist is in full extension and ulnar deviation. The examiner's thumb prevents normal flexion of the scaphoid as the wrist is moved from ulnar to radial deviation and pressure is maintained over the tubercle on the volar aspect. The movement is then reversed. As the rest of the carpus moves, the restrained scaphoid has to "catch up" with the lunate and other bones. This occurs gradually if ligament integrity is normal. If the scapholunate ligament is damaged, or another disruption to carpal integration is present, the scaphoid can be restrained in the abnormal position for a prolonged period and palpated as a bulge on the dorsum of the wrist. As the other carpal bones move, the scaphoid has to jump back into position in the scaphoid fossa of the radius. This usually reproduces pain or a "clunk." However, a slight clunk or discomfort can occur even in individuals with normal ligament integrity.[1-2]

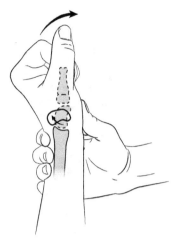

Fig. 74.4   Watson (scaphoid shift) test.

REFERENCES

1. Garcia-Elias M, Geissler WB. Carpal instability. In: Green DP, Hotchkiss RN, Pederson WC, et al, eds. Green's Operative Hand Surgery. 5th ed. Philadelphia: Churchill Livingstone; 2005
2. Lane LB. The scaphoid shift test. J Hand Surg Am 1993;18(2):366–368

WRIST INJURY ASSESSMENT

8. A patient is referred with a stage III perilunate injury after a fall on the outstretched hand. *Which one of the following findings is least likely to be present?*

D. Lunate dislocation into the carpal tunnel

Mayfield et al[1] described four stages of progressive perilunate injury:

Stage I: Scapholunate diastasis
Stage II: Dorsal dislocation of capitate
Stage III: Lunotriquetral dissociation
Stage IV: Dislocation of the lunate volarly

Any of the features described in options A through E may be seen in a stage III injury with the exception of dislocation of the lunate into the carpal tunnel, which would render this a stage IV injury. Median nerve paresthesias are common following perilunate injury and extended carpal tunnel decompression is frequently required as a result. Purely ligamentous injuries occur along the lesser arc, while fracture dislocations such as with a styloid or scaphoid fracture occur along the greater arc. As such, a radial styloid fracture or lunotriquetral ligament rupture could be seen in a stage III injury. The space of Poirier represents a weak zone in the volar wrist capsule and is usually torn in perilunate injuries.[1]

REFERENCE

1. Mayfield JK, Johnson RP, Kilcoyne RK. Carpal dislocations: pathomechanics and progressive perilunar instability. J Hand Surg Am 1980;5(3):226–241

LIGAMENTS OF THE WRIST

9. You are opening a wrist to reduce and repair a perilunate dislocation. *Which one of the following statements is correct?*

C. The dorsal scapholunate ligament usually requires repair.

Unless there is a transscaphoid fracture dislocation, there is always some scapholunate ligament damage in perilunate injuries. A dorsal ligament-sparing capsular flap has been described by Berger[1] which comprises a chevron with the apex ulnarward over the triquetrum to preserve integrity of the dorsal radiocarpal and dorsal intercarpal ligament fibers (**Fig. 74.5**). While this approach is popular with many surgeons, there is insufficient outcome data to prove superiority over a simple dorsal capsular incision and some would argue that the wrist will be immobilized anyway for a sufficient period to avoid subsequent instability due to dorsal ligament insufficiency.

The lunate is found only in the carpal tunnel in stage IV injuries. A volar incision is often employed to decompress the median nerve, to repair the volar capsule, and to aid in relocation of a completely dislocated lunate.[1,2]

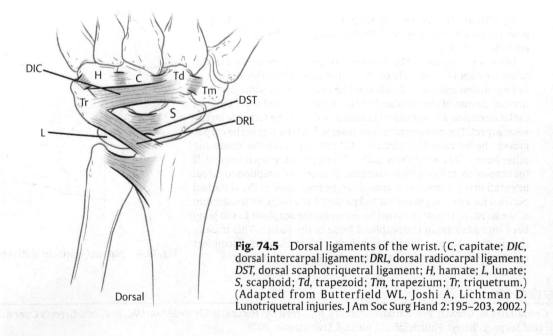

Fig. 74.5 Dorsal ligaments of the wrist. (*C*, capitate; *DIC*, dorsal intercarpal ligament; *DRL*, dorsal radiocarpal ligament; *DST*, dorsal scaphotriquetral ligament; *H*, hamate; *L*, lunate; *S*, scaphoid; *Td*, trapezoid; *Tm*, trapezium; *Tr*, triquetrum.) (Adapted from Butterfield WL, Joshi A, Lichtman D. Lunotriquetral injuries. J Am Soc Surg Hand 2:195–203, 2002.)

REFERENCES

1. Berger RA. A method of defining palpable landmarks for the ligament-splitting dorsal wrist capsulotomy. J Hand Surg Am 2007;32(8):1291–1295
2. Mayfield JK, Johnson RP, Kilcoyne RK. Carpal dislocations: pathomechanics and progressive perilunar instability. J Hand Surg Am 1980;5(3):226–241

MANAGEMENT OF CARPAL INSTABILITY

10. A young patient presents with persistent wrist pain and instability 6 months after a closed wrist injury. A scapholunate ligament disruption is confirmed. *Which one of the following is the most likely treatment?*

   C. Flexor carpi radialis (FCR) ligament reconstruction
   Brunelli and Brunelli[1] described using a distally based strip of half of the FCR tendon passed volar to dorsal through the scaphoid and anchored onto the distal radius. This has since been modified by several authors. Six months after the injury is too late to undertake successful K-wire stabilization or direct ligament repair with a bone anchor. A ligament reconstruction with FCR or extensor carpi radialis longus (ECRL) should be considered only if the joint surfaces are healthy. If degenerative changes are seen, denervation of the wrist or various methods of intercarpal fusion may be considered instead. A radiolunate fusion is employed to reduce pain from the radiolunate articulation. A radioscapholunate fusion addresses pain from the radioscaphoid articulation. Both procedures are used in the setting of degenerative arthritis rather than an acute ligament injury.

REFERENCE

1. Brunelli GA, Brunelli GR. A new technique to correct carpal instability with scaphoid rotary subluxation: a preliminary report. J Hand Surg Am 1995;20(3, Pt 2):S82–S85

WRIST ARTHROSCOPY

11. You are performing arthroscopy to investigate chronic wrist pain in a 40-year-old woman. *Which one of the following is correct?*

   D. Ligamentous injuries should be graded according to the Geissler system.
   The Geissler grading system is based on the appearance of the scapholunate ligament, the alignment of the carpus, and the ability to pass a probe between the scaphoid and lunate:
   Grade 1: There is attenuation or hemorrhage of the scapholunate interosseous ligament (SLIL) and there is no midcarpal malalignment.
   Grade II: Attenuation/hemorrhage of the SLIL and step-off/incongruency of carpal alignment. A slight gap between carpals (less than width of probe)

Grade III: Step-off/incongruency of carpal alignment (and scapholunate gap large enough to pass probe between carpals

Grade IV: Step-off/incongruency of carpal alignment, gross instability and 2.7-mm arthroscope can pass through the gap between the scaphoid and lunate.

The usual equipment for a wrist arthroscopy is a 2.7-mm, 30-degree viewing scope with traction apparatus and a wet technique to aid inspection of the tightly packed carpus. The numbered portals are described according to the extensor compartments. Therefore, the 3–4 portal lies between the third and fourth compartments. The 3–4 portal is the most common first portal, and this is where the extensor pollicis longus (EPL) tendon is at most risk. It is also the most common viewing portal.[1]

REFERENCE

1. Geissler WB, Freeland AE. Arthroscopically assisted reduction of intraarticular distal radial fractures. Clin Orthop Relat Res 1996; (327):125–134

RECOGNITION OF A CARPAL INJURY

12. Which one of the following statements is correct regarding assessment of a plain radiograph of an injured wrist?

C. Volar angulation of the lunate implies disruption of the lunotriquetral ligament.

A flexed scaphoid gives a cortical ring appearance in the anteroposterior (AP) view (**Fig. 74.6**).

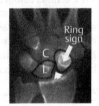

The proximal carpal row includes the scaphoid, lunate, and triquetrum. The lunate is referred to as the *intercalated segment*, because its movements are heavily influenced by the ligamentous complexes between these three bones. When the lunotriquetral ligament complex is disrupted, the lunate becomes volarly angulated giving a scapholunate angle of less than 30 degrees. When the scapholunate ligament complex is disrupted, the lunate becomes more dorsally angulated under the influence of the lunotriquetral ligament complex. This increases the scapholunate angle to more than 60 degrees in the lateral view. Progressive perilunate injuries may be purely ligamentous, passing along the lesser arc, or when fractures of the radial styloid, scaphoid, capitate, or triquetrum occur, this is considered a greater arc injury. A proximal pole capitate fracture is usually part of a greater arc injury and therefore not an isolated injury. The Terry Thomas sign is a radiographic finding where there is an increase scapholunate gap secondary to scapholunate ligament disruption. The cortical ring sign represents hyperflexion of the scaphoid.[1]

Fig. 74.6 Cortical ring sign seen with dorsal intercalated segment instability (DISI). The *arrowhead* points to an increased scapholunate gap. (*C,* capitate; *L,* lunate.)

REFERENCE

1. Garcia-Elias M, Geissler WB. Carpal instability. In: Green DP, Hotchkiss RN, Pederson WC, et al, eds. Green's Operative Hand Surgery. 5th ed. Philadelphia: Churchill Livingstone; 2005

75. Distal Radius Fractures

See *Essentials of Plastic Surgery*, third edition, pp. 1052–1067

DISTAL RADIUS FRACTURE NOMENCLATURE

1. *When describing the radiographic appearance of a distal radius fracture, which one of the following is correct?*
   A. A die punch fracture is characterized by depression of the scaphoid fossa.
   B. A Barton's fracture is characterized by a volarly displaced distal radius fracture with shortening.
   C. A Colles' fracture is dorsally angulated distal radius fracture with shortening and dorsal comminution.
   D. A Smith's fracture is a displaced intra-articular oblique fracture of the radial styloid.
   E. A chauffeur's fracture is characterized by depression of the lunate fossa.

IMAGING OF THE DISTAL RADIUS

2. *When reviewing radiographs for signs of injury to the distal radius, which one of the following is correct?*
   A. A true lateral view of the wrist shows a 50% overlap of the pisiform and distal pole of the scaphoid.
   B. The normal distal radius has an average dorsal tilt of 10 degrees.
   C. The distal ulnar articular surface is in negative variance when sitting distal to the radial articular surface.
   D. The average radial inclination is 10 degrees on a posteroanterior (PA) radiograph of the wrist.
   E. The minimum clinically significant articular step-off for intervention is 2 mm.

NONOPERATIVE MANAGEMENT OF DISTAL RADIAL FRACTURES

3. You are discussing the merits of nonoperative management of a Colles fracture with a fit 52-year-old patient. The radiograph confirms 20-degree dorsal angulation of the articular surface. *Which one of the following is correct?*
   A. This is an absolute indication for surgical management of the fracture.
   B. If the postreduction views are satisfactory, a review with repeat imaging at 1 month is important.
   C. An intra-articular step is likely and will require accurate reduction.
   D. If the fracture has moved again at 1 week, re-manipulation and splinting should be attempted.
   E. There is a risk of extensor pollicis longus tendon rupture with both operative and nonoperative management.

EXTERNAL FIXATION IN A COLLES FRACTURE OF THE WRIST

4. You are planning percutaneous fixation to stabilize a Colles fracture in a frail, osteoporotic 70-year-old woman. *Which one of the following statements is true?*
   A. K-wire fixation will allow earlier mobilization than nonoperative care.
   B. Percutaneous wiring alone should be adequate.
   C. If the dorsal angulation is 10 to 20 degrees, further intervention is not required.
   D. External fixation is contraindicated in this scenario.
   E. Splinting beyond 4 weeks should be avoided to minimize stiffness.

INTERNAL FIXATION OF DISTAL RADIUS FRACTURES

5. *When planning fixation of a comminuted distal radius fracture, which one of the following is correct?*
   A. Conventional spanning plates rely on purchase on the near cortex.
   B. Locking plates rely on purchase on the far cortex.
   C. Buttress plates have an antiglide effect to support intra-articular fractures.
   D. Dorsal plating is more popular than volar plating because it involves a simpler anatomic approach.
   E. Bone grafting and substitutes should not be used in osteoporotic distal radius fractures.

COMPLICATIONS FOLLOWING DISTAL RADIUS FRACTURES

6. *When discussing open fixation of a distal radius fracture with a patient, which one of the following is correct?*
   A. The risk of chronic regional pain syndrome is approximately 40%.
   B. If the patient is a child, volar plating is as likely as if they are an adult.
   C. Wrist strength will reach its maximum at 6 months with physiotherapy.
   D. The postoperative splint may include the elbow, leading to stiffness.
   E. The risk of malunion is avoided by operative intervention.

DISTAL RADIUS FRACTURE OUTCOMES

7. *Which one of the following is true regarding outcomes following distal radius fracture care?*
   A. Functional outcomes are better with percutaneous pinning than volar plating.
   B. External fixation gives superior rates of union to reduction and casting.
   C. Volar locking plates are more likely to require supplementary bone grafting.
   D. Volar nonlocking plates are superior to locking plates in osteoporotic bone.
   E. Restoring volar cortical continuity may best predict final carpal alignment.

Answers

DISTAL RADIUS FRACTURE NOMENCLATURE

1. When describing the radiographic appearance of a distal radius fracture, which one of the following is correct?

C. A Colles' fracture is a dorsally angulated distal radius fracture with shortening and dorsal comminution.
Colles' original 1814 description is reported to be a low-energy extra-articular fracture of the distal radius, as described earlier, occurring in elderly individuals. It may be associated with an ulnar styloid or triangular fibrocartilage complex (TFCC) injury. A die punch fracture is a depression of the lunate fossa from impaction of the lunate into the distal radius. A Barton's fracture is an unstable volar or dorsally displaced intra-articular fracture-subluxation of the distal radius with displacement of the carpus along with the fracture fragment. A Smith's fracture is referred to as a reverse Colles' fracture (i.e., with volar angulation and displacement). A chauffeur's fracture features an intra-articular shear fracture of the distal radius fracture where the fragment includes the radial styloid, which displaces with the carpus (**Fig. 75.1**).[1,2]

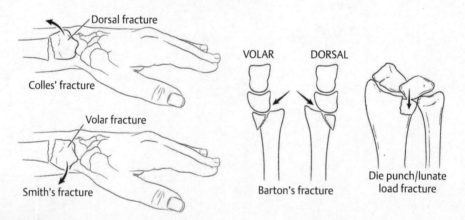

Fig. 75.1 Types of fractures. (Adapted from Berger RA, Weiss APC. Hand Surgery. Philadelphia: Lippincott Williams & Wilkins, 2004.)

REFERENCES

1. Berger RA, Weiss APC. Hand Surgery. Philadelphia: Lippincott Williams & Wilkins; 2004
2. Wong PK, Hanna TN, Shuaib W, Sanders SM, Khosa F. What's in a name? Upper extremity fracture eponyms (Part 1). Int J Emerg Med 2015;8(1):75

IMAGING OF THE DISTAL RADIUS

2. When reviewing radiographs for signs of injury to the distal radius, which one of the following is correct?

A. A true lateral view of the wrist shows a 50% overlap of the pisiform and distal pole of the scaphoid.
The quality of a lateral radiograph can be assessed in part by referencing the relative position of the pisiform to the distal pole of the scaphoid. In a true lateral view, they will overlap by 50%. A rough guide to interpretation of distal radius fracture radiographs is given by the "Rule of 11's":
Average volar tilt: 11 degrees (not dorsal)
Average radial height: 11 mm
Average radial inclination: 22 degrees (e.g., double 11)
Radial height refers to the distance that the radial styloid projects beyond the sigmoid notch (at the distal tip of ulnar articulation) and is usually 11 to 12 mm. Ulnar variance describes the position of the transverse distal ulnar joint surface relative to the distal radius joint surface at the wrist. Positive variance is present if the ulnar sits greater than 2 mm more distally than the radius, and in negative variance if the ulnar surface sits greater than 2 mm more proximally (**Fig. 75.2**). Most surgeons consider a 1-mm intra-articular step-off to be sufficient to indicate intervention.[1,2]

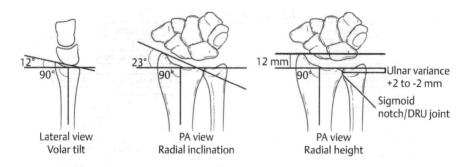

Fig. 75.2 Normal anatomic parameters of the distal radius. (DRU, distal radioulnar; PA, posteroanterior.) (Adapted from Smith DW, Brou KE, Henry MH. Early active rehabilitation for operatively stabilized distal radius fractures. J Hand Ther 17:43–49, 2004.)

REFERENCES

1. Wolfe SW, Pederson WC, Hotchkiss RN, et al, eds. Green's Operative Hand Surgery. 6th ed. Philadelphia: Elsevier; 2011
2. Medoff RJ. Essential radiographic evaluation for distal radius fractures. Hand Clin 2005;21(3):279–288

NONOPERATIVE MANAGEMENT OF DISTAL RADIAL FRACTURES

3. You are discussing the merits of nonoperative management of a Colles fracture with a fit 52-year-old patient. The radiograph confirms 20-degree dorsal angulation of the articular surface. *Which one of the following is correct?*

    E. There is a risk of extensor pollicis longus tendon rupture with both operative and nonoperative management.

    Attrition rupture of the extensor pollicis longus tendon can occur with either operative or nonoperative management of distal radius fractures. It may be due to ischemia from pressure within the rigid tunnel under extensor retinaculum, or direct trauma from a fracture spike/ridge.

    A Colles fracture is an extra-articular injury. All displaced extra-articular fractures would normally be manipulated and placed in a splint in the first instance. If the position is satisfactory following this, a trial of nonoperative management is warranted. If the fracture is behaving in an unstable fashion at 1 week, particularly in a fairly young, active patient, it should be formally stabilized rather than making further attempts at nonoperative management (**Fig. 75.3**).[1,2]

REFERENCES

1. Wolfe SW, Pederson WC, Hotchkiss RN, et al, eds. Green's Operative Hand Surgery. 6th ed. Philadelphia: Elsevier; 2011
2. Medoff RJ. Essential radiographic evaluation for distal radius fractures. Hand Clin 2005;21(3):279–288

EXTERNAL FIXATION IN A COLLES FRACTURE OF THE WRIST

4. You are planning percutaneous fixation to stabilize a Colles fracture in a frail, osteoporotic 70-year-old woman. *Which one of the following statements is true?*

    C. If the dorsal angulation is 10 to 20 degrees, further intervention is not required.

    While dorsal angulation greater than 10 degrees and radial shortening greater than 3 mm after reduction are usually an indication for intervention, up to 20 degrees dorsal angulation and 5 mm shortening can be tolerated in elderly inactive patients.

    K-wire fixation in osteoporotic bone is not sufficiently stable to allow early mobilization. Furthermore, it would usually be supplemented with an external fixator. Four weeks of splint age, either in the form of a plaster splint or external fixator, would be insufficient for healing. A minimum of 6 weeks is required.[1,2]

REFERENCES

1. Medoff RJ. Essential radiographic evaluation for distal radius fractures. Hand Clin 2005;21(3):279–288
2. Garrett WE, Swiontkowski MF, Weinstein JN. The Treatment of Distal Radius Fractures. Guidelines and Evidence Report. Rosemont, IL: American Academy of Orthopaedic Surgeons; 2009

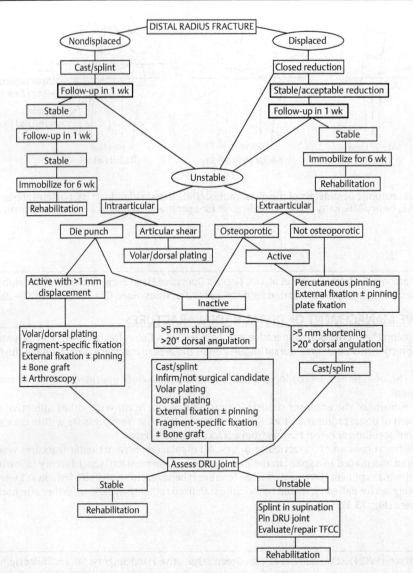

Fig. 75.3 Treatment algorithm for distal radius fracture. (*DRU joint*, distal radioulnar joint; *TFCC*, triangular fibrocartilage complex.)

INTERNAL FIXATION OF DISTAL RADIUS FRACTURES

5. *When planning fixation of a comminuted distal radius fracture, which one of the following is correct?*

C. **Buttress plates have an antiglide effect to support intra-articular fracture fragments.**

Conventional spanning plates rely on purchase into the far cortex, whereas locking plates may be adequate with only the near cortex. Volar plating is preferred to dorsal plating because there are fewer associated complications, and there is a more favorable surface contour to the radius. Bone grafting with autologous or substitute materials is important where there are metaphyseal defects following disimpaction. This can be useful in osteoporotic bone where additional strength may be conferred by use of a substitute.[1]

REFERENCE

1. Garrett WE, Swiontkowski MF, Weinstein JN. The Treatment of Distal Radius Fractures. Guidelines and Evidence Report. Rosemont, IL: American Academy of Orthopaedic Surgeons; 2009

COMPLICATIONS FOLLOWING DISTAL RADIUS FRACTURES

6. *When discussing open fixation of a distal radius fracture with a patient, which one of the following is correct?*

D. **The postoperative splint may include the elbow, leading to stiffness.**

A sugar-tong splint is sometimes required following surgery to prevent forearm rotation when the distal radio-ulnar joint needs to be immobilized, for example, if there has been an associated triangular fibrocartilage complex (TFCC) injury. This interferes with elbow movements and can lead to stiffness, which usually settles with physiotherapy. Although chronic regional pain syndrome has been reported to be as high as 40% with distal radius fractures in the past, it is currently thought to be less common at a rate of less than 3% after surgery.[1] Internal fixation with plates is generally avoided in children because of potential problems with subsequent growth. Wrist strength may continue to improve over the first year with physiotherapy. Patients should always be aware that malunion and nonunion can both still occur despite surgical intervention.

REFERENCE

1. Johnson NA, Cutler L, Dias JJ, Ullah AS, Wildin CJ, Bhowal B. Complications after volar locking plate fixation of distal radius fractures. Injury 2014;45(3):528–533

DISTAL RADIUS FRACTURE OUTCOMES

7. *Which one of the following is true regarding outcomes following distal radius fracture care?*

E. **Restoring volar cortical continuity may best predict final carpal alignment.**

Restoring volar cortical continuity may best predict final carpal alignment.[1] Volar locking plate open reduction internal fixation has been shown to give superior functional outcomes to percutaneous pinning.[2] When reduction and casting was compared to external fixation, all patients achieved union.[3] Locking plates can reduce the requirement for bone graft.[4] Locking plates have superior purchase to nonlocking plates in osteoporotic bone. Extra-articular fractures in patients with good bone stock will often do well with manipulation and splinting, or a variety of fixations, and there is no conclusive evidence to mandate one option over another. The treatment is tailored to the patient's requirements, their health status, and the skill set of the treating surgeon. For a treatment algorithm for distal radius fractures, see **Fig. 75.3**).

REFERENCES

1. LaMartina J, Jawa A, Stucken C, Merlin G, Tornetta P III. Predicting alignment after closed reduction and casting of distal radius fractures. J Hand Surg Am 2015;40(5):934–939
2. McFadyen I, Field J, McCann P, Ward J, Nicol S, Curwen C. Should unstable extra-articular distal radial fractures be treated with fixed-angle volar-locked plates or percutaneous Kirschner wires? A prospective randomised controlled trial. Injury 2011;42(2):162–166
3. Aktekin CN, Altay M, Gursoy Z, Aktekin LA, Ozturk AM, Tabak AY. Comparison between external fixation and cast treatment in the management of distal radius fractures in patients aged 65 years and older. J Hand Surg Am 2010;35(5):736–742
4. Osti M, Mittler C, Zinnecker R, Westreicher C, Allhoff C, Benedetto KP. Locking versus nonlocking palmar plate fixation of distal radius fractures. Orthopedics 2012;35(11):e1613–e1617

76. Metacarpal and Phalangeal Fractures

See *Essentials of Plastic Surgery*, third edition, pp. 1068–1087

FRACTURE TERMINOLOGY

1. *Which one of the following is a fracture type that results in more than two bone fragments?*
   A. Spiral
   B. Greenstick
   C. Intra-articular
   D. Comminuted
   E. Avulsion

FRACTURE TERMINOLOGY

2. *Which one of the following represents a fracture that occurs in elderly females after minimal trauma?*
   A. Spiral
   B. Impaction
   C. Pathologic
   D. Stress
   E. Greenstick

SALTER-HARRIS CLASSIFICATION SYSTEM

3. You are referred a child with a phalangeal fracture passing through both the epiphysis and physis. *According to the Salter-Harris classification system, what type of fracture does this represent?*
   A. Type I
   B. Type II
   C. Type III
   D. Type IV
   E. Type V

FRACTURE HEALING

4. *Which one of the following medications may be best avoided in the early phases of fracture healing?*
   A. Acetaminophen
   B. Ibuprofen
   C. Codeine
   D. Tramadol
   E. Gabapentin

SAFE SPLINTING FOR HAND INJURIES

5. *When applying a splint after closed reduction of a hand fracture, which one of the following is correct?*
   A. The wrist should be placed in neutral.
   B. The interphalangeal (IP) joints should be flexed.
   C. The metacarpophalangeal (MCP) joints should be extended.
   D. The thumb should be abducted from the palm.
   E. The wrist should be placed in ulnar deviation.

HAND INJURIES DUE TO PUNCHING

6. *Which one of the following hand injuries is most commonly observed in professional boxers?*
   A. Metacarpal neck fracture
   B. Metacarpal shaft fracture
   C. Damage to the extensor mechanism
   D. Damage to the collateral ligaments
   E. Phalangeal shaft fracture

CLOSED REDUCTION OF HAND FRACTURES

7. *For which one of the following displaced fracture types is the Jahss maneuver useful?*
   A. Metacarpal neck
   B. Metacarpal base
   C. Proximal phalanx condyles
   D. Proximal phalanx shaft
   E. Proximal phalanx base

DEFORMING FORCES IN HAND FRACTURES

8. Most metacarpal fractures result in apex dorsal angulation. *Which one of the following anatomic features is usually responsible?*
   A. The fracture pattern
   B. The extensor tendons
   C. The flexor tendons
   D. The shape of the bone
   E. The intrinsic muscles

METACARPAL FRACTURES

9. You are seeing a patient 1 week after a punch injury leading to a closed, 40-degree apex dorsally angulated fifth metacarpal neck fracture. *Which one of the following statements is correct?*
   A. This degree of angulation mandates surgical intervention.
   B. This fracture is likely to be unstable and require careful splinting.
   C. There is unlikely to be any associated extensor lag.
   D. Functional outcomes following this injury are usually poor.
   E. This can be treated with buddy taping to the ring finger and mobilization.

METACARPAL FRACTURES

10. A 30-year-old woman presents with an acute spiral fracture of the fifth metacarpal shaft with 4 mm shortening and scissoring of the digits. *Which one of the following statements is correct?*
    A. Closed reduction with transverse K-wires is unsuitable for treating this fracture.
    B. The digital overlap on flexion suggests rotation at the fracture site.
    C. Manipulation and splinting in a resting volar cast are adequate to maintain correction.
    D. Fixation with a lag screw and compression plate should be used for this fracture.
    E. Intramedullary K-wires should be used to treat this fracture.

METACARPAL FRACTURES

11. When considering fractures of the metacarpal base which one of the following statements is correct?
    A. When stabilizing a closed Bennett fracture with percutaneous wires, the proximal fragment needs to be captured by at least one wire.
    B. A reverse Bennett fracture involves the distal shaft of the first metacarpal and usually requires fixation.
    C. Rolando fractures of the first metacarpal are extra-articular basal fractures best treated with K-wires.
    D. Intra-articular fracture dislocations of the fourth and fifth metacarpal bases are inherently unstable and require stabilization into the carpus.
    E. Fracture dislocations of the second and third metacarpal bases are common following axial loading and require external fixation devices.

SEYMOUR FRACTURES

12. In which one of the following scenarios can a Seymour fracture be present?
    A. A 30-year-old man with a distal phalanx crush injury
    B. A 10-year-old girl with a nail bed injury
    C. A 45-year-old woman with a rotational deformity
    D. A 7-year-old boy with a proximal interphalangeal (PIP) joint extensor lag
    E. A 14-year-old boy with loss of distal interphalangeal (DIP) joint flexion

PHALANGEAL FRACTURES

13. Which one of the following is correct regarding intra-articular fractures of the proximal interphalangeal (PIP) joint?
    A. Pilon fractures result in two main fragments with dorsal subluxation of the middle phalanx shaft.
    B. A hemi-hamate bone graft may be used to resurface the middle phalanx base after intra-articular fractures.
    C. Dynamic external fixators require a minimum of three wires in order to adequately stabilize the middle phalanx shaft.
    D. A volar plate avulsion fracture with 10% of the articular surface and no subluxation should initially be splinted in extension.
    E. Open reduction and internal fixation is generally preferable to closed methods to ensure accurate reduction.

FRACTURES OF THE PHALANGES

14. *When considering whether a phalangeal fracture is stable, which one of the following is correct?*
    A. Fractures of the base of the proximal phalanx base tend to angulate apex dorsal because of the pull of the interossei on the proximal fragment.
    B. Oblique fractures are unlikely to lead to sufficient shortening to interfere with tendon balance.
    C. Volar avulsion fractures of the base of the middle phalanx remain stable even where more than 40% of the articular surface is avulsed.
    D. Fractures of the middle phalanx shaft angulate apex volar if the fracture is distal to the flexor digitorum superficialis (FDS) tendon insertion.
    E. Oblique unicondylar fractures tend to be very stable, so rarely lead to lateral deviation or rotational deformities.

FRACTURES OF THE PHALANGES

15. A 30-year-old man has sustained a displaced transverse extra-articular fracture of the ring finger middle phalanx base. There is angulation with the apex dorsal and there are no visible wounds. *Which one of the following statements is correct?*
    A. Internal fixation with lag screws is the best option for this fracture.
    B. This fracture is stable and should be manipulated and buddy taped to the ring finger.
    C. The basal (proximal) fragment is being displaced by the FDS tendon.
    D. A dynamic external fixator is required to enable ligamentotaxis to reduce the deformity.
    E. Crossed K-wires should provide a satisfactory method for stabilizing this fracture.

HAND FRACTURE MANAGEMENT

16. You are discussing treatment options with a patient who has a 40-degree angulated (apex volar) extra-articular transverse basal fracture of the ring finger proximal phalanx. The patient is reluctant to have any manipulation or surgery. *Which one of the following is correct?*
    A. Nonoperative management in this position will give near normal function.
    B. Closed reduction followed by a dorsal metacarpophalangeal (MCP) joint extension blocking splint may be sufficient.
    C. Risk of tendon adhesions is avoided with nonoperative management.
    D. Failed nonoperative management can only be salvaged in the first week.
    E. The risks of infection and nerve injury are less with percutaneous pins than with internal fixation.

Answers

FRACTURE TERMINOLOGY

1. *Which one of the following is a fracture type that results in more than two bone fragments?*

D. Comminuted

Correct fracture terminology aids communication and can help guide treatment. Simple fractures contain two bone fragments, while comminuted fractures have multiple fragments. Spiral fractures have an oblique rotating plane, and greenstick fractures involve only one cortex, occurring in children. Intra-articular fractures extend into a joint surface and may have any number of fragments. Avulsion fractures involve a bone chip caused by distraction forces on a tendon or ligament.[1,2]

REFERENCES

1. Day CS, Stern PJ. Fractures of the metacarpals and phalanges. In: Wolfe SW, Hotchkiss RN, Pederson WC, et al, eds. Green's Operative Hand Surgery. 6th ed. Philadelphia: Churchill Livingstone; 2011
2. Zenn MR, Jones G. Reconstructive Surgery: Anatomy, Technique, and Clinical Applications. St Louis: Quality Medical Publishing; 2012

FRACTURE TERMINOLOGY

2. *Which one of the following represents a fracture that occurs in elderly females after minimal trauma?*

C. Pathologic

Fractures that occur in weakened or abnormal bone are classified as pathologic fractures. These include bones weakened by tumor or osteoporosis. Stress fractures occur in normal bone in response to cyclical loading. Greenstick fractures occur in children where the cortices are more pliable and the periosteum is thicker, tending to lead to buckling or unicortical rather than complete fractures. The radiologic appearance of a fracture can be described as transverse, oblique, spiral, longitudinal, or impacted. Spiral fractures have an oblique fracture plane with rotation. Impacted fractures occur secondary to end on stress causing compression.[1,2]

REFERENCES

1. Haase SC. Treatment of pathologic fractures. Hand Clin 2013;29(4):579–584
2. Nellans KW, Chung KC. Pediatric hand fractures. Hand Clin 2013;29(4):569–578

SALTER-HARRIS CLASSIFICATION SYSTEM

3. You are referred a child with a phalangeal fracture passing through both the epiphysis and physis. *According to the Salter-Harris classification system, what type of fracture does this represent?*

C. Type III

This fracture represents a Salter-Harris type III injury.[1] The Salter-Harris classification applies to fractures that occur at the growth plate (physis) in developing limbs. The classification system is well known and is often tested in examination settings. The most common fracture pattern is a type II injury which involves the metaphysis and physis. These fractures can result in abnormal growth if the epiphyseal plates are permanently damaged (**Fig. 76.1**).[1,2]

REFERENCES

1. Salter RB, Harris WR. Injuries involving the epiphyseal plate. J Bone Joint Surg 1963;45:587–622
2. Nellans KW, Chung KC. Pediatric hand fractures. Hand Clin 2013;29(4):569–578

FRACTURE HEALING

4. *Which one of the following medications may be best avoided in the early phases of fracture healing?*

B. Ibuprofen

There is mixed evidence on the effects of nonsteroidal anti-inflammatory drugs (NSAIDs) on fracture healing, but a number of animal studies suggest that healing is adversely affected by the administration of NSAIDs. In addition, some clinical studies in humans also support this finding. NSAIDs interfere with the inflammatory stage of bone healing. Based on current evidence, they may be best avoided in patients with acute fractures.[1,2]

However, many surgeons do routinely prescribe them in patients following hand fractures.[3]

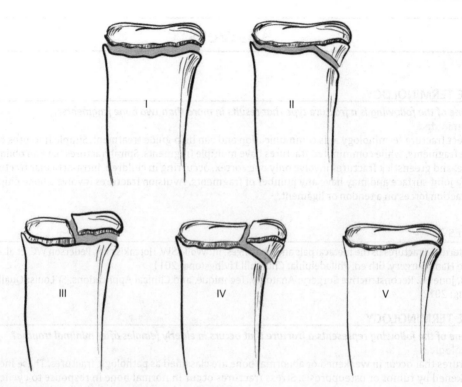

Fig. 76.1   Salter-Harris classification system of pediatric fractures. (Adapted from PediatricEducation.org. Available at: http://www.pediatriceducation.org. March 10, 2005.)

REFERENCES

1. Pountos I, Georgouli T, Calori GM, Giannoudis PV. Do nonsteroidal anti-inflammatory drugs affect bone healing? A critical analysis. ScientificWorldJournal 2012;2012:606404
2. Kurmis AP, Kurmis TP, O'Brien JX, Dalén T. The effect of nonsteroidal anti-inflammatory drug administration on acute phase fracture-healing: a review. J Bone Joint Surg Am 2012;94(9):815–823
3. Marquez-Lara A, Hutchinson ID, Nuñez F Jr, Smith TL, Miller AN. Nonsteroidal anti-inflammatory drugs and bone-healing: a systematic review of research quality. JBJS Rev 2016;4(3)

SAFE SPLINTING FOR HAND INJURIES

5. *When applying a splint after closed reduction of a hand fracture, which one of the following is correct?*

   D. The thumb should be abducted from the palm.

   The safe position for hand splinting involves interphalangeal (IP) joints fully extended, MCP joints flexed to 70 to 90 degrees, and the wrist in slight extension. This places the MCP joint collateral ligaments and IP joint volar plates under maximal stretch and decreases subsequent joint stiffness. It also maximizes function if stiffness persists. The thumb should be abducted from the palm as if holding a beer glass; otherwise it may be more difficult to subsequently regain full range of motion (**Fig. 76.2**).[1,2]

REFERENCES

1. Day CS, Stern PJ. Fractures of the metacarpals and phalanges. In: Green DP, Hotchkiss RN, Pederson WC, eds. Green's Operative Hand Surgery. 6th ed. Philadelphia: Elsevier; 2011
2. Richards T, Clement R, Russell I, Newington D. Acute hand injury splinting - the good, the bad and the ugly. Ann R Coll Surg Engl 2018;100(2):92–96

HAND INJURIES DUE TO PUNCHING

6. *Which one of the following hand injuries is most commonly observed in professional boxers?*

   C. Damage to the extensor mechanism

   The term "boxer's" fracture is used to describe a fifth metacarpal neck fracture occurring during a punch injury. This is a misnomer because professional boxers rarely sustain such an injury. True boxers are more likely to sustain

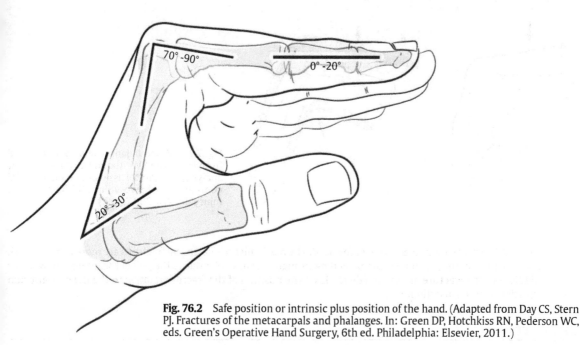

Fig. 76.2   Safe position or intrinsic plus position of the hand. (Adapted from Day CS, Stern PJ. Fractures of the metacarpals and phalanges. In: Green DP, Hotchkiss RN, Pederson WC, eds. Green's Operative Hand Surgery, 6th ed. Philadelphia: Elsevier, 2011.)

sagittal band ruptures at the MCP joint, resulting in extensor tendon subluxation known as "boxer's knuckle," or fractures affecting the index and middle rays.[1,2]

REFERENCES

1. Dunn JC, Kusnezov N, Orr JD, Pallis M, Mitchell JS. The boxer's fracture: splint immobilization is not necessary. Orthopedics 2016;39(3):188–192
2. Day CS, Stern PJ. Fractures of the metacarpals and phalanges. In: Wolfe SW, Hotchkiss RN, Pederson WC, et al, eds. Green's Operative Hand Surgery. 6th ed. Philadelphia: Churchill Livingstone; 2011

CLOSED REDUCTION OF HAND FRACTURES

7. *For which one of the following displaced fracture types is the Jahss maneuver useful?*
   A. Metacarpal neck
   The Jahss maneuver is used to reduce a metacarpal neck fracture, for example, if malrotation or pseudoclawing is present. It is performed under local anesthetic block by flexing the MCP joints to 90 degrees and applying force to the metacarpal head in a dorsal direction through the proximal phalanx, while stabilizing the metacarpal shaft. Holding the MCP joint in flexion relaxes the intrinsic muscles while tightening the collateral ligaments and locates the proximal phalanx base under the metacarpal head such that reduction may be achieved (**Fig. 76.3**).[1,2]

REFERENCES

1. Jahss SA. Fractures of the metacarpals: a new method of reduction and immobilization. J Bone Joint Surg. 1938;20:178–186
2. Hamilton SW, Aboud H. Finite element analysis, mechanical assessment and material comparison of two volar slab constructs. Injury 2009;40(4):397–399

DEFORMING FORCES IN HAND FRACTURES

8. Most metacarpal fractures result in apex dorsal angulation. *Which one of the following anatomic features is usually responsible?*
   E. The intrinsic muscles
   Most metacarpal fractures display apex dorsal angulation because of the intrinsic muscles. For example, metacarpal neck fractures angulate apex dorsally because the intrinsic muscles lie volar to the axis of rotation

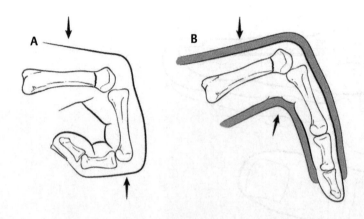

Fig. 76.3 *A* and *B,* Jahss maneuver. (Adapted from Hamilton SW, Aboud H. Finite element analysis, mechanical assessment and material comparison of two volar slab constructs. Injury 40:397–399, 2009.)

of the MCP joint, maintaining flexion of the head. The mechanics of phalangeal fractures are more complex with basal fractures of the proximal phalanx tending to angulate apex volar due to the pull of the interossei, whereas middle phalanx fracture angulation depends on the position of the fracture relative to the flexor digitorum superficialis (FDS) insertion.[1,2]

REFERENCES

1. Stern PJ. Fractures of the metacarpals and phalanges. In: Green DP, Hotchkiss RN, Pederson WC, eds. Green's Operative Hand Surgery. 4th ed. Philadelphia: Churchill Livingstone; 1999
2. Lee SG, Jupiter JB. Phalangeal and metacarpal fractures of the hand. Hand Clin 2000;16(3):323–332, vii

METACARPAL FRACTURES

9. You are seeing a patient 1 week after a punch injury leading to a closed, 40-degree apex dorsally angulated fifth metacarpal neck fracture. *Which one of the following statements is correct?*
    E. This can be treated with buddy taping to the ring finger and mobilization.
    Fifth metacarpal neck fractures are usually very stable after a punch injury, as the distal fragment is highly impacted. A significant degree of apex dorsal angulation can be tolerated without functional deficit and 40-degree angulation is unlikely to cause a functional problem in the little finger.[1] Due to the blunt impact over a flexed MCP joint, there may be an associated injury to the extensor apparatus. Extensor lag is often present initially and is usually due to altered joint mechanics and relative shortening of the bony skeleton versus the tendon. On occasion, the extensor apparatus is also injured, or may be tethered by a bony spicule. Although functional outcomes are good, patients will be left with the appearance of a depressed knuckle. There is no clear consensus on the best nonoperative management of fifth metacarpal fractures and patients tend to do well with either early mobilization with buddy strapping or short-term casting.[2]

REFERENCES

1. Hunter JM, Cowen NJ. Fifth metacarpal fractures in a compensation clinic population. A report on one hundred and thirty-three cases. J Bone Joint Surg Am 1970;52(6): 1159–1165
2. Statius Muller MG, Poolman RW, van Hoogstraten MJ, Steller EP. Immediate mobilization gives good results in boxer's fractures with volar angulation up to 70 degrees: a prospective randomized trial comparing immediate mobilization with cast immobilization. Arch Orthop Trauma Surg 2003;123(10):534–537

METACARPAL FRACTURES

10. A 30-year-old woman presents with an acute spiral fracture of the fifth metacarpal shaft with 4 mm shortening and scissoring of the digits. *Which one of the following statements is correct?*
    B. The digital overlap on flexion suggests rotation at the fracture site.
    While there can sometimes be a mild degree of pseudo-rotation with fifth metacarpal neck fractures as a result of swelling of the interosseous muscles, malrotation seen in the context of a spiral fracture is much more likely to be of clinical significance. The shortening seen makes true malrotation likely, as shortening along a spiral fracture line will generate rotation. Frank scissoring of the digits is always abnormal.
    Closed reduction and transverse percutaneous wires may provide relative stability for this fracture, provided that accurate reduction is produced during manipulation and adequate stabilization against the fourth metacarpal

is provided. This will require two to three transverse wires through the fifth into the fourth metacarpal. A protective splint is still required for the initial 1 to 2 weeks. Some surgeons find this method unacceptable and prefer not to pass K-wires through the interossei.

Internal fixation with multiple lag screws or a lag screw and neutralization plate (not a compression plate) provides a more rigid fixation than K-wires, but at the expense of visible scarring, a palpable plate, and potentially extensive soft-tissue dissection. Early mobilization is preferred following internal fixation to minimize adhesion of gliding surfaces. The choice between multiple lag screws or a screw and plate is determined by the length of the fracture relative to the width and length of the bone. A shorter fracture is unlikely to be stable with screws alone. A noncompressing neutralization plate is applied to support lag screw fixation of a short spiral fracture rather than a compression plate, which would place strain on the lag screw fixation and potentially cause rotation. While intramedullary K-wires can be useful for transverse fifth metacarpal shaft and neck fractures, they cannot control rotation.[1–3]

REFERENCES

1. Day CS, Stern PJ. Fractures of the metacarpals and phalanges. In: Green DP, Hotchkiss RN, Pederson WC, eds. Green's Operative Hand Surgery. 6th ed. Philadelphia: Elsevier; 2011
2. Weinstein LP, Hanel DP. Metacarpal fractures. J Hand Surg Am 2002;2:168–180
3. Freeland AE, Jabaley ME, Hughes JL. Stable Fixation of the Hand and Wrist. New York: Springer-Verlag; 1986

METACARPAL FRACTURES

11. When considering fractures of the metacarpal base which one of the following statements is correct?

D. Intra-articular fracture dislocations of the fourth and fifth metacarpal bases are inherently unstable and require stabilization into the carpus.

Fracture dislocations of the fourth and fifth metacarpals may be termed "reverse Bennett fractures" and can occur following axial loading such as during a punch injury. They are relatively common injuries and may be associated with a fracture of the hamate, which can be missed on plain radiographs. The metacarpal bases can dislocate dorsally and should be reduced and stabilized with percutaneous K-wires into the carpus and adjacent metacarpal.

A Bennett fracture is a two-part fracture of the first metacarpal base that leaves a small fragment attached to the carpus due to the strong volar beak ligament. The remainder of the metacarpal shaft is displaced and requires reduction and stabilization with K-wires, usually passing into the trapezium and often into the index metacarpal base. The proximal fragment is usually small and stable. It is used as a guide to ensure adequate reduction of the metacarpal base but does not have to be included in the K-wire passes (**Fig. 76.4**).

Rolando fractures are comminuted intra-articular fractures of the first metacarpal. They are treated with either open reduction and plate fixation of larger fragments or closed K-wiring. The second and third carpometacarpal (CMC) joints are very stable and are rarely fractured or dislocated.[1–4]

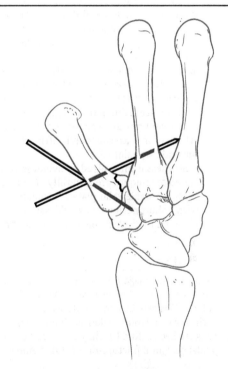

Fig. 76.4 Reduction and stabilization of Bennett's fracture using Kirschner's wires into the trapezium and index metacarpal base.

REFERENCES

1. Weinstein LP, Hanel DP. Metacarpal fractures. J Hand Surg Am 2002;2:168–180
2. Kamath JB, Harshvardhan, Naik DM, Bansal A. Current concepts in managing fractures of metacarpal and phalanges. Indian J Plast Surg 2011;44(2):203–211
3. Wong PK, Hanna TN, Shuaib W, Sanders SM, Khosa F. What's in a name? Upper extremity fracture eponyms (Part 1). Int J Emerg Med 2015;8(1):75
4. Freeland AE, Jabaley ME, Hughes JL. Stable Fixation of the Hand and Wrist. New York: Springer-Verlag; 1986

SEYMOUR FRACTURES

12. In which one of the following scenarios can a Seymour fracture be present?

B. A 10-year-old girl with a nail bed injury

A Seymour fracture is an open epiphyseal injury of the distal phalanx. When assessing a child in clinic with a nail bed injury, it is important to look for the presence of a Seymour fracture, which can be mistaken for a simple mallet deformity or soft-tissue swelling after a crush injury. This is an open Salter-Harris type fracture where a nail bed injury and distal phalanx fracture coexist. The clue is that the nail plate usually lies superficial to the nail fold, rather than tucked underneath it. If the fracture is not reduced, there may be subsequent growth disturbance. Furthermore, part of the proximal nail bed may flip into the fracture site, preventing healing or closed reduction. These injuries are more likely to be treated surgically to ensure that the fracture is properly reduced and stabilized, in addition to cleaning and repairing the nail bed.[1,2]

REFERENCES

1. Seymour N. Juxta-epiphysial fracture of the terminal phalanx of the finger. J Bone Joint Surg Br 1966;48(2):347–349
2. Krusche-Mandl I, Köttstorfer J, Thalhammer G, Aldrian S, Erhart J, Platzer P. Seymour fractures: retrospective analysis and therapeutic considerations. J Hand Surg Am 2013;38(2):258–264

PHALANGEAL FRACTURES

13. Which one of the following is correct regarding intra-articular fractures of the PIP joint?

B. A hemi-hamate bone graft may be used to resurface the middle phalanx base after intra-articular fractures.

Not all intra-articular PIP joint fractures are pilon fractures. A pilon fracture occurs following an axial load, causing impaction and comminution of the base of the middle phalanx, often with splaying of the fragments. Treatment options for intra-articular fractures range from simple buddy taping to dynamic external fixators (e.g., Suzuki pins and rubber band system), which use ligamentotaxis to hold the joint space open while allowing movement to encourage a better final joint surface and minimize stiffness.[1,2] While a third transverse pin/wire is sometimes needed to control dorsal subluxation of the middle phalanx shaft in flexion, it is often possible to achieve adequate control with two pins/wires. Open reduction and fixation may be required to achieve accurate joint surface reduction through either a volar or dorsal approach.

In select circumstances, a bone/cartilage graft may be harvested from the dorsal aspect of the hamate articulation with the fourth/fifth metacarpal bases and used to replace the damaged volar PIP joint surface of the middle phalanx.[3]

Stiffness is minimized by avoiding additional soft-tissue injury and encouraging early movement; therefore, closed techniques are generally preferred where possible for fractures involving the PIP joint.

Minor, stable volar plate avulsion fractures may be managed with either buddy strapping and mobilization or with a short period using a dorsal extension blocking splint and active flexion exercises. Splinting in extension will tend to distract the bony fragment and lead to delayed healing and stiffness.[1-3]

REFERENCES

1. Suzuki Y, Matsunaga T, Sato S, Yokoi T. The pins and rubbers traction system for treatment of comminuted intraarticular fractures and fracture-dislocations in the hand. J Hand Surg [Br] 1994;19(1):98–107
2. Ruland RT, Hogan CJ, Cannon DL, Slade JF. Use of dynamic distraction external fixation for unstable fracture-dislocations of the proximal interphalangeal joint. J Hand Surg Am 2008;33(1):19–25
3. Yang DS, Lee SK, Kim KJ, Choy WS. Modified hemihamate arthroplasty technique for treatment of acute proximal interphalangeal joint fracture-dislocations. Ann Plast Surg 2014;72(4):411–416

FRACTURES OF THE PHALANGES

14. When considering whether a phalangeal fracture is stable, which one of the following is correct?

D. Fractures of the middle phalanx shaft angulate apex volar if the fracture is distal to the flexor digitorum superficialis (FDS) tendon insertion.

Proximal phalangeal shaft fractures usually angulate apex volar because of flexion of the proximal fragment by the interossei. However, middle phalanx shaft fractures can angulate either apex volar or apex dorsal, depending on the location of the fracture in relation to the insertion of the FDS tendon. Oblique phalangeal shaft fractures have a tendency to shorten as the bone fragments slide relative to one another because of the surrounding soft-tissue forces. This can lead to shortening which may interfere with tendon balance.

Volar avulsion fractures at the base of the middle phalanx are commonly stabilized by the intact collateral ligaments (**Fig. 76.5**). While the accessory collateral ligaments attach to the volar plate and therefore cannot exert any stabilizing force on the middle phalanx once the volar plate attachment is avulsed, the true collateral

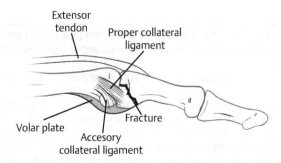

Fig. 76.5 Volar avulsion fracture at the base of the middle phalanx.

ligaments insert broadly onto the volar 40% of the proximal phalanx. Therefore, if some of the true collateral ligament insertion is preserved, the joint may remain fairly stable, but if more than 40% of the middle phalanx is avulsed, there is no longer any stabilizing force from these ligaments acting on the distal fragment, which then usually subluxes dorsally. Oblique unicondylar fractures tend to be very unstable, so they can commonly lead to lateral deviation or rotational deformities.[1-3]

REFERENCES

1. Lögters TT, Lee HH, Gehrmann S, Windolf J, Kaufmann RA. Proximal phalanx fracture management. Hand (N Y) 2018;13(4):376–383
2. Stern PJ. Fractures of the metacarpals and phalanges. In: Green DP, Hotchkiss RN, Pederson WC, eds. Green's Operative Hand Surgery. 4th ed. Philadelphia: Churchill Livingstone; 1999
3. Barton N. Internal fixation of hand fractures. J Hand Surg [Br] 1989;14(2):139–142

FRACTURES OF THE PHALANGES

15. A 30-year-old man has sustained a displaced transverse extra-articular fracture of the ring finger middle phalanx base. There is angulation with the apex dorsal and there are no visible wounds. *Which one of the following statements is correct?*

E. **Crossed K-wires should provide a satisfactory method for stabilizing this fracture.**

The apex dorsal angulation suggests that the proximal (basal) fragment is being pulled by the insertion of the central slip while the distal (shaft) fragment is being pulled by the strong FDS insertion. This is likely to be unstable after reduction and therefore liable to fall into the same position when the patient flexes the fingers. Closed reduction and percutaneous K-wires should stabilize the fracture adequately. Crossed wires from each midlateral line could be used, either antegrade or retrograde (**Fig. 76.6**). Opening the digit to use plate fixation increases the soft-tissue injury and the likelihood of postoperative adhesions but could be considered for this fracture if the basal fragment is of sufficient size. Lag screws are not suited to transverse fractures and are used for oblique or spiral fracture patterns. Dynamic external fixators are generally reserved for intra-articular fractures of the phalanges.[1-4]

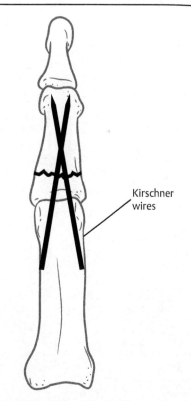

Kirschner wires

Fig. 76.6 Crossed K-wires for stabilization of a middle phalanx fracture.

REFERENCES

1. Burkhalter WE. Closed treatment of hand fractures. J Hand Surg Am 1989;14(2, Pt 2): 390–393
2. Hornbach EE, Cohen MS. Closed reduction and percutaneous pinning of fractures of the proximal phalanx. J Hand Surg [Br] 2001;26(1):45–49
3. Greene TL, Noellert RC, Belsole RJ, Simpson LA. Composite wiring of metacarpal and phalangeal fractures. J Hand Surg Am 1989;14(4):665–669
4. Stern PJ. Fractures of the metacarpals and phalanges. In: Green DP, Hotchkiss RN, Pederson WC, eds. Green's Operative Hand Surgery. 4th ed. Philadelphia: Churchill Livingstone; 1999

HAND FRACTURE MANAGEMENT

16. You are discussing treatment options with a patient who has a 40-degree angulated (apex volar) extra-articular transverse basal fracture of the ring finger proximal phalanx. The patient is reluctant to have any manipulation or surgery. *Which one of the following is correct?*

    B. **Closed reduction followed by a dorsal metacarpophalangeal (MCP) joint extension blocking splint may be sufficient.**

    The pull of the flexor tendons will tend to help maintain the correction, provided an extension block is in place to prevent re-displacement in the early stages. Pseudo-clawing occurs when a basal proximal phalanx fracture unites in apex–volar angulation. This may result in reduced composite flexion of the digit, and also lead to an extensor lag. Tendon adhesions can occur with nonoperative and operative management, but they are most common following open internal fixation. Failed nonoperative management can be salvaged at most stages, but re-manipulation and fixation of the original fracture is easiest in the first 10 to 14 days. There may be a greater risk of nerve injury if care is not taken during closed cutaneous pinning, because the tip of the wire can easily slide off the small, curved phalanx (particularly at the narrow phalangeal neck), whereas the digital nerves can be readily seen and protected during open fixation. There is also a higher risk of infection at pin track sites with external wires than with internal fixation.[1]

REFERENCE

1. Day CS, Stern PJ. Fractures of the metacarpals and phalanges. In: Wolfe SW, Hotchkiss RN, Pederson WC, et al, eds. Green's Operative Hand Surgery. 6th ed. Philadelphia: Churchill Livingstone; 2011

77. Phalangeal Dislocations

See *Essentials of Plastic Surgery*, third edition, pp. 1088–1096

CLINICAL EVALUATION OF THE SMALL JOINTS OF THE HAND

1. *When assessing the small joints of the hand for evidence of a ligamentous injury, which one of the following is correct?*
   A. A grade I collateral ligament tear will be grossly unstable during lateral stress testing.
   B. Lateral stability in extension does not exclude the presence of a collateral ligament tear.
   C. Stener lesions are nonspecific to a particular small joint and can occur with all injury grades I through III.
   D. Dislocations are described according to the position of the proximal bone to normal joint alignment.
   E. Two radiographic views are required involving joints proximal and distal to the injury.

FINGER MCP JOINT ANATOMY

2. *Which one of the following is responsible for the cam effect in metacarpophalangeal (MCP) joint flexion?*
   A. Volar plate
   B. Flexor tendons
   C. Collateral ligaments
   D. Joint contour
   E. Deep transverse metacarpal ligament

DORSAL DISLOCATION OF THE FINGER MCP JOINT

3. You assess a young man with a dorsal index finger MCP joint dislocation after a fall. The MCP joint is in 70 degrees of extension and the interphalangeal (IP) joint is flexed. There are no fractures seen on three plain radiograph views. *Which one of the following is correct?*
   A. Wrist and MCP joint extension will aid closed reduction.
   B. The metacarpal head may be trapped between the long flexor tendons and the lumbrical.
   C. It can be reliably assumed that the collateral ligaments are intact.
   D. If an open reduction is required, a dorsal approach is best.
   E. If an open reduction is required, the A1 pulley must be preserved.

THUMB MCP JOINT INJURY

4. A patient has sustained a closed injury to the thumb during a fall onto an outstretched hand. Ligamentous damage is suspected. *Which one of the following is correct regarding thumb MCP joint collateral ligament injuries?*
   A. Ulnar collateral ligament (UCL) injuries are twice as common as radial collateral ligament (RCL) or volar plate injuries.
   B. UCL tears are most likely to occur at the proximal origin from the metacarpal.
   C. Complete RCL and UCL injuries need operative intervention because of the risk of a Stener lesion.
   D. Grade II UCL and RCL injuries are treated similarly, with 4 weeks of immobilization in a cast.
   E. UCL injuries involving avulsion fractures are most commonly intra-articular and require surgical intervention.

CHRONIC MCP JOINT INJURY OF THE THUMB

5. A 59-year-old man complains of pain and weakness affecting his dominant thumb, which has been getting worse over 5 years. On examination, the interphalangeal (IP) joint and carpometacarpal (CMC) joint are unremarkable. The MCP joint sits in radial deviation, but there is an endpoint on radial stressing at 45 degrees. The radial collateral ligament (RCL) is intact. There is sclerosis and a small radial osteophyte on radiographs. *Which one of the following is correct?*
   A. Fusion of the MCP joint may be the most appropriate long-term solution.
   B. Repeated steroid injections may be all that is required for symptomatic management.
   C. A palmaris longus tendon graft should be used to reconstruct the ulnar collateral ligament (UCL).
   D. If the patient cannot recall a specific injury, it is unlikely that the UCL is the problem.
   E. A period of 8 to 12 weeks in a thumb spica cast should allow this injury to stabilize.

ANATOMY OF THE PIP JOINT

6. *Which one of the following is correct regarding proximal interphalangeal (PIP) joint?*
   A. The ligament box complex comprises two key elements; the volar plate and true collateral ligaments.
   B. The PIP joint is less commonly dislocated than the distal interphalangeal (DIP) joint.
   C. A normal PIP joint range of motion involves a 70-degree arc of rotation.
   D. Dorsal dislocation of the PIP joint is most common, given the joint anatomy.
   E. Volar plate avulsion usually occurs at the proximal phalanx.

CLASSIFICATION OF DORSAL PIP JOINT DISLOCATIONS

7. A patient presents with a type II dorsal dislocation of the PIP joint. *What does this description suggest?*
   A. That there is an associated bony injury.
   B. That some joint congruity is maintained.
   C. That the volar plate is still intact.
   D. That the collateral ligaments are still intact.
   E. That both volar plate and collateral ligaments are injured.

TREATMENT OF ACUTE PIP JOINT DISLOCATIONS

8. You see a patient in the hand trauma clinic following reduction of a dorsal dislocation of the ring finger PIP joint. Post reduction radiographs reveal a 30% volar articular fragment at the base of the middle phalanx that is well aligned. *Which one of the following is the most appropriate management plan?*
   A. Mobilize with buddy strapping to the middle finger and see again in 2 to 3 weeks.
   B. Immobilize for 2 to 3 weeks in extension to prevent joint contracture, then progressively mobilize with buddy strapping.
   C. Protect and mobilize within a dorsal blocking splint at 20 to 30 degrees for 3 weeks, reducing the splint angle weekly.
   D. Perform open reduction and mini-lag screw fixation of the bony fragment and begin early mobilization.
   E. Apply a dynamic skeletal traction frame across the PIP joint and begin early mobilization.

TREATMENT OF ACUTE PIP JOINT DISLOCATIONS

9. A patient presents after a fall during which he injured his little finger PIP joint. He states that immediately after the fall his finger was pointing away from the ring finger at about 60 degrees, but he was able to manipulate the finger back into place. Examination shows a residual 30 degrees of lateral instability on stress testing. Radiographs are all normal. *Which one of the following is correct?*
   A. Although the RCL will have been injured, the volar plate will be spared.
   B. This injury will require surgical intervention with a bone anchor device.
   C. Buddy taping to the ring finger and mobilization may be all that is required.
   D. The outcome following this injury is likely to be excellent with normal function by 6 weeks.
   E. This mechanism of injury is less common than a volar dislocation of the PIP joint.

DIP JOINT DISLOCATIONS

10. *Which one of the following is true with regard to DIP joint injuries?*
    A. They represent the most commonly dislocated small joint of the hand.
    B. They are most commonly closed injuries when they do occur.
    C. They can often be associated with tendon insertion injuries.
    D. When surgery is required this is best undertaken under general anesthesia.
    E. Early mobilization following reduction is generally advised.

Answers

CLINICAL EVALUATION OF THE SMALL JOINTS OF THE HAND

1. *When assessing the small joints of the hand for evidence of a ligamentous injury, which one of the following is correct?*
   B. **Lateral stability in extension does not exclude the presence of a collateral ligament tear.**
   When assessing the stability of the small joints of the hand, stress testing should be performed in both flexion and extension to ensure that the collateral ligaments and volar plate are independently and accurately tested. For example, the proximal interphalangeal (PIP) joint can remain stable in extension despite a collateral ligament tear because of volar plate stability. Flexion of the joint relaxes the volar plate and facilitates assessment of the collateral ligaments. Local anesthetic blocks are often required to perform this assessment.
   Collateral ligament injuries are graded I through III, according to increasing instability. A grade I injury is grossly stable with only a microscopic tear. A grade II injury results in relative instability in lateral stress testing (around 20 degrees), but with a definite endpoint. A grade III injury results in gross instability with no firm endpoint. Only grade III injuries (complete) lead to a Stener lesion which is specific to the thumb metacarpophalangeal (MCP) joint.[1,2]
   Dislocations are described according to the position of the distal bone (not proximal) relative to normal joint alignment. While the joints proximal and distal to the injury must be imaged, this must be in three (not two) views.

REFERENCES

1. Glickel SZ, Barron OA, Catalano LW. Dislocations and ligament injuries in the digits. In: Green DP, Hotchkiss RN, Pederson WC, et al, eds. Green's Operative Hand Surgery. 5th ed. Philadelphia: Churchill Livingstone; 2005
2. Stener B. Skeletal injuries associated with rupture of the ulnar collateral ligament of the metacarpophalangeal joint of the thumb. A clinical and anatomical study. Acta Chir Scand 1963;125:583–586

FINGER MCP JOINT ANATOMY

2. *Which one of the following is responsible for the cam effect in metacarpophalangeal (MCP) joint flexion?*
   D. **Joint contour**
   All of the listed options contribute to the stability of the MCP joint, but during flexion it is particularly stable from the *cam effect* of the joint. A cam effect converts a rotational motion into a linear one (**Fig. 77.1**). The metacarpal head is nonspherical, and when flexion occurs the collateral ligaments are placed on stretch. This explains why splints are designed to maintain the joint in flexion, and why Dupuytren's contractures can be left longer before treatment when involving this joint. There is also more stable bony contact when the MCP joint is placed in 70 degrees or more of flexion, which also contributes to overall stability.[1–3]

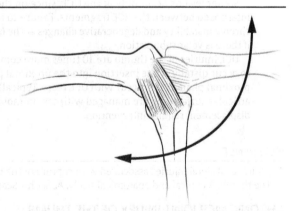

Fig. 77.1 The *cam effect* is created by eccentric movement of the proximal phalanx on the metacarpal head, causing a dynamic change in collateral ligament length.

REFERENCES

1. Minami A, An KN, Cooney WP III, Linscheid RL, Chao EY. Ligamentous structures of the metacarpophalangeal joint: a quantitative anatomic study. J Orthop Res 1984;1(4): 361–368
2. Eaton RG, Littler JW. Joint injuries and their sequelae. Clin Plast Surg 1976;3(1):85–98
3. Minami A, An KN, Cooney WP III, Linscheid RL, Chao EY. Ligament stability of the metacarpophalangeal joint: a biomechanical study. J Hand Surg Am 1985;10(2):255–260

DORSAL DISLOCATION OF THE FINGER MCP JOINT

3. You assess a young man with a dorsal index finger MCP joint dislocation after a fall. The MCP joint is in 70 degrees of extension and the interphalangeal (IP) joint is flexed. There are no fractures seen on three plain radiograph views. *Which one of the following is correct?*
   B. **The metacarpal head may be trapped between the long flexor tendons and the lumbrical.**

The head of the metacarpal is commonly found to be trapped between the lumbrical radially and the flexor tendons ulnarly and this is often a reason why reduction is challenging. Closed reduction is most likely to be successful if the wrist is flexed, because this will slacken off the long flexors. This is a fairly high-energy injury and the radial collateral ligament may have been avulsed. A volar approach provides the best access to the key structures during open reduction. Either the radial digital nerve to the index finger or the lumbrical may lie very superficially over the metacarpal head; so, care must be taken when elevating the skin flaps and exploring the joint to avoid damage.

Dividing the A1 pulley is sometimes used to slacken off the flexor pull and give more flexibility to the volar joint structures during reduction. Loss of this pulley would not have any negative functional consequences. Dorsal subluxations may also be complicated by the volar plate becoming trapped within the joint. In these circumstances, this must be removed from the joint intraoperatively and followed up with joint immobilization in flexion for the first few weeks.[1]

REFERENCE

1. Dinh P, Franklin A, Hutchinson B, Schnall SB, Fassola I. Metacarpophalangeal joint dislocation. J Am Acad Orthop Surg 2009;17(5):318–324

THUMB MCP JOINT INJURY

4. A patient has sustained a closed injury to the thumb during a fall onto an outstretched hand. Ligamentous damage is suspected. *Which one of the following is correct regarding thumb MCP joint collateral ligament injuries?*

D. Grade II UCL and RCL injuries are treated similarly with 4 weeks of immobilization in a cast.

Grade II RCL/UCL injuries of the thumb are treated similarly, with cast immobilization for 4 weeks then protected mobilization for a further 2 weeks. This is because there remains some continuity of the ligaments and in each scenario there will be the potential for adequate healing. In contrast, grade III injuries are treated differently due the risk of a Stener lesion. A Stener lesion is where the adductor aponeurosis becomes interposed between the distal UCL and base of the proximal phalanx. In this situation, primary repair of the ligament cannot occur.

Stener lesions occur only at the UCL, since on the radial side the abductor insertion is too wide to become interposed between the RCL fragments. Failure to recognize and treat a Stener lesion of the UCL may result in chronic instability and degenerative changes at the MCP joint. Surgical repair of RCL injures will need repair only if there is volar subluxation.[1]

UCL injuries of the thumb are 10 times more common than RCL injuries. UCL tears are five times more likely to occur distally at the insertion into the proximal phalanx than at the proximal site. Avulsion fractures of the proximal phalanx can occur with UCL tears. Typically, they are small fracture fragments that do not involve the articular surface and are managed with cast immobilization. Large fracture fragments with more than 2 mm of displacement require intervention.

REFERENCE

1. Stener B. Skeletal injuries associated with rupture of the ulnar collateral ligament of the metacarpophalangeal joint of the thumb. A clinical and anatomical study. Acta Chir Scand 1963;125:583–586

CHRONIC MCP JOINT INJURY OF THE THUMB

5. A 59-year-old man complains of pain and weakness affecting his dominant thumb, which has been getting worse over 5 years. On examination, the interphalangeal (IP) joint and carpometacarpal (CMC) joint are unremarkable. The MCP joint sits in radial deviation, but there is an endpoint on radial stressing at 45 degrees. The radial collateral ligament (RCL) is intact. There is sclerosis and a small radial osteophyte on radiographs. *Which one of the following is correct?*

A. Fusion of the MCP joint may be the most appropriate long-term solution.

Gamekeeper's thumb is a term used for chronic thumb MCP joint UCL injuries. It may be the result of a missed grade III UCL rupture with a Stener lesion, or it may be caused by repeated minor injuries that culminate in gradual attrition of the ligament. Either way, direct delayed repair of the UCL is not usually possible. The joint should always be assessed for signs of osteoarthritis before considering UCL reconstruction. If arthritis is present, it is usually more appropriate to fuse the MCP joint instead of reconstructing the UCL. Fusion of this joint is well tolerated if there is good IP joint and carpometacarpal (CMC) joint function.[1]

REFERENCE

1. Campbell CS. Gamekeeper's thumb. J Bone Joint Surg Br 1955;37-B(1):148–149

ANATOMY OF THE PIP JOINT

6. *Which one of the following is correct regarding proximal interphalangeal (PIP) joint?*

   D. Dorsal dislocation of the PIP joint is most common, given the joint anatomy.

   The PIP joint is the most commonly dislocated small joint in the hand, and dorsal dislocation, because of hyperextension, is the most common mechanism. The joint is normally very stable because of the anatomy of the ligament box complex which comprises the volar plate as well as the proper and accessory collateral ligaments (**Fig. 77.2**).

   This ligament complex must be disrupted in at least two planes for dislocation to occur. The volar plate most commonly (80%) avulses distally from the middle phalanx, and when it avulses proximally it can become trapped within the joint necessitating open reduction. The collateral ligaments usually avulse proximally (85%). The normal range of PIP joint motion varies between digits, but is typically more than 100 degrees. The arc of rotation of the DIP joint is usually 90 degrees.[1-3]

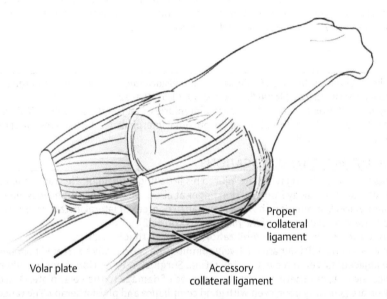

Proper collateral ligament

Volar plate

Accessory collateral ligament

Fig. 77.2   The ligament box complex provides joint stability to the proximal interphalangeal joint.

REFERENCES

1. Freiberg A. Management of proximal interphalangeal joint injuries. Can J Plast Surg 2007;15(4):199–203
2. McElfresh EC, Dobyns JH, O'Brien ET. Management of fracture-dislocation of the proximal interphalangeal joints by extension-block splinting. J Bone Joint Surg Am 1972;54(8):1705–1711
3. Aladin A, Davis TRC. Dorsal fracture-dislocation of the proximal interphalangeal joint: a comparative study of percutaneous Kirschner wire fixation versus open reduction and internal fixation. J Hand Surg [Br] 2005;30(2):120–128

CLASSIFICATION OF DORSAL PIP JOINT DISLOCATIONS

7. A patient presents with a type II dorsal dislocation of the PIP joint. *What does this description suggest?*

   E. That both volar plate and collateral ligaments are injured.

   The classification system for dorsal dislocations of the PIP joint has three categories. The system is useful as it guides treatment. Injury types I and II are soft-tissue injuries only. Type III injuries have associated fractures. Types I and II differ in the degree of soft-tissue damage and joint congruity. Type I is a hyperextension injury with either partial or complete volar plate avulsion and partial articulation of the joint remains intact. Type II is also a hyperextension injury but results in complete dorsal dislocation of the middle phalanx. The volar plate must be completely divided for this to occur and the collateral ligaments must also be damaged.[1-3]

REFERENCES

1. Freiberg A. Management of proximal interphalangeal joint injuries. Can J Plast Surg 2007;15(4):199–203
2. Joyce KM, Joyce CW, Conroy F, Chan J, Buckley E, Carroll SM. Proximal interphalangeal joint dislocations and treatment: an evolutionary process. Arch Plast Surg 2014;41(4):394–397

3. McElfresh EC, Dobyns JH, O'Brien ET. Management of fracture-dislocation of the proximal interphalangeal joints by extension-block splinting. J Bone Joint Surg Am 1972;54(8):1705–1711

TREATMENT OF ACUTE PIP JOINT DISLOCATIONS

8. You see a patient in the hand trauma clinic following reduction of a dorsal dislocation of the ring finger PIP joint. Post reduction radiographs reveal a 30% volar articular fragment at the base of the middle phalanx that is well aligned. *Which one of the following is the most appropriate management plan?*

   C. Protect and mobilize within a dorsal blocking splint at 20 to 30 degrees for 3 weeks, reducing the splint angle weekly.

   Following adequate reduction of a dorsal PIP joint dislocation, the size of any volar fragment at the middle phalanx base tends to indicate the degree of stability and subsequent treatment. Fragments less than 40% of the articular surface, as in this case, are often stable. This is because a portion of the true collateral ligament insertion to the base of the middle phalanx is preserved on each side. If the injury is stable with good alignment of the fragment, operative intervention is not required. A splint regimen should protect against recurrent dorsal dislocation, while mobilizing the joint early to reduce subsequent fibrosis and stiffness.[1–3]

REFERENCES

1. Deitch MA, Kiefhaber TR, Comisar BR, Stern PJ. Dorsal fracture dislocations of the proximal interphalangeal joint: surgical complications and long-term results. J Hand Surg Am 1999;24(5):914–923
2. Freiberg A. Management of proximal interphalangeal joint injuries. Can J Plast Surg 2007;15(4):199–203
3. Eaton RG, Malerich MM. Volar plate arthroplasty of the proximal interphalangeal joint: a review of ten years' experience. J Hand Surg Am 1980;5(3):260–268

TREATMENT OF ACUTE PIP JOINT DISLOCATIONS

9. A patient presents after a fall during which he injured his little finger PIP joint. He states that immediately after the fall his finger was pointing away from the ring finger at about 60 degrees, but he was able to manipulate the finger back into place. Examination shows a residual 30 degrees of lateral instability on stress testing. Radiographs are all normal. *Which one of the following is correct?*

   C. Buddy taping to the ring finger and mobilization may be all that is required.

   Lateral dislocations of the PIP joint are relatively common and can usually be treated nonoperatively with buddy taping to the adjacent finger and early mobilization. Surgical intervention is not usually required. The main injury involves the RCL, but there will also be a degree of damage to the volar plate. Outcomes following PIP joint dislocation are generally poor, even with good compliance and physiotherapy. The range of movement may take several months to recover and may not return to normal. There is often some long-term residual thickening around the PIP joint because of fibrosis after an injury, which some patients find distressing. Lateral dislocations of the little finger PIP joint are more common than volar dislocations, which are rare.[1]

REFERENCE

1. Joyce KM, Joyce CW, Conroy F, Chan J, Buckley E, Carroll SM. Proximal interphalangeal joint dislocations and treatment: an evolutionary process. Arch Plast Surg 2014;41(4):394–397

DIP JOINT DISLOCATIONS

10. *Which one of the following is true with regard to DIP joint injuries?*

    C. They can often be associated with tendon insertion injuries.

    Trauma to the DIP joint can result in fractures, dislocations, and associated tendon injuries. For example, the flexor digitorum profundus (FDP) or flexor pollicis longus (FPL) tendons can be avulsed from the bone during dislocation or fractures of the distal phalanx and DIP joint. If these do become detached, then they must be reattached surgically with either a bone anchor or bone tunnel and a pull-out suture. Although the anatomy of the DIP joint shares characteristics with the PIP joint, and the fingertip is very commonly injured, the DIP joint is still less commonly injured than the PIP, especially with regard to dislocations.

    When DIP joint injuries do occur, they are frequently open injuries and when surgery is required, they usually are undertaken under local anesthetic rather than general anesthetic or regional block. After reduction, it is usual practice to immobilize the DIP joint in slight flexion for a number of weeks. It generally tolerates immobilization well.[1]

REFERENCE

1. Chung S, Sood A, Lee E. Principles of management in isolated dorsal distal interphalangeal joint dislocations. Eplasty 2014;14:ic33

78. Fingertip Injuries

See *Essentials of Plastic Surgery*, third edition, pp. 1097–1113

ANATOMY OF THE FINGERTIP

1. *Which one of the following statements is true regarding the vascular anatomy of the fingertip?*
   A. The volar venous supply is usually dominant.
   B. The proper digital artery bifurcates at the proximal interphalangeal (PIP) joint.
   C. Most digits have a dominant radial digital arterial supply.
   D. Arterial blood supply is received from the distal transverse palmar arch.
   E. The digital nerves are located deep to the digital arteries.

GOALS OF FINGERTIP RECONSTRUCTION

2. *What is generally considered to be the primary goal in fingertip reconstruction?*
   A. Preserve length and range of motion.
   B. Achieve a painless, durable, and sensate tip.
   C. Minimize time off work.
   D. Minimize intraoperative theatre time.
   E. Optimize aesthetic outcomes.

HEALING BY SECONDARY INTENTION IN FINGERTIP INJURIES

3. *You are discussing the merits of leaving a fingertip injury to heal by secondary intention with a patient following a door shut injury. Which one of the following is true?*
   A. It will usually involve bone shortening.
   B. The healing time is usually 6 to 8 weeks.
   C. Weekly dressing changes will normally be required.
   D. Return to work will be significantly delayed.
   E. Near-normal long-term sensitivity can normally be expected.

SKIN GRAFTING IN FINGERTIP INJURIES

4. *What is the main disadvantage of using a split-skin graft for a fingertip injury compared with a full-thickness alternative?*
   A. Reduced chances of graft take
   B. Reduced long-term durability and padding
   C. Technical challenge of graft harvest
   D. Increased healing time
   E. Increased primary graft contraction

HOMODIGITAL SKIN FLAPS

5. *Which one of the following is an oblique triangular V-Y flap based on a single neurovascular pedicle that is useful for reconstructing larger volar oblique injuries of the fingertip?*
   A. Atasoy V-Y advancement
   B. Furlow V-Y advancement
   C. Kutler V-Y advancement
   D. Venkataswami V-Y advancement
   E. Souquet advancement

THE MOBERG (VOLAR ADVANCEMENT) FLAP

6. *Why are Moberg-type advancement flaps usually avoided in the fingers?*
   A. Subsequent interphalangeal (IP) joint stiffness
   B. Cold intolerance to the fingertip
   C. Abnormal sensation to the fingertip
   D. Dorsal skin necrosis
   E. Partial flap failure

THE MOBERG (VOLAR ADVANCEMENT) FLAP

7. *What is the main benefit of using a "V-Y modification" when using a Moberg flap to reconstruct a thumb defect?*
    A. Flap viability is increased
    B. Flap reach is increased
    C. Both digital blood vessels are preserved
    D. Both digital nerves are preserved
    E. The surgical time is reduced

HETERODIGITAL SKIN FLAPS

8. *What is the main drawback of using the cross-finger flap to reconstruct an index fingertip volar defect?*
    A. The limited availability of donor tissue
    B. The technical difficulty of elevating the flap
    C. The lack of postoperative protective sensation
    D. The lack of postoperative tactile sensation
    E. The high risk of long-term postoperative stiffness

HETERODIGITAL SKIN FLAPS

9. *Which one of the following flaps cannot be used to reconstruct finger or thumb tip defects?*
    A. First dorsal metacarpal artery perforator flap (Quaba)
    B. First dorsal metacarpal artery flap (Foucher)
    C. Heterodigital neurovascular pedicled island flap (Littler)
    D. Cross-finger flap
    E. Volar advancement flap (Moberg)

THE LITTLER FLAP FOR FINGERTIP RECONSTRUCTION

10. *Which one of the following statements is true of the pedicled island flap described by Littler?*
    A. It is most commonly used for radial thumb tip defects.
    B. It is consistently harvested from the middle finger.
    C. It involves extended dissection into the palm.
    D. The donor defect can normally be closed directly.
    E. It preserves the normal vascular supply to the donor digit.

THE THENAR FLAP IN FINGERTIP RECONSTRUCTION

11. *What is the main problem with using a thenar flap to reconstruct a volar oblique injury to the index or middle finger?*
    A. The limited availability of donor tissue
    B. The high flap failure rate
    C. The need for a second stage
    D. The risk of postoperative stiffness
    E. The need for a donor-site skin graft

RECONSTRUCTIVE PRINCIPLES

12. *Why is it particularly important to maintain joint mobility in the ring and little fingers?*
    A. To maintain the aesthetic balance of the hand
    B. To maintain pinch grip strength
    C. To maintain power grip strength
    D. To maintain key pinch strength
    E. To maintain support grip

COMPOSITE GRAFTING

13. You are considering using a composite graft in a patient with a fingertip injury. *Which one of the following statements is true regarding composite grafts in this setting?*
    A. Microsurgical skills are required to perform them.
    B. They are primarily indicated for use in adults.
    C. They can be useful as biologic dressings even where they fail.
    D. Successful graft take is improved by postoperative warming.
    E. They are generally useful after crush injuries.

RECONSTRUCTION OF THE FINGERTIP

14. *Which one of the following is the best reconstructive option for a volar oblique middle fingertip amputation, 1 cm², no exposed bone?*
    A. Healing by secondary intention
    B. Split-thickness skin graft
    C. Full-thickness skin graft
    D. Neurovascular pedicled island flap (Littler)
    E. Homodigital neurovascular island flap (Venkataswami)

RECONSTRUCTION OF THE FINGERTIP

15. *Which one of the following is the best reconstructive option for a 2-cm lateral oblique index fingertip amputation from the distal interphalangeal (DIP) joint crease distally on the radial side with exposed bone?*
    A. Volar V-Y advancement flap (Atasoy)
    B. Neurovascular pedicle island flap (Littler)
    C. Homodigital neurovascular island flap (Venkataswami)
    D. Cross-finger flap
    E. Kutler V-Y flap

MANAGEMENT OF THUMB TIP INJURIES

16. *Which one of the following is the best reconstructive option for a pulp defect of the thumb, 1.7 × 3 cm in diameter. The flexor pollicis longus (FPL) tendon is exposed but intact, and the distal phalanx is exposed to the tip. The dorsal aspect is completely intact, with the nail complex unaffected?*
    A. Dorsal metacarpal artery flap (Foucher)
    B. V-Y advancement flap (Atasoy)
    C. Groin flap
    D. Reverse cross-finger flap
    E. Terminalization at interphalangeal (IP) joint

Answers

ANATOMY OF THE FINGERTIP

1. *Which one of the following statements is true regarding the vascular anatomy of the fingertip?*

D. Arterial blood supply is received from the distal transverse palmar arch.

The arterial supply to the fingertip arises from the proper digital arteries which divide into three branches (not two) at the level of the distal interphalangeal (DIP) (not proximal interphalangeal [PIP]) joint. Then at the level of the lunula, the distal transverse palmar arch (DTPA) is formed, and central arteries branch off this to supply the fingertip and pulp. The digital nerves are located superficial to the digital arteries more proximally in the digit, so frequently are divided where arterial injury has occurred. The ulnar digital artery is dominant in the radial three digits (thumb, index, and long fingers), while the radial digital artery is dominant in the little and ring fingers. This is due to the embryological development of the limb from the median artery.

The dorsal (not volar) venous supply is dominant in the digit and veins around the lateral nail wall and distal pulp also form an arch over the distal phalanx. A second arch is formed more proximally over the middle phalanx. The presence of these arches is relevant to distal tip replantation surgery.[1,2]

REFERENCES

1. Scheker LR, Becker GW. Distal finger replantation. J Hand Surg Am 2011;36(3):521–528
2. Nam YS, Jun YJ, Kim IB, Cho SH, Han HH. Anatomical study of the fingertip artery in Tamai zone I: clinical significance in fingertip replantation. J Reconstr Microsurg 2017;33(1): 45–48

GOALS OF FINGERTIP RECONSTRUCTION

2. *What is generally considered to be the primary goal in fingertip reconstruction?*

B. Achieve a painless, durable, and sensate tip.

There are many important considerations in fingertip reconstruction, but in general, the primary goal is to have a painless fingertip which is sensate and has durable soft-tissue coverage. This serves to optimize functional outcomes and minimize morbidity. Preservation of length and range of motion is also important, although achieving these at the expense of the other parameters described would be futile. Pain is a major issue to patients especially in the fingertip where the nerve supply is dense and the areas are exposed to mild trauma on a regular basis. Furthermore, poor vascularity and poor soft-tissue cover can accentuate the discomfort for patients following fingertip injury.

Minimizing time off work and from leisure activities is also important. Individuals who are self-employed will often be particularly motivated to return to work early. In some cultures, the aesthetics of the fingertip are especially important, though in most cases function still assumes the highest aim.[1]

REFERENCE

1. Germann G, Rudolf KD, Levin SL, Hrabowski M. Fingertip and thumb tip wounds: changing algorithms for sensation, aesthetics, and function. J Hand Surg Am 2017;42(4):274–284

HEALING BY SECONDARY INTENTION IN FINGERTIP INJURIES

3. *You are discussing the merits of leaving a fingertip injury to heal by secondary intention with a patient following a door shut injury. Which one of the following is true?*

E. Near-normal long-term sensitivity can normally be expected.

Allowing fingertip injuries to heal by secondary intention is often the best choice for a number of reasons, providing the defect is relatively small. First, it can avoid the need for surgery and additional donor-site morbidity to the same or adjacent fingers where flaps would otherwise be harvested. Second, it avoids the need for a skin graft donor site and for dermal substitutes, which can be expensive. Third, the outcomes are usually good with durable sensate tips achieved. Digit length is also well preserved and although in some cases there needs to be shortening of the bone, this is certainly not required in all cases and even when it is necessary, only minimal amounts generally need removal and this is easily undertaken under local anesthetic.

Initially, dressings are left for 1 week in most cases, but beyond this patients are generally encouraged to change the dressings on a daily basis and wash the digit with soap and water. Low adherence dressings can be used to protect the healing area. Healing time in most cases is around 4 weeks. Return to work is expected to be as quick, if not quicker, than where grafts or flaps are used for fingertip repair. The caveat of allowing healing by secondary intent is that in larger defects, scar contraction and deformity may occur with problems such as a hook nail or reduced range of motion.[1]

REFERENCE

1. Krauss EM, Lalonde DH. Secondary healing of fingertip amputations: a review. Hand (N Y) 2014;9(3):282–288

SKIN GRAFTING IN FINGERTIP INJURIES

4. *What is the main disadvantage of using a split-skin graft for a fingertip injury compared with a full-thickness alternative?*

  B. **Reduced long-term durability and padding**

  Defects of the fingertip may rarely be reconstructed using skin grafts, and it is far more common to allow things to heal by secondary intent. The theoretical advantage of using skin grafts is that larger defects can be reconstructed with accelerated healing, reduced scar contraction, and low donor-site morbidity. However, most authorities would generally avoid grafts for fingertip reconstruction as healing by secondary intent or flap reconstruction each is associated with better outcomes, particularly where sensibility is concerned. Where grafts are used, full-thickness grafts are preferable for the fingertip, as they have a number of advantages. First, the cover provided is more durable and thicker than with split grafts. Second, the color match tends to be better, and third, the donor site may be closed directly. Split grafts are probably more likely to take than full-thickness grafts and are simple to harvest. The healing time is likely to be similar with split- versus full-thickness grafts. Split grafts will have less primary contraction but have more secondary contraction than full-thickness grafts. In general, grafts are to be avoided in fingertip injuries.[1,2]

REFERENCES

1. Holm A, Zachariae L. Fingertip lesions. An evaluation of conservative treatment versus free skin grafting. Acta Orthop Scand 1974;45(3):382–392

2. Pederson WC. Nonmicrosurgical coverage of the upper extremity. In Wolfe SW, Hotchkiss RN, Pederson WC, Kozin SH, Cohen MS, eds. Green's Operative Hand Surgery, 7th ed. Philadelphia, PA: Elsevier. 1528–1573, 2017

HOMODIGITAL SKIN FLAPS

5. *Which one of the following is an oblique triangular V-Y flap based on a single neurovascular pedicle that is useful for reconstructing larger volar oblique injuries of the fingertip?*

  D. **Venkataswami V-Y advancement**

  The Venkataswami flap[1] is an oblique triangular V-Y advancement flap used for reconstructing volar oblique injuries of the fingertip. It is based on a single neurovascular pedicle and is generally designed to extend proximally from the PIP joint to the defect, but some surgeons prefer to have a longer flap length beginning proximal to the PIP joint, while others prefer to extend the proximal incision in a linear fashion only to facilitate flap reach (**Fig. 78.1**).

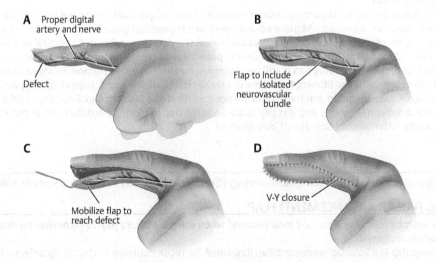

Fig. 78.1 Venkataswami flap. (Germann G, Sherman R, Levin LS. Reconstructive Surgery of the Hand and Upper Extremity. Thieme, 2017.)

Another similar flap is the Segmuller flap, which is a smaller version and is therefore useful for smaller defects.[2]

The Kutler V-Y advancement flap[3] is a bilateral technique that was described for transverse amputations but may be more suited to lateral oblique injuries of the digits. Two triangular flaps are designed and centrally placed to cover the defect (**Fig. 78.2**). The problem with these flaps is that they do not have much movement and can lead to scarring of the fingertip, hence the reason why the Venkataswami and the Segmuller have become popular.

Both the Atasoy[4] and the Furlow[5] flaps are types of volar advancement flaps that are indicated for reconstructing dorsal oblique and some transverse injuries. They are not based on the neurovascular pedicle; so, again advancement is far more limited.

The Souquet flap is a rectangular flap not a V-Y flap, rotated so that the free edge advances to cover a defect in the fingertip. It is based on the neurovascular bundle but does not advance

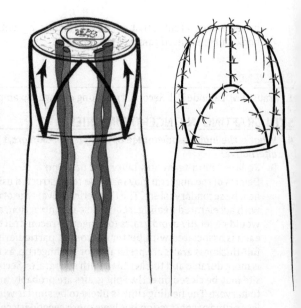

Fig. 78.2   Kutler flap dissection.

especially well. It has been modified by Lloyd and Sammut to maintain sensation and yet improve reach.[6]

REFERENCES

1. Venkataswami R, Subramanian N. Oblique triangular flap: a new method of repair for oblique amputations of the fingertip and thumb. Plast Reconstr Surg 1980;66(2):296–300
2. Smith KL, Elliot D. The extended Segmüller flap. Plast Reconstr Surg 2000;105(4):1334–1346
3. Kutler W. A new method for finger tip amputation. J Am Med Assoc 1947;133(1):29–30
4. Atasoy E, Ioakimidis E, Kasdan ML, Kutz JE, Kleinert HE. Reconstruction of the amputated finger tip with a triangular volar flap. A new surgical procedure. J Bone Joint Surg Am 1970;52(5):921–926
5. Furlow LT Jr. V-Y "Cup" flap for volar oblique amputation of fingers. J Hand Surg [Br] 1984;9(3):253–256
6. Lloyd N, Sammut D. A modification of the Souquet advancement flap in fingertip reconstruction. J Hand Surg Eur Vol 2013;38(4):395–398

THE MOBERG (VOLAR ADVANCEMENT) FLAP

6. *Why are Moberg-type advancement flaps usually avoided in the fingers?*

   D. Dorsal skin necrosis

   The Moberg flap is used for thumb tip defects because of the unique dual dorsal and volar blood supply which the thumb possesses. Although a Moberg advancement flap is potentially feasible for reconstruction of the index fingertip, it is not recommended, as it requires division of the dorsal branches of the digital vessels, and this can lead to subsequent dorsal skin necrosis. While it is possible to preserve many of these branches using a tissue-spreading technique, the Moberg flap is still best reserved for thumb reconstruction. Following reconstruction of a thumb tip defect using the Moberg flap, there is a small risk of subsequent IP joint stiffness, partial flap failure, and cold intolerance to the tip, but these risks are not specific to the Moberg flap. Ensuring careful and adequate flap mobilization can limit this and it is key to advance the flap to the thumb defect rather than the other way around, as the latter would cause the IP joint flexion.[1]

REFERENCE

1. Moberg E. Aspects of sensation in reconstructive surgery of the upper extremity. J Bone Joint Surg Am 1964;46:817–825

THE MOBERG (VOLAR ADVANCEMENT) FLAP

7. *What is the main benefit of using a "V-Y modification" when using a Moberg flap to reconstruct a thumb defect?*

   B. Flap reach is increased

   The Moberg flap is a volar advancement flap described for reconstruction of thumb tip defects. It has a robust vascularity because it is elevated on both neurovascular pedicles simultaneously. It is useful for closing volar soft-tissue defects of the thumb 1 to 1.5 cm in diameter. There are some modifications that can be incorporated to increase flap reach. These include the use of a V-Y advancement technique or by using a transverse incision at the base to create an island flap, which needs to be allowed to heal by secondary intent or skin grafted. Dellon's modification involves extension of the flap base into the first web space and this can increase advancement to around 3 cm. The surgical time is most likely to be slightly increased (not decreased) in modifications of the flap, as a result of the extended dissection involved.[1-3]

REFERENCES

1. Moberg E. Aspects of sensation in reconstructive surgery of the upper extremity. J Bone Joint Surg Am 1964;46:817–825
2. Dellon AL. The extended palmar advancement flap. J Hand Surg Am 1983;8(2):190–194
3. Thibaudeau S, Tremblay DM, Tardif M, Chollet A. Moberg modification using the first web space: thumb reconstruction following distal amputation. Hand (N Y) 2012;7(2):210–213

HETERODIGITAL SKIN FLAPS

8. *What is the main drawback of using the cross-finger flap to reconstruct an index fingertip volar defect?*

D. The lack of postoperative tactile sensation

The main drawback to using the cross-finger flap to reconstruct an index fingertip defect is the postoperative lack of tactile gnosis, which is reported to occur in all patients.[1] Normal tactile gnosis is very important to maintain in the index finger, given its key role in pinch grip, key grip, and precision activity. Protective sensation is generally well maintained with this flap, although it requires cortical relearning. There is plenty of donor soft tissue available from the cross-finger flap in most cases, as this is harvested from the dorsum of the middle finger. It is a technically straightforward procedure that can be accomplished under local anesthetic in a few minutes. The risk of long-term postoperative stiffness is low because splinting can be achieved in the safe position (or close to it) with the IP joints in full extension. In patients of darker skin tone, transfer of dorsal skin to the volar surface results in poor aesthetic outcomes with obvious visible scarring due to the differences in pigmentation between the volar and dorsal skin surfaces.

REFERENCE

1. Nishikawa H, Smith PJ. The recovery of sensation and function after cross-finger flaps for fingertip injury. J Hand Surg [Br] 1992;17(1):102–107

HETERODIGITAL SKIN FLAPS

9. *Which one of the following flaps cannot be used to reconstruct finger or thumb tip defects?*

A. First dorsal metacarpal artery perforator flap (Quaba)

The Quaba flap is not useful for fingertip reconstruction because it does not have sufficient reach to move much beyond the PIP joint. Flow can be antegrade through perforators from the dorsal metacarpal artery (DMA) or retrograde from the volar system or the dorsal digital arteries. Perforators are primarily distal to the junctura tendinea in the distal third of the dorsum of the hand. All of the other flaps are useful for thumb or fingertip reconstruction (see Fig. 78.12).[1,2]

REFERENCES

1. Bailey SH, Andry D, Saint-Cyr M. The dorsal metacarpal artery perforator flap: a case report utilizing a Quaba flap harvested from a previously skin-grafted area for dorsal 5th digit coverage. Hand (N Y) 2010;5(3):322–325
2. Couceiro J, de Prado M, Menendez G, Manteiga Z. The first dorsal metacarpal artery flap family: a review. Surg J (NY) 2018;4(4):e215–e219

THE LITTLER FLAP FOR FINGERTIP RECONSTRUCTION

10. *Which one of the following statements is true of the pedicled island flap described by Littler?*

C. It involves extended dissection into the palm.

The pedicled island flap described by Littler[1] is used to reconstruct large defects of the thumb tip and is most commonly used for ulnar (not radial) pulp defects. It can be harvested from either the ring or middle fingers and involves sacrifice of one of the digital arteries and nerves to the donor digit. It involves significant dissection into the palm in order to obtain sufficient reach and to tunnel the pedicle. The donor defect requires a skin graft.

REFERENCE

1. Littler JW. The neurovascular pedicle method of digital transposition for reconstruction of the thumb. Plast Reconstr Surg (1946) 1953;12(5):303–319

THE THENAR FLAP IN FINGERTIP RECONSTRUCTION

11. *What is the main problem with using a thenar flap to reconstruct a volar oblique injury to the index or middle finger?*

    D. **The risk of postoperative stiffness**

        The thenar flap involves a two-stage process. In the first stage, an area of skin and subcutaneous fat is raised from the thenar eminence and inset into a volar defect of the index (or middle) fingertip. In the second stage, at 10 to 14 days, the flap is divided and inset is completed. The donor site is closed, grafted, or left to heal by secondary intention. The main problem with this flap is that the index finger is flexed at the PIP joint between the first and second stages. This can result in stiffness and loss of motion to the PIP joint secondary to collateral ligament and volar plate tightening that may not fully recover. For this reason, it should be avoided in older patients and those with comorbidities such as arthritis and Dupuytren's disease. The flap has a low failure rate and availability of suitable (glabrous) tissue is good for fingertip reconstruction. The need for a second stage and the potential for a donor-site graft represent limitations, but these are less of a problem (**Fig. 78.3**).[1-4]

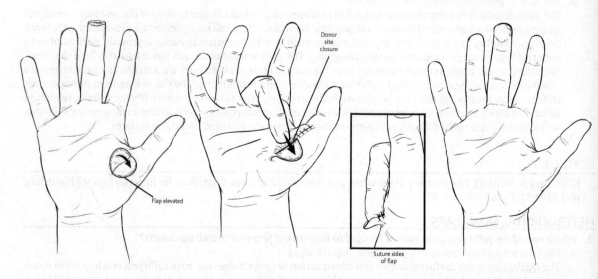

Fig. 78.3   Thenar flap.

REFERENCES

1. Flatt AE. The thenar flap. J Bone Joint Surg Br 1957;39-B(1):80–85
2. Rinker B. Fingertip reconstruction with the laterally based thenar flap: indications and long-term functional results. Hand (N Y) 2006;1(1):2–8
3. Barbato BD, Guelmi K, Romano SJ, Mitz V, Lemerle JP. Thenar flap rehabilitated: a review of 20 cases. Ann Plast Surg 1996;37(2):135–139
4. Melone CPJ Jr, Beasley RW, Carstens JH Jr. The thenar flap--an analysis of its use in 150 cases. J Hand Surg Am 1982;7(3):291–297

RECONSTRUCTIVE PRINCIPLES

12. *Why is it particularly important to maintain joint mobility in the ring and little fingers?*

    C. **To maintain power grip strength**

        The ring and little fingers have an important functional role in the power grip of the hand. For this reason, it is important to maintain joint mobility (flexion, in particular, combines with wrist extension) while minimizing pain. Sensibility and aesthetics are generally less important features.[1]

REFERENCE

1. Landsmeer JM. Power grip and precision handling. Ann Rheum Dis 1962;21(2):164–170

COMPOSITE GRAFTING

13. You are considering using a composite graft in a patient with a fingertip injury. *Which one of the following statements is true regarding composite grafts in this setting?*

C. They can be useful as biologic dressings even where they fail.

Non-microsurgical replantation of the amputated fingertip is known as composite grafting and is not usually recommended in adults. The main indication is in children younger than 6 years. Some authorities think that composite grafts act only as biologic dressings that allow granulation and healing from underneath, while others believe they are able to successfully act as true grafts. Attempts have been made to improve graft take by cooling (not warming) the grafts postoperatively. In spite of recommendations to reserve the technique for use in children, there have been successful reports of their use in adults. Graft survival has been improved by excision of bone, defatting, tie over-suturing, and finger splinting.[1,2] Composite grafting is best suited to clean sharp lacerations rather than crush injuries.

REFERENCES

1. Elsahy NI. When to replant a fingertip after its complete amputation. Plast Reconstr Surg 1977;60(1):14–21
2. Moiemen NS, Elliot D. Composite graft replacement of digital tips. 2. A study in children. J Hand Surg [Br] 1997;22(3): 346–352

RECONSTRUCTION OF THE FINGERTIP

14. *Which one of the following is the best reconstructive option for a volar oblique middle fingertip amputation, 1 cm², no exposed bone?*

A. Healing by secondary intention

In this scenario, no critical structures are exposed, and the defect is no more than 1 cm² in size; so, healing by secondary intention should be fairly quick, easy, and give good cover, color, contour, and sensation to the finger over time. The use of skin grafts would be undesirable, as each would give a worse outcome than healing by secondary intent and also involve a donor site. The Littler neurovascular island flap is indicated as a heterodigital flap, for example, to reconstruct the thumb. Using the Venkataswami neurovascular island flap would be unnecessary for this case, as the defect is small and there is no exposed bone.[1]

REFERENCE

1. Krauss EM, Lalonde DH. Secondary healing of fingertip amputations: a review. Hand (N Y) 2014;9(3):282–288

RECONSTRUCTION OF THE FINGERTIP

15. *Which one of the following is the best reconstructive option for a 2-cm lateral oblique index fingertip amputation from the distal interphalangeal (DIP) joint crease distally on the radial side with exposed bone?*

C. Homodigital neurovascular island flap (Venkataswami)

The Venkataswami flap is well suited to reconstruct larger volar oblique defects of the fingertip such as this case. A unilateral triangular island flap is designed as a V-Y based on a single neurovascular pedicle. The apex of the flap is located proximal to the PIP joint and can be extended even more proximally if required to further increase flap reach.[1] The Atasoy flap is a volar V-Y flap useful for dorsal oblique fingertip injuries and some transverse injuries. This flap is designed to match the width of the nail bed with the volar wound edge as the base of the flap. This flap can advance only up to 1 cm and involves skin-only incisions with tissue spreading action to release the subcutaneous tissues. The Littler neurovascular pedicled flap maybe used to reconstruct thumb tip defects on the ulnar side. The donor is normally from the ulnar pulp of the ring finger. This flap does require extended dissection into the palm and tunneling over to the thumb to be successful. For this reason, it is not frequently used in most units.[2] The cross-finger flap uses dorsal skin to reconstruct volar skin on the adjacent digit. It could be used in this scenario but can lead to stiffness, as the two adjacent digits must be immobilized together postoperatively. The Kutler V-Y flap is described for transverse fingertip amputations and some lateral oblique injuries. It is designed as bilateral lateral V-Y flaps advanced distally and centrally; however, there is limited reach available with these flaps.[3]

REFERENCES

1. Venkataswami R, Subramanian N. Oblique triangular flap: a new method of repair for oblique amputations of the fingertip and thumb. Plast Reconstr Surg 1980;66(2):296–300
2. Littler JW. The neurovascular pedicle method of digital transposition for reconstruction of the thumb. Plast Reconstr Surg (1946) 1953;12(5):303–319
3. Kutler W. A new method for finger tip amputation. J Am Med Assoc 1947;133(1):29

MANAGEMENT OF THUMB TIP INJURIES

16. *Which one of the following is the best reconstructive option for a pulp defect of the thumb, 1.7 × 3 cm in diameter.*
   The flexor pollicis longus (FPL) tendon is exposed but intact, and the distal phalanx is exposed to the tip. The dorsal
   aspect is completely intact, with the nail complex unaffected?
   A. Dorsal metacarpal artery flap (Foucher)

   The options for this patient include a cross-finger flap from the index finger or a Foucher flap. Of these, the Foucher flap would be preferable due to the robust soft-tissue coverage and the potential for sensory relearning. A Moberg flap would not be large enough. A Littler flap would leave a large defect on the donor finger and is perhaps better suited to smaller defects. A cross-finger flap would fail to provide adequate sensation, which is a key requirement for the thumb pulp. The common principle in thumb reconstruction is maintenance of length; so, with bone length preserved in these scenarios, the aim should be to find soft-tissue cover.[1-3]

REFERENCES

1. Gregory H, Heitmann C, Germann G. The evolution and refinements of the distally based dorsal metacarpal artery (DMCA) flaps. J Plast Reconstr Aesthet Surg 2007;60(7):731–739
2. Rehim SA, Chung KC. Local flaps of the hand. Hand Clin 2014;30(2):137–151, v
3. Delikonstantinou IP, Gravvanis AI, Dimitriou V, Zogogiannis I, Douma A, Tsoutsos DA. Foucher first dorsal metacarpal artery flap versus littler heterodigital neurovascular flap in resurfacing thumb pulp loss defects. Ann Plast Surg 2011;67(2):119–122

79. Nail Bed Injuries

See *Essentials of Plastic Surgery*, third edition, pp. 1114–1123

DEMOGRAPHICS OF NAIL BED INJURIES

1. *Which one of the following is correct regarding nail bed injuries?*
   A. They most commonly occur in children under 2 years of age.
   B. The border digits are most commonly affected.
   C. More than 90% have a concomitant distal phalanx fracture.
   D. Most injuries spare the soft tissues of the fingertip.
   E. They account for two-thirds of hand injuries in children.

NAIL BED ANATOMY

2. *Label the five marked regions of the nail bed complex using the options listed (Fig. 79.1). (Each option may be used once only or not at all.)*
   Options:
   A. Paronychia
   B. Paronychium
   C. Perionychium
   D. Hyponychium

   E. Eponychium
   F. Sterile matrix
   G. Germinal matrix
   H. Extensor origin

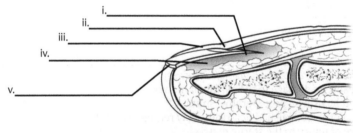

Fig. 79.1 Anatomy of the fingertip and nail bed.

NORMAL NAIL GROWTH

3. *Which one of the following is the key site for nail growth through the process of gradient parakeratosis?*
   A. Lunula
   B. Nail fold
   C. Sterile matrix

   D. Hyponychium
   E. Germinal matrix

NAIL GROWTH RATES

4. You see a patient following avulsion of the nail plate. She asks how long it will take for the nail to regrow and what factors may affect this. *Which one of the following is associated with increased nail growth?*
   A. Winter season
   B. Older age
   C. Female sex

   D. Shorter digits
   E. Onychophagia

CLASSIFICATION OF NAIL BED INJURIES

5. The Van Beek classification is commonly used to describe nail bed injuries. *What is the clinical relevance of a type I or II nail bed injury?*
   A. That no intervention is required.
   B. That splinting is required.
   C. That nail trephination is required.
   D. That nail bed repair is required.
   E. That nail bed grafting is required.

NAIL BED REPAIR

6. You are planning to undertake a nail bed repair on a 5-year-old child following a "door shut injury" which has resulted in a comminuted tuft fracture and nail bed laceration distal to the lunula. *Which one of the following is correct regarding the procedure?*
   A. Neither postoperative antibiotics nor a finger tourniquet are warranted.
   B. Reliable bony stabilization will require a Kirschner wire.
   C. Wound extension is required proximal to the nail fold for access.
   D. Repair outcomes using tissue glue are poor and should be avoided.
   E. The nail bed should be minimally debrided and repaired with a 6-0 or 7-0 suture.

PERFORMING A STANDARD NAIL BED REPAIR

7. When performing a nail bed repair, use of the nail plate as a postoperative splint is often advocated. *What is the other key benefit to replacing the nail plate?*
   A. To prevent subsequent nail ridging
   B. To increase nail regrowth
   C. For improved cosmesis until a new nail has formed
   D. To decrease postoperative pain
   E. To reduce rates of infection

SEYMOUR FRACTURES

8. *What is the key long-term risk of failing to recognize and adequately treat a Seymour fracture of the distal phalanx?*
   A. Distal interphalangeal (DIP) joint stiffness
   B. Fingertip numbness
   C. Inability to flex the DIP joint
   D. Growth arrest of the digit
   E. Complete failure of nail growth

HOOK-NAIL DEFORMITY

9. *Which one of the following is true of the hook-nail deformity?*
   A. It is primarily because of damage to the germinal matrix.
   B. It is best prevented by using a postoperative splint.
   C. Surgical correction of an established deformity may require a local flap.
   D. It is a consequence of injury to the sterile matrix.
   E. It can be corrected with placement of a skin graft under the distal nail bed.

Answers

DEMOGRAPHICS OF NAIL BED INJURIES

1. Which one of the following is correct regarding nail bed injuries?

E. **They account for two-thirds of hand injuries in children.**

Nail bed injuries are extremely common in children and young adults, with most occurring in males between the ages of 4 and 30 years. The middle finger is most commonly affected because of its increased length compared with the other digits. Most injuries involve the nail bed and soft tissue of the fingertip. Many (50%) also involve fractures of the distal phalanx. One of the core procedures first learned in plastic surgery is repair of the nail bed which typically involves removal of the nail plate (if not already removed) cleansing of the area, minimal debridement, and placement of absorbable sutures to tack the nail bed and/or pulp together. Most surgeons will then replace the nail plate as a splint, although there is no strong evidence to support this approach over leaving the nail off. A randomized control trial exists in the United Kingdom called the NINJA trial to evaluate the two options. The pilot study suggested that more complications and infections were seen when the nail plate was replaced.[1,2]

REFERENCES

1. Jain A, Sierakowski A, Gardiner MD, et al. Nail bed INJury Assessment Pilot (NINJA-P) study: should the nail plate be replaced or discarded after nail bed repair in children? Study protocol for a pilot randomised controlled trial. Pilot Feasibility Stud 2015;1:29
2. Greig A, Gardiner MD, Sierakowski A, et al; NINJA Pilot Collaborative. Randomized feasibility trial of replacing or discarding the nail plate after nail-bed repair in children. Br J Surg 2017;104(12):1634–1639

NAIL BED ANATOMY

2. Label the five marked regions of the nail bed complex using the options listed (Fig. 79.1). (Each option may be used once only or not at all.)

Options:

For Fig. 79.2, the anatomic components of the nail bed complex are as follows:

The fingertip includes the volar pulp and dorsal nail complex. The perionychium is a collective description of the nail bed, nail plate, hyponychium, and eponychium. The paronychial regions are the lateral borders adjacent to the nail plate; i.e., they run parallel to the nail edge. The hyponychium is the area between the distal nail and pulp and has a keratin plug that acts as a mechanical barrier. It represents the junction of the sterile matrix and fingertip skin. The eponychium is the distal portion of the nail fold where it is attached to the nail plate. Paronychia refers to an infection of the soft tissues surrounding the nail complex. Treatment normally involves removal of the nail plate to drain the abscess collection. The germinal and sterile matrices are both important in nail growth.[1,2]

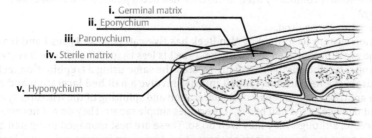

i. Germinal matrix
ii. Eponychium
iii. Paronychium
iv. Sterile matrix
v. Hyponychium

Fig. 79.2 Anatomy of the fingertip and nail bed.

REFERENCES

1. Sommer NZ, Brown RE. The perionychium. In: Wolfe SW, Hotchkiss RN, Pederson WC, et al, eds. Green's Operative Hand Surgery. 6th ed. Philadelphia: Elsevier; 2011
2. Zook EG. Anatomy and physiology of the perionychium. Hand Clin 2002;18(4):553–559, v

NORMAL NAIL GROWTH

3. *Which one of the following is the key site for nail growth through the process of gradient parakeratosis?*

    E. Germinal matrix

        Nail growth occurs at three key sites: the germinal matrix, the dorsal roof of the nail fold, and the sterile matrix. Of these, the germinal matrix is the most important area, as it is responsible for 90% of nail production. It lies immediately distal to the extensor tendon insertion. Nail production occurs through gradient parakeratosis with cells initially moving in a volar–dorsal direction before growing in a proximal–distal direction. The lunula is a white arc just distal to the eponychium that represents the distal part of the germinal matrix. It is white because of the presence of nail cell nuclei within it. The nail fold has a ventral floor and dorsal roof, both of which are involved in nail growth. The ventral floor is the site of the distal germinal matrix and the dorsal roof hosts cells that impart nail shine. The sterile matrix is important for contributing to nail strength and thickness by adding squamous cells to the nail plate. The hyponychium represents the junction of the sterile matrix and the fingertip skin beneath the nail and is not involved in the nail growth but does represent a high concentration of dermal lymphatics.[1,2]

REFERENCES

1. Sommer NZ, Brown RE. The perionychium. In: Wolfe SW, Hotchkiss RN, Pederson WC, et al, eds. Green's Operative Hand Surgery. 6th ed. Philadelphia: Elsevier; 2011
2. Zook EG. Anatomy and physiology of the perionychium. Hand Clin 2002;18(4):553–559, v

NAIL GROWTH RATES

4. You see a patient following avulsion of the nail plate. She asks how long it will take for the nail to regrow and what factors may affect this. *Which one of the following is associated with increased nail growth?*

    E. Onychophagia

        Normal nail growth is variable but is typically 3 to 4 mm per month.[1,2] It therefore takes about 4 months to regrow a nail fully. Factors that seem to increase growth include greater digital length (the nail of the middle finger grows faster than that of the little finger), time of year (growth is increased in the summer), younger age, and a nail-biting habit (onychophagia). There may be a slight sex difference, with growth in males being greater than in females, although this is not confirmed and may simply be a factor of differences in digit length.

REFERENCES

1. Yaemsiri S, Hou N, Slining MM, He K. Growth rate of human fingernails and toenails in healthy American young adults. J Eur Acad Dermatol Venereol 2010;24(4):420–423
2. Wu Z-W, Xu J-Y, Jiao Y, Fan SJ, He K, Qin LQ. Fingernail growth rate and macroelement levels determined by ICP-OES in healthy Chinese college students. Pol J Environ Stud 2012;21:1067–1070

CLASSIFICATION OF NAIL BED INJURIES

5. The Van Beek classification is commonly used to describe nail bed injuries. *What is the clinical relevance of a type I or II nail bed injury?*

    C. That nail trephination is required.

        The classification system described by Van Beek has five categories.[1] Types I and II are both subungual hematomas and are differentiated by their size. Type I is less than 25% and type II is greater than 50%. The difference is arbitrary, since both are usually treated the same using a trephination technique under local anesthetic to drain the hematoma. Type III injuries involve a nail bed laceration and a distal phalangeal fracture. These are treated with repair of the laceration and splinting of the fracture. Types IV and V involve more significant damage to the nail bed that precludes simple repair. They do not necessarily involve a distal phalangeal fracture, although they may well do so. These are best managed using nail bed grafts from the same digit or the great toe, because leaving them to heal by secondary intention will lead to misshapen and nonadherent nail plates.

REFERENCE

1. Van Beek AL, Kassan MA, Adson MH, Dale V. Management of acute fingernail injuries. Hand Clin 1990;6(1):23–35, discussion 37–38

NAIL BED REPAIR

6. You are planning to undertake a nail bed repair on a 5-year-old child following a "door shut injury" which has resulted in a comminuted tuft fracture and nail bed laceration distal to the lunula. *Which one of the following is correct regarding the procedure?*

   E. The nail bed should be minimally debrided and repaired with a 6–0 or 7–0 suture.
   Nail bed tissue is highly specialized, and debridement must be minimal to optimize preserved tissue. Furthermore, crushed and bruised nail bed tissue often survives. Following debridement, careful repair of the nail bed should be performed with a fine absorbable suture (e.g., 6–0 or 7–0 rapidly absorbable suture) under loupe magnification. A finger tourniquet should be used to provide a blood-free field and the application and removal times must be noted by the surgeon and documented by the operating room staff. Strict adherence to this will reduce the chances of inadvertently leaving a tourniquet in situ. A general rule of thumb is to prescribe a short course of antibiotics for nail bed injuries that have a distal phalanx fracture, but not for those without. Tuft fractures do not require K-wire stabilization, as the nail plate and soft tissues provide adequate support. Unstable shaft fractures close to the distal interphalangeal (DIP) joint will, however, normally require K-wiring. Wound extension proximal to the nail fold is required only when access to the germinal matrix is required. Use of glue instead of sutures has shown comparable results for nail bed repair and may be considered.[1]

REFERENCE

1. Strauss EJ, Weil WM, Jordan C, Paksima N. A prospective, randomized, controlled trial of 2-octylcyanoacrylate versus suture repair for nail bed injuries. J Hand Surg Am 2008;33(2):250–253

PERFORMING A STANDARD NAIL BED REPAIR

7. When performing a nail bed repair, use of the nail plate as a postoperative splint is often advocated. *What is the other key benefit to replacing the nail plate?*

   A. To prevent subsequent nail ridging
   The main theoretical benefit of replacing the nail plate within the nail fold is to keep the fold open in the early stages of regrowth and prevent nail fold adhesions (synechiae). Nail fold adhesions are thought to lead to ridging of the nail. There is no effect on nail regrowth, postoperative pain, or rates of infection. Although cosmesis may be improved in the short term, the nail plate remains in situ only for a short period of time and will not remain in place until a new nail has completely regrown.[1,2]

REFERENCES

1. Tos P, Titolo P, Chirila NL, Catalano F, Artiaco S. Surgical treatment of acute fingernail injuries. J Orthop Traumatol 2012;13(2):57–62
2. Jain A, Sierakowski A, Gardiner MD, et al. Nail bed INJury Assessment Pilot (NINJA-P) study: should the nail plate be replaced or discarded after nail bed repair in children? Study protocol for a pilot randomised controlled trial. Pilot Feasibility Stud 2015;1:29

SEYMOUR FRACTURES

8. *What is the key long-term risk of failing to recognize and adequately treat a Seymour fracture of the distal phalanx?*

   D. Growth arrest of the digit
   Originally described in 1966, a Seymour fracture is an open distal phalanx fracture involving the physis with an associated nail bed injury. Special consideration must be taken, as these injuries have interposed soft tissue, including germinal matrix, within the fracture site so a failure to recognize this may result in fracture nonunion, physeal arrest, nail plate deformity, and/or chronic osteomyelitis.

   These injuries can easily be overlooked as a minor injury to the nail bed but clinical suspicion should be raised where there appears to be a mallet deformity with a nail bed injury in children. The difference between a normal mallet deformity and a Seymour fracture is that the mallet deformity occurs through the distal phalanx growth plate rather than through the DIP joint. A good lateral radiograph should clearly allow differentiation between a typical mallet and a Seymour fracture. Treatment involves surgical removal of the soft-tissue interposition, reduction, and stabilization of the fracture, possibly with a K-wire.

   The DIP joint should not be directly affected and because the flexor tendon insertion remains in continuity, DIP joint flexion should be retained. Normal nail growth could be affected, but there should not be a complete failure. Sensation to the fingertip should be unaffected.[1]

REFERENCE

1. Nellans KW, Chung KC. Pediatric hand fractures. Hand Clin 2013;29(4):569–578

HOOK-NAIL DEFORMITY

9. *Which one of the following is true of the hook-nail deformity?*

   C. Surgical correction of an established deformity may require a local flap.

   The hook-nail deformity is caused by a lack of distal phalanx bone support beneath the nail bed which continues to grow distally over the top of the short bone end. It is best prevented by matching bone length and nail bed length so that underlying support is achieved for the full length of the nail bed. Therefore, preservation of distal phalanx length and primary shortening of the nail bed during a revision amputation may avoid subsequent development of this deformity. Neither germinal or sterile matrix damage is the cause of a hook-nail deformity as evidenced by continued growth of the nail, and splinting alone will not prevent it. Once established, the deformity may be corrected using the antennae procedure, which was described by Atasoy et al.[1] This is a two-stage procedure that addresses the lack of support for the nail bed and the relative lack of volar soft tissue. In the first stage, the pulp and nail bed are elevated off the distal phalanx and the nail bed is then splinted in a straight position with two or three small K-wires (hence the term "antennae"). The residual soft-tissue pulp deficit is then reconstructed using a cross-finger flap from the adjacent index finger.

REFERENCE

1. Atasoy E, Godfrey A, Kalisman M. The "antenna" procedure for the "hook-nail" deformity. J Hand Surg Am 1983;8(1):55–58

80. Flexor Tendon Injuries

See *Essentials of Plastic Surgery*, third edition, pp. 1124–1141

FLEXOR TENDON ANATOMY

1. *Which one of the following is true regarding the anatomy of the flexor tendons?*
   A. The flexor digitorum superficialis (FDS) tendons insert into the distal phalanges.
   B. The flexor digitorum profundus (FDP) tendons are attached to the lumbricals in the palm.
   C. Camper's chiasm lies at the level of the proximal interphalangeal (PIP) joint.
   D. At the wrist, the index and little FDS tendons lie most superficial.
   E. Flexor pollicis longus (FPL) originates from the lateral epicondyle of the humerus.

INNERVATION TO THE LONG FLEXORS OF THE HAND

2. *Which of the following flexor muscles receives its innervation entirely from the anterior interosseous nerve?*
   A. FDS
   B. FDP
   C. FPL
   D. FDS and FDP
   E. FDP and FPL

PULLEY SYSTEM OF THE FLEXOR TENDONS IN THE HAND

3. *When repairing a digital flexor tendon injury, which combination of pulleys is most important to preserve?*
   A. A1 and A3
   B. A2 and A4
   C. A3 and A5
   D. A1 and A4
   E. A2 and A5

FLEXOR TENDON NUTRITION

4. *Which one of the following represents the major nutritional supply to the flexor tendons within the digits?*
   A. Sharpey's fibers at the bony tendon insertion
   B. Blood vessels at the myotendinous junction
   C. Vinculum longus and vinculum brevis to each tendon
   D. Synovial diffusion from the flexor sheath
   E. Axial nutrient vessels in the palmar surface of the tendon

ANATOMY OF THE LUMBRICALS

5. *What is the unique feature of the lumbrical muscles?*
   A. They originate and insert solely into bone.
   B. They originate and insert solely into tendon.
   C. They are all bipennate muscles.
   D. They make no discernible contribution to hand function.
   E. They all share a common innervation.

DIGITAL FLEXOR TENDON ZONES

6. *Which one of the flexor tendon zones is known as "no man's" land?*
   A. Zone I
   B. Zone II
   C. Zone III
   D. Zone IV
   E. Zone V

FLEXOR ZONES OF THE THUMB

7. *A patient sustains an injury to the FPL tendon located over the thenar eminence. Within which zone of injury is this located?*
   A. TI
   B. TII
   C. TIII
   D. TIV
   E. TV

PRINCIPLES OF FLEXOR TENDON REPAIR

8. **What represents the traditionally recommended threshold for performing formal repair using a core suture in partially divided flexor tendon injuries?**
   A. Any degree of division
   B. 15% division
   C. 25% division
   D. 50% division
   E. 75% division

ZONE I FLEXOR TENDON INJURIES

9. A 20-year-old rugby player is seen 1 day after sustaining a closed injury while grabbing the shirt of an opponent during a game. He is unable to flex the distal interphalangeal (DIP) joint of his right ring finger but is able to flex the PIP joint. A radiograph confirms the presence of a bony fragment at the level of the PIP joint. **Which one of the following best describes this injury?**
   A. Leddy type I
   B. Leddy type II
   C. Leddy type III
   D. Leddy type IV
   E. Leddy type V

ZONE I FLEXOR TENDON INJURIES

10. **Which one of the following is correct regarding zone I digital flexor tendon injuries?**
    A. Bone anchor devices may be useful for primary repair.
    B. A braided suture is best for a pull-out suture repair.
    C. 10 mm of distal stump is the minimum required to perform a primary repair.
    D. Repair needs to be performed within 1 week of injury.
    E. In sharp injuries, the tendon usually retracts into the palm.

ZONE II FLEXOR TENDON INJURIES

11. **When repairing a zone II digital flexor tendon injury, which one of the following is correct?**
    A. The core suture should lie as dorsal as possible within the tendon to preserve vascularity.
    B. A continuous two-strand repair is recommended to facilitate early rehabilitation.
    C. The core suture should pass 5 mm proximal and distal to the repair.
    D. A Pulvertaft weave should be used, as it is stronger than other suture techniques.
    E. An epitendinous suture can add up to 50% strength to the core suture repair.

TENDON REPAIR WITHIN DIFFERENT FLEXOR ZONES

12. Different zones of flexor tendon injury require different principles of management. **Which one of the following statements is correct?**
    A. The use of epitendinous sutures is necessary for all injury zones.
    B. FDS and FDP should always be individually repaired.
    C. Zone III injuries are traditionally associated with the poorest functional outcomes.
    D. The carpal ligament should not be repaired following zone IV repair.
    E. The oblique pulley is most important to preserve during FPL repairs.

FLEXOR TENDON INJURY MANAGEMENT

13. You are assessing a 23-year-old patient who is no longer able to flex the DIP joint of his dominant ring finger 5 weeks after a game of rugby. A lateral radiograph is unremarkable. **When discussing treatment options with him, which one of the following is correct?**
    A. The proximal tendon end may have to be retrieved at the level of the wrist crease.
    B. Direct repair should not present a problem in this case.
    C. An immediate palmaris longus tendon graft may be required.
    D. Consent should be obtained for both primary and staged repair.
    E. A single-stage direct repair under tension is preferable to a staged reconstruction.

FLEXOR TENDON INJURY MANAGEMENT

14. **In which one of the following intraoperative scenarios should delayed primary tendon repair at a second operation be considered?**
    A. Zone I middle FDP division from a glass injury 3 days earlier
    B. Zone III index FDS division from a knife wound 12 days earlier
    C. Zone II ring FDS and FDP division from a circular saw injury that day
    D. Zone I index FDP division from a human bite wound the previous night
    E. Zone II middle FDP division from a knife wound 2 days earlier with clear, pale fluid in the sheath

FLEXOR TENDON INJURIES

15. A 53-year-old man sustains a stab injury to the volar aspect of his palm in line with the ring finger at the distal palmar crease. On examination, he is able to flex the ring finger at both the PIP and DIP joints, but this is painful on resisted flexion of either joint when tested independently. *What is the most likely diagnosis?*
    A. Partial Zone II FDS injury
    B. Partial Zone III FDP injury
    C. Partial Zone II FDP injury
    D. Partial Zone II FDS and FDP injury
    E. Partial Zone III FDS and FDP injury

MANAGEMENT OF LACERATIONS TO THE WRIST

16. *An 18-year-old girl falls onto glass while on a night out. She sustains a 1-cm laceration over the radial aspect of the wrist. Clinical examination reveals no significant neurovascular or functional deficit, except she is unable to flex the little finger PIP joint independently. What is the next step in management?*
    A. Exploration under local anesthesia
    B. Exploration under general anesthesia
    C. Ultrasound investigation of the wrist
    D. Clinical examination of the contralateral hand
    E. Hand therapy review

REVIEW FOLLOWING FLEXOR TENDON REPAIR

17. *A 25-year-old patient is seen in clinic after occupational therapy following repair of a partial FPL zone II tendon division. Her thumb flexion is good, and she is pain free, but she is unable to flex the thumb without the index finger DIP joint flexing. Which of the following best describes this finding?*
    A. Linburg-Comstock anomaly
    B. Adhesions secondary to repair
    C. Wartenburg's sign
    D. Absent flexor tendon
    E. Intersection syndrome

POSTOPERATIVE CARE FOLLOWING FLEXOR TENDON REPAIR

18. *When applying a splint after flexor tendon repair, which one of the following is correct?*
    A. The metacarpophalangeal (MCP) joints should all be flexed to 90 degrees.
    B. The splint should be placed on the volar aspect.
    C. The wrist should be flexed to 45 degrees.
    D. The interphalangeal (IP) joints should be almost fully extended.
    E. Elastic band traction should routinely be used.

COMPLICATIONS FOLLOWING FLEXOR TENDON REPAIR

19. *Which one of the following is correct regarding outcomes after flexor tendon repair?*
    A. Rupture after primary repair occurs in 15% of cases.
    B. Contractures after primary repair occur in 60% of cases.
    C. FPL is the most frequently ruptured flexor tendon after primary repair.
    D. Most contractures that occur after flexor repair require tenolysis.
    E. Poor surgical technique is usually to blame for rupture.

Answers

FLEXOR TENDON ANATOMY

1. *Which one of the following is true regarding the anatomy of the flexor tendons?*

   B. **The flexor digitorum profundus (FDP) tendons are attached to the lumbricals in the palm.**

   Flexion of the digits is controlled by the flexor digitorum superficialis (FDS), flexor digitorum profundus (FDP), and flexor pollicis longus (FPL) muscles. The FDP originates from the proximal ulna and interosseous membrane and inserts into the distal phalanges to provide flexion at the distal interphalangeal (DIP) joints and contributes to proximal interphalangeal (PIP) joint flexion. It is also attached to the lumbricals in the palm, and this is important after flexor tendon division, as the proximal end of the FDP tendon will therefore not retract further proximal than the midpalm. The FDS originates from the medial epicondyle of the humerus and coronoid process of the ulna and inserts into the middle phalanges to provide flexion at the PIP joints. The FPL originates at the proximal radius, interosseous membrane, and the accessory head (known as Gantzer's muscle) and arises from the coronoid process and the medial epicondyle of the humerus. It inserts into the distal phalanx of the thumb to provide flexion of the interphalangeal (IP) joint as well as the metacarpophalangeal (MCP) joint. Camper's chiasm represents the union of the two slips of FDS over the distal aspect of the proximal phalanx after they have divided into two slips to pass either side of the FDP tendon just distal to the level of the MCP joint. The two slips of FDS insert separately to the middle phalanx. Knowledge of the anatomic position of the FDS tendons at the wrist is useful during spaghetti wrist repair, as this can help identify the tendons accurately. The index and little finger FDS tendons lie deep, not superficial to the ring and middle FDS tendons.[1-3]

REFERENCES

1. Idler RS. Anatomy and biomechanics of the digital flexor tendons. Hand Clin 1985;1(1):3–11
2. Doyle JR, Blythe WF. Anatomy of the flexor tendon sheath and pulleys of the thumb. J Hand Surg Am 1977;2(2):149–151
3. Strickland JW. Development of flexor tendon surgery: twenty-five years of progress. J Hand Surg Am 2000;25(2):214–235

INNERVATION TO THE LONG FLEXORS OF THE HAND

2. *Which of the following flexor muscles receives its innervation entirely from the anterior interosseous nerve?*

   C. **FPL**

   The anterior interosseous nerve is a branch of the median nerve in the forearm. It supplies the FPL, the pronator quadratus, and the radial two FDP tendons. The ulnar two FDP tendons are supplied by the ulnar nerve and the FDS are supplied by the median nerve directly. When not due to neuritis, anterior interosseous nerve palsy can occur secondary to compression of the nerve by the tendinous edge of the deep head of the pronator teres, the tendinous origin of FDS, or an abnormal accessory head of FPL (Gantzer's muscle). Patients with this condition cannot flex the index DIP joint or thumb IP joint normally, resulting in an abnormal tip pinch grip. Furthermore, patients cannot make the "OK" sign where a closed ring shape is made using the index and thumb. There is no sensory deficit present because the anterior interosseous has no cutaneous sensory branches.[1-3]

REFERENCES

1. Idler RS. Anatomy and biomechanics of the digital flexor tendons. Hand Clin 1985;1(1): 3–11
2. Doyle JR. Anatomy of the flexor tendon sheath and pulley system: a current review. J Hand Surg Am 1989;14(2, Pt 2): 349–351
3. Moore KL, Dalley AF, eds. Clinically Oriented Anatomy. 4th ed. New York, NY: Lippincott Williams & Wilkins; 1999

PULLEY SYSTEM OF THE FLEXOR TENDONS IN THE HAND

3. *When repairing a digital flexor tendon injury, which combination of pulleys is most important to preserve?*

   B. **A2 and A4**

   The flexor tendon pulley system in the digits involves five annular pulleys and three cruciate pulleys. The annular pulleys are located along the flexor sheath starting at the MCP joint with A1. The even numbered annular pulleys are located over the phalangeal shafts (A2-proximal phalanx and the A4-middle phalanx), while the odd numbered pulleys are located over the small joints (A1-MCP, A3-PIP, A5-DIP). Their collective function is to prevent bowstringing of the tendon during flexion and provide a mechanical advantage. Ideally, they should be preserved during flexor tendon repair. However, the A2 and A4 pulleys are thought to be the most important. The cruciate pulleys allow for compression and expansion of the flexor sheath during motion without bunching. C1/2/3 lies between A2 and A3, A3 and A4, and A4 and A5, respectively.[1,2]

REFERENCES

1. Doyle JR. Anatomy of the flexor tendon sheath and pulley system: a current review. J Hand Surg Am 1989;14(2, Pt 2): 349–351
2. Doyle JR. Anatomy of the finger flexor tendon sheath and pulley system. J Hand Surg Am 1988;13(4):473–484

FLEXOR TENDON NUTRITION

4. Which one of the following represents the major nutritional supply to the flexor tendons within the digits?

   D. Synovial diffusion from the flexor sheath

   Tendon nutrition in the digits depends significantly on diffusion from the synovial sheath. The other sources of nutrition listed each make a variable contribution to tendon nutrition, but the vascular network within the digital flexor tendons is sparse. The bony insertion and musculotendinous junction blood supply is limited to around 1 cm of tendon length at each site, with the remaining blood supply arising from the vincula. In the forearm and proximal digit, there is also a vascular supply from segmental vessels in the paratenon.[1]

   Axial blood supply within the flexors tends to be located in the dorsal portion of the tendon; so, many surgeons prefer to place sutures in the volar portion during repair in the hope of maximizing blood supply. In contrast, there is some evidence that placing the core sutures dorsally within the tendon may be biomechanically advantageous.[2,3]

REFERENCES

1. Venkatramani H, Varadharajan V, Bhardwaj P, Vallurupalli A, Sabapathy SR. Flexor tendon injuries. J Clin Orthop Trauma 2019;10(5):853–861
2. Komanduri M, Phillips CS, Mass DP. Tensile strength of flexor tendon repairs in a dynamic cadaver model. J Hand Surg Am 1996;21(4):605–611
3. Fenwick SA, Hazleman BL, Riley GP. The vasculature and its role in the damaged and healing tendon. Arthritis Res 2002;4(4):252–260

ANATOMY OF THE LUMBRICALS

5. What is the unique feature of the lumbrical muscles?

   B. They originate and insert solely into tendon.

   The unique feature of the lumbrical muscles is that they each originate and insert into tendon without inserting or originating from bone at either end. There are four lumbricals, with the index and long (middle) finger lumbricals being unipennate and the ring and small (little) finger lumbricals being bipennate. The lumbricals originate from the FDP tendons in the midpalm and insert onto the lateral bands of the extensor mechanism. This means they serve to flex the MCP joints while extending the PIP and DIP joints (intrinsic positive position). The lumbricals do not share a common nerve supply. The ulnar two lumbricals receive innervation from the ulnar nerve and the radial two lumbricals are innervated by the median nerve.[1,2]

REFERENCES

1. Moore KL, Dalley AF, eds. Clinically Oriented Anatomy. 4th ed. New York, NY: Lippincott Williams & Wilkins; 1999
2. Wang K, McGlinn EP, Chung KC. A biomechanical and evolutionary perspective on the function of the lumbrical muscle. J Hand Surg Am 2014;39(1):149–155

DIGITAL FLEXOR TENDON ZONES

6. Which one of the flexor tendon zones is known as "no man's" land?

   B. Zone II

   There is a universal nomenclature for flexor tendon injuries first described by Verdan.[1,2] This categorizes the zone of injury into five areas:

   Zone I: Distal to insertion of the FDS tendon
   Zone II: From proximal edge of A1 pulley to FDS insertion (a.k.a. "no man's land")
   Zone III: From distal end of the carpal tunnel to proximal edge of A1 pulley
   Zone IV: Within the carpal tunnel
   Zone V: Proximal to the carpal tunnel

   This has clinical relevance as the approach to repair and functional outcome will differ according to the zone involved. Zone II has been described as "no man's land" because historically the results following repair were poorest in this zone. This zone is complicated because there are multiple flexors within the tight space of the flexor sheath, i.e., two FDS slips and one FDP. Therefore, achieving a functional repair without damage to the vincula blood supply, the sheath itself or the pulley system is challenging. Beyond this, achieving satisfactory rehabilitation without adhesions and tendon re-injury are also difficult.[3]

REFERENCES

1. Verdan CE. Half a century of flexor-tendon surgery. Current status and changing philosophies. J Bone Joint Surg Am 1972;54(3):472–491
2. Strickland JW. Flexor tendon repair. Hand Clin 1985;1(1):55–68
3. Hage JJ. History off-hand: Bunnell's no-man's land. Hand (N Y) 2019;14(4):570–574

FLEXOR ZONES OF THE THUMB

7. A patient sustains an injury to the FPL tendon located over the thenar eminence. *Within which zone of injury is this located?*

   C. TIII

   The thumb has five flexor zones, but these are different to the flexor zones for the other digits:
   - Zone T I: Distal to IP joint
   - Zone T II: From proximal edge of A1 pulley to IP joint
   - Zone T III: Over thenar eminence
   - Zone T IV: Within the carpal tunnel
   - Zone T V: Proximal to the carpal tunnel

   The anatomy of the thumb flexor mechanism differs to that of the digits in a number of ways. First, there is only a single flexor (the FPL); so, even a zone II injury involves only one tendon repair and thereby reduces some of the complexities of injury in this area despite it running within the flexor sheath. Second, there is only a single IP joint and some degree of stiffness or flexion of the thumb IP joint is far better tolerated than it is at PIP joint in the fingers. The pulley system is different too with just two annular pulleys and one intervening oblique pulley. The A1 pulley is over the MCP joint and the A2 pulley is over the IP joint. The pulleys should ideally be preserved during repair to avoid bowstringing, with the oblique pulley being most important.[1]

REFERENCE

1. Doyle JR, Blythe WF. Anatomy of the flexor tendon sheath and pulleys of the thumb. J Hand Surg Am 1977;2(2):149–151

PRINCIPLES OF FLEXOR TENDON REPAIR

8. *What represents the traditionally recommended threshold for performing formal repair using a core suture in partially divided flexor tendon injuries?*

   D. 50% division

   The management of partial flexor tendon repairs will depend on a number of factors such as the location, the flexor tendon involved, and the type of injury sustained. It will also be affected by surgeon and patient preferences. While there is some biomechanical evidence that shows larger tendon lacerations can still withstand protected active mobilization without repair, most agree that tendon lacerations involving more than 50% of the tendon diameter should be formally repaired with core and epitendinous sutures. Lesser divisions should be smoothed off or repaired with simple sutures to avoid the edges catching and to ensure the tendon ends are neatly apposed.[1–4]

REFERENCES

1. Venkatramani H, Varadharajan V, Bhardwaj P, Vallurupalli A, Sabapathy SR. Flexor tendon injuries. J Clin Orthop Trauma 2019;10(5):853–861
2. Manning DW, Spiguel AR, Mass DP. Biomechanical analysis of partial flexor tendon lacerations in zone II of human cadavers. J Hand Surg Am 2010;35(1):11–18
3. Hariharan JS, Diao E, Soejima O, Lotz JC. Partial lacerations of human digital flexor tendons: a biomechanical analysis. J Hand Surg Am 1997;22(6):1011–1015
4. Lineberry KD, Shue S, Chepla KJ. The management of partial zone II intrasynovial flexor tendon lacerations: a literature review of biomechanics, clinical outcomes and complications. Plast Reconstr Surg 2018;141(5):1165–1170

ZONE I FLEXOR TENDON INJURIES

9. A 20-year-old rugby player is seen 1 day after sustaining a closed injury while grabbing the shirt of an opponent during a game. He is unable to flex the distal interphalangeal (DIP) joint of his right ring finger but is able to flex the PIP joint. A radiograph confirms the presence of a bony fragment at the level of the PIP joint. *Which one of the following best describes this injury?*

   B. Leddy type II

   Zone I closed avulsion injuries of the FDP were classified by Leddy and Packer in 1977 into three categories based on the presence of a bony fragment on radiograph, the blood supply, and the position of the retracted proximal tendon end.[1] Additional fourth and fifth categories were subsequently added.[2] The classification is useful to guide management. The patient described has a type II injury based on the bony fragment position and should undergo an open repair using a pull-out suture or bone anchor device.

The modified Leddy-Packer classification includes the following:

Type I: The FDP tendon retracts into the palm with rupture of both vincula.

Type II: The FDP tendon avulses with a small fragment of distal phalanx, the long vinculum remains intact, and the tendon retracts to the level of the PIP joint (A3 pulley).

Type III: A large bony fragment is avulsed with the tendon and is prevented from retraction beyond the middle phalanx by the A4 pulley.

Type IV: An avulsion fracture of the distal phalanx combines with tendon avulsion from the fragment, along with tendon retraction.

Type V: A bony avulsion of the FDP is coupled with a distal phalanx fracture (either intra-articular or extra-articular).

REFERENCES

1. Leddy JP, Packer JW. Avulsion of the profundus tendon insertion in athletes. J Hand Surg Am 1977;2(1):66–69
2. Al-Qattan MM. Type 5 avulsion of the insertion of the flexor digitorum profundus tendon. J Hand Surg [Br] 2001;26(5):427–431

ZONE I FLEXOR TENDON INJURIES

10. *Which one of the following is correct regarding zone I digital flexor tendon injuries?*

A. Bone anchor devices may be useful for primary repair.

Bone anchor devices may be used successfully in primary tendon repairs. The outcomes using bone anchors are comparable to pull-out suture techniques. The recommended technique is to insert either a mini-Mitek or two micro-Mitek anchors at a 45-degree angle from distal/volar to proximal/dorsal, while taking care not to violate the DIP joint surface or nail bed.[1,2]

When using a pull-out suture technique where the core suture is passed externally over the nail, a monofilament such as nylon or polypropylene is preferred. Braided sutures glide less well, are difficult to remove, and are also more prone to infection. FDP avulsion may also be repaired by drilling a small hole transversely through the distal phalanx for the core suture to pass through, enabling a fully internal repair. Although the normal recommendation for core suture repair is that there is 10 mm of tendon proximal and distal to the repair, a distal stump of 5 mm is considered sufficient for standard core suture repair of zone I flexor tendon injuries. For most flexor tendon injuries, repair within a week of injury is recommended. However, some injuries that involve avulsion of the tendon insertion from the distal phalanx, with minimal proximal retraction (due to either intact vincula or a bony fragment anchored against a pulley) may still be repaired after several weeks. A delay in repairing a retracted tendon can lead to shortening, a quadriga effect, and constriction of the flexor sheath.

REFERENCES

1. Brustein M, Pellegrini J, Choueka J, Heminger H, Mass D. Bone suture anchors versus the pullout button for repair of distal profundus tendon injuries: a comparison of strength in human cadaveric hands. J Hand Surg Am 2001;26(3):489–496
2. McCallister WV, Ambrose HC, Katolik LI, Trumble TE. Comparison of pullout button versus suture anchor for zone I flexor tendon repair. J Hand Surg Am 2006;31(2):246–251

ZONE II FLEXOR TENDON INJURIES

11. *When repairing a zone II digital flexor tendon injury, which one of the following is correct?*

E. An epitendinous suture can add up to 50% strength to the core suture repair.

The main benefit of using an epitendinous suture is that it adds between 10 and 50% additional strength to the repair. In addition, it helps smooth the repair and improve gliding within the flexor sheath. A meta-analysis of complications after flexor tendon repair also suggested that the rate of reoperation is reduced by 84% if an epitendinous suture is used.[1]

There is debate surrounding the optimal positioning of core sutures with volar positioning considered to be best for tendon vascularity and dorsal positioning considered more biomechanically favorable during active flexion. In reality, many tendons are sufficiently thin that reliably placing the suture anywhere other than centrally is challenging.

A minimum of four-strand (not two) core suture repair is required in order to commence early active mobilization. This may be undertaken as a two-strand core suture combined with a two-strand mattress, as two separate two-strand core sutures, or as a single four-strand core suture repair. There is no definitive evidence that a four-strand single-knot technique is superior to two adjacent two-strand core sutures. Some surgeons prefer to use a six-strand technique when the tendon diameter is sufficient to allow this. The core suture should ideally have 10 mm (not 5 mm) proximal and distal to the repair. A Pulvertaft weave is not used in primary tendon repair in the digit, as it would entail significant tendon shortening and would create too much bulk to fit within the tendon sheath. It is reserved for tendon transfer cases outside a tendon sheath, such as the extensor indices transfer to extensor pollicis longus.[1-4]

REFERENCES

1. Dy CJ, Hernandez-Soria A, Ma Y, Roberts TR, Daluiski A. Complications after flexor tendon repair: a systematic review and meta-analysis. J Hand Surg Am 2012;37(3):543–551.e1
2. Savage R, Tang JB. History and nomenclature of multistrand repairs in digital flexor tendons. J Hand Surg Am 2016;41(2):291–293
3. Papandrea R, Seitz WH Jr, Shapiro P, Borden B. Biomechanical and clinical evaluation of the epitenon-first technique of flexor tendon repair. J Hand Surg Am 1995;20(2):261–266
4. Hardwicke JT, Tan JJ, Foster MA, Titley OG. A systematic review of 2-strand versus multistrand core suture techniques and functional outcome after digital flexor tendon repair. J Hand Surg Am 2014;39(4):686–695.e2

TENDON REPAIR WITHIN DIFFERENT FLEXOR ZONES

12. Different zones of flexor tendon injury require different principles of management. *Which one of the following statements is correct?*

E. The oblique pulley is most important to preserve during FPL repairs.

The most important pulley to preserve in the thumb is the oblique pulley. This is done to avoid bowstringing. Although the use of an epitendinous suture can add a further 10 to 50% strength to a flexor tendon repair, it is not necessary for zone V repairs. A four- or six-strand core repair is advocated for most injuries. Zone II injuries have the poorest functional outcomes. This zone was previously termed "no man's land" because of the difficulties with achieving satisfactory repair and outcomes. The carpal ligament should be repaired in zone IV injuries to prevent bowstringing during rehabilitation.

In most cases, it is best to repair both FDS and FDP. However, many people do not have an FDS in the little finger and the FDS may not always be repaired in zone II if it is very small and likely to interfere with satisfactory movement of the FDP repair. Where there is a problem with bulk, some surgeons opt to repair only one slip of FDS and trim the other in zone II.[1-3]

REFERENCES

1. Doyle JR, Blythe WF. Anatomy of the flexor tendon sheath and pulleys of the thumb. J Hand Surg Am 1977;2(2):149–151
2. Bayat A, Shaaban H, Giakas G, Lees VC. The pulley system of the thumb: anatomic and biomechanical study. J Hand Surg Am 2002;27(4):628–635
3. Papandrea R, Seitz WH Jr, Shapiro P, Borden B. Biomechanical and clinical evaluation of the epitenon-first technique of flexor tendon repair. J Hand Surg Am 1995;20(2):261–266

FLEXOR TENDON INJURY MANAGEMENT

13. You are assessing a 23-year-old patient who is no longer able to flex the DIP joint of his dominant ring finger 5 weeks after a game of rugby. A lateral radiograph is unremarkable. *When discussing treatment options with him, which one of the following is correct?*

D. Consent should be obtained for both primary and staged repair.

This is likely to be a Leddy-Packer type I FDP tendon avulsion injury, with the tendon end lying in the palm. The FDP tendon does not usually retract to the wrist because of the lumbrical attachments.

In this scenario, the window for successful direct repair is reduced to 7 to 10 days compared to type II and III injuries, because the tendon has lost both the vincula and synovial nutrient supplies, and the flexor sheath is largely empty and able to shrink down. There is a slim chance that this will actually be a type II injury, with an intact vinculum longum and the tendon end at the A3 pulley, in which case a direct repair might still be possible. However, this is much less likely, and beyond 4 weeks there may have been sufficient musculotendinous contraction to lead to an excessively tight repair, causing a troublesome quadriga effect. A quadriga effect occurs when shortening or tethering of one FDP tendon reduces power and excursion in the remaining three healthy tendons, as described by Verdan.[1]

If a primary repair is not possible in a delayed presentation, it is not advisable to perform an immediate palmaris graft, because the sheath is usually scarred and contracted. Even if there is adequate space for a primary graft, the risk of adhesions is much higher than if a staged approach is used. A silicone (Hunter) rod spacer is usually placed to generate a pseudosheath for subsequent tendon grafting from 8 to 12 weeks later.[2-4]

REFERENCES

1. Verdan C. Syndrome of the quadriga. Surg Clin North Am 1960;40:425–426
2. Lehfeldt M, Ray E, Sherman R. MOC-PS(SM) CME article: treatment of flexor tendon laceration. Plast Reconstr Surg 2008;121(4, Suppl):1–12
3. Momeni A, Grauel E, Chang J. Complications after flexor tendon injuries. Hand Clin 2010;26(2):179–189
4. Griffin M, Hindocha S, Jordan D, Saleh M, Khan W. An overview of the management of flexor tendon injuries. Open Orthop J 2012;6(01):28–35

FLEXOR TENDON INJURY MANAGEMENT

14. *In which one of the following intraoperative scenarios should delayed primary tendon repair at a second operation be considered?*

D. **Zone I index FDP division from a human bite wound the previous night**

Immediate repair is not recommended in bite wounds because of contamination and an element of crush injury. A thorough debridement and washout in addition to antibiotic therapy is preferable, followed by a delayed primary tendon repair if the wound is clean at 48 to 72 hours. When exploring an open tendon injury, serous fluid in the sheath is not uncommon; however, turbid or frankly purulent fluid is a contraindication to immediate repair. In the other scenarios, it is optimal to repair the divided tendon as soon as possible after presentation.[1,2]

REFERENCES

1. Lehfeldt M, Ray E, Sherman R. MOC-PS(SM) CME article: treatment of flexor tendon laceration. Plast Reconstr Surg 2008;121(4, Suppl):1–12
2. Elliot D, Giesen T. Avoidance of unfavourable results following primary flexor tendon surgery. Indian J Plast Surg 2013;46(2):312–324

FLEXOR TENDON INJURIES

15. A 53-year-old man sustains a stab injury to the volar aspect of his palm in line with the ring finger at the distal palmar crease. On examination, he is able to flex the ring finger at both the PIP and DIP joints, but this is painful on resisted flexion of either joint when tested independently. *What is the most likely diagnosis?*

E. **Partial Zone III FDS and FDP injury**

The patient in this scenario has sustained an injury in flexor tendon zone III, which lies in the palm distal to the carpal tunnel until the distal palmar crease and MCP joint. There are two possible explanations for his pain on flexion. Either there is a partial flexion tendon injury or a hematoma from the injury causing discomfort. The safest management is to proceed with formal exploration to confirm the nature of the injury. Although many partial flexor tendon injuries do not require repair, exploration is warranted, because the tendon may subsequently rupture or cause triggering without repair.[1-3]

REFERENCES

1. Duci SB, Ahmeti HR. Partially divided flexor tendon injuries: Should they be repaired or not? Surg J (NY) 2016;2(3): e89–e90
2. Schlenker JD, Lister GD, Kleinert HE. Three complications of untreated partial laceration of flexor tendon–entrapment, rupture, and triggering. J Hand Surg Am 1981;6(4):392–398
3. Lineberry KD, Shue S, Chepla KJ. The management of partial zone II intrasynovial flexor tendon lacerations: a literature review of biomechanics, clinical outcomes and complications. Plast Reconstr Surg 2018;141(5):1165–1170

MANAGEMENT OF LACERATIONS TO THE WRIST

16. An 18-year-old girl falls onto glass while on a night out. She sustains a 1-cm laceration over the radial aspect of the wrist. Clinical examination reveals no significant neurovascular or functional deficit, except she is unable to flex the little finger PIP joint independently. *What is the next step in management?*

D. **Clinical examination of the contralateral hand**

The patient in this scenario is at risk of flexor carpi radialis and radial artery injury given the anatomic site involved, but clinically these structures do not appear to be injured. The chances of her sustaining an isolated FDS little finger injury are slim given the site of injury. It is far more likely that she has a congenital absence of the FDS; this occurs in approximately 20% of the population. It is important therefore to first assess the contralateral limb, since the condition may well be bilateral. It is good to do this as a standard practice when assessing hand function. In this scenario, consideration should still be given to formal wound exploration because glass injuries often penetrate to the bone. Where there is no functional loss and therefore no concern about tendon retraction of the forearm, local anesthesia is a reasonable option for this. Hand therapy is not indicated in this scenario given the current functional state. Ultrasound investigation can be useful to assess damaged tendons or the thumb MCP joint ulnar collateral ligament but would not be indicated as a first-line investigation in this scenario.[1-3]

REFERENCES

1. Townley WA, Swan MC, Dunn RL. Congenital absence of flexor digitorum superficialis: implications for assessment of little finger lacerations. J Hand Surg Eur Vol 2010;35(5): 417–418
2. Tan JS, Oh L, Louis DS. Variations of the flexor digitorum superficialis as determined by an expanded clinical examination. J Hand Surg Am 2009;34(5):900–906
3. Yammine K, Erić M. Agenesis, functional deficiency and the common type of the flexor digitorum superficialis of the little finger: a meta-analysis. Hand Surg Rehabil 2018;37(2): 77–85

REVIEW FOLLOWING FLEXOR TENDON REPAIR

17. *A 25-year-old patient is seen in clinic after occupational therapy following repair of a partial FPL zone II tendon division. Her thumb flexion is good, and she is pain free, but she is unable to flex the thumb without the index finger DIP joint flexing. Which of the following best describes this finding?*

A. **Linburg-Comstock anomaly**

The patient in this scenario displays the Linburg-Comstock anomaly, in which there are attachments between the FPL and index FDP tendons in the carpal tunnel. This occurs in up to a third of the population and will have been present before the tendon repair but may not have been recognized or documented. Where this condition is associated with pain, i.e., it becomes a functional problem, it is described as Linburg-Comstock syndrome.[1-3]

Adhesions occur in approximately 4% of all flexor tendon repairs and can result in limited active range of motion caused by scar tissue forming between tendon and surrounding structures.[4] Wartenburg's sign relates to a situation where the small finger is held in abduction secondary to unopposed action of the extensor digiti minimi and may be due to ulnar nerve injury with intrinsic muscle weakness. Absence of the little finger FDS is demonstrated by an inability to flex the PIP joint when the adjacent digits are held extended to eliminate FDP function.

REFERENCES

1. Gancarczyk SM, Strauch RJ. Linburg-Comstock anomaly. J Hand Surg Am 2014;39(8): 1620–1622
2. Yammine K, Erić M. Linburg-Comstock variation and syndrome. A meta-analysis. Surg Radiol Anat 2018;40(3):289–296
3. Linburg RM, Comstock BE. Anomalous tendon slips from the flexor pollicis longus to the flexor digitorum profundus. J Hand Surg Am 1979;4(1):79–83
4. Dy CJ, Hernandez-Soria A, Ma Y, Roberts TR, Daluiski A. Complications after flexor tendon repair: a systematic review and meta-analysis. J Hand Surg Am 2012;37(3):543–551.e1

POSTOPERATIVE CARE FOLLOWING FLEXOR TENDON REPAIR

18. *When applying a splint after flexor tendon repair, which one of the following is correct?*

D. **The interphalangeal (IP) joints should be almost fully extended.**

Precise postoperative care after flexor tendon repair is critical to achieving a good outcome. The patient must be placed in a dorsal blocking splint to prevent excessive extension of the repair. The wrist is commonly placed in neutral or slight flexion, as this weakens the flexor tendons and can reduce the risk of postoperative rupture. However, many surgeons prefer slight wrist extension, as this is a more natural posture for digital flexion and is thought to improve range of glide and reduce excessive strain in attempted active digital flexion.[1]

The dorsal blocking splint should usually maintain the MCP joints in approximately 60 to 70 degrees of flexion. There is a wide range of preferred MCP joint splint angles reported (20–90 degrees); however, most authors agree that the IP joints should be able to straighten fully, otherwise flexion contractures will develop. Trying to force all four MCP joints into 90 degrees of flexion often results in an MCP joint angle of around 70 degrees and unintended flexion at the IP joints. Most techniques do not require elastic band use in conjunction with the splint. The Kleinert protocol uses elastic band traction to facilitate active extension and passive flexion after repair. Other techniques rely on early active mobilization and splinting alone.[2,3]

REFERENCES

1. Tang JB. New developments are improving flexor tendon repair. Plast Reconstr Surg 2018;141(6):1427–1437
2. Matarrese MR, Hammert WC. Flexor tendon rehabilitation. J Hand Surg Am 2012;37(11):2386–2388
3. Chesney A, Chauhan A, Kattan A, Farrokhyar F, Thoma A. Systematic review of flexor tendon rehabilitation protocols in zone II of the hand. Plast Reconstr Surg 2011;127(4): 1583–1592

COMPLICATIONS FOLLOWING FLEXOR TENDON REPAIR

19. Which one of the following is correct regarding outcomes after flexor tendon repair?

C. **FPL is the most frequently ruptured flexor tendon after primary repair.**

The most commonly re-ruptured flexor tendon is the FPL, but ring and little finger FDP tendons also have high rates of re-rupture. The overall rate of re-rupture after primary flexor tendon repair is around 5% (not 15%). Although re-rupture can be due to poor surgical technique during the repair, the main factors tend to be related to the postoperative care, such as patients removing the splint or not complying with rehabilitation advice. Contractures occur in around 20% of cases, and again this is affected by the rehabilitation and aftercare provided and patient compliance. Few patients require joint release (capsulotomy) for managing this complication. Tenolysis may be required in patients with adhesions that are unresponsive to focused hand therapy. These patients typically display an intact tendon repair with good passive range of motion but poor active range of motion.[1]

REFERENCE

1. Dy CJ, Hernandez-Soria A, Ma Y, Roberts TR, Daluiski A. Complications after flexor tendon repair: a systematic review and meta-analysis. J Hand Surg Am 2012;37(3):543–551.e1

81. Extensor Tendon Injuries

See *Essentials of Plastic Surgery*, third edition, pp. 1142–1152

EXTENSOR TENDON ANATOMY

1. *Which one of the following is correct regarding extensor tendon anatomy?*
   A. The extensor digitorum communis (EDC) to little finger is absent in 10% of patients.
   B. The extensor carpi ulnaris (ECU) is the only extensor with a true sheath.
   C. The EDC is the only structure within the fourth compartment.
   D. The extensor pollicis longus (EPL) travels in the same compartment as the extensor pollicis brevis (EPB).
   E. The extensor carpi radialis longus (ECRL) and extensor carpi radialis brevis (ECRB) insert into the same metacarpal.

EXTENSOR COMPARTMENTS OF THE WRIST

2. *Which one of the following is true of the extensor compartments at the wrist?*
   A. There are five extensor compartments at the wrist.
   B. Three tendons run in the first compartment.
   C. Two tendons run in the second compartment.
   D. Extensor indices run in the third compartment.
   E. ECU and extensor digiti minimi (EDM) run in the fifth compartment.

INTRINSIC MUSCLES OF THE HAND

3. *Which one of the following is correct regarding the intrinsic muscles of the hand?*
   A. There are eight interossei, all innervated by the ulnar nerve.
   B. The sole function of the interossei is adduction and abduction of the digits.
   C. The lumbricals originate from the flexor digitorum profundus (FDP) tendons and are all innervated by the ulnar nerve.
   D. The lumbricals facilitate extension at the interphalangeal (IP) joints and are weak metacarpophalangeal (MCP) joint flexors.
   E. The intrinsic muscles all share a similar bipennate structure.

DIGITAL EXTENSOR TENDON ANATOMY

4. *Correctly identify the anatomic components of the extensor mechanism on the diagram below (Fig. 81.2). Five of the nine options will be used.*
   Options:
   A. Extrinsic extensor
   B. Central slip
   C. Oblique retinacular ligament
   D. Triangular ligament
   E. Interosseous muscle/tendon
   F. Lumbrical
   G. Sagittal band
   H. Bare triangle
   I. Lateral band

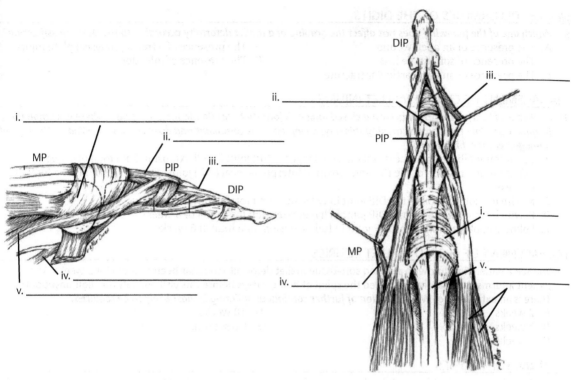

Fig. 81.2 Anatomy of the extensor mechanism of the finger.

VASCULAR ANATOMY OF THE EXTENSOR TENDONS

5. *Which one of the following provides a source of blood supply in flexor but not extensor tendons?*
A. Myotendinous junction
B. Bony insertion
C. Paratenon
D. Synovial fluid
E. Vincula

EXTENSOR TENDON ZONES OF INJURY

6. *A patient sustains a transverse laceration to the dorsal aspect of the wrist when falling through a glass door. How best should this extensor injury be described?*
A. Zone I injury
B. Zone III Injury
C. Zone VI Injury
D. Zone VII Injury
E. Zone IX Injury

SEYMOUR FRACTURES

7. *Which extensor zone of injury is a Seymour fracture sometimes mistaken for?*
A. Zone I
B. Zone II
C. Zone III
D. Zone IV
E. Zone V

EXTENSOR TENDON INJURIES

8. *Which extensor tendon zone of injury does the term "fight bite" usually refer to?*
A. Zone II
B. Zone III
C. Zone IV
D. Zone V
E. Zone VI

MALLET DEFORMITIES OF THE DIGITS

9. *Which one of the following does* not *affect the grading of a mallet deformity according to the Doyle classification?*
   A. The presence of an open wound
   B. The presence of soft-tissue loss
   C. The presence of an intra-articular fracture
   D. The presence of a transepiphyseal plate injury
   E. The presence of infection

MANAGEMENT OF CLOSED MALLET INJURIES

10. *A 39-year-old carpenter presents with a closed mallet deformity to his dominant index finger. There is a small bony fragment on plain radiographs making this a type I injury. He is compliant and does not smoke. What is the typical management for this patient?*
    A. Splint immobilization of the distal interphalangeal (DIP) joint in full extension for a total of 4 weeks.
    B. Splint immobilization of the DIP and proximal interphalangeal (PIP) joints in full extension for a total of 4 weeks.
    C. K-wire immobilization of the DIP joint in extension for a total of 6 weeks.
    D. K-wire immobilization of the DIP joint in hyperextension for a total of 6 weeks.
    E. Splint immobilization of the DIP joint in full extension for a total of 6 weeks.

MANAGEMENT OF CLOSED MALLET INJURIES

11. You see a patient in clinic with a closed soft-tissue mallet deformity that has been splinted for 3 weeks. The patient informs you that they removed the splint at home 2 days before this visit and left the digit unsupported. There is an extensor lag. *What duration of further continuous splinting is most likely to be required?*
    A. 2 weeks
    B. 3 weeks
    C. 6 weeks
    D. 10 weeks
    E. No set time

CENTRAL SLIP INJURIES

12. A young diabetic patient has sustained a closed soft-tissue injury to the index finger PIP joint which has resulted in a new boutonniere deformity. There is no fracture present. *What is the best initial management of the PIP joint in this scenario?*
    A. Active mobilization
    B. External splinting in extension
    C. K-wire stabilization in extension
    D. Open suture repair
    E. Reconstruction with a flap of proximal tendon

ZONE III EXTENSOR TENDON INJURIES

13. A patient presents with a healing 3-day-old transverse incised wound from glass over the dorsum of the PIP joint. Active extension against resistance is preserved, and radiographs reveal that there is no foreign body. *Which one of the following is correct?*
    A. The wound should be left to heal without further intervention.
    B. Full, active extension against resistance implies that the central slip is intact.
    C. The PIP joint capsule is unlikely to be injured.
    D. A turnover tendon flap will be needed if the tendon is divided.
    E. A bone anchor may be required to repair the central slip.

CLINICAL PROBLEMS WITH DIGITAL EXTENSION

14. A 65-year-old woman presents complaining of recurrent problems extending her middle finger. On examination, she is able to fully flex the MCP joint with some discomfort beyond 45 degrees but is unable to then actively extend the joint. She can passively straighten the finger and hold it straight against resistance. The joint appears swollen, but there is no subluxation or dislocation. *What is the most likely cause of her problem?*
    A. Intrinsic muscle tightness interfering with the extensor mechanism balance
    B. An osteophyte tethering the MCP joint collateral ligament in flexion
    C. Radial sagittal band rupture of the middle finger EDC tendon
    D. A dorsal MCP joint capsular tear
    E. A loose osteochondral body in the MCP joint caused by osteoarthritis

CLOSED EXTENSOR TENDON RUPTURES

15. *Which one of the following closed extensor tendon injuries is most likely to require operative intervention?*
    A. A mallet deformity of the ring finger with a 2 × 2 mm bony avulsion fragment from the distal phalanx
    B. An acute soft-tissue central slip injury following a blow from a cricket ball
    C. An acute ECU injury with a small bony avulsion fragment after digging frozen ground with a spade
    D. An acute central slip injury with a 2 × 1 mm bony avulsion fragment from the base of the middle phalanx
    E. A soft-tissue mallet deformity of the thumb after a distal radius fracture

CLINICAL CONCEPTS IN EXTENSOR TENDON MANAGEMENT

16. *How should the hand be placed in a splint following repair of multiple zone VIII extensor tendon injuries that involve the myotendinous junction?*
    A. Wrist neutral, MCP joints extended
    B. Wrist neutral, MP joints flexed 20 degrees
    C. Wrist extended 70 degrees, MP joints flexed 70 degrees
    D. Wrist extended 20 degrees, MP joints flexed 40 degrees
    E. Wrist extended 40 degrees, MP joint flexed 25 degrees

MANAGEMENT OF EXTENSOR TENDON INJURIES

17. *When managing extensor tendon injuries, which one of the following is correct?*
    A. Acute sagittal band ruptures should always be managed nonoperatively.
    B. A swan neck deformity may develop secondary to a zone I extensor rupture.
    C. EPL ruptures are more common at the IP joint than at the wrist.
    D. Tendon ruptures in rheumatoid arthritis can generally be repaired directly.
    E. Extensor tendon repairs are less vulnerable than flexor tendon repairs and require less strict splinting regimens.

EXTRINSIC AND INTRINSIC EXTENSOR PROBLEMS

18. You are asked by the senior hand therapist to give a second opinion on a patient who has difficulty flexing his little and ring fingers 6 months after repair of divided EDC tendons in zone V. When you passively flex the MCP joints, he is unable to flex the IP joints. When you extend the MCP joints, he is able to flex the IP joints. *What is the recommendation that will most likely address this issue?*
    A. Release of the tight intrinsic muscle insertions from the extensor mechanism
    B. An intensive period of active and passive physiotherapy without splints
    C. Extensor tenolysis around the site of repair only
    D. Extensor tenolysis around the site of repair and into the finger as required
    E. An intensive period of active and passive physiotherapy with an MCP joint blocking splint

ABNORMALITIES AFFECTING THE EXTENSOR MECHANISM

19. A patient is seen in clinic following amputation of a digit secondary to trauma at the mid portion of the middle phalanx. They now find this digit extending at the IP joint when attempting to flex into a fist. *Which one of the following anatomic structures most likely accounts for this?*
    A. Lumbricals
    B. Palmar interossei
    C. Dorsal interossei
    D. EDC
    E. extensor indicis proprius

Answers

EXTENSOR TENDON ANATOMY

1. *Which one of the following is correct regarding extensor tendon anatomy?*

   B. **The extensor carpi ulnaris (ECU) is the only extensor with a true sheath.**

   The fact that the ECU has a true sheath has clinical relevance, since a tear to the sheath can lead to ulnar-side wrist pain and subluxation of the ECU with forearm rotation. Absence of the extensor digitorum communis (EDC) to the little finger is surprisingly common and is evident in up to half of the population (not 10%). Extension of the little finger is achieved by the extensor digiti minimi (EDM) alone in these patients. The fourth compartment contains the EDC and extensor indicis proprius (EIP). In addition, the posterior interosseous nerve lies in the floor of the fourth compartment. It is a useful potential donor site for nerve grafts for digital nerve defects, because harvest incurs minimal donor-site morbidity and the nerve diameter is similar to that of the digital nerves.[1,2] The extensor pollicis longus (EPL) and extensor pollicis brevis (EPB) are located in different extensor compartments. The EPL is within the third compartment and has a path that passes around Lister's tubercle. This useful bony landmark is found between the second and third compartments. The EPL is angled around the tubercle as it passes through the compartment and this is a potential site of friction and subsequent attrition rupture (as seen in rheumatoid arthritis or distal radius fractures). The EPB is within the first compartment with the APL. This compartment is positioned on the radial aspect of the wrist and may be spared in dorsal lacerations. The extensor carpi radialis longus (ECRL) and extensor carpi radialis brevis (ECRB) both insert into different metacarpals. The ECRL inserts into the base of the index metacarpal, and the ECRB inserts into the base of the middle metacarpal.

REFERENCES

1. Reissis N, Stirrat A, Manek S, Dunkerton M. The terminal branch of posterior interosseous nerve: a useful donor for digital nerve grafting. J Hand Surg [Br] 1992;17(6):638–640
2. Waters PM, Schwartz JT. Posterior interosseous nerve: an anatomic study of potential nerve grafts. J Hand Surg Am 1993;18(4):743–745

EXTENSOR COMPARTMENTS OF THE WRIST

2. *Which one of the following is true of the extensor compartments at the wrist?*

   C. **Two tendons run in the second compartment.**

   There are six (not five) extensor compartments at the wrist. Knowledge of the extensor compartments of the wrist is often tested in clinical exams and is highly relevant to hand trauma and tendon transfer procedures. In the second compartment, there are two tendons: ECRL and ECRB. Although they both pass through the same compartment, their insertions differ with ECRL inserting into the second metacarpal and the ECRB inserting into the third metacarpal.

   The first compartment contains two tendons (APL and EPB). APL inserts into the first metacarpal, and EPB inserts variably into the thumb proximal phalanx, metacarpophalangeal (MCP) joint extensor hood, terminal phalanx, or is sometimes absent.[1] The third compartment contains just one tendon, the EPL, which inserts into the distal phalanx of the thumb. The fourth compartment contains both the EIP and EDC tendons, which insert into the extensor mechanisms of the digits. The posterior interosseous nerve, which supplies sensation to the wrist, is also found in this compartment. The fifth compartment contains the EDM only, which inserts into the small finger extensor mechanism. The sixth compartment also contains a single tendon, which is the ECU that inserts into the base of the fifth metacarpal base. **Fig. 81.1** shows the various compartments and the structures, which they contain.

REFERENCE

1. Lonne M, Sparks DS, Stephan C, Wagels M, Berger A. Clinical examination of the extensor pollicis brevis: anatomical study and description of a novel clinical sign. J Hand Surg Asian Pac Vol 2018;23(3):330–335

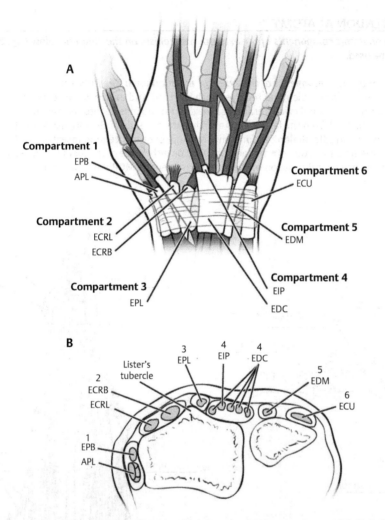

Fig. 81.1   Extensor compartments. (*APL*, abductor pollicis longus; *ECRB*, extensor carpi radialis brevis; *ECRL*, extensor carpi radialis longus; *EDC*, extensor digitorum communis; *ECU*, extensor carpi ulnaris; *EDM*, extensor digiti minimi; *EIP*, extensor indicis proprius; *EPB*, extensor pollicis brevis; *EPL*, extensor pollicis longus.)

INTRINSIC MUSCLES OF THE HAND

3. *Which one of the following is correct regarding the intrinsic muscles of the hand?*

   D. The lumbricals facilitate extension at the IP joints and are weak MCP joint flexors.

   The intrinsic muscles of the hand include the lumbricals and interossei. There are seven interossei (four dorsal and three palmar), all of which are innervated by the ulnar nerve. Their main purpose is abduction (dorsal) and adduction (palmar) of the digits, but they also contribute to MCP flexion and interphalangeal (IP) joint extension. The lumbricals do originate from the FDP tendons and insert on the extensor hood but have dual innervation with the ulnar two receiving innervation from the ulnar nerve and the radial two receiving innervation from the median nerve. The palmar interossei are unipennate, while the dorsal interossei are bipennate.[1,2]

REFERENCES

1. Moore KL, Dalley AF, eds. Clinically Oriented Anatomy. 4th ed. New York, NY: Lippincott Williams & Wilkins; 1999
2. Green DP, Hotchkiss RN, Pederson WC, et al., eds. Green's Operative Hand Surgery. 5th ed. Philadelphia: Churchill Livingstone; 2005

DIGITAL EXTENSOR TENDON ANATOMY

4. *Correctly identify the anatomic components of the extensor mechanism on the diagram below (Fig. 81.2). Five of the nine options will be used.*

   Answer:

   For Fig. 81.3, the anatomic components of the extensor mechanism are as follows:

   The extensor mechanism is complex and receives both intrinsic and extrinsic muscle contribution. The EDC trifurcates into the central slip and two lateral slips. The central slip inserts into the base of the middle phalanx. The lateral bands are formed from the lateral slips and the lateral bands of the intrinsics, and these reunite over the distal portion of the middle phalanx to form the terminal extensor tendon inserting at the distal phalanx. The sagittal bands originate from the intermetacarpal plate on either side of the metacarpal head to form a dorsal hood. They maintain the central position of the extensors over the MCP joint, preventing lateral subluxation during joint flexion.[1-3]

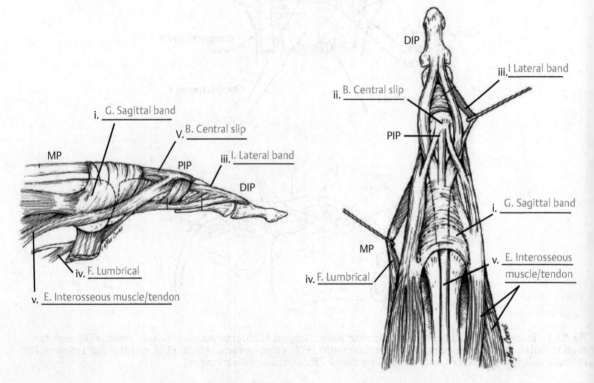

Fig. 81.3   Anatomy of the extensor mechanism of the finger.

REFERENCES

1. Moore KL, Dalley AF, eds. Clinically Oriented Anatomy. 4th ed. New York, NY: Lippincott Williams & Wilkins; 1999
2. Green DP, Hotchkiss RN, Pederson WC, et al, eds. Green's Operative Hand Surgery. 5th ed. Philadelphia: Churchill Livingstone; 2005
3. Rockwell WB, Butler PN, Byrne BA. Extensor tendon: anatomy, injury, and reconstruction. Plast Reconstr Surg 2000;106(7):1592–1603, quiz 1604, 1673

VASCULAR ANATOMY OF THE EXTENSOR TENDONS

5. *Which one of the following provides a source of blood supply in flexor but not extensor tendons?*

   E. Vincula

   The extensor tendons receive blood supply from a number of sources as do the flexor tendons. These include the myotendinous junction, the bony insertion, the paratenon along the length of the tendon, and synovial lined tissue (such as under the retinaculum). Unlike the flexor tendons, however, there are no vincular vessels supplying the extensor tendons.[1]

REFERENCE

1. Gajisin S, Zbrodowski A. Vascular anatomy of the digital extensors. Ann Chir Main 1986;5(2):105–112

EXTENSOR TENDON ZONES OF INJURY

6. *A patient sustains a transverse laceration to the dorsal aspect of the wrist when falling through a glass door. How best should this extensor injury be described?*

 D. Zone VII Injury

 The established nomenclature for extensor tendons contains nine different zones for the fingers and five zones for the thumb starting with zone I most distal over the distal interphalangeal (DIP) joint or IP joint, respectively. The finger zones can then be counted as odd numbers over the joints (DIP, proximal interphalangeal [PIP], MCP, and carpus I, III, V, and VII, respectively.) The even numbers refer to the middle phalanx, proximal phalanx, metacarpal, and distal forearm (II, IV, VI, and VIII, respectively). Zone IX refers to the proximal forearm where muscle bellies are present (**Fig. 81.4**).[1,2]

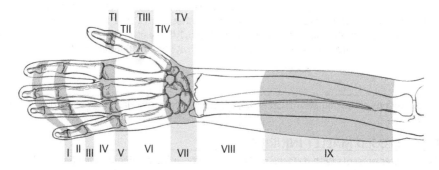

Fig. 81.4 The extensor tendon zones are numbered I through IX, with odd numbers overlying joints. Thumb extensor tendon zones have a separate numbering system.

REFERENCES

1. Kleinert HE, Verdan C. Report of the Committee on Tendon Injuries (International Federation of Societies for Surgery of the Hand). J Hand Surg Am 1983;8(5, Pt 2):794–798
2. Rockwell WB, Butler PN, Byrne BA. Extensor tendon: anatomy, injury, and reconstruction. Plast Reconstr Surg 2000;106(7):1592–1603, quiz 1604, 1673

SEYMOUR FRACTURES

7. *Which extensor zone of injury is a Seymour fracture sometimes mistaken for?*

 A. Zone I

 Zone I injuries involve the extensor tendon near the DIP joint. A Seymour fracture is a type of open fracture with the nail bed trapped in the physis. It often presents with the nail plate sitting on top of the nail fold and is mistaken for a simple nail bed or mallet zone I extensor injury. It requires careful management, because without treatment the nail bed will remain in the physis and affect healing and growth. The extensor tendon inserts on the epiphysis, therefore, is intact in this injury.[1,2]

REFERENCES

1. Lin JS, Popp JE, Balch Samora J. Treatment of acute Seymour fractures. J Pediatr Orthop 2019;39(1):e23–e27
2. Kiely AL, Nolan GS, Cooper LRL. The optimal management of Seymour fractures in children and adolescents: a systematic review protocol. Syst Rev 2020;9(1):150

EXTENSOR TENDON INJURIES

8. *Which extensor tendon zone of injury does the term "fight bite" usually refer to?*

 D. Zone V

 Open zone V extensor tendon injuries commonly occur following a punch injury to the face where the attacker's fist contacts the tooth of the other person during the punch. It is effectively a self-inflicted human bite injury, hence the term "fight bite." This injury mechanism often results in partial division of the extensor over the MCP joint and also involves the joint itself. Presentation is typically delayed until infection begins with swelling, inflammation, and pain in the joint. Management involves admission for intravenous antibiotics, surgical exploration, and wash out of the wound including the joint. The extensor should be repaired, if necessary, only once infection is controlled. The wound may be left to heal by secondary intention or closed as a delayed additional procedure. In some cases, the same mechanism of injury can lead to PIP joint involvement, although this is less common. The treatment principles remain the same.[1]

REFERENCE

1. Shewring DJ, Trickett RW, Subramanian KN, Hnyda R. The management of clenched fist 'fight bite' injuries of the hand. J Hand Surg Eur Vol 2015;40(8):819–824

MALLET DEFORMITIES OF THE DIGITS

9. *Which one of the following does* not *affect the grading of a mallet deformity according to the Doyle classification?*

E. The presence of infection

A mallet injury is a zone I extensor injury with loss of continuity of the extensor close to the DIP joint. A clear classification system is clinically relevant to a mallet injury, as it guides treatment and enables comparison of clinical outcomes between patients. Mallet injuries are open or closed, can involve a fracture or soft-tissue injury, and in some circumstances both are present. The Doyle classification has four grades. Type I is a closed injury with or without a small bony avulsion. Type II is an open injury with a laceration close to the DIP joint that results in a loss of tendon continuity. Type III is an open injury with soft-tissue loss. Type IV injuries are subclassified as types A, B, and C. IVA is a transepiphyseal plate fracture in children, IVB is a fracture of the articular surface between 20 and 50%, and IVC is a fracture >50% of the articular surface with volar subluxation of the distal phalanx.[1]

REFERENCE

1. Doyle JR. Extensor tendons-acute injuries. In: Green DP, ed. Green's Operative Hand Surgery. 3rd ed. New York: Churchill Livingstone; 1993

MANAGEMENT OF CLOSED MALLET INJURIES

10. *A 39-year-old carpenter presents with a closed mallet deformity to his dominant index finger. There is a small bony fragment on plain radiographs making this a type I injury. He is compliant and does not smoke. What is the typical management for this patient?*

E. Splint immobilization of the DIP joint in full extension for a total of 6 weeks.

Most closed mallet injuries can be satisfactorily managed nonoperatively with external splinting. The splint may be placed volar or dorsal and should hold the DIP joint in extension for at least 6 weeks, then a night splint should be used for another 2 weeks. The PIP and MCP joints should be free to mobilize. K-wire immobilization should be reserved for patients where compliance is not possible, for patients with occupations that may find continuous external splinting unacceptable, or in cases where reduction with splinting alone is inadequate. Open mallet injuries should be treated operatively with repair of the damaged structure (e.g., the extensor tendon and soft tissue) followed by splintage. Those where bony injury is present may benefit from K-wire stabilization too.[1,2]

REFERENCES

1. Doyle J. Extensor tendons: acute injuries. In: Green's Operative Hand Surgery. Churchill Livingstone; 1999:195–198
2. Wehbé MA, Schneider LH. Mallet fractures. J Bone Joint Surg Am 1984;66(5):658–669

MANAGEMENT OF CLOSED MALLET INJURIES

11. You see a patient in clinic with a closed soft-tissue mallet deformity that has been splinted for 3 weeks. The patient informs you that they removed the splint at home 2 days before this visit and left the digit unsupported. There is an extensor lag. *What duration of further continuous splinting is most likely to be required?*

C. 6 weeks

The normal duration of splinting following a mallet deformity is 6 weeks of continuous splinting followed by 2 weeks of nighttime splinting. The patient must understand that the splint is to be worn continuously for the entire 6 weeks, and that removal resulting in DIP joint flexion, at any stage before this, will restart the clock and a minimum of an additional 6 weeks of splinting will be required. In general, soft-tissue mallet injuries take longer to heal than bony mallet injuries and this must be kept in mind when selecting a suitable management plan. Patients should be shown how to safely remove and reapply the splint for skin care without flexing the DIP joint.[1,2]

REFERENCES

1. Doyle J. Extensor tendons: acute injuries. In: Green's Operative Hand Surgery. Churchill Livingstone; 1999:195–198
2. Wehbé MA, Schneider LH. Mallet fractures. J Bone Joint Surg Am 1984;66(5):658–669

CENTRAL SLIP INJURIES

12. A young diabetic patient has sustained a closed soft-tissue injury to the index finger PIP joint which has resulted in a new boutonniere deformity. There is no fracture present. *What is the best initial management of the PIP joint in this scenario?*

    B. External splinting in extension

    The boutonniere deformity occurs secondary to injury to the digital extensor in zone III. A closed avulsion can occur following trauma and is often misdiagnosed as a sprained finger. The deformity develops as the lateral bands migrate volarly, changing their vector of pull, to cause PIP joint flexion and DIP joint hyperextension. Closed zone III avulsion injuries are best treated nonoperatively with external splinting of the PIP joint in extension. Regimens vary, but a typical example is 6 weeks of continuous splinting and another 2 weeks of splinting at night only. It is important to keep the remaining finger joints free to actively mobilize throughout, in order to avoid stiffness. K-wires are not normally required to hold the PIP joint in extension and are best avoided, as they can cause damage to the articular surface and also carry a risk of infection. Extra care should be taken to avoid their use in higher risk patients such as diabetics. Active mobilization is not required until the period of splinting is complete. It is, however, very important at this stage in order to minimize subsequent joint stiffness. Some regimens include early graduated flexion with flexion blocking splints, or active flexion and passive extension in a Capener splint, which is a type of dynamic spring-loaded splint that holds the PIP joint in extension but allows flexion against resistance. Capener first described the splint; the Capener splint has now become a generic term used by many manufacturers and hand therapists.[1] Specialized surgical repair is usually required only in open injuries. A proximal extensor tendon turnover flap may be used where there is substance loss.[2]

REFERENCES

1. Capener N. Lively splints. Physiotherapy 1967;53(11):371–374
2. Snow JW. Use of a retrograde tendon flap in repairing a severed extensor in the pip joint area. Plast Reconstr Surg 1973;51(5):555–558

ZONE III EXTENSOR TENDON INJURIES

13. A patient presents with a healing 3-day-old transverse incised wound from glass over the dorsum of the PIP joint. Active extension against resistance is preserved, and radiographs reveal that there is no foreign body. *Which one of the following is correct?*

    E. A bone anchor may be required to repair the central slip.

    Glass injuries often penetrate easily until resistance is met, usually against bone. At PIP joint level, the dorsal soft tissues and tendon are thin; therefore, the joint capsule may well have been injured. At 3 days, the wound has barely started healing and the benefits of identifying and repairing a central slip injury early (avoiding a boutonniere deformity) outweigh the downsides of exploring the wound under a local anesthetic block.

    If the central slip is divided, the patient may well be able to fully extend against resistance. Two intact lateral bands will still give strong extension, and a single intact lateral band is enough to fully extend in the early stages. If a central slip injury is missed, the finger will gradually collapse into a boutonniere deformity as the lateral bands sublux volar to the pivot point of the PIP joint. Contracture of the volar plate and joint capsule can develop quickly, and the central slip remnants become retracted and scarred, making delayed repair more challenging.

    With an acute, sharp division of the central slip, direct repair will normally be possible, but a bone anchor or drill hole through the middle phalanx may be required if the distal stump is insufficient to hold a suture. Turnover flaps, such as described by Snow,[1] are reserved for occasions where a gap prevents direct repair, such as circular saw or abrasive central slip injuries.

REFERENCE

1. Snow JW. Use of a retrograde tendon flap in repairing a severed extensor in the pip joint area. Plast Reconstr Surg 1973;51(5):555–558

CLINICAL PROBLEMS WITH DIGITAL EXTENSION

14. A 65-year-old woman presents complaining of recurrent problems extending her middle finger. On examination, she is able to fully flex the MCP joint with some discomfort beyond 45 degrees but is unable to then actively extend the joint. She can passively straighten the finger and hold it straight against resistance. The joint appears swollen, but there is no subluxation or dislocation. *What is the most likely cause of her problem?*

    C. Radial sagittal band rupture of the middle finger EDC tendon

    This patient's symptoms are associated with a sagittal band rupture, which can present acutely or as a chronic problem. This injury allows the EDC tendon to sublux into the gutters on either side of the prominent metacarpal head when the MCP joint is flexed. When the patient tries to extend the MCP joint from full flexion, this can be difficult because the EDC has lost its tension by slipping off the metacarpal head and its line of pull is no longer dorsal to the pivot point of the MCP joint; therefore, its mechanical advantage is lost.

Another typical scenario for this injury is a young male boxer or fighter with an acutely painful and swollen dorsal aspect of the MCP joint after a punch injury. There will be pain with increasing flexion and a point beyond which the tendon visibly slips into the gutter.[1-3]

REFERENCES

1. Ishizuki M. Traumatic and spontaneous dislocation of extensor tendon of the long finger. J Hand Surg Am 1990;15(6):967–972
2. Rayan GM, Murray D. Classification and treatment of closed sagittal band injuries. J Hand Surg Am 1994;19(4):590–594
3. Catalano LW III, Gupta S, Ragland R III, Glickel SZ, Johnson C, Barron OA. Closed treatment of nonrheumatoid extensor tendon dislocations at the metacarpophalangeal joint. J Hand Surg Am 2006;31(2):242–245

CLOSED EXTENSOR TENDON RUPTURES

15. Which one of the following closed extensor tendon injuries is most likely to require operative intervention?

   E. A soft-tissue mallet deformity of the thumb after a distal radius fracture

   A distal radius fracture is a risk factor for an EPL attrition rupture, which usually occurs around Lister's tubercle. It is important not to miss this diagnosis by mistaking a proximal injury for a simple zone I mallet injury, as the patient may end up with weeks of unnecessary splinting to no avail and will be better served by an EIP to EPL tendon transfer. Closed zone I EPL ruptures can, of course, occur, but these are rare. A combination of the clinical findings (such as swelling and tenderness around either the IP joint or Lister's tubercle) and ultrasound may be helpful in distinguishing the different levels of injury. Many authors advocate a similar management plan for zone I EPL ruptures to finger mallet injuries, i.e., splinting of closed soft-tissue injuries.[1] However, there are also concerns that the EPL tendon tends to retract more than the lateral bands of the fingers, and many patients normally have significant hyperextension possible at the thumb IP joint; so, some authors would advocate surgical repair regardless of zone in the thumb. There is no strong evidence either way in zone I EPL injuries, and imaging may be helpful to identify those whose tendon has retracted more and who may therefore fail nonoperative management.

REFERENCE

1. Tabbal GN, Bastidas N, Sharma S. Closed mallet thumb injury: a review of the literature and case study of the use of magnetic resonance imaging in deciding treatment. Plast Reconstr Surg 2009;124(1):222–226

CLINICAL CONCEPTS IN EXTENSOR TENDON MANAGEMENT

16. How should the hand be placed in a splint following repair of multiple zone VIII extensor tendon injuries that involve the myotendinous junction?

   E. Wrist extended 40 degrees, MP joint flexed 25 degrees

   The correct position of postoperative splinting following repair of the extensor tendons is dependent on the zone of injury involved. The normal "safe" position for splinting is the wrist in slight extension, MCP joints flexed between 70 and 90 degrees, and IP joints in extension. This position is modified following extensor repair in order to minimize tension across the repair sites. For example, the recommended position following a zone VIII repair is to have the wrist extended 40 degrees, the MCP joints flexed 20 degrees, and the fingers free to mobilize into active extension within the splint.[1-3]

REFERENCES

1. Purcell T, Eadie PA, Murugan S, O'Donnell M, Lawless M. Static splinting of extensor tendon repairs. J Hand Surg [Br] 2000;25(2):180–182
2. Yoon AP, Chung KC. Management of acute extensor tendon injuries. Clin Plast Surg 2019;46(3):383–391
3. Crosby CA, Wehbé MA. Early protected motion after extensor tendon repair. J Hand Surg Am 1999;24(5):1061–1070

MANAGEMENT OF EXTENSOR TENDON INJURIES

17. When managing extensor tendon injuries, which one of the following is correct?

   B. A swan neck deformity may develop secondary to a zone I extensor rupture.

   Swan neck deformities may result from a chronic zone 1 extensor tendon rupture or from pathology around the PIP joint, such as volar plate laxity or an FDS tendon rupture.

While acute closed sagittal band ruptures may be managed with an MCP joint flexion blocking splint if they are identified within the first 2 weeks, there is still a risk of subsequent extensor tendon subluxation. Furthermore, delayed presentations and open injuries should ideally be repaired. Surgical treatment involves either directly repairing the sagittal band or re-anchoring the EDC tendon to a firm structure, such as the volar plate or volar transverse metacarpal ligament. This may be achieved with either a suturing technique or a strip of EDC tendon used as a lasso (Watson technique).[1] Operative treatment requires a similar method of splinting to nonoperative care but should give a greater chance of subsequent tendon stability. Extensor tendon repairs in the flat tendon zones within the fingers are more vulnerable to stretching and rupture in the early stages than flexor tendon repairs. Careful protection with splints is required following extensor tendon injury and is equally important as it is in flexor tendon injuries.[1,2]

REFERENCES

1. Watson HK, Weinzweig J, Guidera PM. Sagittal band reconstruction. J Hand Surg Am 1997;22(3):452–456
2. Yoon AP, Chung KC. Management of acute extensor tendon injuries. Clin Plast Surg 2019;46(3):383–391

EXTRINSIC AND INTRINSIC EXTENSOR PROBLEMS

18. You are asked by the senior hand therapist to give a second opinion on a patient who has difficulty flexing his little and ring fingers 6 months after repair of divided EDC tendons in zone V. When you passively flex the MCP joints, he is unable to flex the IP joints. When you extend the MCP joints, he is able to flex the IP joints. *What is the recommendation that will most likely address this issue?*

    D. Extensor tenolysis around the site of repair and into the finger as required

    The scenario given is typical of extrinsic extensor tethering. When the MCP joints are in extension, the extrinsic mechanism is slackened, and the patient is able to flex the IP joints. If the problem was of intrinsic tightness, extending the MCP joints would make the problem worse and prevent IP joint flexion. Accepting this diagnosis and the fact that the patient is already seeing a senior therapist, it is unlikely that further physiotherapy and splinting is going to correct this 6 months after repair. An extensor tenolysis will require release of the expected adhesions around the site of repair, but also usually requires a more extensive release into the surrounding extensor zones due to additional adhesion formation.[1]

REFERENCE

1. Desai MJ, Wanner JP, Lee DH, Gauger EM. Failed extensor tendon repairs: extensor tenolysis and reconstruction. J Am Acad Orthop Surg 2019;27(15):563–574

ABNORMALITIES AFFECTING THE EXTENSOR MECHANISM

19. A patient is seen in clinic following amputation of a digit secondary to trauma at the mid portion of the middle phalanx. They now find this digit extending at the IP joint when attempting to flex into a fist. *Which one of the following anatomic structures most likely accounts for this?*

    A. Lumbricals

    The scenario describes the lumbrical plus finger deformity which occurs where the FDP shortens (e.g., after finger amputation beyond the FDS insertion), and causes lumbrical tension such that paradoxical joint extension occurs when an attempt is made to flex. This is because the lumbricals run between the FDP tendons and the extensor mechanism of the digits. The EDC is not primarily implicated as it is the lumbricals inserting into this common mechanism that are the problem.[1–3]

REFERENCES

1. Chinchalkar SJ, Larocerie-Salgado J, Suh N. Pathomechanics and management of secondary complications associated with tendon adhesions following flexor tendon repair in zone II. J Hand Microsurg 2016;8(2):70–79
2. Parkes A. The "lumbrical plus" finger. J Bone Joint Surg Br 1971;53(2):236–239
3. Green DP, Hotchkiss RN, Pederson WC, et al, eds. Green's Operative Hand Surgery. 5th ed. Philadelphia: Churchill Livingstone; 2005

82. Tendon Transfers

See *Essentials of Plastic Surgery*, third edition, pp. 1153–1162

BOX 82.1 *FOREARM AND HAND MUSCLE ABBREVIATIONS*

ADM: Abductor digiti minimi	**EIP:** Extensor indicis proprius	**FPL:** Flexor pollicis longus
APB: Abductor pollicis brevis	**EPB:** Extensor pollicis brevis	**ODM:** Opponens digiti minimi
APL: Abductor pollicis longus	**EPL:** Extensor pollicis longus	**OP:** Opponens pollicis
BR: Brachioradialis	**FCR:** Flexor carpi radialis	**PL:** Palmaris longus
ECRB: Extensor carpi radialis brevis	**FCU:** Flexor carpi ulnaris	**PQ:** Pronator quadratus
ECRL: Extensor carpi radialis longus	**FDM:** Flexor digiti minimi	**PT:** Pronator teres
ECU: Extensor carpi ulnaris	**FDP:** Flexor digitorum profundus	**SORL:** Spiral oblique retinacular
EDC: Extensor digitorum communis	**FDS:** Flexor digitorum superficialis	ligament
EDM: Extensor digiti minimi	**FPB:** Flexor pollicis brevis	

PRINCIPLES OF TENDON TRANSFER

1. *Which one of the following is a usual feature of a donor muscle selected for tendon transfer?*
   A. A power grading greater than the muscle it is replacing
   B. A synergistic action to the muscle it is replacing
   C. The potential to perform multiple new functions
   D. A greater excursion than the muscle it is replacing
   E. A different vector to the muscle it is replacing

INDICATIONS FOR TENDON TRANSFER

2. *What is the most common indication for tendon transfer?*
   A. Nerve injury alone
   B. Tendon injury alone
   C. Combined nerve and tendon injuries
   D. Spasticity
   E. Muscle injury

CONTRAINDICATIONS FOR TENDON TRANSFER

3. *Which one of the following conditions is the most significant contraindication to tendon transfer?*
   A. Diabetes mellitus
   B. Fluctuating spasticity
   C. Stabilized function following poliomyelitis
   D. Rheumatoid arthritis
   E. Failure of prior tendon grafting

INDICATIONS FOR TENDON TRANSFER

4. *In which one of the following scenarios might an immediate tendon transfer be indicated in a young, otherwise healthy patient?*
   A. Active leprosy with clawing of the hand
   B. Untreated carpal tunnel syndrome with thenar wasting
   C. Radial nerve repair at midhumeral level
   D. Resurfacing of scarred forearm after trauma
   E. Recent ulnar nerve repair at wrist level

TRANSFERS IN MEDIAN NERVE PALSY

5. You see a 20-year-old patient with poor recovery following a median nerve division at the wrist 2 years earlier. She asks about potential reconstructive options. *Which one of the following tendon transfers would best address thenar muscle denervation?*
   A. An EIP transfer around the ulnar border of the wrist
   B. A ring finger FDP transfer through a flexor retinaculum window
   C. An abductor digiti minimi transfer across the palm
   D. A palmaris longus plus fascial strip transfer around an FCU pulley
   E. An FDS ring transfer around an FCR pulley

TRANSFERS IN ULNAR NERVE PALSY

6. A patient presents with full FCU (MRC grade V) and incomplete FDP (MRC grade IV) recovery but persistent clawing 18 months after an ulnar nerve repair at the elbow. *Which one of the following is contraindicated in this case?*
   A. An MCP joint hyperextension-blocking splint for the long term
   B. A ring finger FDS tendon transfer to the lateral bands to correct the clawing
   C. An FCR transfer with PL grafts to the A1/A2 pulleys to correct the clawing
   D. Postponement of tendon transfers until clawing is passively correctable
   E. An ECRB transfer with PL graft to aid thumb adduction

TENDON TRANSFERS IN RADIAL NERVE PALSY

7. You are considering tendon transfers for a young, healthy man 4 months after repair of a radial nerve injury at the elbow. *Which one of the following statements is correct?*
   A. Recovery of some wrist extension would be expected by this stage.
   B. If there is no sign of EPL recovery by now, a tendon transfer will be needed.
   C. An EMG is unlikely to be helpful this long after injury.
   D. Recovery of strong digital extension would be expected by this stage.
   E. If motor recovery is seen, but is slower than expected, re-repair of the nerve may be required.

TENDON TRANSFER IN RADIAL NERVE INJURY

8. *When treating a radial nerve palsy, which one of the following is most likely to cause a functional problem when planning a combined transfer with PT to ECRB?*
   A. PT to ECRB, FDS ring to EDC, FDS middle to EPL/EIP
   B. PT to ECRB, FCR to APL, FDS ring to EDC, FDS middle to EPL
   C. PT to ECRL, FCR to EDC, PL to EPL
   D. PT to ECRB, FCR to APL, FCU to EDC, PL to EPL
   E. PT to ECRL, FCR to EDC, PL to EPL

TRANSFERS IN COMBINED NERVE PALSIES

9. You have a patient with persistent wasting of the thenar eminence muscle group and mild clawing of the digits after a mid-forearm laceration that required repair of both the median and ulnar nerves 4 years earlier. *Which one of the following is correct when considering tendon transfers for this patient?*
   A. Previous compliance with physiotherapy is no longer relevant to this scenario.
   B. One single tendon transfer can be used to address the deficits described.
   C. An EIP tendon transfer is more likely to be successful than a PL (Camitz) or FDS tendon transfer for thumb opposition.
   D. An ADM (Huber) transfer is more likely to be successful than a PL (Camitz) or FDS tendon transfer for thumb opposition.
   E. Previously denervated MRC grade III muscles may be used as donors for transfer.

COMPLICATIONS AFTER TENDON TRANSFERS

10. *Which one of the following scenarios is most likely to lead to a failed tendon transfer?*
    A. A PT to ECRB transfer at the same time as radial nerve exploration in the arm
    B. An EIP to EPL transfer 3 months after a distal radius fracture
    C. A tibialis posterior to tibialis anterior transfer at the same time as a tumor excision from the common peroneal nerve
    D. A tendon transfer in the forearm under a mature, pliable ALT flap
    E. A lateral band transfer to correct a stiff swan neck deformity

TENDON TRANSFERS IN RHEUMATOID ARTHRITIS

11. A patient with rheumatoid arthritis presents with spontaneous inability to extend the IP joint of the thumb. The remaining digits are unaffected. *Which one of the following tendons is commonly transferred to reinstate function in this situation?*
    A. FCR
    B. EDC
    C. APL
    D. EIP
    E. FDP

Answers

PRINCIPLES OF TENDON TRANSFER

1. *Which one of the following is a usual feature of a donor muscle selected for tendon transfer?*

   B. A synergistic action to the muscle it is replacing

   When considering tendon transfers it is vital that passive motion of any joints involved is optimized and the soft-tissue envelope is supple. Beyond this, there are six key principles that underpin tendon transfer in relation to the donor and recipient muscles. These can be remembered with the mnemonic SPEEPS: **S**ingle function, **P**ower (adequate), **E**xpendable, **E**xcursion, **P**ull, **S**ynergistic.

   When considering a transfer, each transferred tendon should ideally restore a single function. The donor must be adequately powered; so, ideally the transferred muscle/tendon will have similar power to the unit being replaced. Medical Research Council (MRC) grade for the donor muscle should ideally be grade V, although grade IV can also be adequate. The donor muscle must be expendable (e.g., one wrist flexor or extensor should be preserved). The excursion or amplitude of the transferred tendon should be similar to the excursion being replaced, but it does not have to be greater. The line of pull or vector should be similar between donor and recipient action and avoid pulleys wherever possible. The transferred donor and recipient muscles should ideally be synergistic. For example, finger flexion is optimal with wrist extension; so, using a wrist extensor for finger flexion is advantageous when it comes to rehabilitation.[1,2]

REFERENCES

1. Beasley RW. Principles of tendon transfer. Orthop Clin North Am 1970;1(2):433–438
2. Richards RR. Tendon transfers for failed nerve reconstruction. Clin Plast Surg 2003;30(2):223–245, vi

INDICATIONS FOR TENDON TRANSFER

2. *What is the most common indication for tendon transfer?*

   A. Nerve injury alone

   The most common indication for tendon transfer is nerve injury. This may be required because repair or grafting of the nerve is not possible, due to delay or extent of injury, or because the distance to reinnervation is too long (e.g., some brachial plexus injuries). Tendon transfer may also be indicated when previous attempts at repair have failed, or to reduce the need for splinting when nerve recovery is awaited (e.g., PT to ECRB for wrist control while a radial nerve repair recovers). The other options listed each represent potential reasons for tendon transfer. Medical diseases where limb function is impaired, such as poliomyelitis or leprosy, represent potential indications for tendon transfer, but the disease must be well controlled before undertaking surgery.[1,2]

REFERENCES

1. Beasley RW. Principles of tendon transfer. Orthop Clin North Am 1970;1(2):433–438
2. Richards RR. Tendon transfers for failed nerve reconstruction. Clin Plast Surg 2003;30(2):223–245, vi

CONTRAINDICATIONS FOR TENDON TRANSFER

3. *Which one of the following conditions is the most significant contraindication to tendon transfer?*

   B. Fluctuating spasticity

   Although sometimes very useful, tendon transfers can also be unpredictable in spasticity, such as in cerebral palsy. This is particularly true where spasticity is variable, such as in athetoid movements. Where a deficit or ability is variable, tendon transfer should be avoided.

   Diabetes mellitus is not a significant contraindication to tendon transfer, but glycemic control should be optimized as for any surgery. A stable deficit post-poliomyelitis can respond well to a tendon transfer where a suitable donor is available; however, sufficient recovery time should have elapsed before surgery is considered.

   Rheumatoid arthritis can provide many opportunities for a tendon transfer, such as EIP to EPL or crossed intrinsic transfer during MCP joint realignment. It is important to address the underlying cause first by controlling the disease medically, debriding active synovitis and excising osteophytes, or addressing other bony prominences (such as a prominent ulnar head). A tendon transfer can be helpful if repair or grafting of a tendon defect has failed; however, any causes for the first failure should be addressed (e.g., prominent hardware, abnormal bony prominences, poor patient compliance with therapy, or infection).[1–3]

REFERENCES

1. Phalen GS, Miller RC. The transfer of wrist extensor muscles to restore or reinforce flexion power of the fingers and opposition of the thumb. J Bone Joint Surg Am 1947;29(4): 993–997
2. Sammer DM, Chung KC. Tendon transfers: part I. Principles of transfer and transfers for radial nerve palsy. Plast Reconstr Surg 2009;123(5):169e–177e
3. Sammer DM, Chung KC. Tendon transfers: Part II. Transfers for ulnar nerve palsy and median nerve palsy. Plast Reconstr Surg 2009;124(3):212e–221e

INDICATIONS FOR TENDON TRANSFER

4. *In which one of the following scenarios might an immediate tendon transfer be indicated in a young, otherwise healthy patient?*

   C. Radial nerve repair at midhumeral level

   Tendon transfers are more commonly performed as delayed procedures, as there are many factors to optimize before surgery, such as allowing any recovery to develop, allowing scar tissue to improve, or infection to settle. One good indication for an immediate tendon transfer is to augment function while waiting for prolonged nerve recovery, or where the prognosis for nerve or muscle recovery is poor. A good example of this is using a PT to ECRB transfer to act as an internal wrist splint for a patient with a high radial nerve injury while recovery is awaited. This potentially frees the patient from an external splint and puts the hand in a better position for using the remaining median and ulnar innervated muscles.[1]

   Tendon transfers can be helpful in leprosy, but the disease must be controlled first.[2,3] An immediate PL transfer for thumb abduction/opposition (Camitz procedure) is sometimes used in carpal tunnel syndrome with thenar wasting, which is more common in elderly patients or others expected to make a poor recovery. In a young, healthy patient with only partial thenar wasting, it would be more common to simply decompress the carpal tunnel and allow a period of recovery before considering a tendon transfer.

   When resurfacing a scarred limb, it is usual to allow the soft-tissue envelope to mature and soften before undertaking tendon transfers, as there is a high risk of adhesions and poor excursion if an immediate transfer is done. Following an immediate distal nerve repair, such as the ulnar nerve at the wrist, recovery is expected to occur much sooner than with a proximal injury, so tendon transfer in this setting is unlikely to be required. It is usual to perform these transfers with regional block; however, there are reports of doing this safely and effectively under local anesthetic, the so-called wide awake local anesthetic surgery (WALANT).[2,3]

REFERENCES

1. Sammer DM, Chung KC. Tendon transfers: part I. Principles of transfer and transfers for radial nerve palsy. Plast Reconstr Surg 2009;123(5):169e–177e
2. Mohammed AK, Lalonde DH. Wide awake tendon transfers in leprosy patients in India. Hand Clin 2019;35(1):67–84
3. Abdullah S, Ahmad AA, Lalonde D. Wide awake local anesthesia no tourniquet forearm triple tendon transfer in radial nerve palsy. Plast Reconstr Surg Glob Open 2020;8(8):e3023

TRANSFERS IN MEDIAN NERVE PALSY

5. You see a 20-year-old patient with poor recovery following a median nerve division at the wrist 2 years earlier. She asks about potential reconstructive options. *Which one of the following tendon transfers would best address thenar muscle denervation?*

   A. An EIP transfer around the ulnar border of the wrist

   Common options for restoration of thumb opposition/flexion include a radial innervated EIP transfer around the ulnar border of the hand, or a proximal median nerve innervated ring finger FDS transfer. The FDP should not be sacrificed because of the unacceptable digital flexion deficit that would result.

   The Huber transfer uses abductor digiti minimi as a transfer across the palm to restore thumb abduction/opposition. It is more commonly performed in children, where it can be helpful in addressing thumb hypoplasia. It is less common in adults, as there are other options which may be simpler, and the cosmetic appearance can be disappointing because of the bridge of muscle crossing the palm.

   The PL can also be transferred with a strip of palmar fascia to augment length (Camitz transfer). However, the vector would be poor and the length insufficient if passed around the FCU, and in this scenario the PL may well have been injured. The FCR is not a good pulley to route an FDS transfer for thumb opposition/abduction around as the vector is incorrect.[1-4]

REFERENCES

1. Beasley RW. Principles of tendon transfer. Orthop Clin North Am 1970;1(2):433–438
2. Huber E. Hilfsoperation bei Medianuslähmung. Deutsche Zeitschrift für Chirurgie 1921;162:271–275
3. Littler JW, Cooley SG. Opposition of the thumb and its restoration by abductor digiti quinti transfer. J Bone Joint Surg Am 1963;45:1389–1396
4. Burkhalter WE. Early tendon transfer in upper extremity peripheral nerve injury. Clin Orthop Relat Res 1974;(104):68–79

TRANSFERS IN ULNAR NERVE PALSY

6. A patient presents with full FCU (MRC grade V) and incomplete FDP (MRC grade IV) recovery but persistent clawing 18 months after an ulnar nerve repair at the elbow. *Which one of the following is contraindicated in this case?*

    B. A ring finger FDS tendon transfer to the lateral bands to correct the clawing

    Although a transfer of the ring finger FDS tendon to the lateral bands could provide good correction of clawing, it would leave the ring finger unacceptably weak, since the FDP to this digit has been denervated and is not fully recovered. Many patients manage perfectly well with a long-term ulnar claw splint, or with no intervention at all; so, it is important to check whether they are content with a splint before embarking on complex reconstruction. Options C and E can also be used successfully in ulnar palsy.[1]

REFERENCE

1. Sammer DM, Chung KC. Tendon transfers: Part II. Transfers for ulnar nerve palsy and median nerve palsy. Plast Reconstr Surg 2009;124(3):212e–221e

TENDON TRANSFERS IN RADIAL NERVE PALSY

7. You are considering tendon transfers for a young, healthy man 4 months after repair of a radial nerve injury at the elbow. *Which one of the following statements is correct?*

    A. Recovery of some wrist extension would be expected by this stage.

    When considering tendon transfers, it is important to understand the expected timescale for nerve regeneration after repair/graft and the likely extent of nerve and muscle recovery, otherwise an unnecessary transfer might be undertaken. The ECRL and the ECRB are supplied very proximally; hence, there should be some wrist extension by 4 months. Although there may be signs of EDC reinnervation, it is unlikely to be strong at this stage. EPL recovery occurs late and may still remain sufficient up to 1 year after injury, as the PIN motor branch enters the muscle more distally in the forearm. Nerve recovery is typically 1 mm/day. EMG studies can be helpful to demonstrate early signs of reinnervation before significant clinical signs of recovery. If EPL displayed early recovery on EMG, a transfer would usually be postponed. Re-repair of a recovering nerve will sacrifice the recovered function and prolong the time to reinnervation of distal muscles. It is therefore unlikely to produce a superior outcome.[1]

REFERENCE

1. Bumbasirevic M, Palibrk T, Lesic A, Atkinson H. Radial nerve palsy. EFORT Open Rev 2017;1(8):286–294

TENDON TRANSFER IN RADIAL NERVE INJURY

8. *When treating a radial nerve palsy, which one of the following is most likely to cause a functional problem when planning a combined transfer with PT to ECRB?*

    D. PT to ECRB, FCR to APL, FCU to EDC, PL to EPL

    Tendon transfers are tailored to each individual patient and according to surgeon experience and preference. One of the core principles is to avoid creating an unacceptable donor deficit. Scenario D would give good wrist and digital extension but at the unacceptable cost of preventing adequate wrist flexion, because both wrist flexors have been used (FCU and FCR). All of the other combinations address the deficits following radial nerve palsy without severe donor morbidity. PT is usually transferred to ECRB in radial nerve injuries to provide wrist extension, but ECRL and ECU are not usually reconstructed. FCR may be transferred to EPB and APL together to provide thumb extension and abduction. FCU or FCR may be used to provide digital extension by transfer to EDC; however, it is preferable not to sacrifice FCU in most scenarios. PL or FDS ring may be used to provide thumb extension by transfer to EPL.[1-4]

REFERENCES

1. Ropars M, Dréano T, Siret P, Belot N, Langlais F. Long-term results of tendon transfers in radial and posterior interosseous nerve paralysis. J Hand Surg [Br] 2006;31(5):502–506

2. Sammer DM, Chung KC. Tendon transfers: part I. Principles of transfer and transfers for radial nerve palsy. Plast Reconstr Surg 2009;123(5):169e–177e
3. Krishnan KG, Schackert G. An analysis of results after selective tendon transfers through the interosseous membrane to provide selective finger and thumb extension in chronic irreparable radial nerve lesions. J Hand Surg Am 2008;33(2):223–231
4. Kruft S, von Heimburg D, Reill P. Treatment of irreversible lesion of the radial nerve by tendon transfer: indication and long-term results of the Merle d'Aubigné procedure. Plast Reconstr Surg 1997;100(3):610–616, discussion 617–618

TRANSFERS IN COMBINED NERVE PALSIES

9. You have a patient with persistent wasting of the thenar eminence muscle group and mild clawing of the digits after a mid-forearm laceration that required repair of both the median and ulnar nerves 4 years earlier. *Which one of the following is correct when considering tendon transfers for this patient?*

C. **An EIP tendon transfer is more likely to be more successful than a PL (Camitz) or FDS tendon transfer for thumb opposition.**

A radial nerve-innervated EIP transfer[1] will be preferable to either a PL or FDS transfer for thumb opposition/abduction, as these muscles are innervated by the median nerve and may also have had direct damage to the muscle belly at the time of injury. A Huber transfer,[2,3] which uses the abductor digiti minimi muscle, is innervated by the ulnar nerve and is unlikely to have recovered well, given that the patient still has other signs of intrinsic muscle denervation.

"One tendon transfer, one function" is one of the core principles when planning a series of transfers, and it is always sensible to review compliance with physiotherapy before undertaking complex upper limb reconstruction. While previously denervated muscles may be used if adequately recovered, it is preferable to use an uninjured donor where possible and MRC grade III power is insufficient for use as a transfer.

REFERENCES

1. Burkhalter WE. Early tendon transfer in upper extremity peripheral nerve injury. Clin Orthop Relat Res 1974; (104):68–79
2. Beasley RW. Principles of tendon transfer. Orthop Clin North Am 1970;1(2):433–438
3. Huber E. Hilfsoperation bei Medianuslähmung. Deutsche Zeitschrift für Chirurgie 1921;162:271–275

COMPLICATIONS AFTER TENDON TRANSFERS

10. *Which one of the following scenarios is most likely to lead to a failed tendon transfer?*

E. **A lateral band transfer to correct a stiff swan neck deformity**

Scenario E demonstrates a violation of one of the core principles of tendon transfer, that is, joints must already be supple enough for functional range of motion before tendon transfer is undertaken. There will likely be a failure to correct, an early recurrence of the original deformity, or adhesions leading to stiffness if a transfer is performed in this scenario. Therefore, the PIP joint should be released as a first stage, with a delayed lateral band transfer once a stable range of joint movement is obtained and the soft-tissue envelope has settled again.[1,2]

Scenarios A through D demonstrate tendon transfers that may be appropriate. It is often sensible to perform an early tendon transfer, despite anticipated nerve recovery to improve quality of life, if this spares the patient from requiring an external splint and the recovery time is likely to be prolonged. As such, PT to ECRB transfer can allow a patient with radial nerve palsy to manage without a bulky wrist splint; likewise, a tibialis posterior to anterior transfer can obviate the need for a foot drop splint in patients with common peroneal nerve injury.[3] EPL rupture can occur with distal radius fractures due to direct injury or ischemia in the third extensor compartment. The EIP passes through a different compartment and is therefore unlikely to rupture following transfer to the EPL. Transfers can be routed beneath a flap reconstruction, but the soft-tissue envelope must be soft and pliable.

REFERENCES

1. de Bruin M, van Vliet DC, Smeulders MJ, Kreulen M. Long-term results of lateral band translocation for the correction of swan neck deformity in cerebral palsy. J Pediatr Orthop 2010;30(1):67–70
2. Foucher G, Tilquin B, Lenoble E. Treatment of post-traumatic swan-neck deformities of the fingers. Apropos of a series of 43 patients [in French]. Rev Chir Orthop Repar Appar Mot 1992;78(8):505–511
3. Krishnamurthy S, Ibrahim M. Tendon transfers in foot drop. Indian J Plast Surg 2019;52(1):100–108

TENDON TRANSFERS IN RHEUMATOID ARTHRITIS

11. A patient with rheumatoid arthritis presents with spontaneous inability to extend the IP joint of the thumb. The remaining digits are unaffected. *Which one of the following tendons is commonly transferred to reinstate function in this situation?*

    D. EIP

       This patient demonstrates spontaneous rupture of the EPL tendon with inability to extend the IP joint. This can occur in advanced rheumatoid arthritis where attrition rupture develops from synovitis or abrasion on bony spurs along the course of the EPL, particularly under the extensor retinaculum and over the carpus. The advantage of using the EIP tendon is that index finger extension can be maintained by the EDC and the path of the tendon transfer avoids some of the areas of previous damage. It is a straightforward procedure to undertake with minimal exposure required. The distal EPL is identified by making a longitudinal incision over the first metacarpal. The EIP is identified at the index MCP joint and is differentiated from the EDC tendon by its more ulnar position and insertion. A small incision allows this tendon to be divided at the extensor expansion. A second, proximal incision over the base of the second metacarpal allows the tendon to be retrieved before being rerouted subcutaneously to the distal stump of the EPL. A Pulvertaft weave is performed with the thumb and wrist in full extension. It is, of course, important to ensure that the EDC to the index finger is intact before transferring the EIP, as there may be multiple tendon ruptures in rheumatoid arthritis. Other tendon transfers for EPL rupture include ring finger FDS and palmaris longus. The FCR is sometimes used for APL and EPB but not EPL. The EDC is usually avoided, as this would give a mass extension action to the digits and thumb. The FDP tendon harvest would sacrifice the DIP joint flexion, which is not generally acceptable.[1]

REFERENCE

1. Biehl C, Rupp M, Kern S, Heiss C, ElKhassawna T, Szalay G. Extensor tendon ruptures in rheumatoid wrists. Eur J Orthop Surg Traumatol 2020;30(8):1499–1504

83. Nerve Transfers

See *Essentials of Plastic Surgery*, third edition, pp. 1163–1174

PRINCIPLES OF NERVE TRANSFER

1. A patient presents with a large neuroma in continuity with little evidence of distal nerve recovery 6 months following a grafted segmental median nerve injury in the upper arm due to impaling. You are looking for a suitable more distal nerve transfer to restore some hand function. *Which one of the following is an ideal characteristic in a donor nerve for transfer in this case?*
   A. A mixed motor and sensory nerve to provide recovery of both functions
   B. A small number of axons dedicated to the desired functional reinnervation
   C. A nerve with postinjury recovery to at least Medical Research Council (MRC) grade 4 motor function
   D. A smaller diameter than the recipient nerve to minimize axonal loss during regeneration
   E. Sufficient proximity to the recipient nerve to avoid using a nerve graft

PRINCIPLES OF NERVE TRANSFER

2. A young woman has a complete right-side brachial plexus avulsion with spinal accessory nerve palsy. *Which one of the following principles of nerve transfer is applied when using the phrenic nerve as a donor to restore elbow flexion in this case?*
   A. A synergistic donor and recipient nerve function
   B. A primary coaptation without need for an intervening nerve graft
   C. An ability to shorten the reinnervation distance
   D. A fully expendable donor nerve function
   E. Selection of an uninjured nerve for transfer

INDICATIONS FOR NERVE TRANSFER

3. *Which one of the following represents a key indication for nerve transfer following an upper limb motor nerve injury?*
   A. A complete distal nerve transection
   B. A complete nerve gap of 2 cm
   C. A recovering motor nerve palsy at 4 weeks postinjury
   D. Minimal evidence of motor nerve recovery 20 months postinjury
   E. A long distance between injury level and motor endplates

UPPER LIMB NERVE TRANSFER TECHNIQUES

4. You have opted for early surgical management of a closed C5/6 root avulsion with surgery planned for 2 months postinjury. *Which one of the following is the preferred technique when transferring the spinal accessory nerve to the suprascapular nerve to restore shoulder abduction?*
   A. Reverse end-to-side (supercharged) coaptation
   B. End-to-end coaptation
   C. End-to-side coaptation
   D. Combined nerve graft and end-to-end coaptation
   E. Combined nerve graft and end-to-side coaptation

NERVE TRANSFERS FOR SHOULDER FUNCTION

5. A 32-year-old man presents with isolated serratus anterior palsy causing symptomatic winging of the scapular. *Which one of the following is a common nerve transfer that might stabilize his scapula with minimal donor nerve morbidity?*
   A. Intercostal nerves to long thoracic nerve transfer
   B. Thoracodorsal nerve to long thoracic nerve transfer
   C. Medial pectoral nerve to long thoracic nerve transfer
   D. Thoracodorsal nerve to axillary nerve transfer
   E. Spinal accessory nerve to suprascapular nerve transfer

NERVE TRANSFERS FOR SHOULDER FUNCTION

6. A 24-year-old man takes a fall at high speed from his motorcycle and presents with evidence of a C5/6 root avulsion. *Which one of the following would be a common procedure to restore effective shoulder abduction for him?*
   A. Single nerve transfer coapting spinal accessory to suprascapular nerve.
   B. Single nerve transfer coapting medial triceps nerve branch to axillary nerve.
   C. Single nerve transfer coapting thoracodorsal nerve to axillary nerve.
   D. Combined nerve transfer coapting spinal accessory to suprascapular and triceps nerve branch to axillary nerve.
   E. Combined nerve transfer coapting spinal accessory to suprascapular and thoracodorsal to axillary nerve.

PRIORITY FOR FUNCTION IN THE UPPER LIMB

7. *Following a brachial plexus injury, which one of the following is generally the first priority for restoration of function?*
   A. Elbow flexion
   B. Elbow extension
   C. Shoulder stabilization
   D. Wrist extension
   E. Digital flexion

NERVE TRANSFERS FOR ELBOW FLEXION

8. A 40-year-old female sustains a C5/6 root avulsion falling from her horse. *Which one of the following is considered to be the "gold standard" nerve transfer to restore her elbow flexion?*
   A. Phrenic nerve to brachialis branch of musculocutaneous nerve
   B. Spinal accessory nerve to biceps branch of musculocutaneous nerve
   C. Flexor carpi ulnaris fascicle to biceps branch of musculocutaneous nerve
   D. Supinator nerve branch to brachioradialis branch of radial nerve
   E. Flexor carpi radialis (FCR) fascicle to brachialis branch of musculocutaneous nerve

WRIST AND DIGIT EXTENSION IN BRACHIAL PLEXUS INJURY

9. *Which one of the following nerve transfers would be indicated to restore both wrist and digit extension following delayed presentation of a radial nerve injury at the proximal humerus?*
   A. Single nerve transfer of flexor digitorum superficialis (FDS) nerve branches to extensor carpi radialis brevis
   B. Single nerve transfer of FCR nerve branches to posterior interosseous nerve
   C. Single nerve transfer of supinator motor branch to posterior interosseous nerve
   D. Dual nerve transfer with FDS nerve branches to extensor carpi radialis brevis combined with FCR branch to posterior interosseous nerve.
   E. Dual nerve transfer with pronator quadratus nerve branches to posterior interosseous nerve and supinator nerve branches to extensor carpi ulnaris.

NERVE TRANSFER FOR INTRINSIC HAND FUNCTION

10. *Which one of the following is generally considered the "gold standard" donor for nerve transfer restoration of intrinsic hand function following ulnar nerve injury in the proximal forearm or arm?*
    A. Posterior interosseous nerve branch to extensor carpi radialis brevis
    B. Musculocutaneous nerve branch to brachialis
    C. Anterior interosseous branch to pronator quadratus
    D. Median nerve motor branch to flexor carpi radialis (FCR)
    E. Radial nerve branch to medial triceps

Answers

PRINCIPLES OF NERVE TRANSFER

1. A patient presents with a large neuroma in continuity with little evidence of distal nerve recovery 6 months following a grafted segmental median nerve injury in the upper arm due to impaling. You are looking for a suitable more distal nerve transfer to restore some hand function. *Which one of the following is an ideal characteristic in a donor nerve for transfer in this case?*

   E. Sufficient proximity to the recipient nerve to avoid using a nerve graft

   In this scenario, there is no realistic prospect of meaningful distal motor reinnervation from revision of the neuroma given the distance and the time since injury. The time elapsed is of less relevance for sensory function. Nerve transfers could be used to shorten the reinnervation distance, provided a suitable expendable donor is available which is distal enough to allow reinnervation before motor end plate degeneration, is close enough to coapt directly without grafting, and is ideally synergistic in function to aid rehabilitation. The ideal donor should be predominantly motor or sensory to match the desired outcome, it should have a large axon count (particularly in a motor transfer), it should be well matched in size to the recipient to facilitate an accurate coaptation, and it should ideally have normal function with no previous injury. Example donors in this case would be branches of the radial nerve (extensor carpi radialis brevis [ECRB]/supinator) or the brachialis branch of the musculocutaneous nerve onto the anterior interosseous nerve (AIN).[1-3]

REFERENCES

1. Weber RV, Davidge KM. Nerve transfer for the forearm and hand. In: Mackinnon S, ed. Nerve Surgery. New York: Thieme; 2015
2. Lee SK, Wolfe SW. Nerve transfers for the upper extremity: new horizons in nerve reconstruction. J Am Acad Orthop Surg 2012;20(8):506–517
3. Tung TH, Mackinnon SE. Nerve transfers: indications, techniques, and outcomes. J Hand Surg Am 2010;35(2):332–341

PRINCIPLES OF NERVE TRANSFER

2. A young woman has a complete right-side brachial plexus avulsion with spinal accessory nerve palsy. *Which one of the following principles of nerve transfer is applied when using the phrenic nerve as a donor to restore elbow flexion in this case?*

   E. Selection of an uninjured nerve for transfer

   A key principle for selection of a donor nerve for nerve transfer is that it is uninjured and has a full MRC grade 5 function. In this case, this does apply to the phrenic nerve. However, it is still generally reserved for last resort reconstructive reinnervation procedures, as it has both a significant donor-site deficit (albeit usually transient) and is not synergistic to upper limb motor function, and therefore can be more difficult to rehabilitate. Its use would usually reflect there being very few suitable donor nerves available, such as a situation with complete root avulsion C5–T1 and where the spinal accessory nerve has also been injured. Many surgeons would prefer to use intercostal nerves rather than the phrenic nerve to reinnervate the elbow flexors because of the limitations described.

   A key element of any donor nerve is that it is expendable and while the phrenic nerve is considered to be expendable when required in scenarios of last resort, which does rely on the patient having sufficient respiratory reserve to withstand 1 to 2 years of measurably reduced respiratory function and a permanent reduction in inspiratory force generated.[1] The negative effects on respiratory function seem to be much greater when the right phrenic nerve is used rather than the left.[2] Its use is therefore not recommended in the presence of multiple rib fractures, significant underlying lung disease, or where there are problems with the contralateral hemidiaphragm. In patients with no underlying respiratory problems, the measurable reduction in lung function does not necessarily correspond to a clinical problem, even if both phrenic and some intercostal nerves are harvested.[3]

   Because the phrenic nerve in the neck is proximal/medial and short in length, an intervening nerve graft is usually required to transfer its function to that of elbow flexion.[4] It therefore does not facilitate shortening of the reinnervation distance that would have been achieved if direct repair or nerve grafting of the plexus injury had been possible to restore elbow flexion. There are, however, thoracoscopic techniques reported to harvest the phrenic nerve distally at its insertion to the diaphragm, greatly increasing its length and facilitating direct coaptation.[5,6]

REFERENCES

1. Xu WD, Gu YD, Lu JB, Yu C, Zhang CG, Xu JG. Pulmonary function after complete unilateral phrenic nerve transection. J Neurosurg 2005;103(3):464–467
2. Luedemann W, Hamm M, Blömer U, Samii M, Tatagiba M. Brachial plexus neurotization with donor phrenic nerves and its effect on pulmonary function. J Neurosurg 2002;96(3):523–526
3. Malungpaishope K, Leechavengvongs S, Ratchawatana P, et al. Simultaneous phrenic and intercostal nerves transfer for elbow flexion and extension in total brachial plexus root avulsion injury. J Hand Surg Asian Pac Vol 2018;23(4):496–500
4. Siqueira MG, Martins RS. Phrenic nerve transfer in the restoration of elbow flexion in brachial plexus avulsion injuries: how effective and safe is it? Neurosurgery 2009;65(4, Suppl):A125–A131
5. Xu WD, Gu YD. Clinical application report of phrenic nerve transfer for treatment of brachial plexus injury through thoracoscopy. Chin J Hand Surg 2000;16:94–97
6. Xu WD, Gu YD, Xu JG, Tan LJ. Full-length phrenic nerve transfer by means of video-assisted thoracic surgery in treating brachial plexus avulsion injury. Plast Reconstr Surg 2002;110(1):104–109, discusion 110–111

INDICATIONS FOR NERVE TRANSFER

3. *Which one of the following represents a key indication for nerve transfer following an upper limb motor nerve injury?*

   E. **A long distance between injury level and motor endplates**

   There are a number of key indications for nerve transfer following motor nerve injury in the upper limb, for example, in cases where a primary nerve repair is not possible, a nerve graft is unlikely to be successful, and where there is a long distance between the level of injury and the target muscle. In cases where nerve grafts greater than 7 cm are required, the outcomes tend to be poor. The benefit of using a nerve transfer in cases where there is a long distance between the injury and the target muscle is that it may prevent irreversible changes to the motor endplates which will occur if they remain denervated for more than about 14 months. By shortening the distance required for nerve recovery, this can sometimes be avoided. This is particularly important in cases where there is a delayed presentation following nerve injury. Nerve transfers are less often used in more distal nerve injuries, as the distance to nerve recovery is shorter and hence there is less of a time constraint in relation to the motor end plates. In these scenarios, nerve repair or grafting is generally preferred. Most nerve gaps of 2 cm can be repaired effectively with nerve grafts. A nerve injury with early signs of recovery does not usually warrant nerve or tendon transfer, as this suggests a neuropraxia and that recovery will continue. In some cases, a tendon transfer may be considered (e.g. pronator teres to ECRB end to side in a high radial nerve injury) in order to provide wrist extension as an alternative to an external splint in the interim, while recovery occurs.

   If there is no evidence of recovery at 20 months post–motor nerve injury, then the motor endplates are unlikely to remain functional; so, the window of opportunity has been missed in terms of benefits of nerve transfer. Contraindications to nerve transfer include an extended time interval between injury and transfer (usually more than 14–18 months is considered too long), where there is no expendable donor, and where the donor nerve has a motor strength below MRC grade M4.[1,2]

REFERENCES

1. Tung TH, Mackinnon SE. Nerve transfers: indications, techniques, and outcomes. J Hand Surg Am 2010;35(2):332–341
2. Mackinnon SE, Colbert SH. Nerve transfers in the hand and upper extremity surgery. Tech Hand Up Extrem Surg 2008;12(1):20–33

UPPER LIMB NERVE TRANSFER TECHNIQUES

4. You have opted for early surgical management of a closed C5/6 root avulsion with surgery planned for 2 months postinjury. *Which one of the following is the preferred technique when transferring the spinal accessory nerve to the suprascapular nerve to restore shoulder abduction?*

   B. **End-to-end coaptation**

   In general, there are some key technical principles in nerve transfer surgery which need to be adhered to in order to optimize functional outcomes.

   In this example, when considering reinnervation of the suprascapular nerve territory to restore glenohumeral stability, initiation of shoulder abduction and external rotation of the upper limb, the maximum number of motor fascicles available should be directed into the recipient nerve. This is generally achieved by having the shortest distance for reinnervation to occur, with the least coaptation possible and by performing the most direct repair which will normally be an end-to-end coaptation. Any interposed nerve graft requires an additional coaptation, increases length of the reinnervation pathway, and reduces the number of axons reaching the target muscles, as there will always be losses crossing even the most technically excellent coaptation site.[1] In this scenario, as the recipient nerve is completely denervated with no prospect of recovery, an end-to-end coaptation will be preferred especially as this will not be sacrificing any residual function that might have been spared by a supercharged reverse end-to-side technique, and will target a greater number of regenerating axons to the distal target than an end-to-side technique. A supercharged reverse end-to-side technique would involve dividing the spinal accessory nerve and coapting it end to side onto an epineurial window in the suprascapular nerve. Conversely, an end-to-side coaptation would involve suturing the distal divided stump of the nonfunctioning suprascapular nerve onto the side of the intact spinal accessory nerve, and has not been demonstrated to be reliable, particularly if no donor axonal injury is induced (**Fig. 83.1**).[2]

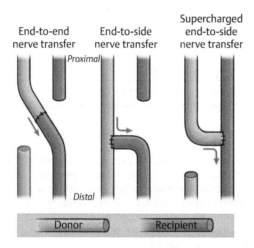

Fig. 83.1: Three types of nerve coaptations. End-to-end is the gold standard for all transfers and the only functional anastomosis for motor nerve transfers. End-to-side is preferred for sensory nerve transfers. Reverse end-to-side, or supercharged, coaptations are utilized to provide small but quick reinnervation of motor endplates while primary or transferred nerve axons regenerate.

REFERENCES

1. Tung TH, Mackinnon SE. Nerve transfers: indications, techniques, and outcomes. J Hand Surg Am 2010;35(2):332–341
2. Pienaar C, Swan MC, De Jager W, Solomons M. Clinical experience with end-to-side nerve transfer. J Hand Surg [Br] 2004;29(5):438–443

NERVE TRANSFERS FOR SHOULDER FUNCTION

5. A 32-year-old man presents with isolated serratus anterior palsy causing symptomatic winging of the scapular. *Which one of the following is a common nerve transfer that might stabilize his scapula with minimal donor nerve morbidity?*

B. Thoracodorsal nerve to long thoracic nerve transfer

Isolated long thoracic nerve palsy resulting in serratus anterior paralysis and scapula winging is usually a closed traction injury related to exercise. Initial management is most commonly nonoperative with physiotherapy to reduce abnormal adaptive movements and reduce stretching out of the weak or paralyzed serratus anterior muscle. In those patients who are not progressing with a recovery of function, a nerve transfer using the thoracodorsal nerve as a donor coapted end-to-end onto the long thoracic nerve to serratus anterior can restore function over a short reinnervation distance. It is technically fairly straightforward as the two nerves are in close proximity either side of a relatively bloodless dissection plane on an accessible area of the chest wall.[1]

Transfer of the medial pectoral nerve has also been described for long thoracic nerve palsy, but is much less common, involves more dissection, and may require interpositional grafting to achieve reach.[2] There has been a cadaveric study supporting intercostal nerve transfer.

This study showed that the size match was reasonable between the donor and recipient nerves and that the required donor site nerve length was adequate to perform direct end-to-end coaptation. This would not be a synergistic transfer.[3] A thoracodorsal nerve to axillary nerve transfer can be used to improve shoulder function by reinnervating the deltoid and teres minor but is not relevant in this scenario.[4] A spinal accessory nerve to suprascapular nerve transfer would be indicated to reinnervate the infraspinatus and supraspinatus muscles in order to improve shoulder abduction following plexus injury but again is not relevant in this scenario.[5]

REFERENCES

1. Mackinnon SE, Yee A. 2011 Thoracodorsal to long thoracic nerve transfer. Video at: https://surgicaleducation.wustl.edu/thoracodorsal-long-thoracic-nerve-transfer/. Accessed December 2020
2. Tomaino MM. Neurophysiologic and clinical outcome following medial pectoral to long thoracic nerve transfer for scapular winging: a case report. Microsurgery 2002;22(6): 254–257
3. Louis RG Jr, Whitesides JD, Kollias TF, Iwanaga J, Tubbs RS, Loukas M. Intercostal nerve to long thoracic nerve transfer for the treatment of winged scapula: a cadaveric feasibility study. Cureus 2017;9(11):e1898
4. Samardzic MM, Grujicic DM, Rasulic LG, Milicic BR. The use of thoracodorsal nerve transfer in restoration of irreparable C5 and C6 spinal nerve lesions. Br J Plast Surg 2005;58(4): 541–546
5. Bertelli JA, Ghizoni MF. Results of spinal accessory to suprascapular nerve transfer in 110 patients with complete palsy of the brachial plexus. J Neurosurg Spine 2016;24(6): 990–995

NERVE TRANSFERS FOR SHOULDER FUNCTION

6. A 24-year-old man takes a fall at high speed from his motorcycle and presents with evidence of a C5/6 root avulsion. *Which one of the following would be a common procedure to restore effective shoulder abduction for him?*

  D. Combined nerve transfer coapting spinal accessory to suprascapular and triceps nerve branch to axillary nerve.

  When a patient sustains a C5/6 root avulsion, there is a significant impact on their upper limb function with loss of shoulder control and elbow flexion. Specific nerves which are targeted for reinnervation include the suprascapular and axillary nerves. The suprascapular nerve normally innervates the supraspinatus and infraspinatus muscles which abduct and externally rotate the upper arm, respectively. The suprascapular nerve also has a role in proprioception of the glenohumeral joint, acromioclavicular joint, the subacromial bursa, and the scapula. The axillary nerve normally innervates deltoid and teres minor muscles. These serve to abduct the shoulder and externally rotate the upper limb, respectively. Each also helps stabilize the glenohumeral joint and shoulder. When a root avulsion occurs, there is no way to directly repair this and nerve transfers are therefore indicated to try and regain innervation to these key muscles. Combining a nerve transfer to each nerve is believed to optimize functional outcome and is currently considered to be the "gold standard" with superior results being shown compared with either transfer alone. The spinal accessory is transferred to the suprascapular nerve and a triceps nerve branch to the axillary nerve.[1–3]

  The most distal branch of the spinal accessory nerve to the lower trapezius is ideally used to minimize morbidity of the nerve sacrifice. Coaptation with the suprascapular nerve is performed as close to the suprascapular notch as possible and this may be undertaken with either an anterior or posterior approach. The radial nerve is used to reinnervate the axillary nerve and most commonly the branch to the long head of triceps is chosen as it contains more motor axons. Alternatively, the branch to the medial head may be used as it is longer and easier to isolate. These can also be performed via anterior or posterior approaches.[1–3]

REFERENCES

1. Merrell GA, Barrie KA, Katz DL, Wolfe SW. Results of nerve transfer techniques for restoration of shoulder and elbow function in the context of a meta-analysis of the English literature. J Hand Surg Am 2001;26(2):303–314
2. Garg R, Merrell GA, Hillstrom HJ, Wolfe SW. Comparison of nerve transfers and nerve grafting for traumatic upper plexus palsy: a systematic review and analysis. J Bone Joint Surg Am 2011;93(9):819–829
3. Bertelli JA, Ghizoni MF. Reconstruction of C5 and C6 brachial plexus avulsion injury by multiple nerve transfers: spinal accessory to suprascapular, ulnar fascicles to biceps branch, and triceps long or lateral head branch to axillary nerve. J Hand Surg Am 2004;29(1):131–139

PRIORITY FOR FUNCTION IN THE UPPER LIMB

7. *Following a brachial plexus injury, which one of the following is generally the first priority for restoration of function?*

  A. Elbow flexion

  The clinical priority for restoration of upper limb function following a brachial plexus injury is elbow flexion in most situations. The second target is usually achieving shoulder stability combined with abduction and external rotation of the shoulder. This combination allows a hand to mouth action that can be a useful adjunct to the contralateral uninjured limb even if no further functional recovery is achieved. Lack of shoulder stability results in poor upper limb function, and a lot of the power generated for elbow flexion can be wasted in relocating a subluxated glenohumeral joint. There is also usually long-term discomfort associated with an unstable scapulothoracic interface and glenohumeral joint. Wrist extension is important for passive tenodesis hand grip or to increase the power of active finger flexion. Hand and wrist function are of limited use if shoulder and elbow paresis leave the patient unable to position the hand in space. Elbow extension is generally assisted by gravity and so is less important to correct with surgery, provided at least one arm has active elbow extension for activities such as pushing up to standing from a seated position, reaching overhead objects, and chair to bed transfers in spinal cord injury patients. In cases where nerve transfer is performed for elbow extension, it is usually coapted to the nerve branch to long head of triceps and the "gold standard" donor is to use the teres major motor branch.[1–5]

REFERENCES

1. Gutowski KA, Orenstein HH. Restoration of elbow flexion after brachial plexus injury: the role of nerve and muscle transfers. Plast Reconstr Surg 2000;106(6):1348–1357, quiz 1358, discussion 1359
2. Brophy RH, Wolfe SW. Planning brachial plexus surgery: treatment options and priorities. Hand Clin 2005;21(1):47–54
3. Tung TH, Mackinnon SE. Nerve transfers: indications, techniques, and outcomes. J Hand Surg Am 2010;35(2):332–341
4. Mackinnon SE, Colbert SH. Nerve transfers in the hand and upper extremity surgery. Tech Hand Up Extrem Surg 2008;12(1):20–33
5. Bertelli JA, Ghizoni MF, Tacca CP. Transfer of the teres minor motor branch for triceps reinnervation in tetraplegia. J Neurosurg 2011;114(5):1457–1460

NERVE TRANSFERS FOR ELBOW FLEXION

8. A 40-year-old female sustains a C5/6 root avulsion falling from her horse. *Which one of the following is considered to be the "gold standard" nerve transfer to restore her elbow flexion?*

   C. Flexor carpi ulnaris fascicle to biceps branch of musculocutaneous nerve
   Elbow flexion is key to upper limb function and is lost in a C5/6 plexus injury. The Oberlin procedure remains the "gold standard" for restoration of elbow flexion by transfer of an expendable ulnar motor fascicle of the flexor carpi ulnaris onto the biceps branch of the musculocutaneous nerve (**Fig. 83.2**).[1]
   It is possible to further augment the Oberlin procedure with additional transfer of an expendable median nerve motor fascicle, such as to flexor carpi radialis (FCR) or flexor digitorum superficialis (FDS), onto the brachialis branch of the musculocutaneous nerve.[2] There is, however, debate as to whether this double fascicular modification to the Oberlin procedure makes a significant difference to the functional outcomes and indeed it may not do so (**Fig. 83.3**).[3,4]
   Other options for restoration of elbow flexion in the brachial plexus injury patient include intercostal nerve transfer, thoracodorsal nerve transfer, and medial pectoral nerve transfer. The intercostal nerve transfer shows inferior results to the Oberlin transfer but is indicated in five root plexus avulsions. Two to three nerves must be transferred. The thoracodorsal nerve is recommended if the Oberlin transfer is not possible but is contraindicated if shoulder adduction is weak. The medial pectoral nerve transfer is used for C5–C6 nerve root injuries as pectoralis function is preserved. Unfortunately, nerve grafting is also required in many cases which impairs overall outcomes.[5,6]

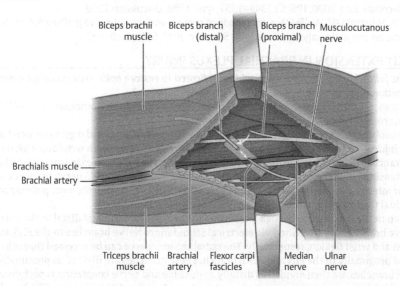

Biceps brachii muscle — Biceps branch (distal) — Biceps branch (proximal) — Musculocutanous nerve

Brachialis muscle
Brachial artery

Triceps brachii muscle — Brachial artery — Flexor carpi fascicles — Median nerve — Ulnar nerve

Fig. 83.2: Oberlin transfer involves coapting flexor carpi ulnaris motor fascicles from the ulnar nerve to the biceps branch of musculocutaneous. The double fascicular transfer combines this with transfer of flexor carpi radialis motor fascicles from the median nerve to brachialis branch.

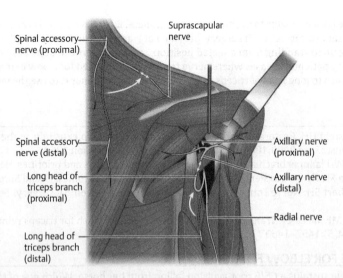

Fig. 83.3: Double nerve transfer for shoulder abduction showing distal branches of spinal accessory nerve to trapezius transferring to suprascapular nerve and motor branch to the long head of the triceps (radial nerve) transferring to the axillary nerve.

REFERENCES

1. Oberlin C, Béal D, Leechavengvongs S, Salon A, Dauge MC, Sarcy JJ. Nerve transfer to biceps muscle using a part of ulnar nerve for C5-C6 avulsion of the brachial plexus: anatomical study and report of four cases. J Hand Surg Am 1994;19(2):232–237
2. Mackinnon SE, Novak CB, Myckatyn TM, Tung TH. Results of reinnervation of the biceps and brachialis muscles with a double fascicular transfer for elbow flexion. J Hand Surg Am 2005;30(5):978–985
3. Carlsen BT, Kircher MF, Spinner RJ, Bishop AT, Shin AY. Comparison of single versus double nerve transfers for elbow flexion after brachial plexus injury. Plast Reconstr Surg 2011;127(1):269–276
4. Martins RS, Siqueira MG, Heise CO, Foroni L, Teixeira MJ. A prospective study comparing single and double fascicular transfer to restore elbow flexion after brachial plexus injury. Neurosurgery 2013;72(5):709–714, discussion 714–715, quiz 715
5. Gutowski KA, Orenstein HH. Restoration of elbow flexion after brachial plexus injury: the role of nerve and muscle transfers. Plast Reconstr Surg 2000;106(6):1348–1357, quiz 1358, discussion 1359
6. Garg R, Merrell GA, Hillstrom HJ, Wolfe SW. Comparison of nerve transfers and nerve grafting for traumatic upper plexus palsy: a systematic review and analysis. J Bone Joint Surg Am 2011;93(9):819–829

WRIST AND DIGIT EXTENSION IN BRACHIAL PLEXUS INJURY

9. *Which one of the following nerve transfers would be indicated to restore both wrist and digit extension following delayed presentation of a radial nerve injury at the proximal humerus?*

D. Dual nerve transfer with FDS nerve branches to extensor carpi radialis combined with FCR branch to posterior interosseous nerve.

There are a number of different transfers that can be used to restore wrist and digit extension following proximal radial nerve injury. A dual nerve transfer approach is preferred to address both wrist and digital extension. Ideally, two nerve branches to flexor digitorum superficialis (FDS) are transferred to extensor carpi radialis brevis (ECRB) for wrist extension while flexor carpi radialis (FCR) and palmaris longus (PL) nerve branches are transferred to the posterior interosseous nerve (PIN) for finger extension. With this approach, most patients are able to recover from individual finger extension.[1]

The median nerve is accessed through an incision in the volar forearm just distal to the antecubital fossa. All median nerve branches are identified via electrical stimulation. Nerve branches to the FDS and FCR will cause finger flexion and wrist flexion, respectively. The radial sensory nerve can be accessed through the same incision and followed proximally to the PIN and ECRB branch. These branches are divided as proximally as possible. The FDS and FCR branches are then divided as distally as possible and nerve coaptation is performed.

An alternative is to use pronator quadratus motor branch of the AIN transfer to PIN, but this is technically more difficult than dual nerve transfer.[2] Transfer of the supinator motor branch onto the PIN is indicated in cases of C7–T1 nerve root injuries and can provide excellent results, as supinator innervation (C6) is preserved.[3,4] It involves the transfer of one or both nerve branches to supinator and helps recover function of extensor pollicis longus and extensor digitorum communis muscles. Nerve transfers for wrist extension tend to target the ECRB to give a more balanced centralized extension of the wrist, rather than ECU or ECRL.

REFERENCES

1. Mackinnon SE, Roque B, Tung TH. Median to radial nerve transfer for treatment of radial nerve palsy. Case report. J Neurosurg 2007;107(3):666–671
2. Bertelli JA, Tacca CP, Winkelmann Duarte EC, Ghizoni MF, Duarte H. Transfer of the pronator quadratus motor branch for wrist extension reconstruction in brachial plexus palsy. Plast Reconstr Surg 2012;130(6):1269–1278
3. Bertelli JA, Ghizoni MF. Transfer of supinator motor branches to the posterior interosseous nerve in C7-T1 brachial plexus palsy. J Neurosurg 2010;113(1):129–132
4. Dong Z, Gu YD, Zhang CG, Zhang L. Clinical use of supinator motor branch transfer to the posterior interosseous nerve in C7-T1 brachial plexus palsies. J Neurosurg 2010;113(1):113–117

NERVE TRANSFER FOR INTRINSIC HAND FUNCTION

10. *Which one of the following is generally considered the "gold standard" donor for nerve transfer restoration of intrinsic hand function following ulnar nerve injury in the proximal forearm or arm?*

    C. Anterior interosseous branch to pronator quadratus

Intrinsic muscle innervation is critical to balancing the extrinsic flexor and extensor tendons when opening and closing the hand, and to most types of grip. The majority of the intrinsic muscles are innervated by the ulnar nerve, and by the T1 nerve root. The median innervated intrinsics can be remembered by "LOAF" (lateral 2 lumbricals, opponens, abductor, and flexor pollicis brevis). A hand without good intrinsic function tends to adopt a claw position. In a proximal ulnar nerve lesion, the reinnervation distance and therefore time may exceed viability of the motor endplates in the hand, leading to little or no functional recovery. The "gold standard" nerve transfer for this scenario is to use the AIN terminal branch to pronator quadratus transferred either end to end or supercharged reverse end to side onto the motor branch of the ulnar nerve, according to whether a late motor recovery is anticipated or not.

The posterior interosseous nerve branch to extensor carpi radialis brevis, musculocutaneous nerve branch to brachialis, median nerve motor branch to flexor carpi radialis, and radial nerve branch to medial triceps are all nerves that can be sacrificed for nerve transfers in the arm, but are all a more significant distance from the intended recipient muscles than the distal pronator quadratus anterior interosseous branch.[1–3]

REFERENCES

1. Wang Y, Zhu S. Transfer of a branch of the anterior interosseus nerve to the motor branch of the median nerve and ulnar nerve. Chin Med J (Engl) 1997;110(3):216–219
2. Haase SC, Chung KC. Anterior interosseous nerve transfer to the motor branch of the ulnar nerve for high ulnar nerve injuries. Ann Plast Surg 2002;49(3):285–290
3. Davidge KM, Yee A, Moore AM, Mackinnon SE. The supercharge end-to-side anterior interosseous-to-ulnar motor nerve transfer for restoring intrinsic function: clinical experience. Plast Reconstr Surg 2015;136(3):344e–352e

84. Hand and Finger Amputations

See *Essentials of Plastic Surgery*, third edition, pp. 1175–1182

DIGITAL AMPUTATIONS

1. You have evaluated a 28-year-old manual worker for acute revision of a traumatic amputation of the ring finger after a circular saw injury. The amputation is at the level of the middle phalanx just proximal to the flexor digitorum superficialis (FDS) insertion. *Which one of the following is correct regarding the surgical procedure?*
   A. The digital nerve stumps should be buried subperiosteally.
   B. The proximal flexor digitorum profundus tendon end should be secured to the bone.
   C. The amputation level should remain at the base of the middle phalanx.
   D. The dorsal and volar skin flaps should be of equal length.
   E. Articular cartilage at the proximal interphalangeal (PIP) joint will need to be removed.

RAY AMPUTATIONS IN THE HAND

2. *Which one of the following improvements is a benefit of performing a ray amputation of the ring finger after traumatic amputation through the proximal phalanx?*
   A. Power grip
   B. Key pinch
   C. Pronation
   D. Interdigital gap
   E. Supination

RAY AMPUTATION OF THE DIGIT

3. *At what level should the index finger metacarpal normally be resected during a ray amputation?*
   A. Neck
   B. Distal shaft
   C. Midshaft
   D. Metacarpal base
   E. Entire metacarpal should be removed

RAY AMPUTATION OF THE DIGIT

4. *In which ray amputations might you consider metacarpal transposition?*
   A. Index or middle finger
   B. Index or ring finger
   C. Index or little finger
   D. Middle or ring finger
   E. Ring or little finger

WRIST AND FOREARM AMPUTATIONS

5. When treating patients with traumatic amputations at the wrist or forearm, *which one of the following is correct?*
   A. Transection of the radius and ulnar in the forearm should be performed at different levels.
   B. Preservation of the radiocarpal joint at the wrist may allow a functional prosthesis to be used.
   C. Fusion of the distal radioulnar joint should be performed during a radiocarpal amputation for improved stability.
   D. Tendon length in the forearm can be minimized if hand transplantation is felt to be a viable future option.
   E. The minimum recommended forearm length for a useful forearm prosthesis is 15 cm.

COMPLICATIONS FOLLOWING DIGITAL AMPUTATION

6. A 28-year-old man complains of an unpleasant tingling and burning sensation with light touch over his amputated index finger stump 6 weeks after surgery. *Which one of the following is the most likely cause?*
   A. A neuroma of the digital nerve
   B. A mild postoperative infection
   C. Complex regional pain syndrome
   D. Allodynia caused by nerve injury and reinnervation
   E. Cold intolerance caused by sympathetic denervation

REVISION AMPUTATION OF THE DIGIT

7. Three months after a revision amputation through the distal interphalangeal (DIP) joint of the middle finger, a patient is unable to actively flex his PIP joint. Each time he tries to do so, the PIP joint extends instead. *What is the correct term used to describe this problem?*

   A. Interosseous plus
   B. Intrinsic minus
   C. Quadriga effect
   D. Lumbrical plus
   E. Lumbrical minus

THE QUADRIGIA EFFECT

8. You receive a call about a patient who has undergone revision amputation by one of your residents and now has problems with hand function. The caller described the dysfunction as a quadriga effect. *Does this term mean the patient will be unable to perform normally?*

   A. Flex the digits
   B. Extend the digits
   C. Abduct the digits
   D. Adduct the digits
   E. Feel the fingertip

Answers

DIGITAL AMPUTATIONS

1. You have evaluated a 28-year-old manual worker for acute revision of a traumatic amputation of the ring finger after a circular saw injury. The amputation is at the level of the middle phalanx just proximal to the flexor digitorum superficialis (FDS) insertion. *Which one of the following is correct regarding the surgical procedure?*

   E. Articular cartilage at the proximal interphalangeal (PIP) joint will need to be removed.

   With no flexor tendon attachment, there is little point in keeping the residual middle phalanx. The proximal phalanx must be shortened to at least remove all articular cartilage in order to avoid a pseudobursa, and more commonly to the neck of the proximal phalanx to avoid the stump being too long when the patient makes a fist. During initial amputation, the digital nerves should simply be divided proximal to the skin flaps and allowed to retract back into the soft tissues. If a subsequent neuroma develops, that can be dealt with by a number of techniques. The flexor and extensor tendon ends should be allowed to retract in order to avoid a quadriga effect. In cases where the FDS insertion remains intact, there may be useful PIP joint flexion, in which case it may be worth using a local flap to preserve digital length. FDP retraction may result in paradoxical extension of the injured digit when trying to flex the fingers caused by tension through the lumbrical. This is uncommon and is dealt with on an elective basis with division of the lumbrical. The fish-mouth incision should be designed to provide a longer volar skin flap, as this is sensate and provides better soft-tissue padding for the new fingertip (**Fig. 84.1**).[1-3]

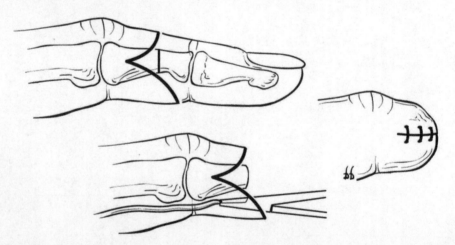

Fig. 84.1   A "fish-mouth" incision design creates volar and dorsal skin flaps for amputation stump coverage. The volar skin flap should be designed slightly longer, such that it can be wrapped over the distal stump, to provide more durable and sensate coverage.

REFERENCES

1. Adamson GJ, Palmer RE. Amputations. In: Achauer BM, Erikson E, Guyuron B, et al, eds. Plastic Surgery: Indications, Operations, and Outcomes. St Louis: Mosby–Year Book; 2000
2. Louis DS, Jebson PJ, Graham T. Amputations. In: Green DP, Hotchkiss RN, Pederson WC, eds. Green's Operative Hand Surgery. 4th ed. Philadelphia: Churchill Livingstone; 1999
3. Kakar S. Digital amputations. In: Wolfe SW, Hotchkiss RN, Pederson WC, Kozin SH, Cohen MS, eds. Green's Operative Hand Surgery. 7th ed. Philadelphia, PA: Elsevier; 2017: 1708–1752

RAY AMPUTATIONS IN THE HAND

2. *Which one of the following improvements is a benefit of performing a ray amputation of the ring finger after traumatic amputation through the proximal phalanx?*

   D. Interdigital gap

   Revision ray amputation is usually an elective procedure following initial care of a more distal digital amputation. The main purpose is to close the interdigital gap to stop objects falling through. A secondary potential benefit is an improvement in cosmesis. Power grip, key grip, pronation, and supination power are usually reduced after ray amputation, so must be considered when pursuing a ray amputation for cosmetic reasons.[1-3]

Ray amputation may also be used primarily in trauma and tumor management, or for removal of a poorly functioning previously reconstructed digit.

REFERENCES

1. Murray JF, Carman W, MacKenzie JK. Transmetacarpal amputation of the index finger: a clinical assessment of hand strength and complications. J Hand Surg Am 1977;2(6): 471–481
2. Garcia-Moral CA, Putman-Mullins J, Taylor PA, et al. Ray resection of the index finger. Orthop Trans 1991;15:71
3. Melikyan EY, Beg MS, Woodbridge S, Burke FD. The functional results of ray amputation. Hand Surg 2003;8(1):47–51

RAY AMPUTATION OF THE DIGIT

3. *At what level should the index finger metacarpal normally be resected during a ray amputation?*

D. Metacarpal base

When performing a ray amputation of the index or little fingers, the osteotomy is usually made at the metacarpal base (metaphyseal flare), preserving tendon attachments to the base and maintaining carpometacarpal joint integrity. The tendon insertions for the index finger are flexor carpi radialis (FCR) and extensor carpi radialis longus (ECRL), while those for the little finger are flexor carpi ulnaris (FCU) and extensor carpi ulnaris (ECU). Preservation of these is important. The bony amputation level for a middle or ring finger may also be through the base, but some surgeons prefer a total base resection.[1]

REFERENCE

1. Blazar PE, Garon MT. Ray resections of the fingers: indications, techniques, and outcomes. J Am Acad Orthop Surg 2015;23(8):476–484

RAY AMPUTATION OF THE DIGIT

4. *In which ray amputations might you consider metacarpal transposition?*

D. Middle or ring finger

The border digits can be transposed to close the gap from the third or fourth ray amputations.[1] The base of the fifth metacarpal should still be preserved in order to protect the insertions of the ECU and FCU tendons. Likewise, the index metacarpal base should be preserved to protect the ECRL and FCR tendon insertions. The osteotomy is performed at the metaphyseal flare. Ray amputations usually result in 15 to 20% reduction in grip strength and narrowing of the palm.[2–4]

REFERENCES

1. Carroll RE. Transposition of the index finger to replace the middle finger. Clin Orthop 1959;15(15):27–34
2. Murray JF, Carman W, MacKenzie JK. Transmetacarpal amputation of the index finger: a clinical assessment of hand strength and complications. J Hand Surg Am 1977;2(6): 471–481
3. Garcia-Moral CA, Putman-Mullins J, Taylor PA, et al. Ray resection of the index finger. Orthop Trans 1991;15:71
4. Melikyan EY, Beg MS, Woodbridge S, Burke FD. The functional results of ray amputation. Hand Surg 2003;8(1):47–51

WRIST AND FOREARM AMPUTATIONS

5. When treating patients with traumatic amputations at the wrist or forearm, *which one of the following is correct?*

B. Preservation of the radiocarpal joint at the wrist may allow a functional prosthesis to be used.

Transection of the radius and ulna should be at the same level. The distal radioulnar joint should be preserved rather than fused where possible to allow pronation and supination. While the tendons are often divided under traction to allow proximal retraction, this is not appropriate if future hand transplantation is a possibility as length should be preserved in this scenario. The minimum length considered useful for a forearm prosthesis is 8 to 10 cm of residual radius and ulna length.[1–3]

REFERENCES

1. Cioffi WG. Upper Extremity Amputations. Philadelphia, PA: Elsevier/Saunders; 2014: 297–320
2. Cuccurullo S. Physical Medicine and Rehabilitation Board Review. New York, NY: Demos Medical; 2004
3. Wright TW, Hagen AD, Wood MB. Prosthetic usage in major upper extremity amputations. J Hand Surg Am 1995;20(4):619–622

COMPLICATIONS FOLLOWING DIGITAL AMPUTATION

6. A 28-year-old man complains of an unpleasant tingling and burning sensation with light touch over his amputated index finger stump 6 weeks after surgery. *Which one of the following is the most likely cause?*

D. Allodynia caused by nerve injury and reinnervation

Allodynia is the perception of a painful sensation following what is normally a non-noxious stimulus, such as a burning sensation in response to a light touch. Mild symptoms can be quite common after digital amputation during the early stages of scar maturation and reinnervation; however, this usually settles with desensitization exercises. If allodynia persists, becomes severe, or is associated with trophic changes to the soft tissues, it may be part of a complex regional pain syndrome.

Six weeks is too early for formation of a neuroma, and this would usually present as a pinpoint site of tenderness over the digital nerve stump or external scar, leading to an "electric shock" sensation or "shooting pain." It is rather late for development of a postoperative infection and if infection was present the digit would usually be painful, swollen, tender, and warm. Cold intolerance is a recognized complication of digital amputation but would not present in this way.[1–3]

REFERENCES

1. Dellon AL, Mackinnon SE. Treatment of the painful neuroma by neuroma resection and muscle implantation. Plast Reconstr Surg 1986;77(3):427–438
2. Buonocore M, Gagliano MC, Bonezzi C. Dynamic mechanical allodynia following finger amputation: unexpected skin hyperinnervation. World J Clin Cases 2013;1(6):197–201
3. Tupper JW, Booth DM. Treatment of painful neuromas of sensory nerves in the hand: a comparison of traditional and newer methods. J Hand Surg Am 1976;1(2):144–151

REVISION AMPUTATION OF THE DIGIT

7. Three months after a revision amputation through the distal interphalangeal (DIP) joint of the middle finger, a patient is unable to actively flex his proximal interphalangeal (PIP) joint. Each time he tries to do so, the PIP joint extends instead. *What is the correct term used to describe this problem?*

D. Lumbrical plus

The lumbrical plus deformity may occur following a partial amputation of the finger. The PIP joint extends during attempts to actively flex the joint because the retracted FDP tendon remains attached to the lumbrical muscles in the palm. FDP contraction, therefore, pulls on the lumbrical muscle, causing flexion of the metacarpophalangeal (MCP) joint and extension of the IP joint. The lumbrical plus deformity can be prevented by securing the FDP to the A4 pulley during revision amputation; however, care must be taken when performing such a procedure as there is a risk of causing a quadriga effect instead. For this reason, it is not commonly performed. If the FDP tendon is overly advanced or tensioned in the injured digit, the action of FDP in the remaining digits is compromised. This is because the FDP tendons share a common muscle belly and if one is significantly tighter than the others, normal flexion in the remaining digits is restricted. Intrinsic minus deformity is a condition where the finger MCP joints are hyperextended and the PIP joints are flexed. This is because the normal function of the intrinsics is restricted, causing an imbalance between the strong extrinsics and the deficient intrinsics. It is typically observed in association with an ulnar nerve motor branch injury.[1]

REFERENCE

1. Parkes A. The "lumbrical plus" finger. J Bone Joint Surg Br 1971;53(2):236–239

THE QUADRIGIA EFFECT

8. You receive a call about a patient who has undergone revision amputation by one of your residents and now has problems with hand function. The caller described the dysfunction as a quadriga effect. *Does this term mean the patient will be unable to perform normally?*

A. Flex the digits

The quadriga effect is where one of the FDP tendons is functionally shorter than the others. As this muscle group has a mass action, when the tightest FDP fully flexes, the remaining digits cannot fully flex and consequently display an active flexion lag or reduced power in grip. The main causes of this are either an overly tight FDP tendon repair to a single digit or after digital terminalization where the FDP is sutured to the extensor tendon or pulleys during the amputation procedure.

Patients tend to complain of weak grip with an inability to actively make a full fist.

Therefore, it is important when performing digital terminalization that the FDP is allowed to retract into the palm without distal tethering. One potential issue with doing so, however, is that the FDP may then pull on the lumbricals proximally and cause an lumbrical plus deformity. These risks have to be balanced when performing such surgery; however, lumbrical plus is uncommon and readily dealt with if it arises by release of the lumbrical in the palm; so, this may be preferable to producing a quadriga effect.[1-3]

REFERENCES

1. Kakar S. Digital amputations. In: Wolfe SW, Hotchkiss RN, Pederson WC, Kozin SH, Cohen MS, eds. Green's Operative Hand Surgery. 7th ed. Philadelphia, PA: Elsevier; 2017: 1708–1752
2. Schreuders TA. The quadriga phenomenon: a review and clinical relevance. J Hand Surg Eur Vol 2012;37(6):513–522
3. Neu BR, Murray JF, MacKenzie JK. Profundus tendon blockage: quadriga in finger amputations. J Hand Surg Am 1985; 10(6, Pt 1):878–883

85. Replantation

See *Essentials of Plastic Surgery*, third edition, pp. 1183–1198

INDICATIONS FOR DIGITAL REPLANTATION

1. *Which one of the following represents a relative contraindication to digital replantation in an adult because of likely poor long-term function?*
   A. Middle finger amputation through neck of middle phalanx
   B. Ring finger amputation through neck of proximal phalanx
   C. Little finger amputation through the distal interphalangeal joint
   D. Thumb amputation through midshaft proximal phalanx
   E. Thumb amputation through the interphalangeal joint

CLASSIFICATION OF DIGITAL AMPUTATIONS

2. A neighboring hospital refers a patient with multiple fingertip amputations. The injury is described according to the Tamai classification system. *On which one of the following is this classification based?*
   A. Mechanism of injury
   B. Level of injury
   C. Time since injury
   D. Predicted outcome after replantation
   E. Number of digits involved

PRESERVATION OF AMPUTATED DIGITS

3. *When arranging transport of an amputated digit, which one of the following is correct?*
   A. The digit should be placed in saline-soaked gauze in a bag or specimen container.
   B. The bag containing the digit should be transported on dry ice.
   C. The optimal temperature for storage of the amputated digit is approximately 4°C.
   D. The maximum cold ischemia time for a digit is 12 hours.
   E. The maximum warm ischemia time for a digit is 3 hours.

PREOPERATIVE WORKUP FOR DIGITAL REPLANTATION

4. *Which one of the following is correct when preparing a patient for replantation of a digit?*
   A. A local anesthetic ring block is advisable to ensure patient comfort.
   B. Plain radiographs of the hand and the amputated digit are required.
   C. Tetanus prophylaxis is required only if surgery will be delayed.
   D. Aspirin 150 mg should be given in the emergency room to improve distal circulation.
   E. Oral antibiotics are indicated only in contaminated injuries.

MANAGEMENT OF PROXIMAL LIMB AMPUTATIONS

5. A patient sustains a midhumeral guillotine amputation. *Which one of the following is correct when undertaking replantation in this case?*
   A. Fasciotomies are not required and risk further unnecessary tissue injury.
   B. Skeletal stabilization need not be achieved before creating a vascular shunt.
   C. Carpal and cubital tunnel decompression is generally discouraged.
   D. The maximum warm ischemia time is 2 hours.
   E. The maximum cold ischemia time is 12 hours.

SURGICAL PRINCIPLES OF REPLANTATION

6. *Which one of the following is correct when performing an upper limb replantation?*
   A. Regional anesthesia should be avoided as it may compromise blood flow.
   B. Use of a tourniquet should be avoided to reduce ischemia time.
   C. The full arm and a leg should be prepared for nerve or vein graft harvest.
   D. The maximum tourniquet time allowed is 90 minutes at 250 mm Hg.
   E. A two-team approach is rarely justified for proximal amputations.

OPERATIVE SEQUENCE IN REPLANTATION

7. In what order should structures usually be repaired when replanting a digit?
A. Bone, tendon, nerve, vessel
B. Bone, vessel, nerve, tendon
C. Vessel, bone, tendon, nerve
D. Vessel, nerve, bone, tendon
E. Bone, vessel, tendon, nerve

MICROSURGERY VESSEL INJURY ASSESSMENT

8. When assessing vessels for replantation of a digit, which one of the following is correct?
A. A pearly gray translucent appearance indicates a friable vessel wall.
B. A tortuous "corkscrew" appearance indicates an intraluminal thrombus.
C. The presence of a terminal thrombus means that the vessel is unsalvageable.
D. A "red-line" appearance along the distal vessel makes salvage less likely.
E. The *sausage sign* requires further vessel resection and a vein graft will be required.

PHARMACOLOGIC ADJUNCTS IN REPLANT SURGERY

9. There are a number of useful pharmacologic agents to improve the success rate in replantation. *Which one of the following is correct?*
A. Topical papaverine may be used to aid vascular anastomosis.
B. If leech therapy is required, amoxicillin prophylaxis is indicated.
C. Systemic heparinization is recommended for distal amputations.
D. Systemic prostaglandin therapy is commonly used after replantation.
E. Oral aspirin should be delayed for 48 hours to reduce bleeding.

OUTCOMES OF LIMB AND DIGITAL REPLANTATION

10. Before replantation of a digit, you are discussing likely outcomes with a patient. *Which one of the following is correct?*
A. Fewer than 50% of replanted digits survive the first 24 hours after surgery, irrespective of injury mechanism or replantation technique.
B. Arterial insufficiency is the main reason for early failure and requires an urgent return to the operating room.
C. Most patients will regain normal fingertip two-point discrimination by 6 months.
D. Cold intolerance is common in many patients and is usually a permanent feature.
E. Few patients will require subsequent secondary surgery providing an adequate rehabilitation protocol is followed.

SECONDARY PROCEDURES FOLLOWING DIGITAL REPLANT

11. Following digital replantation, which one of the following is the most likely secondary procedure a patient will subsequently require?
A. Joint fusion
B. Neurolysis
C. Tenolysis
D. Web space release
E. Correction of nonunion

Answers

INDICATIONS FOR DIGITAL REPLANTATION

1. *Which one of the following represents a relative contraindication to digital replantation in an adult because of likely poor long-term function?*

   B. **Ring finger amputation through neck of proximal phalanx**

   A single digit amputation in flexor tendon zone II is a relative contraindication to replantation, since there is a high likelihood of poor functional outcome because of stiffness and immobility. Almost all patients are likely to require secondary surgery to release tendon adhesions or joint contractures. A detailed discussion with the patient regarding the likely outcome following replantation should be undertaken before proceeding with surgery. In many cases, a single digit amputation proximal to the flexor digitorum profundus insertion is best managed with a revision amputation rather than replantation.

   However, there may still be reasons to pursue replantation in this scenario: for example, the patient may prefer a stiff, potentially painful digit to an absent digit for social, aesthetic, or psychological reasons. In Japan, for example, a missing digit has criminal connotations. In many patients, preservation of length in the left ring finger may be preferred for wearing or receiving a wedding or engagement band. In children, zone II single-digit injuries should still be replanted where possible, as children tend to have significantly better outcomes after surgery with regard to mobility and sensation.

   In contrast to zone II flexor level replants, zone I flexor level replants tend to have far better outcomes even when distal interphalangeal joint motion is not preserved.[1] Therefore, replantation of these is often indicated. All traumatic thumb amputations should be replanted where possible, given the importance of thumb function in opposition. The thumb remains functionally very useful even when it is stiff and relatively immobile.[1-4]

REFERENCES

1. O'Brien BM. Replantation surgery. Clin Plast Surg 1974;1(3):405–426
2. Higgins JP. Replantation. In: Wolfe SW, Hotchkiss RN, Pederson WC, Kozin SH, Cohen MS, eds. Green's Operative Hand Surgery. 7th ed. Philadelphia, PA: Elsevier; 2017:1476–1485
3. Pederson WC. Replantation. Plast Reconstr Surg 2001;107(3):823–841
4. Saint-Cyr M, Wong C, Buchel EW, Colohan S, Pederson WC. Free tissue transfers and replantation. Plast Reconstr Surg 2012;130(6):858e–878e

CLASSIFICATION OF DIGITAL AMPUTATIONS

2. A neighboring hospital refers a patient with multiple fingertip amputations. The injury is described according to the Tamai classification system. *On which one of the following is this classification based?*

   B. **Level of injury**

   The two main classification systems for fingertip amputation are the Tamai[1] and Sebastin and Chung[2] classifications. Both the classifications are based on the level of injury and the clinical relevance of this is in relation to the anticipated difficulty of vascular repair, in particular the venous outflow. For example, in injuries distal to the lunula (Tamai zone I and Chung zone IA), direct anastomosis of venous outflow is not possible. Instead, anastomosis to the volar venous plexus may sometimes be performed; otherwise, leech therapy, nail bed bleed, or heparin therapy is required to provide adequate venous drainage. In more proximal injuries, it may be possible to repair both arteries and veins, but this is still very difficult beyond the FDP insertion. The zones of these two classification systems are shown in **Figs. 85.1** and **85.2**. The mechanism of injury and degree of soft-tissue damage is more relevant to the Urbaniak[3] classification. This is a classification of ring avulsion injuries and does not relate to level of injury. The time since injury and the number of digits involved do not form part of any of these classification systems.

REFERENCES

1. Tamai S. Twenty years' experience of limb replantation–review of 293 upper extremity replants. J Hand Surg Am 1982;7(6):549–556
2. Sebastin SJ, Chung KC. A systematic review of the outcomes of replantation of distal digital amputation. Plast Reconstr Surg 2011;128(3):723–737
3. Urbaniak JR, Evans JP, Bright DS. Microvascular management of ring avulsion injuries. J Hand Surg Am 1981;6(1):25–30

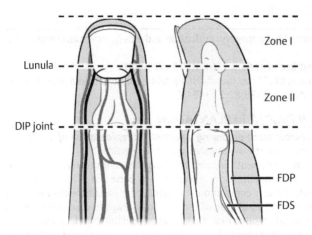

Fig. 85.1 Tamai's classification of fingertip amputation. *(DIP joint*, distal interphalangeal joint; *FDP*, flexor digitorum profundus; *FDS*, flexor digitorum superficialis.)

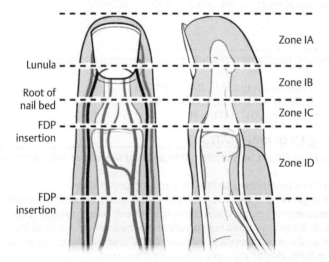

Fig. 85.2 Chung's classification of digital amputations.

PRESERVATION OF AMPUTATED DIGITS

3. *When arranging transport of an amputated digit, which one of the following is correct?*
   C. The optimal temperature for storage of the amputated digit is approximately 4°C.
   The optimal storage temperature for an amputated digit is 4°C, which can be achieved by refrigeration of the transport container. The digit is preferably wrapped in damp gauze and placed in a bag, which may then be kept on iced water. Heavily soaked gauze may result in waterlogging of the tissues and should be avoided. It is essential to avoid the error of allowing contact between the tissues and ice, which may result in freezing and subsequent cell necrosis.[1,2]

   In general, revascularization of amputated parts should be achieved as soon as possible. Digits are more tolerant of warm ischemia than the hand or forearm, as they contain no muscle. Warm ischemia times for digits should ideally be less than 6 hours. Cold ischemia times should be less than 24 hours.

   In spite of these guidance figures, successful digital replantation has been reported in several cases after up to 30 hours of cold ischemia, with one procedure after 94 hours.[3] Such prolonged ischemia times are not generally recommended.

REFERENCES

1. Tosti R, Eberlin KR. "Damage control" hand surgery: evaluation and emergency management of the mangled hand. Hand Clin 2018;34(1):17–26
2. Pederson WC. Replantation. Plast Reconstr Surg 2001;107(3):823–841
3. Wei FC, Chang YL, Chen HC, Chuang CC. Three successful digital replantations in a patient after 84, 86, and 94 hours of cold ischemia time. Plast Reconstr Surg 1988;82(2):346–350

PREOPERATIVE WORKUP FOR DIGITAL REPLANTATION

4. *Which one of the following is correct when preparing a patient for replantation of a digit?*

  B. Plain radiographs of the hand and the amputated digit are required.

  Preoperative imaging of both the patient's injured hand and the amputated part is important to anticipate the functional outcome, plan skeletal stabilization, and assess any bone loss. A local anesthetic ring block may seem a good idea for patient comfort but is contraindicated because it can decrease vascular flow or risk damage to proximal vessels. Also, repeated manipulation of the digit may result in vasospasm, so it should be avoided. This is particularly relevant to partial amputations. In contrast a regional block can be helpful to alleviate pain and promote vasodilatation. The patient should be kept warm and well perfused with adequate intravenous fluids before, during, and after surgery. All patients should receive both tetanus and intravenous antibiotic prophylaxis in the ER. Aspirin is not required before surgery but is commonly given during or after at a dose of 325 mg PR or PO, as it inhibits platelet aggregation at the anastomosis at this dose level.[1–3]

REFERENCES

1. Tosti R, Eberlin KR. "Damage control" hand surgery: evaluation and emergency management of the mangled hand. Hand Clin 2018;34(1):17–26
2. Pederson WC. Replantation. Plast Reconstr Surg 2001;107(3):823–841
3. Higgins JP. Replantation. In: Wolfe SW, Hotchkiss RN, Pederson WC, Kozin SH, Cohen MS, eds. Green's Operative Hand Surgery. 7th ed. Philadelphia, PA: Elsevier; 2017:1476–1485

MANAGEMENT OF PROXIMAL LIMB AMPUTATIONS

5. A patient sustains a midhumeral guillotine amputation. *Which one of the following is correct when undertaking replantation in this case?*

  B. Skeletal stabilization need not be achieved before creating a vascular shunt.

  It is perfectly reasonable to proceed with a temporary vascular shunt before bony stabilization to minimize ischemia time, while careful debridement is undertaken, or a difficult bony fixation planned. This is particularly relevant where the amputated part contains a high proportion of muscle which will be less tolerant of ischemia.[1] Although the most common shunt is a specifically designed PVC vascular shunt, other materials such as chest drains or pediatric feeding tubes may be used as a substitute if required.

  There is always a degree of edema and relative ischemia following a major replantation, in part because only the major inflow and outflow are restored and also because of the vascular response to ischemia. As such, it is prudent to decompress major nerves at their common sites of compression to minimize further insults.

  Fasciotomy is recommended for the same reason to decompress the forearm and intrinsic hand muscle compartments following a major replantation. Tolerable ischemia times vary according to the proportion of muscle in the amputated part and whether appropriate cooling has occurred. For an arm or forearm amputation, a maximum of 4 to 6 hours warm ischemia and a maximum of 10 to 12 hours cold ischemia are generally quoted.

REFERENCE

1. Subramanian A, Vercruysse G, Dente C, Wyrzykowski A, King E, Feliciano DV. A decade's experience with temporary intravascular shunts at a civilian level I trauma center. J Trauma 2008;65(2):316–324, discussion 324–326

SURGICAL PRINCIPLES OF REPLANTATION

6. *Which one of the following is correct when performing an upper limb replantation?*

  C. The full arm and a leg should be prepared for nerve or vein graft harvest.

  When planning an upper limb replantation, the possibility of vessel and nerve gaps should be anticipated; therefore, the full arm and at least one leg should be adequately prepared for donor tissue harvest. In digital replantation, the posterior interosseous nerve can be a useful donor graft for the digital nerves with minimal donor-site disturbance. It is found in the fourth extensor compartment at the wrist. Suitable donor vessel grafts include both volar and dorsal wrist veins for digital vessels. Suitable leg grafts for larger structures in proximal replantations include the sural nerve and dorsal foot or saphenous veins. Graft harvest can proceed while other repairs are performed at the replantation site.

Regional anesthesia is a useful adjunct to general anesthesia, as it improves postoperative comfort and reduces vasospasm. It can also reduce the anesthetic agent requirement, thereby reducing nausea and vomiting. Use of a tourniquet is standard practice for exploration and debridement of any upper limb wound, as it provides a clear blood-free field, making surgery more efficient and reducing blood loss. Inflation of the tourniquet should be avoided once revascularization has been performed, as stopping flow may increase thrombosis at the anastomotic site. The standard pressure used for an adult upper limb is 250 mm Hg and a safe maximum continuous time is 120 minutes. After this time, the tourniquet must be deflated, and the arm allowed to perfuse for at least 20 minutes. Where possible, a two-team approach is recommended for replantation, so one team can prepare the amputated part while the other prepares the injured digit and harvests grafts. This approach should minimize further ischemia time.[1-4]

REFERENCES

1. Maricevich M, Carlsen B, Mardini S, Moran S. Upper extremity and digital replantation. Hand (N Y) 2011;6(4):356–363
2. Ono S, Chung KC. Efficiency in digital and hand replantation. Clin Plast Surg 2019;46(3):359–370
3. Prucz RB, Friedrich JB. Upper extremity replantation: current concepts. Plast Reconstr Surg 2014;133(2):333–342
4. Iorio ML. Hand, wrist, forearm, and arm replantation. Hand Clin 2019;35(2):143–154

OPERATIVE SEQUENCE IN REPLANTATION

7. In what order should structures usually be repaired when replanting a digit?

A. Bone, tendon, nerve, vessel

The usual order for digital replant is bone first in order to set length and provide a stable functional base for further reconstruction. The tendons should be repaired second, as these will take tension off and set the length for nerve and vessel repairs. Leaving tendon repairs until after the microsurgery risks inadvertent damage to delicate nerve and vessel repairs. Repairing the nerves before the vessels is often recommended, as it keeps the operating field clear of blood for longer and ensures that following revascularization no other structural repair is required. It would still be reasonable to repair the vessels before the nerves, especially when ischemia time is already extended, and many surgeons would do so routinely, thereby leaving the nerves until last.[1-4]

REFERENCES

1. Higgins JP. Replantation. In: Wolfe SW, Hotchkiss RN, Pederson WC, Kozin SH, Cohen MS, eds. Green's Operative Hand Surgery. 7th ed. Philadelphia, PA: Elsevier; 2017:1476–1485
2. Tamai S. Twenty years' experience of limb replantation–review of 293 upper extremity replants. J Hand Surg Am 1982;7(6):549–556
3. Sebastin SJ, Chung KC. A systematic review of the outcomes of replantation of distal digital amputation. Plast Reconstr Surg 2011;128(3):723–737
4. Chao JJ, Castello JR, English JM, Tittle BJ. Microsurgery: free tissue transfer and replantation. Sel Read Plast Surg 2000;9:1–32

MICROSURGERY VESSEL INJURY ASSESSMENT

8. When assessing vessels for replantation of a digit, which one of the following is correct?

D. A "red-line" appearance along the distal vessel makes salvage less likely.

A normal, clean digital vessel appears somewhat translucent and gray. The red-line sign along the distal neurovascular bundle may indicate damage to the vessel and is associated with a poorer prognosis. In this situation, revascularization may be futile. The "corkscrew" appearance usually indicates a traction injury, which also makes successful revascularization a challenge. A terminal thrombus may be evacuated, leaving a potentially healthy vessel end. A sausage appearance occurs when the vessel is blocked with a thrombus, which may be evacuated. Where there is doubt about the quality of the vessels further trimming should be considered and where inadequate length is an issue, a vessel graft should be used. The volar wrist is often a useful donor site for digital vessel grafts.[1,2]

REFERENCES

1. Callico CG. Replantation and revascularization of the upper extremity. In: May JW Jr, Littler JW, eds. McCarthy's Plastic Surgery, Vol. 7. The Hand. Philadelphia: WB Saunders; 1990
2. Chao JJ, Castello JR, English JM, Tittle BJ. Microsurgery: free-tissue transfer and replantation. Sel Read Plast Surg 2000;9:1–32

PHARMACOLOGIC ADJUNCTS IN REPLANT SURGERY

9. There are a number of useful pharmacologic agents to improve the success rate in replantation. *Which one of the following is correct?*

   A. Topical papaverine may be used to aid vascular anastomosis.

   Papaverine is a potent smooth muscle relaxant that appears to work through inhibition of phosphodiesterases and by influencing calcium channels. It may be used topically during microsurgery to dilate arteries and veins before and after anastomosis. Other agents used for this purpose include the calcium channel blocker verapamil and the local anesthetic sodium channel blocker lidocaine. Leech therapy is useful for venously congested digits, but carries a small risk of infection with *Aeromonas hydrophila*.[1] The usual prophylaxis for this is ciprofloxacin or a third-generation cephalosporin (although one must consider the possibility of resistant organisms, which is becoming more common). Although systemic heparinization might occasionally be used where there is greater concern than usual regarding thrombosis, this has to be balanced against the risk of hemorrhage and is not routine. Systemic prostaglandin therapy has been used by some microsurgeons, but this is not commonplace.[2] Oral aspirin therapy is regularly administered after replantation and may be given PR during the procedure or by mouth postoperatively, as the antiplatelet effect can reduce platelet aggregation at the anastomosis site.[3-5]

REFERENCES

1. Hackenberger PN, Janis JE. A comprehensive review of medicinal leeches in plastic and reconstructive surgery. Plast Reconstr Surg Glob Open 2019;7(12):e2555
2. Rodríguez Vegas JM, Ruiz Alonso ME, Terán Saavedra PP. PGE-1 in replantation and free tissue transfer: early preliminary experience. Microsurgery 2007;27(5):395–397
3. Maricevich M, Carlsen B, Mardini S, Moran S. Upper extremity and digital replantation. Hand (N Y) 2011;6(4):356–363
4. Buckley T, Hammert WC. Anticoagulation following digital replantation. J Hand Surg Am 2011;36(8):1374–1376
5. Reissis D, Geoghegan L, Sarsam R, Young Sing Q, Nikkhah D. Perioperative thromboprophylaxis in digital replantation: a systematic review. Plast Reconstr Surg Glob Open 2020;8(5):e2806

OUTCOMES OF LIMB AND DIGITAL REPLANTATION

10. Before replantation of a digit, you are discussing likely outcomes with a patient. *Which one of the following is correct?*

   B. Arterial insufficiency is the main reason for early failure and requires an urgent return to the operating room.

   The main reason for early replantation failure is arterial insufficiency (up to 60% of cases). This presents with a pale, cold finger with no bleeding on pinprick testing. Patients must be warned about the risk of both an extended initial procedure time and a potential return to the operating room following replantation. Unfortunately, digits that struggle to survive tend to have poor long-term function with atrophy, reduced sensation, and stiffness.

   Survival rates following digital replantation are generally well above 50% and will depend on factors such as injury mechanism, digit involved, level of injury, timing of replantation, and surgical skill. The overall survival for distal digital amputation was 86%, according to a systematic review published in 2011.[1] Other published success rates range from 54 to 84%, and, as expected, the success for guillotine-type injuries is much better than for crush injuries (77 vs. 49%).[2]

   Most patients do regain useful sensation, but this does not regularly reach normal two-point discrimination. A normal two-point discrimination is 3 mm for dynamic and 6 mm for static. A review of 293 distal replants showed two-point discrimination at less than 15 mm. In the systematic review, mean two-point discrimination was 7 mm. While cold intolerance is common and should be explained to the patient preoperatively, it will usually improve over time (2 years). A large number of patients will require secondary surgery even when the vascularity of the digit remains satisfactory.[3]

REFERENCES

1. Sebastin SJ, Chung KC. A systematic review of the outcomes of replantation of distal digital amputation. Plast Reconstr Surg 2011;128(3):723–737
2. Wilhelmi BJ, Lee WP, Pagenstert GI, May JW Jr. Replantation in the mutilated hand. Hand Clin 2003;19(1):89–120
3. Tamai S. Twenty years' experience of limb replantation–review of 293 upper extremity replants. J Hand Surg Am 1982;7(6):549–556

SECONDARY PROCEDURES FOLLOWING DIGITAL REPLANT

11. *Following digital replantation, which one of the following is the most likely secondary procedure a patient will subsequently require?*

   C. Tenolysis

   More than half of patients undergoing digital replantation are likely to require secondary surgery. This will be affected by the nature of the original injury and rehabilitation protocol. For example, secondary surgery is more likely in zone II flexor level replantations. The most common procedures are flexor or extensor tenolysis and/or release of joint contractures. This is probably because newly revascularized digits are often immobilized longer than in the early postoperative phase, and subsequent stiffness soon develops as the requirements of the extensor and flexor tendon repairs and the fracture union compete in the rehabilitation regimen. Other common secondary procedures are revision fixation of a nonunion, neurolysis and/or nerve grafting, web-space release, and amputation where function remains poor.[1-3]

REFERENCES

1. Cho HE, Kotsis SV, Chung KC. Outcomes following replantation/revascularization in the hand. Hand Clin 2019;35(2):207–219
2. Chinta MS, Wilkens SC, Vlot MA, Chen NC, Eberlin KR. Secondary surgery following initial replantation/revascularization or completion amputation in the hand or digits. Plast Reconstr Surg 2018;142(3):709–716
3. Fufa D, Lin CH, Lin YT, Hsu CC, Chuang CC, Lin CH. Secondary reconstructive surgery following major upper extremity replantation. Plast Reconstr Surg 2014;134(4):713–720

86. Hand Transplantation

See *Essentials of Plastic Surgery*, third edition, pp. 1199–1208

LEVELS OF AMPUTATION AND PROSTHETIC LIMBS

1. A patient is referred for consideration of hand transplantation and currently uses a prosthesis. *Which one of the following amputation levels is optimal for an upper limb prosthesis?*
   A. Transmetacarpal
   B. Radiocarpal
   C. Midforearm
   D. Proximal forearm
   E. Transhumeral

INDICATIONS AND CONTRAINDICATIONS TO HAND TRANSPLANT

2. A 21-year-old right-hand-dominant patient had a left transmetacarpal amputation following meningococcal septicemia 12 months ago. He would like a hand transplant. *What is the main contraindication to hand transplant in this case?*
   A. Age
   B. Level of injury
   C. Hand dominance
   D. Mechanism of injury
   E. Time interval since injury

MEDICAL CONTRAINDICATIONS TO HAND TRANSPLANT

3. There are a number of medical contraindications to hand transplant. *In which one of the following scenarios may transplant still be indicated?*
   A. During early pregnancy
   B. Following medical treatment for hepatitis A infection
   C. A year after mastectomy and radiotherapy
   D. In a healthy patient with symbrachydactyly
   E. In a patient with well-controlled HIV

HAND TRANSPLANTATION CRITERIA

4. *Why is it particularly important for one of the hand transplant team to physically meet a potential donor before embarking on a hand transplant?*
   A. Confirm ABO blood type
   B. Confirm a positive crossmatch
   C. Meet the donor family members
   D. Assess donor limb integrity, size, and appearance
   E. Take written informed consent for limb donation

OPERATIVE STEPS IN HAND TRANSPLANT

5. *When performing a distal forearm hand transplant, which one of the following is correct?*
   A. The donor limb is removed with a humeral fishmouth incision and a trans-elbow amputation.
   B. A single-team approach to transplantation is preferable for optimal matching of nerve, vessel, and tendon length.
   C. The sequence of reconstruction is bone, extensor tendons, flexor tendons, arteries, veins, and nerves.
   D. Tension should be set for the extensors so that the fingers are extended when the wrist is extended.
   E. Epineurial repair is the preferred technique for the ulnar and median nerves at this level.

IMMUNOSUPPRESSION FOLLOWING HAND TRANSPLANT

6. *Which one of the following is correct regarding immunosuppressive therapy in hand transplantation?*
   A. Tacrolimus is normally used as a depletion agent before a transplant.
   B. The most common maintenance regimen is rapamycin with corticosteroids.
   C. Mycophenolate mofetil is restricted to cases with late rejection due to hepatotoxicity.
   D. Antihypertensive and hypoglycemic agents are commonly required.
   E. Metabolic complications of immunosuppressive therapy are permanent.

TISSUE ANTIGENICITY IN RELATION TO HAND TRANSPLANT

7. *Which one of the following is the most antigenic tissue?*

A. Fat

B. Muscle

C. Endothelium

D. Bone

E. Skin

OUTCOMES FOLLOWING HAND TRANSPLANTATION

8. *Which one of the following is true regarding hand transplantation performed at forearm level?*

A. Proximal forearm transplants tend to provide the best extrinsic motor function.

B. Distal forearm transplants consistently provide near-normal intrinsic motor function.

C. Tactile and discriminative sensation are regained in most transplant cases.

D. Peak functional recovery can be expected at 1 year after surgery.

E. Functional outcome is best measured using the DASH (disability of arm and shoulder) score which specifically relates to hand transplant.

OUTCOMES AFTER HAND TRANSPLANT

9. *Which one of the following is expected at 6 months after hand transplantation?*

A. 5% risk of medication-induced diabetes

B. 10% chance of acute rejection

C. 25% chance of opportunistic infection

D. 50% chance of graft loss

E. 75% chance of patient satisfaction

MANAGEMENT OF COMPLICATIONS AFTER HAND TRANSPLANT

10. You are asked to assess a patient following hand transplantation as there are concerns regarding acute rejection. *In order to assess rejection according to the Banff classification, what test will be required?*

A. MRI

B. Blood sample

C. Doppler ultrasound

D. Cytology sample

E. Skin biopsy

MANAGEMENT OF ACUTE REJECTION FOLLOWING HAND TRANSPLANT

11. You have confirmed the presence of acute rejection clinically by using the Banff scoring system in a patient following hand transplant. *Which one of the following represents the first-line agent you should use to manage this rejection?*

A. Tacrolimus

B. Sulfasalazine

C. Mycophenolate mofetil

D. Corticosteroid

E. Monoclonal antibodies

Answers

LEVELS OF AMPUTATION AND PROSTHETIC LIMBS

1. A patient is referred for consideration of hand transplantation and currently uses a prosthesis. *Which one of the following amputation levels is optimal for an upper limb prosthesis?*

   C. Midforearm

   When considering the merits of hand transplantation, the ability to successfully use a prosthesis must first be considered. There are many options for a prosthesis in patients with a midforearm amputation. Patients with a transmetacarpal stump are usually able to use their wrists well to perform many activities and the additional values of a prosthesis can be limited. Amputations at the radiocarpal level preserve length well but have very little function without a prosthetic; yet fitting a useful prosthesis at this level can be difficult. A transhumeral amputation can work well with a prosthesis, but the success of this is dependent on shoulder mobility, and overall function is likely to be poorer than a midforearm prosthesis.[1]

REFERENCE

1. Wright TW, Hagen AD, Wood MB. Prosthetic usage in major upper extremity amputations. J Hand Surg Am 1995;20(4):619–622

INDICATIONS AND CONTRAINDICATIONS TO HAND TRANSPLANT

2. A 21-year-old right-hand-dominant patient had a left transmetacarpal amputation following meningococcal septicemia 12 months ago. He would like a hand transplant. *What is the main contraindication to hand transplant in this case?*

   C. Hand dominance

   Transplantation is considered for traumatic amputations (as opposed to congenital absences) with strict inclusion criteria. The main indication for hand transplantation is a bilateral upper or quadrimembral amputee, or an amputee who has lost their dominant upper limb. Indications for single upper limb amputations are less clear-cut. This patient has retained his dominant upper limb so is very unlikely to warrant the risks associated with the procedure and lifelong immunosuppression. Other criteria include older than 18 years, a good state of general health, and an adequate period of using a prosthesis (which can be arranged after the initial assessment if not already undertaken). He would therefore not be excluded on these grounds. Each case must be judged on its own merits and due thought also given to the quality of the remaining tissues at the stump, which is influenced by the mechanism of injury. Level of injury is important, as removal of a failed transplanted limb should ideally not leave the patient in a worse functional position than when they started; this is difficult to avoid in a transmetacarpal amputation.[1–3]

REFERENCES

1. Kaufman CL, Breidenbach W. World experience after more than a decade of clinical hand transplantation: update from the Louisville hand transplant program. Hand Clin 2011;27(4):417–421, vii–viii
2. Gordon CR, Siemionow M. Requirements for the development of a hand transplantation program. Ann Plast Surg 2009;63(3):262–273
3. Hollenbeck ST, Erdmann D, Levin LS. Current indications for hand and face allotransplantation. Transplant Proc 2009;41(2):495–498

MEDICAL CONTRAINDICATIONS TO HAND TRANSPLANT

3. There are a number of medical contraindications to hand transplant. *In which one of the following scenarios may transplant still be indicated?*

   B. Following medical treatment for hepatitis A infection

   Hepatitis A is an acute, self-limiting viral infection that does not lead to chronic infection. Although there may be liver damage if the initial infection is severe, this can be screened for during assessment for transplant. Active hepatitis infection or HIV represent contraindications to transplant as do a current diagnosis of cancer, high risk of cancer recurrence (such as shortly after mastectomy and radiotherapy), pregnancy, immunologic dysfunction, and hypercoagulable states.

   Hand transplantation is generally contraindicated in the management of congenital limb anomalies. In congenital limb absence, the patient will have no prior experience of a functioning limb at the defect site and will have lifelong learned behavior patterns and cortical representation that are based on the limb deficit being their normal state. Also, in the trauma setting there are predictable recipient structures to unite, which is often not the case in congenital anomalies.[1-3]

REFERENCES

1. Nassimizadeh M, Nassimizadeh AK, Power D. Hand transplant surgery. Ann R Coll Surg Engl 2014;96(8):571–574
2. Hollenbeck ST, Erdmann D, Levin LS. Current indications for hand and face allotransplantation. Transplant Proc 2009;41(2):495–498
3. Elliott RM, Tintle SM, Levin LS. Upper extremity transplantation: current concepts and challenges in an emerging field. Curr Rev Musculoskelet Med 2014;7(1):83–88

HAND TRANSPLANTATION CRITERIA

4. *Why is it particularly important for one of the hand transplant team to physically meet a potential donor before embarking on a hand transplant?*

D. **Assess donor limb integrity, size, and appearance**

Assessment of the physical characteristics of the limb is critical in achieving a good outcome following hand transplant. This affects the functional, cosmetic, and psychological outcome, and also affects practical steps such as completing osteosynthesis of the radius and ulna in the forearm. It is the responsibility of the transplant team to optimize this match and therefore they will be closely involved in selection. Skin tone, hair density, and overall physical match with the recipient are important, so even when there may be a suitable donor match in terms of blood grouping, etc., transplant may be stopped based on physical criteria.

While correct ABO typing and crossmatching are key to a successful transplant, the surgical team does not need to meet the donor to gather this information. During immunological screening, a positive crossmatch is a major problem as it means that the recipient has preformed antibodies to the donor tissue and will likely undergo a hyperacute rejection.

In many transplant programs, contact with the donor family is through the specialist in organ donation who is seeking consent for donation of all (or selected) organs. The upper limb transplant team will usually have made arrangements for the additional consent elements to be included in this process (such as pointing out that the donated limbs will be visible, and that media attention is not always avoidable).[1-3]

REFERENCES

1. Gordon CR, Siemionow M. Requirements for the development of a hand transplantation program. Ann Plast Surg 2009;63(3):262–273
2. Petruzzo P, Lanzetta M, Dubernard JM, et al. The international registry on hand and composite tissue transplantation. Transplantation 2008;86(4):487–492
3. Elliott RM, Tintle SM, Levin LS. Upper extremity transplantation: current concepts and challenges in an emerging field. Curr Rev Musculoskelet Med 2014;7(1):83–88

OPERATIVE STEPS IN HAND TRANSPLANT

5. *When performing a distal forearm hand transplant, which one of the following is correct?*

A. **The donor limb is removed with a humeral fishmouth incision and a trans-elbow amputation.**

This method of removing the donor limb is swift, minimizing the impact on solid-organ retrieval. It also preserves all the required distal tissues with excess length to allow accurate preparation in the recipient operating room.

A two-team approach is preferred within the recipient operating room area, so the ischemic time is kept to a minimum. The teams must coordinate closely to ensure matched osteotomies and clear tagging of important structures at an appropriate length. The sequence of reconstruction varies according to amputation level and tissue type. The urgency to revascularize depends on composite tissue types included, with greater urgency in grafts having a significant muscle component (in more proximal transplants). For a distal forearm transplantation, a typical sequence would be bony fixation, extensor tendons (set to full extension with the wrist flexed), dorsal veins, nerves, arteries, and flexor tendons. This ensures that the dorsal structures are all repaired first prior to supinating for volar structure repairs; therefore, the limb does not require repeated manipulation back and forth during revascularization. At this level, a grouped fascicular nerve repair technique is recommended over an epineural repair where possible to facilitate better matching of predominantly motor and sensory bundles.[1-3]

REFERENCES

1. Azari KK, Imbriglia JE, Goitz RJ, et al. Technical aspects of the recipient operation in hand transplantation. J Reconstr Microsurg 2012;28(1):27–34
2. Kaufman CL, Breidenbach W. World experience after more than a decade of clinical hand transplantation: update from the Louisville hand transplant program. Hand Clin 2011;27(4):417–421, vii–viii
3. Hartzell TL, Benhaim P, Imbriglia JE, et al. Surgical and technical aspects of hand transplantation: is it just another re-plant? Hand Clin 2011;27(4):521–530, x

IMMUNOSUPPRESSION FOLLOWING HAND TRANSPLANT

6. *Which one of the following is correct regarding immunosuppressive therapy in hand transplantation?*

   D. Antihypertensive and hypoglycemic agents are commonly required.

      Patients taking immunosuppressive drugs for transplant surgery may develop hypertension or hyperglycemia as a consequence, often requiring medications to address this.[1] Gastroprotective medication may also be required as a result of prolonged corticosteroid use. Metabolic complications reported following hand transplant in a 28-patient review included hyperglycemia in 13 patients (46.42%), hypertension in 7 patients (25%), and hyperlipidemia in 4 patients (14.28%).[2] Preparation for this is an important component of the preoperative counseling and consent process. While metabolic complications are a common side effect of immunosuppressive regimens, these changes are usually reversed as immunosuppressive medication doses are reduced or stopped.

      Induction immunotherapy is performed before surgery to prevent acute rejection. Lymphocyte depleting agents are used and include antithymocyte globulin and alemtuzumab. Tacrolimus (Prograf) is also used in the induction phase; however, it is a calcineurin inhibitor that reduces lymphocyte activation and not a depleting agent. Tacrolimus also appears to have an additional secondary beneficial effect on nerve recovery/regeneration.[3]

      The most common maintenance regimen is triple therapy with tacrolimus, mycophenolate mofetil (MMF), and corticosteroids. Many protocols attempt to reduce tacrolimus and it may be replaced by rapamycin. MMF is a common component of both induction and maintenance regimens, having a role in B- and T-lymphocyte suppression. It is considered to be much less hepatotoxic than its predecessors: cyclophosphamide and azathioprine.[2-5]

REFERENCES

1. Crutchlow MF, Bloom RD. Transplant-associated hyperglycemia: a new look at an old problem. Clin J Am Soc Nephrol 2007;2(2):343–355
2. Petruzzo P, Lanzetta M, Dubernard JM, et al. The international registry on hand and composite tissue transplantation. Transplantation 2008;86(4):487–492
3. Brandacher G, Lee WP, Schneeberger S. Minimizing immunosuppression in hand transplantation. Expert Rev Clin Immunol 2012;8(7):673–683, quiz 684
4. Landin L, Bonastre J, Casado-Sanchez C, et al. Outcomes with respect to disabilities of the upper limb after hand allograft transplantation: a systematic review. Transpl Int 2012;25(4):424–432
5. Siemionow M, Klimczak A. Basics of immune responses in transplantation in preparation for application of composite tissue allografts in plastic and reconstructive surgery: part I. Plast Reconstr Surg 2008;121(1):4e–12e

TISSUE ANTIGENICITY IN RELATION TO HAND TRANSPLANT

7. *Which one of the following is the most antigenic tissue?*

   E. Skin

      Vascularized composite allografts contain a number of different tissue types such as skin, bone, muscle, and nerve within a single graft. Of these tissue components, skin is the most antigenic and, as a result, direct inspection is important to identify acute rejection. This will manifest as erythematous macules, diffuse redness, or asymptomatic papules. For this reason, patients should be seen in clinic on a regular basis after transplant and must be educated in reporting potential signs of rejection.[1-5]

REFERENCES

1. Cendales LC, Kanitakis J, Schneeberger S, et al. The Banff 2007 working classification of skin-containing composite tissue allograft pathology. Am J Transplant 2008;8(7): 1396–1400
2. Kaufman CL, Marvin MR, Chilton PM, et al. Immunobiology in VCA. Transpl Int 2016;29(6):644–654
3. Issa F. Vascularized composite allograft-specific characteristics of immune responses. Transpl Int 2016;29(6):672–681
4. Siemionow M, Klimczak A. Basics of immune responses in transplantation in preparation for application of composite tissue allografts in plastic and reconstructive surgery: part I. Plast Reconstr Surg 2008;121(1):4e–12e
5. Etra JW, Raimondi G, Brandacher G. Mechanisms of rejection in vascular composite allotransplantation. Curr Opin Organ Transplant 2018;23(1):28–33

OUTCOMES FOLLOWING HAND TRANSPLANTATION

8. Which one of the following is true regarding hand transplantation performed at forearm level?

C. Tactile and discriminative sensation are regained in most transplant cases.

It is reasonable to expect a good sensory recovery after hand transplant, with more than 90% reported rates of return for tactile, pain, and temperature sensation. While extrinsic motor function is expected in all cases, the rate of intrinsic recovery is less predictable. A midforearm transplant is more likely to produce a good result than a more proximal transplant; there is a shorter distance for nerve recovery to reinnervate distal muscles, there is a functioning elbow, and there is the possibility of strong Pulvertaft tendon weaves for uniting the extrinsic motor units (rather than muscle belly repairs). Peak recovery is not at 1 year, as recovery is expected to continue for several years.

The DASH score is a well-regarded scoring system used for upper limb function. However, it is not specific to hand transplantation. A hand transplantation score has been developed (HTSS) and this has six key areas: appearance, sensibility, movement, psychological and social acceptance, activities of daily living, and patient satisfaction.[1-5]

REFERENCES

1. Shores JT, Malek V, Lee WPA, Brandacher G. Outcomes after hand and upper extremity transplantation. J Mater Sci Mater Med 2017;28(5):72
2. Kaufman CL, Breidenbach W. World experience after more than a decade of clinical hand transplantation: update from the Louisville hand transplant program. Hand Clin 2011;27(4):417–421, vii–viii
3. Brandacher G, Ninkovic M, Piza-Katzer H, et al. The Innsbruck hand transplant program: update at 8 years after the first transplant. Transplant Proc 2009;41(2):491–494
4. Ninkovic M, Weissenbacher A, Gabl M, et al. Functional outcome after hand and forearm transplantation: what can be achieved? Hand Clin 2011;27(4):455–465, viii–ix
5. Petruzzo P, Lanzetta M, Dubernard JM, et al. The international registry on hand and composite tissue transplantation. Transplantation 2008;86(4):487–492

OUTCOMES AFTER HAND TRANSPLANT

9. Which one of the following is expected at 6 months after hand transplantation?

E. 75% chance of patient satisfaction

In spite of the rigorous medical regimen, the side effects from medications, and the intrusive therapy and monitoring schedule, more than 75% of patients have a subjective improvement in quality of life after a hand transplant. Most patients perform activities of daily living independently and some have returned to full employment. The risk of metabolic complications is approximately 70%. The risk of hyperglycemia-induced problems secondary to immunotherapy is around 45%.

Acute rejection has been a consistent problem after limb transplant, with 85% incidence within the first year. These episodes are, however, usually treatable with immunotherapy modification. The risk of opportunistic infection is high because of immunosuppression. This is estimated to be approximately 60 to 65%. Infections include cytomegalovirus, herpes, and bacterial subtypes. Appropriate prophylaxis is required, particularly in the first 6 to 12 months. The risk of graft loss is low across all series of vascularized transplant, although the Chinese series on limb transplant reported losses over 40% because of poor postoperative compliance with medical therapy.[1]

REFERENCE

1. Pei G, Xiang D, Gu L, et al. A report of 15 hand allotransplantations in 12 patients and their outcomes in China. Transplantation 2012;94(10):1052–1059

MANAGEMENT OF COMPLICATIONS AFTER HAND TRANSPLANT

10. You are asked to assess a patient following hand transplantation as there are concerns regarding acute rejection. In order to assess rejection according to the Banff classification, what test will be required?

E. Skin biopsy

Vascularized composite allograft rejection is graded according to the Banff classification,[1] which is based on the histological appearances of a 4-mm punch biopsy specimen. The grades of rejection range from 0 to 4 based on evidence of the extent and severity of inflammatory change and the presence or absence of cell necrosis.

REFERENCE

1. Cendales LC, Kanitakis J, Schneeberger S, et al. The Banff 2007 working classification of skin-containing composite tissue allograft pathology. Am J Transplant 2008;8(7): 1396–1400

MANAGEMENT OF ACUTE REJECTION FOLLOWING HAND TRANSPLANT

11. You have confirmed the presence of acute rejection clinically by using the Banff scoring system in a patient following hand transplant. *Which one of the following represents the first-line agent you should use to manage this rejection?*

D. Corticosteroid

The first-line agent in an acute rejection episode is a high-dose corticosteroid (prednisolone/hydrocortisone), while ensuring that tacrolimus or MMF doses are optimized. Second-line agents include high-dose tacrolimus, monoclonal antibodies, and sirolimus.[1]

REFERENCE

1. Fischer S, Lian CG, Kueckelhaus M, et al. Acute rejection in vascularized composite allotransplantation. Curr Opin Organ Transplant 2014;19(6):531–544

87. Targeted Muscle Reinnervation

See *Essentials of Plastic Surgery*, third edition, pp. 1209–1215

DEMOGRAPHICS OF LIMB AMPUTATIONS

1. *Which one of the following is true regarding limb amputations and their sequelae?*
   A. In the United States there are typically 40,000 new limb amputations performed per annum.
   B. The most common reason for limb amputation is poorly managed diabetes.
   C. More than three quarters of all limb amputees experience chronic localized phantom or residual limb pain.
   D. Neuromas represent disorganized nerve fibers and are reliably treated with traditional surgical techniques.
   E. Stump neuromas can have profoundly negative effects on the overall functional ability of a limb amputee.

INDICATIONS FOR TARGETED MUSCLE REINNERVATION

2. *Which one of the following was the original primary indication for targeted muscle reinnervation (TMR)?*
   A. Reduce chronic pain after limb amputation
   B. Provide intuitive control of upper limb prostheses
   C. Accelerate wound healing after limb amputation
   D. Enhance residual muscle function after limb amputation
   E. Provide a more robust soft-tissue cover for the amputated limb

APPROACHES TO NEUROMA MANAGEMENT FOLLOWING AMPUTATION

3. *What is the critical element of TMR that differentiates it from other neuroma operations?*
   A. It uses a minimally invasive approach.
   B. It restores normal localized sensation.
   C. It promotes organized nerve regeneration.
   D. It promotes growth factors for accelerated healing.
   E. It relies on the principles of Wallerian degeneration.

PREOPERATIVE ASSESSMENT IN TARGETED MUSCLE REINNERVATION

4. *Prior to undertaking TMR in a limb amputee with neuroma pain, which one of the following would be most likely to help assess whether treatment will be effective?*
   A. Obtaining a magnetic resonance imaging scan (MRI).
   B. Eliciting a Tinel's sign in the affected limb during clinical examination.
   C. Performing a steroid injection at the suspected neuroma site.
   D. Injecting botulinum toxin to the suspected neuroma site.
   E. Injecting lidocaine at the suspected neuroma site.

SURGICAL TECHNIQUE FOR TARGETED MUSCLE REINNERVATION

5. *When performing TMR which one of the following is true?*
   A. A nerve stimulator should be used to identify the peripheral nerve for transfer.
   B. Nerve coaptation is best performed 1 cm proximal to the target muscle.
   C. Care must be taken to avoid division of the target muscle nerve.
   D. The nerve coaptation is best performed with individual fascicular repair.
   E. A peripheral to motor nerve size discrepancy is generally well tolerated.

OUTCOMES FOLLOWING TARGETED MUSCLE REINNERVATION

6. *When considering the outcomes of TMR, which one of the following is true?*
   A. Phantom limb sensation should progressively disappear postoperatively.
   B. Phantom limb pain usually starts to improve 12 months postsurgery.
   C. Analgesic requirements normally increase in the first few months postsurgery.
   D. Evidence supports the incorporation of TMR at the time of primary amputation.
   E. The need for a prosthesis following amputation is frequently reduced after TMR.

TARGETED MUSCLE REINNERVATION IN BELOW-KNEE AMPUTATION

7. You are performing an elective below-knee amputation (BKA) in a 38-year-old patient following longstanding problems with foot and ankle instability and pain after major trauma. You decide to take a TMR approach in this case. *Which one of the following muscles would be ideally indicated for nerve transfer of the tibial nerve?*
   A. Medial gastrocnemius
   B. Semitendinosus
   C. Gracilis
   D. Peroneus brevis
   E. Adductor longus

Answers

DEMOGRAPHICS OF LIMB AMPUTATIONS

1. *Which one of the following is true regarding limb amputations and their sequelae?*

    E. Stump neuromas can have profoundly negative effects on the overall functional ability of a limb amputee.
    In the United States, there are approximately 185,000 amputations each year (not 40,000) and there are nearly 2 million amputees in total. Nearly half of all amputations occur following trauma or as part of oncologic treatment. The remaining cases are secondary to vascular disease, diabetes, infection, sepsis, and other vasculopathies.[1] Between a quarter and a half of all amputee patients experience chronic localized pain secondary to symptomatic neuromas and/or phantom limb pain (PLP).[2-6]

    Neuromas are disorganized bundles of nerve fibers that form at the end of a divided or damaged nerve secondary to aberrant nerve fiber regeneration. Their development can have a significant negative impact on the functional rehabilitation and overall outcome of patients with amputations because of chronic pain and subsequent problems with fitting of prosthetics. Management of troublesome neuromas and the pain they cause can be challenging with traditional medical and surgical approaches.

REFERENCES

1. Ziegler-Graham K, MacKenzie EJ, Ephraim PL, Travison TG, Brookmeyer R. Estimating the prevalence of limb loss in the United States: 2005 to 2050. Arch Phys Med Rehabil 2008;89(3):422–429
2. Jensen TS, Krebs B, Nielsen J, Rasmussen P. Phantom limb, phantom pain and stump pain in amputees during the first 6 months following limb amputation. Pain 1983;17(3):243–256
3. Jensen TS, Krebs B, Nielsen J, Rasmussen P. Immediate and long-term phantom limb pain in amputees: incidence, clinical characteristics and relationship to pre-amputation limb pain. Pain 1985;21(3):267–278
4. Pierce RO Jr, Kernek CB, Ambrose TA II. The plight of the traumatic amputee. Orthopedics 1993;16(7):793–797
5. Ducic I, Mesbahi AN, Attinger CE, Graw K. The role of peripheral nerve surgery in the treatment of chronic pain associated with amputation stumps. Plast Reconstr Surg 2008;121(3):908–914, discussion 915–917
6. Harris AM, Althausen PL, Kellam J, Bosse MJ, Castillo R; Lower Extremity Assessment Project (LEAP) Study Group. Complications following limb-threatening lower extremity trauma. J Orthop Trauma 2009;23(1):1–6

INDICATIONS FOR TARGETED MUSCLE REINNERVATION

2. *Which one of the following was the original primary indication for targeted muscle reinnervation (TMR)?*

    B. Provide intuitive control of upper limb prostheses
    TMR is a surgical procedure that was originally designed to provide intuitive control of upper limb prostheses following amputation, through transfer of residual nerves to otherwise redundant denervated target muscle. It was noticed early on that many TMR patients noted a reduction in pain, sometimes with complete resolution of neuroma-related pain in an affected limb following this procedure.[1-6] A rabbit amputation model was subsequently developed to study the effects of TMR. This showed that after 10 weeks, transferred nerves were found to more closely resemble that of their uninjured counterparts than that of a neuroma.[7] Since then, multicenter patient trials have shown that TMR provides a consistent long-term benefit of pain relief and symptoms associated with both symptomatic neuroma and phantom limb pain.[8]

REFERENCES

1. Kuiken TA, Dumanian GA, Lipschutz RD, Miller LA, Stubblefield KA. The use of targeted muscle reinnervation for improved myoelectric prosthesis control in a bilateral shoulder disarticulation amputee. Prosthet Orthot Int 2004;28(3):245–253
2. Hijjawi JB, Kuiken TA, Lipschutz RD, Miller LA, Stubblefield KA, Dumanian GA. Improved myoelectric prosthesis control accomplished using multiple nerve transfers. Plast Reconstr Surg 2006;118(7):1573–1578
3. Kuiken TA, Miller LA, Lipschutz RD, et al. Targeted reinnervation for enhanced prosthetic arm function in a woman with a proximal amputation: a case study. Lancet 2007;369(9559): 371–380
4. O'Shaughnessy KD, Dumanian GA, Lipschutz RD, Miller LA, Stubblefield K, Kuiken TA. Targeted reinnervation to improve prosthesis control in transhumeral amputees. A report of three cases. J Bone Joint Surg Am 2008;90(2):393–400
5. Dumanian GA, Ko JH, O'Shaughnessy KD, Kim PS, Wilson CJ, Kuiken TA. Targeted reinnervation for transhumeral amputees: current surgical technique and update on results. Plast Reconstr Surg 2009;124(3):863–869
6. Kuiken TA, Li G, Lock BA, et al. Targeted muscle reinnervation for real-time myoelectric control of multifunction artificial arms. JAMA 2009;301(6):619–628
7. Kim PS, Ko JH, O'Shaughnessy KK, Kuiken TA, Pohlmeyer EA, Dumanian GA. The effects of targeted muscle reinnervation on neuromas in a rabbit rectus abdominis flap model. J Hand Surg Am 2012;37(8):1609–1616

8. Valerio IL, Dumanian GA, Jordan SW, et al. Preemptive treatment of phantom and residual limb pain with targeted muscle reinnervation at the time of major limb amputation. J Am Coll Surg 2019;228(3):217–226

APPROACHES TO NEUROMA MANAGEMENT FOLLOWING AMPUTATION

3. *What is the critical element of TMR that differentiates it from other neuroma operations?*

    C. It promotes organized nerve regeneration.

        Coaptation of the amputated nerve stumps to recipient motor nerve branches in TMR encourages organized nerve regeneration into the denervated target muscles, thus preventing the chaotic and misdirected nerve growth that typically leads to neuroma formation. This critical element of nerve-to-nerve coaptation differentiates TMR from other neuroma operations where nerve ends may be buried in muscle or bone or left to retract in other soft tissue. The central principle underlying the nerve transfers in TMR surgery is to reestablish a function for the divided nerve. This surgery uses a normal open surgical approach and is not minimally invasive. It does not restore normal localized function, nor promote growth factors for healing. Wallerian degeneration occurs when a nerve is divided and there is degeneration of the proximal nerve back to the next node of Ranvier. This is a process that occurs predictably in peripheral nerve divisions irrespective of subsequent surgery. It is after this point that the TMR process and principles differ.[1–4]

REFERENCES

1. Kim PS, Ko JH, O'Shaughnessy KK, Kuiken TA, Pohlmeyer EA, Dumanian GA. The effects of targeted muscle reinnervation on neuromas in a rabbit rectus abdominis flap model. J Hand Surg Am 2012;37(8):1609–1616
2. Souza JM, Fey NP, Cheesborough JE, et al. Advances in transfemoral amputee rehabilitation: early experience with targeted muscle reinnervation. Curr Surg Rep 2014;2:51
3. Bowen JB, Wee CE, Kalik J, Valerio IL. Targeted muscle reinnervation to improve pain, prosthetic tolerance, and bioprosthetic outcomes in the amputee. Adv Wound Care (New Rochelle) 2017;6(8):261–267
4. Ducic I, Mesbahi AN, Attinger CE, Graw K. The role of peripheral nerve surgery in the treatment of chronic pain associated with amputation stumps. Plast Reconstr Surg 2008;121(3):908–914, discussion 915–917

PREOPERATIVE ASSESSMENT IN TARGETED MUSCLE REINNERVATION

4. *Prior to undertaking TMR in a limb amputee with neuroma pain, which one of the following would be most likely to help assess whether treatment will be effective?*

    E. Injecting lidocaine at the suspected neuroma site.

        There are a number of things that are useful in the preoperative workup for TMR in patients with a painful neuroma. These start with an office consultation to discuss the procedure with the patient and set their expectations as well as perform a physical examination. A useful and reliable way to assess whether neuroma surgery is likely to be beneficial is to inject local anesthetic into the area where pain originates, i.e., around the presumed neuroma to assess the effects of doing so. Physical examination and palpation can guide the injection to the site of a neuroma. Tinel's sign or ultrasound guidance can help with this. In essence, if the block proves effective, i.e., it alleviates the patient's usual pain, then they may be a good candidate for TMR. This is probably the most useful single test to be performed preoperatively.

        An MRI may also be ordered if further visualization and characterization of the neuroma is required. It is useful for the patient to record a pain and medication diary, documenting daily symptoms, duration, intensity, and type of pain. This can help assess the effectiveness of surgery postoperatively by repeating the diary exercise. Neither injection of steroid or botulinum toxin would be helpful in this setting.[1,2]

REFERENCES

1. Pet MA, Ko JH, Friedly JL, Mourad PD, Smith DG. Does targeted nerve implantation reduce neuroma pain in amputees? Clin Orthop Relat Res 2014;472(10):2991–3001
2. Souza JM, Cheesborough JE, Ko JH, Cho MS, Kuiken TA, Dumanian GA. Targeted muscle reinnervation: a novel approach to postamputation neuroma pain. Clin Orthop Relat Res 2014;472(10):2984–2990

SURGICAL TECHNIQUE FOR TARGETED MUSCLE REINNERVATION

5. *When performing TMR which one of the following is true?*

    E. A peripheral to motor nerve size discrepancy is generally well tolerated.

        When performing TMR during or following amputation, there is normally a size discrepancy between the donor and target nerves because the motor nerve branches tend to be small, whereas the peripheral nerves tend to be far larger as they would originally have divided distally to form different individual nerves. This size discrepancy is generally well tolerated and the key point is to reestablish the higher-level functions of the major amputated peripheral nerve by giving this nerve somewhere to go.

The peripheral nerves which are to be transferred are identified visually by careful dissection and without a nerve stimulator, but it is the target motor nerves which are identified with the aid of a nerve stimulator following their visualization.

The motor nerve target is transected near its entry point to muscle, preserving only enough length to perform suture neurorrhaphy (~2 mm), as this gives the shortest distance for nerve regeneration to occur. The neurorrhaphy is performed end to end with an epineural suture technique. Individual fascicular or group fascicular coaptation is not normally required.[1]

REFERENCE

1. Bowen JB, Wee CE, Kalik J, Valerio IL. Targeted muscle reinnervation to improve pain, prosthetic tolerance, and bioprosthetic outcomes in the amputee. Adv Wound Care (New Rochelle) 2017;6(8):261–267

OUTCOMES FOLLOWING TARGETED MUSCLE REINNERVATION

6. **When considering the outcomes of TMR, which one of the following is true?**
   D. **Evidence supports the incorporation of TMR at the time of primary amputation.**
   The rates of neuroma formation and the severity of the neuroma which develops are reduced when TMR is performed as part of a primary limb amputation. For this reason, it should be considered in primary amputation cases. Alternatively, where there has been neuroma development postamputation, TMR is indicated to address pain.
   Phantom limb sensation will remain following TMR; however, phantom limb pain should improve in the first 3 months following surgery. Analgesic requirements, particularly for opiates, normally decrease in the first few months following TMR surgery. The use of a prosthesis is increased following TMR (not decreased) because of the reduction in pain.[1,2]

REFERENCES

1. Bowen JB, Wee CE, Kalik J, Valerio IL. Targeted muscle reinnervation to improve pain, prosthetic tolerance, and bioprosthetic outcomes in the amputee. Adv Wound Care (New Rochelle) 2017;6(8):261–267
2. Valerio IL, Dumanian GA, Jordan SW, et al. Preemptive treatment of phantom and residual limb pain with targeted muscle reinnervation at the time of major limb amputation. J Am Coll Surg 2019;228(3):217–226

TARGETED MUSCLE REINNERVATION IN BELOW-KNEE AMPUTATION

7. **You are performing an elective below-knee amputation (BKA) in a 38-year-old patient following longstanding problems with foot and ankle instability and pain after major trauma. You decide to take a TMR approach in this case. Which one of the following muscles would be ideally indicated for nerve transfer of the tibial nerve?**
   A. **Medial gastrocnemius**
   There are a number of recommended nerve transfer combinations in TMR in order to reduce the likelihood of symptomatic end neuroma. These relate to each individual amputation level. The recommended muscle sites for the tibial nerve in BKA are the soleus, tibialis posterior, and gastrocnemius. The semitendinosus is recommended for the common peroneal component of the sciatic nerve during above knee amputation, the gracilis is recommended for the saphenous nerve in the above knee amputation, and the peroneus brevis is indicated for the deep peroneal nerve in a BKA. However, many combinations of nerve transfer can provide the divided nerve with a target muscle and maintain the central principle of TMR: to reestablish the higher level functions of the major amputated peripheral nerve by giving this nerve a direction and function. Other popular combinations include those shown in **Tables 87.1** through **87.5**

Table 87.1 *Nerve Transfers for Below-Knee Amputation TMR*

Donor Nerve	Target Motor Nerve Branch
Tibial	Medial or lateral gastrocnemius Tibialis posterior Medial or lateral soleus
Deep peroneal	Tibialis anterior Peroneus longus Peroneus brevis
Superficial peroneal	Medial soleus Peroneus longus Peroneus brevis
Sural	Tibialis posterior Soleus

Table 87.2 *Nerve Transfers for Above-Knee Amputation TMR*

Donor Nerve	Target Motor Nerve Branch
Tibial component of sciatic nerve	Biceps femoris
Common peroneal component of sciatic nerve	Semitendinosus
Saphenous	Gracilis

Table 87.3 *Nerve Transfers for Forequarter Amputation TMR*

Donor Nerve	Target Motor Nerve Branch
Median nerve	Pectoralis major
Musculocutaneous nerve	Clavicular head nerve branch of pectoralis major
Ulnar nerve	Pectoralis minor
Radial nerve	Long thoracic
	Thoracodorsal

Table 87.4 *Nerve Transfers for Transhumeral Amputation TMR*

Donor Nerve	Target Motor Nerve Branch
Medial antebrachial cutaneous nerve	End-to-side to motor nerve branch of distal brachialis
Lateral antebrachial cutaneous nerve	Motor nerve branch of radial nerve innervating brachialis (where present) or brachioradialis
Median nerve	Musculocutaneous nerve motor branch to short head of biceps brachii
Ulnar nerve	Musculocutaneous nerve motor branch to brachialis
Musculocutaneous nerve	End-to-side to musculocutaneous nerve motor nerve branch of long head of biceps brachii
Radial nerve	Motor nerve branch of lateral head of triceps

Table 87.5 *Nerve Transfers for Transradial Amputation TMR*

Donor Nerve	Target Motor Nerve Branch
Median nerve	Flexor digitorum superficialis
Ulnar	Flexor carpi ulnaris
Superficial radial nerve	Anterior interosseous nerve
	Flexor digitorum profundus

88. Hand Rehabilitation

See *Essentials of Plastic Surgery*, third edition, pp. 1216–1229

THE SAFE HAND SPLINTING POSITION

1. *Which one of the following describes the key elements of the "safe" or "intrinsic plus" hand position? (Numbers refer to wrist extension, and MCP/IP joint flexion, respectively)*
   A. Wrist 0 degrees, metacarpophalangeal (MCP) 80 degrees, interphalangeal (IP) 0 degrees
   B. Wrist 20 degrees, MCP 80 degrees, IP 10 degrees
   C. Wrist 30 degrees, MCP 100 degrees, IP 20 degrees
   D. Wrist 50 degrees, MCP 70 degrees, IP 30 degrees
   E. Wrist 70 degrees, MCP 90 degrees, IP 10 degrees

HAND AND FINGER SPLINTS

2. *Which one of the following would be the most appropriate in the management of a swan-neck deformity of the finger?*
   A. Buddy taping
   B. Figure-of-eight splint
   C. Hyperextension splint
   D. Dorsal blocking splint
   E. Ulnar gutter splint

PRINCIPLES OF HAND SPLINTING

3. *Which one of the following is true regarding hand splinting following injury?*
   A. Dynamic splints are contraindicated in intra-articular fractures.
   B. The joints either side of a fracture site should normally be immobilized.
   C. A short-arm cast is used to stabilize the humerus.
   D. The sugar tong splint is most useful for thumb metacarpal injuries.
   E. The ulnar gutter splint is mainly used for mid shaft ulna fractures.

REHABILITATION FOLLOWING FLEXOR TENDON INJURY

4. *When managing a patient postoperatively following a two-strand zone I flexor tendon repair, which one of the following is true?*
   A. The hand should be rested in a forearm-based volar splint for 4 weeks.
   B. The injured digit should remain immobilized for the first 2 weeks.
   C. The patient should commence an early active mobilization program.
   D. The patient should commence an early passive mobilization program.
   E. This requires more intensive physiotherapy than other flexor zones of injury.

SAFE SPLINTING AFTER EXTENSOR TENDON REPAIR

5. Following repair of multiple extensor tendons in zones 5 and 6, you decide to immobilize the hand and wrist completely for the first week. *How should the splint used differ from the traditionally described "intrinsic plus position"?*
   A. The angle of wrist position
   B. The angle of the MCP joint position
   C. The angle of the proximal interphalangeal joint position
   D. The angle of the distal interphalangeal joint position
   E. The length of the splint

MANAGEMENT OF SCAPHOID FRACTURES

6. *When managing a patient nonoperatively with a scaphoid fracture, which one of the following is correct?*
   A. They should be placed in a forearm-based thumb spica for 4 weeks.
   B. They should commence active assist range of motion (ROM) at 4 weeks.
   C. They should commence passive ROM exercises at 6 weeks.
   D. They should commence active ROM exercises at 8 weeks.
   E. They should commence strengthening exercises at 10 weeks.

PATIENT ASSESSMENT FOLLOWING HAND INJURY REHABILITATION

7. *When assessing patients in clinic following hand injury, which one of the following will provide the best indication of grip strength?*
   A. Goniometer
   B. Semmes-Weinstein monofilament
   C. Rubber band traction
   D. Dynamometer
   E. 2-point discriminator

MANAGEMENT OF THE INJURED WRIST

8. *When managing a distal radius fracture, which one of the following is true?*
   A. A small proportion of patients will need hand therapy.
   B. Where hand therapy is indicated, it typically involves two to three sessions per week.
   C. Where hand therapy is indicated, it usually involves a 12-week program.
   D. Hand therapy beyond 12 weeks is still beneficial in this setting.
   E. In older patients returning directly to activities of daily living is discouraged.

MANAGEMENT OF BENNETT'S FRACTURE OF THE THUMB

9. *Which one of the following is true when managing a Bennett fracture of the thumb?*
   A. The rehabilitation protocol is the same whether surgery has been performed or not.
   B. Surgery will be required in all cases for this type of injury pattern.
   C. Splinting is limited to 2 to 3 weeks in order to optimize postoperative ROM.
   D. Active ROM is restricted until after 6 weeks postinjury.
   E. A dorsal blocking splint is usually preferred to immobilize these fractures.

METACARPAL AND PHALANGEAL FRACTURE MANAGEMENT

10. *What is the main benefit of treating metacarpal or phalangeal fractures with open reduction and internal fixation (ORIF) as opposed to nonoperative treatment?*
    A. Superior functional outcome
    B. Ability to mobilize earlier
    C. A reduction in postinjury pain
    D. A reduction in postinjury swelling
    E. Better aesthetic outcomes

Answers

THE SAFE HAND SPLINTING POSITION

1. *Which one of the following describes the key elements of the "safe" or "intrinsic plus" hand position? (Numbers refer to wrist extension, and metacarpophalangeal (MCP)/interphalangeal (IP) joint flexion, respectively)*

    B. Wrist 20 degrees, MCP 80 degrees, IP 10 degrees

        The "safe" position for splinting of the hand is also known as "intrinsic plus" and involves placing the joints into positions which will minimize stiffness and loss of motion based on hand anatomy principles. The position includes the wrist at 20 to 30 degrees of extension, the MCP joints at 70 to 90 degrees of flexion, and the IP joints at 0 to 20 degrees of flexion. This position is also sometimes known as the Edinburgh position as originally described by James.[1,2]

        This position ensures appropriate tension on the collateral ligaments and volar plates of the wrist and finger joints so that shortening and subsequent flexion contractures are less likely to occur. It also maximizes function if stiffness persists in the splinted position (**Fig. 88.1**).

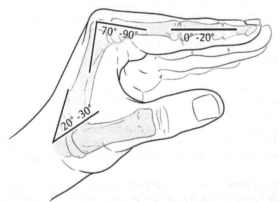

Fig. 88.1 Safe position for splinting of the hand (also known as intrinsic plus position).

REFERENCES

1. James JIP. Fractures of the proximal and middle phalanges of the fingers. Acta Orthop Scand 1962;32:401–412
2. James JIP. The assessment and management of the injured hand. Hand 1970;2(2):97–105

HAND AND FINGER SPLINTS

2. *Which one of the following would be the most appropriate in the management of a swan-neck deformity of the finger?*

    B. Figure-of-eight splint

        The figure-of-eight splint is shown in **Fig. 88.2**.

        This is useful in cases of swan-neck deformity. The swan-neck deformity is characterized by hyperextension at the proximal interphalangeal (PIP) joint combined with flexion at the distal interphalangeal (DIP) joint. It is caused by an imbalance of muscle and tendon forces within the digit and can occur as a result of many different problems, including but not limited to: volar plate injury at the PIP joint, generalized hyperextensibility, MCP joint volar subluxation (as occurs in rheumatoid arthritis), flexor digitorum superficialis (FDS) tendon injury, intrinsic muscle contractures, and chronic mallet finger. The primary problem is often disruption of the volar plate at the PIP joint which allows the joint to slide into hyperextension. A chronic mallet injury can lead to transference of DIP joint extension forces into PIP extension forces. An FDS rupture can lead to unopposed PIP joint extension with gradual attenuation of volar plate integrity, or unmasking of underlying volar plate

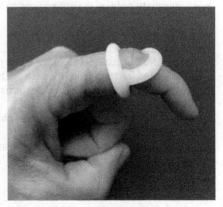

Fig. 88.2 Figure-of-eight splint.

laxity. When the PIP joint hyperextends, tethering of the lateral bands by the transverse retinacular ligament at PIP joint level restricts their transmission of force to the terminal tendon, i.e., DIP joint extension; so, the DIP joint tends to exhibit an extension lag and the PIP joint extension may be further exaggerated. The figure-of-eight splint serves to restrain the extending PIP joint in a mild degree of flexion while still allowing active flexion and extension without a cumbersome dorsal splint or adhesive tapes; therefore, it is usually readily tolerated. In fact, some companies manufacture ornamental swan-neck splints that serve as functional jewelry.

Buddy taping is useful for managing collateral ligament injuries of the digit as well as some closed fractures of the digits and hand. It relies on the principle that the adjacent uninjured digit supports the injured digit through a safe range of movement to minimize stiffness while protecting any healing structures. Hyperextension splints are static splints used for the management of terminal extensor tendon disruption (mallet finger). Holding the DIP joint in hyperextension can help maximize approximation of the tendon end to its bony insertion. Dorsal blocking splints can be made for many purposes. For example, they are useful short-term for volar plate injuries to facilitate early mobilization while avoiding hyperextension. The splint angle is usually progressively reduced as weeks go by. They are also useful for flexor tendon repair protocols. Ulnar gutter splints are useful for 4th and 5th ray injuries, such as metacarpal fractures and carpometacarpal (CMC) joint fracture dislocations to immobilize the injured digits whilst allowing movement of the uninjured digits.[1-3]

REFERENCES

1. Richards T, Clement R, Russell I, Newington D. Acute hand injury splinting - the good, the bad and the ugly. Ann R Coll Surg Engl 2018;100(2):92–96
2. Chan DY. Management of simple finger injuries: the splinting regime. Hand Surg 2002;7(2):223–230
3. Lalonde D. Managing Boutonniere and swan-neck deformities. BMC Proc 2015;9(Suppl 3):A50

PRINCIPLES OF HAND SPLINTING

3. *Which one of the following is true regarding hand splinting following injury?*

   B. The joints either side of a fracture site should normally be immobilized.

One of the key principles in fracture management using splints is that the joint proximal and the joint distal to the fracture site should be immobilized within the splint. As with many rules in medicine, there are exceptions. For example, in some metacarpal injuries the MCP joints are left free. However, this is a general principle that is usually followed.

Dynamic splints are useful for managing some intra-articular joint fractures, as they can be used to hold the joint out to length (i.e., distract it), while facilitating early range of motion (ROM) to reduce long-term stiffness and to encourage healing of a damaged joint surface in a functional contour. Examples include the Suzuki frame and the Giddins frame; each used for PIP joint injuries.[1,2]

The short-arm splint is used for wrist and metacarpal stabilization, as opposed to the humerus. The sugar tong splint is so named because of its similarity to tongs used to pick up sugar cubes. It prevents forearm supination and pronation; so, for example, it can be useful for some distal radius, ulnar styloid, and carpal bone fractures, along with elective procedures involving the distal radioulnar joint. The free ends are volar and dorsal at the level of the metacarpal heads, with a continuous slab passing along the dorsal and volar aspects of the forearm and around the elbow (which is flexed at 90 degrees). The ulnar gutter splint is generally used to immobilize the 4th and 5th metacarpals after injury rather than the ulnar itself. One key element to ensure when applying splints is that superficial nerve locations are well padded to prevent neuropraxia. Splint materials are exothermic; so, adequate padding is also required to avoid contact burns.[3,4]

REFERENCES

1. Suzuki Y, Matsunaga T, Sato S, Yokoi T. The pins and rubbers traction system for treatment of comminuted intraarticular fractures and fracture-dislocations in the hand. J Hand Surg [Br] 1994;19(1):98–107
2. Hynes MC, Giddins GEB. Dynamic external fixation for pilon fractures of the interphalangeal joints. J Hand Surg [Br] 2001;26(2):122–124
3. Hardy MA. Principles of metacarpal and phalangeal fracture management: a review of rehabilitation concepts. J Orthop Sports Phys Ther 2004;34(12):781–799
4. Bullocks J, Hsu P, Izaddoost S, et al, eds. Plastic Surgery Emergencies. Principles and Techniques. 2nd ed. New York, NY: Thieme; 2017

REHABILITATION FOLLOWING FLEXOR TENDON INJURY

4. *When managing a patient postoperatively following a two-strand zone I flexor tendon repair, which one of the following is true?*

D. The patient should commence an early passive mobilization program.

This patient should be placed in a forearm-based **dorsal** blocking splint (not volar) which should pass distally to just beyond the fingertips. This is to protect the repair from excessive extension and should be worn for 4 to 6 weeks. Patients with such injuries usually need to be mobilized early to prevent adhesions and stiffness, and this can be done using either an active or a passive program, depending on strength of repair, and surgeon, therapist preferences. This patient has only a two-strand repair. It would be most appropriate to undertake an early passive mobilization program such as the modified Duran protocol.[1] This involves passive flexion of all digits combined with active extension of all digits to the limits of the splint in week 1 and 2. Then in week 3, a place and hold approach is used to facilitate limited isometric flexion of all digits. At week 6, active ROM of all digits can be commenced and from weeks 8 to 12, further strengthening exercises are undertaken. Active motion protocols, such as the Indiana protocol, can incur a higher incidence of rupture, but an improved ROM compared with passive motion protocols.[2] However, these should be reserved for four strand (or greater) flexor tendon repair techniques.[3] Of all the flexor tendon zones, it is zone 2 that would typically require the most intensive physiotherapy, although zone 1 injures will still require intensive and meticulous care (**Table 88.1**).

Table 88.1 *Modified Duran Protocol for Flexor Tendon Rehabilitation*

Modified Duran Protocol	
Orthosis: Forearm-based dorsal block splint, wrist in 20-degree flexion, MCPs at 40–50 degrees and IPs straight for 4–6 weeks	Week 1: passive flexion of all digits and active extension to the limits of the splint
	Week 3: place and hold—limited isometric flexion of all digits using rubber band traction
	Week 6: active range of motion (AROM) of all digits
	Weeks 8–12: strengthening
Thumb FPL (early passive motion protocol)	
Orthosis: Forearm-based dorsal block for thumb only, wrist in neutral, thumb MP at 30-degree flexion, thumb IP at 20-degree flexion	Days 3–5: thumb passive flexion and active extension within the limits of the splint
	Week 3–4: thumb AROM
	Week 6: strengthening

REFERENCES

1. Duran RJ, Houser RG. Controlled passive motion following flexor tendon repair in zones two and three. In: American Association of Orthopedic Surgeons Symposium on Tendon Surgery in the Hand. St. Louis, MO: C.V. Mosby Company, 1975
2. Trumble TE, Vedder NB, Seiler JG III, Hanel DP, Diao E, Pettrone S. Zone-II flexor tendon repair: a randomized prospective trial of active place-and-hold therapy compared with passive motion therapy. J Bone Joint Surg Am 2010;92(6):1381–1389
3. Starr HM, Snoddy M, Hammond KE, Seiler JG III. Flexor tendon repair rehabilitation protocols: a systematic review. J Hand Surg Am 2013;38(9):1712–7.e1, 14

SAFE SPLINTING AFTER EXTENSOR TENDON REPAIR

5. Following repair of multiple extensor tendons in zones 5 and 6, you decide to immobilize the hand and wrist completely for the first week. *How should the splint used differ from the traditionally described "intrinsic plus position"?*

B. The angle of the MCP joint position

The traditional "intrinsic plus" hand position is designed to keep collateral ligaments and flexible joint structures in a suitably stretched position so that flexion contractures and subsequent stiffness are minimized. The wrist is held in 20 to 30 degrees of extension, the MCP joints in 70 to 90 degrees of flexion, and the IP joints in (or near to) extension. Following zone 5, 6, or 7 extensor tendon injury repair, the "safe" position is modified slightly to protect the repair at the MCP joint level. Therefore, while the wrist and IP joint angles are maintained, the MCP joint position is more extended at between 0- and 30-degree flexion according to surgeon and therapist preference. Some surgeons and therapist prefer to leave the IP joints free for early motion while the MCP joint is immobilized, whereas others use exercises within a full length splint to keep the IP joints mobile and allow some active MCP joint extension. Active ROM at the wrist is usually commenced at 4 weeks (**Table 88.2**).[1]

Table 88.2 *Extensor Tendon Injury*

Zone of Injury	Orthosis	Protocol
Zone 1 Mallet finger	DIP in full extension or slight hyperextension, PIP free	6-week full-time wear
Zone 2 Non-op and post-op	Finger splint in full extension for 6–8 weeks	Weeks 6–8: active range of motion (AROM) Week 12: passive range of motion (PROM), strengthening if indicated
Zone 3/4 Boutonniere non-op	Central slip injury: PIP extension splint full time for 4 weeks Central slip + lateral band injury: PIP + DIP extension splint full time for 4 weeks	Central slip injury: Week 1: DIP A/PROM Central slip + lateral band injury: Week 4: DIP AROM
Zone 3/4 Boutonniere post-op	Finger splint in full extension until 6 weeks; Exercise template splint may also be fabricated allowing gradual PIP and DIP flexion	Central slip repair: week 1: AROM of DIP Central slip + lateral band repair: limit DIP flexion 35 degrees Week 5: full digit flexion and strengthening
Zone 5/6/7 post-op	Forearm-based volar splint wrist in 30-degree extension; MPs at 0-degree extension, IPs free for 4 weeks	Week 4: AROM wrist and digits Week 8: strengthening

REFERENCE

1. Comer GC, Gordon C, Yao J. Hand therapy modalities following extensor mechanism surgery. J Hand Surg Am 2015;40(10):2081–2084

MANAGEMENT OF SCAPHOID FRACTURES

6. *When managing a patient nonoperatively with a scaphoid fracture, which one of the following is correct?*

   D. They should commence active ROM exercises at 8 weeks.

   Rehabilitation for scaphoid fractures will differ depending on whether the treatment is operative or nonoperative. For nonoperative cases such as low-risk stable scaphoid waist fractures, most U.S. protocols involve 8 weeks of immobilization within a forearm-based thumb spica, followed by active ROM exercises from weeks 8 to 12. Formal strengthening exercises can be commenced at 12 weeks. Many European protocols would instead use 6 weeks' immobilization in a short-arm cast with the thumb free for a low-risk stable scaphoid fracture.[1]

   In contrast, the other options listed all relate to the postsurgical management of scaphoid injuries, which can be mobilized earlier than nonoperatively managed fractures. In this scenario, the forearm-based thumb spica is used for the first 4 weeks. Then assisted active ROM can commence at 4 weeks, passive ROM at 6 weeks, and strengthening exercises at 10 weeks (**Table 88.3**).[1–3]

Table 88.3 *Comparison of Scaphoid Fracture Management: Non versus Operatively (USA)*

Scaphoid	Nonoperative	Postoperative
Orthosis	Forearm-based thumb spica splint/cast full time 8 weeks	Forearm-based thumb spica splint 4 weeks
	Weeks 8–12: AROM	Week 2: wrist and thumb AROM
	Week 12+: strengthening	Week 4: AAROM
		Week 6: PROM
		Weeks 10–12: strengthening

REFERENCES

1. Clementson M, Björkman A, Thomsen NOB. Acute scaphoid fractures: guidelines for diagnosis and treatment. EFORT Open Rev 2020;5(2):96–103

2. Jones NF, Jupiter JB, Lalonde DH. Common fractures and dislocations of the hand. Plas Recon Surg 2012;130(5):722e–736e

3. Watson NJ, Martin SA, Keating JL. The impact of wrist fracture, surgical repair and immobilization on patients: a qualitative study. Clin Rehabil 2018;32(6):841–851

PATIENT ASSESSMENT FOLLOWING HAND INJURY REHABILITATION

7. **When assessing patients in clinic following hand injury, which one of the following will provide the best indication of grip strength?**

   D. Dynamometer

   There are a number of key elements to assess during hand therapy after injury. These can be considered as those affecting range of motion (both active and passive), sensation, and strength. The dynamometer allows assessment of grip strength or pinch strength depending on the instrument used. Static grip strength (measured in pounds) is based on average consecutive trials and the recording is compared with non-injured hand. This can be used to determine return to work limitations as well as progression in recovery. Static pinch grip strength is also measured in pounds, and is performed in three positions: chuck, lateral, and tip.[1] The passive and active ROM is measured using a goniometer, a device with two moveable limbs that facilitates measuring internal angles of joints in the lateral view. Again, joint function can be compared with the contralateral hand or standard values expected for any given joint. Semmes-Weinstein monofilaments are used to assess sensation by applying light touch to fingertips using five different thickness filaments, starting from thinnest to thickest and noting the first perception of touch. Muscle group strength may be tested against gravity using rubber bands. This is measured by strength scale (0/5–5/5): 0 = no movement; 3 = movement against gravity; 5 = movement against resistance. Precision of fingertip sensation can be assessed with two-point discrimination. With vision occluded, the ability to sense one as opposed to two points is assessed. It is usual to start 5 mm apart and increase as needed to record two-point sensation. In the normal uninjured hand, it is possible to discriminate less than 6 mm distances.[1–4]

REFERENCES

1. Bohannon RW. Test-retest reliability of measurements of hand-grip strength obtained by dynamometry from older adults: a systematic review of research in the PubMed database. J Frailty Aging 2017;6(2):83–87
2. Gilbert M, Thomas JJ, Pinardo A. Adult grip and pinch strength norms for the baseline digital dynamometer and baseline digital pinch gauge. Am J Occup Ther 2016;70:7011500055
3. Dent JA, Orr MM. Which tests to choose when assessing hand function. J R Coll Surg Edinb 1993;38(5):315–319
4. Fonseca MCR, Elui VMC, Lalone E, et al. Functional, motor, and sensory assessment instruments upon nerve repair in adult hands: systematic review of psychometric properties. Syst Rev 2018;7(1):175

MANAGEMENT OF THE INJURED WRIST

8. **When managing a distal radius fracture, which one of the following is true?**

   B. Where hand therapy is indicated, it typically involves two to three sessions per week.

   Eighty percent of patients with distal radius fracture require hand therapy[1] and common treatment plans include two to three sessions for a 6-week period.[2,3]

   It is unclear if therapy beyond 12 weeks is beneficial after surgical intervention, although it may be for nonsurgical cases. Patients treated nonsurgically and those older than 65 years may simply benefit from being encouraged to return to activities of daily living as soon as possible.[4]

   The protocols following distal radius fracture are shown in **Table 88.4**.

Table 88.4 *Distal Radius Fracture Management*

Distal Radius Fracture	Nonoperative	Postoperative
Orthosis	Sugar tong or Muenster splint 4–6 weeks then transition to a wrist splint for another 2–4 weeks	Wrist splint for 4–6 weeks
	Week 1: digit and uninvolved joint A/AAROM in splint	Week 1: digit and uninvolved joint A/AAROM
	Weeks 4–6: wrist, forearm, elbow AROM	Week 2: wrist AROM, may want to hold forearm AROM depending on ulna
	Weeks 6–8: AAROM	Week 4: AAROM
	Week 8: PROM, strengthening	Week 6: PROM, strengthening

REFERENCES

1. Handoll HH, Elliott J. Rehabilitation for distal radial fractures in adults. Cochrane Database Syst Rev 2015;(9):CD003324
2. Watson NJ, Martin SA, Keating JL. The impact of wrist fracture, surgical repair and immobilization on patients: a qualitative study. Clin Rehabil 2018;32(6):841–851

3. Gruber G, Zacherl M, Giessauf C, et al. Quality of life after volar plate fixation of articular fractures of the distal part of the radius. J Bone Joint Surg Am 2010;92(5):1170–1178
4. Chung KC, Malay S, Shauver MJ; Wrist and Radius Injury Surgical Trial Group. The relationship between hand therapy and long-term outcomes after distal radius fracture in older adults: evidence from the randomized wrist and radius injury surgical trial. Plast Reconstr Surg 2019;144(2):230e–237e

MANAGEMENT OF BENNETT'S FRACTURE OF THE THUMB

9. *Which one of the following is true when managing a Bennett fracture of the thumb?*
    A. The rehabilitation protocol is the same whether surgery has been performed or not.
    A Bennett fracture is a two-part fracture of the thumb metacarpal base that extends into the CMC joint.[1] There is a volar fragment which is attached to the volar stabilizing ligament complex of the CMC joint, and the main metacarpal fragment tends to be pulled dorsally and radially with flexion of the shaft by forces from abductor pollicis longus and the thenar muscles in particular. It is the most common intra-articular fracture of the thumb and typically involves some form of hyper abduction of the thumb. Treatment may be operative or nonoperative depending on the fracture pattern stability. Reduction and stabilization is most often with K-wires and splint but may be performed with open reduction and internal fixation using screws or plates.
    Splinting the thumb is unlikely to lead to significant stiffness and even where stabilized with screws or plates, external splinting is still usually indicated. Therefore, protocol is normally the same whether operative or nonoperative treatment undertaken (**see Fig. 88.3** and **Table 88.5**).

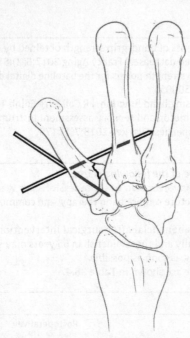

Fig. 88.3 Reduction and stabilization of Bennett's fracture using K-wires into the trapezium and index metacarpal base.

Table 88.5   *Bennett's and Reverse Bennett's Fracture*

Bennett's (1st CMC) Reverse Bennett's (5th CMC)	Nonoperative	Postoperative
Orthosis: Bennett's—thumb spica *Orthosis: reverse Bennett's—ulnar gutter*	Forearm-based thumb spica/ulnar gutter splint × 4 weeks	Forearm-based thumb spica/ulnar gutter splint × 4 weeks
	Week 4: AROM	AROM after pin removal
	Week 6: AAROM	AAROM
	Week 8: strengthening	Strengthening

REFERENCE

1. Guss MS, Kaye D, Rettig M. Bennett fractures a review of management. Bull Hosp Jt Dis (2013) 2016;74(3):197–202

METACARPAL AND PHALANGEAL FRACTURE MANAGEMENT

10. *What is the main benefit of treating metacarpal or phalangeal fractures with open reduction and internal fixation (ORIF) as opposed to nonoperative treatment?*

B. Ability to mobilize earlier

Fractures of the metacarpals and phalanges can very often be managed nonoperatively with good functional results. Many fractures are minimally displaced and will not often need reduction. Where reduction is required, splint stabilization may be sufficient, but if not then K-wire fixation is often a good minimally invasive choice. A downside is that postoperative splinting is usually still required.

In contrast, fractures that are stabilized with ORIF in the form of screws and/or plates can often be managed without external splintage and should be mobilized early postsurgery to reduce the risk of adhesions forming to the plate and cutaneous scar. The ability to mobilize early depends on many factors such as stability of the fixation, the quality/stability of the soft tissues, and the reliability of the patient. While mobilization can commence earlier, there is no certainty that outcomes will be better in the longer term. Postinjury pain and swelling are probably increased by the trauma of surgery and aesthetically ORIF can often be worse; e.g., a dorsal approach to a metacarpal fracture will leave a permanent and visible scar and the plate may be palpable or even visible. Patients should be counseled that ORIF may require secondary surgery in the form of tenolysis or removal of hardware in the future (**Table 88.6**).[1]

Table 88.6 *Metacarpal and Phalangeal Fractures*

Metacarpal	Nonoperative	Postoperative
Orthosis	Distal: MPs at 70 degrees, IPs free Proximal: forearm-based radial/ulnar gutter, MPs at 70 degrees, IPs free	Distal: MPs at 70 degrees, IPs free Proximal: forearm-based radial/ulnar gutter, MPs at 70 degrees, IPs free
	Week 3—AROM	Week 3—AROM after pin removal
	Week 6—PROM, strengthening	Week 6—PROM, strengthening
Proximal phalanx	**Nonoperative**	**Postoperative (pinning)**
Orthosis	Hand-based ulnar/radial gutter MPs at 70 degrees and IPs straight for 4 weeks	Hand-based ulnar/radial gutter MPs at 70 degrees and IPs straight for 3 weeks
	Week 3: AROM of MPs and IPs	Week 1: AROM of uninvolved MPs and IPs
	Week 4: AAROM of MPs and IPs, buddy taping when out of the splint	Week 2: AAROM of uninvolved MPs and IPs
	Week 6: strengthening	Week 3: AROM of fractured joint once pin is removed
		Week 6: strengthening
Middle phalanx	**Nonoperative**	**Postoperative (pinning)**
Orthosis	Hand-based radial/ulnar gutter MPs at 70 degrees and IPs straight for 3–4 weeks; may consider finger splint in full extension for 4 weeks	Hand-based radial/ulnar gutter splint MPs at 70 degrees and PIP in pinned position
	Week 1: AROM of uninvolved MPs and IPs	Week 1: AROM of uninvolved MPs and DIPs
Metacarpal	**Nonoperative**	**Postoperative**
	Weeks 4–6: AROM of involved IPs when stable	Week 3: AROM of PIP once pin is removed
	Week 8: PROM, strengthening	Week 4: AAROM
		Week 6: PROM, strengthening
Distal phalanx, bony and soft-tissue mallet finger injuries	**Nonoperative**	**Postoperative (pinning)**
Orthosis	Finger splint with DIP in full extension or slight hyperextension, PIP free, **full-time wear** for 6 weeks	Finger splint to protect pin, PIP free
	6 months*—wean to wear orthosis only at night, PIP AROM	**Days 3–5: PIP AROM**
		Week 3: AROM of DIP once pin is removed Week 6: gradual strengthening if required, care must be taken to ensure that DIP remains in extension and does not lag

*Skin care important during this time.

REFERENCE

1. Kollitz KM, Hammert WC, Vedder NB, Huang JI. Metacarpal fractures: treatment and complications. Hand (N Y) 2014;9(1):16–23

89. Thumb Reconstruction

See *Essentials of Plastic Surgery*, third edition, pp. 1230–1245

GENERAL CONSIDERATIONS IN THUMB AMPUTATION

1. *When considering traumatic amputation of the thumb, which one of the following is correct?*
   A. Acquired thumb loss would be expected to reduce hand function by 70 to 75%.
   B. Thumb injuries are most commonly classified by the mechanism of injury.
   C. Traumatic amputation of the thumb is most commonly seen in children.
   D. Replanting an amputated thumb achieves superior results to reconstruction.
   E. Thumb reconstruction is best performed early following traumatic injury.

RECONSTRUCTIVE OPTIONS IN THE THUMB

2. *Which one of the following statements is correct when considering thumb reconstruction?*
   A. An index finger cross-finger flap is ideal for a 2 · 2 cm volar defect over the metacarpophalangeal (MCP) joint and proximal phalanx.
   B. A full-thickness skin graft will ultimately achieve similar sensation to a homodigital flap on the thumb pulp.
   C. The wraparound procedure is ideal for children, because it expands well with growth.
   D. A great toe transfer is the preferred option for carpometacarpal (CMC) joint amputations to achieve ideal length and aesthetics.
   E. Free toe transfer can be carried out as a single stage immediately after the initial debridement.

VOLAR ADVANCEMENT FLAPS TO THE THUMB

3. You have a patient with a 1.5 · 1.5 cm defect of the thumb pulp with exposed bone. *Which one of the following is correct when using a Moberg flap to reconstruct this defect?*
   A. This flap may be based on either the radial or ulnar digital vessels.
   B. Midlateral incisions should form a "zigzag" to improve flap advancement.
   C. Release of skin proximally should be undertaken to achieve adequate flap advancement.
   D. The interphalangeal and MCP joints should be held in full extension during wound closure.
   E. The patient should be warned that long-term sensory function will be poor.

MANAGEMENT OF THE FIRST WEB SPACE

4. You are planning to release a contracted first web space 18 months after a crush injury to the thumb that resulted in amputation through the proximal phalanx and has left the patient with a stiff CMC joint and a short thumb. *Which one of the following is correct?*
   A. The optimal Z-plasty design involves multiple 30-degree flaps.
   B. The longitudinal axis for the Z-plasty should be perpendicular to the web space ridge.
   C. Providing the skin is released properly, deeper structures need not be disturbed.
   D. Partial adductor pollicis release would be contraindicated in this case.
   E. The first dorsal interosseous muscle may need to be released.

HETEROTOPIC DIGIT TRANSFER IN THUMB RECONSTRUCTION

5. *When undertaking delayed reconstruction of a middle third amputation of the thumb, which one of the following digits is the preferred donor choice for heterotopic digit transfer if no other digits are injured?*
   A. Index
   B. Middle
   C. Ring
   D. Small
   E. All equally preferred

LENGTHENING OF THE THUMB METACARPAL FOLLOWING TRAUMATIC AMPUTATION

6. *When considering distraction osteogenesis to lengthen the metacarpal of a partially amputated thumb, which one of the following is correct?*
   A. A minimum of 50% of the metacarpal is required.
   B. Up to 5 cm of lengthening can be reliably produced.
   C. Approximately 2 mm of advancement per week is optimal for lengthening.
   D. Bone grafting may still be required in patients over 25 years of age.
   E. The soft-tissue envelope is unlikely to need any surgical intervention.

POLLICIZATION FOR THUMB RECONSTRUCTION

7. *When pollicizing the index finger, which one of the following is correct?*
   A. The index CMC joint becomes the new thumb CMC joint.
   B. The first dorsal interosseous muscle becomes the new APL.
   C. The FDS tendon becomes the new FPL tendon.
   D. The proximal phalanx becomes the middle phalanx.
   E. The EIP tendon becomes the new EPL tendon.

FREE TOE TRANSFER TO THE THUMB

8. *When planning a free toe transfer for thumb reconstruction, which one of the following is correct?*
   A. Second toe transfers are equal in strength to great toe transfers.
   B. An oblique osteotomy through the toe metatarsal can improve function in the new thumb.
   C. The arterial supply to the great toe is consistently from the first metatarsal artery arising from dorsalis pedis.
   D. The contralateral great toe is preferred to favorably align the arterial anastomosis in the first web space.
   E. The second toe donor site often requires skin grafting for closure.

TYPES OF TOE TRANSFER

9. *Which one of the following toe transfers for a distal metacarpal level thumb amputation typically requires an additional iliac bone graft?*
   A. Great toe
   B. Second toe
   C. Wraparound toe
   D. Trimmed toe
   E. Partial toe

Answers

GENERAL CONSIDERATIONS IN THUMB AMPUTATION

1. **When considering traumatic amputation of the thumb, which one of the following is correct?**

   D. **Replanting an amputated thumb achieves superior results to reconstruction.**

   Optimal thumb function is achieved with the original thumb itself; so, where possible replantation remains the ideal option for an amputated thumb in all but the most distal cases. Even a stiff replanted thumb is normally superior in aesthetics and function to an alternative reconstruction. However, there are always exceptions to any rule, and each case should be assessed individually (e.g., the amputated part may be too damaged and some patients may opt for terminalization to facilitate a speedier return to work, especially where the amputation is fairly distal).

   The importance of the thumb in overall hand function is well recognized and estimated as 40% (not 75%) of total hand function. It is required for many simple and complex hand movements acting as a post for opposition against the other digits.

   Thumb injuries are classified as proximal, middle, and distal third injuries (rather than by mechanism) and their management is typically guided by this classification (**Fig. 89.1**).

   Trauma in young adult males represents the most common etiology for acquired thumb loss. Although replantation should be performed as an emergency, definitive secondary reconstruction need not be done so urgently and can be delayed until the soft tissues

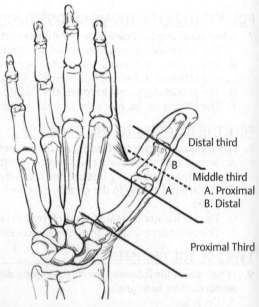

Fig. 89.1   Areas of thumb loss: distal third, middle third, and proximal third. The middle third is subdivided into proximal (*A*) and distal (*B*).

have stabilized and the patient has had sufficient time to assess their own function and give thought to their reconstructive options. In order to facilitate the optimum secondary reconstruction, there may need to be an acute partial reconstruction, for example, free tissue transfer to preserve first web and cover remaining thumb metacarpal prior to subsequent definitive reconstruction.[1–5]

REFERENCES

1. Parvizi D, Koch H, Friedl H, et al. Analysis of functional outcome after posttraumatic thumb reconstruction in comparison to nonreconstructed amputated thumbs at the proximal phalanx of the thumb ray: a mid-term follow-up with special attention to the Manchester-modified M2 DASH questionnaire and effect size of Cohen's d. J Trauma Acute Care Surg 2012;72(2):E33–E40
2. Shale CM, Tidwell JE III, Mulligan RP, Jupiter DC, Mahabir RC. A nationwide review of the treatment patterns of traumatic thumb amputations. Ann Plast Surg 2013;70(6):647–651
3. Friedrich JB, Vedder NB. Thumb reconstruction. Clin Plast Surg 2011;38(4):697–712
4. Haas F, Hubmer M, Rappl T, Koch H, Parvizi I, Parvizi D. Long-term subjective and functional evaluation after thumb replantation with special attention to the Quick DASH questionnaire and a specially designed trauma score called modified Mayo score. J Trauma 2011;71(2):460–466
5. Pet MA, Ko JH, Vedder NB. Reconstruction of the traumatized thumb. Plast Reconstr Surg 2014;134(6):1235–1245

RECONSTRUCTIVE OPTIONS IN THE THUMB

2. **Which one of the following statements is correct when considering thumb reconstruction?**

   E. **Free toe transfer can be carried out as a single stage immediately after the initial debridement.**

   Free toe transfer is more commonly used for delayed reconstructions, but it may be carried out acutely if there are suitable recipient soft tissues and bone, the wound is clean and healthy, and appropriate informed consent has been obtained.

A cross-finger flap from the index finger would not reach the proximal or radial extent of a defect overlying the proximal phalanx and metacarpophalangeal (MCP) joint. This flap is better suited to defects over the distal phalanx and interphalangeal (IP) joint.

Full-thickness skin grafts are sometimes used for pulp defects, but sensory return is better with split-thickness grafts, healing by secondary intent, or homodigital flaps. Wraparound flaps are more likely to be performed urgently than full toe transfers, such as when there is exposed bone and immediate soft-tissue cover is required, but are not usually recommended for young children because of subsequent growth restriction. An amputation through the carpometacarpal (CMC) joint might be better reconstructed with pollicization. The great toe would not provide sufficient length and, because it is usually around 20% wider than the thumb, the aesthetic outcome is not ideal. The donor site is also not aesthetically pleasing, may require skin grafting, and can cause functional problems for some patients.[1-4]

REFERENCES

1. Lin PY, Sebastin SJ, Ono S, Bellfi LT, Chang KW, Chung KC. A systematic review of outcomes of toe-to-thumb transfers for isolated traumatic thumb amputation. Hand (N Y) 2011;6(3):235–243
2. Waljee JF, Chung KC. Toe-to-hand transfer: evolving indications and relevant outcomes. J Hand Surg Am 2013;38(7): 1431–1434
3. Rui Y, Mi J, Shi H, Zhang Z, Yan H. Free great toe wrap-around flap combined with second toe medial flap for reconstruction of completely degloved fingers. Microsurgery 2010;30(6):449–456
4. Morrison WA, O'Brien BM, MacLeod AM. Thumb reconstruction with a free neurovascular wrap-around flap from the big toe. J Hand Surg Am 1980;5(6):575–583

VOLAR ADVANCEMENT FLAPS TO THE THUMB

3. You have a patient with a 1.5 × 1.5 cm defect of the thumb pulp with exposed bone. *Which one of the following is correct when using a Moberg flap to reconstruct this defect?*

C. Release of skin proximally should be undertaken to achieve adequate flap advancement.

The Moberg advancement flap may be used for thumb tip defects of up to 50% of the volar pulp surface. The standard Moberg flap can be advanced about 1 cm but requires further release at the base of the flap to move the 1.5 cm required in this case (**Fig. 89.2**). A number of modifications of the Moberg flap have been described to increase flap reach. These include advancing the flap in a V-Y fashion, or transversely releasing the proximal skin and applying a full-thickness skin graft to the donor site. Straight midlateral incisions are made to elevate the flap and the volar skin is advanced with both ulnar and radial neurovascular bundles superficial to the flexor tendon sheath. This generally requires some flexion of both the MCP and IP joints during inset, which is not always fully corrected with physiotherapy. The thumb is functionally most useful with some flexion at the IP and MCP joints anyway, so a small loss of extension is generally of little concern.[1-5]

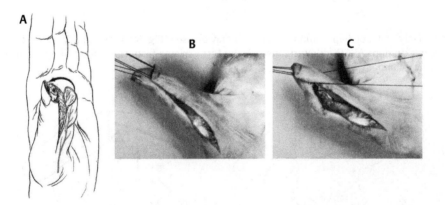

Fig. 89.2   Volar advancement flap (Moberg flap). **A,** Arc to the distal phalanx of the thumb. **B,** Elevation of the flap. **C,** Coverage of the distal phalanx of the thumb.

REFERENCES

1. Moberg E. Aspects of sensation in reconstructive surgery of the upper extremity. J Bone Joint Surg Am 1964;46:817–825
2. Baumeister S, Menke H, Wittemann M, Germann G. Functional outcome after the Moberg advancement flap in the thumb. J Hand Surg Am 2002;27(1):105–114

3. Mutaf M, Temel M, Günal E, Işık D. Island volar advancement flap for reconstruction of thumb defects. Ann Plast Surg 2012;68(2):153–157

4. Foucher G, Delaere O, Citron N, Molderez A. Long-term outcome of neurovascular palmar advancement flaps for distal thumb injuries. Br J Plast Surg 1999;52(1):64–68

5. Bang H, Kojima T, Hayashi H. Palmar advancement flap with V-Y closure for thumb tip injuries. J Hand Surg Am 1992;17(5):933–934

MANAGEMENT OF THE FIRST WEB SPACE

4. You are planning to release a contracted first web space 18 months after a crush injury to the thumb that resulted in amputation through the proximal phalanx and has left the patient with a stiff CMC joint and a short thumb. *Which one of the following is correct?*

E. The first dorsal interosseous muscle may need to be released.

Deepening the first web space can help increase thumb excursion, specifically palmar and radial abduction with improvement in opposition and grasp. It can provide an apparent or relative lengthening of the thumb. Techniques to do this involve skin repositioning with flaps and or grafts and often deeper tissue release is also required.[1]

If the CMC joint is stiff and the web space contracted as in this case, it is unlikely that skin release alone will be sufficient. It may be necessary to release both the first dorsal interosseous and adductor pollicis muscles, often reinserting the adductor muscle more proximally. When using a Z-plasty technique for first web release, a 60-degree Z-plasty is preferred with the longitudinal axis of the Z-plasty on the dorsal ridge of the first web space (**Fig. 89.3**).

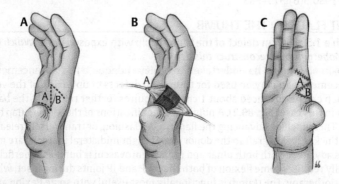

Fig. 89.3   Dorsal metacarpal artery flap. (From Germann G, Sherman R, Levin AS. Reconstructive Surgery of the Hand and Upper Extremity. Thieme, 2017.)

Alternatively, the four-flap "jumping man" flap may be used (**Fig. 89.4**). "CADBury" refers to the order of the transposed skin flaps ABCD following inset. It is a term arising from the United Kingdom from the popular confectionary company Cadbury's.[2]

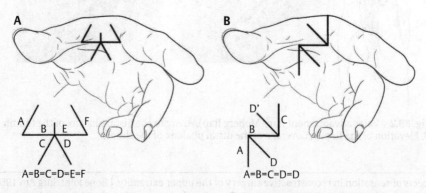

Fig. 89.4   Thumb–index web space deepening with **A,** double opposing Z or **B,** four-flap reconstruction.

REFERENCES

1. Muzaffar AR, Chao JJ, Friedrich JB. Posttraumatic thumb reconstruction. Plast Reconstr Surg 2005;116(5):103e–122e
2. Fraulin FO, Thomson HG. First webspace deepening: comparing the four-flap and five-flap Z-plasty. Which gives the most gain? Plast Reconstr Surg 1999;104(1):120–128

HETEROTOPIC DIGIT TRANSFER IN THUMB RECONSTRUCTION

5. *When undertaking delayed reconstruction of a middle third amputation of the thumb, which one of the following digits is the preferred donor choice for heterotopic digit transfer if no other digits are injured?*

    C. Ring

    Heterotopic digit transfer is a potential solution for patients who have sustained a middle third, or more proximal, thumb injury that requires bone and soft-tissue reconstruction. This is most often applicable to cases where there are multiple injured digits and the transfer can essentially use "spare parts" from an injured digit to reconstruct the amputated thumb. In this setting, the index is the usual donor when already injured, as thumb to middle finger pinch grip works well and patients often bypass a repaired index finger anyway. However, in cases where all other digits are completely preserved (noninjured), the ring finger is considered the best digit to harvest and use for thumb reconstruction, as it plays a lesser overall role in hand function than the others. This transfer is termed an "on top plasty" and can be used in both the acute and elective settings without significant functional loss overall.[1-4] A downside is, of course, the cosmesis and some patients may be keen to avoid loss of part of the ring finger on this basis, for example, those interested in wearing a wedding band and those from societies which place a particularly high importance on the hand and digit appearance (e.g., Japan).

REFERENCES

1. Bravo CJ, Horton T, Moran SL, Shin AY. Traumatized index finger pollicization for thumb reconstruction. J Hand Surg Am 2008;33(2):257–262
2. Foucher G, Rostane S, Chammas M, Smith D, Allieu Y. Transfer of a severely damaged digit to reconstruct an amputated thumb. J Bone Joint Surg Am 1996;78(12):1889–1896
3. Haddock NT, Ehrlich DA, Levine JP, Saadeh PB. The crossover composite filet of hand flap and heterotopic thumb replantation: a unique indication. Plast Reconstr Surg 2012;130(4):634e–636e
4. Kokkoli E, Spyropoulou GA, Shih HS, Feng GM, Jeng SF. Heterotopic procedures in mutilating hand injuries: a synopsis of essential reconstructive tools. Plast Reconstr Surg 2015;136(5):1015–1026

LENGTHENING OF THE THUMB METACARPAL FOLLOWING TRAUMATIC AMPUTATION

6. *When considering distraction osteogenesis to lengthen the metacarpal of a partially amputated thumb, which one of the following is correct?*

    D. Bone grafting may still be required in patients over 25 years of age.

    Lengthening of the thumb metacarpal with distraction osteogenesis can be useful to provide an increased total thumb length following injury in the proximal third. In order to perform this, two-thirds of the metacarpal must be remaining (not 50%) and a robust soft-tissue envelope must be present. When using this technique, up to 3.5 cm of lengthening can be expected over a 4- to 6-week period at a rate of 1 mm lengthening per day. Many patients over 25 years of age may benefit from additional bone grafting at the site of distraction osteogenesis to improve the rate of union.[1] The soft-tissue envelope may not tolerate distraction if there is scarring or previous skin-grafted tissue and this may require revision prior to distraction. Most patients will need a subsequent web space deepening procedure as part of this reconstructive approach.

REFERENCE

1. Matev I. Thumb metacarpal lengthening. Tech Hand Up Extrem Surg 2003;7(4):157–163

POLLICIZATION FOR THUMB RECONSTRUCTION

7. *When pollicizing the index finger, which one of the following is correct?*

    E. The EIP tendon becomes the new EPL tendon.

    Pollicization is a useful and reliable procedure for complete thumb reconstruction. It results in minimal sacrifice of hand function and can provide excellent cosmetic and functional results when performed well. The index finger is classically used and the EIP (extensor indicis proprius) becomes the new EPL (extensor pollicis longus). The MCP joint (not CMC joint) becomes the new thumb CMC joint as the digit is shortened. The first dorsal interosseous muscle becomes the new abductor pollicis brevis (not the APL [abductor pollicis longus]), the flexor digitorum profundus (not FDS [flexor digitorum superficialis]) becomes the new FPL (flexor pollicis longus), and the proximal phalanx becomes the metacarpal. The key structures involved in converting the index finger to a thumb are shown below (**Table 89.1**). Kozin[1] presented his modifications of the concept, technical details, and outcome of pollicization. The original concept was brought to prominence by Buck-Gramcko in 1971[2] after his experience treating patients affected by thalidomide.

Table 89.1   *Structural Changes During Pollicization*

Initial Index Finger Structure	Reconstructed Thumb Structure
Metacarpal head	Trapezium
Proximal phalanx	Metacarpal
Middle phalanx	Proximal phalanx
Distal phalanx	Distal phalanx
Extensor digitorum communis	Abductor pollicis longus
Extensor indices proprius	Extensor pollicis longus
First dorsal interosseous	Abductor pollicis brevis
First palmar interosseous	Adductor pollicis

REFERENCES

1. Kozin SH. Pollicization: the concept, technical details, and outcome. Clin Orthop Surg 2012;4(1):18–35
2. Buck-Gramcko D. Pollicization of the index finger. Method and results in aplasia and hypoplasia of the thumb. J Bone Joint Surg Am 1971;53(8):1605–1617

FREE TOE TRANSFER TO THE THUMB

8. *When planning a free toe transfer for thumb reconstruction, which one of the following is correct?*

B. **An oblique osteotomy through the toe metatarsal can improve function in the new thumb.**

Toe to thumb transfer is an effective way to reconstruct an absent or deficient thumb and has become the standard of care for amputations distal to the CMC joint. The choices for toe to hand include great or second toe. The great toe is historically the most common choice and has some advantages and disadvantages as compared with the second toe. There are a number of technical points to consider in planning and performing surgery.[1,2]

There is often sufficient length in a transferred toe without using the metatarsal, but if required, a second toe donor site is usually better tolerated than a great toe due to the role of the great toe metatarsal in weight bearing. An oblique osteotomy through the metatarsal helps improve alignment and range of motion in the new thumb, as the toe metatarsophalangeal (MTP) joints naturally tend to hyperextend a great deal, which can be undesirable in the reconstructed thumb.

Great toe transfers are generally stronger than second toe transfers. Although there is debate about which is more aesthetically pleasing, the great toe is usually about 20% broader than the thumb which it is replacing, whereas the second toe is usually noticeably thinner with a short nail. This is variable between individuals. The arterial supply to both is most commonly via the first dorsal metatarsal artery; however, there is considerable variation. An ipsilateral great toe orientates the first dorsal metatarsal artery more favorably in the first dorsal web space for anastomosis. The second toe donor site usually closes directly, but the great toe may require skin grafting.

REFERENCES

1. Lin PY, Sebastin SJ, Ono S, Bellfi LT, Chang KW, Chung KC. A systematic review of outcomes of toe-to-thumb transfers for isolated traumatic thumb amputation. Hand (N Y) 2011;6(3):235–243
2. Waljee JF, Chung KC. Toe-to-hand transfer: evolving indications and relevant outcomes. J Hand Surg Am 2013;38(7): 1431–1434

TYPES OF TOE TRANSFER

9. *Which one of the following toe transfers for a distal metacarpal level thumb amputation typically requires an additional iliac bone graft?*

C. **Wraparound toe**

There are numerous ways to transfer different components of the great toe and second toes. All of the above options involve harvesting bone and soft tissues with the exception of the wraparound technique which is a soft tissue plus nail-only flap that is transferred from the great toe. Osseous support, as required in this case, is provided by a bone graft such as that from the iliac crest. The advantages of this flap are that it provides good sensation, adequate strength, better aesthetics, and less donor site morbidity. It is therefore particularly useful in cases where there is exposed retained bone length to cover, or less overall length required such that a nonvascularized bone graft within the wraparound flap will suffice. The disadvantages of this flap are that it is technically demanding to raise, and where a bone graft is used there is a risk of bone resorption and no joint for motion within the reconstructed length. This flap should be avoided in children because of growth restriction.

The trimmed toe technique can be an elegant method for thumb reconstruction that harvests bone but involves a longitudinal osteotomy with trimming of the toe such that the size match is better than a traditional great toe transfer. Again, this is a more complicated procedure and should be avoided in children. A partial toe transfer is indicated in partial thumb defects, which may be bony or soft tissue related.

Current evidence suggests there is no significant difference in outcomes between different toe transfer techniques[1]; so, reconstruction selection should be individualized to the patient, the defect, and the expertise of the treating surgeon. The following summary from the parent text is a useful guide to different toe transfer options:

At or distal to IP joint
- Partial toe transfer or free neurovascular island flap from first webspace.

Through proximal phalanx with intact MCP joint
- Wraparound transfer (better appearance than great toe)
- Trimmed toe provides better aesthetics with preservation of joint mobility
- Great toe provides best strength.

Distal half of metacarpal
- Great toe is an excellent option, harvested at MTP joint.
- If the great toe is too short, then the second toe should be used.

Proximal half of metacarpal with CMC joint preserved
- Second toe is the best option due to additional metatarsal length.
- Second toe is skin deficient proximally over metatarsal; secondary coverage procedure may be required.

REFERENCE

1. Lin PY, Sebastin SJ, Ono S, Bellfi LT, Chang KW, Chung KC. A systematic review of outcomes of toe-to-thumb transfers for isolated traumatic thumb amputation. Hand (N Y) 2011;6(3):235–243

90. Soft-Tissue Coverage of the Hand and Upper Extremity

See *Essentials of Plastic Surgery*, third edition, pp. 1246–1259

SKIN GRAFTS ON THE HAND

1. *Which one of the following is correct when using a skin graft in the hand?*
   A. Full-thickness grafts are best harvested from the contralateral upper limb.
   B. The heel is a good donor site for glabrous skin graft harvest.
   C. Split-thickness skin grafts should be meshed to improve graft take.
   D. It is normal for glabrous skin grafts to appear sloughy at 1 to 2 weeks.
   E. Split-thickness skin grafts will contract more immediately after harvest than full-thickness grafts.

LOCAL FLAPS FOR FINGER RECONSTRUCTION

2. *Which one of the following is correct regarding local flaps used to reconstruct the digit?*
   A. The Kutler bilateral V-Y flaps are best applied to large dorsal oblique fingertip amputations.
   B. The Atasoy V-Y flap is ideal for reconstructing volar oblique fingertip injuries.
   C. The reverse cross-finger flap is mainly indicated for volar defects over the phalanges.
   D. Homodigital island flaps are contraindicated for fingertip reconstruction following digital vessel injury.
   E. The Moberg flap is ideal for reconstruction of volar defects of the middle finger pulp.

LOCAL FLAPS FOR THUMB TIP RECONSTRUCTION

3. A 21-year-old man presents with a transverse soft-tissue tip amputation to his dominant thumb at the level of the lunula. There is exposed distal phalanx and the soft-tissue defect measures 2 × 1 cm. He is generally healthy and a nonsmoker. *Which one of the following would be the best reconstructive option in this case?*
   A. Healing by secondary intention
   B. Revision amputation
   C. Distally based dorsal hand flap (Quaba)
   D. Thenar flap
   E. Neurovascular island flap (Littler)

FLAP RECONSTRUCTION OF THE HAND

4. A 40-year-old woman sustains an 8 × 7 cm degloving injury to the dorsum of her right hand, leaving exposed extensor tendons without paratenon. She is generally healthy and of slim build. *Which one of the following is correct regarding reconstruction in her case?*
   A. A pedicled posterior interosseous artery flap could cover this defect, but will leave an EPL weakness as the posterior interosseous nerve is sacrificed.
   B. A reverse radial forearm flap could comfortably cover this defect but will give a poor cosmetic outcome.
   C. Free tissue transfer for reconstruction of this defect with an anterolateral thigh flap would be unnecessary and is best avoided in this patient.
   D. An Allen's test should be performed before using a radial forearm flap to reconstruct the defect to ensure flap flow is adequate.
   E. Centering the skin paddle for a reverse radial forearm flap in the middle third of the forearm would provide the most reliable skin perfusion for reconstruction.

THE REVERSE RADIAL FOREARM FLAP

5. *When reconstructing a soft-tissue defect of the hand using the reverse radial forearm flap, which one of the following is true?*
   A. The flap design should be checked for adequate reach, assuming the pivot point is the radial styloid.
   B. The radial artery is found within an intramuscular septum between the flexor digitorum superficialis and the FCR.
   C. The cephalic vein is usually incorporated within the flap to aid venous drainage.
   D. The donor site is best closed with meshed split-thickness graft.
   E. The radial artery is routinely reconstructed with a vein graft after flap harvest.

THE POSTERIOR INTEROSSEUS FLAP

6. *When reconstructing a soft-tissue defect of the hand using a pedicled posterior interosseous flap, which one of the following is true?*

A. The flap is centered on a line between the wrist and medial epicondyle.

B. Flap markings should be performed with the elbow in extension.

C. The PIA is located distally between the ECU and EDM tendons.

D. The flap pivot point is 1 cm distal to the ulnar styloid.

E. The PIA arises from the radial artery at the level of the antecubital fossa.

FLAPS USED FOR ELBOW SOFT-TISSUE COVERAGE

7. *Which one of the following flaps is based on the posterior radial collateral artery and can only provide coverage of a distal elbow defect if used as a free tissue transfer?*

A. Reverse lateral arm flap

B. Flexor carpi ulnaris flap

C. Radial forearm flap

D. Lateral arm flap

E. Brachioradialis flap

VASCULAR SUPPLY TO FREE FLAPS USED IN THE UPPER LIMB

8. *Which one of the following soft-tissue flaps may be useful as a free flap for upper limb reconstruction and is based on the circumflex scapular vessels?*

A. The serratus anterior flap

B. The latissimus dorsi flap

C. The scapula/parascapular flap

D. The pectoralis major flap

E. The gracilis flap

Answers

SKIN GRAFTS ON THE HAND

1. *Which one of the following is correct when using a skin graft in the hand?*

   D. **It is normal for glabrous skin grafts to appear sloughy at 1 to 2 weeks.**

   The appearance of a glabrous graft can be concerning at 1 to 2 weeks as the thick stratum corneum sloughs. This can give the impression that the graft has failed to take. It does, however, regrow in most cases, so it may be helpful to warn the patient and the nursing staff about this before surgery. Glabrous skin grafts can be useful for defects on the palm. They should be harvested from the hypothenar eminence or from a non–weight-bearing part of the foot such as the instep (rather than the heel).

   Split-thickness skin grafts are best used as sheet grafts to minimize contraction and improve cosmesis when reconstructing the hand. This is especially true for larger areas on the dorsum, such as burns where early grafting is also prioritized over many other body areas. There are benefits to using split- versus full-thickness grafts in general. Split-thickness grafts show less primary contraction than full-thickness grafts, but are more prone to later secondary contraction. Full-thickness grafts are the reverse, so they provide less secondary contraction over time. Split-thickness graft donor sites have to heal by the process of reepithelialization, where full-thickness graft donor sites are closed directly. Split-thickness grafts can provide cover for much larger defects and graft take can be more predictable. Smaller defects are best reconstructed with full-thickness grafts where possible, as a better color and texture match is achieved. Furthermore, the skin cover is likely to be more robust which is highly relevant to the hand and upper limb. Most potential full-thickness graft donor sites are suitable, provided hair-bearing skin is avoided. Common sites include the upper arm, forearm, groin, and supraclavicular fossa. The contralateral upper limb should generally be avoided as both limbs will have temporary limited function which makes activities of daily living difficult for the patient. It is often possible to use the same limb as a donor for smaller grafts by harvesting skin from the forearm or medial arm.[1-3]

REFERENCES

1. Milner CS, Thirkannad SM. Resurfacing glabrous skin defects in the hand: the thenar base donor site. Tech Hand Up Extrem Surg 2014;18(2):89–91
2. Thorne CH, ed. Grabb and Smith's Plastic Surgery. 7th ed. Philadelphia: Lippincott Williams & Wilkins; 2014
3. Hallock GG, Morris SF. Skin grafts and local flaps. Plast Reconstr Surg 2011;127(1):5e–22e

LOCAL FLAPS FOR FINGER RECONSTRUCTION

2. *Which one of the following is correct regarding local flaps used to reconstruct the digit?*

   D. **Homodigital island flaps are contraindicated for fingertip reconstruction following digital vessel injury.**

   Homodigital island flaps require sacrifice of one digital vessel; therefore, they are contraindicated in single-vessel digits. They can be useful for reconstructing fingertip defects unsuitable for skin grafts or healing by secondary intention. The neurovascular bundle is dissected proximally to the basal digital crease or into the palm and the flap is advanced in a V-Y or step-cut fashion. Kutler[1] flaps are two small lateral V-Y flaps that are usually indicated in selected cases for primary repair of transverse or lateral oblique injuries. A good indication is for secondary revision of fingertip amputations. The Atasoy[2] flap is a small volar V-Y advancement flap indicated for dorsal oblique injuries and some transverse amputations. It is contraindicated in volar oblique injuries, as the flap should not extend proximal to the distal interphalangeal joint crease. It should be elevated in the plane just above the periosteum in order to preserve vascularity.

   The reverse cross-finger flap usually involves raising a thin (subdermal) skin flap away from the defect site (which is later replaced in situ) followed by raising a subcutaneous flap in the opposite direction at the level of paratenon to cover the defect. Alternatively a de-epithelialized skin flap can be raised toward the defect. It is indicated for coverage of exposed tendon or bone on the dorsum of an adjacent digit. A standard cross-finger flap is used for volar defects. The Moberg flap is contraindicated in finger reconstruction because of the risk to the blood supply of the dorsal skin. It is generally indicated for volar defects of the thumb tip/pulp.[3]

REFERENCES

1. Kutler W. A new method for finger tip amputation. J Am Med Assoc 1947;133(1):29–30
2. Atasoy E, Ioakimidis E, Kasdan ML, Kutz JE, Kleinert HE. Reconstruction of the amputated finger tip with a triangular volar flap. A new surgical procedure. J Bone Joint Surg Am 1970;52(5):921–926
3. Moberg E. Aspects of sensation in reconstructive surgery of the upper extremity. J Bone Joint Surg Am 1964;46:817–825

LOCAL FLAPS FOR THUMB TIP RECONSTRUCTION

3. A 21-year-old man presents with a transverse soft-tissue tip amputation to his dominant thumb at the level of the lunula. There is exposed distal phalanx and the soft-tissue defect measures 2 × 1 cm. He is generally healthy and a nonsmoker. *Which one of the following would be the best reconstructive option in this case?*

E. Neurovascular island flap (Littler)

The Littler[1] neurovascular island flap is useful for the reconstruction of thumb soft-tissue defects. It involves elevation of a flap from the middle or ring finger hemi-pulp based on one neurovascular bundle. Dissection of the bundle is performed proximally into the palm and tunneled radially across to the thumb (**Fig. 90.1**). The donor site is skin grafted.

The key principles in thumb reconstruction are to preserve length and achieve sensate, durable soft-tissue cover. Reconstruction is therefore often (but not always) best achieved with a local flap. Other options depend on the level of injury and the amount of bone exposed, but range from trimming of the exposed bone and leaving to heal by secondary intention to burying the thumb temporarily in the groin or performing free toe or soft-tissue transfer in larger defects. Given that this is a young patient and the dominant thumb is involved, preservation of length with sensation is important, so neither revision amputation nor healing by secondary intention is appropriate given the defect size and location in this case.

A first dorsal metacarpal artery perforator flap (Quaba flap)[2] would not reach the thumb tip and is usually used for reconstructing the dorsum of the hand and proximal digits. A first dorsal metacarpal artery flap (Foucher)[3] could, however, be used with a skin flap harvested from the dorsum of the index finger.

The thenar flap is occasionally used to reconstruct volar defects of the digits as a two-stage procedure. However, in adults it results in significant stiffness at the IP joints, given that the finger is held in flexion for 2 weeks before flap division and it is therefore mainly reserved for children. It would not be possible to cover the defect described in this scenario using a thenar flap, as the thumb would not flex sufficiently to enable flap reach. Even if it could, the stiffness incurred would be counterproductive. The Moberg[4] flap might also be able to cover this defect but may struggle to reach even with Dellon's modification. This involves extension of the flap proximally onto the thenar eminence, and incorporation of two local rotation flaps to close the donor defect.[5]

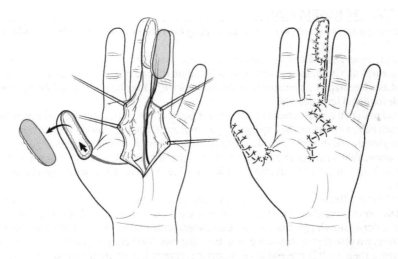

Fig. 90.1   Littler neurovascular island flap, for thumb reconstruction.

REFERENCES

1. Littler JW. The neurovascular pedicle method of digital transposition for reconstruction of the thumb. Plast Reconstr Surg (1946) 1953;12(5):303–319
2. Quaba AA, Davison PM. The distally-based dorsal hand flap. Br J Plast Surg 1990;43(1): 28–39
3. Foucher G, Braun JB. A new island flap transfer from the dorsum of the index to the thumb. Plast Reconstr Surg 1979;63(3):344–349
4. Moberg E. Aspects of sensation in reconstructive surgery of the upper extremity. J Bone Joint Surg Am 1964;46:817–825
5. Dellon AL. The extended palmar advancement flap. J Hand Surg Am 1983;8(2):190–194

FLAP RECONSTRUCTION OF THE HAND

4. A 40-year-old woman sustains an 8 × 7 cm degloving injury to the dorsum of her right hand, leaving exposed extensor tendons without paratenon. She is generally healthy and of slim build. *Which one of the following is correct regarding reconstruction in her case?*

   B. **A reverse radial forearm flap could comfortably cover this defect but will give a poor cosmetic outcome.**
   This defect may be adequately reconstructed using a reverse radial forearm flap, but the donor-site scarring is a real disadvantage in a young female patient.[1] Other locoregional reconstructive options for this defect include the posterior interosseous and ulnar artery–based flaps, such as the Becker[2] flap, but each of these are also likely to require a skin graft to the donor site. For this reason, free tissue transfer with a thin pliable fasciocutaneous flap such as an anterolateral thigh flap or scapula flap may be better for this patient.

   The posterior interosseous flap[3] may leave a numb patch on the forearm if the posterior, medial, or lateral antebrachial cutaneous nerves are divided during flap harvest. The posterior interosseous nerve should not be divided when using this flap.

   An Allen test is performed to confirm that the hand is perfused independently by the radial and ulnar arteries. It involves manually occluding the radial and ulnar arteries at the wrist, then releasing them in turn while assessing perfusion of the digits. It is not a test of flap viability.

   When designing the reverse radial forearm flap, it is important to remember that skin perforators are predominantly found in the proximal and distal forearm with a relative paucity in the middle, so ideally the skin paddle should avoid the middle third.

REFERENCES

1. Becker C, Gilbert A. The ulnar flap—description and applications. Eur J Plast Surg 1988;11:79–82
2. Biswas D, Wysocki RW, Fernandez JJ, Cohen MS. Local and regional flaps for hand coverage. J Hand Surg Am 2014;39(5):992–1004
3. Angrigiani C, Grilli D, Dominikow D, Zancolli EA. Posterior interosseous reverse forearm flap: experience with 80 consecutive cases. Plast Reconstr Surg 1993;92(2):285–293

THE REVERSE RADIAL FOREARM FLAP

5. *When reconstructing a soft-tissue defect of the hand using the reverse radial forearm flap, which one of the following is true?*

   A. **The flap design should be checked for adequate reach, assuming the pivot point is the radial styloid.**
   The radial forearm flap is a fasciocutaneous flap based on the radial artery and associated venae comitantes. It may be used as a free flap or a pedicled flap. When pedicled, it may be used-based antegrade for elbow defects or retrograde for distal limb defects.

   The reverse pedicled radial forearm has its pivot point at the radial styloid, and it is important to confirm adequate reach before elevating the flap by using a template. Good perforating vessels supplying the skin paddle are found proximally and this will provide a long flap reach. Venous outflow is generally adequate using the venae comitantes alone. When raising the antegrade flow radial forearm flap as a free flap, it is common practice to include the cephalic vein, as this can also provide a reliable venous outflow with a good size vein for subsequent anastomosis.

   The radial artery lies within an intramuscular septum between the flexor carpi radialis (FCR) and brachioradialis. Retracting these two muscles gives a clear view of the pedicle during flap dissection. Closure of radial forearm donor sites larger than a few centimeters wide will usually require a skin graft. A full-thickness graft from the groin provides reasonable donor-site cosmesis. Meshed split grafts should be avoided. Where split grafts are used, a sheet graft is preferable for superior cosmesis. It is unusual to reconstruct the radial artery after flap harvest and this should not be necessary, provided the distal perfusion was checked first with an Allen test. However, in cases where the hand is compromised after tourniquet release, either replacement of a pedicled flap or reconstruction of the radial artery with a vein graft would be indicated. The long saphenous vein is a suitable donor.[1,2]

REFERENCES

1. Biswas D, Wysocki RW, Fernandez JJ, Cohen MS. Local and regional flaps for hand coverage. J Hand Surg Am 2014;39(5):992–1004
2. Yannascoli SM, Thibaudeau S, Levin LS. Management of soft tissue defects of the hand. J Hand Surg Am 2015;40(6):1237–1244, quiz 1245

THE POSTERIOR INTEROSSEUS FLAP

6. When reconstructing a soft-tissue defect of the hand using a pedicled posterior interosseous flap, which one of the following is true?

C. The PIA is located distally between the ECU and EDM tendons.

The posterior interosseous artery (PIA) flap was originally described in 1985 and some modifications have been presented.[1,2] When used as a pedicled flap to cover defects in the hand, the PIA flap is based on reverse flow in the posterior interosseous artery. The PIA courses between the extensor carpi ulnaris (ECU) and extensor digiti minimi (EDM) in the forearm, and proximally this course is oblique. This means that dissection is safer and easier from distal to proximal to reduce the chance of injuring the perforators supplying the proximal skin flap. The skin paddle is designed over the dorsal forearm at around the junction between the proximal and middle third along a line made between the distal radioulnar joint and the lateral (not medial) epicondyle (**Fig. 90.2**).

The donor site is highly visible. Flaps up to 5 cm in width will usually close directly, otherwise a skin graft is required. The markings should be performed with the elbow *flexed*, not extended. The pivot point for this flap is 2 cm *proximal to* the ulnar styloid, so adequate reach must be confirmed before flap elevation. The PIA emerges on the interosseous membrane 5 to 6 cm distal to the lateral epicondyle. It arises from the ulnar and not the radial artery.

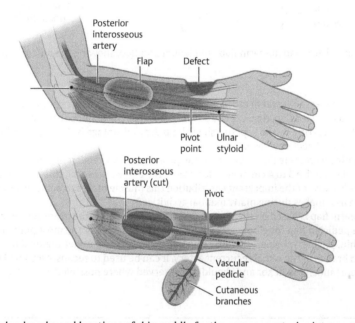

Fig. 90.2   Bony landmarks and locations of skin paddle for the reverse posterior interosseous artery flap.

REFERENCES

1. Angrigiani C, Grilli D, Dominikow D, Zancolli EA. Posterior interosseous reverse forearm flap: experience with 80 consecutive cases. Plast Reconstr Surg 1993;92(2):285–293
2. Costa H, Gracia ML, Vranchx J, Cunha C, Conde A, Soutar D. The posterior interosseous flap: a review of 81 clinical cases and 100 anatomical dissections--assessment of its indications in reconstruction of hand defects. Br J Plast Surg 2001;54(1):28–33

FLAPS USED FOR ELBOW SOFT-TISSUE COVERAGE

7. Which one of the following flaps is based on the posterior radial collateral artery and can only provide coverage of a distal elbow defect if used as a free tissue transfer?

D. Lateral arm flap

The lateral arm flap is based on the posterior radial collateral artery (**Fig. 90.3**).

It can be pedicled to cover defects of the shoulder and proximal arm. It is also a popular choice for free tissue transfer to the hand because it restricts surgery to a single limb and the donor site can be closed directly. Because of its reach, reconstruction of elbow defects could only be undertaken as a free tissue transfer.

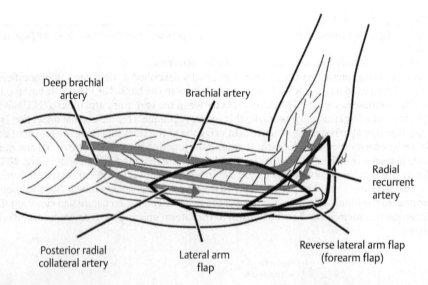

Fig. 90.3 The reverse lateral arm flap (forearm flap) and lateral arm flap, showing the different vascular supplies.

In contrast, the reverse lateral arm flap is based on the radial recurrent artery and is useful for elbow reconstruction as a pedicled flap. Again, a key advantage is that the donor site is within the same operative field, as the defect and the scarring can be kept to a single limb. A disadvantage is that the arc of rotation may not always allow complete elbow defect coverage.[1]

A flexor carpi ulnaris muscle flap is based on the posterior ulnar recurrent artery and can be useful in some elderly patients who require 3 to 4 cm of muscle cover at the elbow. However, this flap should be avoided in young or active patients because of the important contribution this muscle makes to power grip and the "dart-throwing" motion that the wrist makes during many manual activities.[2]

The radial forearm flap is based on the main radial artery rather than the posterior radial collateral artery. This can be used as a pedicled flap for elbow reconstruction and is probably the most popular choice for significant defects as it is thin, pliable, reliable, and fairly quick to perform, even under regional block. The brachioradialis flap is based on a branch of the radial recurrent artery. It can be used to reconstruct small elbow defects, but this muscle is an important elbow flexor and should be preserved where possible.[2–4]

REFERENCES

1. Tung TC, Wang KC, Fang CM, Lee CM. Reverse pedicled lateral arm flap for reconstruction of posterior soft-tissue defects of the elbow. Ann Plast Surg 1997;38(6):635–641
2. Kelley BP, Chung KC. Soft-tissue coverage for elbow trauma. Hand Clin 2015;31(4):693–703
3. Yannascoli SM, Thibaudeau S, Levin LS. Management of soft tissue defects of the hand. J Hand Surg Am 2015;40(6):1237–1244, quiz 1245
4. Masquelet AC, Gilbert A. An Atlas of Flaps of the Musculoskeletal System. Boca Raton, FL: CRC Press; 2001

VASCULAR SUPPLY TO FREE FLAPS USED IN THE UPPER LIMB

8. *Which one of the following soft-tissue flaps may be useful as a free flap for upper limb reconstruction and is based on the circumflex scapular vessels?*

C. The scapula/parascapular flap

The scapular and parascapular flaps are reliable, thin, pliable fasciocutaneous flaps useful for upper limb reconstruction. They are both supplied by cutaneous branches of the circumflex scapular vessels and differ slightly in their skin paddle location and precise blood supply. The scapular flap is supplied by the transverse branch of the circumflex scapular artery, while the parascapular flap is supplied by the descending branch. The skin paddle for the scapular flap is therefore positioned transversely over the middle part of the scapula, while the parascapular flap skin paddle is positioned along the lower lateral border of the scapula. The donor site is generally closed directly and is well hidden in clothing. The lateral border of the scapula may be harvested where bone is needed.

The serratus muscle flap is more commonly harvested in conjunction with a latissimus dorsi or bony scapular flap but can be harvested individually where a small muscle flap is required. This muscle is important in the stabilization of the scapula, so must not be sacrificed in its entirety. However, the last three digitations can safely be raised without functional impairment. The serratus receives its blood supply from a number of different sources, but the component harvested for free tissue transfer is based on the serratus branch of the thoracodorsal artery. This is why it can be raised along with a latissimus dorsi flap.

The gracilis flap is a real workhorse flap for both static and functional reconstruction in the upper limb. It is an excellent flap for achieving dynamic elbow flexion following brachial plexus injury. It is generally raised as a muscle-only flap and is an ideal donor because morbidity is low, with no discernible functional loss and a well-hidden scar passing along the medial thigh. The blood supply to the gracilis is the medial femoral circumflex (which is a branch of the profunda femoris). The muscle differs in size according to age and sex but typically provides 6×20 cm of muscle in adult males. It is possible to take a skin paddle with the gracilis, although a longitudinal paddle is generally considered to be unreliable. A transverse proximal skin paddle may be taken as a transverse upper gracilis flap when skin is required. This is more often used for breast or perineal reconstruction.

Other useful free flaps for upper limb reconstruction include the anterolateral thigh flap (lateral circumflex femoral vessels), the pectoralis major and pectoralis minor muscle flaps (thoracoacromial vessels), and the rectus abdominis muscle flap (deep inferior epigastric vessels).[1,2]

REFERENCES

1. Masquelet AC, Gilbert A. An Atlas of Flaps of the Musculoskeletal System. Boca Raton, FL: CRC Press; 2001
2. Kelley BP, Chung KC. Soft-tissue coverage for elbow trauma. Hand Clin 2015;31(4):693–703

91. Compartment Syndrome

See *Essentials of Plastic Surgery*, third edition, pp. 1260–1271

INTRACOMPARTMENTAL PRESSURES

1. *What is the threshold intracompartmental pressure that would require intervention when a potential compartment syndrome is being assessed?*
    A. An absolute pressure of 10 mm Hg
    B. An absolute pressure of 20 mm Hg
    C. An absolute pressure of 30 mm Hg
    D. Within 40 mm Hg of systolic pressure
    E. Within 80 mm Hg of diastolic pressure

LOWER LIMB COMPARTMENTS

2. You are asked to review a patient following a tibial fracture because there is concern regarding compartment syndrome. *Which one of the following lower leg compartments is most likely to develop compartment syndrome in this scenario?*
    A. Deep posterior
    B. Superficial posterior
    C. Lateral
    D. Anterior
    E. Medial

FOREARM COMPARTMENTS

3. *Which one of the following muscles is most likely to be damaged by a forearm compartment syndrome?*
    A. Flexor digitorum superficialis
    B. Flexor pollicis longus
    C. Flexor carpi radialis
    D. Flexor carpi ulnaris
    E. Pronator teres

CLINICAL ASSESSMENT IN SUSPECTED COMPARTMENT SYNDROME

4. The six Ps are often described for the assessment of an awake patient with suspected compartment syndrome. *Which one of these is the best early indicator of this condition?*
    A. Pallor
    B. Pulselessness
    C. Paresthesia
    D. Pain
    E. Poikilothermia

INDICATIONS FOR FASCIOTOMY

5. A patient sustains a high-voltage electrical injury stealing copper wire from a substation. He complains of pain in his right forearm. *In addition to the history, which one of the following is the strongest indicator for prompt fasciotomies?*
    A. Three consecutive intracompartmental pressure (ICP) readings of 20 mm Hg
    B. Paresthesia in the median nerve distribution
    C. Severe pain on passive finger extension
    D. A circumferential superficial burn to the forearm
    E. Radius and ulna fractures on plain radiographs

DELAYED PRESENTATION OF COMPARTMENT SYNDROME

6. A 40-year-old man crushed his arm at work 3 days ago and has been referred from a peripheral hospital because his hand has markedly reduced sensation and power, despite his pain improving. The working diagnosis had been neurapraxia; however, a blood creatinine phosphokinase (CPK/CK) level was checked and is 21,000. His hand is well perfused and his forearm is a little firm and tender. *Which one of the following is correct?*
    A. He should have prompt fasciotomies to the forearm.
    B. His renal function should be checked, then he should have prompt fasciotomies to the forearm.
    C. Serial observation and measurement of ICPs should be initiated.
    D. He should be closely observed, with the hand elevated, hand therapy, and maintenance of good urine output.
    E. He should undergo urgent ultrasonography of the forearm.

PERFORMING A LEG FASCIOTOMY

7. There are a number of accepted approaches to fasciotomies in the lower leg. *When undertaking a combined lateral and medial two-incision approach, which one of the following is correct?*
   A. The superficial and deep peroneal nerves are at high risk of damage during the lateral release.
   B. Flexor hallucis longus is the first muscle encountered after the lateral incision.
   C. The interosseous membrane must be divided after locating the tibialis anterior.
   D. The medial approach risks damage to the posterior tibial vessels and nerve.
   E. The medial incision should be placed 10 cm behind the tibial border.

COMPARTMENTS OF THE LEG

8. *Which one of the following nerves is found in the anterior compartment of the leg?*
   A. Superficial peroneal nerve
   B. Common peroneal nerve
   C. Deep peroneal nerve
   D. Anterior tibial nerve
   E. Saphenous nerve

FASCIOTOMIES IN DIFFERENT ANATOMIC SITES

9. *Which one of the following is correct regarding fasciotomies?*
   A. The arm is decompressed using volar and dorsal incisions.
   B. The 10-hand compartments are decompressed using two dorsal and one midpalmar incision.
   C. All four of the major foot compartments can be decompressed through a single medial approach.
   D. The thigh has three compartments traditionally decompressed through a single medial approach.
   E. A single medial approach remains popular for decompression of the four-leg compartments.

Answers

INTRACOMPARTMENTAL PRESSURES

1. *What is the threshold intracompartmental pressure that would require intervention when a potential compartment syndrome is being assessed?*

    C. An absolute pressure of 30 mm Hg

    The normal intracompartmental pressure (ICP) is less than 10 mm Hg. Elevated compartment pressure occurs when either the contents of an osseofascial compartment increase in volume or when the compartment itself reduces in volume (e.g., after a circumferential deep burn, or secondary to external constriction). In compartment syndrome, elevated interstitial pressure overwhelms perfusion pressure. As the ICP rises, venous pressure rises. When venous pressure is higher than capillary perfusion pressure, the capillaries collapse. The accepted threshold above which there is occlusion of capillary flow is 30 mm Hg, or a relative difference between the ICP and the diastolic blood pressure of less than 30 mm Hg. Both of these are very important parameters to be aware of.[1-3]

REFERENCES

1. Velmahos GC, Toutouzas KG. Vascular trauma and compartment syndromes. Surg Clin North Am 2002;82(1):125–141, xxi
2. McQueen MM, Gaston P, Court-Brown CM. Acute compartment syndrome. Who is at risk? J Bone Joint Surg Br 2000;82(2):200–203
3. Matsen FA III, Winquist RA, Krugmire RB Jr. Diagnosis and management of compartmental syndromes. J Bone Joint Surg Am 1980;62(2):286–291

LOWER LIMB COMPARTMENTS

2. You are asked to review a patient following a tibial fracture because there is concern regarding compartment syndrome. *Which one of the following lower leg compartments is most likely to develop compartment syndrome in this scenario?*

    D. Anterior

    The anterior compartment is most likely to be involved in a lower limb compartment syndrome. McQueen et al[1] reviewed 59 cases of leg compartment syndrome that included both open and closed tibial injuries. They found that all cases involved the anterior compartment but only 18 involved all four compartments. For ICP monitoring, the anterior compartment is easy to access. The deep posterior compartment is probably the most difficult to reliably decompress but is the second most at-risk compartment. In 6 of the 59 cases, the lateral compartment was also involved, and in 5 cases the deep posterior compartment was also involved. The deep posterior compartment is probably the most difficult to reliably assess and is the second most at-risk compartment. A more recent study by McQueen et al retrospectively reviewed 1,407 patients who had sustained an open tibial shaft fracture, in order to identify predictors of compartment syndrome. Their analysis showed that the main predictor was age, with males between the ages of 12 and 29 to be most at risk. They did not comment on the compartment involved in this study; however, they postulated that the increased risk in younger patients is due to the increased physical size of muscles in this patient group. The anterior compartment may be most at risk of developing compartment syndrome because it is a particularly tight compartment with well-developed musculature. The close proximity to the tibia is also likely to be a factor.[2]

REFERENCES

1. McQueen MM, Gaston P, Court-Brown CM. Acute compartment syndrome. Who is at risk? J Bone Joint Surg Br 2000;82(2):200–203
2. McQueen MM, Duckworth AD, Aitken SA, Sharma RA, Court-Brown CM. Predictors of compartment syndrome after tibial fracture. J Orthop Trauma 2015;29(10):451–455

FOREARM COMPARTMENTS

3. *Which one of the following muscles is most likely to be damaged by a forearm compartment syndrome?*

    B. Flexor pollicis longus (FPL)

    Compartment syndrome affects the deep muscles of the volar compartment (flexor digitorum profundus and FPL) most significantly. They are more susceptible to damage, since they are compressed against the radius, the ulna, and interosseous membrane (**Fig. 91.1**). A retrospective study on acute compartment syndrome of the forearm

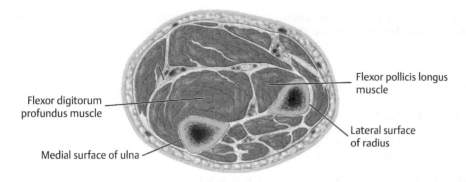

Fig. 91.1   Cross-sectional view of the right proximal forearm.

in 93 patients by Duckworth et al[1] showed that the volar compartment was most commonly decompressed (99% of cases), and this included the carpal tunnel in around half of these cases. The decision on which compartment to decompress was based on clinical examination and intracompartmental measurement. The most common complication was a neurological deficit (18%) followed by contracture (4%). Muscle necrosis with associated weakness was observed in around 3% of cases in this series.

REFERENCE

1. Duckworth AD, Mitchell SE, Molyneux SG, White TO, Court-Brown CM, McQueen MM. Acute compartment syndrome of the forearm. J Bone Joint Surg Am 2012;94(10):e63

CLINICAL ASSESSMENT IN SUSPECTED COMPARTMENT SYNDROME

4. **The six Ps are often described for the assessment of an awake patient with suspected compartment syndrome.** *Which one of these is the best early indicator of this condition?*
   D. Pain
   The six Ps (**p**ain, **p**allor, **p**oikilothermia, **p**ressure, **p**aralysis/paresthesias, **p**ulselessness) are useful to consider in suspected compartment syndrome. They must be placed in the context of the injury and patient history. Pain is the single most important early finding and will be disproportionate to the expected pain from injury and exacerbated by passive extension of the affected compartmental muscles. Progressive loss of nerve function begins with sensory nerves and progresses to motor nerves and is usually a later sign. Pulselessness is another late sign of compartment syndrome, and if present early in the episode, a vascular injury or occlusion is more likely to be the underlying cause. The presence of one of the six Ps alone remains a poor indicator of compartment syndrome. When more than two features coexist in the lower leg, the likelihood increases to above 90%.[1]

REFERENCE

1. Ulmer T. The clinical diagnosis of compartment syndrome of the lower leg: are clinical findings predictive of the disorder? J Orthop Trauma 2002;16(8):572–577

INDICATIONS FOR FASCIOTOMY

5. **A patient sustains a high-voltage electrical injury stealing copper wire from a substation. He complains of pain in his right forearm.** *In addition to the history, which one of the following is the strongest indicator for prompt fasciotomies?*
   C. Severe pain on passive finger extension
   Pain on passive stretch of the muscles in a compartment is one of the cardinal signs of compartment syndrome. Patients who suffer a high-voltage electrical injury are at risk of developing acute compartment syndrome. The bone has a high resistance and becomes disproportionately hot during electrical current conduction. The surrounding muscle is damaged by both the electrical current itself and the heat from the underlying bone. This leads to a massive amount of swelling, which may result in compartment syndrome.
      An ICP reading of 30 mm Hg (not 20 mm Hg) or above would indicate a compartment syndrome, as would a series of rising pressure readings in association with clinical signs.
      Tingling in the median nerve distribution can be an early indicator of rising pressure in the volar compartment of the forearm, but the strongest indication in this scenario is the pain on passive muscle stretch. The presence

of radius and ulna fractures indicates that significant force has been applied to the arm, increasing the risk of elevated compartment pressures, but this is not necessarily an indication for decompression in isolation.[1-3]

REFERENCES

1. Doyle JR. Compartment syndrome. In: Doyle JR, ed. Hand and Wrist. 1st ed. Philadelphia: Lippincott Williams &Wilkins; 2006
2. Chandraprakasam T, Kumar RA. Acute compartment syndrome of forearm and hand. Indian J Plast Surg 2011;44(2):212–218
3. Boccara D, Lavocat R, Soussi S, et al. Pressure guided surgery of compartment syndrome of the limbs in burn patients. Ann Burns Fire Disasters 2017;30(3):193–197

DELAYED PRESENTATION OF COMPARTMENT SYNDROME

6. A 40-year-old man crushed his arm at work 3 days ago and has been referred from a peripheral hospital because his hand has markedly reduced sensation and power, despite his pain improving. The working diagnosis had been neurapraxia; however, a blood creatinine phosphokinase (CPK/CK) level was checked and is 21,000. His hand is well perfused and his forearm is a little firm and tender. *Which one of the following is correct?*

   D. **He should be closely observed, with the hand elevated, hand therapy, and maintenance of good urine output.**
   This man has several features of missed compartment syndrome, with a high-risk mechanism of injury. The elevated CPK/CK levels are concerning, and it is important to maintain good diuresis and monitor renal function while he clears myoglobinuria to avoid renal injury. Unfortunately, the window of opportunity to decompress his forearm has passed. Late decompression converts a closed injury with nonviable muscle into an open injury with little additional benefit, running the risk of secondary infection, compartmentectomy, and, in some case series, death. If he still had worsening or static levels of pain, this might indicate viable muscle that could still be salvaged, but as his pain has largely subsided this does not apply. Ultrasonography is not helpful in the diagnosis of compartment syndrome, although it can help eliminate other diagnoses. In the absence of raised CPK/CK, but with a swollen limb, a scan may be indicated to exclude deep venous thrombosis or other soft-tissue swelling. A key step in the management of patients with missed compartment syndrome is to ensure physical therapy commences early to minimize swelling, stiffness, and long-term dysfunction.[1,2]

REFERENCES

1. Glass GE, Staruch RM, Simmons J, et al. Managing missed lower extremity compartment syndrome in the physiologically stable patient: a systematic review and lessons from a Level I trauma center. J Trauma Acute Care Surg 2016;81(2):380–387
2. Lundy DW, Bruggers JL. Management of missed compartment syndrome. In: Mauffrey C, Hak DJ, Martin III MP, eds. Compartment Syndrome: A Guide to Diagnosis and Management [Internet]. Cham (CH): Springer; 2019

PERFORMING A LEG FASCIOTOMY

7. There are a number of accepted approaches to fasciotomies in the lower leg. *When undertaking a combined lateral and medial two-incision approach, which one of the following is correct?*

   D. **The medial approach risks damage to the posterior tibial vessels and nerve.**
   The two-incision approach to leg fasciotomy involves a posteromedial incision combined with either a lateral or anterolateral incision (**Fig. 91.2**). This access facilitates decompression of the two posterior and anterior/lateral compartments, respectively.[1] The medial incision is generally placed 1 to 2 cm posterior to the tibial border to preserve perforating skin vessels from the posterior tibial artery that may be required for local transposition flaps. The incision passes into the superficial posterior compartment and dissection continues around the soleus to access the deep compartment. During this dissection, care must be taken to avoid damage to the posterior tibial neurovascular bundle.

   The lateral incision is placed anterior to the fibula border and the first compartment entered would be either the lateral or anterior depending on the incision location; therefore, the peroneal or anterior compartment muscles (not FHL) would be seen first. The anterolateral incision is commonly placed 2 cm posterior to the lateral tibial border, and the first muscle encountered in this approach is the tibialis anterior as the anterior compartment is entered. Dissection then continues subfascially in a lateral direction toward the peroneal septum, which is then divided to release the lateral compartment. The superficial and deep peroneal nerves lie within these two compartments (depending on the level) but are unlikely to be damaged using these approaches. The interosseous membrane, separating the anterior and deep posterior compartments, does not need to be divided.

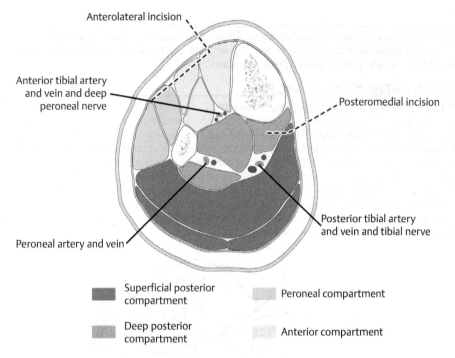

Fig. 91.2   Incisions and anatomic structures for leg fasciotomies.

REFERENCE

1. Standards for the Management of Open Fractures of the Lower Limb. London: British Orthopaedic Association and British Association of Plastic Reconstructive and Aesthetic Surgeons; 2009

COMPARTMENTS OF THE LEG

8. Which one of the following nerves is found in the anterior compartment of the leg?

C. Deep peroneal nerve

The anterior compartment of the leg contains the anterior tibial vessels and deep peroneal nerve. There is no anterior tibial nerve. It also contains the following four muscles: the tibialis anterior; the extensor hallucis longus; the extensor digitorum longus; and the peroneus tertius, which runs with the digitorum longus (**Fig. 91.3**). The saphenous nerve is located on the medial aspect of the leg and lies superficial to the leg compartments. The superficial peroneal nerve is located in the lateral compartment along with peroneus longus and brevis, emerging superficially at the junction of the middle and distal third of the leg. The tibial nerve is located in the posterior compartment with the posterior tibial vessels, the gastrocnemius, soleus, tibialis posterior, and the long flexors.[1,2]

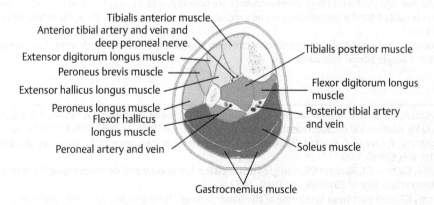

Fig. 91.3   Cross-section of the lower leg.

REFERENCES

1. Moore KL, Dalley AF, eds. Clinically Oriented Anatomy. 4th ed. New York, NY: Lippincott Williams & Wilkins; 1999
2. Standards for the Management of Open Fractures of the Lower Limb. London: British Orthopaedic Association and British Association of Plastic Reconstructive and Aesthetic Surgeons; 2009

FASCIOTOMIES IN DIFFERENT ANATOMIC SITES

9. *Which one of the following is correct regarding fasciotomies?*

   C. **All four of the major foot compartments can be decompressed through a single medial approach.**

     The foot is considered to have either four or nine compartments (depending on how they are classified), all of which can be decompressed using a single medial incision along the plantar border of the first metatarsal (**Fig. 91.4**).[1-3]

     The arm is considered to have two or three compartments (anterior, posterior, +/– deltoid) that are usually decompressed through one medial, or two (medial and posterolateral) incisions (see Fig. 91.6, *Essentials of Plastic Surgery*, third edition).[4] The hand is normally considered to have 10 compartments and is commonly decompressed using two dorsal and two volar incisions. The dorsal incisions are placed over the index and ring metacarpals, while the volar incisions are placed on the ulnar and radial borders of the glabrous palmar skin (see Fig. 91.8, *Essentials of Plastic Surgery*, third edition).[5]

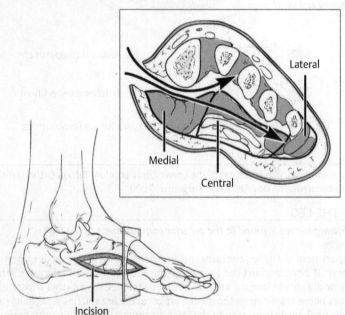

Fig. 91.4 Foot fasciotomy by medial incision. To decompress the four compartments of the foot using a medial approach, an incision is made along the plantar border of the first metatarsal, allowing access to all four compartments. The incision can be extended proximally if the posterior tibial neurovascular bundle requires decompression as well.

     The anterior and posterior thigh compartments are decompressed using a lateral incision. A separate medial incision is required for decompression of the medial compartment (see Fig. 91.5, *Essentials of Plastic Surgery*, third edition).[6]

     The common options for decompression of the four-leg compartments include combined medial and lateral incisions or a single lateral approach.

REFERENCES

1. Fulkerson E, Razi A, Tejwani N. Review: acute compartment syndrome of the foot. Foot Ankle Int 2003;24(2):180–187
2. Kamel R, Sakla FB. Anatomical compartments of the sole of the human foot. Anat Rec 1961;140:57–60
3. Frink M, Hildebrand F, Krettek C, Brand J, Hankemeier S. Compartment syndrome of the lower leg and foot. Clin Orthop Relat Res 2010;468(4):940–950
4. Ojike NI, Alla SR, Battista CT, Roberts CS. A single volar incision fasciotomy will decompress all three forearm compartments: a cadaver study. Injury 2012;43(11):1949–1952
5. Oak NR, Abrams RA. Compartment syndrome of the hand. Orthop Clin North Am 2016;47(3):609–616
6. Ojike NI, Roberts CS, Giannoudis PV. Compartment syndrome of the thigh: a systematic review. Injury 2010;41(2):133–136

92. Upper Extremity Compression Syndromes

See *Essentials of Plastic Surgery*, third edition, pp. 1272–1286

MEDIAN NERVE PATHOLOGY

1. A patient presents with isolated abnormal sensation to the thenar eminence. The forearm and digits are spared. Motor function of the digits and wrist is normal. *Where is the median nerve most likely to be compressed in this case?*
   A. Proximal forearm
   B. Midforearm
   C. Distal forearm
   D. Wrist
   E. Distal end of carpal tunnel

RADIAL NERVE PATHOLOGY

2. *What is the most common site for compression of the radial nerve?*
   A. Proximal to the radial tunnel
   B. The vascular leash of Henry
   C. Proximal margin of ECRB
   D. Arcade of Frohse
   E. Biceps tendon

ULNAR NERVE PATHOLOGY

3. *Which one of the fo llowing represents a simple test for ulnar nerve motor function?*
   A. Making a thumb's-up sign
   B. Making an "OK" ring sign
   C. Crossing the index and middle fingers
   D. Abducting the thumb
   E. Extending the index finger

NERVE COMPRESSION PHYSIOLOGY

4. *Which one of the following is correct regarding nerve compression?*
   A. Axonal damage is always the first sign of a nerve compression injury.
   B. Compressive forces of more than 10 mm Hg are sufficient to impair nerve function.
   C. Symptoms of nerve compression can be caused by adhesions rather than pressure.
   D. Demyelination is an isolated and late sign following chronic nerve compression.
   E. Reduced sensory latency in a nerve conduction study indicates reduced salutatory conduction.

CARPAL TUNNEL SYNDROME

5. *Which one of the following is true regarding carpal tunnel syndrome?*
   A. The prevalence of carpal tunnel syndrome is 1% of the adult population.
   B. Only adults are affected by carpal tunnel syndrome.
   C. Sensory disturbance is limited to the thumb, index, and middle fingers.
   D. More than 90% of patients with proven carpal tunnel syndrome improve after surgical release.
   E. The main advantage of endoscopic carpal tunnel release is reduced nerve injury risk.

CARPAL TUNNEL SYNDROME

6. An obese 30-year-old office worker presents with symptoms of carpal tunnel syndrome. His symptoms include discomfort radiating up the forearm. Nerve conduction studies (NCS) show moderate median nerve compression in the carpal tunnel. *Which one of the following is correct?*
   A. Use of a wrist splint at night may be effective at reducing his symptoms.
   B. Frequent use of a computer keyboard is likely to be causing his symptoms.
   C. His weight is not a relevant contributory factor to his carpal tunnel syndrome.
   D. His forearm discomfort is unlikely to be improved by carpal tunnel release.
   E. Carpal tunnel release would be contraindicated if he also has cervical nerve root compression.

PRONATOR SYNDROME

7. *Which one of the following is true of a patient with pronator syndrome?*
   A. Sensation to the thenar eminence will usually be normal.
   B. The site of compression is likely to be pronator quadratus at the wrist.
   C. Motor weakness of the digits and wrist will generally be evident.
   D. Pain on resisted FDS contraction is a characteristic finding.
   E. Resolution of symptoms is unlikely after surgical decompression.

ANTERIOR INTEROSSEOUS SYNDROME

8. *What is a typical clinical finding in anterior interosseous syndrome?*
   A. Abnormal sensation to the thenar eminence
   B. Abnormal sensation to the radial digits
   C. Weakness of little finger flexion
   D. Weakness of thumb IP joint flexion
   E. Weakness of thumb abduction

RADIAL NERVE PATHOLOGY

9. A patient has paralysis of the digital and thumb extensors, but some preservation of wrist extension. *Which of the following is the most likely cause of his radial nerve palsy?*
   A. Plating of a humeral shaft fracture
   B. Posterior dislocation of the shoulder
   C. Dislocation of the radial head
   D. Plating of a distal radius fracture
   E. An antecubital fossa lipoma

RADIAL TUNNEL SYNDROME

10. A patient is referred with a diagnosis of radial tunnel syndrome. *What is the most likely differential diagnosis or coexisting condition?*
   A. Lateral epicondylitis (tennis elbow)
   B. Medial epicondylitis (golfer's elbow)
   C. Anterior interosseous nerve syndrome
   D. Posterior interosseous nerve syndrome
   E. Wartenberg's syndrome

WARTENBERG'S SYNDROME

11. *What is a typical finding in Wartenberg's syndrome?*
   A. Inability to extend the thumb
   B. Inability to extend the index finger
   C. Abnormal dorsal sensation over the fifth metacarpal
   D. Pain over the dorsoradial aspect of the hand
   E. Inability to adduct the little finger

ULNAR NERVE COMPRESSION AT THE ELBOW

12. *When exploring a compressed ulnar nerve at the elbow, which one of the following is least likely to be a site of compression?*
   A. The origin of flexor carpi ulnaris
   B. The roof of the cubital tunnel/Osborne's ligament
   C. The medial intermuscular septum of the arm
   D. Lesions in the floor of the cubital tunnel (e.g., osteophytes)
   E. The vascular leash of Henry

MANAGEMENT OF CUBITAL TUNNEL SYNDROME

13. *Which one of the following is correct regarding the management of cubital tunnel syndrome?*
   A. Medial epicondylectomy is always superior to in situ decompression.
   B. Submuscular nerve transposition is usually reserved for recurrent cases.
   C. Medial epicondylectomy requires complete resection of the epicondyle.
   D. Splint therapy is well tolerated and should always be tried before surgery.
   E. Results of surgical decompression are highly predictable.

ULNAR NERVE COMPRESSION IN GUYON'S CANAL

14. *Which one of the following is correct regarding ulnar nerve compression in Guyon's canal?*
   A. Ulnar nerve compression here will only produce motor symptoms and signs.
   B. Guyon's canal is divided into two zones related to the ulnar nerve branches.
   C. The underlying cause may be an aneurysm of the ulnar artery.
   D. Surgical release requires a different incision to that of a carpal tunnel release.
   E. Imaging is not required if nerve conduction studies show ulnar nerve compression in Guyon's canal.

UPPER LIMB COMPRESSION SYNDROMES

15. An elderly patient complains that his little finger sticks out all the time and his grip on his walking stick is weak. *What is the most likely diagnosis?*
   A. Radial tunnel syndrome
   B. Cubital tunnel syndrome
   C. Pronator syndrome
   D. Ulnar tunnel syndrome
   E. Wartenberg's syndrome

Answers

MEDIAN NERVE PATHOLOGY

1. A patient presents with isolated abnormal sensation to the thenar eminence. The forearm and digits are spared. Motor function of the digits and wrist is normal. *Where is the median nerve most likely to be compressed in this case?*

   C. Distal forearm

   This patient has dysfunction of the thenar sensory branch (palmar cutaneous branch) of the median nerve. This arises from the main nerve approximately 5 cm proximal to the wrist and initially runs parallel to the main nerve before passing volarly to the skin. It may be compressed by localized swellings such as hematoma, lipoma, or ganglion cysts. It may also be injured following penetrating trauma to the distal forearm. Further investigation or exploration is warranted in either scenario.[1,2]

REFERENCES

1. Eversmann WW Jr. Entrapment and compression neuropathies. In: Green DP, Hotchkiss RN, Pederson WC, eds. Green's Operative Hand Surgery. 4th ed. Philadelphia: Churchill Livingstone; 1998
2. Meyer P, Lintingre PF, Pesquer L, Poussange N, Silvestre A, Dallaudière B. The median nerve at the carpal tunnel … and elsewhere. J Belg Soc Radiol 2018;102(1):17

RADIAL NERVE PATHOLOGY

2. *What is the most common site for compression of the radial nerve?*

   D. Arcade of Frohse

   The Arcade of Frohse refers to the proximal edge of the superficial supinator muscle and is the most common site of radial nerve compression. Radial nerve compression is much less common than ulnar or median nerve compression. The radial nerve passes through the radial tunnel, which is formed by the radiocapitellar joint bursa, the brachioradialis tendon, the extensor carpi radialis longus (ECRL) and the extensor carpi radialis brevis (ECRB) tendons, and the biceps tendon and brachialis muscle. There are three other key sites of compression and these are fibrous bands anterior to the radiocapitellar joint (just proximal to the radial tunnel), the vascular leash of Henry (which represents the radial recurrent artery), and the proximal tendon of the ECRB.[1-3] Saturday night palsy is a condition with signs of a new sudden-onset radial nerve compression following prolonged pressure overnight typically with the arm resting over a chair and often associated with intoxication. This is due to compression of the radial nerve at the spiral groove of the humerus.[4]

REFERENCES

1. Moore KL, Dalley AF, eds. Clinically Oriented Anatomy. 4th ed. New York, NY: Lippincott Williams & Wilkins; 1999
2. Eversmann WW Jr. Compression and entrapment neuropathies of the upper extremity. J Hand Surg Am 1983;8(5, Pt 2): 759–766
3. Latef TJ, Bilal M, Vetter M, Iwanaga J, Oskouian RJ, Tubbs RS. Injury of the radial nerve in the arm: a review. Cureus 2018;10(2):e2199
4. Lotem M, Fried A, Solzi P, Natanson T. Saturday night palsy [in Hebrew]. Harefuah 1972;83(8):328

ULNAR NERVE PATHOLOGY

3. *Which one of the following represents a simple test for ulnar nerve motor function?*

   C. Crossing the index and middle fingers

   Ulnar nerve motor palsy is demonstrated by the inability to cross the index and middle fingers or to deviate the extended middle finger ulnarly or radially when the hand is placed on a flat surface. Both of these tests are quick and simple to perform in clinic.

   These clinical findings are because the intrinsic muscles (dorsal and palmar interossei) are paralyzed. In addition, the flexor digitorum profundus (FDP) to the little and ring fingers may be affected, depending on compression/injury level. Making a thumb's-up sign relies on radial nerve innervation of the extensor pollicis longus, extensor pollicis brevis (EPB), and abductor pollicis longus (APL). The "OK" ring sign requires anterior interosseous nerve innervation of the flexor pollicis longus (FPL) and FDP index finger. Thumb abduction requires innervation of the abductor pollicis brevis by the median nerve.[1-3]

REFERENCES

1. Spinner M, Spencer PS. Nerve compression lesions of the upper extremity. A clinical and experimental review. Clin Orthop Relat Res 1974;(104):46–67
2. Dellon AL. Patient evaluation and management considerations in nerve compression. Hand Clin 1992;8(2): 229–239
3. Eversmann WW Jr. Entrapment and compression neuropathies. In: Green DP, Hotchkiss RN, Pederson WC, eds. Green's Operative Hand Surgery. 4th ed. Philadelphia: Churchill Livingstone; 1998

NERVE COMPRESSION PHYSIOLOGY

4. *Which one of the following is correct regarding nerve compression?*

    C. Symptoms of nerve compression can be caused by adhesions rather than pressure.

        Although external compression is readily considered as a cause of nerve pathology, common symptoms (such as those of carpal or cubital tunnel syndrome) may arise from repeated traction on a nerve. Adhesions may limit nerve excursion, such as around the medial epicondyle during elbow flexion. One study demonstrated that while isolated elbow flexion from 10 to 90 degrees requires only 5 mm of ulnar nerve excursion, combined movements of the shoulder, elbow, and wrist can require up to 22 mm excursion at the cubital tunnel.[1] When this movement is prevented by adhesions, repeated traction insults may lead to the same changes of vascular injury, inflammation, and fibrosis with demyelination or axonal degeneration that may occur with recurrent compression. If adhesions are the cause of nerve pathology, it can be difficult to prevent a recurrence. This may be why gliding exercises can be useful for some nerve compression symptoms. For example, stretching adhesions within the carpal tunnel is thought to reduce synovial edema, and improve venous return within nerve bundles.[2]

        Demyelination occurs early in repeatedly compressed nerve segments, whereas axonal damage is a later finding. Compressive forces above 20 mm Hg are considered to be sufficient to impair many aspects of nerve function. Reduced saltatory nerve conduction would be reflected by reduced conduction speeds and prolonged latencies in a nerve conduction study.

REFERENCES

1. Wright TW, Glowczewskie F Jr, Cowin D, Wheeler DL. Ulnar nerve excursion and strain at the elbow and wrist associated with upper extremity motion. J Hand Surg Am 2001;26(4):655–662
2. Rozmaryn LM, Dovelle S, Rothman ER, Gorman K, Olvey KM, Bartko JJ. Nerve and tendon gliding exercises and the conservative management of carpal tunnel syndrome. J Hand Ther 1998;11(3):171–179

CARPAL TUNNEL SYNDROME

5. *Which one of the following is true regarding carpal tunnel syndrome?*

    D. More than 90% of patients with proven carpal tunnel syndrome improve after surgical release.

        Carpal tunnel syndrome is a compression neuropathy of the median nerve at the wrist within the carpal tunnel. Surgical treatment is most commonly an open release of the transverse carpal ligament. More than 90% of patients with confirmed carpal tunnel syndrome will have an improvement in their symptoms after adequate median nerve decompression.

        Carpal tunnel syndrome represents the most common upper extremity compression neuropathy and prevalence is estimated to be between 3 and 4%.[1] The condition is not restricted to adults, as children can occasionally develop carpal tunnel syndrome too. The main concern in children is that symptoms tend to present late, often with bilateral disease and established thenar wasting. It is treated in the same way as adult carpal tunnel syndrome.

        In addition to altered sensation in the radial three digits, the radial border of the ring finger is also commonly affected by sensory changes. The thenar eminence is spared because the palmar cutaneous branch is given off proximal to the carpal tunnel. The main reported advantages of endoscopic carpal tunnel release are an earlier return to work and reduced scar sensitivity; however, there are higher rates of neuropraxia and of recurrent symptoms as a result of incomplete release.[1,2]

REFERENCES

1. Papanicolaou GD, McCabe SJ, Firrell J. The prevalence and characteristics of nerve compression symptoms in the general population. J Hand Surg Am 2001;26(3):460–466
2. Singh I, Khoo KMA, Krishnamoorthy S. The carpal tunnel syndrome: clinical evaluation and results of surgical decompression. Ann Acad Med Singap 1994;23(1):94–97

CARPAL TUNNEL SYNDROME

6. An obese 30-year-old office worker presents with symptoms of carpal tunnel syndrome. His symptoms include discomfort radiating up the forearm. Nerve conduction studies (NCS) show moderate median nerve compression in the carpal tunnel. *Which one of the following is correct?*

A. Use of a wrist splint at night may be effective at reducing his symptoms.

Neutrally positioned wrist splints can be very effective for relieving symptoms of carpal tunnel syndrome and are usually tolerated best at night. In mild to moderate carpal tunnel syndrome, many patients may choose to avoid surgery after a trial of splint therapy. Splints may also help with symptom management while a patient is waiting for surgery. If splints are helpful but are difficult to tolerate, steroid injection into the tunnel may be an effective alternative to surgery for some patients. However, only around one-fifth of patients will have a sustained improvement in symptoms after a steroid injection.

The frequency of carpal tunnel syndrome in keyboard workers with variable intensity of use has been reviewed and found to be most common in workers with low-intensity keyboard activity.[1] Obesity is recognized as a common association with carpal tunnel syndrome, along with pregnancy, diabetes, and thyroid disorders.[2]

Although forearm discomfort is not a classic feature of carpal tunnel syndrome, many patients experience this. Following carpal tunnel release, many such patients report improvement in their pain symptoms. This is thought to be a result of the "multiple crush phenomenon" in which there are multiple additive insults influencing axonal transport along the length of a nerve.[3] Relieving one factor may sufficiently improve overall nerve function such that symptoms relating to other segments of the nerve are also improved. This is not a predictable outcome and patients should not be led to expect an improvement in symptoms, which are not directly attributable to compression of the median nerve at the wrist following carpal tunnel release. However, in a patient with coexisting nerve root or thoracic outlet nerve compression and peripheral nerve compression, it is prudent to relieve the peripheral compression in the first instance, as this may give sufficient relief to obviate the need for more complex proximal surgery.[3]

REFERENCES

1. Atroshi I, Gummesson C, Ornstein E, Johnsson R, Ranstam J. Carpal tunnel syndrome and keyboard use at work: a population-based study. Arthritis Rheum 2007;56(11):3620–3625
2. Dellon AL. Patient evaluation and management considerations in nerve compression. Hand Clin 1992;8(2):229–239
3. Upton AR, McComas AJ. The double crush in nerve entrapment syndromes. Lancet 1973;2(7825):359–362

PRONATOR SYNDROME

7. *Which one of the following is true of a patient with pronator syndrome?*

D. Pain on resisted FDS contraction is a characteristic finding.

Pronator syndrome is a nerve compression affecting the median nerve in the forearm. It presents with forearm and hand pain, paresthesia, and hypoesthesia including the thenar eminence. It is often worse during resisted flexor digitorum superficialis (FDS) contraction, particularly of the middle finger. This is because the compression commonly occurs proximally within the forearm at the fibrous arch of FDS. Other key sites of compression include pronator teres (not pronator quadratus, which is deep at the wrist), the ligament of Struthers (ligament between the distal humerus and pronator teres fascia) just proximal to the elbow, and the bicipital aponeurosis (lacertus fibrosus) at the elbow. Compression may also be due to abnormal vasculature in the distal forearm.

Pronator syndrome is predominantly a sensory pathology with no motor weakness usually evident. Occasionally, however, there may be additional signs of weak flexion of the thumb and index finger. Diagnosis is confirmed by history and examination which can show increased tingling on elbow flexion, forearm pronation, resisted FDS contraction, and tapping over the pronator teres. Surgical decompression is usually very successful with resolution of symptoms.[1–3]

REFERENCES

1. Olehnik WK, Manske PR, Szerzinski J. Median nerve compression in the proximal forearm. J Hand Surg Am 1994;19(1):121–126
2. Morris HH, Peters BH. Pronator syndrome: clinical and electrophysiological features in seven cases. J Neurol Neurosurg Psychiatry 1976;39(5):461–464
3. Dang AC, Rodner CM. Unusual compression neuropathies of the forearm, part II: median nerve. J Hand Surg Am 2009;34(10):1915–1920

ANTERIOR INTEROSSEOUS SYNDROME

8. *What is a typical clinical finding in anterior interosseous syndrome?*

    D. Weakness of thumb IP joint flexion

The anterior interosseous nerve is a branch of the median nerve that supplies the radial slips of the FDP, FPL, and pronator quadratus. Compression of the nerve is therefore characterized by loss of thumb flexion at the interphalangeal (IP) joint and index/middle finger distal interphalangeal (DIP) joint flexion. Cutaneous sensation is unaffected. Compression can occur at the tendinous edge of the pronator teres (deep head) or the tendinous origin of the FDS. However, there is also the possibility of other noncompressive causes such as an inflammatory cause (amyotrophy). Diagnosis involves clinical assessment of pinch strength and the OK sign. Nerve compression and EMG studies are often useful. Surgical decompression with neurolysis at the antecubital fossa and proximal forearm is considered by some to be highly effective but may not always be so. For example, a study reviewing a case series of 16 patients found that resolution of symptoms following decompression was similar to patients who were managed nonoperatively, and the authors suggested that surgery should be restricted to those patients with isolated and complete anterior interosseous motor loss that is persistent at 6 months.[1]

REFERENCE

1. Sood MK, Burke FD. Anterior interosseous nerve palsy. A review of 16 cases. J Hand Surg [Br] 1997;22(1):64–68

RADIAL NERVE PATHOLOGY

9. A patient has paralysis of the digital and thumb extensors, but some preservation of wrist extension. *Which of the following is the most likely cause of his radial nerve palsy?*

    C. Dislocation of the radial head

The motor branches to the ECRL usually arise before the radial nerve splits around the supinator muscle into the posterior interosseous nerve (PIN) and the superficial radial nerve. Therefore, following an injury or compression at or around the region of the supinator muscle (such as a dislocation of the radial head), there is likely to be preservation of some wrist extension as a result of ECRL function. More proximal injuries to the radial nerve, such as secondary to a humeral shaft fracture or posterior dislocation of the shoulder, would be likely to affect brachioradialis, ECRL +/- triceps function as well. Plating of a distal radius fracture should not cause a loss of digital or wrist extension as a result of nerve injury, as the muscles will have been innervated proximal to this level. There could, however, be direct injury to the extensor tendons.[1,2]

REFERENCES

1. Eversmann WW Jr. Compression and entrapment neuropathies of the upper extremity. J Hand Surg Am 1983;8(5, Pt 2):759–766
2. Latef TJ, Bilal M, Vetter M, Iwanaga J, Oskouian RJ, Tubbs RS. Injury of the radial nerve in the arm: a review. Cureus 2018;10(2):e2199

RADIAL TUNNEL SYNDROME

10. A patient is referred with a diagnosis of radial tunnel syndrome. *What is the most likely differential diagnosis or coexisting condition?*

    A. Lateral epicondylitis (tennis elbow)

Patients with radial tunnel syndrome experience pain in the proximal forearm on movement at the elbow, wrist, or digits similar to tennis elbow, with radiation distally to the dorsum of the hand. There is often tingling of the hand and a secondary weakness of grip due to pain. The pain is typically more distal to that of lateral epicondylitis and is described as being induced by resisted middle finger extension.

Medial epicondylitis or golfer's elbow is similar but affects the ulnar aspect of the forearm. Anterior interosseous syndrome is a motor condition with weakness of the FPL and FDP to index. Posterior interosseous syndrome is predominantly a motor weakness with difficulty extending the wrist and digits because of nerve compression or traction neuropraxia along the path of the nerve in the forearm. Pain can be a feature, but normal sensation is preserved. Wartenberg's syndrome involves pain over the radial aspect of the hand and wrist due to compression of the superficial radial nerve. There is no motor weakness.[1,2]

REFERENCES

1. Dang AC, Rodner CM. Unusual compression neuropathies of the forearm, part I: radial nerve. J Hand Surg Am 2009;34(10):1906–1914
2. Eversmann WW Jr. Entrapment and compression neuropathies. In: Green DP, Hotchkiss RN, Pederson WC, eds. Green's Operative Hand Surgery. 4th ed. Philadelphia: Churchill Livingstone; 1998

WARTENBERG'S SYNDROME

11. What is a typical finding in Wartenberg's syndrome?

D. Pain over the dorsoradial aspect of the hand

Wartenberg's syndrome is compression of the superficial radial nerve as it emerges from beneath brachioradialis, resulting in pain and paresthesia to the dorsoradial aspect of the hand and wrist. On examination, there will usually be a positive Tinel's sign over the superficial radial nerve proximal to the radial styloid. Differential diagnoses include intersection syndrome, which is tenosynovitis caused by friction between the tendons of the first and second extensor compartments (APL and EPB over ECRL and ECRB). Initial treatment includes splinting, activity modification, and steroid injections. These modalities may be sufficient for most patients. Some patients may go on to benefit from surgical release of the surrounding fascia. Motor function of the index and thumb will be preserved in Wartenberg's syndrome.[1] In contrast, this function will be reduced in PIN compression. The PIN is primarily a motor nerve to the extensor compartment of the forearm with no cutaneous sensory supply. However, patients may complain of unpleasant sensations or pain in the forearm or wrist due to the nociceptive and proprioceptive roles of the PIN. Sensation will be preserved over the fifth MCP joint dorsally in either condition, as this is ulnar nerve territory. The inability to adduct the little finger is called Wartenberg's sign and is due to ulnar nerve palsy with intrinsic muscle weakness, which leaves the slightly abducting line of pull of the EDM tendon unopposed.

REFERENCE

1. Lanzetta M, Foucher G. Entrapment of the superficial branch of the radial nerve (Wartenberg's syndrome). A report of 52 cases. Int Orthop 1993;17(6):342–345

ULNAR NERVE COMPRESSION AT THE ELBOW

12. When exploring a compressed ulnar nerve at the elbow, which one of the following is least likely to be a site of compression?

E. The vascular leash of Henry

The vascular leash of Henry is formed by the radial recurrent artery in the antecubital fossa and is a potential site of radial rather than ulnar nerve compression. The other sites are all potential places for the ulnar nerve to be compressed during its course in the arm. The five potential sites of compression affecting the ulnar nerve at the elbow are, from proximal to distal:

1. Medial intermuscular septum
2. Arcade of Struthers
3. Ligament of Osbourne
4. Proximal fascia between the two heads of FCU
5. Fascial bands within the FCU tunnel

Preoperatively, to justify this exploration, the patient would be expected to have symptoms and signs of ulnar nerve compression that are not responding to nonoperative care, usually supported by NCS/EMG findings. Symptoms and signs include ulnar-side forearm tingling and pain extending to the ulnar half of the ring finger, the entire little finger, and the ulnar dorsal half of the hand. This may be associated with weakness +/– atrophy of the ulnar forearm and finger flexors and the hand intrinsics.[1]

REFERENCE

1. Eversmann WW Jr. Compression and entrapment neuropathies of the upper extremity. J Hand Surg Am 1983;8(5, Pt 2):759–766

MANAGEMENT OF CUBITAL TUNNEL SYNDROME

13. Which one of the following is correct regarding the management of cubital tunnel syndrome?

B. Submuscular nerve transposition is usually reserved for recurrent cases.

The results of ulnar nerve decompression at the elbow are less predictable than those following median nerve decompression at the wrist. There is considerable debate regarding the optimal surgical intervention,[1] with many preferring to perform a simple in situ decompression in the first instance and reserve transposition procedures for recurrent cases. Others are strongly in favor of medial epicondylectomy as the primary surgical procedure. Where epicondylectomy is preferred, a partial bony resection is undertaken, rather than complete resection of the epicondyle, to reduce the risk of valgus instability of the elbow following surgery. In recurrent cases, submuscular nerve transposition may be indicated[2,3]; however, this is not common, and many surgeons prefer a subcutaneous transposition[4] if the nerve is to be relocated. An intramuscular pocket is also described. Submuscular transposition is more complex to perform than a subcutaneous pocket and has a much longer recovery period while the divided flexor-pronator mass heals. Both transposition procedures require great care to ensure that new areas of tension and compression along the nerve are avoided throughout the range of elbow motion, e.g., by resection of components of the intermuscular septum and FCU fascia.

Although some patients find splinting of the elbow helpful, this prevents elbow flexion and interferes with activities and is therefore used only at night and generally less well tolerated than splinting in carpal tunnel syndrome. In severe ulnar nerve compression, splinting has not been shown to be beneficial, and surgery should not be delayed by a trial of conservative therapy.

REFERENCES

1. Boone S, Gelberman RH, Calfee RP. The management of cubital tunnel syndrome. J Hand Surg Am 2015;40(9):1897–1904, quiz 1904
2. Learmonth JR. A technique for transplanting the ulnar nerve. Surg Gynecol Obstet 1942;75:792
3. Amadio PC, Beckenbaugh RD. Entrapment of the ulnar nerve by the deep flexor-pronator aponeurosis. J Hand Surg Am 1986;11(1):83–87
4. Harrison MJ, Nurick S. Results of anterior transposition of the ulnar nerve for ulnar neuritis. BMJ 1970;1(5687):27–29

ULNAR NERVE COMPRESSION IN GUYON'S CANAL

14. *Which one of the following is correct regarding ulnar nerve compression in Guyon's canal?*

C. The underlying cause may be an aneurysm of the ulnar artery.

One of the recognized causes of ulnar nerve compression in Guyon's canal is an aneurysm of the ulnar artery, as can occur in occupations such as carpentry as a result of repetitive motion (hypothenar hammer syndrome). However, there are many potential causes, including a ganglion, lipoma, fracture of the hook of hamate, and synovial inflammation. Thus, plain radiographs, ultrasound with or without Doppler imaging, and even CT/MRI can be important to determine the specific cause before surgery, as the management may involve more than a simple decompression. If there is an aneurysm, the involved segment of the artery will be resected and replaced with a vein graft; so, the patient must be warned about a donor-site scar and the possibility of ischemic complications.

Guyon's canal can be superficially decompressed at the same time as a carpal tunnel release through the same incision. Alternatively, a more ulnar incision can be used in order to more easily access and release the deep motor branch. A standard carpal tunnel release can alter the shape of Guyon's canal and reduce ulnar nerve compression without any direct dissection.[1,2]

Ulnar nerve compression in Guyon's canal may present with mixed or isolated motor or sensory signs due to the branching pattern of the nerve at this site (**Fig. 92.1**). In zone I, the ulnar nerve has not yet bifurcated and there will be motor and sensory disturbance. In zone II, the deep motor branch is affected in isolation. In zone

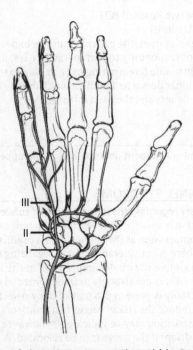

Fig. 92.1   Zones of ulnar nerve compression within Guyon's canal.

III, only the superficial sensory branch to the hypothenar skin and ulnar one and a half digits are affected. Zone III compression is the least common.

REFERENCES

1. Ginanneschi F, Filippou G, Reale F, Scarselli C, Galeazzi M, Rossi A. Ultrasonographic and functional changes of the ulnar nerve at Guyon's canal after carpal tunnel release. Clin Neurophysiol 2010;121(2):208–213
2. König PS, Hage JJ, Bloem JJ, Prosé LP. Variations of the ulnar nerve and ulnar artery in Guyon's canal: a cadaveric study. J Hand Surg Am 1994;19(4):617–622

UPPER LIMB COMPRESSION SYNDROMES

15. An elderly patient complains that his little finger sticks out all the time and his grip on his walking stick is weak. *What is the most likely diagnosis?*

B. Cubital tunnel syndrome

In this scenario, the patient is exhibiting Wartenberg's sign, which has nothing to do with Wartenberg's syndrome. Wartenberg's sign is abduction of the little finger caused by intrinsic muscle weakness that leaves the abducting force of the EDM unopposed. The weak grip is also in keeping with ulnar nerve palsy, the most common cause of which would be cubital tunnel syndrome.

Radial tunnel syndrome would present with pain during movement at the elbow secondary to radial nerve compression in the proximal forearm. Pronator syndrome results in proximal forearm pain with paresthesia over pronator teres, extending distally onto the thenar eminence and radial digits. It is caused by median nerve compression in the forearm. Ulnar tunnel syndrome refers to ulnar nerve compression within Guyon's canal at the wrist/hand. Patients present with ulnar sensory and/or motor deficits in the hand. Wartenberg's syndrome is compression of the superficial radial nerve in the proximal forearm. This leads to pain and numbness to the dorsal radial aspect of the distal forearm and hand.[1,2]

REFERENCES

1. Eversmann WW Jr. Compression and entrapment neuropathies of the upper extremity. J Hand Surg Am 1983;8(5, Pt 2): 759–766
2. O'Driscoll SW, Horii E, Carmichael SW, Morrey BF. The cubital tunnel and ulnar neuropathy. J Bone Joint Surg Br 1991;73(4):613–617

93. Brachial Plexus

See *Essentials of Plastic Surgery*, third edition, pp. 1287–1302

BRACHIAL PLEXUS ANATOMY

1. *Which one of the following statements is correct?*
   A. The roots of the brachial plexus are C5–T1 and are found between the middle and posterior scalene muscles.
   B. The three trunks are upper, middle, and lower and are found in the anterior triangle of the neck.
   C. The cords are named according to their position in relation to the axillary vein (lateral, posterior, and medial).
   D. The lateral cord contains contributions from C5, C6, and C7 and is the only cord forming the musculocutaneous/myocutaneous nerve.
   E. The medial cord contains contributions from C7, C8, and T1 and is the only cord forming the median nerve.

PERIPHERAL NERVE BRANCHES FROM THE BRACHIAL PLEXUS

2. *When exploring the brachial plexus, which of the following branches should arise at or near the Erb point?*
   A. Suprascapular
   B. Long thoracic
   C. Dorsal scapular
   D. Upper subscapular
   E. Lower subscapular

PERIPHERAL NERVE BRANCHES FROM THE BRACHIAL PLEXUS

3. *Which one of the following clinical findings suggests a root avulsion injury?*
   A. Deltoid wasting
   B. Trapezius wasting
   C. Exophthalmos
   D. Scapular winging
   E. Pectoralis major wasting

ERB'S POINT

4. *Which one of the following is most suggestive of a brachial plexus injury at Erb's point?*
   A. Weakness of the small muscles of the hand
   B. Horner's syndrome in association with upper limb weakness
   C. Loss of elbow and wrist extension
   D. Loss of elbow flexion and shoulder external rotation
   E. Arm weakness following forced elevation with traction

THE MEDIAL CORD OF THE BRACHIAL PLEXUS

5. *Which one of the following movements most specifically tests medial cord function?*
   A. Elbow flexion
   B. Wrist flexion
   C. Little finger abduction
   D. Thumb abduction
   E. Forearm pronation

NERVE ROOT INJURIES IN THE BRACHIAL PLEXUS

6. *Which one of the following statements is correct regarding nerve root injuries?*
   A. A root avulsion is a postganglionic injury.
   B. Intact paracervical muscles suggest a preganglionic injury.
   C. A C5–C6 avulsion will result in Horner's syndrome.
   D. It is easier to repair a preganglionic than postganglionic injury.
   E. Wallerian degeneration does not occur in a preganglionic injury.

BRACHIAL PLEXUS BIRTH PALSY

7. *Which one of the following statements is correct regarding brachial plexus birth injury?*
   A. The incidence in the developed world is 1 per 100,000 term births.
   B. Most cases present with isolated C8–T1 injuries (Klumpke's palsy).
   C. Shoulder dystocia is one of the most common risk factors.
   D. Spontaneous recovery is rare following these injuries.
   E. Exploration is recommended if no biceps function is observed by 1 month.

MANAGING THE SHOULDER IN BRACHIAL PLEXUS BIRTH INJURIES

8. *Which one of the following is correct when managing the shoulder in brachial plexus birth injuries?*
   A. Botulinum toxin injections to rotator cuff contractures may be useful.
   B. Plain radiographs are important to monitor deformity of the glenohumeral joint.
   C. Spinal accessory to suprascapular nerve transfer is contraindicated.
   D. The Waters classification relates to the degree of plexus injury.
   E. Shoulder capsular release should be avoided in obstetric brachial plexus injury.

TREATMENT OPTIONS IN OBSTETRIC BRACHIAL PLEXUS INJURY

9. An otherwise healthy newborn baby is brought to your clinic with the classic signs of upper trunk Erb-Duchenne palsy. The parents want an early intervention with the best possible outcome. *Which of the following is the most appropriate initial management plan?*
   A. Physiotherapy and observation with follow-up by the age of 6 months
   B. Physiotherapy and observation with follow-up by the age of 3 months
   C. Exploration and sural nerve grafting within 6 weeks
   D. Exploration and nerve transfers within 6 weeks
   E. MRI and nerve conduction studies within 6 weeks

TRAUMATIC BRACHIAL PLEXUS INJURY

10. *Which one of the following statements is correct when considering injury mechanisms in brachial plexus?*
   A. Traumatic injuries are most often caused by deep lacerations or crush injuries.
   B. Open injuries, while less common, are often associated with vascular injury.
   C. A violent shoulder abduction beyond 90 degrees is likely to injure C5–C7.
   D. Violent shoulder depression causes isolated FCU and hand intrinsic weakness.
   E. Immediate repair of open injuries is contraindicated due to risk of infection.

ASSESSING BRACHIAL PLEXUS INJURIES

11. *When examining a patient with a suspected brachial plexus injury, which one of the following is correct?*
   A. Weak digital flexion and extension suggests a T1 nerve root lesion.
   B. Weak rhomboids and serratus anterior suggest an injury at Erb's point.
   C. Pectoralis major contraction assesses both the posterior and lateral cords.
   D. Root injury is more likely with shoulder dislocation than cord/branch injury.
   E. Paralysis of the latissimus dorsi would indicate a posterior cord injury.

GRADING MUSCLE POWER WHEN ASSESSING THE BRACHIAL PLEXUS

12. A patient with a C5/C6 injury is able to flex the elbow in the horizontal plane when resting on a table but is unable to elevate his forearm off the table against gravity. *What is the Medical Research Council (MRC) grade for the biceps in this patient?*
   A. 1   D. 4
   B. 2   E. 5
   C. 3

ELECTROPHYSIOLOGIC TESTING IN BRACHIAL PLEXUS INJURY

13. *When planning electrophysiological testing for a patient with a brachial plexus injury, which one of the following statements is correct?*
   A. Intraoperative nerve testing offers no additional benefit to direct visualization and palpation of the nerves.
   B. Somatosensory evoked potentials are detected through the digits and help rule out preganglionic injury.
   C. Motor evoked potentials are detected through the paraspinous muscles and help to rule out postganglionic injury.
   D. EMG is useful within the first 2 weeks to give a baseline assessment of function.
   E. Intact SNAPs and normal peripheral sensory conduction velocity with paralyzed muscles implies a preganglionic injury.

PRIORITIES FOR RECONSTRUCTION IN BRACHIAL PLEXUS INJURY

14. *When managing a patient with a brachial plexus injury, which one of the following is usually the first priority?*
   A. Shoulder abduction   D. Wrist extension
   B. Wrist flexion   E. Finger flexion
   C. Elbow flexion

SURGICAL INTERVENTION IN BRACHIAL PLEXUS INJURY

15. A 27-year-old man presents with no recovery evident either clinically or on nerve conduction studies (NCS)/EMG studies 6 months after a C5–C7 injury. Root avulsions are demonstrated on MRI. *How could you best restore elbow flexion?*
    A. Sural nerve grafting from the C5 nerve root to the anterior division of C5/C6
    B. Sural nerve grafting from the C8 nerve root to the musculocutaneous nerve
    C. Ulnar nerve fascicle to musculocutaneous branch nerve transfer
    D. Intercostal nerve to musculocutaneous nerve transfer
    E. Free functional gracilis muscle flap coapted to an ulnar nerve fascicle

MANAGEMENT OF BRACHIAL PLEXUS INJURIES

16. A 60-year-old woman presents 10 years after a complete brachial plexus injury from a horse-riding accident. She is well known to the pain team and is struggling with her shoulder brace and a dragging sensation from her paralyzed arm. She has good scapulothoracic control. *Which of the following is most likely to improve her symptoms?*
    A. Insertion of a spinal cord stimulator
    B. Neurotization
    C. Shoulder fusion
    D. Insertion of a plexus catheter for local anesthetic infusion
    E. Below-elbow amputation

NERVE TRANSFERS FOR SHOULDER FUNCTION

17. *Which one of the following is the preferred nerve transfer for restoring shoulder stability in brachial plexus palsy?*
    A. Spinal accessory nerve onto suprascapular nerve
    B. Intercostal nerves onto suprascapular nerve
    C. Thoracodorsal nerve onto axillary nerve
    D. Medial pectoral nerve onto axillary nerve
    E. Thoracodorsal nerve onto long thoracic nerve

Answers

BRACHIAL PLEXUS ANATOMY

1. *Which one of the following statements is correct?*
   D. The lateral cord contains contributions from C5, C6, and C7 and is the only cord forming the musculocutaneous/myocutaneous nerve.

   The musculocutaneous nerve is also known as the myocutaneous nerve and supplies the biceps, coracobrachialis, and brachialis muscles. It also supplies sensation to the upper limb through the lateral cutaneous nerves of the arm and forearm, respectively.

   The brachial plexus comprises roots, trunks, divisions, cords, and terminal branches, and typically arises from C5–T1, but may be supplemented by significant contributions from C4 or T2 nerve roots. The roots pass between the anterior and middle scalene muscles (not the middle and posterior) and split into trunks as follows: C5–C6 becomes the upper trunk, C7 the middle trunk, and C8–T1 the lower trunk. The three trunks lie in the posterior (not anterior) triangle of the neck and each splits into anterior and posterior divisions. The upper (C5, C6) and middle (C7) trunk anterior divisions form the lateral cord, while the lower trunk (C8, T1) anterior division forms the medial cord. All three posterior divisions combine to form the posterior cord. The cords are named in relation to the axillary artery, not the vein. The lateral and medical cords subsequently rejoin to form the median nerve. The medial cord is formed by the C8 and T1 roots only, and although it is a significant contributor to the median nerve, the median nerve also receives a major contribution from the lateral cord (C5–C7) (**Fig. 93.1**).[1–3]

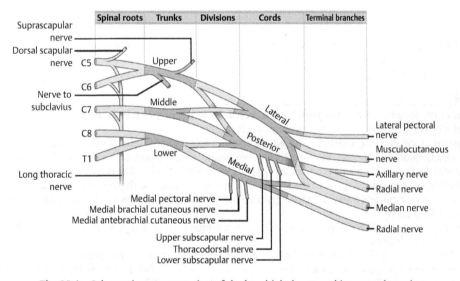

Fig. 93.1 Schematic representation of the brachial plexus and its nerve branches

REFERENCES

1. Moore KL, Dalley AF, eds. Clinically Oriented Anatomy. 4th ed. New York, NY: Lippincott Williams & Wilkins; 1999
2. ASSH Manual of Hand Surgery. Philadelphia: Lippincott Williams & Wilkins; 2010
3. Tung THH, Moore A. Brachial plexus injuries. In: Mackinnon S. Nerve Surgery. New York: Thieme; 2015

PERIPHERAL NERVE BRANCHES FROM THE BRACHIAL PLEXUS

2. *When exploring the brachial plexus, which of the following branches should arise at or near the Erb point?*
   A. Suprascapular

   Knowledge of the branches of the brachial plexus is important, particularly during surgical exploration. The suprascapular nerve supplies the supraspinatus and infraspinatus muscles and is a key target for reinnervation procedures. Erb's point is the confluence of the C5 and C6 nerve roots as the upper trunk. The suprascapular nerve usually arises in this zone. During surgical reconstruction, the suprascapular nerve is prioritized as a recipient for C5 grafting or for a spinal accessory nerve transfer in order to restore shoulder stability along with initiation of abduction and external rotation. There is one other nerve arising from the trunks: the nerve to subclavius, which innervate the subclavius muscles.

There are two nerves arising from the roots. These are the long thoracic and dorsal scapular nerves, which innervate the serratus anterior and rhomboids/levator scapulae, respectively. There are no nerve branches that arise directly from the divisions of the brachial plexus (see **Fig. 93.1**).[1–3]

REFERENCES

1. Moore KL, Dalley AF, eds. Clinically Oriented Anatomy. 4th ed. New York, NY: Lippincott Williams & Wilkins; 1999
2. Russell S, ed. Examination of Peripheral Nerve Injuries: An Anatomical Approach. 2nd ed. Thieme; 2015
3. Spinner RJ, Shin AY, Hebert-Blouin M, et al. Green's Operative Hand Surgery. 6th ed. Philadelphia: Elsevier; 2010

PERIPHERAL NERVE BRANCHES FROM THE BRACHIAL PLEXUS

3. *Which one of the following clinical findings suggests a root avulsion injury?*

D. Scapular winging

Scapular winging occurs most commonly with serratus anterior weakness, and occasionally with trapezius or rhomboid palsy. Serratus anterior is supplied by the long thoracic nerve which arises from the C5, C6, and C7 nerve roots. Therefore, serratus weakness is suggestive of a very proximal root level injury. Other signs of a root avulsion include rhomboid paralysis, paraspinal muscle paralysis, phrenic palsy, and Horner's syndrome (miosis, ptosis, and anhidrosis). Horner's syndrome is due to disruption of the sympathetic chain and can also result in a degree of apparent enophthalmus. Deltoid is supplied by the axillary nerve from the posterior cord. Trapezius is supplied by the spinal accessory nerve and is not a part of the brachial plexus territory. Pectoralis major is supplied by the medial and lateral pectoral nerves which are branches of the medial and lateral cords.[1–3]

REFERENCES

1. Gooding BW, Geoghegan JM, Wallace WA, Manning PA. Scapular winging. Shoulder Elbow 2014;6(1):4–11
2. Moore KL, Dalley AF, eds. Clinically Oriented Anatomy. 4th ed. New York, NY: Lippincott Williams & Wilkins; 1999
3. ASSH Manual of Hand Surgery. Philadelphia: Lippincott Williams & Wilkins; 2010

ERB'S POINT

4. *Which one of the following is most suggestive of a brachial plexus injury at Erb's point?*

D. Loss of elbow fixation and shoulder external rotation

Erb's point represents the anatomic site where the C5 and C6 nerve roots converge to form the upper trunk and is also the point where the suprascapular nerve usually arises. Injury at this level typically produces loss of shoulder abduction and external rotation, along with loss of elbow flexion. The classic appearance of an Erb's palsy reflects this, i.e., the arm hangs with the shoulder internally rotated and the elbow extended. This is sometimes termed a "waiter's tip deformity" and may also include more prominent loss of wrist extension when there is an associated C7 injury.

The upper trunk C5/C6 +/–C7 pattern of injury is a common pattern of injury and occurs in both obstetric and adult traumatic plexus patients.

Weakness of the small muscles of the hand and upper eyelid ptosis with constriction of the pupil is a feature of lower nerve root injury with damage to the stellate ganglion (C8–T1). This pattern of injury is more typical of the scenario in option E. Elbow and wrist extensions are predominantly C7 or radial nerve functions.[1–3]

REFERENCES

1. Mackinnon SEDA. Surgery of the Peripheral Nerve. New York: Thieme; 1988
2. Terzis JK, Kostopoulos VK. The surgical treatment of brachial plexus injuries in adults. Plast Reconstr Surg 2007;119(4):73e–92e
3. Tung THH, Moore A. Brachial plexus injuries. In: Mackinnon S. Nerve Surgery. New York: Thieme; 2015

THE MEDIAL CORD OF THE BRACHIAL PLEXUS

5. *Which one of the following movements most specifically tests medial cord function?*

C. Little finger abduction

The medial cord contributes to the median nerve along with the lateral cord, but it is the only cord contributing to the ulnar nerve; therefore, assessing movement in an ulnar innervated muscle such as the abductor digiti minimi will test the medial cord most reliably. Elbow flexion is provided predominantly by the biceps and brachialis, with initiation assisted by brachioradialis. These muscles are innervated by the musculocutaneous and radial nerves, respectively. Therefore, there is lateral and posterior cord involvement with this action. Wrist flexion is provided by the flexor carpi ulnaris (FCU) and the flexor carpi radialis (FCR) which are innervated by the median and ulnar nerves, respectively. It will therefore not usually discriminate between the medial and lateral cords. Thumb abduction is median nerve innervated through the abductor pollicis brevis, as is forearm pronation, which is provided by the pronator teres and pronator quadratus.[1–3]

REFERENCES

1. Brunelli GA, Brunelli GR. Preoperative assessment of the adult plexus patient. Microsurgery 1995;16(1):17–21
2. Tung THH, Moore A. Brachial plexus injuries. In: Mackinnon S. Nerve Surgery. New York: Thieme; 2015
3. Moore KL, Dalley AF, eds. Clinically Oriented Anatomy. 4th ed. New York, NY: Lippincott Williams & Wilkins; 1999

NERVE ROOT INJURIES IN THE BRACHIAL PLEXUS

6. *Which one of the following statements is correct regarding nerve root injuries?*

   E. Wallerian degeneration does not occur in a preganglionic injury.

   In a root avulsion, there is a preganglionic injury where the cell bodies in the dorsal root ganglia are still in continuity with the axons; therefore, there is no Wallerian degeneration. This is why somatosensory evoked potentials are preserved and a NCS/electromyography (EMG) report may state that sensory nerve action potentials (SNAPs) are preserved despite a severe sensory deficit clinically; the EMG component would demonstrate severe abnormalities in the affected nerve root territory. Root avulsions are preganglionic injuries and may be accompanied by signs of proximal injury such as paracervical muscle paralysis or Horner's syndrome (C8 or T1 avulsion affecting the sympathetic supply). Preganglionic injuries are not amenable to direct repair or grafting.[1,2]

REFERENCES

1. Giuffre JL, Kakar S, Bishop AT, Spinner RJ, Shin AY. Current concepts of the treatment of adult brachial plexus injuries. J Hand Surg Am 2010;35(4):678–688, quiz 688
2. Alnot JY. Traumatic brachial plexus lesions in the adult. Indications and results. Hand Clin 1995;11(4):623–631

BRACHIAL PLEXUS BIRTH PALSY

7. *Which one of the following statements is correct regarding brachial plexus birth injury?*

   C. Shoulder dystocia is one of the most common risk factors.

   The U.S. incidence of obstetric brachial plexus injury is reported as between 1 and 1.5 per 1,000 live births depending on source reviewed, and the most common presentation is Erb-Duchenne palsy with C5–C6 upper root/trunk pathology. The mechanism of injury is commonly shoulder dystocia, in which the fetus becomes stuck by one shoulder at the pelvic inlet and the advancing head and neck are forced into lateral flexion away from this shoulder. Other common associations include breech birth, forceps delivery, and vacuum extraction. Gestational diabetes and macrosomia are also risk factors. Spontaneous recovery is common, and in some studies 50% have achieved a full recovery by 6 months with the remainder making a partial recovery. Exploration should be considered after 3 months if biceps and deltoid function are still absent.[1–4]

REFERENCES

1. Waters PM. Pediatric brachial plexus palsy. In: Wolfe SW, Hotchkiss RN, Pederson WC, et al, eds. Green's Operative Hand Surgery. 6th ed. Philadelphia: Elsevier; 2010
2. Shenaq SM, Kim JY, Armenta AH, Nath RK, Cheng E, Jedrysiak A. The surgical treatment of obstetric brachial plexus palsy. Plast Reconstr Surg 2004;113(4):54E–67E
3. Hale HB, Bae DS, Waters PM. Current concepts in the management of brachial plexus birth palsy. J Hand Surg Am 2010;35(2):322–331
4. ASSH Manual of Hand Surgery. Philadelphia: Lippincott Williams & Wilkins; 2010

MANAGING THE SHOULDER IN BRACHIAL PLEXUS BIRTH INJURIES

8. *Which one of the following is correct when managing the shoulder in brachial plexus birth injuries?*

   A. Botulinum toxin injections to rotator cuff contractures may be useful.

   Infants with brachial plexus injury may develop shoulder weakness, contracture, or joint deformity. Internal rotation contractures are common and caused by weakness of the infraspinatus and teres minor muscles leading to unopposed internal rotation forces from subscapularis and others. Treatment options for the shoulder include physiotherapy, splinting, contracture release, and muscle rebalancing through transfers, such as combined latissimus dorsi and teres major transfer. Rarely, formal joint reduction may be required for dislocation.[1]

Botulinum toxin injections are commonly used to treat a range of pediatric spasticity problems, and these are thought by some surgeons to be helpful as part of the management of rotator cuff contractures. Daily physiotherapy should be undertaken by parents to prevent shoulder contractures developing in the first place and to avoid secondary deformity of the growing glenoid fossa and humeral head. They are given as a standard component of treatment in nonsurgical and surgical care of these patients but are particularly important to maintain the benefits following tendon lengthening/transfer procedures or capsular release.

Brachial plexus birth palsy patients usually also have a degree of glenohumeral joint dysplasia, and this is assessed using the Waters classification, which grades the degree of abnormality at this joint.[2] Plain radiographs are not particularly helpful in young children, because there is a predominantly cartilaginous component to the immature glenohumeral joint that is better assessed by a skilled ultrasonographer or MRI/CT.[1]

If the trapezius, the rhomboids, and the serratus anterior are functioning, there can be good movement of the scapula, which can allow some compensation for poor shoulder movement. Subscapularis lengthening and greenstick fracture of the coronoid process can sometimes be helpful in the management of a severe internal rotation joint contracture in obstetric brachial plexus palsy. This may be in combination with a limited capsular release; however, care must be taken not to destabilize the glenohumeral joint. Following release, a tendon transfer may be required for active external rotation to maintain the correction, such as combined latissimus dorsi and teres major transfer.

The spinal accessory nerve is a common, useful donor for nerve transfer in both adults and children for shoulder reanimation, often in combination with triceps to axillary nerve transfer, and is usually used in the presence of nerve root avulsions.[3]

REFERENCES

1. Pearl ML. Shoulder problems in children with brachial plexus birth palsy: evaluation and management. J Am Acad Orthop Surg 2009;17(4):242–254
2. Waters PM. Pediatric brachial plexus palsy. In: Wolfe SW, Hotchkiss RN, Pederson WC, et al, eds. Green's Operative Hand Surgery. 6th ed. Philadelphia: Elsevier; 2010
3. Hale HB, Bae DS, Waters PM. Current concepts in the management of brachial plexus birth palsy. J Hand Surg Am 2010;35(2):322–331

TREATMENT OPTIONS IN OBSTETRIC BRACHIAL PLEXUS INJURY

9. An otherwise healthy newborn baby is brought to your clinic with the classic signs of upper trunk Erb-Duchenne palsy. The parents want an early intervention with the best possible outcome. *Which of the following is the most appropriate initial management plan?*

B. Physiotherapy and observation with follow-up by the age of 3 months

An Erb-Duchenne palsy is an upper trunk C5/C6 lesion characterized by loss of shoulder movement and elbow flexion with or without loss of wrist extension (C7 involvement). Pediatric patients with brachial plexus injuries generally recover better function than adults within both nonoperative and operatively managed groups. This is thought to be due to greater potential for recovery in infants, shorter limbs, and greater brain plasticity.[1]

In this scenario, it is appropriate to start with observation, since most obstetric brachial plexus palsies will improve without surgery. Active range of movement scores at 3 months can serve as a useful predictor of which patients might benefit from surgery. Initial management involves gentle range of movement exercises and stretching by the parents under the guidance of a physiotherapist. Particular attention is directed to shoulder external rotation, as internal rotation contractures are common as a result of subscapularis overpowering the weaker or paralyzed external rotators (infraspinatus, teres minor). If deltoid (shoulder abduction) and biceps (elbow flexion) are not recovering by 3 months, then surgery is usually recommended. If there has been a progressive partial recovery, then further observation may be chosen at regular appointments up to 6 months. If satisfactory progress is still not evident by 6 months, such as at least antigravity power in shoulder abduction and elbow flexion, then surgery is again usually recommended.[1,2]

REFERENCES

1. Tse R, Kozin SH, Malessy MJ, Clarke HM. International Federation of Societies for Surgery of the Hand Committee report: the role of nerve transfers in the treatment of neonatal brachial plexus palsy. J Hand Surg Am 2015;40(6):1246–1259
2. Cornwall R, Waters PM. Pediatric brachial plexus palsy. In: Wolfe SW, Pederson WC, Kozin SH. eds. Green's Operative Hand Surgery. 6th ed. Philadelphia: Elsevier; 2010

TRAUMATIC BRACHIAL PLEXUS INJURY

10. Which one of the following statements is correct when considering injury mechanisms in brachial plexus?

B. Open injuries, while less common, are often associated with vascular injury.

Brachial plexus injuries are most commonly closed injuries resulting from excessive traction or compression, but open injuries such as gunshot or stab wounds do occur. Although less common, open injuries are the strongest indication for immediate exploration and repair. The likelihood of an associated vessel injury is high, particularly with sharp penetrating wounds. These wounds should be formally explored, with assessment and repair or tagging of the plexus and other key structures where appropriate. Only in heavily contaminated or infected wounds or gunshot injuries is delayed repair usually indicated. The argument for delayed repair of the plexus after debridement of gunshot injuries is that there is often a complex multilevel injury with profound tissue edema in an extensive zone of injury; therefore, a delay allows edema and neuropraxia to settle and for multiple sites of nerve injury to appear more obvious on inspection and intraoperative neurophysiological testing.

Violent shoulder abduction is most likely to cause a lower (C8, T1) or complete plexus injury than an isolated C5–67 injury. Violent downward shoulder traction will tend to cause an upper plexus injury and would usually spare the FCU and intrinsic muscle innervation unless a pan-plexus injury occurs.[1,2]

REFERENCES

1. Giuffre JL, Kakar S, Bishop AT, Spinner RJ, Shin AY. Current concepts of the treatment of adult brachial plexus injuries. J Hand Surg Am 2010;35(4):678–688, quiz 688
2. Alnot JY. Traumatic brachial plexus lesions in the adult. Indications and results. Hand Clin 1995;11(4):623–631

ASSESSING BRACHIAL PLEXUS INJURIES

11. When examining a patient with a suspected brachial plexus injury, which one of the following is correct?

E. Paralysis of the latissimus dorsi would indicate a posterior cord injury.

The latissimus dorsi is supplied by the posterior cord, along with the deltoid, subscapularis, teres major, and all the muscles innervated by the radial nerve. A T1 lesion will usually produce weak intrinsic muscle function in the hand and a sensory deficit affecting the medial forearm. Digital flexion and extension is usually affected if C8 is also injured. In practice, C8/T1 deficits usually occur together in trauma.

The rhomboid muscles are supplied by the dorsal scapular nerve, which arises early from the C5 nerve root prior to formation of the upper trunk. The nerve to serratus anterior (long thoracic nerve of Bell) arises from the C5–C7 nerve roots. Paralysis of these muscles is indicative of a root-level injury, because they would be preserved if the injury occurred at trunk level or distally.

The pectoralis major is supplied by the medial and lateral pectoral nerves, from the medial and lateral cords of the plexus, respectively, and not by the posterior cord. A shoulder dislocation presenting with neurologic disturbance is usually associated with injuries to the cords or terminal branches.[1,2]

REFERENCES

1. Shin AY, Spinner RJ, Steinmann SP, Bishop AT. Adult traumatic brachial plexus injuries. J Am Acad Orthop Surg 2005;13(6):382–396
2. Fox IK, Mackinnon SE. Adult peripheral nerve disorders: nerve entrapment, repair, transfer, and brachial plexus disorders. Plast Reconstr Surg 2011;127(5):105e–118e

GRADING MUSCLE POWER WHEN ASSESSING THE BRACHIAL PLEXUS

12. A patient with a C5/C6 injury is able to flex the elbow in the horizontal plane when resting on a table but is unable to elevate his forearm off the table against gravity. *What is the Medical Research Council (MRC) grade for the biceps in this patient?*

B. 2

The British Medical Research Council (MRC) grade has five categories (**Table 93.1**). Because this patient is unable to flex the arm against gravity, it is an MRC power grading of 2. This is one of the important classification systems to remember, especially with respect to brachial plexus assessment as it is used internationally. The MRC grade is used to document changes in function following injury and treatment.[1–3]

Although this is the most commonly accepted international classification, there are some others which may be useful. Birch et al[4] presented a further MRC grading system for assessing a particular nerve territory, derived from Highet, that includes categories from M0 to M5. M0 is no contraction, M1 is visible contraction in proximal muscles, M2 is visible contraction in proximal and distal muscles, M3 includes all important muscles and both proximally and distally contract against resistance, M4 is return of function such that synergistic and independent movements are possible, and M5 is complete recovery. Kline and Hudson then titled this system "grading of the entire nerve" and added a sixth category to make it run from M0 to M6.[5]

Table 93.1   *British Medical Research Council Grading System*

Grade	Degree of Strength
1	Muscle contracts, but part does not move
2	Movement with gravity eliminated
3	Movement through full range of motion against gravity
4	Movement through full range of motion against resistance
5	Normal strength

REFERENCES

1. Mackinnon SE, Dellon AL. Surgery of the Peripheral Nerve. New York: Thieme Medical; 1988
2. Fox IK, Mackinnon SE. Adult peripheral nerve disorders: nerve entrapment, repair, transfer, and brachial plexus disorders. Plast Reconstr Surg 2011;127(5):105e–118e
3. Novak CB. Evaluation of the patient with nerve injury or nerve compression. In: Mackinnon S. Nerve Surgery. New York: Thieme; 2015
4. Birch R, Bonney G, Wynn Parry CB. Surgical disorders of the peripheral nerves. London, England. Churchill Livingstone; 1998
5. Kline DG, Hudson AR. Nerve Injuries: Operative Results for Major Nerve Injuries, Entrapments and Tumors. Philadelphia, PA: WB Saunders; 1995

ELECTROPHYSIOLOGIC TESTING IN BRACHIAL PLEXUS INJURY

13. *When planning electrophysiological testing for a patient with a brachial plexus injury, which one of the following statements is correct?*

   E. Intact SNAPs and normal peripheral sensory conduction velocity with paralyzed muscles implies a preganglionic injury.

   Because the cell bodies of the sensory neurons lie within the dorsal root ganglion, a root avulsion (i.e., preganglionic injury) means that the cell body is still in continuity with the axon and therefore there will not be any Wallerian degeneration. During electrophysiological testing, there will therefore be intact sensory nerve action potentials and normal conduction speeds along the peripheral sensory components. This will be accompanied by profound motor abnormalities and clinical sensory deficits.

   Different forms of intraoperative nerve testing can be a useful adjunct to inspection and palpation of the plexus when it can be difficult to come to an accurate diagnosis; for example, in recovering injuries, assessing a neuroma in continuity, and in distinguishing preganglionic from postganglionic injuries. Somatosensory and motor evoked potentials (SSEP and MEPs) can be used intraoperatively to distinguish preganglionic and postganglionic injury. Both SSEP and MEP are detected through the contralateral scalp and their presence rules out preganglionic injury. Not many surgeons use SSEP and MEP tests, but most would use a nerve stimulator in combination with clinical inspection of a nerve and palpation for "empty" or "hard" segments. A nerve stimulator is also helpful in assessing potential donor nerves for transfer, such as the phrenic and spinal accessory nerves. The muscular changes associated with acute denervation take a few weeks to develop; therefore, 3 to 6 weeks is usually allowed before initial EMG testing. A 3-week interval is a sufficient time for most Wallerian degeneration to occur and to demonstrate muscle denervation changes, whereas waiting until 6 to 8 weeks can give the opportunity for early signs of reinnervation to be identified.[1,2]

REFERENCES

1. Ferrante MA, Wilbourn AJ. The electrodiagnostic examination with peripheral nerve injuries. In: Mackinnon S. Nerve Surgery. New York: Thieme; 2015
2. Brunelli GA, Brunelli GR. Preoperative assessment of the adult plexus patient. Microsurgery 1995;16(1):17–21

PRIORITIES FOR RECONSTRUCTION IN BRACHIAL PLEXUS INJURY

14. *When managing a patient with a brachial plexus injury, which one of the following is usually the first priority?*

   C. Elbow flexion

   The first priority in managing a patient with brachial plexus palsy is to achieve elbow flexion so that hand-to-mouth transfer is possible. Achieving shoulder stability is the next priority, since this will support proper elbow function and allow positioning of the forearm and hand in space. A paralyzed hand and forearm can still be very useful with a good shoulder and elbow flexion. Once these areas have been addressed, wrist extension and finger flexion can be considered. In addition to these motor functions, sensation in the median distribution is also a high priority.[1-3]

REFERENCES

1. Brophy RH, Wolfe SW. Planning brachial plexus surgery: treatment options and priorities. Hand Clin 2005;21(1):47–54
2. Sinha S, Khani M, Mansoori N, Midha R. Adult brachial plexus injuries: surgical strategies and approaches. Neurol India 2016;64(2):289–296
3. Terzis JK, Kostopoulos VK. The surgical treatment of brachial plexus injuries in adults. Plast Reconstr Surg 2007;119(4):73e–92e

SURGICAL INTERVENTION IN BRACHIAL PLEXUS INJURY

15. A 27-year-old man presents with no recovery evident either clinically or on NCS/EMG studies 6 months after a C5–C7 injury. Root avulsions are demonstrated on MRI. *How could you best restore elbow flexion?*

C. Ulnar nerve fascicle to musculocutaneous branch nerve transfer

Restoration of hand to mouth elbow flexion is a top treatment priority in the management of brachial plexus injuries. At 6 months postinjury, the absence of any functional recovery clinically and electrophysiologically is very concerning. Where root avulsions have been identified, there will not be any motor recovery, so surgical intervention is warranted early. In general, root avulsions are a good indication for surgery earlier than 6 months, e.g., 6 to 12 weeks postinjury. Other factors such as associated vascular, skeletal, and head injuries along with fitness for surgery must, however, be taken into account and can dictate a delay or change in treatment.

An Oberlin transfer[1] involves selecting a predominantly FCU-activating fascicle in the ulnar nerve within the upper arm and transferring this to the motor branch of the musculocutaneous nerve which supplies biceps brachii. A modification of this technique, the double fascicular transfer (**Fig. 93.2**), includes an additional transfer of a predominantly FCR-activating median nerve fascicle to the motor branch supplying brachialis.[2] These transfers are usually easier to rehabilitate compared to extra-plexus transfers such as an intercostal nerve to musculocutaneous nerve transfer. There can also be a struggle to gain sufficient length with an intercostal transfer such that cable grafting may be required, reducing the likely final amount of distal muscle reinnervation as axons are inevitably lost at each coaptation site due to scarring and misdirection.[3] The reinnervation distance for the Oberlin and modified Oberlin transfers is also much shorter than with an intercostal transfer, so there is a greater chance of more substantial reinnervation. It is also easier to exclude the sensory component of the musculocutaneous nerve from the transfer using the Oberlin technique, as the motor branches to the individual muscles are being directly selected, thus avoiding wasted misdirected axonal regeneration.

An avulsed nerve root cannot be used to reconstruct distal function, and in the presence of C5, C6, C7 avulsions, it would not be advisable to sacrifice remaining C8 function in favor of elbow flexion. Finally, while a free functional gracilis muscle transfer coapted to an FCU ulnar nerve fascicle (i.e., driven by an Oberlin transfer) could

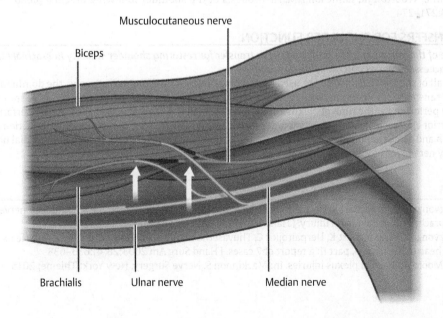

Musculocutaneous nerve

Biceps

Brachialis   Ulnar nerve   Median nerve

Fig. 93.2 The modified Oberlin procedure involves a double fascicular transfer. An FCU ulnar nerve fascicle is transferred to the biceps motor branch of the musculocutaneous nerve and an FCR fascicle from the median nerve is transferred to the motor branch to brachialis.

produce good elbow flexion, at 6 months postinjury this patient should have a healthy biceps and brachialis that are still available for reinnervation. The free muscle option should be reserved for scenarios where reinnervation of native muscle is no longer a good option or has failed to achieve sufficient function.

REFERENCES

1. Oberlin C, Béal D, Leechavengvongs S, Salon A, Dauge MC, Sarcy JJ. Nerve transfer to biceps muscle using a part of ulnar nerve for C5-C6 avulsion of the brachial plexus: anatomical study and report of four cases. J Hand Surg Am 1994;19(2):232–237
2. Mackinnon SE, Novak CB, Myckatyn TM, Tung TH. Results of reinnervation of the biceps and brachialis muscles with a double fascicular transfer for elbow flexion. J Hand Surg Am 2005;30(5):978–985
3. Merrell GA, Barrie KA, Katz DL, Wolfe SW. Results of nerve transfer techniques for restoration of shoulder and elbow function in the context of a meta-analysis of the English literature. J Hand Surg Am 2001;26(2):303–314

MANAGEMENT OF BRACHIAL PLEXUS INJURIES

16. A 60-year-old woman presents 10 years after a complete brachial plexus injury from a horse-riding accident. She is well known to the pain team and is struggling with her shoulder brace and a dragging sensation from her paralyzed arm. She has good scapulothoracic control. *Which of the following is most likely to improve her symptoms?*
    C. Shoulder fusion
    In this scenario, there will be established instability at the shoulder. A shoulder fusion may ameliorate some of this patient's symptoms by better supporting the weight of the limb, but this may cause other difficulties as a result of the fixed position of the joint. If a patient has some scapulothoracic control, as is the case here, this may actually allow a degree of active limb positioning. Amputation is also sometimes indicated to give relief from supporting the dead weight of a paralyzed limb, but it is important to recognize that it may not resolve pain (particularly neuropathic pain related to root avulsion). Local anesthetic catheters and spinal cord stimulators can help some patients with chronic pain after plexus injuries, but this should be a joint undertaking with the pain team and will not necessarily alter the heavy dragging sensation from the weight of the arm.[1,2]

REFERENCES

1. Sousa R, Pereira A, Massada M, Trigueiros M, Lemos R, Silva C. Shoulder arthrodesis in adult brachial plexus injury: what is the optimal position? J Hand Surg Eur Vol 2011;36(7): 541–547
2. Rouholamin E, Wootton JR, Jamieson AM. Arthrodesis of the shoulder following brachial plexus injury. Injury 1991;22(4):271–274

NERVE TRANSFERS FOR SHOULDER FUNCTION

17. *Which one of the following is the preferred nerve transfer for restoring shoulder stability in brachial plexus palsy?*
    A. Spinal accessory nerve onto suprascapular nerve
    While all of the above transfers are used in various scenarios by different surgeons, the dominant first choice nerve transfer to stabilize the shoulder is the spinal accessory nerve to suprascapular nerve transfer. It can be readily performed at the time of plexus exploration through the same approach, or it can be performed through a posterior approach. In addition to shoulder stability, this transfer tries to restore some abduction and external rotation and can be supplemented by additional transfers, such as the triceps branch of the radial nerve onto the axillary nerve.[1-3]

REFERENCES

1. Leechavengvongs S, Witoonchart K, Uerpairojkit C, Thuvasethakul P, Malungpaishrope K. Combined nerve transfers for C5 and C6 brachial plexus avulsion injury. J Hand Surg Am 2006;31(2):183–189
2. Leechavengvongs S, Witoonchart K, Uerpairojkit C, Thuvasethakul P. Nerve transfer to deltoid muscle using the nerve to the long head of the triceps, part II: a report of 7 cases. J Hand Surg Am 2003;28(4):633–638
3. Tung THH, Moore A. Brachial plexus injuries. In: Mackinnon S. Nerve Surgery. New York: Thieme; 2015

94. Nerve Injuries

See *Essentials of Plastic Surgery*, third edition, pp. 1303–1315

NERVE ANATOMY

1. *Which one of the following directly surrounds the axons within a peripheral nerve?*
   A. Schwann cell
   B. Perineurium
   C. Epineurium
   D. Mesoneurium
   E. Endoneurium

ABERRANT NERVE ANATOMY

2. *Which one of the following anatomic abnormalities could account for the ability to abduct some of the fingers, despite complete median and ulnar nerve transection at the wrist?*
   A. Martin-Gruber anastomosis
   B. Riche-Cannieu anastomosis
   C. Froment-Rauber anastomosis
   D. Berrettini connection
   E. Double crush phenomenon

NERVE INJURY

3. *After a peripheral nerve has been divided, which one of the following processes is responsible for guiding the regenerating axon to the correct distal nerve stump?*
   A. Chromatolysis
   B. Neurotropism
   C. Wallerian degeneration
   D. Neurotrophism
   E. Axonal sprouting

PRINCIPLES OF MUSCLE DENERVATION

4. *Following complete transection of the ulnar nerve at the elbow, which one of the following is true with regard to muscle denervation?*
   A. Muscles require 25% of their motor end plates to retain contractile function.
   B. Following direct repair, the nerve should regenerate at a rate of 3 mm/day.
   C. If the intrinsics are not reinnervated within 6 months, they are unlikely to regain normal function.
   D. Reinnervation after ulnar nerve repair is consistent across different age groups.
   E. Hand therapy should be postponed until signs of reinnervation are present.

CLASSIFICATION OF NERVE INJURIES

5. *What is the main clinical relevance of the Sunderland classification of nerve injury?*
   A. It describes the injury mechanism.
   B. It describes the chronicity of injury.
   C. It describes outcomes according to age.
   D. It dictates surgical management.
   E. It provides prognostic information.

ASSESSING SENSATION IN THE HAND

6. *When assessing two-point sensory discrimination in the fingertip, which one of the following is true?*
   A. 6 mm represents a normal static two-point discrimination.
   B. 8 mm represents a normal dynamic two-point discrimination.
   C. Semmes-Weinstein monofilaments should be used for the test.
   D. It is important to cross over the digit during each test.
   E. This assessment forms part of a standard nerve conduction test.

PRIMARY NERVE REPAIR

7. *You are repairing a sharply divided digital nerve 1 week after injury. Which one of the following is correct?*
   A. A direct repair should still be possible at this stage.
   B. Fascicular repair will give a superior result to epineurial repair.
   C. An 8-mm deficit is better repaired directly in flexion than with a nerve graft.
   D. Trimming the nerve ends should be avoided to preserve length.
   E. There is no need to apply a splint after digital nerve repair.

MANAGING A NERVE GAP

8. *You have a patient with a 4-cm gap in the ulnar nerve above the elbow following debridement of a gunshot injury 3 weeks ago.* **Which one of the following is correct?**
   A. Anterior transposition of the nerve to gain length is contraindicated.
   B. One sural nerve would provide sufficient cable grafts for this defect.
   C. This is a good indication for a vascularized nerve transfer.
   D. Neurotization will give as good a functional outcome as grafting.
   E. This defect is too small to justify using a nerve conduit.

NERVE REPAIR TECHNIQUES

9. *Which one of the following techniques would be best indicated for repair of a complete sharp transection of the ulnar nerve in the distal third of the forearm?*
   A. Direct perineural repair
   B. Direct epineurial repair
   C. Direct grouped fascicular repair
   D. Conduit repair to bridge gap
   E. Nerve grafting with sural nerve

NERVE REPAIR TECHNIQUES

10. *Which one of the following would be preferred for repair of a 6-cm midhumeral gap in the radial nerve after debridement of a high-energy open fracture?*
    A. Conduit-only nerve repair
    B. Mobilization and group fascicular repair
    C. Nerve grafting with sural nerve
    D. Nerve grafting with lateral antebrachial cutaneous nerve
    E. Bone shortening and primary nerve repair

ASSESSING OUTCOMES FOLLOWING NERVE INJURY

11. *When assessing for motor and sensory nerve recovery following injury, what grading represents a return to normal function?*
    A. M0, S0
    B. M3, S3
    C. M4, S4
    D. M5, S5
    E. M5, S4

Answers

NERVE ANATOMY

1. *Which one of the following directly surrounds the axons within a peripheral nerve?*

   E. Endoneurium

   The structure of a peripheral is shown in **Fig. 94.1.** The basic structure of a nerve comprises a series of axons which are grouped together to form fascicles. Groups of fascicles together form a complete nerve. The axons are covered by a loose gelatinous collagen matrix called endoneurium. This has minimal tensile strength. Schwann cells surround individual myelinated axons in many peripheral nerves and help insulate the nerve and increase conduction speed. Groups of axons arranged into fascicles are collectively surrounded by perineurium. This is a connective tissue layer with selective permeability that is thin but dense with high tensile strength. The bundles of fascicles are covered by epineurium, which represents the outer layer of the nerve. This contains collagen and elastin fibers and is surrounded by a thin loose areolar tissue called mesoneurium, which is critical for normal nerve excursion during movement. Nerve repair is most commonly performed by suturing the epineurium to reconstitute complete external nerve continuity (an epineurial repair). In some cases, grouped fascicular repair is performed instead. In this case, sutures are placed in the perineurium. When nerve injury occurs, a predictable set of processes are initiated. These are described in **Fig. 94.2.**[1-3]

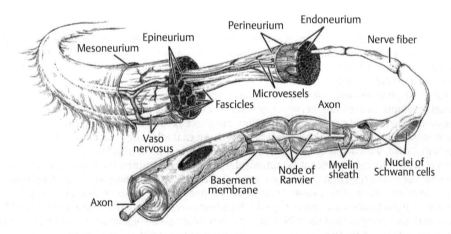

Fig. 94.1 Nerve anatomy. Nerves are formed from multiple axons running in parallel. Axons are grouped together in bundles to form fascicles. Multiple fascicles collectively form the nerve.

REFERENCES

1. Brandt KE, Mackinnon SE. Microsurgical repair of peripheral nerves and nerve grafts. In: Aston JS, Beasley RW, Thorne CM, eds. Grabb and Smith's Plastic Surgery. 5th ed. New York: Lippincott-Raven; 1997
2. Jabaley ME. Current concepts of nerve repair. Clin Plast Surg 1981;8(1):33–44
3. Maggi SP, Lowe JB III, Mackinnon SE. Pathophysiology of nerve injury. Clin Plast Surg 2003;30(2):109–126

ABERRANT NERVE ANATOMY

2. *Which one of the following anatomic abnormalities could account for the ability to abduct some of the fingers, despite complete median and ulnar nerve transection at the wrist?*

   C. Froment-Rauber anastomosis

   The Froment-Rauber anastomosis is a rare condition in which there is a connection between the posterior interosseous nerve (superficial radial nerve) and the ulnar nerve motor branches innervating the dorsal interossei (typically first, second, or third). This could explain why a patient could still have residual finger abduction following median and ulnar nerve division. According to Guo et al,[1] Froment[2] first described the distal continuation of the posterior interosseous nerve (PIN), and Rauber[3] later reported a similar finding. Spinner[4] subsequently referred to this anomalous connection as the Froment-Rauber nerve.

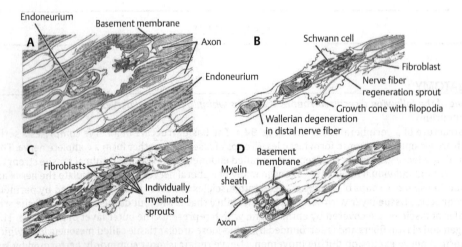

Fig. 94.2   Nerve regeneration. *A,* When a myelinated axon is injured, degeneration occurs distally and for a variable distance proximally. *B,* Multiple regenerating fibers sprout from the proximal axon, forming a regenerating unit. A growth cone at the tip of each regenerating fiber samples the environment and advances the growth process distally. *C,* Schwann cells eventually myelinate the regenerating fibers. *D,* Because it is from a single nerve fiber, a regenerating unit that contains several fibers is formed, and each fiber is capable of functional connections.

The Martin-Gruber and Riche-Cannieu anastomoses involve motor connections between the ulnar and median nerves proximally and distally and lead to diagnostic confusion by masking injury when one but not both nerves is affected. The Berrettini connection is a sensory connection between the ulnar and median nerves, so it would not affect ulnar motor nerve function.

Double-crush phenomenon[5] refers to the scenario where nerve entrapment at one location can predispose an individual to symptoms of clinical nerve compression at another site along that same nerve despite only minimal compression at that second site. Focal compression can affect axoplasmic flow and increase the susceptibility to further minor insults elsewhere along the nerve length. An example is thoracic outlet syndrome (TOS) affecting C8/T1/medial cord, which may lower the threshold for symptoms of ulnar nerve compression at the elbow (or vice versa), producing significant symptoms despite relatively minimal compression at the either site on electrophysiological testing. In such cases, patients often benefit from decompression of the simplest site to treat in the first instance, followed by review of symptoms. Therefore, in the example above, treating the cubital tunnel despite minimal electrophysiological changes at this site may resolve both the cubital tunnel and TOS symptoms and signs without having to treat the TOS. Treatment may no longer be required at the other sites of compression, as overall nerve function is often improved, and the other site becomes asymptomatic.

REFERENCES

1. Guo BY, Ayyar DR, Grossman JA. Posterior interosseus palsy with an incidental Froment-Rauber nerve presenting as a pseudoclaw hand. Hand (N Y) 2011;6(3):344–347
2. Froment JBF. Traité D'Anatomie Humaine. Paris: Mequignon-Marvis; 1846
3. Rauber A. Vatersche Köper der Bänder–und Periostnerven. Munich: Inauug Diss; 1865
4. Spinner M. Injuries to the Major Branches of Peripheral Nerves of the Forearm. 2nd ed. Philadelphia: WB Saunders; 1978
5. Upton AR, McComas AJ. The double crush in nerve entrapment syndromes. Lancet 1973;2(7825):359–362

NERVE INJURY

3. *After a peripheral nerve has been divided, which one of the following processes is responsible for guiding the regenerating axon to the correct distal nerve stump?*

B. Neurotropism

Neurotropism is a process where a chemotactic gradient attracts a regenerating axon toward the correct end target at the distal nerve stump. Initially around half of axonal sprouts will make an incorrect connection and this is subsequently modified such that correct realignment is achieved. Groups of damaged axonal endings form a growth cone and these ends grow toward the distal nerve ends guided by the neurotropic factors.

Neurotrophism is also important in nerve regrowth but more precisely refers to the nutritional support provided to axons connecting with the correct nerve stump. Factors include nerve growth factor, insulin-like growth factor, and epidermal growth factor. When a nerve is divided, the distal stump undergoes Wallerian degeneration. The damaged Schwann cells and macrophages form a neural tube and organize into bands called bands of Bunger. This process forms a scaffold or conduit for nerve regeneration. Proximal to the injury a process called chromatolysis occurs with axon degeneration. The main objective of nerve repair is to return continuity to the framework of damaged nerve such that organized axonal regeneration can proceed along the correct path. When incorrect alignment and excess scarring occur, a neuroma will form with disorganized nerve ends, resulting in pain and dysfunction.[1]

REFERENCE

1. Maggi SP, Lowe JB III, Mackinnon SE. Pathophysiology of nerve injury. Clin Plast Surg 2003;30(2):109–126

PRINCIPLES OF MUSCLE DENERVATION

4. *Following complete transection of the ulnar nerve at the elbow, which one of the following is true with regard to muscle denervation?*
   A. Muscles require 25% of their motor end plates to retain contractile function.
   Following denervation, muscles undergo atrophy and fibrosis. Muscles require 25% of their motor endplates to be intact to contract well, and following denervation these are permanently lost at a rate of 1% per week. For optimal functional outcome, a denervated muscle should be reinnervated within 3 months of injury and directed therapy should be initiated early. Early hand therapy can maintain passive range of motion prior to reinnervation and support function during this period with splints or other adaptations. Functional reinnervation usually remains possible for up to 18 months, but thereafter recovery of muscle function is less likely regardless of the arrival of recovering functional axons and after 2 or 3 years it is no longer possible. Nerve regeneration occurs at a rate of 1 mm/day (not 3 mm/day) following repair, which equates to around 1 inch per month. Therefore, if the ulnar nerve is repaired at the elbow in an adult, it is likely to take at least a year for the regenerating nerve to reach the intrinsic muscles. Consequently, complete reinnervation of the muscles is unlikely in many patients and hand function will be impaired. Outcomes following nerve repair vary across ages with younger adults and children having the best outcomes. In a situation where a muscle is expected to remain denervated for a prolonged time, it may be possible to use a temporary nerve supply to maintain motor endplate function. This forms the basis of the babysitter procedure used in facial nerve injury, or the end-to-side anterior interosseous nerve (AIN) to ulnar motor transfer following a more proximal ulnar nerve repair.[1] In a facial nerve babysitter procedure, part of the hypoglossal nerve is used to innervate the facial muscles while a cross-face nerve graft is placed to regenerate from the contralateral side. In the AIN to ulnar transfer, the functioning distal AIN is redirected at the level of pronator quadratus into the side of the ulnar motor branch in the distal forearm with the intention of more rapid initial intrinsic reinnervation from the AIN while still allowing later recovery from the native proximal ulnar regenerating axons.[1-3]

REFERENCES

1. Barbour J, Yee A, Kahn LC, Mackinnon SE. Supercharged end-to-side anterior interosseous to ulnar motor nerve transfer for intrinsic musculature reinnervation. J Hand Surg Am 2012;37(10):2150–2159
2. Maggi SP, Lowe JB III, Mackinnon SE. Pathophysiology of nerve injury. Clin Plast Surg 2003;30(2):109–126
3. McLeod GJ, Peters BR, Quaife T, Clark TA, Giuffre JL. Anterior interosseous-to-ulnar motor nerve transfers: a single center's experience in restoring intrinsic hand function. Hand (N Y) 2020;22:1558944720928482

CLASSIFICATION OF NERVE INJURIES

5. *What is the main clinical relevance of the Sunderland classification of nerve injury?*
   E. It provides prognostic information.
   The Sunderland classification for nerve injury contains five grades, 1 through 5, and the grade of injury is clinically important as it corresponds to prognosis. A first-degree injury is expected to have complete return of function within days or months. This is where the axon has retained continuity with an intact endoneurium. In contrast, a 5th degree injury involves complete transection of all nerve structures and will have a marked reduction in functional return even after satisfactory repair. The original classification system by Seddon had three categories: neuropraxia, axonotmesis, and neurotmesis. Sunderland[1,2] later expanded this classification into five grades by subclassifying neurotmesis into three further grades (3rd, 4th, and 5th degree). Mackinnon and Dellon[3] later added a sixth category, which represents a mixed nerve injury. These classifications do not describe the mechanism or chronicity of injury. Nor do they relate specific outcomes to age, although younger patients typically achieve the best outcomes after nerve injury. These classifications are often referred to in the conclusion of an Nerve conduction studies (NCS)/electromyography report and can aid surgical decision making (**Table 94.1**).

Table 94.1 *Two Classification Systems of Nerve Injuries*

Seddon	Sunderland	Disrupted Structure	Prognosis
Neurapraxia	1st degree	Axon (minimal)	Complete return in days or months
Axonotmesis	2nd degree	Axon (total, Wallerian degeneration)	Complete return in months
Neurotmesis	3rd degree	Axon, endoneurium	Mild/moderate reduction in function
Neurotmesis	4th degree	Axon, endoneurium, perineurium	Moderate reduction in function
Neurotmesis	5th degree	All structures	Marked reduction in functional return

REFERENCES

1. Sunderland S. A classification of peripheral nerve injuries producing loss of function. Brain 1951;74(4):491–516
2. Sunderland S. The anatomy and physiology of nerve injury. Muscle Nerve 1990;13(9): 771–784
3. Mackinnon SE, Dellon AL. Surgery of the Peripheral Nerve. New York: Thieme; 1988

ASSESSING SENSATION IN THE HAND

6. *When assessing two-point sensory discrimination in the fingertip, which one of the following is true?*

   A. **6 mm represents a normal static two-point discrimination.**

   Two-point discrimination is a test of nerve density most applicable to nerve injuries and less reliable in compression neuropathies. A normal static two-point value is up to 6 mm for the volar fingertip. A moving two-point discrimination is 2 to 3 mm when testing perpendicular to the digit, moving longitudinally from proximal to distal. Specialized calipers are used to test this and the patient is asked to confirm whether they feel one or two pressure points with the caliper tips set apart at differing distances. It is important to stay on the ulna or radial aspect of the digit without crossing over, otherwise a false result will occur with sensation being due to different digital nerves. Semmes-Weinstein monofilaments are not used for two-point discrimination. They are used to measure pressure thresholds and are most applicable to compression neuropathies. They are often used in diabetic patients to assess for protective sensation in the feet. Other tests include vibration thresholds and Tinel's sign, where tapping over a site of nerve degeneration/regeneration produces paresthesia and/or an electrical sensation.[1–3]

REFERENCES

1. Russell S, ed. Examination of Peripheral Nerve Injuries: An Anatomical Approach. 2nd ed. Thieme; 2015
2. Mackinnon SE, Dellon AL. Surgery of the Peripheral Nerve. New York: Thieme Medical; 1988
3. Fox IK, Mackinnon SE. Adult peripheral nerve disorders: nerve entrapment, repair, transfer, and brachial plexus disorders. Plast Reconstr Surg 2011;127(5):105e–118e

PRIMARY NERVE REPAIR

7. *You are repairing a sharply divided digital nerve 1 week after injury. Which one of the following is correct?*

   A. **A direct repair should still be possible at this stage.**

   Although the nerve ends are less amenable to mobilization in the digits than more proximally, it is unlikely that there will be sufficient retraction or fibrosis to prohibit primary repair during the first week. There is no established advantage of one repair over another when comparing epineurial and grouped fascicular repairs; however, there is a balance to be struck between potentially more accurate alignment with a grouped fascicular repair and increased scarring from the foreign body reaction to suture material. In the small digital sensory nerves, it is an accepted practice to use epineurial sutures, as there are few fascicles and good alignment is readily achieved with an epineurial repair. Regardless of the technique used, bulging fascicles should be trimmed to avoid buckling of the repair and subsequent misdirection of the regenerating axons.

   If there is a nerve gap, it is preferable to insert a good quality graft (if >5 mm) or use a conduit to bridge a short gap (<5 mm) than to perform a tight primary repair ameliorated by flexing the digit. The digit will need to be mobilized within a few weeks, at which point there will be tension across the nerve repair site again before regeneration has occurred. Excessive tension is recognized to have a detrimental effect upon nerve regeneration; however, some tension is considered acceptable.[1,2] Use of a postoperative extension blocking splint is common in the first 2 to 3 weeks following digital nerve repair; however, this should not be used as a substitute for a nerve graft or conduit where indicated.

REFERENCES

1. Terzis J, Faibisoff B, Williams B. The nerve gap: suture under tension vs. graft. Plast Reconstr Surg 1975;56(2):166–170
2. Bahm J, Esser T, Sellhaus B, El-kazzi W, Schuind F. Tension in peripheral never suture. In: Vanaclocha V, Saiz-Sapena N, eds. Treatment of Brachial Plexus Injuries. IntechOpen. Available at: http://dx.doi.org/10.5772/intechopen.78722. Accessed January 2, 2020

MANAGING A NERVE GAP

8. You have a patient with a 4-cm gap in the ulnar nerve above the elbow following debridement of a gunshot injury 3 weeks ago. *Which one of the following is correct?*

B. One sural nerve would provide sufficient cable grafts for this defect.

A single sural nerve may provide 30 to 40 cm of suitable nerve graft material. Three to five individual nerve grafts, depending on the cross-sectional size of the graft, might be used in parallel for an ulnar nerve defect (often termed "cable grafting"). Anterior transposition of the ulnar nerve at the elbow can gain a small amount of additional nerve length and may well be indicated, even when nerve grafts are planned as reducing the length of the grafts would be beneficial. While the nerve may have suffered an additional zone of injury to the 4-cm defect, anterior transposition may still be appropriate to both reduce the defect length and to move the nerve repair outside the zone of injury if applicable. Vascularized nerve grafts are not common and are generally reserved for extensively scarred tissues, such as tissues that have undergone radiotherapy, or in longer defects. Nerve conduits generally perform better in smaller nerves over shorter defects, such as a 3-mm digital nerve gap.[1,2]

REFERENCES

1. Millesi H. The nerve gap. Theory and clinical practice. Hand Clin 1986;2(4):651–663
2. Dvali L, Mackinnon S. Nerve repair, grafting, and nerve transfers. Clin Plast Surg 2003;30(2):203–221

NERVE REPAIR TECHNIQUES

9. *Which one of the following techniques would be best indicated for repair of a complete sharp transection of the ulnar nerve in the distal third of the forearm?*

C. Direct group fascicular repair

When performing direct nerve repair, there is no proven advantage in using an epineurial versus grouped fascicular technique, and a perineural technique would be technically difficult to achieve and involve an excess of foreign material. When repairing nerves that have obvious motor and sensory components with consistent topology, such as the ulnar or median nerves in the distal forearm, repairing groups of fascicles may be helpful to more accurately align motor and sensory components.

In this scenario, there is likely to be clean cut with no tissue loss, so neither nerve grafting, a bridging conduit, nor significant mobilization would usually be required.[1-3]

REFERENCES

1. Watchmaker GP, Mackinnon SE. Advances in peripheral nerve repair. Clin Plast Surg 1997;24(1):63–73
2. Brushart T. Nerve repair and grafting. In: Green DP, Hotchkiss RN, Pederson WC, eds. Green's Operative Hand Surgery, Vol. 2. 4th ed. Philadelphia: Churchill Livingstone; 1998
3. Young L, Wray RC, Weeks PM. A randomized prospective comparison of fascicular and epineural digital nerve repairs. Plast Reconstr Surg 1981;68(1):89–93

NERVE REPAIR TECHNIQUES

10. *Which one of the following would be preferred for repair of a 6-cm midhumeral gap in the radial nerve after debridement of a high-energy open fracture?*

C. Nerve grafting with sural nerve

For small nerve gaps in the upper limb, selection of a local nerve graft donor site is preferable; so for radial nerve repair, the lateral antebrachial cutaneous nerve is a good choice and provides 5 to 8 cm total graft length. However, the nerve is variable in cross-sectional size, and in the scenario described the defect is already 6 cm and likely requires further sharp debridement before graft inset, leaving an even longer defect. The multiple lengths of nerve graft required will therefore necessitate sural nerve harvest, which can provide 30 to 40 cm of graft. The PIN is a good option for cases where there is segmental loss of a digital nerve, as the donor site is easily accessed on the same limb, it leaves minimal morbidity, and is a good size match for digital nerves. Mobilization of a transected nerve can avoid nerve grafting, but the length of nerve gap described in this scenario cannot be closed directly unless there is significant shortening of other tissues, i.e., bone, muscle, and tendon as it may sometimes be necessary following major limb trauma. In general, up to 5 cm of humeral shortening can be tolerated in adults without significant problems with musculotendinous unit length.[1] When mobilizing a nerve, it is considered acceptable to do so up to 25% of its length. Beyond this, the vascularity and function could be impaired. Other options to avoid grafting in some settings include transposition of the nerve to shorten this distance required (e.g., ulnar nerve at the elbow) or direct neurotization of the proximal nerve into a target muscle. Nerve conduits are not favored in long defects or in major nerves and are most commonly reserved for short gaps (<5 mm) in small nerves, such as in the finger.[2]

REFERENCES

1. Kusnezov N, Dunn JC, Stewart J, Mitchell JS, Pirela-Cruz M. Acute limb shortening for major near and complete upper extremity amputations with associated neurovascular injury: a review of the literature. Orthop Surg 2015;7(4):306–316
2. Dvali L, Mackinnon S. Nerve repair, grafting, and nerve transfers. Clin Plast Surg 2003;30(2):203–221

ASSESSING OUTCOMES FOLLOWING NERVE INJURY

11. When assessing for motor and sensory nerve recovery following injury, what grading represents a return to normal function?

E. M5, S4

The British Medical Research Council (MRC) grading system is a useful and globally accepted approach to classify nerve function. Highet and Dellon have modified this to relate more specifically to nerve recovery following injury (**Box 94.1**).

Motor recovery has six grades ranging from M0 (no muscle contraction) to M5 (complete recovery). Sensory recovery also has six grades, but these range from S0 (no sensory recovery) to S4 (complete recovery with two-point discrimination 2–6 mm), with S3 being split into two different grades designated S3 and S3+. This terminology allows comparison of results and accurate communication between clinicians regarding outcome following injury.[1]

BOX 94.1   *HIGHET'S METHOD OF END-RESULT EVALUATION AS MODIFIED BY DELLON ET AL*

Motor recovery
M0	No contraction
M1	Return of perceptible contraction on both proximal muscles
M2	Return of perceptible contraction in both proximal and distal muscles
M3	Return of function in both proximal and distal muscles to degree that all important muscles are sufficiently powerful to act against gravity
M4	Return of function as with stage M3; in addition, all synergistic and independent movements possible
M5	Complete recovery

Sensory recovery
S0	Absence of sensory recovery
S1	Recovery of deep cutaneous pain sensibility within autonomous area of nerve
S2	Return of some degree of superficial cutaneous pain and tactile sensibility with autonomous area of nerve
S3	Return of superficial cutaneous pain and tactile sensibility throughout autonomous area, with disappearance of any previous overresponse
S3+	Return of sensibility as with stage S3; in addition, discrimination within autonomous area (7–15 mm)
S4	Complete recovery (two-point discrimination, 2–6 mm)

Note: In the hand, proximal muscles are defined as extrinsic and distal muscles are defined as intrinsic.

REFERENCE

1. Medical Research Council. Memorandum No. 45, Crown Copyright; 1976

95. Hand Infections

See *Essentials of Plastic Surgery*, third edition, pp. 1316–1336

SURGICAL PRINCIPLES IN HAND INFECTIONS

1. *When draining a severe flexor sheath infection with an associated palmar abscess, which one of the following is true?*
   A. An Esmarch bandage is recommended to fully exsanguinate the limb.
   B. Minimal access incisions are required in order to leave wounds open.
   C. An arm tourniquet should be avoided, as bacteremia occurs following release.
   D. Primary amputation should be considered in a diabetic with renal problems.
   E. Bruner incisions are the preferred method of opening up the finger.

PARONYCHIA

2. A patient with a painful swollen fingertip is diagnosed with acute paronychia. *Which one of the following is true?*
   A. This is a common infection originating in the pulp space.
   B. Incision and drainage is the first-line treatment.
   C. Management always requires removal of the nail plate.
   D. Eponychial marsupialization is often required.
   E. *Staphylococcus aureus* is the most likely pathogen.

CLINICAL MANAGEMENT OF A PAINFUL, SWOLLEN FINGER

3. A 30-year-old man presents to the clinic with a swollen, red, painful index pulp and nail fold. It began spontaneously 3 days ago as a burning sensation. Clear fluid is evident under some small superficial blisters that appeared only this morning. He is otherwise healthy, takes no regular medication, and is not a nail biter. *Which one of the following is the best course of action in this case?*
   A. Admit for 24 to 48 hours of intravenous antibiotic therapy with elevation of the hand.
   B. Admit for surgical incision and drainage under local anesthetic.
   C. Debride the finger in clinic and prescribe broad-spectrum oral antibiotics.
   D. Apply a simple dry dressing and follow up in 24 to 48 hours.
   E. Scrape the wound for urgent microbiologic analysis and prescribe acyclovir.

VOLAR/DEEP SPACE ABSCESSES OF THE HAND

4. A female patient presents with exquisite tenderness in the thumb and little finger that is worse with flexion 3 days after sustaining mild trauma to the little finger pulp. The remaining digits are normal. *Which one of the following hand spaces is associated with this clinical presentation?*
   A. Thenar space
   B. Midvolar space
   C. Parona's space
   D. Hypothenar space
   E. Interdigital web space

FLEXOR TENOSYNOVITIS

5. A 45-year-old builder presents with a hot, swollen, painful left middle finger 3 days after stabbing himself in the palm with a screwdriver. His middle finger is flexed and has a fusiform shape. He cannot tolerate passive digital extension or direct, gentle pressure over the volar aspect of the digit. A small bead of pus is expressed at the site of his original injury. *Which one of the following is correct?*
   A. Kanavel's cardinal signs of flexor sheath infection are all present.
   B. This can be adequately managed with high-dose antibiotics and splinting.
   C. This is likely to be polymicrobial and will require at least two antibiotic types.
   D. There are no specific risk factors here for a poor outcome following flexor sheath infection.
   E. Minimal access incisions alone should be adequate for surgical management.

MANAGEMENT OF A "FIGHT BITE"

6. A patient is seen for washout of a wound following a punch injury. There is a 1-cm transverse dorsal wound over the right ring finger metacarpophalangeal (MCP) joint with evidence of pus and surrounding cellulitis. His hand is very swollen, and he is unable to fully extend the ring and middle fingers. Plain radiographs show no evidence of fracture or foreign body. **Which one of the following is correct?**
   A. The wound edges require debridement, but wound extension should be avoided to prevent joint exposure.
   B. After thorough irrigation with saline, any damage to the extensor tendon should be repaired immediately.
   C. It is not necessary to formally explore the MCP joint in this case, given the radiologic findings.
   D. Even if the wound is debrided and irrigated adequately, it should not be closed primarily.
   E. The hand should be splinted with the MCP joints at 20 degrees to relax the joint capsule.

ANIMAL BITES

7. **Which one of the following is correct regarding animal bites?**
   A. Dog bites represent 25% of all reported animal bites in the developed world.
   B. Patients are usually bitten by animals not known to them.
   C. Cat bites are more likely to become infected than dog bites.
   D. Adults are more commonly bitten by animals than children.
   E. Infection from *Pasteurella multocida* occurs exclusively in cat bites.

SEPTIC ARTHRITIS OF THE HAND AND WRIST

8. *In a patient with a suspected wrist septic arthritis, which one of the following is true?*
   A. Joint fluid samples should be taken through the area of greatest erythema.
   B. Synovial fluid analysis with WBC 10,000 cm³ is diagnostic of septic arthritis.
   C. The presence of articular cartilage will prevent osteomyelitis developing.
   D. Crystalline arthropathy is best differentiated from sepsis with radiographs.
   E. In a child this may represent hematogenous spread of another infection.

9. A diabetic patient presents with a rapidly progressing soft-tissue infection of the forearm. There is obvious crepitus within the soft tissues and overlying cellulitis with swelling. A diagnosis of gas gangrene is suspected. **Which one of the following organisms is most likely to be involved?**
   A. *Clostridium perfringens*   D. *Eikenella corrodens*
   B. *S. aureus*   E. *Bacteroides fragilis*
   C. *Streptococcus* spp.

OSTEOMYELITIS IN THE HAND

10. An elderly man with poorly controlled diabetes and chronic renal failure presents with osteomyelitis destroying part of the distal and middle phalanges of his middle finger following a neglected infection of a mucus cyst. **Which of the following best describes this presentation?**
    A. Class D host, type I osteomyelitis
    B. Class C host, type II osteomyelitis
    C. Class D host, type II osteomyelitis
    D. Class C host, type IV osteomyelitis
    E. Class A host, type IV osteomyelitis

MANAGEMENT OF FUNGAL HAND INFECTIONS

11. A 74-year-old avid gardener presents to the clinic with a localized suppurative nodule to the fingertip that has been present for several weeks. He cannot recall any significant trauma to this finger but gets regular thorn pricks and scratches while gardening. **Which one of the following is correct about this condition?**
    A. The diagnosis is onychomycosis and will probably resolve without active intervention.
    B. Best management will involve nail plate removal and a 1-week course of antibiotic therapy.
    C. Application of saturated solution of potassium iodide is the preferred current treatment modality.
    D. An extended course of oral itraconazole or fluconazole is indicated in this case.
    E. *Trichophyton rubrum* is the most common cause of such infections in the United States.

PATHOGENS IN HAND INFECTIONS

12. A 50-year-old pet shop owner sustained a superficial glass injury at work while cleaning an aquarium. The wound has since healed, but he has developed painful superficial erythematous nodules nearby. **What is the most likely pathogen involved?**
    A. *Mycobacterium* spp.   D. Group A *Streptococcus* spp.
    B. *T. rubrum*   E. *E. corrodens*
    C. *P. multocida*

BIOFILMS AND THEIR MANAGEMENT

13. *Why are bacterial biofilms so difficult to treat?*
   A. They usually coexist with fungal spores.
   B. The bacteria have altered genetics.
   C. The bacteria have low adherence to synthetic structures.
   D. The bacteria are protected by a polysaccharide matrix.
   E. They most commonly involve methicillin-resistant *S. aureus* (MRSA).

HIGH-PRESSURE INJECTION INJURIES

14. A patient inadvertently injects an oil-based material into a digit while using a high-pressure tool. *Which one of the following is correct?*
   A. The dominant thumb is the most likely digit to be affected.
   B. Urgent debridement and decompression is required.
   C. Water-based solvents cause similar levels of tissue damage.
   D. The risk of subsequent need for amputation is low.
   E. Soft-tissue damage can be predicted by the size of the entry wound.

Answers

SURGICAL PRINCIPLES IN HAND INFECTIONS

1. **When draining a severe flexor sheath infection with an associated palmar abscess, which one of the following is true?**
   D. Primary amputation should be considered in a diabetic with renal problems.

   Some key principles are relevant when surgically managing infections of the upper limb. The context of the patient's general health status is always important and a diabetic with renal problems is at high risk of systemic complications from a severe hand infection. There is a high likelihood of ending up with amputation of the affected digit anyway with this severe an infection in this patient group[1]; therefore, the option of primary amputation should be considered to reduce overall risk to the patient and to reduce the number of procedures required. Even if a primary amputation is completed, the wounds will still need to be left at least partially open to drain and at least one further procedure is likely to be required to check that there is no progression of tissue changes requiring further debridement and to close wounds where appropriate.

   It is standard practice to use a tourniquet for incision and drainage of an infected upper limb, as this facilitates a clear, blood-free view of structures during debridement. The Esmarch bandage is a rubber band that is used to wrap the hand and forearm for exsanguination before inflation of a tourniquet. Gentle gravity exsanguination is preferred in infected cases to reduce the risk of causing bacteremia.

   Incisions should be designed to allow adequate access while minimize subsequent wound healing and scar complications. In particular, longitudinal incisions across flexion creases should be avoided, as they are likely to lead to scar contractures. As with all hand surgery explorations, incisions should be designed to place scars within skin creases where possible and facilitate good access. Using larger access incisions is generally recommended in severe soft-tissue infections to facilitate accurate debridement and drainage. Some exceptions include mild flexor sheath infections, which can be irrigated with minimal access incisions if not responding to nonoperative management. One proximal incision in the distal palm, and one distally at the level of the DIP joint can be adequate for irrigation if pus is thin.

   Bruner's incisions are commonly used in hand surgery, but in the scenario of a severe hand infection, there is a risk of skin flap necrosis leading to exposure of critical structures and wound healing problems.[2] Therefore, a midlateral approach is preferable if the whole finger needs to be opened. This also has the advantage of less pain and swelling during the early healing period which in turn facilitates more effective early mobilization and reduced stiffness. Popular access incisions for draining hand infections are illustrated in **Fig. 95.1**. Copious

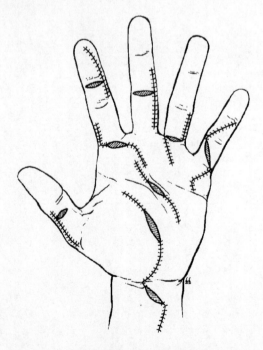

Fig. 95.1   Incision placement for access in the hand.

irrigation of infected wounds is required, and this is often best done with a large saline bag and an intravenous administration set. Following surgery, early active mobilization is optimal to reduce postoperative edema, stiffness, and loss of joint motion.

REFERENCES

1. Francel TJ, Marshall KA, Savage RC. Hand infections in the diabetic and the diabetic renal transplant recipient. Ann Plast Surg 1990;24(4):304–309
2. Osterman M, Draeger R, Stern P. Acute hand infections. J Hand Surg Am 2014;39(8): 1628–1635, quiz 1635

PARONYCHIA

2. *A patient with a painful swollen fingertip is diagnosed with acute paronychia. Which one of the following is true?*

   E. Staphylococcus aureus is the most likely pathogen.

Paronychia is an infection of the soft tissues surrounding the nail and can be acute or chronic. Acute paronychia is generally caused by a bacterial infection with *Staphylococcus aureus* and is associated with nail biting and minor trauma. First-line treatment is oral antibiotics, hand baths, and rest/elevation of the affected digit. In cases unresponsive to conservative management, it is necessary to drain the abscess and/or remove the nail plate. Chronic infections are more likely to be fungal and may require marsupialization or nail ablation in cases resistant to medical management. Pulp space infections are called felons. They can coexist with paronychia but are different entities. They are treated with incision and drainage plus antibiotics.[1]

REFERENCE

1. Franko OI, Abrams RA. Hand infections. Orthop Clin North Am 2013;44(4):625–634

CLINICAL MANAGEMENT OF A PAINFUL, SWOLLEN FINGER

3. A 30-year-old man presents to the clinic with a swollen, red, painful index pulp and nail fold. It began spontaneously 3 days ago as a burning sensation. Clear fluid is evident under some small superficial blisters that appeared only this morning. He is otherwise healthy, takes no regular medication, and is not a nail biter. *Which one of the following is the best course of action in this case?*

   D. Apply a simple dry dressing and follow up in 24 to 48 hours.

The differential diagnosis in this patient is herpetic whitlow or a felon/paronychia. Given the appearance of vesicles, the mild swelling, and the history of prodromal burning provided, herpetic whitlow is the most likely diagnosis. This condition is generally self-limiting and is caused by infection with herpes simplex virus.[1] De-roofing a vesicle allows a Tzanck smear to be performed for diagnostic purposes, but debridement and release of fluid is not recommended because this can lead to viral spread. In severe cases, usually in immunocompromised patients, viral spread can result in encephalitis and even death. Herpetic whitlow should be treated with application of a dry dressing to reduce contact with the lesion, unless there is concern regarding superimposed bacterial infection (which is not evident in this case). There is no indication here for either antibiotics or antiviral medications in an otherwise healthy patient. A secondary bacterial infection would require debridement of purulent vesicles and a course of antibiotics.[2]

REFERENCES

1. Louis DS, Silva J Jr. Herpetic whitlow: herpetic infections of the digits. J Hand Surg Am 1979;4(1):90–94
2. Franko OI, Abrams RA. Hand infections. Orthop Clin North Am 2013;44(4):625–634

VOLAR/DEEP SPACE ABSCESSES OF THE HAND

4. A female patient presents with exquisite tenderness in the thumb and little finger that is worse with flexion 3 days after sustaining mild trauma to the little finger pulp. The remaining digits are normal. *Which one of the following hand spaces is associated with this clinical presentation?*

   C. Parona's space

This patient displays signs of a horseshoe abscess (**Fig. 95.2**). Parona's space is located in the distal forearm between pronator quadratus and the flexor digitorum profundus tendons. An infection of either the little finger or thumb flexor sheaths can spread by a communication through the ulnar and radial bursae into Parona's space. This explains why a patient can have an injury in the little finger presenting with a thumb flexor sheath infection.

Other important spaces in the hand that may become infected are the midvolar, hypothenar, thenar, and interdigital spaces. Midvolar infections present with central palm pain and swelling with loss of concavity between thenar and hypothenar eminences. Thenar space infections present with local swelling and pain, which

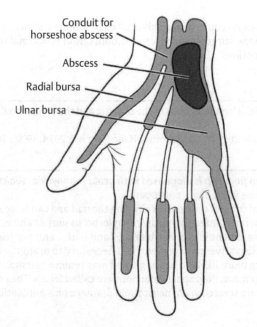

Conduit for horseshoe abscess

Abscess

Radial bursa

Ulnar bursa

Fig. 95.2   Radial and ulnar bursas communicating with Parona's space may cause a horseshoe abscess.

is worse on thumb opposition. Hypothenar space infections are rare and present with swelling and pain on little finger opposition. Collar button abscesses can form in the interdigital web spaces. They present with loss of web space contour and tenderness within the affected web space.

Any suspected infected collections in the hand require urgent surgical drainage, usually supplemented with antibiotics. The normal surgical principles apply.[1]

REFERENCE

1. Franko OI, Abrams RA. Hand infections. Orthop Clin North Am 2013;44(4):625–634

FLEXOR TENOSYNOVITIS

5. A 45-year-old builder presents with a hot, swollen, painful left middle finger 3 days after stabbing himself in the palm with a screwdriver. His middle finger is flexed and has a fusiform shape. He cannot tolerate passive digital extension or direct, gentle pressure over the volar aspect of the digit. A small bead of pus is expressed at the site of his original injury. *Which one of the following is correct?*

A. Kanavel's cardinal signs of flexor sheath infection are all present.

   Kanavel's four cardinal signs of a flexor sheath infection are:
   1. Severe pain on passive extension of the digit
   2. Fusiform swelling of the digit
   3. Tenderness over the flexor tendon sheath
   4. Partially flexed posture of the digit (added later to the original description)
   This patient displays all of these signs, as is quite typical for a more advanced infection.

   Some flexor sheath infections that present early with mild symptoms can be managed adequately with antibiotics, mobilization, and splinting alone.[1] This is not usually effective for infections associated with a penetrating wound. This patient requires urgent surgical drainage because there is pus evident and there has been delayed management of the initial penetrating injury.

   Ideally, minimal access incisions are used for flexor sheath washout, provided the sheath can be irrigated well. This enables a quicker and more comfortable rehabilitation and reduces the likelihood of wound healing problems. At least a degree of palmar wound extension will be required in this case to explore and debride the initial puncture wound. With pus leaking from the palm, there is likely to be thicker pus in the sheath that will require more extensive access than an early infection would in order to irrigate adequately.

   The most common pathogen in flexor sheath infection is *S. aureus* alone, rather than a polymicrobial cause. Polymicrobial infections are more common in diabetic and other immunocompromised patients. Treatment is usually with a single penicillin-based antibiotic such as amoxicillin with clavulanic acid or flucloxacillin. This patient has two risk factors for a poor outcome following flexor sheath infection: age over 43 years and the presence of subcutaneous pus. Level II evidence has shown a number of other risk factors for poor outcome, which include the presence of diabetes, peripheral vascular or renal disease, and the presence of digital ischemia.[1,2]

REFERENCES

1. Steer AC, Lamagni T, Curtis N, Carapetis JR. Invasive group a streptococcal disease: epidemiology, pathogenesis and management. Drugs 2012;72(9):1213–1227
2. Pang HN, Teoh LC, Yam AK, Lee JY, Puhaindran ME, Tan AB. Factors affecting the prognosis of pyogenic flexor tenosynovitis. J Bone Joint Surg Am 2007;89(8):1742–1748

MANAGEMENT OF A "FIGHT BITE"

6. A patient is seen for washout of a wound following a punch injury. There is a 1-cm transverse dorsal wound over the right ring finger metacarpophalangeal (MCP) joint with evidence of pus and surrounding cellulitis. His hand is very swollen, and he is unable to fully extend the ring and middle fingers. Plain radiographs show no evidence of fracture or foreign body. *Which one of the following is correct?*

   D. Even if the wound is debrided and irrigated adequately, it should not be closed primarily.

   Primary wound closure should be avoided in a "fight bite" and is definitely contraindicated if there is frank pus. Any tendon repair should be delayed until the wound is clean, and a monofilament suture is preferred to further reduce the risk of bacterial colonization at the repair site. The risk of joint capsule penetration is very high with these injuries; so, the capsule should be carefully inspected throughout the range of motion. Any resting splint should be in the safe position of immobilization and is particularly important when the hand is swollen. The wrist should be slightly extended, MCP joints flexed to approximately 70 degrees, and the IP joints straight.[1]

   The key principles for managing these injuries are:
   1. Promptly and thoroughly debride the wound edges and extend the wound to ensure adequate inspection of the tendon and joint capsule throughout the range of MCP joint motion.
   2. Send deep specimens for microbiologic analysis.
   3. Thoroughly irrigate the wound. Wash out the joint too if capsule is open or infected.
   4. Do not primarily repair the joint capsule or tendon if there is frank pus.
   5. Leave at least some part of the wound open for drainage. Consider closing the wound extensions using a monofilament nonabsorbable suture.
   6. Dress the wound with a wick/pack to encourage drainage, a low-adherent dressing, gauze, wool, and crepe.
   7. Apply a splint with the hand placed in the "safe" position.
   8. Continue IV antibiotics and hand elevation, then reassess the wound and mobilize/soak in an antiseptic/soapy hand bath at 24 hours.

REFERENCE

1. Joyce CW, O' Regan A, Kelly JL, O' Shaughnessy M. Fight bite injuries: aggressive tendencies associated with smaller second to fourth digit ratio. J Hand Surg Asian Pac Vol 2017;22(4):452–456

ANIMAL BITES

7. *Which one of the following is correct regarding animal bites?*

   C. Cat bites are more likely to become infected than dog bites.

   Dog bites represent 90% of all animal bites in the developed world, whereas cat bites represent just 5%. Despite this massive difference, cat bites represent three quarters of all infected bites. This is probably because their long, thin teeth are more likely to cause narrow, deep puncture wounds prone to infection. Cat bites need early treatment with antibiotics and washout and can still take a prolonged time to settle. In over two-thirds of dog bites, the animal is known to the patient. Children younger than 5 years are at increased risk of dog bites with half of all dog bites occurring in this age group. *P. multocida* is associated with both cat and dog bites. Therefore, antibiotics must be selected to cover these and staphylococcus, streptococcus, and anaerobe pathogens.[1,2]

REFERENCES

1. Kheiran A, Palial V, Rollett R, Wildin CJ, Chatterji U, Singh HP. Cat bite: an injury not to underestimate. J Plast Surg Hand Surg 2019;53(6):341–346
2. Franko OI, Abrams RA. Hand infections. Orthop Clin North Am 2013;44(4):625–634

SEPTIC ARTHRITIS OF THE HAND AND WRIST

8. *In a patient with a suspected wrist septic arthritis, which one of the following is true?*

E. In a child this may represent hematogenous spread of another infection.

Septic arthritis is infection of a joint space and may be primary or represent hematogenous spread from an infective source elsewhere in the body. For this reason, it is important to exclude other sources of infection, particularly in children. *Streptococcus*, *Staphylococcus*, and *Haemophilus influenza* are the most common pathogens involved in joint infections. Diagnosis involves a good history and clinical assessment complemented by microscopy of a joint fluid sample. Plain radiographs, blood inflammatory markers, and urate levels should also usually be requested.

A joint aspirate should ideally be obtained without passing the needle through obviously inflamed or wounded skin in order to avoid seeding of bacteria into a joint which actually is not infected, and to ensure a reliable sample is obtained. Fluid analysis with WBC >50,000 per mm^3 (not 10,000 per cm^3) is strongly suggestive of joint sepsis. An urgent Gram stain should be requested from the lab. Joint fluid also provides the best evidence for or against a crystal arthropathy, such as gout or pseudogout, and some of the fluid should be sent for crystal analysis.

An infected joint requires urgent joint washout and antibiotics. Early mobilization with hand therapy and a resting splint in a safe position is required. Untreated septic arthritis may quickly and irreversibly erode the articular cartilage, resulting in arthritic changes and increasing the risk of progression to osteomyelitis.[1]

REFERENCE

1. Jennings JD, Zielinski E, Tosti R, Ilyas AM. Septic arthritis of the wrist: incidence, risk factors, and predictors of infection. Orthopedics 2017;40(3):e526–e531

9. A diabetic patient presents with a rapidly progressing soft-tissue infection of the forearm. There is obvious crepitus within the soft tissues and overlying cellulitis with swelling. A diagnosis of gas gangrene is suspected. *Which one of the following organisms is most likely to be involved?*

A. *Clostridium perfringens*

Gas gangrene is uncommon in the upper extremity but is a severe life-threatening infection caused by *Clostridium* species. There are more than 60 subtypes of *Clostridium*, but perfringens is most commonly associated with gas gangrene. Clostridia produce multiple toxins which cause local tissue destruction. Management involves rapid diagnosis and early surgical debridement with high-dose antibiotics and general supportive care. Gas gangrene has a high mortality rate (approximately 25%). Necrotizing fasciitis is the main differential diagnosis, and this can either be polymicrobial or caused by group A Streptococci. Many soft-tissue infections are caused by *S. aureus*, including paronychia, flexor sheath infection, and felon. *Eikenella* is implicated in some human bites as are *Streptococcus viridans* and *Bacteroides*.[1]

REFERENCE

1. Leiblein M, Wagner N, Adam EH, Frank J, Marzi I, Nau C. Clostridial gas gangrene - a rare but deadly infection: case series and comparison to other necrotizing soft tissue infections. Orthop Surg 2020;12(6):1733–1747

OSTEOMYELITIS IN THE HAND

10. An elderly man with poorly controlled diabetes and chronic renal failure presents with osteomyelitis destroying part of the distal and middle phalanges of his middle finger following a neglected infection of a mucus cyst. *Which of the following best describes this presentation?*

D. Class C host, type IV osteomyelitis

Cierney et al[1] developed a classification for osteomyelitis that encourages consideration of both host and disease characteristics that can be useful for planning treatment.

Physiologic class (host characteristics)

A host: Normal host with good immune system

B host: Local or systemic compromise

C host: Markedly compromised host. Treatment of disease is more risky than disease itself

Anatomic location

Type I: Medullary osteomyelitis—limited to endosteum, most common is hematogenous cause or intramedullary fixation

Type II: Superficial osteomyelitis—involves surface of bone

Type III: Localized infection—both medullary and superficial; full-thickness sequestrum

Type IV: Diffuse; bony instability

By falling into the group C host, type IV location category of osteomyelitis, assessment of this patient is likely to guide the clinician toward a prompt, simple, low-risk local anesthetic terminalization of the affected digit rather than debridement and prolonged courses of antibiotics.[2]

REFERENCES

1. Cierney GIN, Mader J, Penninck J. A clinical staging system for adult osteomyelitis. Contemp Orthop 1985;10:17–37
2. Pinder R, Barlow G. Osteomyelitis of the hand. J Hand Surg Eur Vol 2016;41(4):431–440

MANAGEMENT OF FUNGAL HAND INFECTIONS

11. A 74-year-old avid gardener presents to the clinic with a localized suppurative nodule to the fingertip that has been present for several weeks. He cannot recall any significant trauma to this finger but gets regular thorn pricks and scratches while gardening. **Which one of the following is correct about this condition?**

D. An extended course of oral itraconazole or fluconazole is indicated in this case.

Common fungal infections of the upper extremity include sporotrichosis and onychomycosis. Sporotrichosis is a granulomatous fungal infection of the skin or subcutaneous tissue, while onychomycosis is a fungal infection of the nail.

The patient in this scenario is most likely to have a soft-tissue fungal infection acquired while gardening. The likely pathogen is *Sporothrix schenckii* which is typically sustained from a puncture wound during contact with rose thorns, moss, or other plants. For this reason, it is often called "rose handler's disease." The classic treatment described is the use of a saturated solution of potassium iodide, but this has now been supplanted by an extended oral course of itraconazole or fluconazole such as 3 to 6 months, or at least 4 weeks after resolution of symptoms. Patients tend to present with a nodule at a puncture site, which later ulcerates. This is followed by nodule formation along lymphatic channels, which then also ulcerate. A definitive diagnosis is made by fungal culture of a nodule aspirate.

Onychomycosis is a fungal condition of the nail most often caused by *T. rubrum*. *C. albicans* is another common cause, particularly in diabetics. This condition results in an abnormal, thickened, and discolored nail plate. Fungal cultures are required to guide selection of antifungal therapies. For example, *T. rubrum* responds best to oral terbinafine, while *C. albicans* may require ketoconazole, itraconazole, or griseofulvin. Removal of the thickened nail plate can be useful, as it can reduce the duration required for oral antifungal therapy. Paronychia is an infection of the soft tissues surrounding the nail and can be acute or chronic. Acute paronychia is normally bacterial, whereas chronic paronychia is normally fungal. Acute paronychia is often best treated with a combination of antibiotics and wound debridement with nail plate removal. Chronic paronychia requires antifungal medication and may need marsupialization of the eponychial fold.

PATHOGENS IN HAND INFECTIONS

12. A 50-year-old pet shop owner sustained a superficial glass injury at work while cleaning an aquarium. The wound has since healed, but he has developed painful superficial erythematous nodules nearby. **What is the most likely pathogen involved?**

A. Mycobacterium spp.

The patient in this scenario has developed an atypical mycobacterial infection, also known as *fish tank granuloma*. It is caused by *Mycobacterium marinum*. Typical and atypical mycobacterial infections are rare and have a broad range of subtypes. These include tuberculous infections and leprosy. The diagnosis should be suspected where there is a chronic skin nodule (as in this case), a draining sinus tract, or another infection that fails to heal within a typical timeframe. A biopsy will show granulomas with negative fungal staining. Cultures can take an extended time to process due to the slow replication of mycobacteria and empiric antibiotic selection may be indicated while these are awaited. Treatment is likely to require surgical debridement followed by an extended course of antibiotics.[1,2]

T. rubrum represents a fungal infection that causes onychomycosis. This is treated with oral terbinafine. *P. multocida* is seen most commonly in cases of infected cat bites. These should be treated with debridement and irrigation in conjunction with amoxicillin and clavulanic acid or clindamycin. Group A *Streptococcus* spp. can cause an aggressive, rapidly progressing soft-tissue infection in previously fit individuals. Early recognition is required alongside prompt treatment with high-dose penicillin antibiotics in the first instance. *E. corrodens* is a common pathogen in human bite injuries and is generally responsive to combined amoxicillin and clavulanic acid.[3]

REFERENCES

1. Veraldi S, Molle M, Nazzaro G. Eczema-like fish tank granuloma: a new clinical presentation of *Mycobacterium marinum* infection. J Eur Acad Dermatol Venereol 2018;32(5): e200–e201
2. Hashish E, Merwad A, Elgaml S, et al. *Mycobacterium marinum* infection in fish and man: epidemiology, pathophysiology and management; a review. Vet Q 2018;38(1):35–46
3. Soldatos T, Omar H, Sammer D, Chhabra A. Atypical infections versus inflammatory conditions of the hand: the role of imaging in diagnosis. Plast Reconstr Surg 2015;136(2): 316–327

BIOFILMS AND THEIR MANAGEMENT

13. *Why are bacterial biofilms so difficult to treat?*

D. The bacteria are protected by a polysaccharide matrix.

Biofilms can be a problem in plastic surgery, most commonly affecting implanted devices and chronic wounds. Biofilms are implicated in a variety of clinical infections, as well as in breast implant capsular contracture.

Biofilms are particularly difficult to treat because they are strongly adherent to implanted devices and less healthy/nonviable tissue. Here, they form multiorganism colonies protected beneath an exopolysaccharide matrix. This isolates them from surrounding tissues and protects them from host defense mechanisms and antibiotics. The biofilm is often inactive for extended periods of time with no evidence of infection present. It can subsequently become activated to release certain free bacteria from beneath the polysaccharide matrix which are described as being in a planktonic state. When a wound is swabbed, it is only these planktonic bacteria that can be detected rather than the true polymicrobial activity going on beneath the matrix. As a result, antibiotic concentrations 1,000 times higher than normal may be required to penetrate a biofilm. Surgical debridement of chronic wounds and removal of nonviable tissue help reduce a biofilm, and prosthetic devices are generally exchanged or removed where a biofilm is present and causing infection. Bacterial biofilms do not usually coexist with fungal spores where the genetics of the bacteria are otherwise normal. MRSA has become increasingly common in recent years as a result of antibacterial resistance; however, this is not the main reason why biofilms are difficult to treat.[1]

REFERENCE

1. Jamal M, Ahmad W, Andleeb S, et al. Bacterial biofilm and associated infections. J Chin Med Assoc 2018;81(1):7–11

HIGH-PRESSURE INJECTION INJURIES

14. A patient inadvertently injects an oil-based material into a digit while using a high-pressure tool. *Which one of the following is correct?*

B. Urgent debridement and decompression is required.

High-pressure injection injuries are a surgical emergency and can cause significant tissue damage through a small entry wound. Material is inadvertently injected into the digit at high pressure (often as high as 7000 psi). The most commonly involved digit is the nondominant index finger as the offending tool tends to be held in the dominant hand with the nondominant hand supporting the target object. These injuries need urgent surgical management with wound extension, irrigation, and tissue debridement. Both oil-based and water-based solvents can cause significant damage, but oil-based injuries tend to be worse and generate greater irritation of the soft tissues. Risk of amputation is high (up to 50%) after an oil-based, high-pressure injury such as paint injection. The entry wound does not provide much information with regard to the zone of tissue damage, so it is easy to underestimate its severity. Debridement often fails to remove all traces of injection material satisfactorily. If the fingertip is the entry point, material can frequently be identified in the forearm where it has been forced under pressure along the tendon sheath. This is in addition to the pressure insult to the soft tissues surrounding the entry point, for example, the fat of the pulp may be completely nonviable due to both barotrauma and foreign material contamination.[1,2]

REFERENCES

1. Amsdell SL, Hammert WC. High-pressure injection injuries in the hand: current treatment concepts. Plast Reconstr Surg 2013;132(4):586e–591e
2. Bekler H, Gokce A, Beyzadeoglu T, Parmaksizoglu F. The surgical treatment and outcomes of high-pressure injection injuries of the hand. J Hand Surg Eur Vol 2007;32(4):394–399

96. Benign and Malignant Masses of the Hand

See *Essentials of Plastic Surgery*, third edition, pp. 1337–1353

GANGLION CYSTS

1. Your resident sees a child with a painless soft-tissue mass on the radial volar aspect of the wrist and diagnoses a ganglion cyst. *Which one of the following is correct?*
   A. Ganglion cysts are the most common benign mass in the upper limb and have an equal sex distribution.
   B. A biopsy will generally be required to confirm the diagnosis.
   C. Wrist ganglia consistently indicate underlying degenerative change in the joint.
   D. The volar wrist is the most common site for ganglia in children.
   E. Prompt surgical excision is still recommended to exclude malignancy.

GANGLION CYSTS OF THE WRIST

2. *Which one of the following ligaments is most commonly associated with symptomatic ganglion cysts in adults?*
   A. Radiolunate
   B. Scapholunate
   C. Radiocapitate
   D. Scaphotriquetral
   E. Radioscaphoid

GIANT CELL TUMORS OF THE TENDON SHEATH

3. A patient is referred with a suspected giant cell tumor of the tendon sheath. *Which one of the following statements is correct?*
   A. It is most likely to affect the little finger.
   B. The patient is most likely to be younger than 20 years.
   C. Hand function is unlikely to be affected.
   D. Previous injury may be a predisposing factor.
   E. Recurrence after surgical excision is unlikely.

FINGERTIP LESIONS

4. A 28-year-old hairdresser presents with a nontender 5-mm soft-tissue mass in the right middle finger pulp. *What is the most likely diagnosis?*
   A. Giant cell tumor
   B. Epidermal inclusion cyst
   C. Glomus tumor
   D. Pyogenic granuloma
   E. Melanoma

FINGERTIP LESIONS

5. A 78-year-old retired schoolteacher presents with a tender soft-tissue swelling between the dorsal nailfold and DIP joint of the right ring finger. It has developed over the past 12 months. She has a groove in the nail plate. *What is the most likely diagnosis?*
   A. Neurofibroma
   B. Enchondroma
   C. Basal cell carcinoma (BCC)
   D. Mucous cyst
   E. Melanoma

TUMORS OF THE HAND AND WRIST

6. A 43-year-old right-hand–dominant carpenter presents with a small soft-tissue swelling over the volar aspect of the right wrist that has developed over 8 months. He complains of altered sensation in the little finger and pain in the ulnar digits while working, especially in cold weather. What is the most likely diagnosis?
   A. Carpal boss
   B. Ulnar artery aneurysm
   C. Ganglion cyst
   D. Chondrosarcoma

GLOMUS TUMORS

7. **A patient is referred with a suspected glomus tumor of the hand. Which one of the following is true?**
    A. It is the most commonly occurring benign hand tumor.
    B. It carries a moderate risk of malignant transformation.
    C. The main symptom is altered sensation in the affected digit.
    D. Use of a tourniquet in clinic can help aid clinical diagnosis.
    E. Radiographic imaging is key to confirming the diagnosis.

SIGNS OF SOFT-TISSUE SARCOMA

8. You are working in the sarcoma clinic, and a 34-year-old patient is referred to you with a soft-tissue mass in the volar compartment of the proximal forearm. It has been present for 16 months, measures 4 cm in diameter, is fixed by resisted elbow flexion, and is nontender. *Which one of the following represents the most significant concern regarding this lesion?*
    A. The size
    B. The lack of pain
    C. The duration of symptoms
    D. The depth of the mass
    E. The patient's age

DIAGNOSING SOFT-TISSUE SARCOMA

9. A young adult patient is referred to the clinic with a deep, rapidly enlarging, painful soft-tissue mass in the left hand. *Which one of the following is the preferred method for obtaining an initial tissue diagnosis in this case?*
    A. Fine-needle aspiration cytology
    B. Incisional biopsy
    C. Excisional biopsy
    D. Core needle biopsy
    E. Marginal excision

IMAGING IN SOFT-TISSUE SARCOMA

10. A patient is referred to the clinic with a suspicious soft-tissue mass in the right upper limb. It has doubled in size over the past month. *Which one of the following is the best imaging modality to use for this patient?*
    A. High-resolution CT
    B. Isotope bone scan
    C. MRI
    D. Ultrasound
    E. PET scan

SARCOMA SUBTYPES

11. *Which one of the following describes a soft-tissue sarcoma seen in patients with immune compromise presenting with dark blue to violaceous firm macules and plaques?*
    A. Kaposi's sarcoma
    B. Epithelioid sarcoma
    C. Clear cell sarcoma
    D. Fibrosarcoma
    E. Synovial sarcoma

MANAGEMENT OF SOFT-TISSUE SARCOMAS

12. *When considering the treatment principles for sarcoma of the hand, which one of the following is correct?*
    A. Wide surgical excision is performed with 1- to 2-cm margins.
    B. Surgical excision is unlikely to require amputation.
    C. Any diagnostic biopsy tract must be excised en bloc with the resection.
    D. All patients will require postsurgical radiotherapy (adjuvant).
    E. All patients are likely to need systemic chemotherapy postsurgery.

BENIGN BONE LESIONS OF THE HAND

13. A 26-year-old woman presents with a fracture of the proximal phalanx of the left ring finger sustained while washing dishes. She is otherwise healthy. A plain radiograph shows a well-demarcated, round, lytic lesion with some areas of calcification within the proximal phalanx. *What is the most likely diagnosis?*
    A. Nora's lesion
    B. Periosteal chondroma
    C. Enchondroma
    D. Maffucci's syndrome
    E. Ollier's disease

MALIGNANT BONE TUMORS OF THE HAND

14. *Which one of the following is the most common primary malignant bone tumor in the hand and tends to occur in middle age patients?*
    A. Ewing's sarcoma
    B. Chondrosarcoma
    C. Osteosarcoma
    D. Malignant giant cell tumor
    E. Osteoblastoma

Answers

GANGLION CYSTS

1. Your resident sees a child with a painless soft-tissue mass on the radial volar aspect of the wrist and diagnoses a ganglion cyst. *Which one of the following is correct?*

   D. The volar wrist is the most common site for ganglia in children.

   The volar wrist is generally thought to be the most common site for ganglion cysts in children. Ganglion cysts are the most common benign mass in the hand and are two or three times more common in females. They are most common in the second to fourth decades. Diagnosis is based on history and clinical examination and may be enhanced by transillumination using a penlight. Radiographs should be obtained to exclude underlying joint pathology or soft-tissue calcification, but these do not usually help diagnose a ganglion. Ultrasonography may be of use when there is doubt about the nature and extent of a probable ganglion cyst and a solid rather than cystic mass may require biopsy or excision to exclude malignancy.

   Two-thirds of ganglia in children are reported to resolve spontaneously,[1] but persistent lesions or those associated with pain or reduced function may require treatment. Aspiration may be sufficient, but patients should be warned there is a 50% recurrence rate. The addition of hyaluronidase or steroid does not offer any additional advantage and the recurrence rate following surgical excision in children is particularly low at 5%[2] compared to 25% on average in adults.[3] This may reflect the greater likelihood of underlying degenerative changes in adults.

REFERENCES

1. Rosson JW, Walker G. The natural history of ganglia in children. J Bone Joint Surg Br 1989;71(4):707–708
2. Simon Cypel TK, Mrad A, Somers G, Zuker RM. Ganglion cyst in children: reviewing treatment and recurrence rates. Can J Plast Surg 2011;19(2):53–55
3. Head L, Gencarelli JR, Allen M, Boyd KU. Wrist ganglion treatment: systematic review and meta-analysis. J Hand Surg Am 2015;40(3):546–53.e8

GANGLION CYSTS OF THE WRIST

2. *Which one of the following ligaments is most commonly associated with symptomatic ganglion cysts in adults?*

   B. Scapholunate

   Dorsal wrist ganglia are the most common symptomatic ganglia in adults and are most frequently identified between the third and fourth extensor compartments. They are most often associated with the scapholunate ligament, which is a key structure in providing carpal stability. Volar wrist ganglion cysts are the most common asymptomatic wrist ganglia in adults and tend to occur between flexor carpi radialis (FCR) and the radial artery. They can arise from the FCR tendon sheath, radiocarpal or scaphotrapezial joints. Many ganglia, such as mucous cysts at the distal interphalangeal (DIP) joint, flexor sheath ganglia and some dorsal wrist ganglia, can comfortably be excised under local anesthesia. Volar wrist ganglia are more commonly excised under regional block or general anesthesia with a tourniquet to aid careful dissection around the radial artery.[1–3]

REFERENCES

1. Nahra ME, Bucchieri JS. Ganglion cysts and other tumor related conditions of the hand and wrist. Hand Clin 2004;20(3):249–260, v
2. Lowden CM, Attiah M, Garvin G, Macdermid JC, Osman S, Faber KJ. The prevalence of wrist ganglia in an asymptomatic population: magnetic resonance evaluation. J Hand Surg [Br] 2005;30(3):302–306
3. Zhang A, Falkowski AL, Jacobson JA, Kim SM, Koh SH, Gaetke-Udager K. Sonography of wrist ganglion cysts: Which location is most common? J Ultrasound Med 2019;38(8):2155–2160

GIANT CELL TUMORS OF THE TENDON SHEATH

3. A patient is referred with a suspected giant cell tumor of the tendon sheath. *Which one of the following statements is correct?*

   D. Previous injury may be a predisposing factor.

   Giant cell tumors of the tendon sheath are also called pigmented villonodular synovitis. They are yellow-brown–colored subcutaneous masses that develop spontaneously and may be a reaction to injury. They are most common between the third and fifth decades of life and may be clinically confused with ganglion cysts. The radial three digits are most frequently affected, although other sites can be involved. Continued growth of the tumor will usually interfere with hand function, particularly with range of motion. Treatment with marginal excision is advocated to preserve function, but recurrence rates are high because of close margins or satellite lesions. Adjunctive radiotherapy is sometimes used to treat recurrent tumors or following incomplete surgical excision.[1-3]

REFERENCES

1. Adams EL, Yoder EM, Kasdan ML. Giant cell tumor of the tendon sheath: experience with 65 cases. Eplasty 2012;12:e50
2. Garg B, Kotwal PP. Giant cell tumour of the tendon sheath of the hand. J Orthop Surg (Hong Kong) 2011;19(2):218–220
3. Errani C, Ruggieri P, Asenzio MA, et al. Giant cell tumor of the extremity: a review of 349 cases from a single institution. Cancer Treat Rev 2010;36(1):1–7

FINGERTIP LESIONS

4. A 28-year-old hairdresser presents with a nontender 5-mm soft-tissue mass in the right middle finger pulp. *What is the most likely diagnosis?*

   B. Epidermal inclusion cyst

   Epidermal inclusion cysts are commonly seen in the palms and fingertips of patients with occupations that predispose them to penetrating injuries, as in this scenario. The penetrating injury causes implantation of epidermal cells into the dermis. This can also occur secondary to surgery at any site if epidermal implantation occurs. For example, leaving epidermal tissue in the wound or dragging it in with sutures. Examination of a patient with an inclusion cyst will typically show evidence of a firm, spherical, painless mass with fixity to skin. Treatment is achieved with complete surgical excision to minimize recurrence.[1]

   A giant cell tumor could also present as a nontender nodule, but these tend to be more proximally located in the digit rather than at the pulp. A glomus tumor is a benign tumor of the arteriovenous anastomosis involved in the regulation of cutaneous circulation in the distal part of the digit. Discoloration (often red/blue tinged) in the presence of exquisite tenderness over the finger or thumb nail is a strong indication for the presence of a glomus tumor. A pyogenic granuloma is another vascular tumor that can occur at the site of minor trauma. They usually present with a friable nodule that bleeds easily. They may be amenable to cauterization or excisional surgery. Melanoma can affect the digits and would tend to be observed as a cutaneous lesion or pigmented area within the nail rather than a mass in the pulp. Pigmentation of the nail is therefore concerning in the absence of trauma and may warrant urgent nail-bed biopsy to exclude a subungual melanoma.[2,3]

REFERENCES

1. Lucas GL. Epidermoid inclusion cysts of the hand. J South Orthop Assoc 1999;8(3):188–192
2. Athanasian EA. Bone and soft tissue tumors. In: Green DP, Hotchkiss RN, Pederson WC, eds. Green's Operative Hand Surgery. 4th ed. Philadelphia, PA: Churchill Livingstone; 1998
3. Fleegler EJ. Skin tumors. In: Green DP, Hotchkiss RN, Pederson WC, eds. Green's Operative Hand Surgery. 4th ed. Philadelphia, PA: Churchill Livingstone; 1998

FINGERTIP LESIONS

5. A 78-year-old retired schoolteacher presents with a tender soft-tissue swelling between the dorsal nailfold and DIP joint of the right ring finger. It has developed over the past 12 months. She has a groove in the nail plate. *What is the most likely diagnosis?*

   D. Mucous cyst

   Mucous cysts are small ganglia that originate from the DIP joint and are associated with osteoarthritis. They may be associated with nail grooving and osteophytes. Treatment is with surgical excision of the cyst and adjacent osteophytes. This is usually performed under local anesthetic and some cases may need excision of skin and a graft or local advancement flap (such as a hatchet based on the middle phalanx). Occasionally joint fusion is required if the mucus cysts are recurrent and bothersome.

   Neurofibromas are common nerve tumors that can proliferate within and along nerve fibres. They can therefore be associated with functional abnormality such as paresthesia or pain, although for the most part they appear as benign, nodular soft-tissue growths within the skin on a background of neurofibromatosis. They may need surgical excision depending on site, size, and symptoms experienced by the patient.

   Enchondromas are benign bone tumors seen in the hand, most often in patients in their third or fourth decade of life. They are well-defined lytic lesions with relative lack of normal bone replaced by aberrant cartilage that can lead to weakness of the bone. Hence, most enchondromas are diagnosed when patients present with pathological fractures or as an incidental finding on X-ray for another reason. Treatment involves curettage and replacing the defect with bone graft or bone graft substitute. This is normally performed in the elective setting once any fractures have healed.

BCCs are slow-growing malignant skin tumors that are relatively common on the hand, but less common on the individual digits themselves. They tend to occur in the age group as in this scenario (i.e., age 60 onward) but are slow growing with typical features including a pearly appearance, pink/red discoloration, telangiectasia, and ulceration. Excision of BCCs on the hand may require reconstruction with a full-thickness skin graft or local flap.

Melanomas are malignant tumors of the skin that are relatively uncommon in the hand. When they do occur on the hand, volar or subungual locations are most common. Acral lentiginous, nodular, and superficial spreading are common subtypes seen. Wide excision may necessitate digital amputation at the next most proximal joint.[1,2]

REFERENCES

1. Athanasian EA. Bone and soft tissue tumors. In: Green DP, Hotchkiss RN, Pederson WC, eds. Green's Operative Hand Surgery. 4th ed. Philadelphia, PA: Churchill Livingstone; 1998
2. Fleegler EJ. Skin tumors. In: Green DP, Hotchkiss RN, Pederson WC, eds. Green's Operative Hand Surgery. 4th ed. Philadelphia, PA: Churchill Livingstone; 1998

TUMORS OF THE HAND AND WRIST

6. A 43-year-old right-hand–dominant carpenter presents with a small soft-tissue swelling over the volar aspect of the right wrist that has developed over 8 months. He complains of altered sensation in the little finger and pain in the ulnar digits while working, especially in cold weather. *What is the most likely diagnosis?*

B. Ulnar artery aneurysm

This patient has symptoms of ulnar nerve compression close to Guyon's canal. This can occur as a result of lesions such as a lipoma or a ganglion cyst, although the latter tends to occur on the radial rather than the ulnar aspect. Furthermore, pain and cold sensitivity on working would fit with an ischemic component to the compression. Palpation of a pulsatile mass would strongly support the diagnosis of an aneurysm, especially in the setting of emboli and digital ischemic changes. This condition is commonly seen in manual laborers, such as builders and carpenters, where it is termed "hypothenar hammer syndrome." It results from repetitive trauma to the ulnar artery at the wrist. Treatment involves resection, ligation, or interposition vein grafting.[1]

Osteoid osteomas are uncommon, benign tumors that typically affect the distal phalanx in young adult patients. They are particularly associated with night pain and this is often relieved by nonsteroidal anti-inflammatory drug use. Chondrosarcoma is a malignant tumor that can present with a mass (often close to the metacarpophalangeal joint) that is usually painful and tends to occur in older individuals. Imaging is important in further characterizing such bony lesions. Carpal bosses are often confused with ganglion cysts on the dorsal wrist, but some key differences are that bosses tend to be painful, do not fluctuate in size, are generally firmer and noncompressible, and are sited distal to the carpus over the metacarpal bases.[2,3]

REFERENCES

1. Ferris BL, Taylor LM Jr, Oyama K, et al. Hypothenar hammer syndrome: proposed etiology. J Vasc Surg 2000;31(1, Pt 1):104–113
2. Athanasian EA. Bone and soft tissue tumors. In: Green DP, Hotchkiss RN, Pederson WC, eds. Green's Operative Hand Surgery. 4th ed. Philadelphia, PA: Churchill Livingstone; 1998
3. Goiney C, Porrino J, Richardson ML, Mulcahy H, Chew FS. Characterization and epidemiology of the carpal boss utilizing computed tomography. J Wrist Surg 2017;6(1):22–32

GLOMUS TUMORS

7. A patient is referred with a suspected glomus tumor of the hand. Which one of the following is true?

D. Use of a tourniquet in clinic can help aid clinical diagnosis.

Glomus tumors are benign vascular tumors of the fingertip and are reasonably common but still represent less than 5% of all hand tumors. The key triad of symptoms are:
1. Stabbing pain in the fingertip
2. Pinpoint tenderness
3. Cold sensitivity

They tend to occur most commonly in females and almost never undergo malignant change. Assessment of patients with suspected glomus tumors would normally show discoloration of the fingertip and pain on pinpoint pressure of the affected region of the finger tip. This is termed *"Love's maneuver."* The use of a tourniquet can be useful because inflation can mitigate the pain caused by this, with recurrence of the pain on deflation. This is termed "Hildreth's sign." Plain radiographs are not especially useful in identifying this condition, but are useful to rule out other diagnoses. Ultrasound with high-frequency transducer or magnetic resonance imaging (MRI) can be helpful. Treatment of glomus tumors involves complete excision through the sterile matrix. Recurrence rates are low provided complete excision is achieved.[1,2]

REFERENCES

1. Lee W, Kwon SB, Cho SH, Eo SR, Kwon C. Glomus tumor of the hand. Arch Plast Surg 2015;42(3):295–301
2. Morey VM, Garg B, Kotwal PP. Glomus tumours of the hand: review of literature. J Clin Orthop Trauma 2016;7(4):286–291

SIGNS OF SOFT-TISSUE SARCOMA

8. You are working in the sarcoma clinic, and a 34-year-old patient is referred to you with a soft-tissue mass in the volar compartment of the proximal forearm. It has been present for 16 months, measures 4 cm in diameter, is fixed by resisted elbow flexion, and is nontender. *Which one of the following represents the most significant concern regarding this lesion?*

   D. The depth of the mass

   This may well be a benign mass such as a lipoma; however, the most concerning feature of this lesion is the tissue depth. Because it is fixed on elbow flexion, this suggests it involves the volar muscle compartment. Being deep to the fascia is one of the key criteria of concern for soft-tissue sarcomas. The other red flags are size greater than 5 cm, pain, and rapid growth. The more of these features that coexist, the more likely it is that malignancy is present. In general, the single most important concern is rapid growth of the lesion (i.e., weeks to months).[1–3]

REFERENCES

1. Grimer R, Judson I, Peake D, Seddon B. Guidelines for the management of soft tissue sarcomas. Sarcoma 2010;2010:506182
2. Stomeo D, Tulli A, Ziranu A, Mariotti F, Maccauro G. Chondrosarcoma of the hand: a literature review. J Cancer Ther 2014;5:403–409
3. Henderson M, Neumeister MW, Bueno RA Jr. Hand tumors: II. Benign and malignant bone tumors of the hand. Plast Reconstr Surg 2014;133(6):814e–821e

DIAGNOSING SOFT-TISSUE SARCOMA

9. A young adult patient is referred to the clinic with a deep, rapidly enlarging, painful soft-tissue mass in the left hand. *Which one of the following is the preferred method for obtaining an initial tissue diagnosis in this case?*

   D. Core needle biopsy

   Patients with suspected soft-tissue sarcomas should undergo triple assessment in a specialist clinic. This involves a history, examination, imaging, and biopsy. Where timing allows, it can be helpful to obtain imaging before biopsy to preserve soft-tissue appearances (e.g., on MRI), or imaging may be used to guide biopsies of deeper lesions. The recommended approach to obtaining a tissue biopsy is to take several core biopsies, because this maximizes diagnostic yield.[1] If the lesion is superficial or small, then incisional or excisional biopsies may occasionally be considered. When a biopsy is obtained, it must be planned in such a way that the biopsy tract can be completely removed en bloc during the subsequent tumor excision; hence, biopsies are generally better performed by the treating surgical team. Fine-needle aspiration cytology is not recommended as a primary diagnostic modality, although it may be useful in confirming disease recurrence. Furthermore, it only provides cells for analysis, rather than formal tissue subtyping.[1,2]

REFERENCES

1. Grimer R, Judson I, Peake D, Seddon B. Guidelines for the management of soft tissue sarcomas. Sarcoma 2010;2010:506182
2. Henderson M, Neumeister MW, Bueno RA Jr. Hand tumors: II. Benign and malignant bone tumors of the hand. Plast Reconstr Surg 2014;133(6):814e–821e

IMAGING IN SOFT-TISSUE SARCOMA

10. A patient is referred to the clinic with a suspicious soft-tissue mass in the right upper limb. It has doubled in size over the past month. *Which one of the following is the best imaging modality to use for this patient?*

C. MRI

An MRI scan is the preferred imaging modality for patients with suspected soft-tissue sarcoma, both for identifying the nature and extent of the lesion and to aid surgical planning. MRI avoids high-dose radiation and provides clear images to help assess soft-tissue and bony changes. That said, it is usual to begin with plain radiographs in the assessment of most soft tissue or bone abnormality of the hand and this will often provide some useful initial information regarding the underlying diagnosis. CT may also be useful especially for the assessment of the bone. Ultrasound is a useful modality for soft-tissue lesions, as it is low cost, noninvasive, and yet can provide valuable information on the characteristics of the mass. It can provide information on whether, for example, the lesion is a lipoma versus a liposarcoma. It also avoids a radiation dose. Once the diagnosis of sarcoma has been confirmed histologically, a high-resolution staging CT scan should be performed to exclude metastatic spread. Isotope bone scans and PET scans are not currently recommended as routine diagnostic or staging investigations for soft-tissue sarcomas.[1-3]

REFERENCES

1. Grimer R, Judson I, Peake D, Seddon B. Guidelines for the management of soft tissue sarcomas. Sarcoma 2010;2010:506182
2. Sobanko JF, Dagum AB, Davis IC, Kriegel DA. Soft tissue tumors of the hand. 2. Malignant. Dermatol Surg 2007;33(7):771–785
3. Patel DB, Matcuk GR Jr. Imaging of soft tissue sarcomas. Linchuang Zhongliuxue Zazhi 2018;7(4):35

SARCOMA SUBTYPES

11. *Which one of the following describes a soft-tissue sarcoma seen in patients with immune compromise presenting with dark blue to violaceous firm macules and plaques?*

A. Kaposi's sarcoma

There are a number of different types of sarcoma. These include epithelioid, clear cell, fibrosarcoma, synovia, and Kaposi's.

Kaposi's sarcoma is a sarcoma subtype which can be aggressive and is seen in immunocompromised patients such as those with AIDS or human herpes virus 8. It tends to present in the fourth or fifth decade of life with a male-to-female preponderance of 15:1. Clinical presentation involves dark blue to violaceous firm macules, which become replaced by infiltrative plaques measuring up to 3 cm in diameter. Treatment includes control of HIV load where applicable, radiotherapy, and chemotherapy. Kaposi's sarcoma cannot be cured but can usually be controlled.

Epithelioid sarcoma is the most common sarcoma subtype occurring in the hand and is insidious, slow growing, and typically originates on the volar surface of the palm or digits. It is treated with wide resection margins. Clear cell sarcoma is rare. It is a slow-growing tumor with a poor prognosis and tends to be a deep mass attached to tendons and aponeuroses or fascia. Fibrosarcoma can occur in the deep subcutaneous space, the facial septa, or muscle. It is insidious in onset and metastasizes by hematogenous spread. Synovial sarcoma originates in soft tissues close to joints (tendon, tendon sheath, bursa). This also has a poor prognosis and a high incidence of metastases. Treatment involves surgery and radiotherapy or chemotherapy.[1-3]

REFERENCES

1. Schneider JW, Dittmer DP. Diagnosis and treatment of Kaposi sarcoma. Am J Clin Dermatol 2017;18(4):529–539
2. Sobanko JF, Meijer L, Nigra TP. Epithelioid sarcoma: a review and update. J Clin Aesthet Dermatol 2009;2(5):49–54
3. Cormier JN, Pollock RE. Soft tissue sarcomas. CA Cancer J Clin 2004;54(2):94–109

MANAGEMENT OF SOFT-TISSUE SARCOMAS

12. *When considering the treatment principles for sarcoma of the hand, which one of the following is correct?*

B. Any diagnostic biopsy tract must be excised en bloc with the resection.

The treatment principles of sarcoma are wide resection with margins typically of 2 to 3 cm of normal tissue, or as an anatomical compartment, and the diagnostic biopsy tract must be excised en bloc with the main resection specimen. This means that in most centers, the biopsy and resection surgery are performed by the same team such that the placement of the core biopsy scar is kept within the planned confines of the final resection margins.

Using margins of 2 to 3 cm in the hand means that the risk of needing amputation is high. However, limb-preserving surgery and reconstruction with free tissue transfer can be utilized. Local recurrence is rare provided adequate margins are achieved in the first instance. Many, but not all, patients will need adjuvant radiotherapy after sarcoma surgery. Chemotherapy is not generally indicated, although it depends on the tumor subtype. Adjuvant treatment is guided by the subtype of tumor, patient's overall health, and the surgical resection margins achieved.[1–3]

REFERENCES

1. Grimer R, Judson I, Peake D, Seddon B. Guidelines for the management of soft tissue sarcomas. Sarcoma 2010;2010:506182
2. Brien EW, Terek RM, Geer RJ, Caldwell G, Brennan MF, Healey JH. Treatment of soft-tissue sarcomas of the hand. J Bone Joint Surg Am 1995;77(4):564–571
3. Nicholson S, Milner RH, Ragbir M. Soft tissue sarcoma of the hand and wrist: epidemiology and management challenges. J Hand Microsurg 2018;10(2):86–92

BENIGN BONE LESIONS OF THE HAND

13. A 26-year-old woman presents with a fracture of the proximal phalanx of the left ring finger sustained while washing dishes. She is otherwise healthy. A plain radiograph shows a well-demarcated, round, lytic lesion with some areas of calcification within the proximal phalanx. *What is the most likely diagnosis?*

C. Enchondroma

The presence of a pathologic fracture and this radiologic appearance is suggestive of an enchondroma. Enchondromas are benign bone tumors that most often occur in the third of fourth decade of life. They result from an aberrant focus of cartilage in the metacarpals or phalanges. Patients often present with a pathological fracture at the enchondroma site and radiographs show a well-defined lytic lesion with stippled calcification. The presence of multiple enchondromas is called *Ollier's disease*, and, when combined with vascular malformations, is termed *Maffucci's syndrome*. Nora's lesion was described by Nora and is also known as *bizarre parosteal osteochondromatous proliferation*.[1] It is a rare lesion affecting the tubular bones of the hand (proximal and middle phalanges and metacarpals). It is thought to be a reactive lesion and develops as an exophytic outgrowth from the cortical surface. It contains bone, cartilage, and fibrous tissue. Typical presentation involves development of an obvious tender mass over a few months. Treatment involves excision using a high-speed burr (saucerization). Periosteal chondromas are also rare and represent surface lesions arising from the periosteum of the tubular bones. They typically present as painful but slow-growing masses.[2,3]

REFERENCES

1. Nora FE, Dahlin DC, Beabout JW. Bizarre parosteal osteochondromatous proliferations of the hands and feet. Am J Surg Pathol 1983;7(3):245–250
2. Feldman F. Primary bone tumors of the hand and carpus. Hand Clin 1987;3(2):269–289
3. Henderson M, Neumeister MW, Bueno RA Jr. Hand tumors: II. Benign and malignant bone tumors of the hand. Plast Reconstr Surg 2014;133(6):814e–821e

MALIGNANT BONE TUMORS OF THE HAND

14. *Which one of the following is the most common primary malignant bone tumor in the hand and tends to occur in middle age patients?*

B. Chondrosarcoma

Chondrosarcoma is the most common primary malignant bone tumor in the hand and may develop de novo or within a benign lesion such as an osteochondroma. Chondrosarcomas represent about one-fifth of the total malignant bone tumors, but of course are not solely restricted to the hand. Overall, this is still a rare disease (1/1000,000) and tends to present in middle age (40–70). This is one area in which it differs from other bone tumors such as Ewing's sarcoma and osteosarcoma which both occur most often in adolescents and young adults. Osteosarcoma can occur in the hand in middle-aged patients but is extremely rare. Early chondrosarcomas tend not to metastasize, and may be responsive to nonsurgical treatment. However, advanced stage tumors are not only more likely to metastasize more readily, they are more resistant to both chemo and radiation therapies. The most common site of metastasis is the lung, hence the reason for regular chest radiographs in these sarcoma patients. Chondrosarcoma of the hand usually occurs in the epiphyseal regions of the phalanges or metacarpals and presents as a destructive bony lesion which is often slow growing. However, the most common anatomic sites are the femur, humerus, and pelvis. Treatment for any site is wide surgical resection. Radiotherapy is sometimes indicated in either the adjunctive setting where margins are close, or in the palliative setting.[1–4]

Ewing's sarcoma, osteosarcoma, and malignant giant cell tumors are less common in the hand. Ewing's sarcoma is an aggressive subtype of sarcoma that occurs in adolescents and young adults. It most commonly affects the femur, although it was first described by Ewing in 1921 within the radius of a 14-year-old girl.[5]

Osteosarcoma management differs from that of Ewing's and chondrosarcoma in that it tends to be very responsive to chemotherapy. Therefore, management usually involves neoadjuvant chemotherapy then surgery and further chemotherapy. Osteoblastoma is usually considered benign, although an aggressive variant has been described.[1,2]

REFERENCES

1. Stomeo D, Tulli A, Ziranu A, Mariotti F, Maccauro G. Chondrosarcoma of the hand: a literature review. J Cancer Ther 2014;5:403–409
2. Sobanko JF, Dagum AB, Davis IC, Kriegel DA. Soft tissue tumors of the hand. 2. Malignant. Dermatol Surg 2007;33(7):771–785
3. Boehme KA, Schleicher SB, Traub F, Rolauffs B. Chondrosarcoma: a rare misfortune in aging human cartilage? The role of stem and progenitor cells in proliferation, malignant degeneration and therapeutic resistance. Int J Mol Sci 2018;19(1):311
4. Riedel RF, Larrier N, Dodd L, Kirsch D, Martinez S, Brigman BE. The clinical management of chondrosarcoma. Curr Treat Options Oncol 2009;10(1-2):94–106
5. Ewing J. Diffuse endothelioma of bone. Proc NY Path Soc 1921;21:17–24

97. Dupuytren's Disease

See *Essentials of Plastic Surgery*, third edition, pp. 1354–1362

ETIOLOGIC FACTORS IN DUPUYTREN'S DISEASE

1. *Which one of the following is correct regarding Dupuytren's disease?*
   A. It occurs almost exclusively in white males over the age of 40.
   B. Excess alcohol intake has no association with its development.
   C. Inheritance is normally autosomal recessive with variable penetrance.
   D. The middle and index fingers are the most commonly affected digits.
   E. No clear correlation exists between the use of vibration tools and cord development.

DUPUYTREN'S DIATHESIS

2. A 38-year-old patient presents to clinic with palpable nontender lumps in both palms affecting the ring finger and thumb. They have been present for 6 months and are now limiting his ability to fully open his hands. His father and grandfather had similar problems, and he would like to discuss treatment options with you. *Which one of the following is correct?*
   A. All of the risk factors for Dupuytren's diathesis are present.
   B. This is a typical age of onset for Dupuytren's contracture.
   C. If he has sisters, they are unlikely to be affected.
   D. His risk of recurrence after treatment is high.
   E. Dorsal knuckle pads would be unusual in this patient.

STRUCTURES AFFECTED BY DUPUYTREN'S DISEASE

3. *Which one of the following structures is typically spared in Dupuytren's contracture?*
   A. Cleland's ligament
   B. Grayson's ligament
   C. Spiral cord
   D. Lateral digital sheet
   E. Natatory ligament

CORD COMPONENTS IN DUPUYTREN'S DISEASE

4. Your resident is presenting a case of Dupuytren's disease to you in clinic and states that the patient has a "spiral cord" on examination. *Which one of the following structures does not form part of the spiral cord?*
   A. Lateral digital sheet
   B. Grayson's ligament
   C. Landsmeer's ligament
   D. Pretendinous band
   E. Spiral band

INDICATIONS FOR SURGERY IN DUPUYTREN'S DISEASE

5. *Which one of the following is most likely to be an indication for surgical intervention in Dupuytren's disease?*
   A. A palpable spiral cord in a straight finger
   B. The presence of Garrod's pads
   C. A PIP joint contracture of 10 degrees
   D. An MCP joint contracture of 20 degrees
   E. A negative Hueston's test

COLLAGENASE INJECTIONS FOR DUPUYTREN'S CONTRACTURE

6. A patient comes to clinic having read about "an enzyme injection therapy" for Dupuytren's disease. He has unilateral disease with palpable pretendinous cords affecting the ring and little fingers. The flexion contractures are 40 degrees at the MCP joint and 10 degrees at the PIP joint. *Which one of the following is correct regarding collagenase injections for this patient?*
   A. Even if full correction is achieved, he has a 75% chance of recurrence within 3 years.
   B. Each cord will require two office visits, and both can be treated simultaneously.
   C. This treatment will avoid the risk of developing a posttreatment wound.
   D. His risk of flexor tendon rupture is approximately 5% following this treatment.
   E. He is likely to develop antibodies to *Streptococcus histolyticus* spp. following this treatment.

THE IP JOINTS IN DUPUYTREN'S DISEASE

7. *When planning a limited fasciectomy for a finger with Dupuytren's causing a PIP joint contracture, which one of the following is correct?*
   A. If a boutonniere deformity is present it is likely that the PIP joint correction will be maintained.
   B. A lazy-S volar incision is the preferred approach.
   C. Contracture of the accessory collateral ligaments and volar plate at the MCP joint is common.
   D. Correction of the PIP joint contracture may be limited by tolerance of the neurovascular bundles.
   E. In severe PIP joint contracture, aggressive joint release gives a better long-term result than fasciectomy alone.

TREATMENT OPTIONS FOR DUPUYTREN'S CONTRACTURE

8. A 55-year-old man has Dupuytren's contractures affecting the ring and little fingers of his right hand. Both MCP joints have contractures of 45 degrees and the ring finger PIP joint has a contracture of 20 degrees. There are pretendinous and spiral cords. *Which one of the following statements is correct?*
   A. Reported recurrence rates after radical fasciectomy are less than 10% at 5 years.
   B. The risk of neurovascular injury during surgery is minimal, given the anatomy of his disease.
   C. Needle fasciotomy may achieve complete correction, but recurrence would be more likely than with fasciectomy.
   D. Because both MCP and PIP joints are affected, a primary dermofasciectomy is recommended.
   E. The PIP joint is unlikely to be fully corrected with limited fasciotomy.

SURGICAL PRINCIPLES IN FASCIECTOMY

9. *When undertaking a fasciectomy for Dupuytren's disease, which one of the following is true?*
   A. Skin flaps are best designed with a narrow base to optimize movement.
   B. Dissection should start in the palm and proceed distally.
   C. All palmar fascia should normally be removed.
   D. Wounds should always be fully closed or otherwise skin grafted.
   E. A tourniquet must remain inflated until the wounds are closed.

COMPLICATIONS FOLLOWING FASCIECTOMY FOR DUPUYTREN'S

10. Following surgery for Dupuytren's disease, a patient develops a disproportionate amount of swelling, redness, and stiffness to the hand in the absence of any signs of clinical infection. *Which one of the following should be initiated in this scenario?*
    A. Splinting in the safe position
    B. Oral antibiotics
    C. Plan to return to theater
    D. A regional block
    E. Steroid and gabapentin

Answers

ETIOLOGIC FACTORS IN DUPUYTREN'S DISEASE

1. *Which one of the following is correct regarding Dupuytren's disease?*
   E. No clear correlation exists between the use of vibration tools and cord development.

   Dupuytren's disease is a benign fibroproliferative disorder that occurs in the palmar fascia leading to nodules, cords, and contractures of the fingers. There is no proven correlation with vibration tools or other manual work in development of Dupuytren's disease, although there are theories that a microtrauma mechanism may act to direct myofibroblast contracture.

   The link between alcohol intake and Dupuytren's disease has been questioned over the years. A review by Hindocha et al[1] concluded that alcohol excess is associated with the disease that is more likely to require surgical correction than conservative management, although the mechanism for this is unclear. A previous study by this group has shown that excess alcohol intake was associated with an increased severity of the disease.[2]

   The inheritance of Dupuytren's disease is thought to be autosomal dominant (not recessive) with variable penetrance. As better epidemiological data emerge, it is recognized that white men of Northern European descent are most commonly affected. The disease is also regularly encountered in women and in other ethnic groups such as Japanese individuals. There appears to be both a genetic and environmental influence on the condition. The ring and little fingers (not the middle and ring) are most commonly affected, followed by the middle finger. The thumb and index finger can be affected, but this is less common.

REFERENCES

1. Hindocha S, McGrouther DA, Bayat A. Epidemiological evaluation of Dupuytren's disease incidence and prevalence rates in relation to etiology. Hand (N Y) 2009;4(3):256–269
2. Hindocha S, Stanley JK, Watson JS, Bayat A. Revised Tubiana's staging system for assessment of disease severity in Dupuytren's disease-preliminary clinical findings. Hand (N Y) 2008;3(2):80–86

DUPUYTREN'S DIATHESIS

2. A 38-year-old patient presents to clinic with palpable nontender lumps in both palms affecting the ring finger and thumb. They have been present for 6 months and are now limiting his ability to fully open his hands. His father and grandfather had similar problems, and he would like to discuss treatment options with you. *Which one of the following is correct?*
   D. His risk of recurrence after treatment is high.

   The presence of multiple Dupuytren's diathesis factors in a patient such as this man increases the risk of recurrent disease by up to approximately 70%, compared with a baseline recurrence risk of 20–25% in patients without diathesis factors.[1] The initial description of Dupuytren's diathesis by Hueston included four factors[2]:
   1. Ethnicity
   2. Family history
   3. Bilateral disease
   4. Ectopic lesions (outside the palm)
   The scenario gives only two of these factors. He may develop ectopic disease, such as dorsal knuckle pads (Garrod's pads) and may also be affected by plantar or penile fibromatosis.

   Subsequent to Hueston's description, additional items have been added by Hindocha et al[1] who suggested two new factors: male sex and age at onset less than 50 years (for which this patient meets both criteria). These authors also proposed that the family history should include one or more affected siblings/parents and that only ectopic lesions in the knuckles (Garrod's pads) should count. Finally, because inheritance is autosomal dominant, any of his siblings including sisters are also at risk, although penetrance of the phenotype is variable.

REFERENCES

1. Hindocha S, Stanley JK, Watson S, Bayat A. Dupuytren's diathesis revisited: evaluation of prognostic indicators for risk of disease recurrence. J Hand Surg Am 2006;31(10): 1626–1634
2. Hueston JT. Dupuytren's Contracture. Edinburgh: E & S Livingstone; 1963

STRUCTURES AFFECTED BY DUPUYTREN'S DISEASE

3. *Which one of the following structures is typically spared in Dupuytren's contracture?*

A. Cleland's ligament

Dupuytren's disease affects much of the palmar fascia, but Cleland's ligaments are usually spared in this condition. These fascial bands pass dorsal to the neurovascular bundles in the fingers from the periosteum and flexor tendon sheath to the lateral skin.

Grayson's ligament passes transversely from the volar aspect of the flexor tendon sheath to the skin. It prevents bowstringing of the neurovascular bundle during digital flexion. In Dupuytren's disease Grayson's ligament is often tightly adherent to the bundle, making dissection more challenging. The natatory ligaments are found just deep to the skin, extending transversely between the web spaces and, when involved in Dupuytren's disease, may restrict both metacarpophalangeal (MCP) joint abduction and proximal interphalangeal (PIP) joint extension. The lateral digital sheet is located lateral to the neurovascular bundles within the digit and, when involved in Dupuytren's disease, can restrict proximal interphalangeal (PIP) and distal interphalangeal (DIP) joint function.[1-3]

REFERENCES

1. McFarlane RM. Patterns of the diseased fascia in the fingers in Dupuytren's contracture. Displacement of the neurovascular bundle. Plast Reconstr Surg 1974;54(1):31–44
2. McFarlane RM. On the origin and spread of Dupuytren's disease. J Hand Surg Am 2002;27(3):385–390
3. Rayan GM. Palmar fascial complex anatomy and pathology in Dupuytren's disease. Hand Clin 1999;15(1):73–86, vi–vii

CORD COMPONENTS IN DUPUYTREN'S DISEASE

4. Your resident is presenting a case of Dupuytren's disease to you in clinic and states that the patient has a "spiral cord" on examination. *Which one of the following structures does not form part of the spiral cord?*

C. Landsmeer's ligament

The presence of a spiral cord can complicate the surgical management of Dupuytren's disease, as the pliable neurovascular bundle can become distorted around the shortened fibrous structures, spiraling around the disease as it tightens up. Great care must therefore be taken when dissecting the Dupuytren's disease from the neurovascular bundle in the presence of a spiral cord, as the abnormal anatomy risks iatrogenic damage to the nerve and vessel which may be displaced to or beyond the midline of the digit. Spiral cords may cause flexion contractures of the PIP joint.

The common components of a spiral cord are:

- Lateral digital sheet
- Pretendinous band
- Spiral band
- Grayson's ligament
- Natatory ligaments (included by many, but not all, authors)

Landsmeer's ligament is not part of the spiral cord. It is also known as the oblique retinacular ligament and originates on the volar aspect of the middle phalanx and inserts on the dorsal aspect of the distal phalanx. It helps coordinate PIP joint and DIP joint motion.[1-3]

REFERENCES

1. Ritter MA. The anatomy and function of the palmar fascia. Hand 1973;5(3):263–267
2. Rayan GM. Palmar fascial complex anatomy and pathology in Dupuytren's disease. Hand Clin 1999;15(1):73–86, vi–vii
3. Macey ARM, Thomas R. "The serpentine zone": a surgeon's guide to the surface anatomy of the digital neurovascular spiral in Dupuytren's contracture. J Hand Microsurg 2018;10(1):54–56

INDICATIONS FOR SURGERY IN DUPUYTREN'S DISEASE

5. *Which one of the following is most likely to be an indication for surgical intervention in Dupuytren's disease?*

C. A PIP joint contracture of 10 degrees

Established flexion contractures of the PIP joint are the most difficult to correct because the volar structures shorten when the joint is left in flexion for a prolonged time. The MCP joint is far more forgiving, as the collateral ligaments are taut when the joint is flexed (i.e., the "safe" position for splinting). MCP joint contractures greater than 30 degrees and any PIP joint contracture are commonly quoted as indications for surgery, although lesser contractures of the MCP joint may be sufficiently troubling to warrant treatment, so the decision is tailored to the individual. Garrod's pads are rarely an indication for surgery but may be so if they are symptomatic. A positive Hueston's test is where the hand cannot be placed flat on a tabletop and may be an indication for surgery if there are associated functional problems.[1-4]

REFERENCES

1. Smith AC. Diagnosis and indications for surgical treatment. Hand Clin 1991;7(4):635–642, discussion 643
2. Rodrigues JN, Becker GW, Ball C, et al. Surgery for Dupuytren's contracture of the fingers. Cochrane Database Syst Rev 2015;(12):CD010143
3. Watt AJ, Leclercq C. Management of Dupuytren's disease. In: Neligan PC, Chang J, Van Beek AL, eds. Plastic Surgery, Vol. 6 – Hand and Upper Extremity. London: Elsevier; 2013:346–362
4. Hueston JT. The table top test. Hand 1982;14(1):100–103

COLLAGENASE INJECTIONS FOR DUPUYTREN'S CONTRACTURE

6. A patient comes to clinic having read about "an enzyme injection therapy" for Dupuytren's disease. He has unilateral disease with palpable pretendinous cords affecting the ring and little fingers. The flexion contractures are 40 degrees at the MCP joint and 10 degrees at the PIP joint. *Which one of the following is correct regarding collagenase injections for this patient?*

B. Each cord will require two office visits, and both can be treated simultaneously.

Collagenase injection for the treatment of Dupuytren's disease has more recently become popular. The treatment involves injecting collagenase into a palpable cord and then allowing it to weaken before physically breaking the cord by external manipulation 24–48 hours later. Initial recommendations were that one cord should be treated at a time, but this has been relaxed and it is considered appropriate to treat the two cords simultaneously. Two office visits remain the minimum per cord, assuming that one injection and one manipulation is sufficient. Some cords require more than one injection/manipulation cycle. Recurrence is dependent on which joint is affected as well as by other factors including disease severity. At 5 years posttreatment, significant recurrence at the MCP joint is reported to be around 20–40%, while this is increased to 60–70% at the PIP joint.[1-3] Collagenase treatment does not obviate any risk of a wound, as skin tears can commonly occur with postinjection manipulation. Therefore, all patients must be warned about wounds due to skin tears developing. These do tend to heal quickly with nonsurgical management and are not usually of great concern.

The collagenase used in Dupuytren's contracture is a blend of two clostridial collagenases, AUX I and AUX II, from *Clostridium histolyticum* (not *Streptococcus*). *Streptococcus pyogenes*, *Staphylococcus aureus*, and *Clostridium perfringens* all produce hyaluronidase (rather than collagenase) as a mechanism of penetrating soft tissues. Methods of producing hyaluronidase (Hyalase) have led to its use in local anesthesia and correction of hyaluronic acid facial fillers.

All patients will have developed antibodies to the injection by their second injection, but this has not been associated with any adverse outcomes. Subsequent tendon rupture is extremely rare, with three reports in 2,600 injections performed within the Collagenase Option for Reduction of Dupuytren's (CORD's) clinical trials.[1-4]

REFERENCES

1. Peimer CA, Blazar P, Coleman S, et al. Dupuytren contracture recurrence following treatment with collagenase clostridium histolyticum (CORDLESS study): 3-year data. J Hand Surg Am 2013;38(1):12–22
2. Werlinrud JC, Hansen KL, Larsen S, Lauritsen J. Five-year results after collagenase treatment of Dupuytren disease. J Hand Surg Eur Vol 2018;43(8):841–847
3. Peimer CA, Blazar P, Coleman S, et al. Dupuytren contracture recurrence following treatment with collagenase clostridium hystolyticum (CORDLESS study): 5-year data. J Hand Surg Am 2015;40(8):1597–1605
4. Hurst LC, Badalamente MA, Hentz VR, et al; CORD I Study Group. Injectable collagenase clostridium histolyticum for Dupuytren's contracture. N Engl J Med 2009;361(10):968–979

THE IP JOINTS IN DUPUYTREN'S DISEASE

7. *When planning a limited fasciectomy for a finger with Dupuytren's causing a PIP joint contracture, which one of the following is correct?*

D. Correction of the PIP joint contracture may be limited by tolerance of the neurovascular bundles.

Following a severe, prolonged contracture, the neurovascular bundles may be restricted and unable to tolerate full extension of the digit. The risk of vascular compromise is also increased in revision surgery.

Although aggressive release of a contracted PIP joint capsule may give improved correction of the finger intraoperatively, this may be at the expense of joint stability, or result in a loss of flexion if care is not taken. Loss of flexion may be more troublesome than loss of extension for most functional activities. Many surgeons advocate careful serial release of the accessory collateral ligaments and volar plate to improve correction, but many would advise against a forced capsulotomy. The reported outcomes are mixed, with some series demonstrating greater early loss of correction with joint release, but comparable outcomes to fasciectomy alone in the longer term.[1,2]

A lazy-S incision is not recommended as it is difficult to deal with a skin deficit using local flaps with this incision pattern. Problems with the MCP joint volar plate or ligaments would be highly unusual. A boutonniere deformity indicates central slip attenuation, and a PIP joint correction is unlikely to be maintained without this being addressed.

REFERENCES

1. Weinzweig N, Culver JE, Fleegler EJ. Severe contractures of the proximal interphalangeal joint in Dupuytren's disease: combined fasciectomy with capsuloligamentous release versus fasciectomy alone. Plast Reconstr Surg 1996;97(3):560–566, discussion 567
2. Ritchie JF, Venu KM, Pillai K, Yanni DH. Proximal interphalangeal joint release in Dupuytren's disease of the little finger. J Hand Surg [Br] 2004;29(1):15–17

TREATMENT OPTIONS FOR DUPUYTREN'S CONTRACTURE

8. A 55-year-old man has Dupuytren's contractures affecting the ring and little fingers of his right hand. Both MCP joints have contractures of 45 degrees and the ring finger PIP joint has a contracture of 20 degrees. There are pretendinous and spiral cords. *Which one of the following statements is correct?*

  C. Needle fasciotomy may achieve complete correction, but recurrence would be more likely than with fasciectomy.

  There are variable recurrence rates reported worldwide following treatment of Dupuytren's disease, and confusion arises because there is debate about whether any recurrence of disease is included in outcome figures, or whether only recurrent disease requiring further treatment should be included.[1,2] Despite these variations, it is generally accepted that needle fasciotomy shows earlier recurrence than fasciectomy. However, the trade-off of greater downtime after fasciectomy means that many surgeons and patients find needle fasciotomy preferable. Some surgeons do report comparable outcome figures with extensive needle fasciotomy. Reported recurrence rates after limited fasciectomy are in the order of 21% at 5 years, compared with 85% for needle fasciotomy.[3]

  Dermofasciectomy is usually reserved for cases with extensive skin involvement or for aggressive or recurrent disease. It is most often required over the proximal phalanx. Wounds are closed with skin grafts or left to heal by secondary intention. Radical fasciotomy involves extensive resection of volar and digital fascia including diseased and nondiseased tissue. It does not decrease the recurrence rate and carries higher rates of complication than limited fasciectomy. In this scenario, the PIP joint contractures are mild, and a full correction is likely whichever technique is performed.

REFERENCES

1. Crean SM, Gerber RA, Le Graverand MP, Boyd DM, Cappelleri JC. The efficacy and safety of fasciectomy and fasciotomy for Dupuytren's contracture in European patients: a structured review of published studies. J Hand Surg Eur Vol 2011;36(5):396–407
2. Werker PM, Pess GM, van Rijssen AL, Denkler K. Correction of contracture and recurrence rates of Dupuytren contracture following invasive treatment: the importance of clear definitions. J Hand Surg Am 2012;37(10):2095–2105.e7
3. van Rijssen AL, Ter Linden H, Werker PMN. Five-year results of a randomized clinical trial on treatment in Dupuytren's disease: percutaneous needle fasciotomy versus limited fasciectomy. Plast Reconstr Surg 2012;129(2):469–477

SURGICAL PRINCIPLES IN FASCIECTOMY

9. *When undertaking a fasciectomy for Dupuytren's disease, which one of the following is true?*

  B. Dissection should start in the palm and proceed distally.

  When undertaking a fasciectomy for Dupuytren's disease, dissection should start in the palm to safely identify the neurovascular bundles. Skin flaps are elevated to expose the normal and abnormal palmar fascia. In the palm the nerves and vessels will be deep to this fascia and, once identified, they can be traced distally under direct vision. As dissection proceeds distally into the digits, the course of the nerves and vessels may be abnormal with them encased in and distorted by disease. The risk of iatrogenic damage is minimized using this approach.

  When designing skin flaps in the palm and digits, a balance must be made between narrow bases that reduce flap vascularity and wide bases that do not transpose well. Z-plasties in the palm need to be small, as there is little movement here, whereas larger Z-plasty flaps can work over the proximal phalanx. Skin flap thickness is carefully judged to minimize residual disease attached to skin while maintaining vascularity. Where there is obvious involvement of disease with the overlying skin, dermofasciectomy should be performed. Only diseased fascia needs to be removed, as there is no benefit in radical fasciectomy, which is now only of historical interest. Complete wound closure on the palm is not necessary and in fact, leaving areas to heal by secondary intent works very well. Grafts may, however, be preferred in larger defects in the digits. Tourniquet release (if used) before wound closure allows assessment of digit vascularity and hemostasis, and reduces the risk of hematoma. Vascularity of each digit must always be checked and if the finger is white secondary to tension on the contracted digital vessels, then splinting the finger in the least amount of flexion that allows it to be pink is advocated. In clinic, extension can be progressively increased over 1–2 weeks.[1,2]

REFERENCES

1. Watt AJ, Leclercq C. Management of Dupuytren's disease. In: Neligan PC, Chang J, Van Beek AL, eds. Plastic surgery, Vol. 6 – Hand and Upper Extremity. London: Elsevier; 2013:346–362
2. Rodrigues JN, Becker GW, Ball C, et al. Surgery for Dupuytren's contracture of the fingers. Cochrane Database Syst Rev 2015;(12):CD010143

COMPLICATIONS FOLLOWING FASCIECTOMY FOR DUPUYTREN'S

10. Following surgery for Dupuytren's disease, a patient develops a disproportionate amount of swelling, redness, and stiffness to the hand in the absence of any signs of clinical infection. *Which one of the following should be initiated in this scenario?*

E. Steroid and gabapentin

The patient in this scenario is displaying signs of a Dupuytren's flare, which is sudden-onset development of swelling, redness, and stiffness to the operated hand similar to, or a subtype of, complex regional pain syndrome. This tends to occur toward the end of the first month following surgery after an apparently normal early healing response. At week 3 or 4 postsurgery, there is typically a deterioration in rehabilitation progression and function which may be linked in some way to therapy and splinting regimens.

The key steps to take are early and frequent hand therapy (not immobilization, which will lead to additional stiffness), together with methylprednisolone (Medrol) and gabapentin (Neurontin). Regular nonsteroidal medications may also be useful where not contraindicated. Sympathetic blockade (stellate ganglion block) may be helpful, rather than a regional nerve anesthetic block. Antibiotics are indicated only in cases where there is evidence of active infection with wound healing issues or erythema and cellulitis. Likewise, a return to theater would only be indicated in this scenario if underlying infection with an abscess requiring drainage was suspected.[1,2]

REFERENCES

1. Rivlin M, Osterman M, Jacoby SM, Skirven T, Ukomadu U, Osterman AL. The incidence of postoperative flare reaction and tissue complications in Dupuytren's disease using tension-free immobilization. Hand (N Y) 2014;9(4):459–465
2. Prosser R, Conolly WB. Complications following surgical treatment for Dupuytren's contracture. J Hand Ther 1996;9(4):344–348

98. Rheumatoid Arthritis

See *Essentials of Plastic Surgery*, third edition, pp. 1363–1376

PATHOPHYSIOLOGY OF RHEUMATOID ARTHRITIS

1. *Which one of the following tissues is primarily affected in rheumatoid arthritis?*
   A. Articular cartilage
   B. Periosteum
   C. Bone
   D. Tendon
   E. Synovium

DIAGNOSING RHEUMATOID ARTHRITIS

2. You see a 50-year-old woman in clinic with a 4-week history of bilateral wrist and elbow joint stiffness that is worse in the morning. She is a nonsmoker and is otherwise healthy. Recent blood tests show her to be seronegative for rheumatoid factor. *Which one of the following is correct?*
   A. She meets the criteria for a diagnosis of rheumatoid arthritis.
   B. Her blood test result excludes a diagnosis of rheumatoid arthritis.
   C. Her risk of developing rheumatoid arthritis is double that of an equivalent male.
   D. Her smoking history is not relevant to a diagnosis of rheumatoid disease
   E. Joint space narrowing on plain radiographs will confirm her diagnosis.

DEFORMITIES IN RHEUMATOID ARTHRITIS

3. *When you examine a patient with rheumatoid arthritis, which one of the following would you expect to observe?*
   A. Weakness of the radial sagittal bands
   B. Ulnar deviation of the wrist
   C. Radial deviation at the metacarpophalangeal (MCP), joints
   D. Dorsal subluxation at the MCP joints
   E. Firm subcutaneous swellings over the distal interphalangeal (DIP) joints

SITES INVOLVED IN RHEUMATOID ARTHRITIS AT THE WRIST

4. *Which one of the following is usually seen only at the wrist in the later stages of rheumatoid arthritis?*
   A. Degenerative change of the scaphoid waist
   B. Scapholunate ligament disruption
   C. Radiocarpal joint involvement
   D. Ulnar styloid involvement
   E. Distal radioulnar joint degenerative change

MCP JOINT DEFORMITY IN RHEUMATOID ARTHRITIS

5. *Which one of the following is not usually implicated in causing the characteristic deformities seen at the MCP joints in rheumatoid patients?*
   A. Radial deviation of the carpus
   B. Pinch forces between the finger and thumb
   C. Attenuation of the radial sagittal bands
   D. Ulnar subluxation of the extensor tendons
   E. Tightness of the flexor tendons

PIP JOINT SURGERY IN RHEUMATOID ARTHRITIS

6. *What is the main reason index PIP joint replacement is avoided in rheumatoid arthritis (RA)?*
   A. The joint is rarely affected by RA.
   B. Surgical access is challenging.
   C. The joint architecture precludes this.
   D. The long-term range of motion is poor.
   E. The joint soft-tissue stability is inadequate.

SWAN NECK DEFORMITY IN RHEUMATOID ARTHRITIS

7. *Which one of the following is correct regarding the swan neck deformity in rheumatoid arthritis?*
   A. Swan neck includes PIP joint flexion with DIP joint hyperextension.
   B. Abnormal PIP joint anatomy is the primary cause.
   C. It is often caused by central slip attenuation with lateral band subluxation.
   D. Function is more significantly impaired than with a boutonniere deformity.
   E. Initial treatment involves a sublimis tendon sling to stabilize the PIP joint.

THE RHEUMATOID THUMB

8. *What is the most common thumb abnormality on examination in rheumatoid arthritis?*
   A. MCP joint hyperextension
   B. Interphalangeal (IP) joint fixed flexion
   C. MCP joint flexion deformity
   D. Carpometacarpal (CMC) joint dislocation
   E. Adduction of the metacarpal

MANAGING RHEUMATOID MEDICATIONS PERIOPERATIVELY

9. You are planning to replace all four digital MCP joints with silicone prostheses in a patient with rheumatoid arthritis. *Which one of the following medications should be stopped during the perioperative period?*
   A. Methotrexate
   B. Naproxen
   C. Sulfasalazine
   D. Etanercept
   E. Prednisolone

SURGICAL PRINCIPLES IN RHEUMATOID ARTHRITIS

10. *When considering surgery in a rheumatoid patient, which one of the following is true?*
    A. Medical management must be in place for 24 months prior to surgery.
    B. Pain management is the most important indication for surgery.
    C. Functional gain is the most predictable outcome of surgery.
    D. Deformity and aesthetics are the main indication for surgery.
    E. Joint involvement in the head and neck region has little impact on surgery.

SURGICAL PROCEDURES IN RHEUMATOID ARTHRITIS

11. *Which one of the following is correct for patients with rheumatoid arthritis?*
    A. Trigger finger should be treated with surgical division of the A1 pulley.
    B. Carpal tunnel syndrome should be treated with a standard approach.
    C. Tenosynovectomy to reduce tendon rupture is increasingly common.
    D. A Mannerfelt lesion may be treated with an FDS tendon transfer.
    E. EPL rupture is the first sign of Vaughn-Jackson syndrome.

MANAGEMENT OF MCP JOINT DEFORMITIES IN RHEUMATOID ARTHRITIS

12. *When correcting severe MCP joint deformities in a patient with rheumatoid arthritis, which one of the following is commonly required?*
    A. Radial collateral release
    B. Cross-intrinsic transfer
    C. Radial sagittal band release
    D. Ulnar sagittal band imbrication
    E. Pyrocarbon MCP joint arthroplasty

UNSALVAGEABLE JOINTS IN RHEUMATOID ARTHRITIS

13 *When addressing advanced wrist and DRUJ deformities in rheumatoid arthritis, which one of the following is correct?*
    A. The Sauve-Kapandji procedure increases the risk of ulnar carpal translocation.
    B. The ulna stump may be unstable following both Darrach and Sauve-Kapandji procedures.
    C. The Darrach procedure relies on good bone stock for success.
    D. When bone stock is poor, a plate is preferable to a Steinmann pin for wrist fusion.
    E. Radioscapholunate arthrodesis may be helpful if the midcarpus is degenerative.

AUTOIMMUNE DISEASES AFFECTING THE HANDS

14. A 40-year-old woman presents with severe arthritic changes affecting both hands. She has pits in her fingernails. *What is the most likely diagnosis?*
    A. Systemic lupus erythematosus
    B. Rheumatoid arthritis
    C. Psoriatic arthritis
    D. Scleroderma
    E. Osteoarthritis

Answers

PATHOPHYSIOLOGY OF RHEUMATOID ARTHRITIS

1. Which one of the following tissues is primarily affected in rheumatoid arthritis?

E. Synovium

Rheumatoid arthritis is a chronic, progressive, systemic autoimmune inflammatory disease that primarily affects the synovium. Synovium is a thin layer of tissue that lines the articular surface of joints and tendon sheaths. It has two main functions: first, it acts as a selectively permeable membrane to control entry and exit of factors to the joint; second, it produces substances that lubricate the joint, e.g., synovial fluid.

In certain disease processes, such as rheumatoid arthritis, there is an abnormal inflammatory response within the synovium. The synovium produces matrix metalloproteinases, collagenases, and cathepsins, which in turn cause damage to the cartilage, bone, and periosteum. The end result is a thickened, inflamed synovium called pannus, with erosion of adjacent soft tissues such as tendon, joint capsule, ligament, and bone.[1-3]

REFERENCES

1. Brown FE, Collins ED, Harmatz AS. Rheumatoid arthritis of the hand and wrist. In: Achauer BM, Elof E, Guyuron B, et al, eds. Plastic Surgery: Indications, Operations, and Outcomes, Vol. 4. St Louis, MO: Mosby-Year Book; 2000
2. Feldon P, Terrono AL, Nalebuff EA. Rheumatoid arthritis in the hand and wrist. In: Green DP, Hotchkiss RN, Pederson WC, eds. Operative Hand Surgery, Vol. 2. 6th ed. Philadelphia, PA: Churchill Livingstone; 2011
3. Ramírez J, Celis R, Usategui A, et al. Immunopathologic characterization of ultrasound-defined synovitis in rheumatoid arthritis patients in clinical remission. Arthritis Res Ther 2016;18:74

DIAGNOSING RHEUMATOID ARTHRITIS

2. You see a 50-year-old woman in clinic with a 4-week history of bilateral wrist and elbow joint stiffness that is worse in the morning. She is a nonsmoker and is otherwise healthy. Recent blood tests show her to be seronegative for rheumatoid factor. Which one of the following is correct?

C. Her risk of developing rheumatoid arthritis is double that of an equivalent male.

The risk for females developing rheumatoid arthritis is two or even three times that of males. The diagnosis of rheumatoid arthritis requires that four of seven key criteria are met and that symptoms have been present for at least 6 weeks. The criteria are as follows:

1. Morning stiffness in joints
2. Soft-tissue swelling at three or more joints
3. Symmetrical involvement of joints
4. Involvement of metacarpophalangeal (MCP), proximal interphalangeal (PIP), or wrist joints
5. Rheumatoid nodules
6. Seropositive for rheumatoid factor (RF)
7. Typical radiographic findings

Therefore, although she has three of the key symptoms, she would need one further feature for the diagnosis, and her symptoms would need to persist for at least another 2 weeks. *Note that a patient being rheumatoid factor negative does **not** exclude a diagnosis of rheumatoid arthritis.* Only 70 to 80% of patients are seropositive, and some may develop positivity later in the disease. In some cases, patients become seropositive prior to experiencing any symptoms.[1,2] There does appear to be an epidemiologic association between smoking and caffeine intake and rheumatoid arthritis, although the latter is not uniformly observed in all studies, and actually decaffeinated coffee may itself be a risk factor. Tea drinking seems to be inversely related to risk of developing rheumatoid.[3] Joint space narrowing is one of the radiologic features of rheumatoid arthritis, but this is also seen in other forms of arthritis and joint spaces are sometimes increased because of swelling in early disease.[1-3]

REFERENCES

1. Arnett FC, Edworthy SM, Bloch DA, et al. The American Rheumatism Association 1987 revised criteria for the classification of rheumatoid arthritis. Arthritis Rheum 1988;31(3):315–324
2. Otón T, Carmona L. The epidemiology of established rheumatoid arthritis. Best Pract Res Clin Rheumatol 2019;33(5):101477
3. Mikuls TR, Cerhan JR, Criswell LA, et al. Coffee, tea, and caffeine consumption and risk of rheumatoid arthritis: results from the Iowa Women's Health Study. Arthritis Rheum 2002;46(1):83–91

DEFORMITIES IN RHEUMATOID ARTHRITIS

3. *When you examine a patient with rheumatoid arthritis, which one of the following would you expect to observe?*
    A. Weakness of the radial sagittal bands
    Some of the common features of established rheumatoid arthritis in the hand are:
    • Attenuation or rupture of the radial sagittal bands of the extensor digiti communis (EDC) mechanism over the MCP joint
    • **Radial** deviation of the wrist
    • **Ulnar** deviation at the MCP joints
    • Volar (not dorsal) subluxation of the MCP joints
    • Rheumatoid nodules around the olecranon and ulnar proximal forearm or other pressure points
    • Swan neck and boutonniere finger deformities
    • • Synovitis with visible swellings from pannus (e.g., around extensor compartments at the wrist)
    Firm subcutaneous swellings over the DIP joint are more characteristic of Heberden's nodes in osteoarthritis.
        It is important to understand the underlying mechanisms for rheumatoid hand deformities. Pannus generally starts to erode supporting soft tissues around joints and the tendency is for the wrist to drift into radial deviation and palmar subluxation. This alters the line of pull of the extrinsic extensor tendons to the digits, which in turn tends to lead to ulnar deviation of the digits at MCP joint level. The radial joint soft tissues are friable from inflammation and as such the dorsoradial joint capsule, radial sagittal bands, and radial collateral ligaments start to give way under this additional mechanical strain quite early in the disease process. The extensor tendons eventually drop into the sulcus between the metacarpal heads to the ulnar aspect of each joint, preventing active extension at the MCP joint and further exacerbating volar subluxation and ulnar drift at this level. Swan neck and boutonniere deformities in the digits follow suit due to the deranged mechanics of the intrinsic and extrinsic tendon mechanisms.[1-3]

REFERENCES

1. Chinchalkar SJ, Pitts S. Dynamic assist splinting for attenuated sagittal bands in the rheumatoid hand. Tech Hand Up Extrem Surg 2006;10(4):206–211
2. Feldon P, Terrono AL, Nalebuff EA. Rheumatoid arthritis in the hand and wrist. In: Green DP, Hotchkiss RN, Pederson WC, eds. Operative Hand Surgery, Vol. 2. 6th ed. Philadelphia, PA: Churchill Livingstone; 2011
3. Sammer DM, Chung KC. Rheumatologic conditions of the hand and wrist. In: Neligan PC, ed. Plastic Surgery, Vol. 6. 3rd ed. London: Elsevier; 2013

SITES INVOLVED IN RHEUMATOID ARTHRITIS AT THE WRIST

4. *Which one of the following is usually seen only at the wrist in the later stages of rheumatoid arthritis?*
    C. Radiocarpal joint involvement
    Early sites of involvement around the wrist in rheumatoid arthritis include the scaphoid waist, scapholunate ligament, ulnar styloid, and distal radioulnar joint (DRUJ). Late changes occur at the radiocarpal joint and midcarpus. Other late findings include erosion of the volar rim of radius, volar subluxation of the carpus, ulnar translocation and radial deviation of carpus, and dorsal prominence of the ulna with carpal supination (caput ulnae).[1,2]

REFERENCES

1. Feldon P, Terrono AL, Nalebuff EA. Rheumatoid arthritis in the hand and wrist. In: Green DP, Hotchkiss RN, Pederson WC, eds. Operative Hand Surgery, Vol. 2. 6th ed. Philadelphia, PA: Churchill Livingstone; 2011
2. Lister G. Rheumatoid arthritis, its variants, and osteoarthritis. In: Smith P, ed. Lister's the Hand: Diagnosis and Indications. 4th ed. London: Churchill Livingstone; 2002

MCP JOINT DEFORMITY IN RHEUMATOID ARTHRITIS

5. *Which one of the following is **not** usually implicated in causing the characteristic deformities seen at the MCP joints in rheumatoid patients?*
    E. Tightness of the flexor tendons
    The characteristic finding at the MCP joints in rheumatoid arthritis is ulnar deviation with volar subluxation. Tightness of the flexor tendons is not usually implicated in this deformity. If, however, an A1 pulley release is considered for triggering, it should be borne in mind that the flexor tendon angle of approach may drift ulnarward and further exacerbate the ulnar deviation deformity already caused by other factors. Tightness of the intrinsics is implicated in the volar subluxation, rather than the flexor tendons, and this is the rationale for releasing the intrinsics at the ulnar aspect of each MCP joint and transferring them to augment the weaker radial aspect of each joint during reconstructive surgery.

There are a number of contributory factors in ulnar deviation at the MCP joint. All of factors A through D are important. Radial deviation of the carpus alters the angle of approach of the extensor tendons to the MCP joints, while pinch forces between the thumb and fingers also push them in an ulnar direction. Pannus stretches and erodes the joint capsule (which tends to erode most dorsoradially because of the other forces in action); and the same factors similarly damage the radial sagittal bands and collateral ligaments. The extensor tendons then subluxate ulnarward into the valleys between the metacarpal heads, further increasing the deforming forces and pulling the digits ulnarward.[1,2]

REFERENCES

1. Feldon P, Terrono AL, Nalebuff EA. Rheumatoid arthritis in the hand and wrist. In: Green DP, Hotchkiss RN, Pederson WC, eds. Operative Hand Surgery, Vol. 2. 6th ed. Philadelphia, PA: Churchill Livingstone; 2011
2. Lister G. Rheumatoid arthritis, its variants, and osteoarthritis. In: Smith P, ed. Lister's the Hand: Diagnosis and Indications. 4th ed. London: Churchill Livingstone; 2002

PIP JOINT SURGERY IN RHEUMATOID ARTHRITIS

6. What is the main reason index PIP joint replacement is avoided in rheumatoid arthritis (RA)?

E. The joint soft-tissue stability is inadequate.

The index PIP joint really has only one option for surgical management in severe rheumatoid arthritis and this is arthrodesis rather than arthroplasty. This joint is subject to significant lateral loading during normal activities such as key pinch and grip, and the surrounding soft-tissue support is inadequate in RA for arthroplasty to succeed. In contrast, the long, ring, or small finger PIP joints can be effectively treated with either arthrodesis or arthroplasty. Arthrodesis can be more predictable with fewer complications, but sacrifices joint motion. Arthroplasty can be less predictable with higher complication rates, but preserves motion. The PIP joints are frequently affected by RA; so, surgery is commonly required. The surgical access is straightforward using a dorsal approach. When arthrodesis surgery is performed to the PIP joints, the joint surfaces are prepared by removing cartilage and subchondral bone, exposing cancellous bone before being stabilized with the surgeon's preferred methods which may include K-wires, a headless compression screw, or (the most common approach) tension band wiring. When PIP joint arthroplasty is performed, cartilage and subchondral bone are removed, the medullary canals are reamed to accept implant stems and a silicone prosthesis is inserted. Pyrocarbon or surface replacement arthroplasties are not good options in RA because of poor soft-tissue support.[1,2]

REFERENCES

1. Longo UG, Petrillo S, Denaro V. Current concepts in the management of rheumatoid hand. Int J Rheumatol 2015;2015:648073
2. Ibrahim MS, Jordan RW, Kallala R, Koris J, Chakrabarti I. Total proximal interphalangeal joint arthroplasty for osteoarthritis versus rheumatoid arthritis--a systematic review. Hand Surg 2015;20(1):181–190

SWAN NECK DEFORMITY IN RHEUMATOID ARTHRITIS

7. Which one of the following is correct regarding the swan neck deformity in rheumatoid arthritis?

D. Function is more significantly impaired than with a boutonniere deformity.

When stiff or fixed, swan neck deformities are much more debilitating than boutonniere deformities. With a boutonniere, patients can grip and pinch. With a swan neck, these motions are difficult or impossible. The swan neck deformity involves PIP joint hyperextension with DIP joint flexion (**Fig. 98.1**).

It can occur secondary to joint abnormalities of the DIP, PIP, or MCP joints. This is in contrast to a boutonniere deformity, which involves PIP joint flexion with DIP joint hyperextension and is always secondary to an abnormality at the level of the PIP joint.

Both boutonniere and swan neck deformities can occur secondary to pannus erosion that weakens joint support. The swan neck deformity can occur from extensor tendon rupture at the DIP joint (leading to a mallet deformity), rupture of the volar plate at the PIP joint, or rupture of the flexor digitorum superficialis (FDS) tendon insertion. Alternatively, a swan neck deformity can begin at the MCP joint secondary to volar subluxation and intrinsic muscle tightening. Central slip attenuation (resulting from pannus erosion) with lateral band subluxation describes the process underlying a boutonniere deformity in RA.

Initial treatment for a swan neck deformity is with a splint, and rebalancing surgery is considered only if this fails, and the PIP joint remains supple. Surgical interventions include using a slip of the FDS tendon or one lateral band to prevent PIP joint hyperextension and may require intrinsic muscle release. PIP joint fusion in a more functional position may also be helpful.[1-3]

REFERENCES

1. Lister G. Rheumatoid arthritis, its variants, and osteoarthritis. In: Smith P, ed. Lister's the Hand: Diagnosis and Indications. 4th ed. London: Churchill Livingstone; 2002
2. Boyer MI, Gelberman RH. Operative correction of swan-neck and boutonniere deformities in the rheumatoid hand. J Am Acad Orthop Surg 1999;7(2):92–100
3. Firpo CA. Correction of swan-neck and boutonnière deformities. Ann Chir Gynaecol Suppl 1985;198:48–53

THE RHEUMATOID THUMB

8. *What is the most common thumb abnormality on examination in rheumatoid arthritis?*

   C. MCP joint flexion deformity

      The most common thumb abnormality in a rheumatoid patient is a boutonniere deformity, which is also termed a Z-deformity. This involves MCP joint flexion with IP joint hyperextension and radial abduction of the metacarpal. It occurs because of dorsal pannus erosion leading to rupture of the EPB insertion and volar subluxation of the extensor pollicis longus (EPL). Swan neck deformity is commonly seen in rheumatoid patients, although less frequent in the thumb. This involves MCP joint hyperextension, IP joint flexion, and adduction contracture of the metacarpal secondary to CMC joint subluxation. This process occurs secondary to volar pannus erosion through the joint capsule and MCP joint volar plate (see **Fig. 98.1**)[1,2]

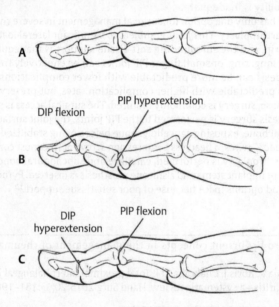

Fig. 98.1 Characteristics of swan neck and boutonniere deformities. *A*, Normal. *B*, Swan neck. *C*, Boutonniere deformity. (Adapted from Smith P, ed. Lister's The Hand, 4th ed. London: Churchill Livingstone, 2002.)

REFERENCES

1. Stein AB, Terrono AL. The rheumatoid thumb. Hand Clin 1996;12(3):541–550
2. Dyer GS, Simmons BP. Rheumatoid thumb. Hand Clin 2011;27(1):73–77

MANAGING RHEUMATOID MEDICATIONS PERIOPERATIVELY

9. You are planning to replace all four digital MCP joints with silicone prostheses in a patient with rheumatoid arthritis. *Which one of the following medications should be stopped during the perioperative period?*

   D. Etanercept

      Pharmacologic agents used in rheumatoid arthritis can be broadly classified as nonsteroidal anti-inflammatory drugs (e.g., naproxen and indomethacin), steroids (e.g., prednisolone) and disease-modifying antirheumatoid drugs (DMARDs). DMARDs are further subdivided into conventional (e.g., methotrexate, sulfasalazine, and gold) and biologic (e.g., etanercept and infliximab).

      As a general guide, most medications used in rheumatoid arthritis can be continued safely during the perioperative period for relatively small procedures like MCP joint replacement. However, there is an exception with the biological DMARDS. These should be stopped for 2 to 4 weeks before and after surgery (depending on the half-life of the drug). The injectable biologic agents are anti-tumor necrosis factor-alpha agents, and their use is associated with increased gram-positive infection.[1] If in doubt, you should discuss the perioperative management of rheumatoid medications with the patient's rheumatologist, because stopping medications can lead to a rheumatoid flare.[1,2]

REFERENCES

1. Dixon WG, Watson K, Lunt M, Hyrich KL, Silman AJ, Symmons DP; British Society for Rheumatology Biologics Register. Rates of serious infection, including site-specific and bacterial intracellular infection, in rheumatoid arthritis patients receiving anti-tumor necrosis factor therapy: results from the British Society for Rheumatology Biologics Register. Arthritis Rheum 2006;54(8):2368–2376
2. Abbasi M, Mousavi MJ, Jamalzehi S, et al. Strategies toward rheumatoid arthritis therapy; the old and the new. J Cell Physiol 2019;234(7):10018–10031

SURGICAL PRINCIPLES IN RHEUMATOID ARTHRITIS

10. *When considering surgery in a rheumatoid patient, which one of the following is true?*

   B. Pain management is the most important indication for surgery.

The most important and predictable indication for surgery in rheumatoid arthritis is pain management. Improved function is also clearly important and therefore an indication in many cases, but is less predictably achieved than pain relief. Neither deformity nor aesthetics alone are strong indications for surgery. For example, deformity can be severe, yet there may be absent pain and good function. Surgery to correct a visible deformity might risk downgrading function. When considering surgery, it is good practice to ensure all nonoperative measures have been explored. It is generally accepted that 6–12 months of medical therapy is adequate time to try before embarking on surgery. There are always exceptions, some of which include transfers for or repair of spontaneous tendon ruptures, nerve decompressions, or early synovectomy to prevent tendon destruction.

The involvement of joints in the head and neck region has significant impact on surgical management of the hands in rheumatoid arthritis, because limited movement at the temporomandibular or atlantoaxial joints can make airway management and safe intubation a challenge in general anesthesia.[1,2]

REFERENCES

1. O'Brien ET. Surgical principles and planning for the rheumatoid hand and wrist. Clin Plast Surg 1996;23(3):407–420
2. Sammer DM, Chung KC. Rheumatologic conditions of the hand and wrist. In: Neligan PC, ed. Plastic Surgery, Vol. 6. 3rd ed. London: Elsevier; 2013

SURGICAL PROCEDURES IN RHEUMATOID ARTHRITIS

11. *Which one of the following is correct for patients with rheumatoid arthritis?*

   D. A Mannerfelt lesion may be treated with an FDS tendon transfer.

A *Mannerfelt lesion* is a spontaneous rupture of the FPL tendon observed in the rheumatoid hand.[1] It is usually caused by osteophytes around the scaphoid, which must be debrided at the time of reconstruction to reduce the risk of recurrent attrition. The FPL is usually reconstructed with an index FDS transfer, tendon graft, or arthrodesis of the thumb IP joint.

Trigger finger and carpal tunnel syndrome are treated differently in rheumatoid patients, because the underlying cause is usually tenosynovitis and there can be adverse mechanical side effects from standard surgical management of these conditions. Carpal tunnel syndrome can result from the compressive effect of thick tenosynovitis/pannus within the carpal tunnel and should generally be treated with an extended carpal tunnel release and synovectomy. Trigger finger results from focal tenosynovitis or a rheumatoid nodule within the sheath or tendon. It should also be treated with synovectomy. Division of the A1 pulley will increase the likelihood of ulnar deviation at the MCP joints, and should be avoided where at all possible. Although early tenosynovectomy can reduce the risk of tendon rupture, it is less commonly required nowadays because of the improved medical control of rheumatoid arthritis.

The term *Vaughn-Jackson syndrome* refers to spontaneous attrition rupture of the extensor tendons, starting with the little finger (not the thumb) and progressing with sequential rupture from ulnar to radial.[2] Isolated EPL rupture may be treated with EIP transfer, but again it is vital that the underlying friction points are excised and covered with capsular flaps where possible to prevent recurrence.[3,4]

REFERENCES

1. Mannerfelt L, Norman O. Attrition ruptures of flexor tendons in rheumatoid arthritis caused by bony spurs in the carpal tunnel. A clinical and radiological study. J Bone Joint Surg Br 1969;51(2):270–277

2. Vaughan-Jackson OJ. Rupture of extensor tendons by attrition at the inferior radio-ulnar joint; report of two cases. J Bone Joint Surg Br 1948;30B(3):528–530
3. O'Brien ET. Surgical principles and planning for the rheumatoid hand and wrist. Clin Plast Surg 1996;23(3):407–420
4. Sammer DM, Chung KC. Rheumatologic conditions of the hand and wrist. In: Neligan PC, ed. Plastic Surgery, Vol. 6. 3rd ed. London: Elsevier; 2013

MANAGEMENT OF MCP JOINT DEFORMITIES IN RHEUMATOID ARTHRITIS

12. *When correcting severe MCP joint deformities in a patient with rheumatoid arthritis, which one of the following is commonly required?*
    B. Cross-intrinsic transfer
    The typical deformity at the MCP joint level in rheumatoid is ulnar deviation, with volar subluxation. This can be corrected with the following maneuvers:
    - Intrinsic muscle release to allow MCP joint extension
    - Cross-intrinsic transfer: The tight intrinsic tendon on the ulnar side is sutured to the radial side of the adjacent digit to relieve ulnar-deviating forces and strengthen corrective radially deviating forces.
    - Ulnar-side sagittal band (which is tight) is released: This helps centralize the subluxed extensor tendon
    - The radial-side sagittal band (which is attenuated) is tightened: This helps centralize the subluxed extensor tendon
    - The radial collateral ligament is tightened or reconstructed: This helps correct the ulnar deviation
    If the joint surface is preserved, an arthroplasty is not required. However, if the joint surface requires replacement, it is important to complete careful soft-tissue rebalancing, since typical flexible silicone prostheses will not be strong enough to realign the joint alone and deviating forces across a prosthesis will also encourage erosion of arthroplasty stems through soft bone. Silicone prostheses are preferred to pyrocarbon in rheumatoid MCP joints due to poor soft-tissue stability.[1,2]

REFERENCES

1. Oster LH, Blair WF, Steyers CM, Flatt AE. Crossed intrinsic transfer. J Hand Surg Am 1989;14(6):963–971
2. Kozlow JH, Chung KC. Current concepts in the surgical management of rheumatoid and osteoarthritic hands and wrists. Hand Clin 2011;27(1):31–41

UNSALVAGEABLE JOINTS IN RHEUMATOID ARTHRITIS

13. *When addressing advanced wrist and DRUJ deformities in rheumatoid arthritis, which one of the following is correct?*
    B. The ulna stump may be unstable following both Darrach and Sauve-Kapandji procedures.
    The Sauve-Kapandji procedure fuses the detached ulnar head to the distal radius, with the aim of relieving pain from a degenerative DRUJ and restoring pro/supination, while stabilizing the triangular fibrocartilage complex (TFCC) and ulnar wrist joint and reducing the risk of ulnarward carpal translocation[1] The Darrach procedure involves excision of the ulnar head and may increase the risk of carpal translocation, despite preservation of the TFCC remnants and ulnar collateral ligament of the wrist.[2] Since there is no element of fusion or fixation in a Darrach procedure, bone stock is not as important as in many other wrist procedures in rheumatoid arthritis. The distal ulna stump may be unstable following both, potentially leading to pain.
    During wrist fusion, a common technique is to insert a Stanley or Steinmann pin (with a single trochar tip) through from the third metacarpal head, along the shaft, through the carpus, and into the radius. This technique has been in use since the 1960s, and a variety of different pins have been used. The original general purpose Steinmann pins have been modified by Stanley et al.[3] Some surgeons insert the pin between, rather than through, the metacarpals, although this is less common. Although plating techniques (often using precontoured compression plates) are also available for wrist fusion, these generally require good bone stock for adequate purchase and are less frequently used in rheumatoid arthritis than in osteoarthritis. Locking plates can ameliorate this problem to a degree. Radioscapholunate arthrodesis is only of use in scenarios where the midcarpal joint surfaces are preserved.

REFERENCES

1. Vincent KA, Szabo RM, Agee JM. The Sauve-Kapandji procedure for reconstruction of the rheumatoid distal radioulnar joint. J Hand Surg Am 1993;18(6):978–983
2. Lee SK, Hausman MR. Management of the distal radioulnar joint in rheumatoid arthritis. Hand Clin 2005;21(4):577–589
3. Stanley JK, Gupta SR, Hullin MG. Modified instruments for wrist fusion. J Hand Surg [Br] 1986;11(2):245–249

AUTOIMMUNE DISEASES AFFECTING THE HANDS

14. A 40-year-old woman presents with severe arthritic changes affecting both hands. She has pits in her fingernails. *What is the most likely diagnosis?*

C. Psoriatic arthritis

Nail pitting is a feature of psoriatic arthritis, which is a seronegative arthropathy. The skin may be minimally affected, with some patients reporting only mild scalp psoriasis rather than florid plaques. The arthritic changes can be severe, with marked dissolution of bone leading to arthritis mutilans. The DIP joints are more often involved than in rheumatoid arthritis.

Nail pitting is not a feature of the other conditions listed. Systemic lupus erythematosus is a multisystem disease found in young women. Hand findings include joint problems without cartilage destruction and with normal joint spaces retained. The hallmark of this condition is ligamentous and volar plate laxity with tendon subluxation. The visual deformity is similar to rheumatoid arthritis but with preservation of joint surfaces. Scleroderma is another multisystem disease that can affect the hand. Key features include fingertip ulceration, Raynaud's phenomenon, and sclerodactyly. The small vessel vasculitis can result in fingertip ulceration, chronic wounds, and amputations. Contractures usually result from skin and soft-tissue changes, with MCP joint hyperextension and PIP joint flexion contractures both common. Osteoarthritis tends to present with pain, swelling, stiffness, and deformity in the small joints of the hand. Characteristic findings include Heberden's nodules near the DIP joint and Bouchard nodes near the PIP joint.[1]

REFERENCE

1. Liu JT, Yeh HM, Liu SY, Chen KT. Psoriatic arthritis: epidemiology, diagnosis, and treatment. World J Orthop 2014;5(4):537–543

99. Osteoarthritis

See *Essentials of Plastic Surgery*, third edition, pp. 1377–1388

DEMOGRAPHICS OF OSTEOARTHRITIS

1. *Which one of the following groups is most likely to have osteoarthritis (OA) of the hand?*
   A. Males between age 30 and 40
   B. Females between age 30 and 40
   C. Males between age 60 and 70
   D. Females between age 60 and 70
   E. Males and females between age 60 and 70

CLINICAL HISTORY IN OSTEOARTHRITIS

2. *When taking a history from a patient with OA of the hands, which one of the following would be unusual?*
   A. Pain that is worse in the morning
   B. Perceived weakness of grip
   C. Pain that affects sleeping patterns
   D. Increased discomfort with joint loading and movement
   E. Involvement of the interphalangeal (IP) joints and wrist

JOINTS AFFECTED BY OSTEOARTHRITIS

3. *Which one of the following joints is most commonly affected by OA in the first ray?*
   A. IP joint
   B. Metacarpophalangeal (MCP) joint
   C. Carpometacarpal (CMC) joint
   D. Scaphoid–trapezium–trapezoid (STT) joint
   E. Midcarpal joint

EXAMINATION OF THE OSTEOARTHRITIC HAND

4. *When examining a patient with OA of the hand, where would you expect to find Heberden's nodes?*
   A. DIP joint
   B. Proximal interphalangeal (PIP) joint
   C. MCP joint
   D. Olecranon
   E. In the palm

PLAIN RADIOGRAPHS IN OSTEOARTHRITIS

5. *Which one of the following tends to be the earliest finding in OA on plain radiographs?*
   A. Joint space narrowing
   B. Joint space widening
   C. Joint subluxation
   D. Subchondral sclerosis/eburnation
   E. Osteophytes and periarticular erosions

IMAGING FOR OSTEOARTHRITIS OF THE THUMB

6. *Which one of the following radiographic views gives a true anteroposterior image of the thumb and allows visualization of all four articulations of the trapezium?*
   A. Waters' view
   B. Bett's view
   C. Robert's view
   D. Eaton's stress view
   E. Towne's view

CLINICAL HISTORY IN HAND OSTEOARTHRITIS

7. A patient with a several year history of OA presents with hand pain and stiffness. He describes particular difficulty pulling his pants up and opening food jars. *Which one of the following joints of the hand is most likely to be affected?*
   A. First CMC
   B. Fifth CMC
   C. First MCP
   D. Fifth MCP
   E. Second PIP

INDICATIONS FOR SURGERY IN HAND OSTEOARTHRITIS

8. *Which one of the following is the main indication for surgery in OA of the hand?*

A. Stiffness

B. Poor aesthetics

C. Pain relief

D. Poor range of motion

E. Deformity

NONOPERATIVE MANAGEMENT OF HAND OSTEOARTHRITIS

9. *Which one of the following treatments should be avoided in patients with OA of the hand?*

A. Rest and heat treatment

B. Nonsteroidal anti-inflammatories

C. Night splinting

D. Steroid injections

E. Disease-modifying drugs (DMARDS)

THUMB CMC JOINT OSTEOARTHRITIS

10. A 60-year-old woman has a 1-year history of increasing pain at the base of her dominant thumb. She takes regular analgesia and has tried a custom thermoplastic splint, but these have not significantly helped her symptoms. Radiographs show Eaton's grade IV arthritic changes affecting the thumb base. *What is the next most likely step in the management for this patient?*

A. Image-guided steroid injection to the CMC and scaphotrapezial (ST) joints

B. First CMC joint fusion

C. First CMC joint arthroplasty

D. Standard trapeziectomy

E. Trapeziectomy with ligament reconstruction and tendon interposition (LRTI)

MANAGING THUMB CMC JOINT OSTEOARTHRITIS

11. A 23-year-old woman presents with painful, subluxing first CMC joints without degenerative changes on X-ray. *How should this best be managed surgically?*

A. Trapeziectomy alone

B. Trapeziectomy plus LRTI

C. Volar beak and intermetacarpal ligament reconstruction

D. First CMC joint fusion

E. Pyrocarbon CMC joint arthroplasty

MCP JOINT OSTEOARTHRITIS

12. *In a young, active patient with severe symptomatic OA in the middle finger MCP joint following trauma, which one of the following is most likely to provide the best result in the medium to long term, assuming that range of motion is 0 to 90 degrees in this joint?*

A. Steroid injection

B. Silastic arthroplasty

C. Arthrodesis

D. Pyrocarbon arthroplasty

E. Ray amputation

PIP JOINT OSTEOARTHRITIS

13. *Which one of the following is most likely to fail in painful OA of the dominant index finger PIP joint?*

A. Denervation of the PIP joint

B. Silastic arthroplasty

C. Arthrodesis–plating

D. Pyrocarbon arthroplasty

E. Arthrodesis–tension band technique

DIP JOINT OSTEOARTHRITIS

14. *Which one of the following is correct regarding DIP joint OA?*

A. Severity of deformity and symptoms are positively correlated.

B. It is frequently seen in association with Notta's nodes.

C. A consistent finding is deformity of the nail plate.

D. Joint fusion is usually indicated.

E. Ideal joint fusion angles are less than for the PIP joint.

Answers

DEMOGRAPHICS OF OSTEOARTHRITIS

1. Which one of the following groups is most likely to have osteoarthritis (OA) of the hand?

D. Females between age 60 and 70

Hand and wrist OA is a common condition that affects patients of varying ages, most typically in middle to older age individuals. It is most commonly seen in patients older than 65 years, and incidence is much higher in women than in men. This gender difference is thought to be related to hormonal influences on the ligamentous support of joints leading to laxity and increased early joint wear. Of the population affected by OA, less than 2% are younger than 45 years, around 30% are between 45 and 64 years, with the remainder being older than 65 years. OA can be classified as either primary or secondary. Primary means idiopathic and is associated with genetic factors combined with cartilage aging secondary to mechanical forces. Secondary means there has been a causative factor which would be trauma, joint infection, or repetitive minor injury. These factors may lead to arthritis through joint instability, abnormal loading, or direct cartilage damage.[1,2]

REFERENCES

1. Johnson VL, Hunter DJ. The epidemiology of osteoarthritis. Best Pract Res Clin Rheumatol 2014;28(1):5–15
2. Neogi T, Zhang Y. Epidemiology of osteoarthritis. Rheum Dis Clin North Am 2013;39(1):1–19

CLINICAL HISTORY IN OSTEOARTHRITIS

2. When taking a history from a patient with OA of the hands, which one of the following would be unusual?

A. Pain that is worse in the morning

The pain experienced by patients with OA of the upper limb is variable. It can be constant or intermittent and ranges from a dull ache to a sharp pain. Pain typically occurs with joint loading and repetitive movement, and it is often better in the morning and worse at night after a day's activities. This is in contrast to rheumatoid arthritis which tends to be more painful in the morning and associated with stiffness that improves as the day progresses. OA frequently affects sleep patterns, and this can be a key factor in determining when surgical intervention is warranted. Subjective weakness is common and may result from a combination of pain and reduced range of motion. OA symptoms such as weakness may be exacerbated by coexisting conditions: for example, many patients, particularly those with first carpometacarpal (CMC) joint arthritis, also have carpal tunnel syndrome.[1]

REFERENCE

1. Haugen IK, Englund M, Aliabadi P, et al. Prevalence, incidence and progression of hand osteoarthritis in the general population: the Framingham Osteoarthritis Study. Ann Rheum Dis 2011;70(9):1581–1586

JOINTS AFFECTED BY OSTEOARTHRITIS

3. Which one of the following joints is most commonly affected by OA in the first ray?

C. CMC joint

Although distal interphalangeal (DIP) joints are the joint most commonly affected by OA in the upper limb overall, the most commonly affected joint in the first ray is the CMC joint rather than the interphalangeal (IP) joint. When considering treatment for first CMC joint arthritis, it is important to look at the scaphoid–trapezium–trapezoid joint at the same time, because there may be disease between the scaphoid and trapezoid that could lead to persistent pain after trapeziectomy if it is not addressed.[1]

The first ray can be regarded as a column based on the radial aspect of the radius from scaphoid, through trapezium, into the metacarpal and phalanges. The midcarpal joint is adjacent to, rather than a component of, this column.

REFERENCE

1. Haugen IK, Englund M, Aliabadi P, et al. Prevalence, incidence and progression of hand osteoarthritis in the general population: the Framingham Osteoarthritis Study. Ann Rheum Dis 2011;70(9):1581–1586

EXAMINATION OF THE OSTEOARTHRITIC HAND

4. *When examining a patient with OA of the hand, where would you expect to find Heberden's nodes?*
   A. DIP joint
      Heberden's nodes are found at the DIP joint in patients with OA, while Bouchard's nodes are located over the PIP joint. They both represent strong markers for underlying IP joint OA and are a familial trait. They were traditionally thought to represent osteophytes but may actually represent traction spurs due to repetitive loading. Heberden's and Bouchard's nodes are sometimes painful and can also be associated with ganglia and mucous cysts. Other characteristic findings in the osteoarthritic hand include swelling and deviation of the digits, particularly at the IP joints and less frequently at the MCP joints. There is usually a reduction in both active and passive joint motion which may be associated with ligament instability or pain.[1]

      Nodules in the palm are more common with Dupuytren's, trigger finger, or a flexor sheath ganglion. Nodules around the olecranon are associated with rheumatoid arthritis.

REFERENCE

1. Alexander CJ. Heberden's and Bouchard's nodes. Ann Rheum Dis 1999;58(11):675–678

PLAIN RADIOGRAPHS IN OSTEOARTHRITIS

5. *Which one of the following tends to be the earliest finding in OA on plain radiographs?*
   B. Joint space widening
      The classic radiographic features of OA are joint space narrowing, subchondral sclerosis, and osteophyte formation (see Fig. 99.1, *Essentials of Plastic Surgery,* third edition).[1] However, the earliest sign is actually joint space widening secondary to inflammation causing an effusion. An example of how these stages are used in classifying osteoarthritic changes is in the Eaton–Littler classification of thumb CMC joint OA.[2] In advanced cases, joint subluxation may occur. Periarticular erosions are associated with rheumatoid arthritis. Progressive subchondral sclerosis can lead to eburnation, which is the degeneration of bone into a hard, ivory-like mass as seen in OA. It explains why breaking up the trapezium during a trapeziectomy can sometimes seem to be disproportionately difficult.

REFERENCES

1. Feydy A, Pluot E, Guerini H, Drapé JL. Role of imaging in spine, hand, and wrist osteoarthritis. Rheum Dis Clin North Am 2009;35(3):605–649
2. Eaton RG, Glickel SZ. Trapeziometacarpal osteoarthritis. Staging as a rationale for treatment. Hand Clin 1987;3(4):455–471

IMAGING FOR OSTEOARTHRITIS OF THE THUMB

6. *Which one of the following radiographic views gives a true anteroposterior image of the thumb and allows visualization of all four articulations of the trapezium?*
   C. Robert's view
      For patients with suspected OA of the first CMC joint, plain radiographs of the hand and wrist in the anteroposterior (AP), lateral, and oblique planes are commonly ordered. Additional views can also be helpful[1]; for example, Robert's view is a true AP view of the thumb and is taken with the hand in hyperpronation and the dorsum of the thumb against the cassette, which allows visualization of all four articulations of the trapezium. Eaton's posteroanterior (PA) stress views are taken with the thumbs pressed together and may be useful to assess increased CMC joint laxity. Bett's/Gedda's view is a PA taken in pronation and flexion that gives a true lateral view of the trapeziometacarpal joint. The other trapezial articulations are also clearly demonstrated. Waters' and Towne's views are both craniofacial radiographs used in the assessment of facial trauma injuries.

REFERENCE

1. Melville DM, Taljanovic MS, Scalcione LR, et al. Imaging and management of thumb carpometacarpal joint osteoarthritis. Skeletal Radiol 2015;44(2):165–177

CLINICAL HISTORY IN HAND OSTEOARTHRITIS

7. A patient with a several year history of OA presents with hand pain and stiffness. He describes particular difficulty pulling his pants up and opening food jars. *Which one of the following joints of the hand is most likely to be affected?*
   A. First CMC
      The first CMC joint is a biconcave saddle joint that allows flexion, extension, and opposition at the thumb base. It has an important role in a number of key power grip functions. It is normally a very stable joint with 16 described ligaments supporting it. The most important of these are thought to be the dorsoradial and deep anterior oblique ligaments.[1]

The first CMC joint is very commonly affected by OA which can develop with advancing age, hormonal influences, or posttrauma.[2] Key findings in the clinical history are pain with or without swelling, a weak lateral pinch (pulling pants up or holding large objects/book) and a weak grip (opening jars/door knobs).

Physical examination will likely demonstrate thumb metacarpal adduction into the palm and dorsal subluxation of the CMC joint, with or without compensatory MCP joint hyperextension. Pain is typically induced by distraction and torque, or joint loading.

REFERENCES

1. Colman M, Mass DP, Draganich LF. Effects of the deep anterior oblique and dorsoradial ligaments on trapeziometacarpal joint stability. J Hand Surg Am 2007;32(3):310–317
2. Haugen IK, Englund M, Aliabadi P, et al. Prevalence, incidence and progression of hand osteoarthritis in the general population: the Framingham Osteoarthritis Study. Ann Rheum Dis 2011;70(9):1581–1586

INDICATIONS FOR SURGERY IN HAND OSTEOARTHRITIS

8. Which one of the following is the main indication for surgery in OA of the hand?

  C. Pain relief

The presence of OA in the hand can present a number of problems for the patient. The most important of these, and the primary reason for undergoing surgery, is pain. This is also true of other joints such as the hip, knee, and shoulder. There may also be loss of function due to stiffness, deformity, and reduced range of joint motion. The overall aim of surgery is to gain a functional advantage for the patient; therefore, there should be a clear goal for each procedure. Two main approaches exist: arthrodesis and arthroplasty. Neither procedure will usually improve range of motion, although the relief of pain following surgery sometimes can increase the useful range at a joint (e.g., thumb base). At best, an arthroplasty will usually provide a similar amount of motion as presurgery but without pain, and arthrodesis will obviously limit movement but relieve pain. Aesthetics are down the list in terms of importance when compared with pain and function for most patients in relation to hand OA, although this is certainly not always the case.[1–3]

REFERENCES

1. Hunter DJ, Felson DT. Osteoarthritis. BMJ 2006;332(7542):639–642
2. Swanson AB, Swanson GD. Osteoarthritis in the hand. J Hand Surg Am 1983;8(5, Pt 2):669–675
3. Lane JCE, Rodrigues JN, Furniss D, Burn E, Poulter R, Gardiner MD. Basal thumb osteoarthritis surgery improves health state utility irrespective of technique: a study of UK Hand Registry data. J Hand Surg Eur Vol 2020;45(5):436–442

NONOPERATIVE MANAGEMENT OF HAND OSTEOARTHRITIS

9. Which one of the following treatments should be avoided in patients with OA of the hand?

  E. Disease-modifying drugs (DMARDS)

There are a number of nonsurgical interventions that may be useful in managing OA of the hand. DMARDS, such as methotrexate, leflunomide, and sulphasalazine, have not been shown to offer any significant improvement in pain in this patient group. DMARDS are best reserved for other hand conditions such as rheumatoid arthritis.

First-line treatment for hand OA is rest and heat. Heat is typically applied by placing the hand in water or wax twice daily, usually initially guided by a hand therapist. Nonsteroidal anti-inflammatory drugs (NSAIDs) such as ibuprofen, diclofenac, or meloxicam can be useful for managing the symptoms of OA; however, caution should be exercised in those with peptic ulcers or asthma, and in the older population where comorbidities may mean NSAIDs are contraindicated. Both topical and systemic NSAIDs have a role. Opioid medications should be minimized where at all possible due to their addictive properties and side effects. Splinting at night can be beneficial for some patients to offload involved joints and relieve sleep disturbance due to painful joint movements. Range-of-motion exercises must be maintained to optimize the movement in associated joints and to avoid deconditioning of muscles. Intra-articular steroid injections can reduce pain in OA and these are often delivered with radiological guidance.

Other treatments that have been tried include autologous fat injections and hyaluronic acid injection. There is some limited evidence of the effectiveness of these interventions.[1,2]

REFERENCES

1. Herold C, Rennekampff HO, Groddeck R, Allert S. Autologous fat transfer for thumb carpometacarpal joint osteoarthritis: a prospective study. Plast Reconstr Surg 2017;140(2): 327–335
2. Figen Ayhan F, Üstün N. The evaluation of efficacy and tolerability of Hylan G-F 20 in bilateral thumb base osteoarthritis: 6 months follow-up. Clin Rheumatol 2009;28(5):535–541

THUMB CMC JOINT OSTEOARTHRITIS

10. A 60-year-old woman has a 1-year history of increasing pain at the base of her dominant thumb. She takes regular analgesia and has tried a custom thermoplastic splint, but these have not significantly helped her symptoms. Radiographs show Eaton's grade IV arthritic changes affecting the thumb base. *What is the next most likely step in the management for this patient?*

A. Image-guided steroid injection to the CMC and ST joints.

This woman has radiographically advanced disease according to Eaton's classification, and is likely to need surgical intervention at some point in the future. However, symptoms do not always correlate with radiologic findings, and nonoperative measures should be explored fully in the first instance. The next step in her management is to trial one or more intra-articular steroid injections. Image guidance can be very helpful in ensuring accurate steroid placement (particularly in the presence of subluxation and osteophyte formation).

Eaton's classification may be used to grade the radiographic changes observed in OA and originally included four grades (**Table 99.1**). Grade IV disease involves degenerative destruction of both the first CMC joint and the ST joint. In this scenario, surgery that only addresses the CMC joint will not resolve the patient's symptoms; therefore, neither CMC joint arthroplasty nor CMC joint fusion is appropriate for this woman. The likely surgical procedure of choice would be a trapeziectomy, and if this is performed, the remaining interface between the scaphoid and trapezoid must be inspected, since there is a likelihood of arthritic changes here too that can lead to persistent pain if left untreated. There is no consistent evidence that LRTI is superior to simple trapeziectomy alone in general. However, there are scenarios where one is more appropriate than the other and most surgeons base their choice upon factors such as functional demands of the patient, best results in that surgeon's hands, and intraoperative instability of the metacarpal following trapeziectomy alone.[1,2]

Table 99.1 *Eaton's Radiographic Stages of CMC Joint Degeneration*[1]

Stage	Radiographic Findings
I	Normal articulations with widening of joint space suggestive of an effusion, less than one-third CMC joint subluxation
II	Slight narrowing of the thumb CMC joint, minimal subchondral sclerosis, debris/osteophytes <2 mm diameter, more than a third of CMC joint subluxation
III	As per stage II, increased sclerosis, subchondral cysts, debris/osteophytes >2 mm diameter
IV	As per stage III, with narrowed ST joint demonstrating sclerosis and cysts
V	Pantrapezial arthritis

CMC, carpometacarpal; *ST*, scaphotrapezial.

REFERENCES

1. Gillis J, Calder K, Williams J. Review of thumb carpometacarpal arthritis classification, treatment and outcomes. Can J Plast Surg 2011;19(4):134–138
2. Bakri K, Moran SL. Thumb carpometacarpal arthritis. Plast Reconstr Surg 2015;135(2):508–520

MANAGING THUMB CMC JOINT OSTEOARTHRITIS

11. A 23-year-old woman presents with painful, subluxing first CMC joints without degenerative changes on X-ray. *How should this best be managed surgically?*

C. Volar beak and intermetacarpal ligament reconstruction

First CMC joint instability can occur in young healthy females who may present with painless, but visible, joint subluxation on thumb loading. Radiographs at rest may be normal, but on pushing the thumbs together during imaging, the dynamic changes may be revealed. Sometimes pain can prevent good stress-view imaging in more severe cases. In first CMC joint laxity, reconstruction of the joint capsule and volar ligamentous support using a partial flexor carpi radialis (FCR) sling has shown good results in many patients, although the procedure is not recommended in the presence of Eaton's grade II–IV arthritis, as the joint surface is not addressed.[1] Some authors have also described good results in patients with early joint changes using extension osteotomy of the metacarpal to alter joint biomechanics.[2]

Patients with isolated first CMC joint degenerative changes can respond well to CMC joint fusion, but that would not be the first-line option in this case provided she has good articular surfaces when inspected. Likewise, a trapeziectomy is not warranted in this scenario as the degenerative process is too mild and there are less aggressive options available. When a trapeziectomy is performed, the degree of metacarpal collapse should be assessed after removal of the trapezium. If there is a good endpoint on loading the thumb axially without abutment against the scaphoid through a range of wrist movements, there is no definitive evidence that a ligament reconstruction with or without a tendon interposition procedure is likely to give additional benefit.[3]

Pyrocarbon hemi-arthroplasty is an option in some patients with severe isolated thumb CMC joint OA. Implant survival rates of 80% have been reported[4] and favorable results in stage III and early-stage IV have also been described.[5]

REFERENCES

1. Freedman DM, Eaton RG, Glickel SZ. Long-term results of volar ligament reconstruction for symptomatic basal joint laxity. J Hand Surg Am 2000;25(2):297–304
2. Parker WL, Linscheid RL, Amadio PC. Long-term outcomes of first metacarpal extension osteotomy in the treatment of carpal-metacarpal osteoarthritis. J Hand Surg Am 2008;33(10):1737–1743
3. Lane LB, Henley DH. Ligament reconstruction of the painful, unstable, nonarthritic thumb carpometacarpal joint. J Hand Surg Am 2001;26(4):686–691
4. Martinez de Aragon JS, Moran SL, Rizzo M, Reggin KB, Beckenbaugh RD. Early outcomes of pyrolytic carbon hemiarthroplasty for the treatment of trapezial-metacarpal arthritis. J Hand Surg Am 2009;34(2):205–212
5. Badia A, Sambandam SN. Total joint arthroplasty in the treatment of advanced stages of thumb carpometacarpal joint osteoarthritis. J Hand Surg Am 2006;31(10):1605–1614

MCP JOINT OSTEOARTHRITIS

12. *In a young, active patient with severe symptomatic OA in the middle finger MCP joint following trauma, which one of the following is most likely to provide the best result in the medium to long term, assuming that range of motion is 0 to 90 degrees in this joint?*
    D. Pyrocarbon arthroplasty
    The MCP joints of the fingers are not commonly affected by symptomatic OA unless, as in this case, the condition is secondary to trauma. The best surgical option is usually arthroplasty in order to preserve joint range of motion, in contrast to the thumb where arthrodesis is usually most successful and well-tolerated. Given that this patient is young, a pyrocarbon arthroplasty is preferable to a Silastic joint as it will have greater stability and should have more long-term component integrity. Silastic implants are usually reserved for older patients with poor soft-tissue stability and lower physical demands. They are most commonly used in rheumatoid arthritis. Steroid injection is only likely to give a very limited, short-term response for this patient, given the extent of his joint disease. A ray amputation would be less favorable in terms of both aesthetics and function in this scenario but might be more relevant if there were other additional problems with the ray related to the original injury.[1,2]

REFERENCES

1. Wall LB, Stern PJ. Clinical and radiographic outcomes of metacarpophalangeal joint pyrolytic carbon arthroplasty for osteoarthritis. J Hand Surg Am 2013;38(3):537–543
2. Morrell NT, Weiss AC. Silicone metacarpophalangeal arthroplasty for osteoarthritis: long-term results. J Hand Surg Am 2018;43(3):229–233

PIP JOINT OSTEOARTHRITIS

13. *Which one of the following is most likely to fail in painful OA of the dominant index finger PIP joint?*
    B. Silastic arthroplasty
    While arthrodesis and steroid injections are widely employed, arthroplasty for the PIP joint is less common. Patient selection and technical excellence are critical for successful PIP joint pyrocarbon arthroplasty and index finger disease is a good indication. A silicone/Silastic implant is unlikely to be able to withstand the lateral stresses through the dominant index finger during pinch and key grips. For these reasons, many surgeons would choose arthrodesis over arthroplasty for the border digits. Good results have been reported following denervation procedures for some small joint arthritis.[1–3]

REFERENCES

1. Lorea P, Ezzedine R, Marchesi S. Denervation of the proximal interphalangeal joint: a realistic and simple procedure. Tech Hand Up Extrem Surg 2004;8(4):262–265
2. Herren D. The proximal interphalangeal joint: arthritis and deformity. EFORT Open Rev 2019;4(6):254–262
3. Morrell NT, Weiss AC. Silicone metacarpophalangeal arthroplasty for osteoarthritis: long-term results. J Hand Surg Am 2018;43(3):229–233

DIP JOINT OSTEOARTHRITIS

14. Which one of the following is correct regarding DIP joint OA?

E. Ideal joint fusion angles are less than for the PIP joint.

The DIP joint is the most commonly affected joint in OA and if arthrodesis is performed, the joint is usually fixed in 0 to 10 degrees of flexion, although more angulation is sometimes preferred in the index finger and the angle selected should take into account individual functional demands (see Fig. 99.3, *Essentials of Plastic Surgery,* third edition). DIP joint angles of fusion are therefore generally less than those for the PIP joints, which are usually fused between 20 and 40 degrees of flexion, depending on the digit and functional requirements of the patient.

In reality, the DIP joint is frequently asymptomatic in OA and clinical and radiological deformities are often unrelated to symptoms. As such, surgery is often not required. A cheilectomy is one surgical option that involves debridement of the osteophyte and joint preservation.

Notta's node refers to a nodule on the thumb of an infant causing triggering of the flexor tendon. It is accredited to the French physician Alphonse Notta who first described the condition of trigger finger. It is Heberden's nodes that are associated with DIP joint OA. These bony swellings are commonly observed but do not usually require treatment.

Nail deformity is often seen in DIP joint OA and is usually related to a mucous cyst. A mucous cyst is a small ganglion associated with DIP joint OA, and surgical excision may be warranted due to pain, impending rupture risking infection, or nail deformity. When this is performed, the use of an **H**-shaped or **Y**-shaped incision over the dorsum of the DIP joint can facilitate access to the full extent of the ganglion and debridement of osteophytes. When an area of skin loss is anticipated, a dorsal advancement flap may be useful.[1-4]

REFERENCES

1. Moberg E, Henrikson B. Technique for digital arthrodesis. A study of 150 cases. Acta Chir Scand 1960;118:331–338
2. Lin EA, Papatheodorou LK, Sotereanos DG. Cheilectomy for treatment of symptomatic distal interphalangeal joint osteoarthritis: a review of 78 patients. J Hand Surg Am 2017;42(11):889–893
3. Mantovani G, Fukushima WY, Cho AB, Aita MA, Lino W Jr, Faria FN. Alternative to the distal interphalangeal joint arthrodesis: lateral approach and plate fixation. J Hand Surg Am 2008;33(1):31–34
4. Jabbour S, Kechichian E, Haber R, Tomb R, Nasr M. Management of digital mucous cysts: a systematic review and treatment algorithm. Int J Dermatol 2017;56(7):701–708

100. Vascular Disorders of the Upper Extremity

See *Essentials of Plastic Surgery*, third edition, pp. 1389–1414

CLINICAL EVALUATION OF THE UPPER LIMB VASCULATURE

1. A 50-year-old man is referred with concerns over the upper limb arterial supply. The referring doctor states that the patient has early fatigue and pallor in the hands with moderate activity and reports a normal (negative) Allen test. *What is the most accurate assessment based on this information?*
   A. That motor and sensory nerve functions are both clinically intact to the distal limb.
   B. That exercise induced ischemia to the hand and forearm can be excluded.
   C. There is adequate blood supply to the hand from either the ulnar or radial arteries at rest.
   D. The referring doctor has already arranged vascular imaging in the form of computed tomography angiography (CTA).
   E. There are no bruits or thrills detectable on clinical examination.

IMAGING OF THE UPPER LIMB VASCULATURE

2. *Which one of the following characteristics of conventional angiography contributes to making it the gold standard for assessing the upper extremity vasculature?*
   A. It negates the risk for intravenous (IV) contrast.
   B. It is quick and noninvasive.
   C. It avoids the need for ionizing radiation.
   D. It is the cheapest imaging modality.
   E. It allows treatment to be given simultaneously.

MANAGEMENT OF THE ACUTELY ISCHEMIC LIMB

3. A patient presents with evidence of a spontaneous acute arterial obstruction to the left upper limb. The hand and forearm are cool, pale, and painful. No distal pulses are palpable. *Which one of the following represents the standard approach to treatment?*
   A. Low-molecular-weight heparin and embolectomy
   B. Embolectomy combined with intra-arterial urokinase
   C. Intra-arterial urokinase followed by a calcium channel blocker
   D. IV heparin and embolectomy followed by outpatient warfarin therapy
   E. IV heparin and open bypass graft followed by outpatient warfarin therapy

MANAGEMENT OF VASCULAR HAND PROBLEMS

4. A patient is seen in hand clinic where she describes episodes where the hand and digits become pale, cool, and painful. These attacks are short lived and following a period of color change in the affected digit from white to blue to red, before things return to normal spontaneously. *Which one of the following would be the next step in the treatment for this patient if calcium channel blockers had failed to help?*
   A. Bleomycin injection
   B. Botulinum toxin injection
   C. Oxymetazoline administration
   D. Cervical sympathectomy
   E. Digital sympathectomy

UPPER EXTREMITY ANEURYSMS

5. *When assessing a patient with a suspected upper limb aneurysm, which one of the following is true?*
   A. It is most likely to be a "true" aneurysm.
   B. It is most likely to be secondary to trauma.
   C. Cold intolerance would be a key pathognomic clinical finding.
   D. Imaging would show a fusiform-shape deformity.
   E. Management would be prescriptive and strongly evidence based.

MANAGEMENT OF SUPRACONDYLAR FRACTURES IN CHILDREN

6. A 7-year-old girl falls from a tree and sustains a left supracondylar humeral fracture. Her left hand is cold and pale on admission and remains this way following closed fracture reduction. She states her finger and thumb feel "fuzzy." *Which one of the following is the next key step in managing this patient?*
   A. Doppler ultrasound
   B. Arteriography
   C. Embolectomy
   D. CT angiography
   E. Open surgical exploration

RAYNAUD'S DISEASE

7. A 50-year-old woman presents with a diagnosis of Raynaud's disease managed by her general practitioner. For the past 5 years she has had episodes in cold weather where her fingers become pale, then blue, before turning bright red. *Which one of the following is correct regarding this woman's condition?*
   A. She will almost certainly have signs of systemic sclerosis.
   B. Her diagnosis forms part of a systemic autoimmune condition.
   C. The age at which she first experienced symptoms is typical of this condition.
   D. Use of regular nifedipine would be contraindicated in this case.
   E. Vasospasm and hyperemia may not be limited to the hands and feet.

THORACIC OUTLET SYNDROME

8. *Which one of the following statements is correct regarding neurologic thoracic outlet syndrome (TOS)?*
   A. The most common cause is a cervical rib.
   B. Males and females are equally affected.
   C. Clinical examination is commonly unremarkable.
   D. Adson's test is a reliable provocative test.
   E. Surgical decompression is performed via an endoscopic approach.

HEMANGIOMAS IN THE UPPER LIMB

9. You are discussing hemangiomas with the parents of a 1-year-old infant with a vascular lesion on their arm. *Which one of the following should you advise the parents?*
   A. They are always present at birth.
   B. They will always eventually spontaneously involute.
   C. There is a high risk of bleeding requiring treatment.
   D. They are a subtype of vascular malformation.
   E. They do not normally require surgical intervention.

ARTERIOVENOUS MALFORMATIONS

10. *Which one of the following statements is correct regarding arteriovenous malformations?*
   A. They develop in utero during the first trimester.
   B. Their causes are well understood.
   C. Most malformations are familial.
   D. Females are more commonly affected than males.
   E. Malformations are clinically evident at birth.

GLOMUS TUMORS

11. *When examining a patient with a suspected glomus tumor, which one of the following is most likely to be true?*
   A. A consistent finding will be a solitary painless vascular lesion on one digit.
   B. Love's sign should be routinely used to establish the diagnosis.
   C. The effects of inflating a tourniquet can reliably aid confirmation of the diagnosis.
   D. Abnormal skin color changes from white to blue then red are characteristically observed.
   E. The condition will be limited to the hand and if similar signs are present elsewhere, they indicate an alternative diagnosis.

COLD INTOLERANCE AND PAIN TO THE UPPER LIMB

12. A right-hand–dominant, self-employed carpenter presents to clinic with chronic cold intolerance and pain to the right little and ring fingers. Examination reveals early signs of ulceration to these digits. He is otherwise well with no other systemic signs of vasculopathy. *Which one of the following represents the most likely diagnosis?*
    A. True aneurysm
    B. False aneurysm
    C. Venous thrombosis
    D. Glomus tumor
    E. Raynaud's phenomenon

VASCULAR CHANGES IN THE FINGERTIPS

13. A 54-year-old woman presents to clinic with a history of cold hypersensitivity and paroxysmal pain affecting the index fingertip. Examination shows a slight blue discoloration to the nail bed. *What is the most likely diagnosis?*
    A. Venous thrombosis
    B. Autoimmune vasculitis
    C. Hemangioma
    D. Lymphangioma
    E. Glomus tumor

DIAGNOSIS OF VASCULAR LIMB DISORDERS

14. A 30-year-old left-hand–dominant soldier presents with a 3-month history of dull ache and weakness in the left arm. The pain is exacerbated by activity and the arm fatigues easily. He has not experienced any altered sensation to the limb. *What is the most likely diagnosis in this case?*
    A. Buerger's disease
    B. Compartment syndrome
    C. Arterial thrombosis
    D. Venous thrombosis
    E. Thoracic outlet syndrome

DIAGNOSIS OF VASCULAR LIMB PROBLEMS

15. A 26-year-old athlete has been working out at the gym and notices that his right arm has become swollen and purple with distended veins. *What is the most likely diagnosis in this case?*
    A. Buerger's disease
    B. Autoimmune vasculitis
    C. Arterial thrombosis
    D. Venous thrombosis
    E. Raynaud's disease

DIAGNOSIS OF VASCULAR LIMB CONDITIONS

16. A 29-year-old man presents to clinic with a few months history of calf pain when walking. He is not diabetic and has no other specific medical comorbidities. Examination reveals cool, pale feet with palpable pulses. His upper limbs are unaffected, but significant digital tar staining is evident. *What is the most likely effective treatment for this patient given his symptoms?*
    A. Smoking cessation
    B. Acetylsalicylic acid
    C. Low-molecular-weight heparin
    D. Nifedipine
    E. Rivaroxaban

DIFFERENTIAL DIAGNOSIS OF VASCULAR ANOMALIES

17. A 10-year-old child is brought to clinic by their parents with a lymphatic malformation to the left upper limb. *Which one of the following would be in keeping with this diagnosis on clinical examination?*
    A. A 15 cm × 20 cm fixed color, deep purple patch of skin to the distal forearm
    B. A soft, fluctuant 15 cm × 5 cm swelling to the mid forearm that remains the same irrespective of arm position
    C. A 5-cm blue colored swelling to the dorsal hand which reduces in volume with elevation
    D. A 2-cm warm swelling to the distal forearm and wrist with a palpable bruit
    E. A 3-cm soft, pale pink swelling to the mid forearm that is nontender with some skin excess

Answers

CLINICAL EVALUATION OF THE UPPER LIMB VASCULATURE

1. A 50-year-old man is referred with concerns over the upper limb arterial supply. The referring doctor states that the patient has early fatigue and pallor in the hands with moderate activity and reports a normal (negative) Allen test. *What is the most accurate assessment based on this information?*

    C. There is adequate blood supply to the hand from either the ulnar or radial arteries at rest.

    In most individuals, the brachial artery divides to form the radial and ulnar arteries just distal to the elbow. These two arteries are joined distally by an extensive collateral network involving the superficial and deep palmar arches. This means that in more than 90% of people, the radial artery can be sacrificed without compromising the blood supply to the hand; therefore, radial artery cannulation and radial artery harvest are usually safe.

    The Allen test was originally described by Dr. Allen in 1929 and in this first description it was used in the diagnosis of ulnar artery occlusion secondary to thromboangiitis obliterans. The test was performed by occluding the radial artery at the wrist after emptying the hand vasculature by clenching the fist for 1 minute.[1,2]

    The test is now widely used to assess independent vascular integrity of the radial and ulnar arteries to the hand as well as their interconnection via the palmar arches. Ideally, the hand should remain well perfused when either the radial or ulnar vessels are occluded providing the palmar arches are intact.

    The Allen test may be described as abnormal in cases where there is ulnar artery occlusion. It is better to describe it as abnormal rather than "positive," as it can be confusing to remember what "positive" or "negative" can mean in such tests. The Allen test is a simple procedure yielding consistent results, and its ability to predict perfusion of the hand following radial artery harvesting has been demonstrated.[2-4] It can be a useful part of the upper limb vascular assessment particularly where there may be signs of decreased perfusion or where the radial or ulnar arteries may be required for harvest.

    A normal Allen test does not exclude exercise-induced ischemia to the limb, as it assesses only perfusion at rest. It may be that there is a partial occlusion/compression of the distal ulnar artery by a mass or fascial band for example, which allows sufficient flow at rest but not during exertion.

    A full physical exam of the upper limb should include assessment of the appearance of the hand and fingers including skin color, temperature, turgor, nails, and capillary refill. It should also include a full assessment of motor and sensory nerve function as well as assessment of distal pulses, any obvious masses, and bruits. Any abnormal findings can direct the examiner to consider more specific tests. The Allen test does not provide information regarding the motor or sensory nerve function, nor whether any imaging has been performed.

REFERENCES

1. Allen EV. Thromboangiitis obliterans. Am J Med Sci 1929;2:1–8
2. Cable DG, Mullany CJ, Schaff HV. The Allen test. Ann Thorac Surg 1999;67(3):876–877
3. Lippert H, Pabst R. Arterial Variations in Man Classification and Frequency. Munich, Germany: JF Bergmann Verlag Munchen; 1985
4. Komeda M, Buxton BF, Raman J, Mullaly L, Hare DL. Allen test — new value of the "old" test. J Am Coll Cardiol 1998;31(Abstract):425

IMAGING OF THE UPPER LIMB VASCULATURE

2. *Which one of the following characteristics of conventional angiography contributes to making it the gold standard for assessing the upper extremity vasculature?*

    E. It allows treatment to be given simultaneously.

    Conventional angiography remains the gold standard for assessing the upper extremity vasculature in most settings. It is an invasive test that requires arterial access (typically in the groin or contralateral radial artery) and catheter placement in the desired location. It remains the best study to determine stenosis and occlusion in small distal vessels, particularly in patients with calcified vessels when artifact may prevent accurate examination by other modalities. A particular strength of this modality is that endovascular intervention can be undertaken at the same time as diagnostic angiogram. Unfortunately, angiography does expose the patient to ionizing radiation and IV contrast dye as well as the possibility of access complications (e.g., hematoma, arteriovenous [AV] fistula formation).[1]

    CTA/computed tomographic venography is another common modality for assessing the upper extremity vasculature, particularly in the setting of trauma. It is quick with high-quality images and may be used in patients in whom magnetic resonance imaging (MRI) is contraindicated. Disadvantages include exposure to ionizing radiation and contrast dye (which can induce contrast nephropathy and acute kidney injury). Usually, iodine-based contrast agents used in CT are responsible for this effect.[2]

In contrast, magnetic resonance angiography (MRA/MRV) does not expose the patient to ionizing radiation and the contrast material (gadolinium) used is less nephrotoxic than the iodine-based materials used in CT. However, MRA is more expensive, time consuming, and does not allow for endovascular intervention. While gadolinium is far less nephrotoxic than iodine-based contrast, it is not risk free. For example, it may carry a risk of deposition in the brain, which as yet has no proven specific morbidity, but may do so in the future.[3]

Ultrasound has a major role in the assessment of upper limb vasculature, especially in vascular malformations. It is pain free, noninvasive, nonionizing, and low cost. Traditionally, it has been limited by the availability of a suitably trained sonographer or radiologist, but with recent advances in technology and equipment availability many surgeons have the potential to develop sonography skills to use in their everyday clinical practice.[1]

REFERENCES

1. Sumner DS. Noninvasive assessment of upper extremity and hand ischemia. J Vasc Surg 1986;3(3):560–564
2. Hasebroock KM, Serkova NJ. Toxicity of MRI and CT contrast agents. Expert Opin Drug Metab Toxicol 2009;5(4):403–416
3. Kanda T, Ishii K, Kawaguchi H, Kitajima K, Takenaka D. High signal intensity in the dentate nucleus and globus pallidus on unenhanced T1-weighted MR images: relationship with increasing cumulative dose of a gadolinium-based contrast material. Radiology 2014;270(3):834–841

MANAGEMENT OF THE ACUTELY ISCHEMIC LIMB

3. A patient presents with evidence of a spontaneous acute arterial obstruction to the left upper limb. The hand and forearm are cool, pale, and painful. No distal pulses are palpable. *Which one of the following represents the standard approach to treatment?*

   D. IV heparin and embolectomy followed by outpatient warfarin therapy

   Emboli to the upper extremity are relatively uncommon representing less than 20% of all embolic events. However, when they do occur, it is a surgical emergency that requires multifaceted management. **The five Ps associated with acute arterial obstruction are: P**ain, **p**allor, **p**ulselessness, **p**aresthesia, **p**oikilothermia) as evident in this case. The standard treatment for acute arterial obstruction is immediate IV heparin therapy in combination with an embolectomy using a Fogarty catheter. This procedure is generally performed by the vascular team. Subsequent anticoagulation treatment with either warfarin or low-molecular-weight heparin is required to prevent recurrence. Other newer alternative medical therapies such as apixaban or rivaroxaban may be considered instead of warfarin. Intra-arterial thrombolysis of the distal upper extremity is not standard practice but has been shown to be effective in select cases. When this is performed, both a thrombolytic agent such as urokinase and a calcium channel blocker are used to achieve simultaneous vasodilation and thrombolysis. Management of emboli secondary to penetrating trauma such as catheter-related brachial artery occlusions is managed differently because many patients will continue to have compromised circulation even once the thrombosis is removed. In these cases, it may be necessary to perform open repair of the involved artery with primary resection and repair, or an interposition vein graft. Long-term anticoagulation is not necessarily required in such cases.[1–3]

REFERENCES

1. Andersen LV, Lip GY, Lindholt JS, Frost L. Upper limb arterial thromboembolism: a systematic review on incidence, risk factors, and prognosis, including a meta-analysis of risk-modifying drugs. J Thromb Haemost 2013;11(5):836–844
2. Koman AL, Smith BP, Smith TL, Ruch DSLZ. Vascular disorders. In: Green's Operative Hand Surgery. 6th ed. Philadelphia, PA: Elsevier Inc.; 2011:2197–2240
3. Lyaker MR, Tulman DB, Dimitrova GT, Pin RH, Papadimos TJ. Arterial embolism. Int J Crit Illn Inj Sci 2013;3(1):77–87

MANAGEMENT OF VASCULAR HAND PROBLEMS

4. A patient is seen in hand clinic where she describes episodes where the hand and digits become pale, cool, and painful. These attacks are short lived and following a period of color change in the affected digit from white to blue to red, before things return to normal spontaneously. *Which one of the following would be the next step in the treatment for this patient if calcium channel blockers had failed to help?*

   B. Botulinum toxin injection

   This patient has Raynaud's disease based on the clinical presentation. This is a condition in which there is spontaneous, self-limiting, reversible vasospasm in the digital vessels leading to rapid-onset ischemia followed by hyperemia.

   Most cases do not require intervention and treatment begins with avoiding cold temperatures and wearing warm, loose-fitting clothing such as hats and gloves. Beyond this, first-line medical management involves calcium channel blockers such as nifedipine for their vasodilatory properties. Phosphodiesterase inhibitors may also be effective, as they can increase the availability or effects of nitric oxide which is a powerful vasodilator.

The next step would be to consider using botulinum toxin injections around the neurovascular bundles of the affected digits, as this has proven to be effective in reducing pain and improving tissue perfusion in such cases.[1]

Botulinum toxin works by preventing neurotransmitter release into the synaptic cleft via the SNAP-25 pathway and is injected on the volar aspect of the digit under the dermis into the interstitial fluid surrounding the digital neurovascular bundles. A typical treatment involves 100 U dissolved in 10 mL of normal saline. The hand is injected in 10 places with 1 mL aliquots of the solution.[1] Studies show that botulinum toxin A injections help with pain relief, increase blood flow to fingers, and can improve overall hand function. Potential side effects include anhidrosis and hand/grip weakness. The long-term effects and toxicity are presently unknown.[1]

Beyond this, potential surgical treatment options include cervical sympathectomy which is still considered controversial and may offer only temporary relief, or digital sympathectomy which may be beneficial for a select number of patients with severe, tissue-threatening disease that is unresponsive to other treatment modalities.[2,3]

Bleomycin is a traditional chemotherapy medication used to treat vascular malformations and some skin cancers with electrochemotherapy. Oxymetazoline is a topical decongestant that acts as a vasoconstrictor and is used in the nasal mucosa. Neither has a role in the management of Raynaud's.

REFERENCES

1. Mannava S, Plate JF, Stone AV, et al. Recent advances for the management of Raynaud phenomenon using botulinum neurotoxin A. J Hand Surg Am 2011;36(10):1708–1710
2. McCall TE, Petersen DP, Wong LB. The use of digital artery sympathectomy as a salvage procedure for severe ischemia of Raynaud's disease and phenomenon. J Hand Surg Am 1999;24(1):173–177
3. Flatt AE. Digital artery sympathectomy. J Hand Surg Am 1980;5(6):550–556

UPPER EXTREMITY ANEURYSMS

5. *When assessing a patient with a suspected upper limb aneurysm, which one of the following is true?*

B. It is most likely to be secondary to trauma

Aneurysms are classified as either true or false according to the layers of the arterial wall involved. True aneurysms involve all three layers of the arterial wall (intima, media, and adventitia) where false aneurysms do not. Instead, they represent a collection of blood leaking out of a vessel that is confined by the surrounding tissue. False aneurysms are far more common in the upper limb and typically result from arterial perforation such as arterial cannulation or blood gas sampling (i.e., iatrogenic injury). Blood leaks into surrounding tissue and the hematoma later resolves and is replaced with scar.

There is no single specific clinical finding with a suspected aneurysm, although frequently a pulsatile painful mass is felt at the site. Other potential signs include cold intolerance, altered sensation, distal embolism, and thrombosis causing critical limb ischemia. Radiologic imaging can help differentiate between true and false aneurysms, which are fusiform or saccular in shape, respectively. There are limited data to guide management of upper extremity aneurysms, but a treatment plan must be individualized to the symptoms of the patient and may include observation only, surgical excision and ligation, or surgical excision and revascularization.[1,2]

REFERENCES

1. Igari K, Kudo T, Toyofuku T, Jibiki M, Inoue Y. Surgical treatment of aneurysms in the upper limbs. Ann Vasc Dis 2013;6(3):637–641
2. Gray RJ, Stone WM, Fowl RJ, Cherry KJ, Bower TC. Management of true aneurysms distal to the axillary artery. J Vasc Surg 1998;28(4):606–610

MANAGEMENT OF SUPRACONDYLAR FRACTURES IN CHILDREN

6. A 7-year-old girl falls from a tree and sustains a left supracondylar humeral fracture. Her left hand is cold and pale on admission and remains this way following closed fracture reduction. She states her finger and thumb feel "fuzzy." *Which one of the following is the next key step in managing this patient?*

E. Open surgical exploration

This patient has sustained a common childhood fracture that can be associated with damage to the brachial artery either during the initial injury or during fracture reduction. Loss of arterial flow can occur due to direct compression of the artery within the fracture site or secondary to arterial thrombosis following intimal damage. A persistent abnormality after fracture reduction requires urgent investigation and warrants operative exploration. Brachial artery thrombectomy with arterial repair or vein grafting should be anticipated. This would normally be undertaken with a multidisciplinary approach involving plastic, orthopaedic, and vascular surgeons. It is vital to assess neurovascular status of these children at multiple stages.

While this child has a frankly ischemic limb and there is no question that this should be explored, there is perhaps unexpectedly greater controversy regarding the pink pulseless limb. Even if the limb is pink, if it remains pulseless postreduction, it is better to avoid missing a treatable arterial injury and explore the limb.[1] An associated neuropathy in a pink pulseless limb, particularly of the median nerve, further increases the likelihood of the brachial artery injury being sufficient to require surgical management and should aid the decision to explore.[2] Intraoperatively, the median nerve should be identified just as carefully as the brachial artery, and normal status documented, or repair undertaken, as this lies in close proximity to the artery and is also at risk of injury in a supracondylar fracture.

No further imaging is required in this case, but noninvasive Doppler studies may be helpful in documenting abnormal pulses in an injured extremity, where there remains uncertainty about distal perfusion. Arteriography is best avoided in children because of the risk of iatrogenic damage. Embolectomy alone would not be recommended as the artery and median nerve need to be visualized along with the fracture site in this case. The cause of the occlusion (the fracture) must also be addressed.[3,4]

REFERENCES

1. Towler R, Corfield L, Carrell T. "The pink pulseless hand"—not a benign condition. Neurovascular compromise in paediatric supracondylar fracture of the humerus. Arch Dis Child 2010;95:A39–A40
2. Mangat KS, Martin AG, Bache CE. The 'pulseless pink' hand after supracondylar fracture of the humerus in children: the predictive value of nerve palsy. J Bone Joint Surg Br 2009;91(11):1521–1525
3. Kumar V, Singh A. Fracture supracondylar humerus: a review. J Clin Diagn Res 2016;10(12):RE01–RE06
4. Vaquero-Picado A, González-Morán G, Moraleda L. Management of supracondylar fractures of the humerus in children. EFORT Open Rev 2018;3(10):526–540

RAYNAUD'S DISEASE

7. A 50-year-old woman presents with a diagnosis of Raynaud's disease managed by her general practitioner. For the past 5 years she has had episodes in cold weather where her fingers become pale, then blue, before turning bright red. *Which one of the following is correct regarding this woman's condition?*

E. Vasospasm and hyperemia may not be limited to the hands and feet.

Raynaud's disease and Raynaud's phenomenon are distinctly different, although the terms are often used interchangeably. Raynaud's disease (primary Raynaud's) is a condition that involves reversible ischemia of peripheral tissues secondary to vasospasm. It is most commonly treated with nifedipine, a calcium channel blocker, although phosphodiesterase inhibitors such as sildenafil may be helpful too. Other medications sometimes prescribed include angiotensin-converting enzyme inhibitors, angiotensin II receptor antagonists, α-blockers, nitrates, and the selective serotonin receptor uptake inhibitor fluoxetine.

Raynaud's phenomenon (secondary Raynaud's) refers to the same vasospasm process in association with another illness, which is most commonly autoimmune. The most common association with Raynaud's phenomenon is scleroderma; however, it is not a given she will have this. Patients first presenting with Raynaud's should be investigated for an autoimmune condition.

In Raynaud's disease, fingers are most commonly affected, but the nose, ears, and toes may also be involved. Raynaud's disease can occur at any age, although commonly begins in the second or third decade and is not the typical age of first presentation in this case (i.e., age 45 years). Raynaud's phenomenon tends to present later in adult life.[1,2]

REFERENCES

1. Wigley FM. Clinical practice. Raynaud's phenomenon. N Engl J Med 2002;347(13):1001–1008
2. Herrick AL. Evidence-based management of Raynaud's phenomenon. Ther Adv Musculoskelet Dis 2017;9(12):317–329

THORACIC OUTLET SYNDROME

8. *Which one of the following statements is correct regarding neurologic thoracic outlet syndrome (TOS)?*

C. Clinical examination is commonly unremarkable.

Clinical examination findings are frequently normal in TOS, although certain provocative tests aim to aid identification, and so a careful history is very important. Although cervical ribs are involved in most arterial cases, they are rarely present in venous and neurologic cases. The most common site of neurologic compression is the scalene triangle (between the anterior scalene, middle scalene, and upper border of the first rib) and many patients have congenital fibromuscular bands in this region. Females are more commonly affected by TOS than males, and this difference is most apparent in neurologic TOS, with a ratio of 3.5:1. Adson's test assesses the radial pulse during compression of the subclavian artery with positional change but is unreliable, as patients without TOS may have considerable positional pulse variation.[1] Surgical decompression is usually performed using an open supraclavicular approach, or less commonly transaxillary.[1]

REFERENCE

1. Plewa MC, Delinger M. The false-positive rate of thoracic outlet syndrome shoulder maneuvers in healthy subjects. Acad Emerg Med 1998;5(4):337–342

HEMANGIOMAS IN THE UPPER LIMB

9. You are discussing hemangiomas with the parents of a 1-year-old infant with a vascular lesion on their arm. *Which one of the following should you advise the parents?*

   E. **They do not normally require surgical intervention.**

   Hemangiomas are a type of vascular tumor that may arise in utero or during the first few weeks of life. They are therefore classified as either infantile or congenital, depending on the time of first presentation. They are distinctly different from vascular malformations.[1] Classic infantile lesions show three phases of growth, with first appearance as a vascular papule followed by rapid growth, then involution. Traditional teaching suggests that by the age of 7, approximately 70% of infantile hemangiomas have spontaneously involuted, but not all subtypes do so. Congenital hemangiomas are mature at birth and are classified by their natural history as either rapidly involuting (RICH) or noninvoluting (NICH). Because most hemangiomas involute, surgical intervention is not usually required. Problematic hemangiomas, such as those that ulcerate or affect function, may be treated with surgery, sclerotherapy, laser therapy, or beta-blocker medication. Those that leave a fibrofatty remnant or skin excess may also benefit from surgical excision.[1-3]

REFERENCES

1. Mulliken JB, Glowacki J. Classification of pediatric vascular lesions. Plast Reconstr Surg 1982;70(1):120–121
2. Couto RA, Maclellan RA, Zurakowski D, Greene AK. Infantile hemangioma: clinical assessment of the involuting phase and implications for management. Plast Reconstr Surg 2012;130(3):619–624
3. Mulliken JB. Diagnosis and natural history of hemangiomas. In: Mulliken JB, Burrows PE, Fishman SJ, eds. Mulliken and Young's Vascular Anomalies: Hemangiomas and Malformations. Oxford University Press; 2013

ARTERIOVENOUS MALFORMATIONS

10. *Which one of the following statements is correct regarding arteriovenous malformations?*

    A. **They develop in utero during the first trimester.**

    Vascular malformations are inborn errors in embryonic development that occur between weeks 4 and 10 of intrauterine growth. The causes are not well understood and most occur spontaneously. Males and females are equally affected, and although all malformations are present at birth, they may not be clinically evident. For example, a triggering stimulus during puberty or pregnancy can precipitate the first clinical signs of the malformation.[1-4]

REFERENCES

1. Mulliken JB, Glowacki J. Classification of pediatric vascular lesions. Plast Reconstr Surg 1982;70(1):120–121
2. Wassef M, Blei F, Adams D, et al; ISSVA Board and Scientific Committee. Vascular anomalies classification: recommendations from the International Society for the Study of Vascular Anomalies. Pediatrics 2015;136(1):e203–e214
3. Ek ET, Suh N, Carlson MG. Vascular anomalies of the hand and wrist. J Am Acad Orthop Surg 2014;22(6):352–360
4. Taghinia AH, Upton J. Vascular anomalies. J Hand Surg Am 2018;43(12):1113–1121

GLOMUS TUMORS

11. *When examining a patient with a suspected glomus tumor, which one of the following is most likely to be true?*

    C. **The effects of inflating a tourniquet can reliably aid confirmation of the diagnosis.**

    Glomus tumors are benign vascular lesions containing cells from the glomus apparatus involved in thermoregulation that commonly affect the nail bed and fingertip. They often present as a bluish discoloration under the nail plate, with or without nail ridging. Although lesions are often painful and solitary, this is not always the case and multiple painful or painless lesions may be present.

Hildreth's sign is observed in patients with glomus tumors of the hand, where pain is abolished on exsanguination of the limb with inflation of a blood pressure cuff. There is supporting evidence to show the efficacy of this test in the diagnosis of glomus tumors, with sensitivity and specificity above 90%.[1]

Love's sign is elicited when point pressure is applied to the nail bed with a pinhead at the site of the tumor, resulting in intense pain. There are usually enough other signs to make a diagnosis without performing this test, which is clearly unpleasant for the patient.

The skin color changes described here are more characteristic of those described by patients with Raynaud's disease, where the hand passes through a series of vascular changes: white (pallor), blue (cyanosis), and red (hyperemia).

Although most cases of glomus tumor (75%) are found in the hand, the condition is not exclusively seen in this site. They may be present in the toes or even in extracutaneous sites such as bone and the gastrointestinal tract. Following examination, further imaging with ultrasound or MRI may be useful. Treatment of upper limb glomus tumors is with surgical excision.[2,3]

REFERENCES

1. Giele H. Hildreth's test is a reliable clinical sign for the diagnosis of glomus tumours. J Hand Surg [Br] 2002;27(2):157–158
2. Vasisht B, Watson HK, Joseph E, Lionelli GT. Digital glomus tumors: a 29-year experience with a lateral subperiosteal approach. Plast Reconstr Surg 2004;114(6):1486–1489
3. Al-Qattan MM, Al-Namla A, Al-Thunayan A, Al-Subhi F, El-Shayeb AF. Magnetic resonance imaging in the diagnosis of glomus tumours of the hand. J Hand Surg [Br] 2005;30(5):535–540

COLD INTOLERANCE AND PAIN TO THE UPPER LIMB

12. A right-hand–dominant, self-employed carpenter presents to clinic with chronic cold intolerance and pain to the right little and ring fingers. Examination reveals early signs of ulceration to these digits. He is otherwise well with no other systemic signs of vasculopathy. *Which one of the following represents the most likely diagnosis?*

A. True aneurysm

This patient has hypothenar hammer syndrome where repetitive blunt trauma to the hypothenar area leads to a true aneurysm (not false) of the ulnar artery in the area of Guyon's canal. This typically occurs in upholsterers, carpenters, and carpet layers. The repetitive trauma results in tunica media damage followed by aneurysm formation and then eventual arterial thrombosis (not venous). Patients present with cold intolerance, pain at night or with repetitive activity, and skin changes to the ulnar digits. If neglected, the digits can ulcerate.[1,2]

Patients with minimal symptoms, but normal flow through the radial artery, and a complete palmar arch can be observed, and symptoms treated medically, with acetylsalicylic acid (ASA) and a calcium channel blocker (nifedipine). However, patients with a proven aneurysm, recurrent embolic events, or persistent symptoms despite medical management require surgical intervention with resection of the affected arterial segment and, most likely, reconstruction of the damaged section of the ulnar artery with a vein graft. This procedure also allows for simultaneous decompression of the ulnar nerve in Guyon's canal which can help alleviate nerve compression symptoms that may also be present secondary to the aneurysm. Unfortunately, repair and revascularization may fail early due to the local anatomy and background cause without lifestyle alteration, i.e., stopping the regular trauma which caused the problem in the first instance.[1,2]

A false aneurysm tends to occur following arterial puncture as an acute trauma and is usually iatrogenic. Most will settle spontaneously, although a minority will also require surgery to excise the damaged section and graft it. Venous thrombosis typically presents with a swollen upper limb with signs of venous congestion such as bluish skin discoloration and altered capillary refill. Glomus tumors affect the digits most usually at the level of the nail bed resulting in painful subcutaneous nodules. Raynaud's phenomenon more typically presents with bilateral bouts of ischemia to the digits, which are self-limiting and resolve spontaneously. Neither of these conditions would present as in this scenario.

REFERENCES

1. Cigna E, Spagnoli AM, Tarallo M, et al. Therapeutic management of hypothenar hammer syndrome causing ulnar nerve entrapment. Plastic Surgery International 2010;2010:Article ID 343820, 1-5 pages
2. Hui-Chou HG, McClinton MA. Current options for treatment of hypothenar hammer syndrome. Hand Clin 2015;31(1):53–62

VASCULAR CHANGES IN THE FINGERTIPS

13. A 54-year-old woman presents to clinic with a history of cold hypersensitivity and paroxysmal pain affecting the index fingertip. Examination shows a slight blue discoloration to the nail bed. *What is the most likely diagnosis?*

E. Glomus tumor

This woman has the typical features of a glomus tumor, which is a benign vascular lesion commonly affecting the fingertip, most often beneath the nail plate. The glomus apparatus contains an AV shunt that contributes to temperature regulation. The classic clinical triad observed with glomus tumors is cold hypersensitivity, paroxysmal pain, and pinpoint tenderness. Glomus tumors may be classified into three groups: solitary lesions, multiple painful lesions, or multiple painless lesions. Imaging can sometimes be useful with MRI or Doppler ultrasound prior to treatment. MRI may typically show a dark, well-defined lesion on T1-weighted images and a bright lesion on T2-weighted images.[1,2] Doppler ultrasound studies can help detect the high blood flow in glomus tumors. Surgical excision of the lesion is generally the treatment of choice, either directly through sterile nail matrix or with a lateral subperiosteal approach.

REFERENCES

1. Al-Qattan MM, Al-Namla A, Al-Thunayan A, Al-Subhi F, El-Shayeb AF. Magnetic resonance imaging in the diagnosis of glomus tumours of the hand. J Hand Surg [Br] 2005;30(5):535–540
2. Drapé JL. Imaging of tumors of the nail unit. Clin Podiatr Med Surg 2004;21(4):493–511, v

DIAGNOSIS OF VASCULAR LIMB DISORDERS

14. A 30-year-old left-hand–dominant soldier presents with a 3-month history of dull ache and weakness in the left arm. The pain is exacerbated by activity and the arm fatigues easily. He has not experienced any altered sensation to the limb. *What is the most likely diagnosis in this case?*

E. Thoracic outlet syndrome

Thoracic outlet syndrome refers to compression of the neurovascular structures of the upper limb as they pass between the neck/thorax and axilla. It can involve variable combinations of neurovascular signs and symptoms. The patient in this scenario is most likely to have TOS with an arterial component. This would explain the exercise-induced ischemic pain he is experiencing and the time frame over which the problems have been present.

The most commonly affected structures in TOS are the brachial plexus (95%), subclavian vein (4%), and subclavian artery (1%). Most presentations are nonemergent and require only symptomatic treatment and referral.

There are a number of potential anatomical compression points including the Scalene triangle (between the anterior scalene, middle scalene, and first rib), cervical ribs, and congenital fibromuscular bands of the cervical transverse processes. Arterial problems tend to be associated with the first two areas of compression.

Treatment in this case will be to address the site of compression and then to address any ongoing vascular abnormalities.[1,2]

Buerger's disease may present in a similar age patient but would tend to affect the lower limb. Compartment syndrome would present with acute-onset pain and swelling to the affected limb, most often after trauma. An arterial thrombosis would tend to present with a pale, cool ischemic limb, while a venous thrombosis would tend to present with a swollen congested limb.[1–3]

REFERENCES

1. Oates SD, Daley RA. Thoracic outlet syndrome. Hand Clin 1996;12(4):705–718
2. Huang JH, Zager EL. Thoracic outlet syndrome. Neurosurgery 2004;55(4):897–902, discussion 902–903
3. Hood DB, Kuehne J, Yellin AE, Weaver FA. Vascular complications of thoracic outlet syndrome. Am Surg 1997;63(10):913–917

DIAGNOSIS OF VASCULAR LIMB PROBLEMS

15. A 26-year-old athlete has been working out at the gym and notices that his right arm has become swollen and purple with distended veins. *What is the most likely diagnosis in this case?*

D. Venous thrombosis

The patient in this scenario has evidence of acute-onset venous thrombosis of the upper limb, most likely the subclavian vein. This is termed *effort vein thrombosis* when associated with vigorous upper limb exercise in a healthy individual, as in this case, and can be caused by an underlying undiagnosed thoracic outlet compression. It is a rare condition that tends to affect young, active, and otherwise healthy people and is also known as Paget–Schröetter syndrome. It is thought to occur as a result of repetitive minor trauma to the subclavian vein where it passes between the first rib and clavicle.

This type of venous thrombosis is distinctly different from other forms of deep vein thrombosis with respect to the underlying pathophysiology, clinical presentation, and functional consequences, so requires swift management of the thrombus in the acute setting followed by addressing the underlying cause. Management will therefore likely involve early catheter-based venography, thrombolytic therapy, and prompt paraclavicular thoracic outlet decompression with direct subclavian vein reconstruction.[1]

Buerger's disease would tend to present in a young patient with signs of limb ischemia similar to an older patient with atherosclerotic disease. An arterial thrombosis would present with a white, cool peripheral limb and would normally be managed with embolectomy. Autoimmune vasculitis can present with numbness and coldness to the affected limb with easy fatigability and altered pulses. There will usually be other systemic clues in the history that raise suspicion of a vasculitis such vascular compromise to internal organs (bowel and kidney), jaw claudication, visual disturbances, and skin changes.[2]

REFERENCES

1. Thompson RW. Comprehensive management of subclavian vein effort thrombosis. Semin Intervent Radiol 2012;29(1):44–51
2. Okazaki T, Shinagawa S, Mikage H. Vasculitis syndrome-diagnosis and therapy. J Gen Fam Med 2017;18(2):72–78

DIAGNOSIS OF VASCULAR LIMB CONDITIONS

16. A 29-year-old man presents to clinic with a few months history of calf pain when walking. He is not diabetic and has no other specific medical comorbidities. Examination reveals cool, pale feet with palpable pulses. His upper limbs are unaffected, but significant digital tar staining is evident. *What is the most likely effective treatment for this patient given his symptoms?*

A. Smoking cessation

The patient in this scenario demonstrates features of Buerger's disease, which includes intermittent claudication of the lower limbs, poor lower limb perfusion, and sparing of the upper limbs in a young person who smokes heavily. The tar staining and lack of other medical comorbidities are strongly suggestive of this diagnosis, which is characterized by inflammatory thrombi affecting both arteries and veins. It typically presents, as in this case, with claudication and later progresses to pain at rest and tissue necrosis. The only proven treatment is complete cessation of smoking; so, support in this is the best management for the scenario given.[1]

Low-molecular-weight heparin and rivaroxaban are used to treat patients who have a history of venous thromboembolism or are at high risk of developing this such as with atrial fibrillation. Rivaroxaban is an alternative to coumarin (warfarin) that is taken as a daily tablet. Where patients are undergoing major surgery, it is usual to request they stop this medication for 48–72 hours to allow reversal of its anticoagulation effects. Acetylsalicylic acid (aspirin) is used as an antiplatelet agent in patients with ischemic heart or peripheral vascular disease. It is also used in the setting of hypothenar hammer syndrome alongside nifedipine, a calcium channel antagonist, which has a powerful vasodilatory effect on the peripheral vasculature. Nifedipine is also used in Raynaud's disease for the same physiologic effects.

REFERENCE

1. Olin JW. Thromboangiitis obliterans (Buerger's disease). N Engl J Med 2000;343(12):864–869

DIFFERENTIAL DIAGNOSIS OF VASCULAR ANOMALIES

17. A 10-year-old child is brought to clinic by their parents with a lymphatic malformation to the left upper limb. *Which one of the following would be in keeping with this diagnosis on clinical examination?*

B. A soft, fluctuant 15 cm × 5 cm swelling to the mid forearm that remains the same irrespective of arm position.

Vascular anomalies are classified as either tumors or malformations. Hemangiomas are tumours, while other benign vascular anomalies are malformations.

Malformations are congenital and comprise of abnormal vessels, be it arteries, veins, capillaries, lymphatics, or a combination of these. They are therefore most commonly described as capillary, venous, lymphatic, arteriovenous, or mixed. They can also be classified according to flow rate: low flow, high flow, or mixed flow. These features can often be identified from the history and examination alone and determine aspects of their management.

Most vascular malformations can be diagnosed on clinical examination alone because of their specific characteristics; however, imaging may assist in the diagnosis and can also useful in determining extent and flow rate.

Lymphatic malformations vary according to whether they are microcystic or macrocystic in nature and according to their location. They may have a soft, fluctuant consistency with minimal change on gravity, or they may be characterized by cutaneous vesicles which may contain clear fluid, or be discolored brown by bleeding. Their color can also vary according to their tissue depth and whether there is any vascular (usually venous) component.

Venous malformations tend to have a blue or purple appearance according to depth, location, and size, and usually deflate with elevation of the limb or expand with dependent positioning or exercise. There may be associated firm lumps palpated due to phleboliths.

Capillary malformations are not usually affected by gravity or exertion and tend to have a characteristic port-wine stain red/purple appearance. They may be smooth in the early years, or become textured (cobblestoned) in later life.

Arteriovenous malformations generally feel warm and have a palpable pulsatility, thrill, or bruit.

The last description above represents a hemangioma. These tend to have a characteristic bright red or "strawberry" appearance at presentation, as they represent an abnormal collection of blood vessels. By the age of 10 years, these have generally involuted spontaneously and if this is incomplete, then the color therefore changes to a paler white/pink. This involution can leave a small excess of skin and fat and this may require surgical correction.[1-4]

REFERENCES

1. Greene AK, Perlyn CA, Alomari AI. Management of lymphatic malformations. Clin Plast Surg 2011;38(1):75–82
2. Mulliken JB. Diagnosis and natural history of hemangiomas. In: Mulliken JB, Burrows PE, Fishman SJ, eds. Mulliken and Young's Vascular Anomalies: Hemangiomas and Malformations. Oxford University Press; 2013
3. Maguiness SM, Liang MG. Management of capillary malformations. Clin Plast Surg 2011;38(1):65–73
4. Greene AK, Alomari AI. Management of venous malformations. Clin Plast Surg 2011;38(1):83–93

PART VII

Aesthetic Surgery

101. Aesthetic Facial Anatomy

See *Essentials of Plastic Surgery*, third edition, pp. 1417–1434

SOFT-TISSUE LAYERS OF THE FACE

1. *When performing surgery on the face, directly under which anatomic layer would the main neurovascular structures normally be located?*
   A. Skin
   B. Subcutaneous tissue
   C. Superficial musculoaponeurotic system (SMAS)
   D. Mimetic muscles
   E. Deep facial fascia

THE SUPERFICIAL MUSCULOAPONEUROTIC SYSTEM

2. *The SMAS is a key structure to understand in rhytidectomy and is continuous with other anatomic fascial planes. Which one of the following layers is distinct from the SMAS layer?*
   A. Temporoparietal fascia
   B. Superficial cervical fascia
   C. Parotidomasseteric fascia
   D. Frontalis and platysmal fascia
   E. Zygomaticus major fascia

THE SUPERFICIAL MUSCULOAPONEUROTIC SYSTEM

3. *Which one of the following represents the site where the SMAS is both thickest and fixed?*
   A. The parotid
   B. The neck
   C. The temple
   D. The midface
   E. The brow

THE FRONTAL BRANCH OF THE FACIAL NERVE

4. *When performing surgery on the temple, just lateral to the brow, running on which structure would you expect to find the frontal branch of the facial nerve?*
   A. Temporoparietal fascia
   B. Parotidotemporal fascia
   C. Superficial layer of the deep temporal fascia
   D. Deep layer of the deep temporal fascia
   E. Superficial temporal fat pad

FACIAL FAT COMPARTMENTS

5. *Which one of the following is true of the facial fat compartments?*
   A. The bulk of facial fat in the cheek is deep to SMAS.
   B. The nasolabial fat compartment loses most of its volume with increasing age.
   C. The buccal fat pad and the malar fat pad are equivalent.
   D. The malar fat pad is formed by the nasolabial and medial cheek fat compartments.
   E. The suborbicularis oculi fat (SOOF) and retro-orbicularis oculi fat (ROOF) both lie superficial to the orbicularis oculi.

RETAINING LIGAMENTS OF THE FACE

6. *Weakening of which facial ligaments are believed to be primarily responsible for the appearance of jowls in the aging face?*
   A. Masseteric
   B. Zygomatic
   C. Mandibular
   D. Orbital
   E. Temporal

MIMETIC MUSCLES OF THE FACE

7. *Which one of the following is true of the facial mimetic muscles*
   A. They are all innervated by the CN VII on their deep surfaces.
   B. They are all innervated by CN VII on their superficial surfaces.
   C. They are arranged into three different layers each innervated by CN VII.
   D. The majority are innervated on their deep surfaces by CN VII.
   E. Only one is not innervated on its deep surface by CN VII.

BLOOD SUPPLY OF THE FACE AND NECK

8. *Which one of the following is true of the vascularity of the face and neck?*
   A. The primary vascular supply arises from the external carotid artery.
   B. The internal carotid makes no significant contribution.
   C. Facial vessels generally lie superficial to the muscles they supply.
   D. The lateral face contains the most robust blood supply in the head and neck.
   E. Areas involving the retaining ligaments tend to be poorly vascularized.

SENSORY DEFICITS AFTER A FACE LIFT

9. A patient has numbness of the lobule of the ear following a SMAS plication face lift. *Injury to which nerve would most likely account for this?*
   A. Lesser occipital
   B. Great auricular
   C. Greater occipital
   D. Auriculotemporal
   E. Zygomaticotemporal

MOTOR DEFICITS AFTER A FACE LIFT

10. Following a combined face- and neck-lift procedure, a patient has a new-onset lower lip asymmetry when performing a full denture smile. He is still able to pucker his lips normally. *Which one of the following facial nerve branches is most likely to be injured?*
    A. Marginal mandibular branch
    B. Cervical branch
    C. Frontal branch
    D. Buccal branch
    E. Zygomatic branch

MOTOR DEFICITS AFTER A FACE LIFT

11. A patient has temporary shoulder weakness after an extended face and neck lift. *Injury to which nerve would likely account for this?*
    A. Spinal accessory nerve
    B. Lesser occipital nerve
    C. Hypoglossal nerve
    D. Facial nerve
    E. Cervical plexus

Answers

SOFT-TISSUE LAYERS OF THE FACE

1. *When performing surgery on the face, directly under which anatomic layer would the main neurovascular structures normally be located?*

E. Deep facial fascia

The soft-tissue layers of the face can be conceptualized as a series of concentric layers from superficial to deep (**Fig. 101.1**). These layers are the skin, subcutaneous tissues, superficial musculoaponeurotic system (SMAS), facial mimetic muscles, deep facial fascia, and bone. The main neurovascular structures lie just deep to the deep facial fascia and include the facial nerve, parotid duct, and facial vessels. This layer also contains the buccal fat pad. However, it is possible to damage the facial nerve intraoperatively when deep to SMAS and medial to the parotid, as the facial nerve becomes more superficial in this area, so care must be taken during sub-SMAS dissection. Retaining ligaments and fascial septa span across these layers to support the soft tissues of the face.[1]

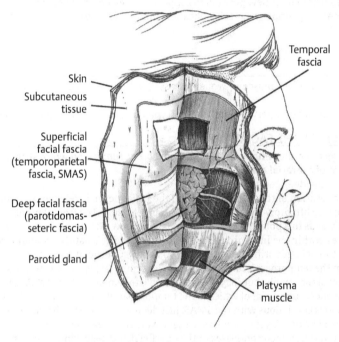

Fig. 101.1 Facial soft-tissue layers.

REFERENCE

1. Nahai F, ed. The Art of Aesthetic Surgery: Principles and Techniques. St Louis, MO: Quality Medical Publishing; 2005

THE SUPERFICIAL MUSCULOAPONEUROTIC SYSTEM

2. The SMAS is a key structure to understand in rhytidectomy and is continuous with other anatomic fascial planes. *Which one of the following layers is distinct from the SMAS layer?*

C. Parotidomasseteric fascia

The SMAS is part of the superficial fascial system of the face and neck, whereas the parotidomasseteric fascia is part of the deep fascial system of the face and neck. The SMAS is highly relevant to face-lift procedures and is often elevated and manipulated to support facial soft-tissue structures during rhytidectomy. It is continuous caudally with the platysma and superficial cervical fascia and cranially with the frontalis, galea, and superficial temporal fascia. At its most anterior extent, the SMAS forms the fascia around zygomaticus major, which can be a tethering point during a face lift requiring release. In contrast, the deep fascia which consists of the masseteric fascia, investing fascia of the parotid, deep temporal fascia, and deep cervical fascia, is not normally manipulated during face-lift procedures.[1–4]

REFERENCES

1. Nahai F, ed. The Art of Aesthetic Surgery: Principles and Techniques. St Louis, MO: Quality Medical Publishing; 2005
2. Gosain AK, Yousif NJ, Madiedo G, Larson DL, Matloub HS, Sanger JR. Surgical anatomy of the SMAS: a reinvestigation. Plast Reconstr Surg 1993;92(7):1254–1263, discussion 1264–1265
3. Mitz V, Peyronie M. The superficial musculo-aponeurotic system (SMAS) in the parotid and cheek area. Plast Reconstr Surg 1976;58(1):80–88
4. Stuzin JM, Baker TJ, Gordon HL. The relationship of the superficial and deep facial fascias: relevance to rhytidectomy and aging. Plast Reconstr Surg 1992;89(3):441–449, discussion 450–451

THE SUPERFICIAL MUSCULOAPONEUROTIC SYSTEM

3. *Which one of the following represents the site where the SMAS is both thickest and fixed?*

A. **The parotid**

The SMAS has both mobile and fixed components. The fixed SMAS overlies the parotid gland and is thickest in this region. The increased thickness at this site provides protection to the main facial nerve and its proximal branches. The mobile SMAS lies beyond the parotid (medially) over the facial mimetic muscles, facial nerves, and parotid duct. It is both thinner and more mobile than the fixed SMAS. This is clinically relevant to face-lifting techniques where the SMAS is mobilized around the parotid region and elevated in a posterior, oblique, or vertical direction. The SMAS is then secured in its new position to support the elevated soft tissues of the face and neck during the rhytidectomy. SMAS suspension can involve plication, imbrication, resection, or advancement techniques using sutures.[1,2]

REFERENCES

1. Mitz V, Peyronie M. The superficial musculo-aponeurotic system (SMAS) in the parotid and cheek area. Plast Reconstr Surg 1976;58(1):80–88
2. Nahai F, ed. The Art of Aesthetic Surgery: Principles and Techniques. St Louis, MO: Quality Medical Publishing; 2005

THE FRONTAL BRANCH OF THE FACIAL NERVE

4. *When performing surgery on the temple, just lateral to the brow, running on which structure would you expect to find the frontal branch of the facial nerve?*

C. **Superficial layer of the deep temporal fascia**

Knowledge of the location of the frontal branch of the facial nerve is relevant to many procedures in plastic surgery including face lift, brow lift, and temporal tumor excision. The frontal branch travels along a line from 0.5 cm below the tragus to a point 1.5 cm above the lateral brow (Pitanguy's line). After crossing the zygomatic arch, which it does within the innominate fascia just deep to SMAS, at the midpoint between the tragus and lateral canthus, it may be identified running on top of the superficial part of the deep temporal fascia, just beneath or within the temporoparietal fascia or parotidotemporal fascia.[1] There is often confusion with regard to the fascial layers of the temple, but they are fairly simple to remember (**Fig. 101.2**). There are four fascial layers in this region. The most superficial of which is the temporoparietal fascia. This is also known as the superficial temporal fascia and is continuous with the SMAS. Just deep to this layer is the parotidotemporal or innominate fascia, which is an additional layer of soft tissue that covers the frontal branch in this area. Beneath this layer is the deep temporal fascia, which comprises both superficial and deep components separated by a fat pad. The temporalis muscle is deep to both of these layers and is adherent to the underlying pericranium. Protection of the frontal branch intraoperatively can be achieved by keeping superficial to the SMAS layer or deep to the deep fascia. At the level of the arch it should still also be safe to carefully elevate SMAS.[1] When dissection is required in the plane just above the superficial layer of the deep fascia, additional care must be taken to protect the nerve branch.[1,2]

REFERENCES

1. Agarwal CA, Mendenhall SD III, Foreman KB, Owsley JQ. The course of the frontal branch of the facial nerve in relation to fascial planes: an anatomic study. Plast Reconstr Surg 2010;125(2):532–537
2. Seckel BR, ed. Facial Danger Zones: Avoiding Nerve Injury in Facial Plastic Surgery. St Louis, MO: Quality Medical Publishing; 1994

FACIAL FAT COMPARTMENTS

5. *Which one of the following is true of the facial fat compartments?*

D. **The malar fat pad is formed by the nasolabial and medial cheek fat compartments.**

The "malar fat pad" is a commonly used term referring to the region of the superficial cheek fat compartments that are thought to play a role in the appearance of the youthful cheek. With age, the malar fat pad loses volume

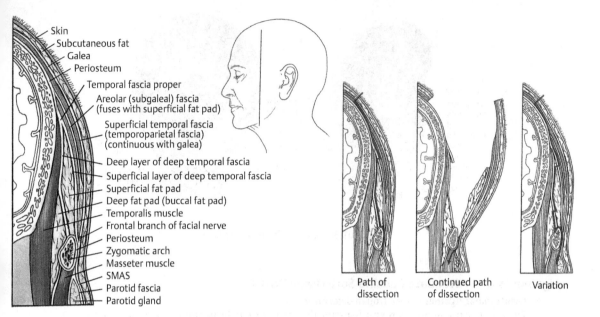

Fig. 101.2 Anatomic layers of the temporal region.

and descends caudally, secondarily creating upper midface emptiness, lower-face fullness, and deepening of the nasolabial folds. The two primary components of the malar fat pad are the nasolabial and medial cheek fat compartments. The inferior orbital fat compartment can also be considered as part of this fat pad. It is separated from the other two components by cutaneous insertions of the zygomaticocutaneous ligaments.

The facial fat compartments are divided into superficial and deep layers according to their relation to the SMAS and facial mimetic muscles. They are further described according to their anatomic subunit location, e.g., cheek, nasolabial, forehead, and orbit. There is a fairly even split between superficial and deep volume proportions in the cheek (54% compared to 46%, respectively). The superficial fat compartments of the cheek include the nasolabial, medial, middle, and lateral cheek fat compartments. The deep parts of the cheek are the buccal fat pad and the deep medial compartment. The superficial parts of the periorbital region are the superior, inferior, and lateral compartments. The deep compartments are the SOOF and the ROOF which are located beneath orbicularis oculi, not superficial to it. Of all the compartments in the face, the nasolabial one is unusual in that its volume remains fairly consistent through life. Fat located in the deep compartments seems to selectively age more than the superficial fat.[1,2]

REFERENCES

1. Rohrich RJ, Pessa JE. The fat compartments of the face: anatomy and clinical implications for cosmetic surgery. Plast Reconstr Surg 2007;119(7):2219–2227
2. Wan D, Amirlak B, Rohrich R, Davis K. The clinical importance of the fat compartments in midfacial aging. Plast Reconstr Surg Glob Open 2014;1(9):e92

RETAINING LIGAMENTS OF THE FACE

6. *Weakening of which facial ligaments are believed to be primarily responsible for the appearance of jowls in the aging face?*
   A. Masseteric

   The retaining ligaments of the face provide support for the facial soft tissues and are implicated in the facial aging process, either from attenuation or tethering. They originate from either bone or fascia and inset into the dermis. It is important to be familiar with them, as some of them must be released and/or repositioned during facial rejuvenation surgery, such as rhytidectomy and brow lift. They include the following:

Ligaments that Cause Soft-Tissue Tethering

- **Mandibular ligament:** Jowls and marionette lines (**Fig. 101.3**)

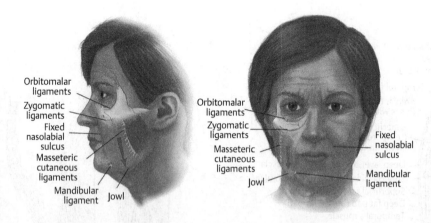

Fig. 101.3   Changes in the aging face.

Ligaments that Attenuate Causing Soft-Tissue Ptosis

• **Orbitomalar ligament**: Tear-trough deformity
• **Zygomaticocutaneous ligament:** Tear-trough deformity and deepening of the nasolabial fold
• **Masseteric ligament:** Formation of jowls and marionette lines [1-4]

REFERENCES

1. Moss CJ, Mendelson BC, Taylor GI. Surgical anatomy of the ligamentous attachments in the temple and periorbital regions. Plast Reconstr Surg 2000;105(4):1475–1490, discussion 1491–1498
2. Furnas DW. The retaining ligaments of the cheek. Plast Reconstr Surg 1989;83(1):11–16
3. Rohrich RJ, Pessa JE. The retaining system of the face: histologic evaluation of the septal boundaries of the subcutaneous fat compartments. Plast Reconstr Surg 2008;121(5): 1804–1809
4. Muzaffar AR, Mendelson BC, Adams WP Jr. Surgical anatomy of the ligamentous attachments of the lower lid and lateral canthus. Plast Reconstr Surg 2002;110(3):873–884, discussion 897–911

MIMETIC MUSCLES OF THE FACE

7. Which one of the following is true of the facial mimetic muscles

D. The majority are innervated on their deep surfaces by CN VII.

There are 23 paired muscles and the single orbicularis oris muscle involved in facial movement. They are grouped into four layers according to depth, not three. Those in layer 1 are the most superficial and include depressor anguli oris, zygomaticus minor, and orbicularis oculi. Those in layer 2 include depressor labii inferioris, risorius, and platysma. Those in layer 3 include orbicularis oris and levator labii superioris. Those in layer 4 include mentalis, levator anguli oris, and buccinator. All muscles are innervated by CN VII. A common examination question is which of the three represents the deep layer. The clinical relevance is that the nerve supply to these three is on their superficial surface rather than the deep surface which is the case with all muscles in the more superficial three layers.[1,2]

REFERENCES

1. Freilinger G, Gruber H, Happak W, Pechmann U. Surgical anatomy of the mimic muscle system and the facial nerve: importance for reconstructive and aesthetic surgery. Plast Reconstr Surg 1987;80(5):686–690
2. Nahai F, ed. The Art of Aesthetic Surgery: Principles and Techniques. St Louis, MO: Quality Medical Publishing; 2005

BLOOD SUPPLY OF THE FACE AND NECK

8. Which one of the following is true of the vascularity of the face and neck?

A. The primary vascular supply arises from the external carotid artery.

The vascular territory of the face and scalp is supplied primarily by the branches of the external carotid artery, with small contributions to the eyelid, brow, forehead, and scalp through the ophthalmic divisions of the internal carotid artery. The eight branches of the external carotid are:

1. Superior thyroid
2. Ascending pharyngeal

3. Lingual
4. Facial
5. Occipital
6. Posterior auricular
7. Maxillary
8. Superficial temporal

The anterior facial arteries include the facial, labial, and supraorbital and supratrochlear vessels. The lateral facial arteries include the submental, zygomatico-orbital, and anterior auricular vessels. The scalp and forehead arteries are the superficial temporal, frontal, and temporal branches of the superficial temporal, posterior auricular, and occipital vessels.

Facial vessels lie in the deepest plane with the parotid duct and buccal and zygomatic branches of the facial nerve. Blood supply to the anterior facial skin is through a dense network of myocutaneous perforators located along the oral commissures and nasolabial folds. The lateral facial skin is supplied by a network of sparsely populated fasciocutaneous perforators. Skin undermining during a face lift divides the fasciocutaneous perforators located laterally; thus, the blood supply of the facial flap is dependent on the medially based myocutaneous perforators. Many of the blood vessels that supply the face tend to travel in proximity to the retaining ligaments. For example, in the area of the zygomatic ligament, McGregor's patch is known to contain a density of blood vessels that often bleed during dissection in that area.[1-3]

REFERENCES

1. Nahai F, ed. The Art of Aesthetic Surgery: Principles and Techniques. St Louis, MO: Quality Medical Publishing; 2005
2. Owsley JQ Jr. Platysma-fascial rhytidectomy: a preliminary report. Plast Reconstr Surg 1977;60(6):843–850
3. Moore KL, Dalley AF, eds. Clinically Oriented Anatomy. 4th ed. New York, NY: Lippincott, Williams & Wilkins; 1999

SENSORY DEFICITS AFTER A FACE LIFT

9. A patient has numbness of the lobule of the ear following a SMAS plication face lift. *Injury to which nerve would most likely account for this?*

B. Great auricular

The great auricular nerve (C2–C3) lies on the sternocleidomastoid (SCM) muscle in the subplatysmal plane and is the most often recognized nerve injury after a face lift (6–7%).[1] It is at greatest risk in its superficial location, which begins along the posterior border of the SCM muscle, 6.5 cm inferior to the tragus. This is known as *McKinney's point.*[2] *Ozturk's* triangle is also a useful topographic marking for this nerve. The triangle is formed by a vertical line through the lobule perpendicular to Frankfurt's horizontal line and then angles at 30 degrees posterior (**Fig. 101.4**).[3]

Division of the nerve or one of its key branches leads to numbness to the lower half of the ear including the lobule on both the medial and lateral surfaces. The lobular branch of the great auricular nerve is, as expected, the main branch responsible for sensation to the lobule. This branch courses within a defined area between vertical lines drawn between the tragus and antitragus (**Fig. 101.5**).[4]

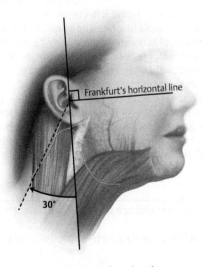

Fig. 101.4 *Ozturk's* triangle.

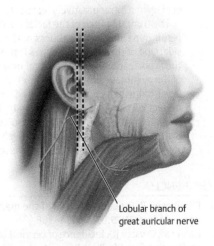

Fig. 101.5 Lobular branch of the great auricular nerve.

The auriculotemporal nerve is a branch of the trigeminal nerve and courses with the superficial temporal artery. It may be inadvertently divided during a face lift. If the auriculotemporal nerve is divided, sympathetic reinnervation can occur, causing gustatory sweating (Frey's syndrome). This is also a potential complication of parotid surgery. The lesser occipital nerve (C2–C3) travels over SCM muscle running between the muscle fascia and superficial fascia. It normally supplies the superior third of the ear and mastoid region. The zygomaticotemporal nerve is another branch of the trigeminal nerve that supplies sensation to a small area of skin in the temple. It is located lateral to the lateral canthus. It may be intentionally avulsed during migraine surgery but is not usually affected in face-lift surgery. The greater occipital nerve supplies the occiput and is also targeted in migraine surgery. It is decompressed rather than avulsed in this situation but is not at risk during face-lift surgery.

REFERENCES

1. Lefkowitz T, Hazani R, Chowdhry S, Elston J, Yaremchuk MJ, Wilhelmi BJ. Anatomical landmarks to avoid injury to the great auricular nerve during rhytidectomy. Aesthet Surg J 2013;33(1):19–23
2. McKinney P, Katrana DJ. Prevention of injury to the great auricular nerve during rhytidectomy. Plast Reconstr Surg 1980;66(5):675–679
3. Ozturk CN, Ozturk C, Huettner F, Drake RL, Zins JE. A failsafe method to avoid injury to the great auricular nerve. Aesthet Surg J 2014;34(1):16–21
4. Sharma V, Wright B, Stephens R, Surek C. What is the lobular branch of the great auricular nerve? Significance in rhytidectomy procedures. Plast Reconstr Surg 2017;139(2):371–379e

MOTOR DEFICITS AFTER A FACE LIFT

10. Following a combined face- and neck-lift procedure, a patient has a new-onset lower lip asymmetry when performing a full denture smile. He is still able to pucker his lips normally. *Which one of the following facial nerve branches is most likely to be injured?*

B. Cervical branch

The facial nerve generally has five main branches. From cranial to caudal these are the frontal (or temporal), zygomatic, buccal, marginal mandibular, and cervical, respectively. Both the marginal mandibular and cervical branches are at risk of injury when the neck is undermined during a face or neck lift particularly when a subplatysmal dissection or muscle division is involved. Injury to either can have some similarity in clinical appearance. Essentially there will be some weakness of the lower lip with either, but there is a subtle difference in appearance and longevity of dysfunction.

Damage to the marginal mandibular branch results in an inability to evert the lower lip, indicating depressor labii inferioris and depressor anguli oris paralysis. These two muscles pull the corners of the lip inferiorly and are supplied purely by the marginal mandibular branch in most cases. Therefore, patients struggle to pout (evert) the lips normally and may well have an asymmetric smile.

The platysma is another lower lip depressor and is supplied by the cervical branches of the facial nerve on its deep surface. In some smile types (typically the full denture smile), the dysfunction of platysma after surgery can lead to new-onset obvious smile asymmetry without the lower lip eversion dysfunction. This is termed *platysma pseudoparalysis*. Patients typically recover completely from this injury within 6 months.[1,2] It is thought to occur where there is division of platysma intraoperatively leading to division or stretching of some of the arborizing branches of the nerve.

The frontal branch of the facial nerve is at risk during surgical procedures including face and brow lift. This can result in permanent weakness of the ipsilateral frontalis muscle and loss of brow elevation and rhytids on this side. One of the buccal branches is probably the most commonly injured motor nerve during a face lift, but given the arborization between buccal branches and zygomatic branches, this could often go unnoticed. Injury to one of the zygomatic branches is therefore similarly affected. This is most at risk of damage during an extended SMAS face lift due to its position deep and close to zygomaticus major. Avoidance of damage can be achieved by keeping dissection superficial to this muscle. Temporary weakness is suggestive of a neuropraxia or the effects of local anesthetic and most likely will resolve spontaneously. Ensuring the potential for motor nerve damage has been discussed with patients preoperatively is paramount, and should nerve injury be evident, regular additional office reviews will often be helpful and necessary to support them through the postoperative process.

REFERENCES

1. Ellenbogen R. Pseudo-paralysis of the mandibular branch of the facial nerve after platysmal face-lift operation. Plast Reconstr Surg 1979;63(3):364–368
2. Daane SP, Owsley JQ. Incidence of cervical branch injury with "marginal mandibular nerve pseudo-paralysis" in patients undergoing face lift. Plast Reconstr Surg 2003;111(7):2414–2418

MOTOR DEFICITS AFTER A FACE LIFT

11. A patient has temporary shoulder weakness after an extended face and neck lift. *Injury to which nerve would likely account for this?*

A. Spinal accessory nerve

The spinal accessory nerve (SAN) or CN XI supplies the SCM and trapezius muscles. It usually passes deep to or through the SCM in the anterior neck and is unlikely to be damaged there during a face lift. It is most at risk in the posterior triangle, passing between the SCM and trapezius, where it lies more superficially just beneath the skin. The anatomical landmark for this nerve has been described as Erb's point which usually is the point at which it leaves SCM en route to trapezius. Erb's point, however, is a term also used to describe the confluence of C5/C6 in the brachial plexus. The two points are distinct from one another.

The SAN is purposefully dissected and preserved where possible during a neck dissection. In a face lift, it is often not seen. When there is injury to it, both SCM and trapezius muscles are affected leading to shoulder dysfunction, including depression of the shoulder girdle, scapular dyskinesis, muscle atrophy, difficulty initiating arm abduction, and some difficulty shrugging of the shoulders. Testing of the upper trapezius by asking the patient to shrug their shoulders alone, however, is unreliable because both the levator scapulae and rhomboid can provide this action. A useful clinical sign to confirm SAN dysfunction is the scapular flip sign. This is when the scapular lifts or flips from the thoracic wall during resisted glenohumeral external rotation. To perform this test, the examiner views the patient from behind and asks the patient to stand with the arm at the side and the elbow flexed to 90 degrees. The examiner resists external rotation at the distal forearm while observing the scapula position. In the presence of a SAN palsy, the unopposed pull of infraspinatus and posterior deltoid are believed to account for this finding.[1,2]

The hypoglossal nerve (CN VII) should not be encountered during a face lift but is seen during neck dissection. Damage to this would cause unilateral weakness of the tongue, as it supplies all of the intrinsic and extrinsic muscles except for the palatoglossus which receives vagal innervation. The facial nerve supplies the mimetic muscles of the face and the posterior belly of digastric muscle. The anterior belly is supplied by the trigeminal nerve (CN VIII) via the mylohyoid nerve of the inferior alveolar nerve. All of the facial nerve branches are at potential risk during face or neck lift surgery to a greater or lesser degree, depending on the technique employed.

REFERENCES

1. Kelley MJ, Kane TE, Leggin BG. Spinal accessory nerve palsy: associated signs and symptoms. J Orthop Sports Phys Ther 2008;38(2):78–86
2. Kelley MJ, Brenneman S. The Scapular Flip Sign: An Examination Sign to Identify the Presence of a Spinal Accessory Nerve Palsy. APTA Combined Sections Meeting. New Orleans, LA: 2000

102. Facial Analysis

See *Essentials of Plastic Surgery*, third edition, pp. 1435–1446

SKIN QUALITY ASSESSMENT

1. A patient is referred to clinic unhappy with their facial appearance. The referring practitioner has assessed this patient using the Glogau classification. *What key information will this provide regarding the patient?*
   A. Their response to sun exposure
   B. Their age and gender
   C. Their degree of photoaging
   D. Their prior treatment
   E. Their required treatment

THE FIBONACCI RATIO

2. When discussing aesthetically pleasing facial proportions, the Fibonacci ratio is often quoted. *Which one of the following numbers represents this "golden ratio"?*
   A. 1:1.33
   B. 1:1.62
   C. 1:2.33
   D. 1:2.62
   E. 1:4.33

FACIAL CANONS OF DIVINE PROPORTION

3. *According to the classical description of facial canons, which one of the following statements is correct?*
   A. The horizontal midpoint of the head is the nasal base.
   B. The length of the ear equals the length of the nose.
   C. The nasal width is one-third of the facial width.
   D. The nose occupies one quarter of the facial height.
   E. The mouth has twice the width of the nose.

ASSESSMENT OF THE FACE FROM THE FRONTAL VIEW

4. *When considering the "ideal" facial proportions in the frontal view, which one of the following is correct?*
   A. The lateral and medial canthi can be used to divide the face into vertical thirds.
   B. The width of the mouth and the vertical stomion-to-menton distance are equal.
   C. The distance between the medial canthi should approximate the width of the mouth.
   D. Facial width at the malar level is similar to the vertical distance from the anterior hairline to the menton.
   E. The upper lip vermilion marks the vertical midpoint of the lower third of the face.

ASSESSMENT OF THE FACE FROM THE LATERAL VIEW

5. *When considering the "ideal" facial proportions in the lateral view, which one of the following is correct?*
   A. The facial profile is usually divided into horizontal fifths.
   B. The vertical hairline-to-menton distance is approximately three times the mandibular angle to the menton distance.
   C. The lower lip should project 2 mm further than the upper lip.
   D. The nasolabial angle is normally more acute in female patients.
   E. The ear lobule and nasal base lie at similar horizontal levels.

ANALYSIS OF THE UPPER EYELID

6. *When assessing a white female patient with normal upper eyelid anatomy in forward gaze, which one of the following is expected?*
   A. A neutral intercanthal axis
   B. An intercanthal distance of 38 mm
   C. Vertical eye opening greater than 15 mm
   D. Upper lid level with the upper limbus
   E. A supratarsal fold 10 mm from the lash line

ANALYSIS OF THE UPPER EYELID

7. **When assessing levator function of the upper eyelid, what would be considered to be a normal amount of excursion?**
   A. 3 mm
   B. 6 mm
   C. 9 mm
   D. 12 mm
   E. 15 mm

FACIAL PROPORTIONS

8. **When considering the relative proportions of the face, which one of the following normally has the same measurement as intercanthal distance?**
   A. Eye width
   B. Ear width
   C. Nose width
   D. Mouth width
   E. Chin width

ANALYSIS OF THE NOSE

9. **When assessing the aesthetics of a Caucasian's nose, which one of the following is correct?**
   A. Deviation is best assessed by drawing a line from the radix to the supratip break.
   B. Nasal length is most accurately measured from the radix to the columella base.
   C. Tip rotation may appear increased secondary to a prominent caudal septum.
   D. Tip projection should be approximately one-third of the nasal length.
   E. The dorsal nasal line lies more anteriorly in females in the lateral view.

ANALYSIS OF THE EXTERNAL EAR

10. **When assessing a patient with normal ears, which one of the following would be expected?**
    A. Posterior inclination of 40 degrees from the vertical in the lateral view
    B. Slight projection of the helix beyond the antihelix in the anterior view
    C. The top of ear site level with the superior brow in the lateral view
    D. Lateral inclination of 5 degrees from the vertical in the anterior view
    E. An ear height-to-width ratio of 3:1 in the lateral view

Answers

SKIN QUALITY ASSESSMENT

1. A patient is referred to clinic unhappy with their facial appearance. The referring practitioner has assessed this patient using the Glogau classification. *What key information will this provide regarding the patient?*

   C. Their degree of photoaging

   When assessing a patient's face during a cosmetic consult, assessment of photoaging is vital, as this can affect treatment selection and outcome following treatment. Photoaging forms a key part of the Glogau classification system,[1] which considers many of the key signs of photoaging including degree of wrinkling, scarring, pigmentary changes, and actinic damage. It also considers the requirement for make-up and the age group, but not gender or specific patient's age. It does not provide information on prior or required treatment, although this would be a useful addition. The ideal classification system should guide treatment and facilitate comparison of results of different treatments between patient groups.

   There are some other useful classification systems other than the Glogau system. These include the Fitzpatrick,[2,3] the Shiftman,[4] and the Ellenbogen[5] systems.

   There are two different Fitzpatrick's classifications relevant to photoaging. The most commonly used system assesses different skin types, ranging from I to VI, with white individuals representing types I to III and those with darker skin tones representing types IV to VI. This system is often used as a measure of patients' susceptibility to sun damage with respect to skin cancer.[2] There is also a separate Fitzpatrick classification (not the same author) for wrinkles that has three grades ranging from fine to deep wrinkles.[3]

   The Shiftman[4] classification is used to assess facial aging and considers four factors: tear-trough depth, cheek fat loss, nasolabial fold depth, and jowl prominence. The Ellenbogen classification considers aspects of the neck that change with age: the cervicomental angle, the inferior mandibular border, the presence of subhyoid depression, and the visibility of thyroid cartilage and sternocleidomastoid.[5,6]

REFERENCES

1. Glogau RG. Aesthetic and anatomic analysis of the aging skin. Semin Cutan Med Surg 1996;15(3):134–138
2. Fitzpatrick TB. The validity and practicality of sun-reactive skin types I through VI. Arch Dermatol 1988;124(6):869–871
3. Fitzpatrick RE, Goldman MP, Satur NM, Tope WD. Pulsed carbon dioxide laser resurfacing of photo-aged facial skin. Arch Dermatol 1996;132(4):395–402
4. Shiftman MA, Mirrafati SJ, Lam SM, eds. Simplified Facial Rejuvenation. New York, NY: Springer; 2008
5. Ellenbogen R, Karlin JV. Visual criteria for success in restoring the youthful neck. Plast Reconstr Surg 1980;66(6):826–837
6. O'Brien M. Plastic and Hand Surgery in Clinical Practice—Classifications and Definitions. New York, NY: Springer; 2009

THE FIBONACCI RATIO

2. When discussing aesthetically pleasing facial proportions, the Fibonacci ratio is often quoted. *Which one of the following numbers represents this "golden ratio"?*

   B. 1:1.62

   The Fibonacci sequence is a set of numbers starting with a 1 or 0. The number sequence proceeds as 1, 2, 3, 5, 8, 13 ..., where two consecutive numbers add up to form the next number. The so-called golden ratio between a given number and the preceding number is 1:1.62. (e.g., 13/8 = 1.62). This ratio, termed *Phi*, is characteristic of forms with aesthetically pleasing proportions and is highly relevant to relative facial proportions. Many examples are found in nature; a good example is the external ear, which displays a spiral pattern conforming to Fibonacci ratios (**Fig. 102.1**).[1]

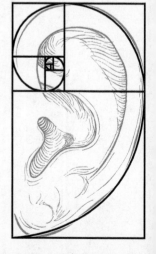

REFERENCE

1. Bashour M. History and current concepts in the analysis of facial attractiveness. Plast Reconstr Surg 2006;118(3):741–756

Fig. 102.1 The external ea
demonstrating the Fibonacci spira

FACIAL CANONS OF DIVINE PROPORTION

3. *According to the classical description of facial canons, which one of the following statements is correct?*

    B. **The length of the ear equals the length of the nose.**

        The facial canons of proportion were formulated and documented by artists of the Renaissance (**Fig. 102.2**). According to these descriptions, the length of the ear and nose is equal. The head can be divided into equal horizontal halves or quarters and the face can be divided into equal horizontal thirds. The horizontal midpoint of the head is the nasal bridge and not the nasal base. Nasal width at the alar base is one quarter of the facial width. The mouth is 1.5 times the width of the nasal base.[1]

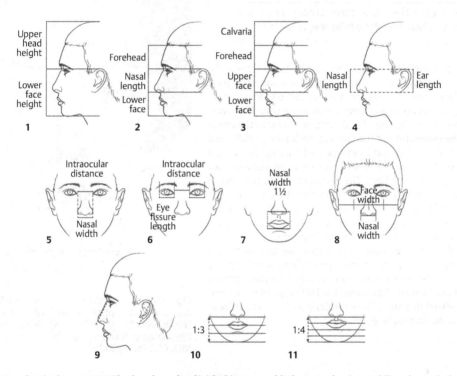

Fig. 102.2 Neoclassical canons. *1,* The head can be divided into equal halves at a horizontal line through the eyes. *2,* The face can be divided into equal thirds, with the nose occupying the middle third. *3,* The head can be divided into equal quarters, with the middle quarters being the forehead and nose. *4,* The length of the ear is equal to the length of the nose. *5,* The distance between the eyes is equal to the width of the nose. *6,* The distance between the eyes is equal to the width of each eye (the face width can be divided into equal fifths). *7,* The width of the mouth is 1½ times the width of the nose. *8,* The width of the nose is one-fourth the width of the face. *9,* The nasal bridge inclination is the same as the ear inclination. *10,* The lower face can be divided into equal thirds. *11,* The lower face can be divided into equal quarters. (From Gunther JP, Rohrich RJ, Adams WP Jr. Dallas Rhinoplasty: Nasal Surgery by the Masters. St. Louis, MO: CRC Press, 2002.)

REFERENCE

1. Bashour M. History and current concepts in the analysis of facial attractiveness. Plast Reconstr Surg 2006;118(3):741–756

ASSESSMENT OF THE FACE FROM THE FRONTAL VIEW

4. *When considering the "ideal" facial proportions in the frontal view, which one of the following is correct?*

    B. **The width of the mouth and the vertical stomion-to-menton distance are equal.**

        Facial proportions, angles, and contours vary with race, age, and sex, but there are certain measurements considered to represent aesthetic ideals. The width of the mouth and the vertical distance between the stomion and menton should be equal in a patient with a normal chin (**Fig. 102.3**). The lateral and medial canthi can be used to divide the face into vertical fifths (not thirds). It is the distance between the medial limbus of each cornea and not the distance between the medial canthi that equates to the mouth width. Mouth width is approximately 1.5 times the width of the intercanthal distance. Facial width at the malar level is similar to the vertical distance from the brows (not the anterior hairline) to the menton. The lower lip vermilion (not the upper) marks the vertical midpoint of the lower third of the face.[1,2]

REFERENCES

1. Rohrich RJ, Adams WP Jr, Amad J, Gunter JP. Dallas Rhinoplasty Nasal Surgery by the Masters. 3rd ed. New York, NY: Thieme; 2014
2. Nahai F, ed. The Art of Aesthetic Surgery: Principles and Techniques. 2nd ed. St Louis, MO: Quality Medical Publishing; 2011

ASSESSMENT OF THE FACE FROM THE LATERAL VIEW

5. *When considering the "ideal" facial proportions in the lateral view, which one of the following is correct?*

   E. **The ear lobule and nasal base lie at similar horizontal levels.**

   The facial profile can be divided into horizontal thirds by drawing transverse lines at the nasal base and nasal root. The desired lip–chin complex relationship is an upper lip that projects approximately 2 mm more than the lower lip. In women, the chin lies slightly posterior to the lower lip. The lower third of the face can be further subdivided into upper third and lower two-thirds by drawing a transverse line at the level of the oral commissure (not the upper lip vermilion). The vertical hairline-to-menton distance is approximately twice (not three times) the mandibular angle to the menton distance (**Fig. 102.4**).

   The nasolabial angle is measured by drawing a straight line through the most anterior and posterior points of the nostrils on lateral view. Where this line bisects with a perpendicular line to the natural horizontal facial plane is the nasolabial angle. Women tend to have more obtuse nasolabial angles than men (95–100 degrees compared with 90–95 degrees). The ear lobule and nasal base lie at similar horizontal levels.[1,2]

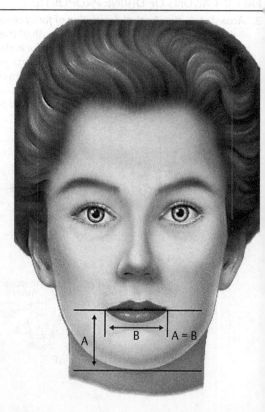

Fig. 102.3   Stomion-to-menton (**A**) distance and the width of the mouth (**B**) are equidistant. (From Gunther JP, Rohrich RJ, Adams WP Jr. Dallas Rhinoplasty: Nasal Surgery by the Masters. St. Louis, MO: CRC Press, 2002.)

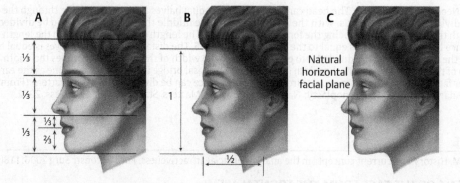

Fig. 102.4   A, Horizontal thirds. **B,** Distance from the mandibular angle to menton is half the distance from the hairline to the menton. **C,** Desired lip–chin complex relationship. (From Gunther JP, Rohrich RJ, Adams WP Jr. Dallas Rhinoplasty: Nasal Surgery by the Masters. St. Louis, MO: CRC Press, 2002.)

REFERENCES

1. Rohrich RJ, Adams WP Jr, Amad J, Gunter JP. Dallas Rhinoplasty Nasal Surgery by the Masters. 3rd ed. New York, NY: Thieme; 2014
2. Nahai F, ed. The Art of Aesthetic Surgery: Principles and Techniques. 2nd ed. St Louis, MO: Quality Medical Publishing; 2011

ANALYSIS OF THE UPPER EYELID

6. *When assessing a white female patient with normal upper eyelid anatomy in forward gaze, which one of the following is expected?*

   E. A supratarsal fold 10 mm from the lash line

   When assessing the normal upper eyelid, the skin quality, fat herniation, and soft tissues should all be assessed. The supratarsal fold is between 7 and 11 mm above the lash line. In women, it is usually between 8 and 10 mm, whereas in men it is slightly lower at 7–8 mm. There will be variability with different ethnic groups and some Asian patients' eyelids have no fold present at all. There is usually a tilt to the intercanthal axis with the lateral canthus sited higher than the medial canthus. A normal intercanthal distance is 31–33 mm; however, a slightly increased distance (33–36 mm) may be considered attractive. Vertical eye opening is normally around 10 mm and the upper eyelid should sit just below (not at the same level as) the upper limbus.[1,2]

REFERENCES

1. McCord CD Jr, Codner MA, eds. Eyelid and Periorbital Surgery. 2nd ed. New York, NY: Thieme; 2016
2. Nahai F, ed. The Art of Aesthetic Surgery: Principles and Techniques. 2nd ed. St Louis, MO: Quality Medical Publishing; 2011

ANALYSIS OF THE UPPER EYELID

7. *When assessing levator function of the upper eyelid, what would be considered to be a normal amount of excursion?*

   E. 15 mm

   Conscious elevation of the upper eyelid is predominantly achieved by levator palpebrae superioris. This muscle originates from the lesser wing of the sphenoid and inserts on the superior edge of the tarsus. It is innervated by the superior division of cranial nerve III. It is assisted by Müller's muscle, which arises from the inferior surface of the levator and inserts onto the superior edge of the tarsus. This has sympathetic innervation.

   Testing of the levator function is performed facing the patient with a thumb gently placed on their brow to limit frontalis function, while asking the patient to look down and then up without moving their head or their brow. Excursion of the upper lid is normally 15 mm or greater. Reduced elevation may be secondary to muscle weakness or disruption of the soft-tissue attachments.[1,2]

REFERENCES

1. McCord CD Jr, Codner MA, eds. Eyelid and Periorbital Surgery. 2nd ed. New York, NY: Thieme; 2016
2. Nahai F, ed. The Art of Aesthetic Surgery: Principles and Techniques. 2nd ed. St Louis, MO: Quality Medical Publishing; 2011

FACIAL PROPORTIONS

8. *When considering the relative proportions of the face, which one of the following normally has the same measurement as intercanthal distance?*

   A. Eye width

   Many facial structures share similar proportions. The intercanthal distance is a good example of this, with a number of other measurements being equal to it. These include eye width, alar base width, nasal projection, and the vertical distance between the infraorbital rim and the nasal base. Ear width is not equivalent to these distances. However, the ear does share some proportions with other facial components; for example, ear length is the same as nose length and ear width is approximately half of ear length in most individuals. Nose width is a nonspecific measurement, as the nose differs in width from root to alar base. The alar base width is the widest part of the nose and this does match the intercanthal distance. The nasal body width is normally 80% of the nasal base width. Mouth and chin widths are essentially the same as one another and are usually 1.5 times the width of the nose at its widest point (i.e., alar base). When any of these typical distances do not match, it is important to identify why this is the case. For example, alar flaring or lack of nasal tip projection can increase the alar base width. Ethnicity also affects these measurements, for example, black patients tend to have broader nasal bridges and more alar flaring.[1–4]

REFERENCES

1. Nahai F, ed. The Art of Aesthetic Surgery: Principles and Techniques. 2nd ed. St Louis, MO: Quality Medical Publishing; 2011

2. Rohrich RJ, Adams WP Jr, Amad J, Gunter JP. Dallas Rhinoplasty Nasal Surgery by the Masters. 3rd ed. New York, NY: Thieme; 2014

3. McCord CD Jr, Codner MA, eds. Eyelid and Periorbital Surgery. 2nd ed. New York, NY: Thieme; 2016

4. Byrd HS, Hobar PC. Rhinoplasty: a practical guide for surgical planning. Plast Reconstr Surg 1993;91(4):642–654, discussion 655–656

ANALYSIS OF THE NOSE

9. *When assessing the aesthetics of a Caucasian's nose, which one of the following is correct?*

   C. **Tip rotation may appear increased secondary to a prominent caudal septum.**

   Tip rotation is determined by the degree of the nasolabial angle. The nasolabial angle is measured by drawing a straight line through the most anterior and posterior points of the nostrils on lateral view and noting the point this bisects with a perpendicular line to the natural horizontal facial plane. The angle between these lines represents the nasolabial angle and varies from 90 to 100 degrees, depending on gender and race (**Fig. 102.5**).

   It is important to be aware of other factors that may give the appearance of increased tip projection. For example, a prominent caudal septum can give this appearance, even when the nasolabial angle is within normal range. Understanding these principles is key to rhinoplasty. Also, a nose with a high dorsum without a supratip break will appear less rotated than one with a low dorsum and supratip break, even though the degree of rotation is the same.

   Nasal deviation is best assessed by drawing a plumb line from the mid-glabellar point to the menton. This line should bisect the nasal bridge, nasal tip, and cupid's bow (**Fig. 102.6**).

   Nasal length is the distance from the radix to the tip and should be 1.5 times the nasal tip projection. The dorsal nasal line typically lies 2 mm posterior to and parallel with a line connecting the nasofrontal angle with the desired tip projection. In men, it lies slightly more anteriorly.[1-3]

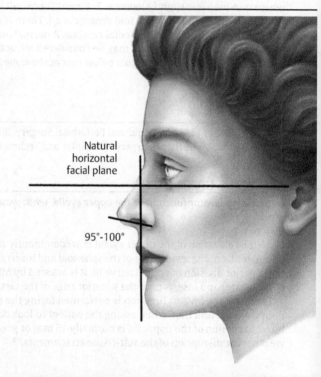

Natural horizontal facial plane

95°–100°

Fig. 102.5 Nasolabial angle. (From Gunther JP, Rohrich RJ, Adams WP Jr. Dallas Rhinoplasty: Nasal Surgery by the Masters. St. Louis, MO: CRC Press, 2002.)

REFERENCES

1. Nahai F, ed. The Art of Aesthetic Surgery: Principles and Techniques. 2nd ed. St Louis, MO: Quality Medical Publishing; 2011

2. Rohrich RJ, Adams WP Jr, Amad J, Gunter JP. Dallas Rhinoplasty Nasal Surgery by the Masters. 3rd ed. New York, NY: Thieme; 2014

3. Byrd HS, Hobar PC. Rhinoplasty: a practical guide for surgical planning. Plast Reconstr Surg 1993;91(4):642–654, discussion 655–656

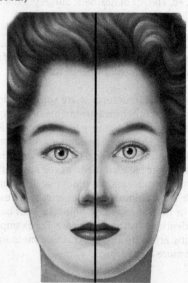

Fig. 102.6 Deviation of the nose is evaluated by drawing a line from the mid-glabella to the menton. (From Gunther JP, Rohrich RJ, Adams WP Jr. Dallas Rhinoplasty: Nasal Surgery by the Masters. St. Louis, MO: CRC Press, 2002.)

ANALYSIS OF THE EXTERNAL EAR

10. *When assessing a patient with normal ears, which one of the following would be expected?*

   B. **Slight projection of the helix beyond the antihelix in the anterior view**

   Understanding of external ear aesthetics is critical to ear reconstruction and correction of ear deformities such as prominent ear. In the anterior view, the helix should be slightly more prominent (approximately 5 mm) than the antehelical fold (**Fig. 102.7**).

   Overcorrection of the prominent ear can leave the antihelix as the most prominent part of the ear, resulting in an unnatural appearance and increased risk of development of pressure damage to the ear that may result in *chondrodermatitis nodularis helicis*. The ear usually measures 5–6.5 cm in height and 2–3.5 cm in width. The ratio of width to height is usually 55–60%. The ear is normally placed with its superior aspect level with the upper eyelid and just below the lateral-most part of the eyebrow and around 5–6 cm posterior to the lateral orbital rim. It is inclined posteriorly in the lateral view about 20 degrees. It is inclined laterally from the scalp in the anterior view (20–30 degrees), and this means that the top of the ear is about 1.5–2 cm from the scalp.[1,2]

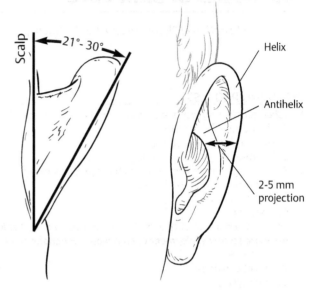

Fig. 102.7 Normal ear aesthetics.

REFERENCES

1. Janis JE, Rohrich RJ, Gutowski KA. Otoplasty. Plast Reconstr Surg 2005;115(4):60e–72e
2. Ha RY, Trovato MJ. Plastic surgery of the ear. Sel Read Plast Surg 2011;11(3):1–16

103. Basics of Skin Care

See Essentials of Plastic Surgery, third edition, pp. 1447–1455

THE AGING PROCESS

1. **When considering intrinsic aging of the skin, which one of the following increases?**
   A. The depth of the dermis
   B. The depth of the epidermis
   C. The ratio of type III to I collagen
   D. The number of melanocytes
   E. The depth of subdermal fat

2. Extrinsic aging is a major factor in the aging process of skin. **Which one of the following is the main cause of this?**
   A. Ultraviolet (UV) A radiation
   B. UVB radiation
   C. Smoking
   D. Dehydration
   E. Poor nutrition

3. There are a number of clinical signs of extrinsic aging. **Which one of the following changes is most specifically associated with development of cutaneous malignancies such as squamous cell carcinomas?**
   A. Keratoses
   B. Loss of elasticity
   C. Fine rhytids
   D. Irregular pigmentation
   E. Telangiectasia

HEALTHY SKIN

4. **When assessing skin health, which one of the following desirable features is most strongly linked to the presence of abundant glycosaminoglycans?**
   A. Smooth skin
   B. Even color
   C. Firmness and tightness
   D. Optimal hydration
   E. Contour fullness

THE KERATINOCYTE MATURATION CYCLE

5. The keratinocyte maturation cycle (KMC) has clinical relevance to skin treatments. **Which one of the following describes its usual duration?**
   A. 12 days
   B. 28 days
   C. 40 days
   D. 52 days
   E. 92 days

DURATION OF SKIN THERAPY

6. A patient is seen in the office requesting skin rejuvenation therapy. **What would be the usual ratio of pretreatment to treatment duration when considering skin rejuvenation therapy with topical agents?**
   A. 1:1
   B. 1:2
   C. 1:3
   D. 1:4
   E. 1:5

EFFECTS OF MOISTURIZERS ON SKIN CELL TURNOVER

7. **How does overuse of skin moisturizers affect the natural skin turnover cycle?**
   A. It speeds it up.
   B. It slows it down.
   C. It improves keratinocyte quality.
   D. It reduces keratinocyte quality.
   E. It both speeds it up and improves keratinocyte quality.

MEDICAL SKIN CARE

8. **Which one of the following is true with regard to medical skin care?**
   A. It will only include topical agents.
   B. It should be available over the counter.
   C. It will avoid the use of sunscreens.
   D. It will comprise a standard recipe.
   E. It will involve prescription-based topicals

SUNSCREENS

9. *Which one of the following agents would most effectively protect the skin from both UVA and UVB with minimal contact sensitivity?*
   A. Titanium dioxide
   B. Padimate A
   C. Padimate O
   D. Avobenzone
   E. Anthranilate

SUNSCREEN AND SPF

10. The terms "Sun Protection Factor" or "SPF" 30, 50, and 60 are often used when describing sunblock medication. *When using a sunblock with an SPF 30, what does this terminology actually mean for the patient?*
    A. That 30% of the sun's UV radiation is blocked by the agent
    B. That the effective duration of sun block is 30 minutes
    C. That the time to burning is 30 times longer than without protection
    D. That only 30% of the atmospheric UV radiation can reach the skin surface
    E. That the percentage of the active ingredient in the product is 30%.

USE OF TRETINOIN

11. A patient is seen in clinic and has a number of questions regarding tretinoin and its use. *Which one of the following is true with regard to tretinoin?*
    A. It is a derivative of vitamin D.
    B. Its use results in rapid changes to the dermis within a few days.
    C. It has little effect on dermal collagen and elastin.
    D. It commonly causes skin irritation and burning.
    E. The most common concentrations used are 5 and 10%.

COMPLICATIONS WITH TOPICAL AGENTS

12. A patient presents to the office while undergoing a topical skin treatment plan designed elsewhere. They find they have developed dark blue-black speckled pigmentation in some treated areas. *Which one of the following agents within their plan is most likely responsible?*
    A. Kojic acid
    B. Hydroquinone
    C. Glycolic acid
    D. α-Tocopherol
    E. coenzyme Q10

CHEMICAL PEEL AGENTS

13. *Which one of the following would be most effective at managing a patient with oily facial skin who wished to have an exfoliant/chemical peel within their treatment program?*
    A. Glycolic acid
    B. Salicylic acid
    C. Lactobionic acid
    D. Alpha-lipoic acid
    E. L-ascorbic acid

EVALUATION OF THE SKIN CARE PATIENT

14. *When considering the Fitzpatrick skin classification in relation to skin care, which one of the following is true?*
    A. It is most useful to guide the selection of antioxidant use.
    B. It is most useful to direct the use of a melanin-modifying agent.
    C. It is limited for use in predicting a patient's response to topical treatment.
    D. It is particularly useful to predict outcomes after facial peels.
    E. It is no longer used in clinical practice.

A TYPICAL SKIN CARE REGIMEN

15. *Which one of the following is true of a typical effective skin care regimen?*
    A. It would usually last for 3 months.
    B. It would usually last for five skin cycles.
    C. It should be continued indefinitely.
    D. It would include tretinoin, hydroquinone, and alpha hydroxy acid (AHA).
    E. Maintenance and therapeutic treatments should run simultaneously.

Answers

THE AGING PROCESS

1. *When considering intrinsic aging of the skin, which one of the following increases?*

   C. **The ratio of type III to I collagen**

   There are a number of changes, which occur within the skin and subcutaneous tissues with increasing age. The majority of these changes relate to atrophy or reduced numbers of cells resulting in a reduction in overall tissue depth. The ratio of collagen subtypes also changes with age. In the skin there is usually a far higher proportion of type I collagen to type III ratio (4:1) with aging; this ratio changes as proportionally more type III collagen is present.

   Other histologic changes in the skin include thinning of both the dermis and epidermis, with flattening of the dermal–epidermal junction. This results from cellular apoptosis and is affected by genetic predisposition. There is also a decrease in the number of Langerhans cells and melanocytes, blood vessels, fibroblasts, and mast cells. The stratum corneum becomes more disorganized, with collagen and elastin becoming less well ordered. Beneath the skin, there is atrophy of the subdermal fat. All of the above contribute to reducing the overall thickness and quality of the skin and subcutaneous tissues with advancing age. This has clinical relevance in many areas of plastic surgery, including approaches to facial rejuvenation.

2. Extrinsic aging is a major factor in the aging process of skin. *Which one of the following is the main cause of this?*

   A. **Ultraviolet (UV) A radiation**

   Extrinsic aging results from skin exposure to a number of environmental factors including UV radiation, dehydration, inadequate nutrition, temperature extremes, physical damage, and traumatic injuries. In addition, smoking will have a profound effect on the extrinsic aging process of the skin. Of all of these factors, actinic damage from **UVA** radiation is the major cause of extrinsic aging. UVB radiation is primarily responsible for sunburns. UV radiation generally results in DNA damage within the nucleus and mitochondria. More specifically, UVA results in damage through the creation of free radicals in the form of reactive oxygen species.

3. There are a number of clinical signs of extrinsic aging. *Which one of the following changes is most specifically associated with development of cutaneous malignancies such as squamous cell carcinomas?*

   A. **Keratoses**

   The extrinsic aging process results in thickening of the stratum corneum, atrophy of the epidermis with cellular atypia, irregular dispersion of melanin, collagen fragmentation, and abnormal deposition of elastin. These changes can be observed clinically with the presence of keratosis, which are associated with actinic damage and development of nonmelanoma skin malignancies such as squamous cell carcinoma. Telangiectasia is a common finding in sun-damaged skin; however, it is not specifically associated with development of cutaneous malignancies. Instead, it is a feature of basal cell carcinomas and can be a distracting finding in such patients. Irregular pigmentation is observed in the aging skin with solar lentigines and freckle development. Almost all adult patients will have a combination of intrinsic and extrinsic aging that can be accelerated by environmental factors and genetic predisposition.[1-3]

REFERENCES

1. Fitzgerald R, Graivier MH, Kane M, et al. Update on facial aging. Aesthet Surg J 2010;30(Suppl):11S–24S
2. Khavkin J, Ellis DAF. Aging skin: histology, physiology, and pathology. Facial Plast Surg Clin North Am 2011;19(2):229–234
3. Farkas JP, Pessa JE, Hubbard B, Rohrich RJ. The science and theory behind facial aging. Plast Reconstr Surg Glob Open 2013;1(1):e8–e15

HEALTHY SKIN

4. *When assessing skin health, which one of the following desirable features is most strongly linked to the presence of abundant glycosaminoglycans?*

   D. **Optimal hydration**

   The appearance of normal skin is poorly defined in classic dermatology and plastic surgery textbooks, but it is an infant's skin qualities that really define and illustrate healthy skin. The skin of an infant and hence healthy skin will have a smooth surface, an even color/pigmentation, firmness and tightness, adequate hydration, and fullness in contour with an absence of static rhytids, scars, and pigmentary imperfections. Collectively, the constituents of the skin and subcutaneous tissues will each impact upon these features. However, glycosaminoglycan content of the tissues will have the most significant impact on skin hydration, as glycosaminoglycans carry a large volume of fluid. Their role as a cosmetic filler takes advantage of this feature such that when such fillers are injected into the tissues, they not only increase volume by their presence, but they also draw in fluid to the area and further plump up the skin and soft tissues. Skin smoothness reflects the surface of the skin and is affected mainly by the effects of exfoliation where soft keratin remains, and harder keratin is removed. Uniform color or pigmentation reflects normal melanocyte function. With aging or unhealthy skin, there is an increase in pigmentation abnormalities. Firmness and tightness of the skin represent healthy elastin and collagen levels and organization, respectively.[1]

REFERENCE

1. Obagi ZE. Principles and objectives of skin health restoration. In: Obagi ZE, ed. The Art of Skin Health Restoration and Rejuvenation. Boca Raton, FL: CRC Press; 2015:17–44

THE KERATINOCYTE MATURATION CYCLE

5. The keratinocyte maturation cycle (KMC) has clinical relevance to skin treatments. *Which one of the following describes its usual duration?*
   C. 40 days
   The KMC is the amount of time for a new keratinocyte to ascend through the epidermis and exfoliate. It is typically 40 days, i.e., 6 weeks' duration. This is an important concept for treating skin with topical agents and chemical peels as pretreatment and treatment durations are both prescribed in units of the KMC. A keratinocyte is formed from mitosis of the basal layer of the skin, and takes approximately 28 days to mature. The keratinocyte then undergoes denucleation to become a corneocyte in the stratum corneum and exfoliates in approximately 12 days. The normal KMC is therefore approximately 6 weeks because it includes both of these phases (28 + 12 days).

DURATION OF SKIN THERAPY

6. A patient is seen in the office requesting skin rejuvenation therapy. *What would be the usual ratio of pretreatment to treatment duration when considering skin rejuvenation therapy with topical agents?*
   C. 1:3
   A skin cycle is defined as the KMC and lasts for 6 weeks. This comprises a 4-week (28-day) process for a keratinocyte to develop and mature, plus a further 12 days (approximately 2 weeks) for it to denucleate and exfoliate. Treatment duration is prescribed in terms of skin cycles. It is usual to pretreat skin with topical agents for at least one skin cycle before peeling or commencing a therapeutic treatment plan. A typical course of medical topicals (therapeutic skin care) without a peel is three skin cycles. Although this is the standard approach, other aspects of the patient's health will need to be considered, as certain disease processes will accelerate or slow down the KMC. For example, KMC is accelerated in psoriasis, skin cancers, and verrucae. Conversely, it is prolonged in intrinsic aging, photoaging, and when using topical moisturizers and steroids. Skin complexion will also impact treatment cycles and patients with darker and complex skin types should be treated with topicals for more than one skin cycle before peeling.

EFFECTS OF MOISTURIZERS ON SKIN CELL TURNOVER

7. *How does overuse of skin moisturizers affect the natural skin turnover cycle?*
   B. It slows it down.
   Overuse of moisturizers can have a number of detrimental effects on skin including a reduction in barrier function and a contribution to development of sensitive skin. In addition, overuse of moisturizers can increase the skin cycle turnover time or KMC which has implications for selecting duration of pretreatment and treatment plans. It is important therefore to educate patients on appropriate use of moisturizers and ensure that overuse is not undertaken as the effectiveness of the topical treatment program may be reduced, prolong the KMC, reduce barrier function, and contribute to "sensitive" skin.

MEDICAL SKIN CARE

8. *Which one of the following is true with regard to medical skin care?*
   E. It will involve prescription-based topicals.
   Medical skin care is the use of prescription-based topicals to induce clinically significant changes in the skin. Prescription-based topicals are primarily tretinoin and hydroquinone.
   These are used in combination with cleansers, toners, alpha hydroxy acids (AHAs), antioxidants, and sunscreens to form a customized regimen for the patient, rather than a "standard recipe." Medical skin care should therefore

be directed by a physician and not available over the counter. Although the majority of the program is delivered topically, oral prescriptions for skin diseases, e.g., isotretinoin or antibiotics for acne or rosacea, may also be added into the medical skin care regimen.

SUNSCREENS

9. *Which one of the following agents would most effectively protect the skin from both UVA and UVB with minimal contact sensitivity?*
   A. Titanium dioxide

   Sunscreens prevent photoaging by reducing UV light absorption through the skin. There are three types of UV light: A, B, and C. However, only UVA and UVB are clinically relevant as UVC does not penetrate the earth's atmosphere. UVA is associated with skin aging leading to formation of rhytids, while UVB is associated with sunburn and skin cancer development.

   Some sunscreen's active ingredients will affect UVA only, such as Avobenzone or Anthranilates, which are both chemical agents that have limited absorption spectrums (320–360 nm). Others affect UVB only such as Padimate A and Padimate O which are chemical agents based on p-aminobenzoic acid and its esters. These agents absorb the entire UVB spectrum (280–320 nm). Avobenzone is tolerated cosmetically but can produce allergic reactions. In contrast, physical sunblocks will reflect or scatter both UVA and UVB spectra. Titanium dioxide and micronized zinc oxide are the most common forms of physical sunblocks and are well tolerated by patients, as they do not produce contact sensitivity, phototoxicity, or photoallergy.

SUNSCREEN AND SPF

10. The terms "Sun Protection Factor" or "SPF" 30, 50, and 60 are often used when describing sunblock medication. *When using a sunblock with an SPF 30, what does this terminology actually mean for the patient?*
    C. That the time to burning is 30 times longer than without protection

    Sun protection factor (SPF) is the ratio of UV radiation dose that produces the first sign of erythema in sunscreen-protected skin to unprotected skin. As the SPF value increases, sunburn protection increases. So for example, SPF 30 blocks 96.7% of UV radiation (not 30 or 70%). If a person develops sunburn in 10 minutes on unprotected skin, then it will take 300 minutes to sunburn with SPF 30 sunscreen, i.e., 30 times longer. In contrast, an SPF 15 blocks 93.3% of UV radiation, and if a person develops sunburn in 10 minutes on unprotected skin, then it will take 150 minutes to sunburn with SPF 15 sunscreen. However, an SPF 30 sunscreen is not active or effective any longer than an SPF 15 sunscreen; therefore, both should be reapplied every 2 hours during direct sun exposure. SPF therefore is primarily showing the level of protection provided against UVB rather than UVA. In addition to the SPF rating, there is also a star rating used for sunscreens. This relates to the UVA protection. The stars range from 0 to 5 and indicate the percentage of UVA radiation absorbed by the sunscreen in comparison to UVB, i.e., the ratio between the level of protection by UVA and UVB. In general, therefore it is both advisable to have a high SPF and a high star rating combined in a single product (http://www.bad.org.uk/skin-cancer/sunscreen-fact-sheet).

USE OF TRETINOIN

11. A patient is seen in clinic and has a number of questions regarding tretinoin and its use. *Which one of the following is true with regard to tretinoin?*
    D. It commonly causes skin irritation and burning.

    Tretinoin is a derivative of vitamin A (not vitamin D) and represents the gold standard for the topical treatment of facial rhytids and photoaging. Unfortunately, while it is an effective medication, it can often cause skin irritation leading to redness, dryness, scaling, burning, and peeling, so patients must be advised of this prior to commencing treatment. Tretinoin induces epidermal hyperplasia and deposition of glycosaminoglycans. It also increases the thickness of the stratum corneum and reduces both keratinocyte and melanocyte atypia. Its use increases collagen types I and III in the papillary dermis through the inhibition of metalloproteinases. Changes within the epidermis are usually seen within 3 to 6 months (not a few days), while dermal changes are seen later at 9 or 12 months. The most common formulations for tretinoin are 0.025, 0.05, and 0.1% concentrations, not 5 or 10%.

COMPLICATIONS WITH TOPICAL AGENTS

12. A patient presents to the office while undergoing a topical skin treatment plan designed elsewhere. They find they have developed dark blue-black speckled pigmentation in some treated areas. *Which one of the following agents within their plan is most likely responsible?*
    B. Hydroquinone

    Hydroquinone (HQ) is a melanin-modifying agent commonly used to treat skin hyperpigmentation such as melasma, solar lentigines, and postinflammatory hyperpigmentation due to injury, acne, dermatitis, lupus, or peels. The mechanism of action is to block conversion of dihydroxyphenylalanine (DOPA) to melanin by inhibition of tyrosine. HQ thereby inhibits melanocytes and prevents formation of melanosomes. It is used in concentrations of 2–4% and is frequently combined with other agents such as tretinoin, glycolic acids, and steroids to improve efficacy and decrease side effects. Side effects, although uncommon, may include redness, dryness, irritation, hypersensitivity, and allergic reactions. Prolonged topical HQ use can induce a condition called "exogenous ochronosis," resulting in dark, blue-black, speckled pigmentation in treated areas. An interruption in HQ therapy is therefore recommended every 5 to 6 months for a minimum period of 3 months before reinitiating therapy.[1]

Kojic acid is another tyrosinase inhibitor with a similar but less effective action than HQ. It is derived from a Japanese mushroom, and side effects include contact dermatitis and hypersensitivity. Glycolic acid is an AHA used to treat acne, keratosis, warts, psoriasis, and photoaging. The mechanism of action is uncertain but may be related to the removal of calcium ions from the epidermal corneocytes producing exfoliation of the stratum corneum. Side effects include burning, pain, and erythema. Coenzyme Q10 (CoQ 10), usually available as alpha-lipoic acid, is a cellular antioxidant, which stabilizes free radicals. Clinically, CoQ 10 reduces UVB-induced erythema and improves photoaging. α-Tocopherol is a form of vitamin E and is used to protect cell membrane viability, which may reduce UV-induced erythema.

REFERENCE

1. Ly F, Soko AS, Dione DA, et al. Aesthetic problems associated with the cosmetic use of bleaching products. Int J Dermatol 2007; 46(1, Suppl 1):15–17

CHEMICAL PEEL AGENTS

13. *Which one of the following would be most effective at managing a patient with oily facial skin who wished to have an exfoliant/chemical peel within their treatment program?*

   B. Salicylic acid

   Hydroxy acids represent a group of compounds (AHAs, beta-hydroxy acids [BHAs], polyhydroxy acids [PHAs], and bionic acids) found in many cosmetic formulations used to treat acne, keratosis, warts, psoriasis, photoaging, and other disorders. They are used as chemical peel/exfoliating agents. BHAs have a hydroxy group in the beta-position and are hydrophobic. Salicylic acid is the most commonly used BHA. BHAs are lipophilic and indicated for use in oily areas of the face such as the chin, nose, and central forehead.

   The AHAs are the most commonly used hydroxy acids overall for skin treatment and include glycolic, lactic, mandelic, malic, and pyruvic acids. Of these, glycolic acid is the most frequently used. AHAs have a hydroxy group in the alpha-position and are water-soluble. The mechanism of action is thought to be related to the removal of calcium ions from the epidermal keratinocytes producing exfoliation of the stratum corneum. Daily application results in epidermal exfoliation, early thinning of the stratum corneum, and late thickening of the skin related to increased glycosaminoglycan and collagen deposition.

   PHAs have limited dermal penetration due to their larger molecular size compared to other AHAs and so are less commonly used; however, they do result in less burning and skin irritation. Common forms of PHAs are gluconolactone and lactobionic acid. They can have improved cell turnover and act as a humectant and antioxidant. Alpha-lipoic acid and L-ascorbic acid are both antioxidants used in topical treatment regimens, but neither are used as chemical peel or exfoliating agents. Alpha-lipoic acid is the most common form of coenzyme Q10 that is a cellular antioxidant, which stabilizes free radicals. Clinically, it reduces UV-induced erythema and improves photoaging. L-ascorbic acid is the active form of vitamin C, which acts as an antioxidant and as a promoter of collagen synthesis. It may be used to improve skin hydration and reduce fine rhytids by reducing inflammation and UV-induced immunosuppression.[1,2]

REFERENCES

1. Kornhauser A, Coelho SG, Hearing VJ. Applications of hydroxy acids: classification, mechanisms, and photoactivity. Clin Cosmet Investig Dermatol 2010;3:135–142
2. Babilas P, Knie U, Abels C. Cosmetic and dermatologic use of alpha hydroxy acids. J Dtsch Dermatol Ges 2012;10(7): 488–491

EVALUATION OF THE SKIN CARE PATIENT

14. *When considering the Fitzpatrick skin classification in relation to skin care, which one of the following is true?*

   C. It is limited for use in predicting a patient's response to topical treatment.

   The Fitzpatrick skin classification is commonly used in dermatology and plastic surgery circles. It describes the skin color and response to sun exposure in terms of tanning. While it may be relevant in skin cancer patient management, its use in skin rejuvenation is limited because it fails to accurately predict a patient's response to topical treatments and peels (**Table 103.1**).

Table 103.1 *Fitzpatrick Skin Type Classification*

Skin Type	Characteristics	Sun Exposure History
I	Pale white, freckles, blue eyes, blond or red hair	Always burns, never tans
II	Fair white, blue/green/hazel eyes, blond or red hair	Usually burns, minimally tans
III	Cream white, any hair or eye color	Sometimes burns, tans uniformly
IV	Moderate brown (Mediterranean)	Rarely burns, always tans well
V	Dark brown (Middle Eastern)	Rarely burns, tans easily
VI	Dark brown to black	Never burns, tans easily

(From Janis JE. Essentials of Aesthetic Surgery, Thieme, 2018.)

A TYPICAL SKIN CARE REGIMEN

15. Which one of the following is true of a typical effective skin care regimen?

   D. It would include tretinoin, hydroquinone, and AHA.

   Following pretreatment, patients will cycle between therapeutic and maintenance skin care and the mainstays of a therapeutic regimen are tretinoin, hydroquinone, and an AHA, such as glycolic acid. These topicals act synergistically to induce visible changes in the skin.

   Therapeutic skin care is usually a 5-month (not 3) regimen (i.e., three skin cycles) to treat a specific skin condition, e.g., hyperpigmentation, photoaging, acne, or rosacea.

   After the skin condition is treated, therapeutic skin care is stopped and maintenance skin care is initiated. If the skin condition recurs, then therapeutic skin care is initiated once again. The clinician should be able to provide both therapeutic and maintenance skin care guidance throughout the lifetime of the patient. Maintenance skin care usually involves weaning a patient from hydroquinone, changing from tretinoin to retinol (if there are patient tolerance issues), and maximizing antioxidant and sun protection use.

104. Neurotoxins

See Essentials of Plastic Surgery, third edition, pp. 1456–1467

NEUROTOXIN SEROTYPES

1. *Which one of the following* Clostridium botulinum *serotypes is predominantly used in clinical practice for the treatment of facial rhytids?*
   A. Serotype A
   B. Serotype B
   C. Serotype D
   D. Serotype E
   E. Serotype G

FOOD AND DRUG ADMINISTRATION (FDA) APPROVAL FOR NEUROTOXIN USE

2. There are three commercially available preparations of C. botulinum toxin used in aesthetic facial rejuvenation. *For which one of the following treatment indications do all three have FDA approval?*
   A. Bunny lines
   B. Glabellar lines
   C. Crow's feet
   D. Nasolabial folds
   E. Marionette lines

COMBINING BOTULINUM TOXIN AND FILLERS IN FACIAL REJUVENATION

3. *When planning nonsurgical treatment for a patient who requests a combination of neurotoxins and fillers, which one of the following is true?*
   A. They must be performed on separate clinic visits.
   B. Marking the injection points with pen beforehand carries no risk.
   C. The filler component should ideally be performed first.
   D. The toxin component should ideally be performed first.
   E. The specific order of injection should be flexible.

DOSING STRATEGY IN NEUROTOXIN USE

4. You normally use Botox for injection and move to a different clinic where the preparation Dysport is used instead. *How will this affect your usual dosing schedule?*
   A. The onset of action will be delayed.
   B. The number of units per treatment area will need to be doubled.
   C. The number of units per treatment area will need to be halved.
   D. The duration between treatments will be reduced.
   E. It will not have any significant effect.

BENEFITS OF USING XEOMIN AS A NEUROMODULATOR

5. *Which one of the following represents a key benefit of using Xeomin as your neurotoxin of choice for aesthetic facial rejuvenation?*
   A. It does not require refrigeration.
   B. It does not cause headaches.
   C. It does not require reconstitution.
   D. It has a low immunogenicity.
   E. It does not require a prescription.

PREPARATION AND DELIVERY OF NEUROTOXINS IN AESTHETIC FACIAL REJUVENATION

6. *When reconstituting botulinum toxin in clinic for the treatment of rhytids, what would be the potential advantage of using preserved saline for this purpose?*
   A. Longer action of product
   B. Reduced immunogenicity
   C. Decreased pain on injection
   D. Reduced bruising risk
   E. Lower financial cost

RISKS IN BOTULINUM TOXIN FACIAL REJUVENATION THERAPY

7. *When a patient requests isolated treatment of their transverse forehead rhytids without treatment for the crow's feet and glabella regions, what is the main risk of doing so?*
   A. There is generally a high risk of dissatisfaction when treating a single area.
   B. There is an increased risk of causing brow ptosis.
   C. There is an increased risk of causing eyelid ptosis.
   D. There is an increased risk of causing ectropion.
   E. There is no specific risk of treating this single area.

MUSCLES TARGETED WITH BOTULINUM TOXIN TREATMENT

8. *Which muscle is targeted when treating bunny lines with C. botulinum toxin?*
   A. Procerus
   B. Orbicularis oculi
   C. Orbicularis oris
   D. Nasalis
   E. Levator labii superioris

AREAS OF THE FACE AND NECK TARGETED WITH BOTULINUM TOXIN TREATMENT

9. *Which one of the following areas may particularly benefit from the use of the "microbotox technique"?*
   A. A dimpled chin
   B. A droopy nasal tip
   C. Marionette lines
   D. Masseteric hypertrophy
   E. Platysmal bands

BOTULINUM TOXIN USE IN FACIAL AESTHETICS

10. Botulinum toxins are derived from the bacterium *C. botulinum*. *Which one of the following statements is correct regarding their use in facial aesthetics?*
    A. Toxin subtypes A, B, and C are commercially available for facial rejuvenation.
    B. All subtypes work through direct interaction with a protein called *SNAP-25*.
    C. Toxins cause temporary chemodenervation by preventing binding and release of acetylcholine.
    D. Subtypes A and B have FDA approval for use in all zones of facial rhytids.
    E. Units are measured in mouse units and are comparable between different manufacturers.

ADMINISTRATION OF BOTOX FOR FACIAL REJUVENATION

11. You are preparing some Botox for a 30-year-old woman who has requested treatment for her frown line (glabellar) region. It is her first experience with Botox injections. *Which one of the following is correct?*
    A. A standard dilution should be 4 units/mL in water for injection.
    B. Reconstitution involves firmly shaking the bottle to mix it fully.
    C. The product should be used within 4 hours of reconstitution.
    D. A typical starting dose for this patient would be 20 units.
    E. Four to six injections should be used, each placed above the orbital rim.

DECISION MAKING IN FACIAL AESTHETICS

12. A 33-year-old woman presents with early dynamic crow's-feet rhytids. *What would be a reasonable total neurotoxin dosing schedule for her to target this area?*
    A. Botox 16–24 units
    B. Dysport 16–24 units
    C. Xeomin 5–10 units
    D. Botox 8–12 units
    E. Dysport 8–12 units

CONSENT IN BOTULINUM TOXIN THERAPY

13. *When consenting a patient pretreatment with botulinum toxin in the glabella region, what risk should you quote them for developing temporary eyelid ptosis?*
    A. 1%
    B. 3%
    C. 5%
    D. 10%
    E. 12%

Answers

NEUROTOXIN SEROTYPES

1. **Which one of the following Clostridium botulinum *serotypes is predominantly used in clinical practice for the treatment of facial rhytids?***

   A. Serotype A

   There are seven botulinum toxin subtypes (A through G) derived from varying strains of the bacterium *Clostridium botulinum* (C. botulinum). Of the seven toxin serotypes, only A and B are commercially available for clinical use.

   Popularity of these toxins in clinical practice has increased dramatically in the past 40 years since their first use for strabismus in children in the 1980s. In 2002, botulinum toxin first gained Food and Drug Administration (FDA) approval for use in glabellar rhytids and has since become one of the most commonly used aesthetic facial nonsurgical interventions since. Type A was initially FDA approved for treatment of glabellar frown lines in patients 65 years or younger and this approval has since expanded to include other indications such as hyperhidrosis, blepharoptosis, and cervical dystonia, as well as other aesthetic indications. Type B is FDA approved only for the treatment of cervical dystonia, so other uses are off label.[1,2]

REFERENCES

1. Carruthers J, Fagien S, Matarasso SL; Botox Consensus Group. Consensus recommendations on the use of botulinum toxin type a in facial aesthetics. Plast Reconstr Surg 2004; 114(6, Suppl):1S–22S
2. Lorenc ZP, Kenkel JM, Fagien S, et al. Consensus panel's assessment and recommendations on the use of 3 botulinum toxin type A products in facial aesthetics. Aesthet Surg J 2013; 33(1, Suppl):35S–40S

FOOD AND DRUG ADMINISTRATION (FDA) APPROVAL FOR NEUROTOXIN USE

2. There are three commercially available preparations of C. botulinum toxin used in aesthetic facial rejuvenation. **For which one of the following treatment indications do all three have FDA approval?**

   B. Glabellar lines

   There are currently three preparations of botulinum toxin A with on and off label indications for facial aesthetics. These preparations are Botox, Xeomin, and Dysport.
   - Botox is **Ona**botulinumtoxinA, manufactured by Allergan, Santa Barbara, CA.
   - Dysport is **Abo**botulinumtoxinA, manufactured by Medicis Aesthetics, Scottsdale, AZ.
   - Xeomin is **Inco**botulinumtoxinA, manufactured by Merz Pharmaceuticals, Greensboro, NC

   All three have FDA approval for the treatment of glabellar lines/rhytids. In addition, Botox has approval for treatment of crow's feet (lateral canthal lines and forehead rhytids). Use of these preparations for other facial areas is therefore technically off label, although each manufacturer gives advice on their use and worldwide each preparation is widely used at all anatomical sites including the forehead, periorbital area, perioral area, neck, and nose.[1,2]

REFERENCES

1. Wu DC, Fabi SG, Goldman MP. Neurotoxins: current concepts in cosmetic use on the face and neck – lower face. Plast Reconstr Surg 2015;136(5, Suppl):76S–79S
2. Walker TJ, Dayan SH. Comparison and overview of currently available neurotoxins. J Clin Aesthet Dermatol 2014;7(2):31–39

COMBINING BOTULINUM TOXIN AND FILLERS IN FACIAL REJUVENATION

3. **When planning nonsurgical treatment for a patient who requests a combination of neurotoxins and fillers, which one of the following is true?**

   E. The specific order of injection should be flexible.

   Neuromodulators and injectable fillers are frequently used together as part of the facial rejuvenation process, as they are complimentary to one another, with neuromodulators addressing dynamic rhytids and fillers treating static ones. When using fillers and neuromodulators in the same location, it is possible to perform the injections in two separate settings with the neuromodulator in the first session to correct the dynamic deformities, and the filler in the second session to correct the residual static ones. Of course, many patients will prefer a single clinic visit and will prefer to combine neuromodulators and fillers in one sitting, for both economic and logistic reasons. In this case, it is preferable to inject the filler first followed by the neuromodulator. This allows fine-tuning massage of the injected filler by the injector but avoids massage to an area, which has just received toxin, as this could potentially displace the toxin to unwanted areas. This highlights the need to be flexible with injections and place them in order according to a specific circumstance. Many clinicians like to mark the proposed sites/areas of injection, but care then must be taken to avoid injection through them in case this results in tattooing.[1]

REFERENCE

1. de Maio M, Swift A, Signorini M, Fagien S; Aesthetic Leaders in Facial Aesthetics Consensus Committee. Facial assessment and injection guide for botulinum toxin and injectable hyaluronic acid fillers: focus on the upper face. Plast Reconstr Surg 2017;140(2):265e–276e

DOSING STRATEGY IN NEUROTOXIN USE

4. **You normally use Botox for injection and move to a different clinic where the preparation Dysport is used instead.** *How will this affect your usual dosing schedule?*

B. **The number of units per treatment area will need to be doubled.**

Dysport (Medicis Aesthetics, Scottsdale, AZ) is the trade name for AbobotulinumtoxinA. and is a popular choice of neuromodulator in aesthetic practice. It received FDA approval in 2009 for the treatment of glabellar rhytids and cervical dystonia. Prior to this, it had been used for nearly two decades outside of the United States for aesthetic facial rejuvenation purposes. It is available in 300- and 500-unit vials and is typically diluted to a final concentration of 10 to 50 unit/0.1 mL.

Units of botulinum toxin A are not directly interchangeable between the three brands. Similar results can be achieved with different preparations using normalized clinical dosing. Consensus recommendations suggest that a **1:1** dosing ratio can be used when switching between Botox and Xeomin, but that a **2:1 or 2.5:1** dosing ratio should be followed when switching to Dysport from either Botox or Xeomin. Indeed, separate dosing and injection guidelines are available for Dysport.[1,2] This highlights that there can be subtle nuances between different injectable products and should be a reminder to be flexible in one's practice if an alternative product is being used compared with what is one's standard usual.

Following injection, the spread of toxin occurs immediately and will be influenced by injection volume and injection technique. Diffusion from the injection site occurs over days and follows a concentration gradient (toxin-dose dependent). The onset of effect following *C. botulinum* injection is fairly uniform for each of the available preparations and begins within 1–3 days. Patients normally notice results by the end of the first week.

Reassessing the patient at 14 days can be useful for neurotoxin injections, especially as this allows touch-ups to be undertaken at that time.

The typical interval for treatment is 3–6 months across the three different brands of toxin, so changing from one brand to another should not make a difference to the frequency of injections required by a patient.[1,2]

REFERENCES

1. Matarasso A, Shafer D. Botulinum neurotoxin type A-ABO (Dysport): clinical indications and practice guide. Aesthet Surg J 2009;29(6, Suppl):S72–S79
2. Lorenc ZP, Kenkel JM, Fagien S, et al. Consensus panel's assessment and recommendations on the use of 3 botulinum toxin type A products in facial aesthetics. Aesthet Surg J 2013; 33(1, Suppl):35S–40S

BENEFITS OF USING XEOMIN AS A NEUROMODULATOR

5. **Which one of the following represents a key benefit of using Xeomin as your neurotoxin of choice for aesthetic facial rejuvenation?**

A. **It does not require refrigeration.**

Xeomin is also known as incobotulinumtoxinA and is manufactured by Merz Pharmaceuticals. It is one of the three key preparations of *C. botulinum* toxin. It has FDA approval for use in glabellar rhytids, cervical dystonia, and blepharoptosis.

It has two key advantages over other preparations:

1. It does not require refrigeration before use.
2. It has a low immunogenicity.

The other preparations (Botox and Dysport) both require refrigeration, which can present a logistical problem in terms of storage and access to toxins in clinic. The reason why Xeomin has the lowest immunogenicity of all preparations is that the amount of complexing proteins is very low and these are believed to be implicated in immune reactions to the injected product.

Botulinum toxin A is expressed as a 150-KDa core toxin within a larger 900-KDa protein complex. The immune system may recognize any component of this complex and trigger an immune reaction. The amount of neurotoxin and complexing protein injected defines the foreign protein load. High or repeat protein loads may trigger toxin A antibody production and secondary nonresponse. Current commercial preparations seek to minimize delivered protein load by eliminating complexing proteins. Xeomin has effectively eliminated complexing proteins during preparation, which may suggest the lowest immunogenicity of the available preparations. Xeomin does have 5% risk of headache following treatment of glabellar lines, although this is slightly lower than a quoted 9% risk for patients having Dysport for example. All of the preparations require reconstitution, as they are stored as powders and all require prescription for use.[1-5]

REFERENCES

1. Lorenc ZP, Kenkel JM, Fagien S, et al. A review of abobotulinumtoxinA (Dysport). Aesthet Surg J 2013;33(1, Suppl): 13S–17S
2. Matarasso A, Shafer D. Botulinum neurotoxin type A-ABO (Dysport): clinical indications and practice guide. Aesthet Surg J 2009;29(6, Suppl):S72–S79
3. Maas C, Kane MA, Bucay VW, et al. Current aesthetic use of abobotulinumtoxinA in clinical practice: an evidence-based consensus review. Aesthet Surg J 2012;32(1, Suppl):8S–29S
4. Lorenc ZP, Kenkel JM, Fagien S, et al. IncobotulinumtoxinA (Xeomin): background, mechanism of action, and manufacturing. Aesthet Surg J 2013;33(1, Suppl):18S–22S
5. Lorenc ZP, Kenkel JM, Fagien S, et al. IncobotulinumtoxinA in clinical literature. Aesthet Surg J 2013;33(1, Suppl):23S–34S

PREPARATION AND DELIVERY OF NEUROTOXINS IN AESTHETIC FACIAL REJUVENATION

6. *When reconstituting botulinum toxin in clinic for the treatment of rhytids, what would be the potential advantage of using preserved saline for this purpose?*
   C. **Decreased pain on injection.**

   Each of the botulinum toxins requires reconstitution before use. This is normally performed with preservative-free 0.9% sodium chloride and once done the product should be clear, colorless, and free from particulate matter. Either preserved or nonpreserved saline may be used, although Botox, Dysport, and Xeomin instructions all describe the use of nonpreserved saline.

   There is evidence that use of preserved saline helps reduce the pain for patients during injections. In one study, both prospective and retrospective approaches were undertaken. In the prospective study, preserved saline was used on one side of the face, while nonpreserved was used on the other. Patients consistently reported less pain on the side treated with preserved saline. In the retrospective study, patients who previously had undergone treatment with nonpreserved saline were treated with preserved saline and described reduced pain with the latter.[1]

   There is no difference to the action of the product, the immunogenicity, or bruising risk due to different saline types. Bruising can be minimized by taking some sensible steps including stopping anticoagulant medication 10–14 days beforehand and taking care to identify and avoid injecting through or past blood vessels. When this does occur, swift application of pressure to the area can help minimize the bruising effects. The cost of using preserved saline may be higher than that of nonpreserved saline, so this would not reduce the business overhead.

REFERENCE

1. Alam M, Dover JS, Arndt KA. Pain associated with injection of botulinum A exotoxin reconstituted using isotonic sodium chloride with and without preservative: a double-blind, randomized controlled trial. Arch Dermatol 2002;138(4): 510–514

RISKS IN BOTULINUM TOXIN FACIAL REJUVENATION THERAPY

7. *When a patient requests isolated treatment of their transverse forehead rhytids without treatment for the crow's feet and glabella regions, what is the main risk of doing so?*
   B. **There is an increased risk of causing brow ptosis.**

   In general, most patients will likely follow a variation of a standard "recipe" for neurotoxin therapy, which tends to most often include treatment of the brow, glabellar region, and crow's feet. Other patients may request treatment to additional areas such as bunny lines, marionette lines, platysmal bands, or the lips. It is therefore important to adapt treatment plans to be individualized to each patient. Despite this, caution must be taken when asked by a patient to perform treatment solely for transverse forehead rhytids, as this risks brow ptosis. The target muscle for transverse forehead rhytids is the frontalis, which is a brow elevator. Treating this area is ideally combined with glabellar treatments to reduce activity in the corrugator and procerus muscles which are brow depressors. Brow ptosis can occur when the brow depressors in the glabella are left at their normal strength while the frontalis (brow elevator) is weakened.

Eyelid ptosis is the most common adverse event of treating the glabellar area rather than treating the forehead and occurs in 3% of patients. To minimize this risk, injections should remain away from the levator palpebrae superioris and lateral corrugator injections should be at least 1 cm above the supraorbital ridge and not less than 1 cm above the central eyebrow.

The risk of ectropion is high where the crow's feet or midface are injected with neurotoxin, especially in the setting of pre-existing lower eyelid laxity. This is therefore not specifically associated with treating a single area alone but injecting in to or beyond an area inappropriately.

Providing the patient has a good understanding of what they are after, there is no other reason for not treating a single area only, in terms of achieving patient satisfaction. For the clinician, it may be difficult to accept that only a single area is treated when they feel the best result would be achieved with more, but the key is that the patient's aims and objectives of treatment are followed and they are satisfied.[1-4]

REFERENCES

1. de Maio M, Swift A, Signorini M, Fagien S; Aesthetic Leaders in Facial Aesthetics Consensus Committee. Facial assessment and injection guide for botulinum toxin and injectable hyaluronic acid fillers: focus on the upper face. Plast Reconstr Surg 2017;140(2):265e–276e
2. Carruthers J, Fagien S, Matarasso SL; Botox Consensus Group. Consensus recommendations on the use of botulinum toxin type a in facial aesthetics. Plast Reconstr Surg 2004;114(6, Suppl):1S–22S
3. Monheit G. Neurotoxins: current concepts in cosmetic use on the face and neck – upper face (glabella, forehead, and crow's feet). Plast Reconstr Surg 2015; 136(5, Suppl):72S–75S
4. Lorenc ZP, Kenkel JM, Fagien S, et al. Consensus panel's assessment and recommendations on the use of 3 botulinum toxin type A products in facial aesthetics. Aesthet Surg J 2013; 33(1, Suppl):35S–40S

MUSCLES TARGETED WITH BOTULINUM TOXIN TREATMENT

8. Which muscle is targeted when treating bunny lines with C. botulinum toxin?

D. Nasalis

Bunny lines refer to wrinkles that appear on the sides of the nose and radiate downward. The target muscles for treating this area are the nasalis and procerus. Two to three injection points are used: one to the dorsal midline of the nose at the level of the medial canthi, and one to each side slightly more caudal. A total of 6 units is usually sufficient when using Botox or Xeomin. To prevent drooping of the upper lip, care should be taken to avoid injecting into levator labii superioris alaeque nasi and levator labii superioris. To prevent botulinum toxin from diffusing into these muscles, vigorous massage should be avoided postinjection.[1,2]

Procerus is targeted during glabellar treatment along with orbicularis oculi and corrugator supercilii. Orbicularis oris is targeted to decrease the appearance of fine vertical wrinkles of the lips, often in combination with lip filler. Levator labii superioris may be targeted for the "gummy smile" where there is excess show of gums and upper dentition while laughing or smiling. Other muscles implicated in the "gummy smile" include levator labii superioris alaeque nasi which elevates the lip and depressor septi nasi which lowers the nasal tip.[1-4]

REFERENCES

1. de Maio M, DeBoulle K, Braz A, Rohrich RJ; Alliance for the Future of Aesthetics Consensus Committee. Facial assessment and injection guide for botulinum toxin and injectable hyaluronic acid fillers: focus on the midface. Plast Reconstr Surg 2017;140(4):540e–550e
2. Carruthers J, Fagien S, Matarasso SL; Botox Consensus Group. Consensus recommendations on the use of botulinum toxin type a in facial aesthetics. Plast Reconstr Surg 2004;114(6, Suppl):1S–22S
3. Kontis T, Lacombe V, eds. Cosmetic Injection Techniques. A Text and Video Guide to Neurotoxins and Fillers. Thieme; 2013
4. Trévidic P, Sykes J, Criollo-Lamilla G. Anatomy of the lower face and botulinum injections. Plast Reconstr Surg 2015; 136(5, Suppl):84S–91S

AREAS OF THE FACE AND NECK TARGETED WITH BOTULINUM TOXIN TREATMENT

9. Which one of the following areas may particularly benefit from the use of the "microbotox technique"?

E. Platysmal bands

The platysma can be targeted with neurotoxin for reducing lines at the jawline or reducing visible bands on animation within the neck. Where skin elasticity is well maintained, or in patients who are post neck-lifting surgery, treatment of platysmal bands can be effective with standard neurotoxin techniques by direct injection into the palpable and visible bands. However, in those with skin laxity, crepey skin, and jowling, who do not wish to undergo surgery, there is a significant risk of increasing the appearance of skin laxity by taking this approach, which patients will dislike. In this setting, the "microbotox technique" can be used instead.

In this technique, microdroplets of 2–4 units of Botox are injected intradermally or just under the skin at 0.8–1.0-cm intervals across the lower face and neck. This produces a smoothing of the skin (atrophy and sweat and sebaceous glands) and weakens the action of the facial muscles where they attach to the skin.[1] Care must be taken with any neurotoxin injection in the neck as going too deep or using too high a dose can lead to dysphagia if the strap muscles are incidentally weakened. Rhytids can occur across the jawline because of contraction of platysma and standard injection approaches can be used, although injection here also risks dysphagia if performed too deep or at too higher dosage (**Fig. 104.1**).

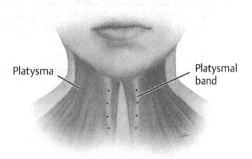

Fig. 104.1   Injection sites for platysmal bands. (From Kontis T, Lacombe V eds. Cosmetic Injection Techniques. A Text and Video Guide to Neurotoxins and Fillers. Thieme, 2013.)

Treatment of the dimpled chin involves neurotoxin delivery to the mentalis muscle. It is important to avoid injecting the depressor labii, as weakening this muscle can result in an asymmetric smile as if there is a marginal mandibular nerve branch palsy. In some patients, the depressor septi nasi can draw the nose downward with smiling and they dislike this appearance. This may be corrected during rhinoplasty by division of the depressor muscle at the columella base but can also be done with neurotoxin. A single injection in the philtrum is usually sufficient but must be avoided in patients with a long upper lip, as this may be accentuated. Treatment of marionette lines with neurotoxin requires delivery to the depressor anguli oris muscle. The injection should not be made too near to the corners of the mouth, as diffusion into orbicularis oris can lead to oral incompetence, which patients find particularly distressing. Treatment of masseteric hypertrophy resulting from jaw clenching can be effective with neurotoxin. Care must be taken to inject deep into masseter to avoid causing inadvertent injection into one of the facial mimetic muscles leading to smile asymmetry. These injections do risk causing deep hematomas.[1–3]

REFERENCES

1. Wu WTL. Microbotox of the lower face and neck: evolution of a personal technique and its clinical effects. Plast Reconstr Surg 2015;136(5, Suppl):92S–100S
2. Kontis T, Lacombe V, eds. Cosmetic Injection Techniques. A Text and Video Guide to Neurotoxins and Fillers. Thieme; 2013
3. Trévidic P, Sykes J, Criollo-Lamilla G. Anatomy of the lower face and botulinum injections. Plast Reconstr Surg 2015; 136(5, Suppl):84S–91S

BOTULINUM TOXIN USE IN FACIAL AESTHETICS

10. Botulinum toxins are derived from the bacterium *C. botulinum*. *Which one of the following statements is correct regarding their use in facial aesthetics?*

C. Toxins cause temporary chemodenervation by preventing binding and release of acetylcholine.

There are seven subtypes of botulinum toxin (A to G), but only two are commercially available (A and B). All of the subtypes cause chemodenervation by blocking the action of acetylcholine at the neuromuscular junction. Type A works on the SNAP-25 protein, and type B on the synaptobrevin protein. Both of these proteins act at the SNARE complex. Only type A is intended for use in facial aesthetics, while type B is for use in cervical dystonia. FDA approval for botulinum toxin A is limited to glabellar rhytids, crow's feet lines, forehead rhytids, cervical dystonia, migraine, or blepharoptosis (depending on brand), so other uses are off-label.

The units of different botulinum toxin preparations are not uniformly comparable, although they are derived from the effects on laboratory mice. One unit is sufficient to cause death in 50% of a specific strain of mouse with intraperitoneal injection. Botox (onabotulinumtoxinA; Allergan, Santa Barbara, CA) and Xeomin (incobotulinumtoxinA; Merz Pharmaceuticals, Greensboro, NC) units are roughly equivalent. Between 2 and 2.5 Dysport (abobotulinumtoxinA; Medicis Aesthetics, Scottsdale, AZ) units are equivalent to a single Botox unit.

The difference in units between products arises from differences in the specifics of the assays used and this has the potential to cause confusion when changing from Botox or Xeomin to Dysport in clinical practice.[1,2]

REFERENCES

1. Lorenc ZP, Kenkel JM, Fagien S, et al. Consensus panel's assessment and recommendations on the use of 3 botulinum toxin type A products in facial aesthetics. Aesthet Surg J 2013;33(1, Suppl):35S–40S
2. Dressler D, Adib Saberi F. Botulinum toxin: mechanisms of action. Eur Neurol 2005;53(1): 3–9

ADMINISTRATION OF BOTOX FOR FACIAL REJUVENATION

11. You are preparing some Botox for a 30-year-old woman who has requested treatment for her frown line (glabellar) region. It is her first experience with Botox injections. *Which one of the following is correct?*

D. A typical starting dose for this patient would be 20 units.

Botox is available in 100- and 200-unit vials and is typically diluted with normal saline to provide 4 units per 0.1 mL. Reconstitution should be performed gently to avoid damage to the product. It should be clear following reconstitution. Consensus opinion suggests it may be stored for up to 6 weeks, providing it is stored at 4°C. However, the manufacturers of botulinum toxins recommend that the product is injected within 4 hours of reconstitution. Because the products do not contain an antimicrobial agent, prolonged storage does not have FDA approval. A typical starting dose would be 20 units placed via five to seven injections. The central injection is placed below the superior orbital rim, but the lateral ones must be placed above.[1,2]

REFERENCES

1. Carruthers J, Fagien S, Matarasso SL; Botox Consensus Group. Consensus recommendations on the use of botulinum toxin type a in facial aesthetics. Plast Reconstr Surg 2004;114(6, Suppl):1S–22S
2. Lorenc ZP, Kenkel JM, Fagien S, et al. Consensus panel's assessment and recommendations on the use of 3 botulinum toxin type A products in facial aesthetics. Aesthet Surg J 2013;33(1, Suppl):35S–40S

DECISION MAKING IN FACIAL AESTHETICS

12. A 33-year-old woman presents with early dynamic crow's-feet rhytids. *What would be a reasonable total neurotoxin dosing schedule for her to target this area?*

A. Botox 16–24 units

This patient could benefit from chemodenervation of the orbicularis oculi muscle; the options include Xeomin, Dysport, or Botox. Treatment of the crow's feet area (lateral canthal lines) is commonly performed, often in conjunction with the brow and glabellar regions. A suggested starting dose for crow's-feet Botox injection is 18–24 units (three injections per side of 4 units each). Since Xeomin units are roughly equivalent, the same dose can be used. The approximate dosing conversion from Botox to Dysport is 2:1 to 2.5:1, so a starting dose would be 36–48 units. The other volumes would be somewhat homeopathic for this patient.

When injecting into the crow's feet or lateral canthal area, three sites are normally injected per side (up to 4 units per injection; **Fig. 104.2**). The first site should be 1.5–2 cm lateral to the lateral canthus, just lateral to the orbital rim. Additional sites should be medial and superior and/or inferior to this depending on whether the lines are distributed above and below the lateral canthus or isolated below the lateral canthus. Injection should be performed with the needle at one-third of its depth. The patient should keep their eyes closed and the injector should use a finger to protect the upper eyelid.

Before injecting this area, a snap test should be performed to the lower lids. If they are lax, there is significant risk for postinjection ectropion, and low injections must be avoided.[1–3]

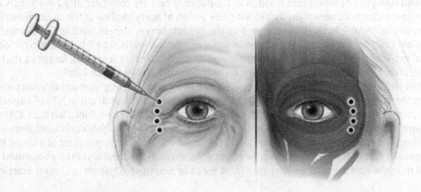

Fig. 104.2 Injection sites for lateral canthal lines. (Adapted from Carruthers J, Fagien S, Matarasso SL; Botox Consensus Group. Consensus recommendations on the use of botulinum toxin type a in facial aesthetics. Plast Reconstr Surg 114(Suppl 6):S1–S22, 2004.)

REFERENCES

1. Lorenc ZP, Kenkel JM, Fagien S, et al. Consensus panel's assessment and recommendations on the use of 3 botulinum toxin type A products in facial aesthetics. Aesthet Surg J 2013;33(1, Suppl):35S–40S
2. Monheit G. Neurotoxins: current concepts in cosmetic use on the face and neck – upper face (glabella, forehead, and crow's feet). Plast Reconstr Surg 2015;136(5, Suppl):72S–75S
3. Carruthers J, Fagien S, Matarasso SL; Botox Consensus Group. Consensus recommendations on the use of botulinum toxin type a in facial aesthetics. Plast Reconstr Surg 2004;114(6, Suppl):1S–22S

CONSENT IN BOTULINUM TOXIN THERAPY

13. When consenting a patient pretreatment with botulinum toxin in the glabella region, what risk should you quote them for developing temporary eyelid ptosis?

B. 3%

Eyelid ptosis is the most common adverse event following botulinum toxin injection to the glabellar region. It occurs in around 3% of cases. In general, accurate and carefully placed injections can help minimize risk of unwanted muscle weakness. For example, eyelid ptosis risk can be minimized by avoiding injecting near the levator palpebrae superioris and by placing lateral corrugator injections at least 1 cm above the supraorbital ridge. In the central eyebrow area, injections must not be placed less than 1 cm of the supraorbital ridge.

The other key risks that must be discussed with patients include pain, bleeding, bruising, swelling, infection, allergic reaction, over- or undercorrection of rhytids, residual static rhytids, headache, eyelid edema, double vision, flulike symptoms, asymmetry, and dissatisfaction with cosmetic result.[1-4]

REFERENCES

1. BOTOX Cosmetic (onabotulinumtoxinA) for injection, for intramuscular use. Food and Drug Administration; 2018
2. de Maio M, Swift A, Signorini M, Fagien S; Aesthetic Leaders in Facial Aesthetics Consensus Committee. Facial assessment and injection guide for botulinum toxin and injectable hyaluronic acid fillers: focus on the upper face. Plast Reconstr Surg 2017;140(2):265e–276e
3. Carruthers J, Fagien S, Matarasso SL; Botox Consensus Group. Consensus recommendations on the use of botulinum toxin type a in facial aesthetics. Plast Reconstr Surg 2004;114(6, Suppl):1S–22S
4. Lorenc ZP, Kenkel JM, Fagien S, et al. Consensus panel's assessment and recommendations on the use of 3 botulinum toxin type A products in facial aesthetics. Aesthet Surg J 2013;33(1, Suppl):35S–40S

105. Soft-Tissue Fillers

See Essentials of Plastic Surgery, third edition, pp. 1468–1475

PATIENT SELECTION IN AESTHETIC INJECTABLES

1. *Which one of the following represents a potential issue for the surgeon performing unnatural, overdone filler injections for patients requesting this look?*
   A. The patients will consistently be unsatisfied with the result.
   B. The patients' risk of complication will be drastically increased.
   C. The risk of a malpractice claim will be significantly elevated.
   D. There may be a consequent negative effect on the surgeon's reputation.
   E. The product will be ineffective at achieving this goal.

MANAGEMENT OF HIV LIPOATROPHY

2. A patient with human immunodeficiency virus (HIV) lipoatrophy presents to clinic. The patient is of slim build and is concerned about the appearance of the cheeks. *Which one of the following fillers may be best suited to address the issues and has specific Food and Drug Administration (FDA) approval for this use?*
   A. Polyether ether ketone
   B. Polyethylene
   C. Polymethylmethacrylate
   D. Low G hyaluronic acid
   E. Poly-L-lactic acid

IDEAL CHARACTERISTICS OF FACIAL FILLERS

3. *Which one of the following desirable qualities of an injectable filler is consistent across all FDA-approved fillers?*
   A. Easy to use
   B. Safe to use
   C. Reversible
   D. Nonallergenic
   E. Temporary

HYALURONIC ACID FOR FACIAL REJUVENATION

4. You are using a hyaluronic acid derivative as an injectable filler in your cosmetic practice. *Which one of the following is true of this filler?*
   A. A pretreatment skin test is normally required.
   B. Further tissue expansion following injection is unlikely.
   C. Effectiveness decreases with repeated injections.
   D. Incorrectly placed product is difficult to correct.
   E. Injections are painful and best combined with lidocaine.

USE OF POLY-L-LACTIC ACID (SCULPTRA) FOR FACIAL REJUVENATION

5. A woman comes to your practice for an injectable filler consultation. On the telephone, she mentioned the nurse that her main concern was superficial upper lip rhytids that were previously treated with hyaluronic acid. You were anticipating using this filler again and had prepared some, along with a range of 20- to 27-gauge needles. When she arrives, you find that the main issue is deep nasolabial folds, and she is dissatisfied that the improvement from her previous injection was relatively short lived. Therefore, she is interested in a longer-lasting improvement. She has been reading about *Sculptra* while in the waiting area and asks if this can be used. *Which one of the following limits your use of Sculptra in this case?*
   A. The nature of the defect
   B. The lack of preparation time
   C. The availability of needles
   D. A lack of skin pretesting
   E. The longevity of Sculptra

USE OF BELLAFILL AS AN INJECTABLE FILLER

6. Your colleague has been advising you of his recent successful outcomes using *Bellafill*. *Which one of the following is correct regarding use of this product?*
   A. It is considered a temporary filler that will require regular reinjections.
   B. It contains absorbable polymethyl acrylate beads that often cause granuloma formation.
   C. It contains collagen that provides the increased volume at the injection site.
   D. It is primarily indicated for use in acne scars and deep nasolabial folds.
   E. The first-line treatment of problematic irregularities after injection is surgical excision.

COMPLICATIONS FOLLOWING INJECTABLE FILLERS

7. A nurse attends your office having undergone injectable filler treatment at another clinic while on vacation. She is concerned about the appearance of a blue discoloration at the injection site and wonders whether this is connected with the injection or a possible vascular lesion. *What is the most likely filler substance she has had injected?*
   A. Juvéderm
   B. Zyderm
   C. Sculptra
   D. Radiesse
   E. Bellafill

PLACEMENT OF INJECTABLE FILLERS IN THE FACE

8. *When performing volume restoration in the malar region, what plane should normally be used for the injection of product?*
   A. Intradermal
   B. Subdermal
   C. Subcutaneous
   D. Intramuscular
   E. Supraperiosteal

TECHNIQUES FOR INJECTION OF FACIAL FILLERS

9. *Which one of the following is consistently advocated during facial aesthetic injections using a nonpermanent filler such as hyaluronic acid?*
   A. To use a 24-gauge needle
   B. To use a cannula instead of a needle
   C. To aspirate before injection
   D. To use a cross-hatching technique
   E. To use a linear deposition technique

COMPLICATIONS OF FACIAL FILLERS

10. *When injecting facial fillers, which anatomic area carries the greatest risk of iatrogenic visual loss?*
    A. Glabellar
    B. Malar
    C. Nasolabial fold
    D. Lips
    E. Lateral brow

POSTINJECTION CARE AFTER FACIAL FILLERS

11. *Following injection of filler to the face, which one of the following should be routinely considered for the first week?*
    A. Oral antibiotics
    B. Antiviral medications
    C. Ice and compression
    D. Regular massage of the area
    E. Regular exercise

EARLY COMPLICATIONS IN FACIAL FILLERS

12. Following injection with hyaluronic acid filler to the face, a patient presents with an area of skin necrosis developing adjacent to the injection site. *Which one of the following is recommended for treatment?*
    A. Surgical debridement
    B. Epinephrine injection
    C. Injection of hyaluronidase
    D. Injection of steroid
    E. Cold compress and ice

INJECTABLES IN THE LIP

13. A 25-year-old patient is seen in the office requesting lip augmentation. *Which one of the following products would be most well suited to this procedure?*
    A. Juvéderm Vobella
    B. Juvéderm Volure
    C. Juvéderm Voluma
    D. Restylane Refine
    E. Sculptra

Answers

PATIENT SELECTION IN AESTHETIC INJECTABLES

1. *Which one of the following represents a potential issue for the surgeon performing unnatural, overdone filler injections for patients requesting this look?*

   D. There may be a consequent negative effect on the surgeon's reputation.

   There will generally be two patient cohorts requesting facial fillers: those who have lost volume with increasing age and or weight loss who require re-volumization and those who are younger and have a "normal" volume but wish to enhance areas that may be naturally deficient for them.

   Within these two groups, there may be patients who seek unnatural and overdone filler. When considering whether to undertake this type of treatment, the surgeon must consider whether they wish to have an association with creation of unnatural or bizarre looks, as this would not be in keeping with the principles of plastic and reconstructive surgery and will likely be a poor advertisement for the surgeon's practice. Patients who do want excessive amounts of filler may actually be very satisfied with this, in spite of the perceived odd looks generated. The complication rate may be higher, but not drastically so by injecting higher volumes of filler. The risk of malpractice claim could be altered but usually when patients know what they want, and a reversible filler is used, then this risk remains relatively low. The product will be able to achieve the goal of creating an unnatural look, hence the need for an objective and common sense approach by the injector. In many countries, medical practitioners are not the sole people performing the injections and a range of other people including beauticians, hairdressers, etc., may be injecting. Nonmedical practitioners may have different principles upon which they operate.[1-3]

REFERENCES

1. Lamb JP, Surek CC. Facial volumization: an anatomic approach. Thieme; 2017
2. Nahai F, ed. The Art of Aesthetic Surgery: Principles and Techniques. 2nd ed. St Louis, MO: Quality Medical Publishing; 2011
3. Homicz MR, Watson D. Review of injectable materials for soft tissue augmentation. Facial Plast Surg 2004;20(1):21–29

MANAGEMENT OF HIV LIPOATROPHY

2. A patient with human immunodeficiency virus (HIV) lipoatrophy presents to clinic. The patient is of slim build and is concerned about the appearance of the cheeks. *Which one of the following fillers may be best suited to address the issues and has specific Food and Drug Administration (FDA) approval for this use?*

   E. Poly-L-lactic acid

   One of the known stigmatizing side effects of HIV antiviral medication is lipoatrophy which can be present at a number of different body sites, but is often most obvious in the malar region giving patients a gaunt, aged appearance. Options for managing this include injectable fillers as well as cheek implants. Fillers may be temporary or permanent.

   Poly-L-lactic acid sold as *Sculptra* has FDA approval specifically for this indication. It is a synthetic polymer, which is biocompatible and nonallergenic. It typically requires reinjection at 24 months. The other temporary injectable that has FDA approval for HIV-associated lipoatrophy is calcium hydroxyapatite, sold as *Radiesse.* This was classically the treatment of choice in this scenario. It is a calcium mineral compound made with human bone. It, too, is biocompatible and nonallergenic. It needs reinjection around 12 months. Low G (more viscous) hyaluronic acid fillers are better suited to superficial placement for treating fine lines and as lip volume fillers, rather than deep volumizers. High G hyaluronic acid fillers like *Juvéderm Voluma* may be suitable for this purpose, but will need more regular reinjection than Sculptra or Radiesse, typically less than 12 months.

   Polyether ether ketone (PEEK sold by Synthes) and polyethylene (sold as Medpor) are both materials used to manufacture solid cheek implants. These may be an alternative to the injectable solution for some patients with HIV. Autologous fat has a role in volumizing the cheeks and other areas of the face; however, the problem for many slim HIV-positive patients such as this patient is that their stores of fat elsewhere are poor for harvest. This is not consistently the case though as the antiviral medications used in HIV (nucleoside reverse transcriptase inhibitors), such as zidovudine and stavudine, can also lead to truncal lipohypertrophy.[1-3]

REFERENCES

1. Available at: https://www.fda.gov/medical-devices/cosmetic-devices/dermal-fillers-approved-center-devices-and-radiological-health. Accessed June 10, 2021

2. Hanke CW, Redbord KP. Safety and efficacy of poly-L-lactic acid in HIV lipoatrophy and lipoatrophy of aging. J Drugs Dermatol 2007;6(2):123–128
3. Silvers SL, Eviatar JA, Echavez MI, Pappas AL. Prospective, open-label, 18-month trial of calcium hydroxylapatite (Radiesse) for facial soft-tissue augmentation in patients with human immunodeficiency virus-associated lipoatrophy: one-year durability. Plast Reconstr Surg 2006;118(3, Suppl):34S–45S

IDEAL CHARACTERISTICS OF FACIAL FILLERS

3. *Which one of the following desirable qualities of an injectable filler is consistent across all FDA-approved fillers?*

   B. Safe to use

   In the United States, FDA approval is required to use facial injectable products. A long list of products has been reviewed and felt to be safe to use, based on available published evidence. These are primarily temporary fillers, although one permanent filler also has approval. The products include hyaluronic acid, polymethylmethacrylate (PMMA), poly-L-lactic acid, calcium hydroxylapatite, and collagen. The other desirable qualities of a filler include being easy to use, being nonallergenic, having predictable and reproducible results with minimal downtime, being reversible if the effects are unwanted, and being nonpalpable and visible. Hyaluronic acid probably comes closest to being the ideal filler, as it has all of the qualities listed earlier (see **Table 105.1**).[1–4]

Table 105.1   *Current FDA-Approved Soft-Tissue Fillers*

Brand Name	Manufacturer	FDA-approved Use
Hyaluronic acid fillers		
BELOTERO Balance	Merz	• Correction of moderate to severe facial wrinkles and folds, mid to deep dermis
Juvéderm Ultra/XC Juvéderm Ultra Plus/XC Restylane Silk Juvéderm Ultra/XC	Allergan	• Deep volume augmentation typically for the midface, supraperiosteal • Correction of moderate to severe facial wrinkles and folds, mid to deep dermis • Lip volume augmentation (Ultra XC)
Juvéderm Volbella XC	Allergan	• Perioral augmentation (i.e., lips)
Juvéderm Vollure XC	Allergan	• Deep volume augmentation typically for the midface, supraperiosteal • Correction of moderate to severe facial wrinkles and folds, mid to deep dermis
Juvéderm Voluma XC	Allergan	• Deep volume augmentation typically for the midface, supraperiosteal
Restylane/Restylane-L	Galderma	• Correction of moderate to severe facial wrinkles and folds, mid to deep dermis
Restylane Defyne	Galderma	• Correction of moderate to severe facial wrinkles and folds, mid to deep dermis
Restylane Lyft	Galderma	• Correction of moderate to severe facial wrinkles and folds, deep dermis to subcutis • Deep volume augmentation typically for the midface, supraperiosteal • Rejuvenation of the dorsum of the hand
Restylane Refyne	Galderma	• Correction of moderate to severe facial wrinkles and folds, mid to deep dermis
Restylane Silk	Galderma	• Lip volume augmentation and fine perioral rhytids, submucosal
Revanesse Versa	Prollenium US	• Correction of moderate to severe facial wrinkles and folds, mid to deep dermis
Calcium hydroxylapatite filler		
Radiesse/Radiesse Plus	Merz	• Correction of moderate to severe facial wrinkles and folds, mid to deep dermis • Hand augmentation to correct volume loss in the dorsum of the hands
Poly-L-lactic acid filler		
Sculptra Aesthetic	Galderma	• Correction of shallow to deep nasolabial fold contour deficiencies and other facial wrinkles, deep dermis • Correction of lipoatrophy in people with HIV
Polymethylmethacrylate filler		
Bellafill	Suneva Medical	• Correction of nasolabial folds and moderate to severe, atrophic, distensible facial acne scars on the cheeks

REFERENCES

1. Available at: https://www.fda.gov/medical-devices/cosmetic-devices/dermal-fillers-approved-center-devices-and-radiological-health. Accessed June 10, 2021
2. Nahai F, ed. The Art of Aesthetic Surgery: Principles and Techniques. 2nd ed. St Louis, MO: Quality Medical Publishing; 2011
3. Homicz MR, Watson D. Review of injectable materials for soft tissue augmentation. Facial Plast Surg 2004;20(1):21–29
4. Lamb JP, Surek CC. Facial Volumization: An Anatomic Approach. Thieme; 2017

HYALURONIC ACID FOR FACIAL REJUVENATION

4. You are using a hyaluronic acid derivative as an injectable filler in your cosmetic practice. *Which one of the following is true of this filler?*

    E. Injections are painful and best combined with lidocaine.

    Hyaluronic acid filler is very popular for facial rejuvenation procedures. Since its FDA approval in 2003, its use has supplanted collagen as the synthetic filler of choice. There are many advantages of using hyaluronic acid as a filler, but injections can be painful, so topical and or injectable local anesthetic agents should be used. Most products also contain lidocaine within the syringe, although for more sensitive areas this alone is not enough to remove pain completely. There is no species specificity and therefore no immunological activity, meaning that skin tests are not required. However, after injection, patients can apply ice packs for the first 24 hours and take antihistamines or anti-inflammatories to settle local reactions and swelling.

    Hyaluronic acid is a normal component of ground substance responsible for dermal hydration, so it absorbs water following injection resulting in further expansion. Injections initially last for 6 to 9 months and subsequent injections actually last longer with lesser volumes usually required. Hyaluronic acid fillers are readily available, reliable to use, and have the added benefit of being reversible if placed incorrectly. This is achieved by injection of hyaluronidase at the previously injected site.[1-3]

REFERENCES

1. Sundaram H, Cassuto D. Biophysical characteristics of hyaluronic acid soft-tissue fillers and their relevance to aesthetic applications. Plast Reconstr Surg 2013;132(4, Suppl 2):5S–21S
2. Gutowski KA. Hyaluronic acid fillers: science and clinical uses. Clin Plast Surg 2016;43(3):489–496
3. Gold MH. Use of hyaluronic acid fillers for the treatment of the aging face. Clin Interv Aging 2007;2(3):369–376

USE OF POLY-L-LACTIC ACID (SCULPTRA) FOR FACIAL REJUVENATION

5. A woman comes to your practice for an injectable filler consultation. On the telephone, she mentioned the nurse that her main concern was superficial upper lip rhytids that were previously treated with hyaluronic acid. You were anticipating using this filler again and had prepared some, along with a range of 20- to 27-gauge needles. When she arrives, you find that the main issue is deep nasolabial folds, and she is dissatisfied that the improvement from her previous injection was relatively short lived. Therefore, she is interested in a longer-lasting improvement. She has been reading about *Sculptra* while in the waiting area and asks if this can be used. *Which one of the following limits your use of Sculptra in this case?*

    B. The lack of preparation time

    Sculptra is a synthetic polymer that would be a good option in this case. It is biodegradable, biocompatible, immunologically inert, and does not require a skin test. It contains Poly-L-lactic acid, which initiates a foreign body reaction and is ultimately replaced with collagen. Therefore, it is not a filler per se, but rather a product that induces volumization by the formation of collagen. Sculptra requires injection with a needle of at least 26 gauge given its viscous nature, and may be combined with local anesthetic. It can provide longer-lasting rhytid correction than hyaluronic acid, although it takes more time to achieve this result. When using this type of filler, patients must be advised that the results will develop over time and this contrasts with other injectables such as hyaluronic acid which can give a rapid-onset change in appearance. This forms part of the initial consultation assessing patients' aims and objectives and setting realistic goals. The limiting factor in this case is the lack of preparation time, as it must be reconstituted at least 2 hours before injection and preferably overnight.[1,2]

REFERENCES

1. Palm M, Chayavichitsilp P. The "skinny" on Sculptra: a practical primer to volumization with poly-L-lactic acid. J Drugs Dermatol 2012;11(9):1046–1052
2. Fitzgerald R, Vleggaar D. Facial volume restoration of the aging face with poly-L-lactic acid. Dermatol Ther (Heidelb) 2011;24(1):2–27

USE OF BELLAFILL AS AN INJECTABLE FILLER

6. Your colleague has been advising you of his recent successful outcomes using *Bellafill*. *Which one of the following is correct regarding use of this product?*

    D. It is primarily indicated for use in acne scars and deep nasolabial folds.

    Bellafill is an example of a permanent filler best used in the nasolabial folds and deep marionette lines. It is also useful to reduce acne scarring. It should be used with caution in thin skin or areas liable to thin with age such as the periorbital and glabellar areas. It is composed of collagen-covered PMMA beads and may require a reinjection. The PMMA beads are permanent but rarely cause granuloma formation. The injected collagen acts as a temporary transport vehicle only and is absorbed during the first 6 weeks post injection. Long-term volume increases are achieved by secondary formation of connective tissue around the beads. First-line treatment of irregularities discovered soon after injection is steroid injection to soften the tissues. Surgical resection is required only in persistent problematic irregularities.[1,2]

REFERENCES

1. Joseph JH, Eaton LL, Cohen SR. Current concepts in the use of Bellafill. Plast Reconstr Surg 2015; 136(5, Suppl):171S–179S
2. Gold MH, Sadick NS. Optimizing outcomes with polymethylmethacrylate fillers. J Cosmet Dermatol 2018;17(3):298–304

COMPLICATIONS FOLLOWING INJECTABLE FILLERS

7. A nurse attends your office having undergone injectable filler treatment at another clinic while on vacation. She is concerned about the appearance of a blue discoloration at the injection site and wonders whether this is connected with the injection or a possible vascular lesion. *What is the most likely filler substance she has had injected?*

   A. Juvéderm

   This woman is most likely to have undergone injection of hyaluronic acid (Juvéderm). Injection of this filler too superficially and with too great a volume can lead to a bluish discoloration. This is described as the Tyndall effect, also known as the Tyndall scattering, and is observed when light is reflected by small particles that are in suspension. It is named after the nineteenth century physicist John Tyndall. As this is a temporary filler, the problem will be self-limiting, but could be treated with an injection of hyaluronidase if the patient is not prepared to wait. Alternative approaches described include firm massage to spread the product more widely or a stab excision using an 18-G needle with expression of the filler to drain the excess. The Nd:YAG laser has also been described to treat this problem. As is the case in all treatments for plastic and aesthetic surgery, it is vital to discuss these risks with patients in advance to set their expectations and reduce anxiety about them posttreatment.[1,2]

REFERENCES

1. King M. Management of Tyndall effect. J Clin Aesthet Dermatol 2016;9(11):E6–E8
2. Hirsch RJ, Narurkar V, Carruthers J. Management of injected hyaluronic acid induced Tyndall effects. Lasers Surg Med 2006;38(3):202–204

PLACEMENT OF INJECTABLE FILLERS IN THE FACE

8. *When performing volume restoration in the malar region, what plane should normally be used for the injection of product?*

   E. Supraperiosteal

   Fillers are generally placed either in the dermis or just below it when used to fill shallow lines and imperfections. Where volumization is being performed, then placing the injections just above periosteum is frequently advocated. The theory behind placement of injections at this level is that small volumes in this location work like "liquid nails" to help suspend tissues and fill them out from deep within. Injections are typically placed on the zygoma and maxilla for volumization of the cheeks. This often has a positive effect on the nasolabial folds and forms part of the so-called liquid facelift. A further benefit of placing the product deep is that it is less likely to be visible or palpable and this plane is safe and avascular. Where more superficial filler is placed, this is often in the dermis or just deep to it.[1-3]

REFERENCES

1. Lamb JP, Surek CC. Facial Volumization: An Anatomic Approach. Thieme; 2017
2. de Maio M. MD codes™: a methodological approach to facial aesthetic treatment with injectable hyaluronic acid fillers. Aesthetic Plast Surg 2020
3. de Maio M. Myomodulation with injectable fillers: an update. Aesthetic Plast Surg 2020;44(4):1317–1319

TECHNIQUES FOR INJECTION OF FACIAL FILLERS

9. *Which one of the following is consistently advocated during facial aesthetic injections using a nonpermanent filler such as hyaluronic acid?*

   C. To aspirate before injection

   There are a number of different approaches to the injection of temporary fillers into the face and these techniques need to be adapted to the situation considering the anatomic area being injected, the intended aim of the injection, and the filler consistency selected.

A consistent requirement is to perform plunger aspiration prior to injection to minimize the risk of inadvertent intravascular injection. Placement of filler into the arterial vasculature can create problems with skin necrosis and even blindness due to filler causing an embolic event. The needle used for injection is usually a 30 gauge, but larger needles such as 27 and 25 gauge may be used. Most products are supplied with the "correct" needle. It is also possible to use a cannula instead, and this will require a larger needle to puncture the skin and soft tissues before switching out to the cannula. The benefit of cannula use is that damage to internal structures is reduced and thus intravascular injury is minimized. Injection techniques may be linear deposition, for example, when filling a deep nasolabial fold or enhancing the white roll of the lips. Alternatively, they may involve a fanning or cross-hatching technique to blend filler over a broader area. When injecting deeply, it is sometimes useful to deposit small blobs of filler as part of the volumizing approach (**Fig. 105.1**).[1,2]

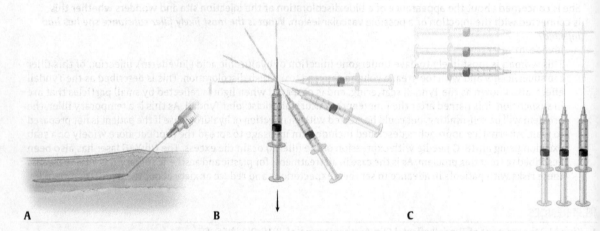

Fig. 105.1 Injection techniques. *A,* Linear deposition. *B,* Fanning. *C,* Cross-hatching.

REFERENCES

1. DeJoseph LM. Cannulas for facial filler placement. Facial Plast Surg Clin North Am 2012;202(2):215–220, vi–vii
2. Chiu A, Fabi S, Dayan S, Nogueira A. Lip injection techniques using small-particle hyaluronic acid dermal filler. J Drugs Dermatol 2016;15(9):1076–1082

COMPLICATIONS OF FACIAL FILLERS

10. *When injecting facial fillers, which anatomic area carries the greatest risk of iatrogenic visual loss?*
  A. Glabellar
      There are two areas of the face, which are associated with a higher risk of blindness where intravascular injection occurs following injectable fillers. These are the glabellar and the nose (a.k.a. liquid rhinoplasty). Liquid rhinoplasty can be helpful as a test prior to or after surgery or used as a definitive treatment instead of surgery. Fillers can be used to augment the nasal tip, adjust the dorsal hump, and address post-rhinoplasty imperfections. The glabella is often first treated with neurotoxins to reduce the dynamic rhytids. However, some patients will also benefit from filler to reduce the static rhytids where there are deep creases. Likewise, the same is true of the transverse forehead rhytids. The malar region is injected as part of a liquid facelift or in isolation to help restore midface volume and cheek projection. The nasolabial and marionette folds are commonly requested sites for treatment. Each of these may be injected directly or indirectly by adding volume more cranially or laterally in the face. The lips can be injected to enhance their appearance. This may be to counteract the appearance of aging or simply to create more lip fullness. Due to the extensive arterial network in the face, each of these areas must still be injected carefully as intravascular injection could result in significant problems.[1,2]

REFERENCES

1. Kapoor K, Kapoor P, Heydenrych I, Bertossi D. Vision loss associated with hyaluronic acid fillers: a systematic review of the literature. Aesthetic Plast Surg 2020;44(3):929–944
2. Moon HJ. Injection rhinoplasty using filler. Facial Plast Surg Clin North Am 2018;26(3):323–330

POSTINJECTION CARE AFTER FACIAL FILLERS

11. *Following injection of filler to the face, which one of the following should be routinely considered for the first week?*

  B. Antiviral medications

There are a number of recommendations for patients undergoing facial injectable therapy. For all patients, it is reasonable to consider whether antiviral prophylaxis is warranted. This will be down to the individual circumstances of the patient and if they have a strong history of herpetic outbreak, then 1200 mg of acyclovir should be prescribed the day before treatment and continued for up to 1 week. In patents with active herpetic outbreaks, then injections should be rescheduled.

Antibiotics should not be routinely prescribed for facial injections, as there is no clinical need and overuse of antibiotics will affect resistance. Some patients and some surgeons have a preference for ice compression following treatment, but this would only be for the first 24 hours and there is no justification for doing this for a full week. In general, patients should be advised to avoid massaging the areas, which have been injected, as this risks displacement of the product from where it was intended. However, some patients may need some gentle massage if there is a particular lump or imperfection, which you and the patient wish to address. For this reason, discussion of this should be made with the patients at the time of injection with advice to make contact if there are any such concerns. Facial fillers do not necessitate a long downtime; however, avoiding strenuous activity is advisable for the first couple of days. There is no justification to undertake exercise posttreatment.[1,2]

REFERENCES

1. De Boulle K, Heydenrych I. Patient factors influencing dermal filler complications: prevention, assessment, and treatment. Clin Cosmet Investig Dermatol 2015;8:205–214
2. Gazzola R, Pasini L, Cavallini M. Herpes virus outbreaks after dermal hyaluronic acid filler injections. Aesthet Surg J 2012;32(6):770–772

EARLY COMPLICATIONS IN FACIAL FILLERS

12. Following injection with hyaluronic acid filler to the face, a patient presents with an area of skin necrosis developing adjacent to the injection site. *Which one of the following is recommended for treatment?*

  C. Injection of hyaluronidase

There are a number of potential complications to consider when injecting facial fillers. Some of these relate to specific products, while others are more broadly applicable.

The scenario described indicates that there has been an intravascular injection leading to an embolic event and consequent ischemia in the surrounding skin. This must be treated urgently with hyaluronidase to breakdown the hyaluronic acid and limit further tissue injury. Management of this problem represents an evolving area of research, but current protocols recommend high dose (450–600 units) and pulsed (hourly) injections of hyaluronidase until clinical improvement is observed.

Allergic reactions are extremely rare with hyaluronic acid or other fillers and the need for epinephrine use to manage anaphylaxis is therefore also extremely unlikely. Surgical debridement is rarely required and even where necrosis of the skin has occurred, conservative measures will be preferred, as they will reduce the sacrifice of potentially viable tissues that may be debrided if surgery was performed. Cold compress and ice are reasonable for moat patients following injections, but cooling the skin would not be of any specific benefit in this scenario. Other things to consider in this setting include things to help cause vasodilatation and blood flow including nitropaste (nitroglycerin), warm compresses, sildenafil, and aspirin for its antiplatelet action.[1]

Steroid is indicated following injection with some fillers, such as PMMA where there is scarring and firmness. However, it is not indicated in this scenario.

REFERENCE

1. DeLorenzi C. New high dose pulsed hyaluronidase protocol for hyaluronic acid filler vascular adverse events. Aesthet Surg J 2017;37(7):814–825

INJECTABLES IN THE LIP

13. A 25-year-old patient is seen in the office requesting lip augmentation. *Which one of the following products would be most well suited to this procedure?*

  A. Juvéderm Vobella

The treatment goal for lips is to add volume and create shape, while respecting the aesthetic proportions. In younger patients, a volume/shape enhancement is typically desired, while in older patients a volume/shape restoration is desired. There are a number of fillers on the market, which are appropriate for use in the lips. These include Juvéderm Vobella and Restylane Silk as well as Juvéderm Ultra/XC. These all have FDA approval for this use.

They are low-molecular-weight hyaluronic acids, i.e., are thinner and less viscous than the other products listed, and so work better in more superficial locations. Lip filler may be placed along the white roll in a retrograde linear deposition fashion to enhance this area. Alternatively, deeper injections in small deposits may be used to help lip eversion and overall fullness. Either way, only small volumes are required to achieve a noticeable effect, and it is advisable to under-correct, rather than overcorrect, as additional top ups may always be considered, where dissolving the product completely is less likely to achieve the desired outcome. Lip injection can be painful and infraorbital nerve blocks can therefore be helpful in addition to the lidocaine contained within these products.[1] Juvéderm Volure is an intermediate filler that can be used for both deep volume augmentation in the midface and correction of moderate to severe facial wrinkles and folds. Juvéderm Voluma is a thicker filler that is also indicated for deep volumization. Restylane has a range of products including "Refyne" and "Defyne" which have similar indications to Volure, i.e., correction of moderate to severe facial wrinkles and folds. Restylane Lyft is indicated for deeper volumization and the dorsal hand.[1,2] Sculptra is indicated for the correction of shallow to deep nasolabial fold contour deficiencies and other facial wrinkles, as well as correction of lipoatrophy in people with HIV (see **Table 105.1**).[3]

REFERENCES

1. Eccleston D, Murphy DK. Juvéderm(®) Volbella™ in the perioral area: a 12-month prospective, multicenter, open-label study. Clin Cosmet Investig Dermatol 2012;5:167–172
2. Rohrich RJ, Bartlett EL, Dayan E. Practical approach and safety of hyaluronic acid fillers. Plast Reconstr Surg Glob Open 2019;7(6):e2172
3. Fitzgerald R, Vleggaar D. Facial volume restoration of the aging face with poly-l-lactic acid. Dermatol Ther (Heidelb) 2011;24(1):2–27

106. Chemical Peels

See Essentials of Plastic Surgery, third edition, pp. 1476–1485

THE BAKER FACIAL PEEL

1. What was the main problem with the original Baker peel for facial rejuvenation?
A. That severe rhytids were not effectively treated
B. That the procedure was too painful to tolerate
C. That the active ingredients were difficult to obtain
D. That patients could be left with significant hypopigmentation
E. That the results were found to be highly variable

PHENOL-BASED FACIAL PEELS

2. What is the main systemic risk to be aware of when using higher concentration phenol peels?
A. Anaphylactic reaction
B. Extensive full-thickness dermal injury
C. Respiratory collapse
D. Gastrointestinal cramps
E. Cardiac arrhythmias

ACTIVE INGREDIENTS IN PHENOL PEELS

3. What has been proposed by Hetter to be the main active ingredient in a Baker-Gordon phenol peel?
A. Phenol
B. Emulsifying agent
C. Croton oil
D. Septisol
E. Acetic acid

CONTRAINDICATIONS TO CHEMICAL PEELS

4. Which one of the following is an absolute rather than a relative contraindication for undertaking a deep chemical peel?
A. Isotretinoin therapy within the last 6 months
B. Deep depth skin resurfacing within the last 6 months
C. Recent facial surgery with skin undermining
D. History of abnormal scar formation or radiation treatment
E. History of rosacea, vitiligo, or psoriasis

CLASSIFICATION OF SKIN TYPES

5. Which one of the following forms part of the Fitzpatrick skin type classification?
A. The degree of wrinkling
B. The use of makeup
C. The presence of actinic damage
D. The response to sun exposure
E. The age of the patient

PRESCRIBING IN CHEMICAL PEELS

6. Which one of the following should be prescribed for all patients prior to undergoing deeper chemical peels for facial rejuvenation?
A. Oral antibiotics
B. Topical steroids
C. Oral nonsteroidal anti-inflammatory drugs (NSAIDs)
D. Oral antivirals
E. Oral antihistamines

PRETREATMENT ASSESSMENT OF PATIENTS CONSIDERING CHEMICAL PEELS

7. What benefit does using a Woods lamp offer in relation to assessing a patient prior to undergoing a chemical peel?
A. To identify the depth of rhytids
B. To identify the extent of rhytids
C. To assess the depth of pigmentation changes
D. To assess the extent of pigmentation changes
E. To instill confidence in them about treatment

SKIN PRECONDITIONING BEFORE A CHEMICAL PEEL

8. A 50-year-old lady is seen in the office requesting a chemical peel. She has type II Fitzpatrick skin and moderate generalized photoaging without significant dyschromia. *Which one of the following should be used as a preconditioner to enhance the effects of the peel?*
   A. Tretinoin
   B. 4% Hydroquinone
   C. 2% Hydroquinone
   D. Glycolic acid
   E. Bupropion

ANALGESIA DURING CHEMICAL PEELS

9. *What is the main caveat of using topical analgesia with a trichloroacetic acid (TCA) chemical peel?*
   A. That the depth of peel may be increased
   B. That the effects of NSAIDs will be reduced
   C. That posttreatment dyschromias may be increased
   D. That they cause vasodilation and subsequent risk of bleeding
   E. That they can cause allergic reactions to the peel

FACTORS AFFECTING THE DEPTH OF A CHEMICAL PEEL

10. *Which one of the following affects the depth of a chemical peel?*
    A. Agent used
    B. Concentration of agent
    C. Length of application
    D. Number of coats applied
    E. All of the above

TRICHLOROACETIC ACID PEELS

11. *What is the clinical appearance during a TCA peel when a mid-reticular dermal injury has been achieved?*
    A. A foggy white frost
    B. A foggy white frost on an erythematous base
    C. An epidermal slide
    D. A grey-white frost
    E. The accordion sign

JESSNER'S SOLUTION

12. *Which one of the following is correct regarding Jessner's solution in relation to facial peels?*
    A. It is used solely as a superficial peel agent.
    B. The solution includes salicylic, trichloroacetic, and lactic acids.
    C. The number of coats has little effect on penetration depth.
    D. It can be combined with TCA for a medium depth peel.
    E. It works in a different manner to that of alpha-hydroxy acids (AHAs).

TRICHLOROACETIC ACID PEELS

13. *What is the main limitation of the TCA peel in clinical practice?*
    A. It needs to be stored in a refrigerator.
    B. It has a short shelf life.
    C. Its use is limited to superficial peels.
    D. It is available only in two different strengths.
    E. It risks poor scarring when used for deeper peels.

ALPHA-HYDROXY ACID PEELS

14. A patient has been using glycolic acid peels at home with modest effects and now wishes to know what benefits an office-based approach may offer her. *What is the main benefit of an office-based approach to glycolic acid peels?*
    A. Multiple coats of the peeling agent can be applied in a single session.
    B. Different acids can be combined to enhance effectiveness.
    C. A local anesthetic is administered.
    D. Higher concentrations of acid can be used.
    E. The peel can be safely left on for a longer duration.

CROTON OIL PEEL

15. *When using a croton oil and phenol peel for a white patient to treat their vertical perioral rhytids, which one of the following is true?*
    A. A concentration of 22% phenol and 1.1 % croton oil would be most appropriate.
    B. The same concentration of preparation could be used to simultaneously treat the lower eyelids.
    C. Hair-bearing areas must be avoided due to the phenol content.
    D. It would be safe to perform this as part of a face-lifting procedure.
    E. The procedure should take less than 10 minutes to perform safely.

Answers

THE BAKER FACIAL PEEL

1. What was the main problem with the original Baker peel for facial rejuvenation?

D. That patients could be left with significant hypopigmentation

Chemical peels were initially used by nonmedical practitioners who used liquid phenol and croton oil as the key ingredients. In the 1960s, Thomas Baker, who was a physician, used a formula containing phenol, croton oil, water, and soap. It was found to be highly effective and reliable in treating severe wrinkles, but carried a high risk of hypopigmentation. It is thought that the reason for this is that the concentration of croton oil was too high. Chemical peels can be uncomfortable but in general are tolerated well with varying degrees of analgesia and the active ingredients are generally available.[1-4]

REFERENCES

1. Baker TJ, Gordon HL. Chemical face peeling and dermabrasion. Surg Clin North Am 1971;51(2):387–401
2. Baker TJ, Gordon HL. Chemical face peeling: an adjunct to surgical facelifting. South Med J 1963;56:412–414
3. Baker TJ, Gordon HL. Chemosurgery of the face: some warnings and misconceptions. J Fla Med Assoc 1962;49: 218–220
4. Baker TJ, Gordon HL, Seckinger DL. A second look at chemical face peeling. Plast Reconstr Surg 1966;37(6):487–493

PHENOL-BASED FACIAL PEELS

2. What is the main systemic risk to be aware of when using higher concentration phenol peels?

E. Cardiac arrhythmias

Phenol has been used as a peeling agent for many years to provide a medium depth peel by the action of protein coagulation. It is, however, a high-risk agent to use, as it is rapidly absorbed through the skin and can lead to renal failure and liver toxicity. It has a direct action on the myocardium which can lead to cardiac arrhythmias. For this reason, patients undergoing a phenol peel require careful cardiac monitoring.[1] To help minimize renal or cardiac toxicity, it is recommended to space peel applications at 10- to 15-minute intervals before applying a new coat in the same aesthetic subunit.[2,3]

REFERENCES

1. Truppman ES, Ellenby JD. Major electrocardiographic changes during chemical face peeling. Plast Reconstr Surg 1979; 63(1):44–48
2. Broughton G, Hashem A, Surek C, Zins J. "Chemical peels" Essentials of Aesthetic Surgery. In: Janis J, ed. 1. Thieme Medical Publishers
3. Hetter GP. An examination of the phenol-croton oil peel: Part I. Dissecting the formula. Plast Reconstr Surg 2000;105(1): 227–239, discussion 249–251

ACTIVE INGREDIENTS IN PHENOL PEELS

3. What has been proposed by Hetter to be the main active ingredient in a Baker-Gordon phenol peel?

C. Croton oil

The Baker-Gordon peel includes phenol, tap water, liquid soap (Septisol), and croton oil. Some authors, such as Hetter,[1,2] believe that the true active ingredient in these peels is the croton oil and that minute changes in the concentration of croton oil can cause very different results. Others such as Stone[3,4] suggest that both the croton oil and phenol more equally affect the peel depth.

The soap is an emulsifying agent that acts as a surfactant to lower surface tension. There is no acetic acid in the preparation. Gregory Hetter diluted the Baker formula and found that his results were very good and patients had less issue with hypopigmentation.[1,2]

REFERENCES

1. Hetter GP. An examination of the phenol-croton oil peel: part IV. Face peel results with different concentrations of phenol and croton oil. Plast Reconstr Surg 2000;105(3):1061–1083, discussion 1084–1087
2. Hetter GP. An examination of the phenol-croton oil peel: Part I. Dissecting the formula. Plast Reconstr Surg 2000;105(1): 227–239, discussion 249–251
3. Stone PA. The use of modified phenol for chemical face peeling. Clin Plast Surg 1998;25(1):21–44

4. Stone PA, Lefer LG. Modified phenol chemical face peels: recognizing the role of application technique. Clin Plast Surg 2001;28(1):13–36

CONTRAINDICATIONS TO CHEMICAL PEELS

4. *Which one of the following is an absolute rather than a relative contraindication for undertaking a deep chemical peel?*

   A. Isotretinoin therapy within the last 6 months

   Indications for undertaking chemical peels include photoaging, deep or superficial rhytids, pigmentary changes, actinic keratosis, solar lentigines, and acne. Before embarking on treatment, it is important to consider the absolute and relative contraindications. Absolute indications to chemical peels include isotretinoin therapy within the last 6 months, active infection, or open wounds. Isotretinoin is thought to increase the risk of wound healing complications and poor scarring especially with invasive surgery and deeper facial rejuvenation techniques. However, current consensus guidelines suggest it is probably safe to continue on this medication where more superficial/less invasive procedures are being performed.[1-3]

   Relative contraindications to chemical peels include medium or deep depth resurfacing procedures (chemical or laser) within the last 3–6 months, recent facial surgery (especially if involved skin undermining to the area being treated), history of abnormal scar formation or radiation therapy, rosacea, vitiligo or psoriasis, and darker skin tones (Fitzpatrick skin type IV, V, and VI)[3-5]

REFERENCES

1. Spring LK, Krakowski AC, Alam M, et al. Isotretinoin and timing of procedural interventions: a systematic review with consensus recommendations. JAMA Dermatol 2017; 153(8):802–809
2. Waldman A, Bolotin D, Arndt KA, et al. ASDS Guidelines Task Force: consensus recommendations regarding the safety of lasers, dermabrasion, chemical peels, energy devices, and skin surgery during and after isotretinoin use. Dermatol Surg 2017;43(10):1249–1262
3. Broughton G, Hashem A, Surek C, Zins J. "Chemical peels" Essentials of Aesthetic Surgery. In: Janis J, ed. 1. Thieme Medical Publishers
4. Rubin MG, ed. Manual of Chemical Peels: Superficial and Medium Depth. Philadelphia, PA: Lippincott Williams & Wilkins; 1995
5. Duffy DM. Avoiding complications with chemical peels. In: Rubin MG, ed. Chemical Peels (Procedures in Cosmetic Dermatology series). Amsterdam: Elsevier; 2006:137–170

CLASSIFICATION OF SKIN TYPES

5. *Which one of the following forms part of the Fitzpatrick skin type classification?*

   D. The response to sun exposure

   The Fitzpatrick skin type classification describes the likely response to sun exposure with six grades and is most relevant to the risk of skin cancer development. It also describes the skin type/ethnicity of the patient ranging from white to brown and black skin types. It is relevant to both an aesthetic consult and one for potential skin cancer given the photoaging effects of UV light.[1]

   Fitzpatrick skin type classification
   Class I: Never tans, burns easily, fair skin
   Class II: Usually burns, tans minimally
   Class III: Burns moderately, tans moderately
   Class IV: Tans moderately and easily, burns minimally
   Class V: Rarely burns, dark brown skin
   Class VI: Never burns, dark brown, or black skin

   The Fitzpatrick classification of facial wrinkling is different and considers perioral and periorbital wrinkling with three classes based on depth of wrinkles and degree of elastosis. This may be a useful system more specifically for an aesthetic facial assessment.[2]

   Fitzpatrick classification of facial wrinkling
   Class I: Fine wrinkles and mild elastosis
   Class II: Fine to moderate wrinkles and moderate elastosis
   Class III: Fine to deep wrinkles and severe elastosis

   The other descriptors (A, B, C, and E) form part of the Glogau classification, which can be used to describe features of photoaging. This contains four categories ranging from mild to severe. Each of these is linked to a typical age range and clinical findings that detail the degree of wrinkles, evidence of actinic sun damage, scarring, and makeup use. Patients are classified into age brackets according to the degree of photoaging. This too is applicable to the assessment of patients before facial rejuvenation.[3]

REFERENCES

1. Fitzpatrick TB. The validity and practicality of sun-reactive skin types I through VI. Arch Dermatol 1988;124(6):869–871
2. Fitzpatrick RE, Goldman MP, Satur NM, Tope WD. Pulsed carbon dioxide laser resurfacing of photo-aged facial skin. Arch Dermatol 1996;132(4):395–402
3. Glogau RG. Aesthetic and anatomic analysis of the aging skin. Semin Cutan Med Surg 1996;15(3):134–138

PRESCRIBING IN CHEMICAL PEELS

6. *Which one of the following should be prescribed for all patients prior to undergoing deeper chemical peels for facial rejuvenation?*

D. Oral antivirals

When considering chemical peels, it is important to evaluate the complete medical history of the patient including other recent treatments, regular medications, and a history of skin disease. Irrespective of their history, when undertaking a medium to deep peel, it is recommended that prophylactic antiviral medication is prescribed to minimize the risk of cold sore development posttreatment. If patients do still develop cold sores posttreatment while on antivirals, it is advisable to double the dose for a short period of time and arrange to see them early in clinic for review.

Patients with history of skin diseases can be an increased risk of postprocedure complications including disease exacerbation, prolonged erythema, and/or healing. Patients with rosacea have a vasomotor instability and may develop an exaggerated inflammatory response after a chemical peel. There is no specific indication for oral antibiotics and if there is evidence of active infection that requires antibiotics, treatment should be postponed as this is an absolute contraindication to treatment. Oral nonsteroidal anti-inflammatory drugs (NSAIDs) are helpful for reducing posttreatment pain and swelling, but do not need to be prescribed pretreatment on a prophylactic basis. Oral antihistamines are not usually part of a chemical peel treatment plan either.[1–3]

REFERENCES

1. Broughton G, Hashem A, Surek C, Zins J. "Chemical peels" Essentials of Aesthetic Surgery. 1. Janis J, ed. Thieme Medical Publishers
2. Rubin MG, ed. Manual of Chemical Peels: Superficial and Medium Depth. Philadelphia, PA: Lippincott Williams & Wilkins; 1995
3. Duffy DM. Avoiding complications with chemical peels. In: Rubin MG, ed. Chemical Peels (Procedures in Cosmetic Dermatology series). Amsterdam: Elsevier; 2006:137–170

PRETREATMENT ASSESSMENT OF PATIENTS CONSIDERING CHEMICAL PEELS

7. *What benefit does using a Woods lamp offer in relation to assessing a patient prior to undergoing a chemical peel?*

D. To assess the depth of pigmentation changes

During the pretreatment evaluation, it is important to identify the location, quantity, and depth of rhytids and the depth of any dyschromias evident. The benefit of using a Woods lamp is that it helps assess the depth of pigmentary changes. The worse the patient looks under a Woods lamp, the more superficial the pigmentation. This can help guide the appropriate treatment plan as to whether a more superficial or deeper peel should be used.[1,2] The use of a Woods lamp has also been described during a superficial peel to help guide the actual treatment so that areas are not missed with the peel application.[3]

Assessment of the rhytids is predominantly clinical. The location and depth of them needs to be assessed as well whether they are static or dynamic in nature. Dynamic rhytids are best managed with an injectable neurotoxin and static rhytids can then be managed with either fillers or resurfacing with laser or a peel.

It is vital to review your clinical findings and discuss them with the patient prior to the procedure. This helps balance realistic treatment expectations for both you and the patients. Be certain to point out gravitational change and skin excess that will not be corrected by chemical peels.

REFERENCES

1. Matarasso SL, Glogau RG, Markey AC. Wood's lamp for superficial chemical peels. J Am Acad Dermatol 1994;30(6):988–992
2. Broughton G, Hashem A, Surek C, Zins J. "Chemical peels" Essentials of Aesthetic Surgery. 1. Janis J, ed. Thieme Medical Publishers
3. Rubin MG, ed. Manual of Chemical Peels: Superficial and Medium Depth. Philadelphia: Lippincott Williams & Wilkins; 1995

SKIN PRECONDITIONING BEFORE A CHEMICAL PEEL

8. A 50-year-old lady is seen in the office requesting a chemical peel. She has type II Fitzpatrick skin and moderate generalized photoaging without significant dyschromia. *Which one of the following should be used as a preconditioner to enhance the effects of the peel?*

   A. Tretinoin

   Use of a pretreatment regimen before performing a chemical peel is essential to prevent complications and optimize outcomes. A standard approach to the pretreatment regimen includes smoking cessation and minimizing sun exposure. A daily skin care program should include a buffing cleanser, an alpha hydroxy acid toner, and a vitamin A conditioner (retinoic acid 0.1%).

   Tretinoin is a synthetic retinoic acid that can stimulate collagen synthesis, exfoliate the stratum corneum, and increase glycosaminoglycan deposition. It does cause increased photosensitivity, so it must be used in conjunction with a sunscreen. It helps precondition the skin and should enhance the effect of the peel and speed epidermal healing.[1–3]

   Tyrosinase inhibitors such as hydroquinone are indicated for use in patients with Fitzpatrick type III, IV, V, or VI skin or where patients have pigment dyschromias to reduce melanin production. This may prevent hyperpigmentation after the peel. Because this patient has pale skin and minimal pigment dyschromia, hydroquinone is not required. When it is used, hydroquinone can be used in 2 or 4% strengths, but the stronger version is available only on prescription. Hydroquinone 2% is sometimes used in combination with glycolic acid gel or kojic acid. A glycolic acid skin-conditioning program may be used 6–8 weeks prior to the peel to enhance overall results. Bupropion is an antidepressant medication that is used to treat both depressive disorders and help with smoking cessation by reducing cravings and withdrawal effects. Smoking cessation is important prior to undergoing a chemical peel but is not the mainstay of cessation therapy and would not be used as a skin preconditioner.

REFERENCES

1. Hevia O, Nemeth AJ, Taylor JR. Tretinoin accelerates healing after trichloroacetic acid chemical peel. Arch Dermatol 1991;127(5):678–682
2. Nemeth AJ, Eaglstein WH, Falanga V, Hevia O, Taylor JR. Methods to speed healing after skin biopsy or trichloroacetic acid chemical peel. Prog Clin Biol Res 1991;365:267–277
3. Mandy SH. Tretinoin in the preoperative and postoperative management of dermabrasion. J Am Acad Dermatol 1986;15(4, Pt 2):878–879, 888–889

ANALGESIA DURING CHEMICAL PEELS

9. *What is the main caveat of using topical analgesia with a trichloroacetic acid (TCA) chemical peel?*

   A. That the depth of peel may be increased

   Superficial chemical peels tend not to cause much patient discomfort and are very well tolerated with little or no analgesia. However, with increasing peel depth comes more patient discomfort; so, anesthesia is often needed. Options include oral analgesics such as NSAIDs, acetaminophen, or opiates. Nerve blocks with local anesthetic can be useful to target the three divisions of the trigeminal nerve. Cooling the face with a fan can also be helpful. Unfortunately, topical agents may be best avoided as, although they can be effective for analgesia, they can induce vasoconstriction and thereby inadvertently increase the depth of a TCA peel. Where topical agents are being used during a TCA peel, it may be wise to reduce the peel strength to account for this. There is no evidence to suggest that topical anesthetic agents will affect the risk of dyschromia, bleeding, or allergic reactions. Their use will be complimentary to the use of NSAIDs.[1,2]

REFERENCES

1. Broughton G, Hashem A, Surek C, Zins J. "Chemical peels" Essentials of Aesthetic Surgery. 1. Janis J, ed. Thieme Medical Publishers
2. Soleymani T, Lanoue J, Rahman Z. A practical approach to chemical peels: a review of fundamentals and step-by-step algorithmic protocol for treatment. J Clin Aesthet Dermatol 2018;11(8):21–28

FACTORS AFFECTING THE DEPTH OF A CHEMICAL PEEL

10. *Which one of the following affects the depth of a chemical peel?*

    E. All of the above

    There are a number of factors which will influence the depth of a chemical peel. These include the agent used, the length of time the agent is in contact with the skin, the number of coats applied, and the pretreatment protocol used. In addition, the depth can be affected by the use of topical anesthetic agents, combining agents, and using occlusive dressings on the area during treatment. It is important to understand how each of these parameters impacts on a peel, as the provider needs to be able to gauge depth according to the desired results and acceptable posttreatment downtime and recovery. A superficial peel results in an epidermal injury, a medium peel results in a superficial dermal injury (papillary dermis), and a deep peel results in an injury into the deep dermis (reticular dermis).

TRICHLOROACETIC ACID PEELS

11. What is the clinical appearance during a TCA peel when a mid-reticular dermal injury has been achieved?

D. A grey-white frost

TCA peels are useful for providing intermediate to deep peels, but in concentrations greater than 45% they risk irregular penetration and scarring. Their effectiveness can be optimized by careful skin preparation. This includes washing and degreasing the skin, mechanically removing surface debris, and applying three or four coats of Jessner's solution. The endpoint for a TCA peel depends on the required depth and can be guided by the appearance of frosting. A pink-white frost suggests injury to the level of the papillary dermis, a dense white frost suggests injury to the superficial reticular dermis, and a dense gray/white frost suggests mid-reticular dermal injury (i.e., a deep peel).

The series of changes during a TCA peel tends to follow the following course. An intermediate peel is a foggy white frost on an erythematous base. A second endpoint is an epidermal slide, which is produced if a cotton tip applicator is applied to the surface of the skin. This is also known as the *accordion sign*. When a deep peel is reached, the epidermal slide will disappear and be replaced by an intense gray-white or yellow blanch.[1-3]

REFERENCES

1. Broughton G, Hashem A, Surek C, Zins J. "Chemical peels" Essentials of Aesthetic Surgery. Vol. 1. Janis J, ed. Thieme Medical Publishers
2. Soleymani T, Lanoue J, Rahman Z. A practical approach to chemical peels: a review of fundamentals and step-by-step algorithmic protocol for treatment. J Clin Aesthet Dermatol 2018;11(8):21–28
3. Nahai F, ed. The Art of Aesthetic Surgery: Principles and Techniques. 2nd ed. St Louis, MO: Quality Medical Publishing; 2011

JESSNER'S SOLUTION

12. Which one of the following is correct regarding Jessner's solution in relation to facial peels?

D. It can be combined with TCA for a medium depth peel.

Jessner's solution includes resorcinol, salicylic acid, lactic acid, and ethanol. It does not contain TCA but is useful when combined with TCA for a medium depth peel. In its own right, it is also a useful peel agent that can provide superficial or intermediate depth treatments, depending on the number of coats applied. It works in a similar way to AHA peels as a keratolytic. A perceived benefit of using this for a chemical peel is that the combination of active agents means each one can be used with a decreased concentration and thereby reduce the risks of unwanted side effects.[1,2]

REFERENCES

1. Broughton G, Hashem A, Surek C, Zins J. "Chemical peels" Essentials of Aesthetic Surgery. 1. Janis J, ed. Thieme Medical Publishers
2. Monheit GD. The Jessner's-trichloroacetic acid peel. An enhanced medium-depth chemical peel. Dermatol Clin 1995; 13(2):277–283

TRICHLOROACETIC ACID PEELS

13. What is the main limitation of the TCA peel in clinical practice?

E. It risks poor scarring when used for deeper peels.

TCA is a derivative of acetic acid and is used for light, intermediate, and deeper peels. It is commonly used in concentrations between 15 and 50%. The problem with using it at the higher concentrations is that it can penetrate the skin in an irregular fashion and cause poor scarring. It is therefore best reserved for superficial and medium-depth peels and when doing so has a relatively short downtime with most of the skin sloughing occurring within a few days. Penetration depth can be improved by washing and cleansing the areas to be treated to remove oil and also mechanically removing surface debris. Chemically disrupting the skin surface barrier with mild acidic solution such as Jessner's can also be helpful. TCA is not light sensitive and so does not need to be refrigerated. It remains stable for at least 23 weeks in an opened container. It is available in multiple different strengths and a 20% concentration can be used for epidermal and papillary dermal peel, with 25–35% concentrations used for upper reticular dermis (medium-depth) penetration.[1-3]

REFERENCES

1. Nahai F, ed. The Art of Aesthetic Surgery: Principles and Techniques. 2nd ed. St Louis, MO: Quality Medical Publishing; 2011
2. Dinner MI, Artz JS. The art of the trichloroacetic acid chemical peel. Clin Plast Surg 1998;25(1):53–62
3. Collins PS. Trichloroacetic acid peels revisited. J Dermatol Surg Oncol 1989;15(9):933–940

ALPHA-HYDROXY ACID PEELS

14. A patient has been using glycolic acid peels at home with modest effects and now wishes to know what benefits an office-based approach may offer her. *What is the main benefit of an office-based approach to glycolic acid peels?*

   D. Higher concentrations of acid can be used.

   AHAs are naturally occurring acids found in citrus fruits. They are used as superficial peel agents and cause exfoliation. They are available as over-the-counter preparations and prescription-only preparations, depending on their concentration and pH values. Higher concentrations of acid will provide a deeper peel. The FDA has limited AHAs for over-the-counter sale to those of maximum 10% concentration (with a pH of >3.5), because more concentrated acids can cause epithelial necrosis instead of exfoliation. Therefore, the benefits of an office-based approach are that a higher concentration of acid may be used to achieve a greater response.[1,2]

REFERENCES

1. Broughton G, Hashem A, Surek C, Zins J. "Chemical peels" Essentials of Aesthetic Surgery. 1. Janis J, ed. Thieme Medical Publishers
2. Sharad J. Glycolic acid peel therapy - a current review. Clin Cosmet Investig Dermatol 2013;6:281–288

CROTON OIL PEEL

15. *When using a croton oil and phenol peel for a white patient to treat their vertical perioral rhytids, which one of the following is true?*

   D. It would be safe to perform this as part of a face-lifting procedure.

   Phenol and croton oil peels are used for achieving deeper peels. Phenol is a derivative of coal tar that causes rapid denaturation and coagulation of surface keratin. Phenol is effective for wrinkles and severe dyschromia and will penetrate to the mid-reticular dermis. Similar to TCA peels, the depth can be affected by skin preparation with washing and degreasing.

   Although deep chemical peeling over undermined skin (i.e., facelift) is not generally recommended, the chemical peeling of non-undermined areas is safe and effective. Therefore, use of this peel at the end of a facelift procedure would be entirely appropriate.

   The most common formulation is the Gordon Baker peel which includes 3 cc of phenol, 2 cc of tap water, 8 drops of liquid soap, and 3 drops of croton oil which is a skin irritant that causes inflammation, vesication (blister formation), and secondary collagen formation.

   When using this preparation to treat vertical perioral rhytids, a common concentration would be 33% phenol and 1.1% croton oil. This concentration is associated with acceptable side effects in Fitzpatrick I and II skin types. In contrast, a common concentration for the treatment of lower eyelid hyperpigmentation and fine lines is lower at 22% phenol and 1.1 % croton oil. Phenol does not affect hair growth; so, the preparation should actually be feathered into hair-bearing areas to ensure optimal blending when treating the forehead and temples. This would not, of course, be relevant to the perioral region. To help minimize renal or cardiac toxicity, it is recommended to space croton peel applications at 10–15 intervals before applying a new coat in the same aesthetic subunit; therefore, it will take longer than 10 minutes to perform this procedure.[1-4]

REFERENCES

1. Hetter GP. An examination of the phenol-croton oil peel: part IV. Face peel results with different concentrations of phenol and croton oil. Plast Reconstr Surg 2000;105(3): 1061–1083, discussion 1084–1087
2. Hetter GP. An examination of the phenol-croton oil peel: Part III. The plastic surgeons' role. Plast Reconstr Surg 2000; 105(2):752–763
3. Ozturk CN, Huettner F, Ozturk C, Bartz-Kurycki MA, Zins JE. Outcomes assessment of combination face lift and perioral phenol-croton oil peel. Plast Reconstr Surg 2013;132(5):743e–753e
4. Bensimon R. The technical use of croton oil peels. In: Tonnard P, Verpaele A, Bensimon R, eds. Centrofacial Rejuvenation. Vol. 1. New York, NY: Thieme Medical Publishing; 2017

107. Fat Grafting

See Essentials of Plastic Surgery, third edition, pp. 1486–1499

GENERAL PRINCIPLES OF FAT GRAFTING

1. *Which one of the following statements is correct regarding fat grafting?*
   A. It involves the transfer of free autografts of vascularized adipose tissue.
   B. It provides predictable results when used to correct soft-tissue contour deformities.
   C. It transfers adipocytes and their surrounding stroma in a single setting.
   D. Only mature adipocytes are able to survive the grafting process.
   E. Preadipocytes are immature fat cells that are poorly tolerant of ischemia.

CLINICAL INDICATIONS FOR FAT GRAFTING

2. A 48-year-old woman is considering fat grafting to the left breast following a wide local excision of a 2-cm breast tumor and subsequent chemoradiotherapy. She dislikes the appearance of the left breast, which has a contour defect with puckered scarring. *In addition to addressing the volume deficiency, what is the main secondary benefit of fat grafting in this patient?*
   A. Tumor recurrence risk will be reduced
   B. Tumor surveillance will be simplified
   C. Breast skin quality will be improved
   D. Wound healing will be enhanced
   E. Postoperative swelling will be avoided

FAT GRAFTING AFTER BREAST RECONSTRUCTION

3. You see a woman in clinic who has undergone breast construction with a free DIEP flap. The lateral part of the flap did not survive, and the patient is now lacking lateral and upper pole fullness. *When discussing risks and benefits of fat grafting to the breast, which one of the following statements is correct?*
   A. Overcorrection of the deficit in the operating room should be avoided.
   B. Multiple fat transfer procedures are likely to be required.
   C. External tissue expansion with the Brava system is needed.
   D. A traditional corrective surgical approach cannot address this problem.
   E. Reconstruction will be unaffected by subsequent fluctuations in weight.

BENEFITS OF FAT GRAFTING

4. You are running a clinic for facial deformity and see a male patient who is interested in fat grafting. He has been taking antiretroviral medications for many years and has been receiving synthetic facial fillers to improve his malar fullness. His CD4 count is normal and his BMI is 20. *In this case, which one of the following is likely to be the greatest challenge of fat grafting?*
   A. Increased risk of rejection
   B. Availability of donor tissue
   C. Low immune status
   D. Unnatural appearance
   E. High donor-site morbidity

FAT HARVEST FOR BREAST SURGERY

5. You are performing fat transfer on a patient following breast reconstruction surgery and want to maximize the viability of the fat cells during harvest. *Which one of the following approaches to harvest has traditionally been associated with improved fat cell viability?*
   A. Ultrasound-assisted liposuction
   B. Power-assisted liposuction
   C. Manual harvest with a large-bore cannula
   D. Use of tumescent infiltration with epinephrine and lidocaine
   E. Use of the central, lower abdomen as a donor site

FAT PROCESSING DURING FAT GRAFTING

6. You are setting up a new practice in fat transfer and have visited a number of units using the technique. You are uncertain which type of fat-processing technique to use and consult the literature. *Which approach to fat processing has been shown to have the best graft retention in* **in vivo** *studies?*
   A. Centrifugation
   B. Washing
   C. Sedimentation
   D. Straining
   E. Cotton-gauze rolling

THE COLEMAN APPROACH TO FAT TRANSFER

7. *When using the Coleman approach to fat processing, which one of the following is correct?*
   A. The lipoaspirate is spun in a centrifuge for 3 minutes at 3000 rpm.
   B. The middle layer of the lipoaspirate is discarded after centrifugation.
   C. The lipoaspirate is washed in sterile water before injection.
   D. Sedimentation and straining of the aspirate through a wire basket is performed.
   E. The lipoaspirate is gently rolled in absorbent gauze before injection.

FAT INJECTION DURING FAT TRANSFER

8. *When injecting fat into the face using the Coleman technique, which one of the following is correct?*
   A. Fat should be injected with 10-cc syringes and a 25-gauge cannula.
   B. Small deposits of fat should be placed during advancement of the cannula.
   C. Pickle fork-style cannulas should be used in most settings.
   D. A cross-hatching technique should be used to evenly distribute fat grafts.
   E. External digital manipulation should be avoided.

CLINICAL TECHNIQUES IN FAT TRANSFER

9. A 25-year-old woman with a body mass index of 30 has small breasts and is interested in enhancing her breast volume without using prosthetic implants. A combined fat transfer and external expansion technique is planned. *Which one of the following is true?*
   A. Fat should be injected into the breast parenchyma but not into the pectoralis major.
   B. Optimal fat retention is achieved where smaller volumes of fat are injected per session.
   C. Graft survival is improved by the use of external expansion with the Brava system.
   D. Fat transfer has now largely replaced the need for prosthetic augmentation.
   E. Cryopreservation of fat in the primary surgery should be strongly considered.

POSTOPERATIVE CARE FOLLOWING FAT TRANSFER

10. *Which one of the following should be avoided during the first week after fat transfer?*
   A. Elevation and ice
   B. Compression garments
   C. Gentle massage
   D. Resumption of full daily activities
   E. Anticoagulant medication

PLACEMENT OF FAT DURING FAT TRANSFER

11. *When performing fat transfer, in which area of the body is it paramount to avoid intramuscular fat injection?*
   A. The breast after LD flap transfer
   B. The breast after free TRAM transfer
   C. The breast during simultaneous implant exchange with fat procedure (SIEF)
   D. The gluteal region during buttock enhancement
   E. The breast during primary augmentation

POSTOPERATIVE FOLLOW-UP AFTER FAT GRAFTING

12. You see a 45-year-old woman 3 months after she underwent fat grafting as a primary breast augmentation procedure. She is feeling very well following her surgery and has been inspired to lose a further 10 pounds. *When examining her, which one of the following is correct?*
   A. There should be no residual swelling.
   B. Her final result should be evident.
   C. Mammography at this stage would be compromised.
   D. About three quarters of the transferred volume will remain.
   E. Firm, palpable areas may represent fat necrosis.

Answers

GENERAL PRINCIPLES OF FAT GRAFTING

1. Which one of the following statements is correct regarding fat grafting?

C. It transfers adipocytes and their surrounding stroma in a single setting.

Fat grafting involves transfer of nonvascularized, but viable, fat cells from one location to another within the same individual. Although fat grafting is generally successful in many circumstances, the results can be unpredictable in terms of volume maintenance. It does transfer fat and stroma in a single setting, although it usually requires multiple stages to achieve satisfactory clinical results, especially when larger contour defects are treated. Both mature adipocytes and preadipocytes can be transferred, but of the two cell types, preadipose cells are more resilient to ischemia and can continue to differentiate and proliferate after regaining a blood supply.[1] Peer's cell survival theory states that the number of viable adipocytes at the time of transplantation correlates with ultimate fat graft survival.[2]

REFERENCES

1. Coleman SR, Mazzola RF. Fat Injection: From Filling to Rejuvenation. St Louis, MO: Quality Medical Publishing; 2009
2. Peer LA. Cell survival theory versus replacement theory. Plast Reconstr Surg (1946) 1955;16(3):161–168

CLINICAL INDICATIONS FOR FAT GRAFTING

2. A 48-year-old woman is considering fat grafting to the left breast following a wide local excision of a 2-cm breast tumor and subsequent chemoradiotherapy. She dislikes the appearance of the left breast, which has a contour defect with puckered scarring. *In addition to addressing the volume deficiency, what is the main secondary benefit of fat grafting in this patient?*

C. Breast skin quality may be improved

One of the main advantages of fat transfer is its beneficial effects on irradiated skin and soft tissue. Although the precise mechanism is not fully understood, fat grafting can soften the skin and allow it to become more pliable. Skin complexion and scar appearance can also be improved. Histologic and electron micrographic evaluation after fat transfer shows progressive regeneration of tissue ultrastructure with a reduction in epidermal thickening, vascular density, and fibrosis. Often, after the first lipofilling procedure, improvements in skin appearance are the most obvious visible benefit. There is no evidence to suggest that tumor recurrence is affected by fat grafting. Concerns have been raised as to whether injection of stem cells places patients at an increased (not decreased) risk of developing further tumors, but this has not been substantiated. Some authors suggest that fat transfer may make tumor surveillance more difficult, rather than simple, due to microcalcification on mammogram, but it should not interfere with detection providing the evaluation is performed by an experienced radiologist. Moderate bruising and swelling to both donor and recipient sites are inevitable following fat grafting, so patients must be aware of this preoperatively.[1-4]

REFERENCES

1. Phulpin B, Gangloff P, Tran N, Bravetti P, Merlin JL, Dolivet G. Rehabilitation of irradiated head and neck tissues by autologous fat transplantation. Plast Reconstr Surg 2009;123(4):1187–1197
2. Rigotti G, Marchi A, Galiè M, et al. Clinical treatment of radiotherapy tissue damage by lipoaspirate transplant: a healing process mediated by adipose-derived adult stem cells. Plast Reconstr Surg 2007;119(5):1409–1422, discussion 1423–1424
3. Delay E, Garson S, Tousson G, Sinna R. Fat injection to the breast: technique, results, and indications based on 880 procedures over 10 years. Aesthet Surg J 2009;29(5):360–376
4. Sultan SM, Stern CS, Allen RJ Jr, et al. Human fat grafting alleviates radiation skin damage in a murine model. Plast Reconstr Surg 2011;128(2):363–372

FAT GRAFTING AFTER BREAST RECONSTRUCTION

3. You see a woman in clinic who has undergone breast construction with a free DIEP flap. The lateral part of the flap did not survive, and the patient is now lacking lateral and upper pole fullness. *When discussing risks and benefits of fat grafting to the breast, which one of the following statements is correct?*

B. Multiple fat transfer procedures are likely to be required.

Use of fat injection (lipomodeling) for refining autologous breast reconstruction has become standard practice for many breast reconstructive surgeons, particularly for the correction of superior and medial pole deficiencies.

Correction in this scenario is possible with fat transfer but will require multiple stages and achieving a perfect contour is challenging. The patient's body habitus will affect outcome, and in thin patients obtaining sufficient volume for transfer can be a challenge. This is exacerbated by the fact that the anterior abdominal wall has already been harvested for the main flap, leaving little fat excess present in this area. Often the flanks are a useful source for fat harvest in these patients. Other suitable donor sites include the thighs and upper central abdomen.

Because up to half of the transferred fat may not survive, it is standard practice to overcorrect defects in the operating room where possible. Quite large volumes of fat (200–300 cc) should be placed at multiple levels within the flap to improve graft take. External expansion with the Brava system is not routinely used in this scenario, although it does represent an uncommon option. It is most commonly indicated for use in primary breast augmentation where a combination of fat transfer and the Brava system may improve outcomes.[1,2]

Although fat transfer is a useful technique in revision reconstructive cases, its limitations must be recognized. Where large deformities are present, standard surgical approaches may be more helpful to inset or recontour the flap. In some cases, where the lateral defect is large, further flap reconstruction with a thoracodorsal artery perforator flap or partial latissimus dorsi (LD) flap may be indicated. A caveat of fat transfer is that fluctuations in weight will affect the recipient area. However, the same is also true of transferred vascularized tissues such as transverse rectus abdominis myocutaneous (TRAM) and deep inferior epigastric perforator (DIEP) flaps, so patients should be advised of this before surgery.[3]

REFERENCES

1. Khouri RK, Eisenmann-Klein M, Cardoso E, et al. Brava and autologous fat transfer is a safe and effective breast augmentation alternative: results of a 6-year, 81-patient, prospective multicenter study. Plast Reconstr Surg 2012;129(5): 1173–1187
2. Del Vecchio DA, Bucky LP. Breast augmentation using preexpansion and autologous fat transplantation: a clinical radiographic study. Plast Reconstr Surg 2011;127(6):2441–2450
3. Delay E, Garson S, Tousson G, Sinna R. Fat injection to the breast: technique, results, and indications based on 880 procedures over 10 years. Aesthet Surg J 2009;29(5):360–376

BENEFITS OF FAT GRAFTING

4. You are running a clinic for facial deformity and see a male patient who is interested in fat grafting. He has been taking antiretroviral medications for many years and has been receiving synthetic facial fillers to improve his malar fullness. His CD4 count is normal and his BMI is 20. *In this case, which one of the following is likely to be the greatest challenge of fat grafting?*
   B. Availability of donor tissue
   Fat transfer has many advantages over synthetic fillers, including low material cost, ready availability, a natural appearance, excellent biocompatibility, permanence, low donor-site morbidity, and the ability to contour donor sites where required. In patients with HIV and subsequent lipodystrophy as a result of taking antiretroviral medications, there is often insufficient fat available for harvest, and these individuals might require a synthetic alternative filler. Some HIV patients can develop fat excess in the posterior neck (buffalo hump appearance) and central regions. In these cases, it may be possible to use these areas for harvest.[1-3]

REFERENCES

1. Uzzan C, Boccara D, Lacheré A, Mimoun M, Chaouat M. Treatment of facial lipoatrophy by lipofilling in HIV infected patients: retrospective study on 317 patients on 9 years [in French]. Ann Chir Plast Esthet 2012;57(3):210–216
2. Martins de Carvalho F, Casal D, Bexiga J, et al. HIV-associated facial lipodystrophy: experience of a tertiary referral center with fat and dermis-fat compound graft transfer. Eplasty 2016;16:e31
3. Fontdevila J, Serra-Renom JM, Raigosa M, et al. Assessing the long-term viability of facial fat grafts: an objective measure using computed tomography. Aesthet Surg J 2008;28(4):380–386

FAT HARVEST FOR BREAST SURGERY

5. You are performing fat transfer on a patient following breast reconstruction surgery and want to maximize the viability of the fat cells during harvest. *Which one of the following approaches to harvest has traditionally been associated with improved fat cell viability?*
   C. Manual harvest with a large-bore cannula
   Atraumatic harvesting, handling, and transfer of fat are key to maximizing fat cell viability during fat grafting. Consequently, minimizing pressure by using a large-bore cannula (e.g., 3, 4, or 5 mm) and low pressure should be beneficial. For this reason, the Coleman technique involves the use of 10-cc syringes for harvest. There is debate regarding the benefits of assisted techniques for fat harvest, such as power-assisted or ultrasound-assisted

liposuction,[1] and traditionally these had been associated with decreased viability of harvested fat. Some evidence has shown high levels of fat cell viability after harvest with ultrasound-assisted liposuction that was at least comparable with or possibly superior to manual harvest.[2] That said, there is usually a larger oil layer when performing suction-assisted fat harvest, which suggests fat cell rupture has occurred. Fat cell viability also seems to correlate with the amount of shear trauma and liposuction circuit pressure. Fat cell rupture is thought to be in part caused by the forces applied while passing through the suction circuit.[3,4] In practice, many surgeons still use suction-assisted liposuction for fat graft harvest especially in larger volume transfers, as this is far more efficient in these settings. Furthermore, there are now some systems that harvest and collect large volumes of fat within a closed system for direct reinjection. Use of a tumescent infiltrate with epinephrine or local anesthetic does not improve viability, although it can reduce bleeding and facilitate ease of harvest. Some evidence suggests that local anesthetics may actually decrease fat cell viability and should ideally be diluted to minimize this.[3,5]

REFERENCES

1. Keck M, Kober J, Riedl O, et al. Power assisted liposuction to obtain adipose-derived stem cells: impact on viability and differentiation to adipocytes in comparison to manual aspiration. J Plast Reconstr Aesthet Surg 2014;67(1):e1–e8
2. Schafer ME, Hicok KC, Mills DC, Cohen SR, Chao JJ. Acute adipocyte viability after third-generation ultrasound-assisted liposuction. Aesthet Surg J 2013;33(5):698–704
3. Cucchiani R, Corrales L. The effects of fat harvesting and preparation, air exposure, obesity, and stem cell enrichment on adipocyte viability prior to graft transplantation. Aesthet Surg J 2016;36(10):1164–1173
4. Lee JH, Kirkham JC, McCormack MC, Nicholls AM, Randolph MA, Austen WG Jr. The effect of pressure and shear on autologous fat grafting. Plast Reconstr Surg 2013;131(5):1125–1136
5. Keck M, Zeyda M, Gollinger K, et al. Local anesthetics have a major impact on viability of preadipocytes and their differentiation into adipocytes. Plast Reconstr Surg 2010;126(5):1500–1505

FAT PROCESSING DURING FAT GRAFTING

6. You are setting up a new practice in fat transfer and have visited a number of units using the technique. You are uncertain which type of fat-processing technique to use and consult the literature. *Which approach to fat processing has been shown to have the best graft retention in* in vivo *studies?*

    E. Cotton-gauze rolling

    The aim of fat processing after harvest is to remove unwanted fluid, cells, and debris from the lipoaspirate, while causing minimal damage to the fat cells. There are different techniques used to achieve this, including centrifugation, sedimentation, straining, rolling, and washing. Cotton gauze rolling has been reported as having the highest graft retention *in vivo*.[1] This technique involves pouring the lipoaspirate from the syringe onto a nonstick absorbent gauze, which is then gently rolled with an instrument handle in order to remove aqueous and oil layers.

    A comparative study by Rose et al[2] compared the other three main processing techniques (centrifugation, washing, and sedimentation) and showed that the number of viable fat cells maintained was highest when sedimentation was used. However, this team did not then assess the outcomes after injection with the different processing techniques. Whether this would translate into a clinical outcome benefit therefore remains unproven. Furthermore, although it may be the least traumatic method of fat processing, it does expose the aspirate to the air and is a relatively slow process which may not be helpful in clinical practice. Based on current clinical data, outcomes appear similar irrespective of processing technique; so, in your practice you should select the one you are most familiar with until stronger evidence is available.

REFERENCES

1. Fisher C, Grahovac TL, Schafer ME, Shippert RD, Marra KG, Rubin JP. Comparison of harvest and processing techniques for fat grafting and adipose stem cell isolation. Plast Reconstr Surg 2013;132(2):351–361
2. Rose JG Jr, Lucarelli MJ, Lemke BN, et al. Histologic comparison of autologous fat processing methods. Ophthal Plast Reconstr Surg 2006;22(3):195–200

THE COLEMAN APPROACH TO FAT TRANSFER

7. *When using the Coleman approach to fat processing, which one of the following is correct?*

    A. The lipoaspirate is spun in a centrifuge for 3 minutes at 3000 rpm.

    There are a number of approaches to processing harvested fat during fat transfer surgery. The Coleman[1] technique uses the centrifugation approach. Centrifugation involves spinning fat in small syringes at speeds of approximately 3000 rpm for up to 3 minutes. This process will separate the harvest into three layers: top (oil), middle (fat cells), and bottom (blood/infiltrate). The middle layer must therefore be kept, as this represents the fat used for grafting.

Centrifugation for longer than this is not recommended, as further separation does not occur and fat cells may be damaged.

When using a washing technique, a number of different solutions may be used including normal saline, 5% glucose, or sterile water. Given the available evidence, saline is preferred compared with water and is common practice. In theory, washing cells in sterile water risks causing cell lysis because of the osmolarity difference. This difference is traditionally related to red blood cells but may also apply to fat cells. Rubin and Hoefflin[2] have an interesting and somewhat controversial "survival of the fittest " view on fat preparation. They use sterile water to wash the fat preparation and combine this with centrifugation at 6000 rpm, reporting satisfactory clinical results. They believe that stressing fat cells before injection results in only the most resilient cells reaching the injection stage. In general, most authorities work to minimize trauma to the fat cells (not increase it) during processing and this would be a more conventional approach.

Sedimentation, decanting, and straining are not part of the Coleman technique, but are thought to represent the least traumatic method of fat processing. The main disadvantage is that this increases processing time and risks prolonged exposure of fat cells to the air, which in turn may lead to desiccation. Handling of the fat is also increased, so it may risk further damage. Cotton-gauze rolling is an alternative low trauma method of fat processing, again not part of the Coleman technique. A potential benefit is that the stromal component is largely retained.

REFERENCES

1. Coleman SR. Structural Fat Grafting. St Louis, MO: Quality Medical Publishing; 2004
2. Rubin A, Hoefflin SM. Fat purification: survival of the fittest. Plast Reconstr Surg 2002;109(4):1463–1464

FAT INJECTION DURING FAT TRANSFER

8. ***When injecting fat into the face using the Coleman technique, which one of the following is correct?***

D. A cross-hatching technique should be used to evenly distribute fat grafts.

When performing fat grafting, it is important to place fat in a cross-hatched pattern using long radial passes from multiple directions. This helps avoid placing an excess of fat in a single place or line. Injection in the face with the Coleman technique involves placement of small aliquots of fat in different tissue layers using 1-cc syringes and a 17-gauge blunt-tipped cannula 7–9 cm long. These are used to minimize trauma to the fat grafts and provide for accurate placement of small fat units; 10-cc syringes are used for harvest only. Fat should be placed on withdrawal, not advancement of the cannula. The pickle fork cannula is used only in areas of scarring and fibrosis where it is useful to break down the tissues and create a space for the fat grafts to sit. External digital manipulation is used to flatten clumps and minor irregularities during fat injection.[1-3]

REFERENCES

1. Coleman SR. Structural Fat Grafting. St Louis, MO: Quality Medical Publishing; 2004
2. Gir P, Brown SA, Oni G, Kashefi N, Mojallal A, Rohrich RJ. Fat grafting: evidence-based review on autologous fat harvesting, processing, reinjection, and storage. Plast Reconstr Surg 2012;130(1):249–258
3. Coleman SR, Mazzola RF. Fat Injection: From Filling to Rejuvenation. St Louis, MO: Quality Medical Publishing; 2009

CLINICAL TECHNIQUES IN FAT TRANSFER

9. **A 25-year-old woman with a body mass index of 30 has small breasts and is interested in enhancing her breast volume without using prosthetic implants. A combined fat transfer and external expansion technique is planned. *Which one of the following is true?***

C. Graft survival is improved by the use of external expansion with the Brava system.

The Brava system is an external tissue expander that has shown promising results when combined with fat transfer for primary breast augmentation. The expander is worn for 4 weeks before fat injection and for 1 week after. Graft survival can be substantially higher when external tissue expansion is used (82% compared to 55%).[1,2] When performing primary breast augmentation with fat grafting, it is generally recommended that fat is injected into three planes: subcutaneously, prepectorally, and intramuscularly. Fat survival is improved when injected into muscle as it has a robust blood supply. However, there have been concerns raised about intramuscular injection of fat in view of the complications of buttock enhancement with fat transfer; so, care should be taken when injecting intramuscularly at any site of the body. Some surgeons will also inject directly into the breast parenchyma, although this does risk leaving small deposits of fat, which can necrose and potentially impact upon imaging for breast cancer further down the line. Long-term fat retention is improved when larger fat volumes are injected at each stage. In this patient with a BMI of 30, she should have a good volume of fat available for transfer (e.g., 300 cc per side), which could give her a meaningful autoaugment. While fat transfer has become very popular, it has not replaced the need for prosthetic breast augmentation, which still remains much more commonly performed. Many patients who wish to have breast augmentation are very slim and have little fat for transfer. Furthermore, because fat transfer often requires multiple stages, the financial implications tend to make it less cost-effective for patients who are self-funding.

Harvesting additional fat and freezing this for future injections has theoretical appeal in that a ready supply of fat for injection in the office setting could provide further enhancement to the breast without the need for additional liposuction. Unfortunately, tissue viability drops with cryopreservation as most cryopreservative agents are also cytotoxic. The adipose-derived stem cell yield is significantly less in cryopreserved fat than from fresh fat; so overall, cryopreservation of fat is not a component of routine clinical practice and would not be indicated in this case.[3,4]

REFERENCES

1. Khouri RK, Eisenmann-Klein M, Cardoso E, et al. Brava and autologous fat transfer is a safe and effective breast augmentation alternative: results of a 6-year, 81-patient, prospective multicenter study. Plast Reconstr Surg 2012;129(5): 1173–1187
2. Del Vecchio DA, Bucky LP. Breast augmentation using preexpansion and autologous fat transplantation: a clinical radiographic study. Plast Reconstr Surg 2011;127(6):2441–2450
3. Lidagoster MI, Cinelli PB, Leveé EM, Sian CS. Comparison of autologous fat transfer in fresh, refrigerated, and frozen specimens: an animal model. Ann Plast Surg 2000;44(5):512–515
4. Matsumoto D, Shigeura T, Sato K, et al. Influences of preservation at various temperatures on liposuction aspirates. Plast Reconstr Surg 2007;120(6):1510–1517

POSTOPERATIVE CARE FOLLOWING FAT TRANSFER

10. Which one of the following should be avoided during the first week after fat transfer?

C. Gentle massage

Massage of the recipient area following fat transfer should be avoided for at least 1 week following surgery, as this risks displacement of the grafts. Compression garments should be worn for a few weeks after surgery at both donor and recipient sites. Edema and bruising may be reduced by application of cool packs. Normal activities of daily living can be resumed early in the postoperative phase and full activities can be resumed after a few weeks. Anticoagulant medication can often be continued throughout the perioperative period or restarted the day after surgery, depending on the indication and medication type.[1,2]

REFERENCES

1. Coleman SR. Structural Fat Grafting. St Louis, MO: Quality Medical Publishing; 2004
2. Simonacci F, Bertozzi N, Grieco MP, Grignaffini E, Raposio E. Procedure, applications, and outcomes of autologous fat grafting. Ann Med Surg (Lond) 2017;20:49–60

PLACEMENT OF FAT DURING FAT TRANSFER

11. When performing fat transfer, in which area of the body is it paramount to avoid intramuscular fat injection?

D. The gluteal region during buttock enhancement

Gluteal fat grafting has become a commonly practiced procedure across the globe and initially fat was purposely injected into both subcutaneous fat and the underlying musculature. The rationale for intramuscular injection was that graft take was enhanced secondarily to the higher vascularity of muscle. Indeed, this practice still continues in breast surgery where it is considered both safe and effective to inject into either transferred or native muscle, be it the rectus abdominis, LD, or the pectoralis major.

In contrast there have been an alarming number of fatalities following gluteal fat grafting for buttock enhancement. These have been in fit, young patients who have succumbed to large fat emboli entering the pulmonary vasculature. The mechanism is thought to be due to direct injection of fat into large vessels within the gluteal muscles that have travelled back to the heart. Subsequent investigations into these deaths and multisociety task force safety meetings have been undertaken.[1]

The recommendations are that fat injections to the buttock must AT ALL TIMES BE SUBCUTANEOUS ONLY. The operators must stay as far away from the gluteal veins and sciatic nerve as possible and ensure they have clear awareness and control of the cannula tip placement throughout the entire procedure to ensure no inadvertent deeper passes are made. Access incisions that facilitate a superficial trajectory for each part of the buttock must also be used. Bendable cannula must not be used, and injection should be performed only when the cannula is moving to avoid high-pressure bolus injections. The risk of death must accordingly be discussed with each patient and the risks of this surgery must be weighed up against the potential benefits.

Injection within the muscle remains an accepted technique in the breast, both in reconstruction and primary autoaugmentation settings. SIEF[2] is a procedure used to allow women to remove their breast implants without losing all of the implanted volume. Fat is injected subcutaneously prior to implant removal and then further fat is injected into the soft tissues once the implants are removed. In primary breast augmentation using a fat transfer technique, fat is injected subcutaneously, prepectorally, and intramuscularly. Following free tissue transfer, fat injection into either fat or muscle is beneficial for contour and volume irregularities. Care, of course, should be taken to avoid the vascular pedicle and implant if there is once in situ.

REFERENCES

1. Mills D, Rubin JP, Saltz R. Multi-Society Gluteal Fat Grafting Task Force issues safety advisory urging practitioners to re-evaluate technique. February 6, 2018. Available at: https://www.surgery.org/sites/default/files/Gluteal-Fat-Grafting-02-06-18_0.pdf. Accessed June 20, 2021
2. Del Vecchio DA. "SIEF"--simultaneous implant exchange with fat: a new option in revision breast implant surgery. Plast Reconstr Surg 2012;130(6):1187–1196

POSTOPERATIVE FOLLOW-UP AFTER FAT GRAFTING

12. You see a 45-year-old woman 3 months after she underwent fat grafting as a primary breast augmentation procedure. She is feeling very well following her surgery and has been inspired to lose a further 10 pounds. *When examining her, which one of the following is correct?*

E. Firm palpable areas may represent fat necrosis.

Fat necrosis is a risk that can occur with breast surgery in general, for example, with reductions, reconstructions, and mastopexy. It is obviously a specific risk of fat transfer where grafts fail to obtain adequate new blood supply and scar tissue is formed. In some cases, it will not significantly affect the outcomes in terms of volume changes, but can leave firm or lumpy areas to the breasts which patients may find distressing. Fat necrosis must always be part of any discussion on breast or major reconstructive plastic surgery with patients during the consenting phase.

The swelling following lipomodeling typically lasts for up to 6 months. At 3 months, the final outcome is unlikely to be apparent and again patients should be advised of this preoperatively. Mammography should not be compromised with an experienced radiologist, providing they understand the treatment she has had. Also given her age, mammography should have been performed preoperatively and is unlikely to be required at this stage.[1] Fat transfers are affected by weight changes and behave as they would have at the donor site. Therefore, as this patient has lost weight, the transferred fat will also be affected, and it is unlikely that three quarters of the transferred volume will remain. This again is one of the key areas that must be discussed with patients preoperatively.

REFERENCE

1. Ihrai T, Georgiou C, Machiavello JC, et al. Autologous fat grafting and breast cancer recurrences: retrospective analysis of a series of 100 procedures in 64 patients. J Plast Surg Hand Surg 2013;47(4):273–275

108. Hair Transplantation

See *Essentials of Plastic Surgery*, third edition, pp. 1500–1512

HAIR ANATOMY

1. *Which one of the following is true with respect to the anatomy of scalp hair?*
   A. Scalp hairs are unusual in that they have a mesodermal origin.
   B. An average scalp contains approximately 200,000 follicular units.
   C. An average scalp contains approximately 350,000 individual hairs.
   D. The total number of hairs is unaffected by natural hair color.
   E. Bald scalps have as many hair follicles as nonbald scalps.

PHYSIOLOGY OF HAIR GROWTH

2. *Which one of the following is correct regarding hair growth?*
   A. It involves four key phases.
   B. Most hairs are usually in the telogen phase.
   C. The catagen phase is the longest phase.
   D. Length of the anagen phase is gender specific.
   E. On average, 20 to 30 hairs are shed daily.

INCIDENCE OF ALOPECIA

3. *In which race is alopecia most common?*
   A. Whites
   B. Blacks
   C. American Indians
   D. Asians
   E. Equal across races

MALE PATTERN BALDNESS

4. A 20-year-old man presents with male pattern baldness. His maternal grandfather lost his hair at a similar age. *Which one of the following is correct regarding his condition?*
   A. The fact that his maternal grandfather also lost his hair is likely to be a coincidence.
   B. His condition will be due to an excess of dihydroxytestosterone (DHT).
   C. He can expect his condition to take a fairly severe course.
   D. Treatment with 5-alpha reductase may be beneficial.
   E. His circulating testosterone will be significantly elevated.

CLASSIFICATION OF MALE PATTERN BALDNESS

5. The Norwood classification is commonly used with reference to male pattern baldness. *What is the clinical relevance of this classification?*
   A. It describes the anatomic location of hair loss.
   B. It describes the physiologic causes of hair loss.
   C. It describes the age of onset of hair loss.
   D. It describes the treatment algorithm for hair loss.
   E. It describes the outcome after surgery for hair loss.

CLINICAL PRESENTATION OF HAIR LOSS

6. A 12-year-old patient presents with a single round bald patch on the scalp with no history of trauma. He has no other obvious signs or symptoms, but his mother has a similar condition. *What is the most likely diagnosis?*
   A. Androgenic alopecia
   B. Traumatic alopecia
   C. Cicatricial alopecia
   D. Alopecia areata
   E. Lichen planopilaris

PHARMACOLOGIC MANAGEMENT OF HAIR LOSS

7. You are considering prescribing finasteride for a patient with significant hair loss. *Which one of the following is correct regarding this treatment?*
   A. It is a topical treatment for hair loss used twice daily.
   B. Side effects such as lethargy and rash are common.
   C. It should be reserved for the treatment of early hair loss in women.
   D. It is particularly effective at treating the temporal region.
   E. The major caveat is that lifelong use is required.

LASER THERAPY IN HAIR LOSS

8. *When using laser therapy for the management of hair loss, which one of the following is correct?*
   A. Wavelengths within the red/infrared spectrum between 600 and 900 nm are used with the intention of inducing hair growth.
   B. The Food and Drug Administration (FDA) has approved laser devices for use in hair loss based on studies demonstrating its efficacy.
   C. Discovery of laser as a modality of treating hair loss was intentional being based on sound scientific theory.
   D. Large multicenter studies have consistently shown improved hair growth following laser therapy.
   E. The mechanism of action is well understood and involves production of dermal inflammation and increased blood flow.

NORMAL HAIR DENSITY

9. When planning a hair transplant procedure, it is important to be aware of the volume of hairs in the normal individual and the density that will appear satisfactory. *What is the normal density of scalp hairs per square centimeter in an average individual?*
   A. 40
   B. 100
   C. 200
   D. 350
   E. 400

SURGICAL MANAGEMENT OF HAIR LOSS

10. *When treating moderate frontotemporal hair loss in a 28-year-old male with hair transplants, which one of the following donor sites should be used?*
    A. Parietal
    B. Temporal
    C. Vertex
    D. Upper occipital
    E. Lower occipital

SURGICAL MANAGEMENT OF HAIR LOSS

11. *Which technique of harvesting in hair transplantation may provide the best donor-site appearance with the least obvious scarring?*
    A. Strip excision
    B. Triple-blade knife
    C. Quadruple-blade knife
    D. Follicular unit extraction
    E. Laser harvest

SURGICAL MANAGEMENT OF HAIR LOSS

12. You are undertaking hair transplantation for a patient with frontotemporal recessions. *Which one of the following is true regarding this procedure?*
    A. The new anterior hairline should start 5 cm above the glabella.
    B. Slit minigrafts will provide the most natural appearance.
    C. Angles selected for hair placement should reflect the anatomic location.
    D. Mixing both slit and hole grafts should be avoided in this area.
    E. Micrografts should be used in preference to minigrafts.

POSTOPERATIVE CARE FOLLOWING HAIR TRANSPLANT

13. *Which one of the following should be part of the typical postoperative care following hair transplant?*
    A. A single overnight stay in the hospital.
    B. A head bandage left undisturbed for 2 weeks.
    C. Daily hair washing with a pouring technique.
    D. Resumption of normal hair washing at day 5.
    E. Two weeks of antibiotic cover.

Answers

HAIR ANATOMY

1. *Which one of the following is true with respect to the anatomy of scalp hair?*

E. Bald scalps have as many hair follicles as nonbald scalps.

Although counterintuitive, there is the same number of hair follicles histologically in a bald scalp as there are in a normal hair-bearing scalp. The difference is that the follicles do not remain in the normal growth cycle within the bald scalp. Scalp hair originates from both ectodermal and mesodermal origins as do hairs on the rest of the body. A normal scalp contains around 100,000 to 150,000 individual hairs. A follicular unit typically contains two hairs; so, there are usually around 50,000 to 75,000 follicular units. It also contains the associated sebaceous glands, the insertions of the erector pili muscles, and the perifollicular nerve and vessel supply. The follicular unit is relevant to hair transplant, as single or multiple units are grafted during this process. Single follicular units containing one or two hairs are termed "micrografts" and those containing more hairs are termed "minigrafts." The total number of scalp hairs is influenced by natural hair color, with blondes having more hairs and redheads having fewer hairs.[1,2]

REFERENCES

1. Orentreich N, Durr NP. Biology of scalp hair growth. Clin Plast Surg 1982;9(2):197–205
2. Barrera A. Hair Transplantation. The Art of Micrografting and Minigrafting. St Louis, MO: Quality Medical Publishing; 2002

PHYSIOLOGY OF HAIR GROWTH

2. *Which one of the following is correct regarding hair growth?*

D. Length of the anagen phase is gender specific.

The process of hair growth has three, not four, phases: anagen, catagen, and telogen. The anagen phase is the active growth phase, and 90% of hairs are usually produced in this phase. It is the longest phase, lasting about 3 years in men and 5 to 8 years in women. The catagen phase (degradation phase) is the shortest, at 2 or 3 weeks, and prepares hairs for shedding by separation of the base from the dermal papilla. The telogen phase is the resting phase and lasts 3 to 4 months. Approximately 10% of hair is in this phase, and within it, 50 to 100 hairs are lost daily. Concurrent shortening of the anagen phase and lengthening of the telogen phase result in hair thinning and the subsequent development of baldness.[1,2]

REFERENCES

1. Orentreich N, Durr NP. Biology of scalp hair growth. Clin Plast Surg 1982;9(2):197–205
2. Orentreich N. Scalp hair replacement in man. In: Oregon Regional Primate Research Center, Montagna W, Dobson RL, eds. Advances on Biology of Skin, Vol 9. Proceedings of the University of Oregon Medical School Symposium on the Biology of Skin. New York, NY: Pergamon Press; 1969

INCIDENCE OF ALOPECIA

3. *In which race is alopecia most common?*

A. Whites

There is a difference in the incidence of alopecia across races, although the mechanism of male pattern baldness remains the same in all groups. Whites are most commonly affected, followed by Asians and blacks. The lowest incidence is seen in American Indians. The reason for these apparent racial differences is not known and may reflect both genetic and environmental factors. In the United States, around 35,000,000 men and 21,000,000 women are affected by scalp hair loss. Onset typically commences in the third and fourth decades, with half of patients affected by the age of 50 years.[1–4]

REFERENCES

1. Norwood OT. Male pattern baldness: classification and incidence. South Med J 1975;68(11):1359–1365
2. Norwood OT, Shiell RC, eds. Hair Transplant Surgery. 2nd ed. Springfield, IL: Charles C Thomas; 1984
3. Hamilton JB. Patterned loss of hair in man; types and incidence. Ann N Y Acad Sci 1951;53(3):708–728
4. Gan DC, Sinclair RD. Prevalence of male and female pattern hair loss in Maryborough. J Investig Dermatol Symp Proc 2005;10(3):184–189

MALE PATTERN BALDNESS

4. **A 20-year-old man presents with male pattern baldness. His maternal grandfather lost his hair at a similar age.** *Which one of the following is correct regarding his condition?*

    C. He can expect his condition to take a fairly severe course.

    Male pattern baldness that occurs at such a young age tends to be more severe in terms of extent and speed of hair loss. Male pattern baldness can be inherited in an X-linked autosomal dominant fashion, therefore coming from the maternal grandfather. Therefore, it is no coincidence that the patient's grandfather is also affected. Not all cases will be inherited this way, however, as there is evidence for several non–X-linked autosomal dominant (variable penetrance) routes of inheritance.

    The mechanism of hair loss in male pattern baldness is thought to be due to the effects of dihydroxytestosterone (DHT) on the growth cycle of scalp hair follicles. However, it is not necessarily an excess of DHT that is responsible. A normal DHT can cause alopecia if the hair follicles are abnormally sensitive to its effects. Likewise, testosterone levels do not need to be elevated to cause androgenic alopecia. Testosterone is normally converted to DHT by the enzyme 5-alpha reductase which is found within the cells of susceptible hair follicles and skin. Therefore, an excess of any of these substances can be responsible for the effects observed in androgenic alopecia, and it is most likely that this patient has both normal testosterone and DHT levels. Treatment with 5-alpha reductase inhibitors, but not 5-alpha reductase itself, may be helpful in some cases to reduce the amount of DHT.[1-3]

REFERENCES

1. Barrera A. Hair Transplantation. The Art of Micrografting and Minigrafting. St Louis, MO: Quality Medical Publishing; 2002
2. Norwood OT. Male pattern baldness: classification and incidence. South Med J 1975;68(11):1359–1365
3. Norwood OT, Shiell RC, eds. Hair Transplant Surgery. 2nd ed. Springfield, IL: Charles C Thomas; 1984

CLASSIFICATION OF MALE PATTERN BALDNESS

5. **The Norwood classification is commonly used with reference to male pattern baldness.** *What is the clinical relevance of this classification?*

    A. It describes the anatomic location of hair loss.

    The Norwood classification[1] is very commonly used and describes the anatomic location and extent of male pattern baldness. It has seven subtypes (I–VII) ranging from mild to severe. It is difficult and unnecessary to memorize the precise details of the classification for daily practice. However, the underlying principles and extremes are worth knowing because male pattern baldness tends to follow relatively predictable patterns in terms of anatomic areas affected. It typically begins affecting only the hairline and frontotemporal areas (type I) and progressively affects the frontotemporal regions and the vertex. Type VII is the most extreme, affecting the hairline, vertex, and frontotemporal areas. Some patients first present with vertex baldness only. Within this classification, there is no subtype for either a normal scalp and hairline or complete baldness. The physiologic causes, age of onset, treatment, and outcomes are not part of this classification system either (**Fig. 108.1**).[1,2]

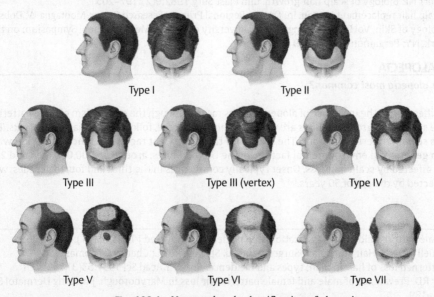

Type I   Type II

Type III   Type III (vertex)   Type IV

Type V   Type VI   Type VII

Fig. 108.1   Norwood male classification of alopecia.

REFERENCES

1. Norwood OT. Male pattern baldness: classification and incidence. South Med J 1975;68(11):1359–1365
2. Norwood OT, Shiell RC, eds. Hair Transplant Surgery. 2nd ed. Springfield, IL: Charles C Thomas; 1984

CLINICAL PRESENTATION OF HAIR LOSS

6. A 12-year-old patient presents with a single round bald patch on the scalp with no history of trauma. He has no other obvious signs or symptoms, but his mother has a similar condition. *What is the most likely diagnosis?*

D. Alopecia areata

Alopecia areata is an autoimmune condition in which hair is randomly lost from small areas of the body, particularly the scalp. It is an inherited condition that can present at any age. It can affect the entire scalp in more extreme cases (alopecia totalis) or even the entire body (alopecia universalis).[1] If this patient was a few years older and had a history of progressive hair loss to the vertex and frontotemporal areas rather than a single patch, then a diagnosis of androgenic alopecia would be more likely, particularly if he was generally fit and well and had siblings with the same condition. Androgenic alopecia involves the conversion of healthy, thick terminal hairs to clear, microscopic vellus hairs. If the patient had learning difficulties with mental illness and had presented with itchiness of the scalp and recent-onset patchy baldness without signs of head lice or inflammation, then a diagnosis of traumatic alopecia could be considered, especially if examination showed evidence of broken hairs in the scalp. In this scenario, patients sustain traumatic alopecia as a result of self-harm by pulling out sections of hair. This condition is more specifically called trichotillomania, and affected individuals feel compelled to pull their hair. Cicatricial alopecia refers to a diverse range of conditions that destroy the hair follicle and replace them with scarring. This normally results in permanent hair loss. Lichen planopilaris refers to hair loss in patients with the inflammatory condition called Lichen planus that progresses to affect the scalp.[1–3]

REFERENCES

1. Messenger AG, McKillop J, Farrant P, McDonagh AJ, Sladden M. British Association of Dermatologists' guidelines for the management of alopecia areata 2012. Br J Dermatol 2012;166(5):916–926
2. Qi J, Garza LA. An overview of alopecias. Cold Spring Harb Perspect Med 2014;4(3):a013615
3. Barrera A. Hair Transplantation. The Art of Micrografting and Minigrafting. St Louis, MO: Quality Medical Publishing; 2002

PHARMACOLOGIC MANAGEMENT OF HAIR LOSS

7. You are considering prescribing finasteride for a patient with significant hair loss. *Which one of the following is correct regarding this treatment?*

E. The major caveat is that lifelong use is required.

Finasteride is a 5-alpha-reductase inhibitor that has been used to treat benign prostatic hypertrophy and male pattern baldness. It is an oral (not topical) medication taken once daily in 1-mg doses. It is most effective on the vertex and frontal region in male pattern baldness and less effective in the temporal region. Side effects are uncommon. The major caveat is that it must be used indefinitely to maintain a response.

Topical solutions of 2 and 5% minoxidil are also used as treatment for baldness. Minoxidil is an antihypertensive medication that causes vasodilation that can also stimulate hair growth. Minoxidil may be useful in both men and women, but at present there is no strong evidence to show a measurable improvement in female hair loss with finasteride. This must also be used indefinitely to maintain a response.[1,2]

REFERENCES

1. McClellan KJ, Markham A. Finasteride: a review of its use in male pattern hair loss. Drugs 1999;57(1):111–126
2. Mysore V, Shashikumar BM. Guidelines on the use of finasteride in androgenetic alopecia. Indian J Dermatol Venereol Leprol 2016;82(2):128–134

LASER THERAPY IN HAIR LOSS

8. *When using laser therapy for the management of hair loss, which one of the following is correct?*

A. Wavelengths within the red/infrared spectrum between 600 and 900 nm are used with the intention of inducing hair growth.

Laser therapy has been promoted as a preventative measure against androgenic alopecia. It is believed that it can help thicken hair and induce growth of existing follicles. Common lasers used for managing alopecia are within the red/infrared spectrum and have wavelengths of between 600 and 900 nm. The mechanism of action of the lasers is not well understood. Theories include provision of an increased blood supply, direct stimulation of hair follicles, an increased and more productive anagen phase, and decreased local DHT levels. The Food and

Drug Administration (FDA) has approved the use of laser for hair loss, but this is based on safety rather than efficacy. Large placebo-controlled trials are lacking. Some smaller studies have shown a benefit of laser on hair growth as have some systematic reviews of case reports, case series, cohort studies and randomized controlled trials (RCTs).[1,2] One meta-analysis containing three RCTs showed that laser treatment promoted hair density in androgenic alopecia.[2]

Laser was originally found to be effective in treating hair loss when used on laboratory mice to initiate skin cancer using a 694-nm ruby laser; hence, its discovery as a modality of treating hair loss was purely accidental rather than a planned deduction.[3]

REFERENCES

1. Adil A, Godwin M. The effectiveness of treatments for androgenetic alopecia: a systematic review and meta-analysis. J Am Acad Dermatol 2017;77(1):136–141.e5
2. Afifi L, Maranda EL, Zarei M, et al. Low-level laser therapy as a treatment for androgenetic alopecia. Lasers Surg Med 2017;49(1):27–39
3. Mester E, Szende B, Tota JG. Effect of laser on hair growth in mice. Kiserl Orvostud 1967;19:628–631

NORMAL HAIR DENSITY

9. When planning a hair transplant procedure, it is important to be aware of the volume of hairs in the normal individual and the density that will appear satisfactory. *What is the normal density of scalp hairs per square centimeter in an average individual?*
    C. 200
      The average number of scalp hairs per unit centimeter is 200. This equates to around 100,000 to 150,000 total hairs. A good visual result can be achieved with a density of around 50 hairs per unit centimeter. This equates to around 25 follicular units per unit centimeter. To treat large areas of hair loss, a few thousand grafts may be required to achieve the required hair density and this is one of the main reasons why the procedure is so time consuming to perform.[1]

REFERENCE

1. Orentreich N, Durr NP. Biology of scalp hair growth. Clin Plast Surg 1982;9(2):197–205

SURGICAL MANAGEMENT OF HAIR LOSS

10. When treating moderate frontotemporal hair loss in a 28-year-old male with hair transplants, which one of the following donor sites should be used?
    E. Lower occipital
      In general, the most popular site for hair harvest is the occipital region. This is commonly used because the donor follicles have decreased or absent DHT and are therefore not influenced by hormonal factors usually associated with hair loss. In addition, providing that the hair is kept above a certain length, the donor scar can be well hidden in this area. The precise level of harvest from the occiput will vary according to age and extent of alopecia. In younger patients such as this man, the donor site is at the junction of the middle and caudal thirds of the vertical distance between the posterior upper healthy fringe and lower hairline (Fig. 108.2).

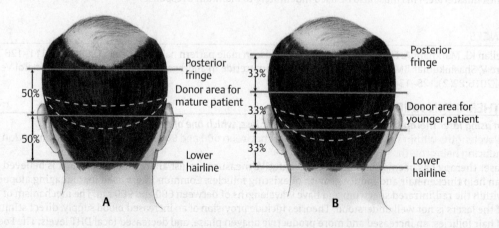

Fig. 108.2 Donor-site locations.

In older patients, the harvest site is placed higher at the midpoint of the healthy fringe and lower hairline. In this patient, who already has frontotemporal hollowing, temple grafts should be avoided. The vertex and parietal regions are not common donor-site areas.[1-4]

REFERENCES

1. Avram MR, Finney R, Rogers N. Hair transplantation controversies. Dermatol Surg 2017;43(Suppl 2):S158–S162
2. Bicknell LM, Kash N, Kavouspour C, Rashid RM. Follicular unit extraction hair transplant harvest: a review of current recommendations and future considerations. Dermatol Online J 2014;20(3):doj_21754
3. Rose PT. Advances in hair restoration. Dermatol Clin 2018;36(1):57–62
4. Vogel JE, Jimenez F, Cole J, et al. Hair restoration surgery: the state of the art. Aesthet Surg J 2013;33(1):128–151

SURGICAL MANAGEMENT OF HAIR LOSS

11. Which technique of harvesting in hair transplantation may provide the best donor-site appearance with the least obvious scarring?

D. Follicular unit extraction

There are a number of ways to harvest hair for hair transplantation and the factors that must be considered include speed of harvest, risk of damage to follicular units, and donor-site scarring. Traditional harvest techniques involve taking a strip of hair (strip excision) with a standard scalpel as a full-thickness graft and then splitting this into smaller mini- and micrografts for transfer. Triple-blade and quadruple-blade knives have been developed so that 2-mm parallel incisions can be made more quickly and accurately to harvest thinner strips of hair-bearing skin. A laser can be used to harvest the skin as an alternative to a blade but appears to offer no advantages.

Because of the problems with donor-site scarring, the technique of follicular unit extraction has been developed. This is a technique that involves harvesting single follicular units individually using a small diameter punch (<1 mm diameter). The advantage of this technique is that linear harvest scars are avoided and instead the harvested areas heal by secondary intention with no visible scarring. The limitations of the technique are that it is blind; so, it risks inadvertent transection of the follicle, it is slow, and it is technically demanding. It may be best suited to treatment of smaller areas in patients who are keen to wear their hair short. It is, however, gaining popularity as powered surgeon/technician handpieces are becoming available and also an automated robot has been developed for this process.[1-4]

REFERENCES

1. Dua A, Dua K. Follicular unit extraction hair transplant. J Cutan Aesthet Surg 2010;3(2):76–81
2. Bicknell LM, Kash N, Kavouspour C, Rashid RM. Follicular unit extraction hair transplant harvest: a review of current recommendations and future considerations. Dermatol Online J 2014;20(3):doj_21754
3. Rose PT. Advances in hair restoration. Dermatol Clin 2018;36(1):57–62
4. Vogel JE, Jimenez F, Cole J, et al. Hair restoration surgery: the state of the art. Aesthet Surg J 2013;33(1):128–151

SURGICAL MANAGEMENT OF HAIR LOSS

12. You are undertaking hair transplantation for a patient with frontotemporal recessions. Which one of the following is true regarding this procedure?

C. Angles selected for hair placement should reflect the anatomic location.

To achieve a natural look after hair transplant surgery, the hairline must be re-created carefully and the grafts should be placed in different formations. The angle of orientation is critical to get right and this varies according to anatomic location. At the anterior hairline, angles of 45 to 60 degrees should be used for hair placement. Posterior to the hairline, the angles should be increased to 75 or 80 degrees. In general, the hairs should be placed to reflect the direction of hair growth if they are to look natural (**Fig. 108.3**).

The anterior hairline should start 7 to 9 cm above the glabella (not 5 cm) and the lateral extent should be in line with the lateral canthus. Grafts can be micro (containing one or two hairs) or mini (containing three to eight hairs). Ideally, a combination of these should be used. Grafts may be placed into small slits or holes. Placing smaller grafts in slits is a good approach, as this is simple and preserves adjacent hair follicles. However, slits do not allow larger grafts to spread out and may give a tufted or "dolls head" appearance. In this instance, it may be preferable to place these in holes instead of slits. In general, a mixture of micrografts and minigrafts should be used. For example, at the anterior hairline, finer grafts are placed first with larger grafts behind them. A combination of slits and holes is probably best to obtain a natural result.[1-5]

REFERENCES

1. Avram MR, Finney R, Rogers N. Hair transplantation controversies. Dermatol Surg 2017;43(Suppl 2):S158–S162
2. Bicknell LM, Kash N, Kavouspour C, Rashid RM. Follicular unit extraction hair transplant harvest: a review of current recommendations and future considerations. Dermatol Online J 2014;20(3):doj_21754

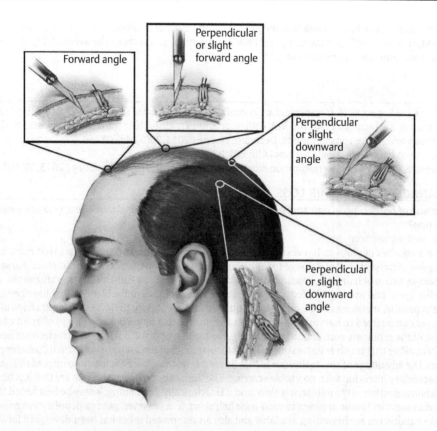

Fig. 108.3   Natural angles in hairline design.

3. Rose PT. Advances in hair restoration. Dermatol Clin 2018;36(1):57–62
4. Vogel JE, Jimenez F, Cole J, et al. Hair restoration surgery: the state of the art. Aesthet Surg J 2013;33(1):128–151
5. Bunagan MJ, Banka N, Shapiro J. Hair transplantation update: procedural techniques, innovations, and applications. Dermatol Clin 2013;31(1):141–153

POSTOPERATIVE CARE FOLLOWING HAIR TRANSPLANT

13. *Which one of the following should be part of the typical postoperative care following hair transplant?*

  C. Daily hair washing with a pouring technique.

  Following a hair transplant, it is important to wash the hair early, but this must be done with a pouring technique using a light mix of shampoo with warm water and no scalp massage, which may risk inadvertent removal of the grafts. Normal hair washing can be resumed after 2 weeks once the grafts have taken. The head is typically wrapped in a turban with a nonstick base layer such as Telfa. Hair transplant is performed as an outpatient procedure without an overnight stay, but it takes a significant length of time to perform; so, it is important to ensure that patients are well hydrated and fed before discharge. They should be accompanied home by a friend or family member. A follow-up appointment should be made for 1 week. There is no reason for patients to have a 2-week course of antibiotics after this surgery.[1–4]

REFERENCES

1. Vogel JE, Jimenez F, Cole J, et al. Hair restoration surgery: the state of the art. Aesthet Surg J 2013;33(1):128–151
2. Harris JA. Conventional FUE. In: Unger W, Shapiro R, Unger R, et al, eds. Hair Transplantation. 5th ed. Informa Healthcare; 2011:291–296
3. Bunagan MJ, Banka N, Shapiro J. Hair transplantation update: procedural techniques, innovations, and applications. Dermatol Clin 2013;31(1):141–153
4. Barrera A. Hair transplantation. The Art of Micrografting and Minigrafting. St Louis, MO: Quality Medical Publishing; 2002

109. Brow Lift

See *Essentials of Plastic Surgery*, third edition, pp. 1513–1524

ANATOMY OF THE FOREHEAD AND BROW

1. *Which one of the following statements is correct regarding brow anatomy?*
   A. The corrugator supercilii muscle has both oblique and vertical heads.
   B. The procerus is the sole muscle responsible for creation of oblique glabellar lines.
   C. The corrugator supercilii would be completely denervated by division of the temporal branch of the facial nerve.
   D. The frontalis is the main brow elevator and is encased within the galeal sheath.
   E. The orbicularis oculi is the main contributor to glabellar rhytids.

BROW PTOSIS

2. *Why does brow ptosis with aging tend to be most evident laterally?*
   A. Because the soft-tissue attachments are strongest medially
   B. Because the soft-tissue attachments are strongest laterally
   C. Because of a lack of frontalis function laterally
   D. Because the lateral brow contains a greater soft-tissue density
   E. It is normally just an illusion created by grooming of the brow

NONSURGICAL MANAGEMENT OF THE BROW

3. A patient attends clinic to consider brow and periorbital rejuvenation. He is most concerned about wrinkles to the brow that occur during animation. You discuss the merits of botulinum toxin therapy. *Which two muscles need to be specifically targeted to eliminate his transverse glabellar and forehead rhytids?*
   A. Frontalis and procerus
   B. Frontalis and corrugator supercilii
   C. Corrugator supercilii and procerus
   D. Orbicularis oculi and procerus
   E. Frontalis and depressor supercilii

SENSATION TO THE BROW

4. *Damage to which one of the following nerves during a brow-lift procedure is responsible for the patient having paresthesia to the central forehead?*
   A. Frontal branch
   B. Zygomaticotemporal
   C. Supraorbital (deep branch)
   D. Supraorbital (superficial branch)
   E. Supratrochlear

AVOIDING BLEEDING DURING AN ENDOSCOPIC BROW LIFT

5. The sentinel vein can be a source of bleeding during an endoscopic brow lift and should be visualized intraoperatively. *What anatomic landmark is particularly useful to guide its location?*
   A. Medial canthus
   B. Midbrow
   C. Glabella
   D. Lateral canthus
   E. Superior orbital ridge

AESTHETIC ASSESSMENT OF THE BROW

6. You assess a 43-year-old beautician who is considering surgical rejuvenation of the brow. When evaluating this woman, you notice she has very thin eyebrows that taper laterally and sit just above the supraorbital ridge. Her anterior hairline is on the vertical aspect of the forehead. *Which one of the following statements is correct?*
   A. Her eyebrows may be artificially lowered, confounding your assessment.
   B. A brow to hairline distance of 5 cm would indicate a low hairline.
   C. The highest point of her eyebrow should be at its midpoint in the frontal view.
   D. A high hairline is likely in this case, given the clinical description.
   E. The description of her eyebrow position is normal for a young woman.

CLINICAL ASSESSMENT OF THE BROW

7. *During assessment of the brow and periorbital region in a white patient, which one of the following vertical distances should normally be approximately 1.5 cm (measured in the midpupillary line during a forward gaze)?*
   A. Brow to the superior orbital rim
   B. Brow to the mid pupil
   C. Brow to the upper lash
   D. Brow to the supratarsal crease
   E. Brow to the lower lash

MANAGEMENT OF BROW RHYTIDS

8. A patient is concerned regarding deep transverse brow rhytids that are present at rest. *How would these best be treated?*
   A. Botulinum toxin injection
   B. Injection of hyaluronic acid filler
   C. Combined botulinum toxin and hyaluronic acid filler
   D. Combined botulinum toxin and laser resurfacing
   E. Surgical muscle weakening and soft-tissue redraping

OPEN CORONAL BROW LIFT

9. *When undertaking an open coronal approach for brow elevation, which one of the following should be avoided to minimize the appearance of a postoperative bald patch or visible scarring?*
   A. Placement of the incision a few centimeters behind the anterior hairline
   B. Beveling the incision at 45 degrees through the skin
   C. Meticulous hemostasis at the skin edges with electrocautery
   D. Closure of the galea with deep sutures combined with skin staples
   E. Avoiding excessive skin resection, particularly in the midline

TECHNIQUE SELECTION FOR BROW PTOSIS

10. You assess a frail 75-year-old man who underwent excision of a basal cell carcinoma from the left temple with a local flap technique 3 months earlier. Histologic analysis confirms the excision margins are complete. On examination, there is an obvious left-side brow ptosis and loss of transverse forehead rhytids. He is distressed by a degree of visual obstruction by the upper eyelid since the procedure. *Which one of the following is the next most appropriate step in management?*
   A. Observe for 6 months
   B. Plan for an endoscopic brow lift under general anesthetic
   C. Plan for a transblepharoplasty brow lift under local anesthetic and sedation
   D. Plan for an upper eyelid blepharoplasty under local anesthetic and sedation
   E. Plan for a direct brow lift under local anesthetic

ENDOSCOPIC BROW LIFTING

11. *Which one of the following is correct when performing an endoscopic brow lift?*
   A. Access should be achieved using just two paramedian incisions placed at the hairline.
   B. Central dissection should proceed in the subcutaneous plane.
   C. Lateral/temporal dissection should pass deep to the deep temporal fascia.
   D. Release of the periorbital septa and associated adhesions should be performed.
   E. Fixation should be achieved using screws rather than sutures or custom-designed products.

TYPES OF BROW LIFTING SURGERY

12. *Which one of the following procedures is best avoided in patients with a high hairline and high forehead?*
   A. Direct brow lift
   B. Coronal brow lift
   C. Endoscopic brow lift
   D. Temporal brow lift
   E. Transpalpebral brow lift

MECHANICS OF BROW ELEVATION SURGERY

13. *What does the elastic band principle refer to with respect to brow lift?*
    A. That brow ptosis will normally recur after a brow lift.
    B. That the soft tissues of the brow have elastic properties.
    C. That fixation in a brow lift should use flexible fixation devices.
    D. That the lift is best when the suspension point is close to the brow.
    E. That the lift is best when the suspension point is further from the brow.

POSTOPERATIVE COMPLICATIONS AFTER BROW LIFT

14. You assess a patient 6 months after performing an endoscopic brow-lift procedure. She has paresthesia at the scar within the hairline. *Which nerve is most likely affected?*
    A. Superficial branch of the supratrochlear nerve
    B. Deep branch of the supratrochlear nerve
    C. Superficial branch of the supraorbital nerve
    D. Deep branch of the supraorbital nerve
    E. Deep branch of the lesser occipital nerve

Answers

ANATOMY OF THE FOREHEAD AND BROW

1. *Which one of the following statements is correct regarding brow anatomy?*
   D. The frontalis is the main brow elevator and is encased within the galeal sheath.

   The frontalis originates at the galea aponeurosis and inserts into the supraorbital dermis and orbicularis oculi to act as the main brow elevator. The galea is an aponeurotic layer that connects the frontalis and the occipitalis muscles over the top of the scalp. It splits into two sheaths around the frontalis, with the deeper layer extending to the periosteum at the supraorbital rim. This attachment needs to be released during a brow lift.

   When closing scalp wounds, such as following an open brow technique, repair of the galeal layer can help reduce skin tension across the wound. It is also a useful layer in general plastic surgery, as it can be resected to provide deep clearance in skin tumor excision or used in the reconstruction of scalp defects as a local flap. In order to enable the frontalis to have mobility to elevate the brow, there is a loose areolar plane beneath the deeper galeal layer and the periosteum.

   The corrugator supercilii has two heads (oblique and transverse, not vertical), which are innervated by the zygomatic and temporal (frontal) branches of the facial nerve, respectively. Therefore, division of the temporal branch will only denervate part of the muscle. Procerus, corrugator, and depressor supercilii muscles all contribute to oblique glabellar lines. The orbicularis oculi muscle has three parts: pretarsal, preseptal, and orbital. The orbital muscle is responsible for forced eye closure and it has a medial and a lateral component. Although the medial portion can cause medial brow depression, it is not a particularly significant contributor to glabellar rhytids. The lateral portion may give rise to crow's feet lines, which are lateral orbital rhytids.[1-5]

REFERENCES

1. Nahai F, Saltz R, eds. Endoscopic Plastic Surgery. 2nd ed. St Louis, MO: Quality Medical Publishing; 2008
2. Mendelson B, Wong CH. Anatomy of the aging face. In: Neligan P, ed. Plastic Surgery. 3rd ed. London: Elsevier; 2013: 78–92
3. Abramo AC. Anatomy of the forehead muscles: the basis for the videoendoscopic approach in forehead rhytidoplasty. Plast Reconstr Surg 1995;95(7):1170–1177
4. Warren RJ. Forehead rejuvenation. In: Neligan P, ed. Plastic Surgery. 3rd ed. London: Elsevier; 2013:93–107
5. Janis JE, Ghavami A, Lemmon JA, Leedy JE, Guyuron B. Anatomy of the corrugator supercilii muscle: part I. Corrugator topography. Plast Reconstr Surg 2007;120(6):1647–1653

BROW PTOSIS

2. *Why does brow ptosis with aging tend to be most evident laterally?*
   C. Because of a lack of frontalis function laterally

   The frontalis muscle is the primary brow elevator, and the remaining muscles of the brow and periorbital region are brow depressors. These include the corrugator, the depressor supercilii, the procerus, and the orbicularis oculi. Therefore, the frontalis is working against both gravity and the brow depressor muscles described. With increasing age, patients frequently activate frontalis to a greater extent to compensate for progressive brow ptosis. This must be checked carefully when considering upper lid blepharoplasty and brow lift. Laterally, because there is no frontalis present, the downward pull of the other muscles, combined with aging soft-tissue ptosis causes the lateral brow to fall more than it does medially. It is not because of the soft tissue or deep attachments. The brow can be manipulated to give the illusion of being higher or lower medially or laterally with neurotoxins and grooming. For example, many female patients will groom the eyebrows to give a more lifted appearance to the lateral brow. Therefore, it would be unlikely that grooming would be causing the lateral brow to be lower.[1]

REFERENCE

1. Warren RJ. Forehead rejuvenation. In: Neligan P, ed. Plastic Surgery. 3rd ed. London: Elsevier; 2013:93–107

NONSURGICAL MANAGEMENT OF THE BROW

3. A patient attends clinic to consider brow and periorbital rejuvenation. He is most concerned about wrinkles to the brow that occur during animation. You discuss the merits of botulinum toxin therapy. *Which two muscles need to be specifically targeted to eliminate his transverse glabellar and forehead rhytids?*
   A. Frontalis and procerus

Neuromodulation of the brow is a simple and effective way to reduce the appearance of dynamic rhytids and also adjust brow position. It can also secondarily lead to improvement in static rhytids, although these often require additional treatment with fillers or skin resurfacing. The main muscle targets for brow and periorbital rejuvenation are the frontalis, orbicularis oculi, procerus, corrugator, and depressor supercilii.

The frontalis is the main brow elevator. Its fibers are vertically oriented so that contraction lifts the brow and results in transverse forehead rhytids. This muscle is targeted to reduce transverse forehead rhytids. Four to eight injections should be placed into the muscle at least 2 cm above the brow to reduce the risk of brow ptosis. Starting doses are between 10 and 30 units in total (Botox or Xeomin). Central injections of the forehead should be avoided, as they can result in a "quizzical" eyebrow appearance with elevation of the lateral brow and central depression.

The procerus muscle is a significant medial brow depressor and is responsible for causing transverse nasal and glabellar lines. This muscle is also targeted to reduce these rhytids. A central medial brow injection directly over procerus with 4–10 units of Botox or Xeomin is usually adequate. However, in most cases, this is combined with injections into the corrugator muscle as well. The corrugator supercilii has two heads, oblique and transverse, and is responsible for creating oblique and vertical glabellar rhytids. It is the transverse head that is predominantly responsible for the vertical lines apparent on frowning, as this passes from the superomedial orbital rim to attach into the dermis in the middle third of the eyebrow, thereby moving the brow medially. The corrugator can be palpated and often visualized when asking a patient to frown. Starting toxin injections involve using a total of 20 to 30 units of Botox or Xeomin placed just above the orbital rim at the medial third of the brow (**Fig. 109.1**).

The orbicularis oculi has three components: pretarsal, preseptal, and orbital. The orbital components are responsible for voluntary movements and cause tight closure of the eye and slight brow depression. The orbital component is subdivided into medial and lateral portions. The lateral portion is responsible for lateral orbital rhytids also known as crow's feet. These may also be treated with botulinum toxin therapy by injecting between 12 and 30 units total at points 1 cm lateral to the bony orbit. Injections must be above the zygomatic arch to avoid inadvertent paralysis of the zygomaticus muscle leading to lip or cheek ptosis (**Fig. 109.2**).[1–7]

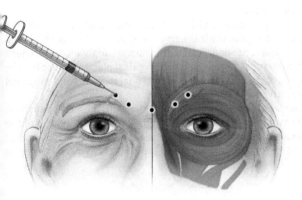

Fig. 109.1 Botulinum toxin injection points for glabellar complex and vertical forehead lines. (Adapted from Carruthers J, Fagien S, Matarasso SL; Botox Consensus Group. Consensus Recommendations on the use of botulinum toxin type A in facial aesthetics. Plast Reconstr Surg 114 (Suppl 6):S1–S22, 2004.)

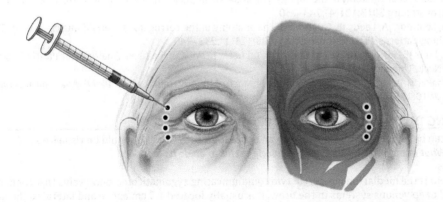

Fig. 109.2 Botulinum toxin injection points for crow's feet. (Adapted from Carruthers J, Fagien S, Matarasso SL; Botox Consensus Group. Consensus Recommendations on the use of botulinum toxin type A in facial aesthetics. Plast Reconstr Surg 114 (Suppl 6):S1–S22, 2004.)

REFERENCES

1. Sundaram H, Signorini M, Liew S, et al; Global Aesthetics Consensus Group. Global Aesthetics Consensus: botulinum toxin type A--evidence-based review, emerging concepts, and consensus recommendations for aesthetic use, including updates on complications. Plast Reconstr Surg 2016;137(3):518e–529e
2. Knize DM. An anatomically based study of the mechanism of eyebrow ptosis. Plast Reconstr Surg 1996;97(7):1321–1333
3. Nahai F. Clinical decision-making in brow lift. In: Nahai F, ed. The Art of Aesthetic Surgery: Principles and Techniques. 2nd ed. St Louis, MO: Quality Medical Publishing; 2011
4. de Maio M, Swift A, Signorini M, Fagien S; Aesthetic Leaders in Facial Aesthetics Consensus Committee. Facial assessment and injection guide for botulinum toxin and injectable hyaluronic acid fillers: focus on the upper face. Plast Reconstr Surg 2017;140(2):265e–276e
5. Carruthers J, Fagien S, Matarasso SL; Botox Consensus Group. Consensus recommendations on the use of botulinum toxin type a in facial aesthetics. Plast Reconstr Surg 2004;114(6, Suppl):1S–22S
6. Lorenc ZP, Kenkel JM, Fagien S, et al. Consensus panel's assessment and recommendations on the use of 3 botulinum toxin type A products in facial aesthetics. Aesthet Surg J 2013; 33(1, Suppl):35S–40S
7. Warren RJ. Forehead rejuvenation. In: Neligan P, ed. Plastic Surgery. 3rd ed. London: Elsevier; 2013:93–107

SENSATION TO THE BROW

4. *Damage to which one of the following nerves during a brow-lift procedure is responsible for the patient having paresthesia to the central forehead?*

E. Supratrochlear

There are a number of nerves, which are at risk during brow lift procedures and the risk is specific to the precise technique and approaches used. The supratrochlear nerve is a terminal branch of the ophthalmic division of the trigeminal nerve. It usually exits the orbit via the frontal notch and passes through or deep to the corrugator, exiting 15 mm superior to the orbital rim before piercing frontalis on its deep surface to supply the central forehead. This nerve is most at risk of damage during corrugator resection, but usually this is of little clinical significance, particularly if discussed with patients in advance.[1,2]

The supraorbital nerve is also a terminal branch of the ophthalmic division of the trigeminal nerve and exits the skull through the supraorbital foramen or notch lateral to supratrochlear nerve and divides into superficial and deep branches. The superficial branch pierces frontalis and runs superficial to the muscle supplying the forehead up to 2 cm beyond the anterior hairline. The deep branch runs laterally in the deep galeal plane and supplies the scalp beyond the hairline up to the vertex. Transection of the deep branch with coronal incisions and subgaleal dissection are believed to be responsible for postoperative scalp paresthesias.[3,4]

The frontal branch is a motor nerve arising from the facial nerve. It innervates the frontalis muscle and division of this nerve leads to brow ptosis. The zygomaticotemporal nerve is a branch of the maxillary division of the trigeminal nerve. It provides sensation to a small area of skin over the temple. It may be inadvertently damaged during an endoscopic brow lift while releasing the lateral orbital adhesions and is purposely avulsed in surgical treatment of migraines.[5]

REFERENCES

1. Moore KL, Dalley AF, eds. Clinically Oriented Anatomy. 4th ed. New York, NY: Lippincott, Williams, & Wilkins; 1999
2. Janis JE, Hatef DA, Hagan R, et al. Anatomy of the supratrochlear nerve: implications for the surgical treatment of migraine headaches. Plast Reconstr Surg 2013;131(4):743–750
3. Janis JE, Ghavami A, Lemmon JA, Leedy JE, Guyuron B. The anatomy of the corrugator supercilii muscle: part II. Supraorbital nerve branching patterns. Plast Reconstr Surg 2008;121(1):233–240
4. Khansa I, Barker JC, Janis JE. Sensory nerves of the head and neck. In: Watanabe K, ed. Anatomy for Plastic Surgery of the Face, Head and Neck. Thieme: 2016
5. Janis JE, Hatef DA, Thakar H, et al. The zygomaticotemporal branch of the trigeminal nerve: Part II. Anatomical variations. Plast Reconstr Surg 2010;126(2):435–442

AVOIDING BLEEDING DURING AN ENDOSCOPIC BROW LIFT

5. The sentinel vein can be a source of bleeding during an endoscopic brow lift and should be visualized intraoperatively. *What anatomic landmark is particularly useful to guide its location?*

D. Lateral canthus

The sentinel vein is the medial (and larger) of two communicating zygomaticotemporal veins that connect the superficial and deep venous systems in the brow. It is usually located 1.5 cm above and lateral to the lateral canthus. It is just lateral to the temporal crest and is itself a useful anatomic landmark, as it represents a key area for release of the periorbital septa and adhesions. It is also related to the frontal branch of the facial nerve, which passes a centimeter above the vein and is therefore a useful guide to avoid injury to this nerve branch. It is

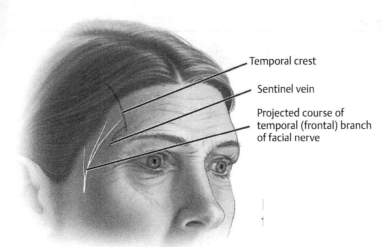

Temporal crest

Sentinel vein

Projected course of
temporal (frontal) branch
of facial nerve

Fig. 109.3   Sentinel vein and frontal branch of facial nerve in relation to the temporal crest. (From Nahai F, ed. The Art of Aesthetic Surgery: Principles and Techniques, 2nd ed. St Louis, MO: CRC Press, 2011.)

important to locate and preserve this vein during a brow lift to avoid bleeding that would obscure the operative view and may lead to a subsequent hematoma formation (**Fig. 109.3**).[1,2]

REFERENCES

1. Nahai F, ed. The Art of Aesthetic Surgery: Principles and Techniques. 2nd ed. St Louis, MO: Quality Medical Publishing; 2011

2. Trinei FA, Januszkiewicz J, Nahai F. The sentinel vein: an important reference point for surgery in the temporal region. Plast Reconstr Surg 1998;101(1):27–32

AESTHETIC ASSESSMENT OF THE BROW

6. You assess a 43-year-old beautician who is considering surgical rejuvenation of the brow. When evaluating this woman, you notice she has very thin eyebrows that taper laterally and sit just above the supraorbital ridge. Her anterior hairline is on the vertical aspect of the forehead. *Which one of the following statements is correct?*

E. The description of her eyebrow position is normal for a young woman.

When assessing a patient's brow during an aesthetic consultation, the brow position at rest and during activation should be assessed. The position of the hairline is also important to ascertain. Although the description of her eyebrow position is normal, women may have an artificially elevated brow position either from chemodenervation with neurotoxin treatment or from brow hair plucking. Either could be giving an appearance of a more elevated brow position. There is individual variation in female brow shape and position, but it should normally form a curve with the medial and lateral ends sitting at roughly the same vertical level. The arch should peak at the junction of the middle and lateral thirds. A high hairline in females is indicated either by a measured distance of greater than 5 cm from the brow to hairline or by an anterior hairline sited on the oblique part of the forehead. This is relevant to correctional surgery, particularly endoscopic brow lifting. This patient would be a fair candidate for an endoscopy-assisted brow lift given her hairline position. The difficulty with performing an endoscopic approach with a high hairline is achieving access to the supraorbital rim "around the corner" with relatively straight instrumentation and small access incisions.[1-5]

REFERENCES

1. Nahai F, ed. The Art of Aesthetic Surgery: Principles and Techniques. 2nd ed. St Louis, MO: Quality Medical Publishing; 2011

2. Byrd HS, Burt JD. Achieving aesthetic balance in the brow, eyelids, and midface. Plast Reconstr Surg 2002;110(3):926–933, discussion 934–939

3. Ellenbogen R. Transcoronal eyebrow lift with concomitant upper blepharoplasty. Plast Reconstr Surg 1983;71(4):490–499

4. McCord CD, Codner MA, eds. Eyelid and Periorbital Surgery. St Louis, MO: Quality Medical Publishing; 2008

5. Janis JE, Potter JK, Rohrich RJ. Brow lift techniques. In: Fahien S, ed. Putterman's Cosmetic Oculoplastic Surgery. 4th ed. Philadelphia, PA: Saunders Elsevier; 2008

CLINICAL ASSESSMENT OF THE BROW

7. *During assessment of the brow and periorbital region in a white patient, which one of the following vertical distances should normally be approximately 1.5 cm (measured in the midpupillary line during a forward gaze)?*

    D. Brow to the supratarsal crease

    The vertical distance from the brow to the supratarsal crease (where the levator muscle inserts into the dermis of the upper eyelid) in the midpupillary line is normally approximately 1.5 cm in a Caucasian patient. Other key measurements in the midpupillary line are as follows:

    Visible pretarsal upper lid skin: 3 to 6 mm

    Supratarsal crease to upper lash line: 8 to 10 mm

    Brow to the superior orbital rim: 10 mm

    Brow to the midpupil: 25 mm

    Brow to the anterior hairline: 5 to 6 cm

    Knowledge of these distances is clinically relevant when assessing patients for brow lift and eyelid rejuvenation surgery. Knowledge of the distance from the upper lash line to the supratarsal crease is important when planning incisions for upper lid blepharoplasty (**Fig. 109.4**).[1,2]

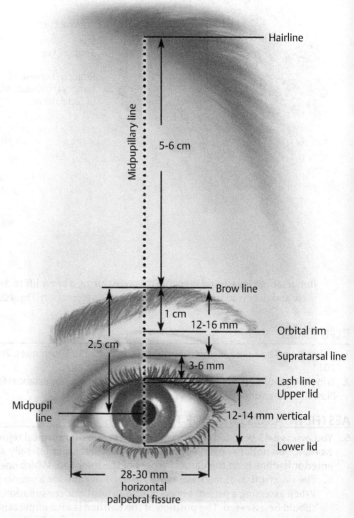

Fig. 109.4   Aesthetic measurements of the brow and periorbital region.

REFERENCES

1. Nahai F, ed. The Art of Aesthetic Surgery: Principles and Techniques. 2nd ed. St Louis, MO: Quality Medical Publishing; 2011
2. McCord CD Jr, Codner MA. Eyelid and Periorbital Surgery. St Louis, MO: Quality Medical Publishing; 2008

MANAGEMENT OF BROW RHYTIDS

8. A patient is concerned regarding deep transverse brow rhytids that are present at rest. *How would these best be treated?*

    E. Surgical muscle weakening and soft-tissue redraping

    Management of rhytids is an important part of brow and periorbital rejuvenation. Rhytids may be classified as static or dynamic and superficial and deep. Static rhytids are present at rest and are due to sustained muscle hyperactivity. They may be partially improved with surgical or chemical muscle weakening but, if deep, as in this case, they will require surgical redraping of the soft tissues. Superficial static rhytids may be improved with fillers such as hyaluronic acid, or resurfacing techniques such as laser or chemical peels.[1,2]

    Dynamic rhytids are present only during animation and are often amenable to botulinum toxin injections. They can also be improved more permanently with surgical weakening during brow-lift procedures. If considering this, it is prudent to trial chemical weakening first as this is temporary, and if the patient does not like the effects, there will be no long-term sequelae. This patient may also benefit from skin resurfacing with laser, chemical peels, and or skin care.

REFERENCES

1. Nahai F, ed. The Art of Aesthetic Surgery: Principles and Techniques. 2nd ed. St Louis, MO: Quality Medical Publishing; 2011
2. Guyuron B, Knize DM. Corrugator supercilii resection through blepharoplasty incision. Plast Reconstr Surg 2001;107(2):606–607

OPEN CORONAL BROW LIFT

9. *When undertaking an open coronal approach for brow elevation, which one of the following should be avoided to minimize the appearance of a postoperative bald patch or visible scarring?*

C. Meticulous hemostasis at the skin edges with electrocautery

Surgery to the scalp can result in hair loss around the incision site, which can be distressing for patients and signposts the fact that patients have undergone treatment. There are a number of techniques that may minimize visible scalp hair loss. It is important to minimize use of electrocautery on the skin edges, as this will damage hair follicles. Raney clips are small **U**-shaped clips that are temporarily placed at the skin edge to gently compress vessel ends and minimize intraoperative bleeding. They are commonly used in neurosurgery and may be useful for coronal approaches to brow lift. Minimizing tension during closure is also important, as excessive tension results in scar stretch and risk of wound dehiscence, each of which result in a more obvious scar with alopecia. For this reason, skin resection should be conservatively performed and the galea should be closed to reduce tension across the skin edges. Staples are useful for scalp closure, as they minimize tissue ischemia. Buried dermal sutures may strangulate the hair follicles and should generally be avoided in the hair-bearing scalp. Thoughtful placement of the scar is important to help camouflage it, although it has no direct effect on the area of hair loss. When performing a traditional coronal approach to the brow, the skin incision is placed at least 3 cm behind the hairline in most cases. If there is a low hairline, this is particularly useful as it can lift the hairline at the same time. (Approximately 1 mm of eyebrow elevation may be expected for every 1.5 mm anterior hairline retrodisplacement.) In patients with a high hairline, it may be preferable to use a hairline incision to reduce the vertical height of the forehead, at the expense of a more visibly located scar. Beveling the skin incision to either avoid follicle damage or encourage hair growth through the scar should help disguise a scar. Use of a zigzag incision can have similar benefits.[1,2]

REFERENCES

1. Ortiz Monasterio F. Aesthetic surgery of the facial skeleton: the forehead. Clin Plast Surg 1991;18(1):19–27
2. Nahai F. Clinical decision-making in brow lift. In: Nahai F, ed. The Art of Aesthetic Surgery: Principles and Techniques. 2nd ed. St Louis, MO: Quality Medical Publishing; 2011

TECHNIQUE SELECTION FOR BROW PTOSIS

10. You assess a frail 75-year-old man who underwent excision of a basal cell carcinoma from the left temple with a local flap technique 3 months earlier. Histologic analysis confirms the excision margins are complete. On examination, there is an obvious left-side brow ptosis and loss of transverse forehead rhytids. He is distressed by a degree of visual obstruction by the upper eyelid since the procedure. *Which one of the following is the next most appropriate step in management?*

E. Plan for a direct brow lift under local anesthetic

This patient has signs and symptoms of frontal nerve injury following his skin cancer excision. Because this is affecting his vision, more immediate surgical intervention is warranted. Given his age, previous scarring, and current symptoms, a direct brow lift would be the most suitable procedure for him. This technique has a reliable outcome, is quick and simple to perform, can be achieved under local anesthetic, and has minimal risk of complications. The incision can be placed just above the eyebrow such that the final scar is hidden at the junction of the eyebrow and adjacent skin, or it can be placed higher within one of the static residual brow rhytids. In this setting, the functional elements probably rate more highly with the patient anyway and this approach will give a good functional benefit.[1,2]

REFERENCES

1. Ortiz Monasterio F. Aesthetic surgery of the facial skeleton: the forehead. Clin Plast Surg 1991;18(1):19–27
2. Janis JE, Potter JK, Rohrich RJ. Brow lift techniques. In: Fahien S, ed. Putterman's Cosmetic Oculoplastic Surgery. 4th ed. Philadelphia, PA: Saunders Elsevier; 2008

ENDOSCOPIC BROW LIFTING

11. Which one of the following is correct when performing an endoscopic brow lift?

  D. Release of the periorbital septa and associated adhesions should be performed.

A key part of performing an endoscopic brow lift is to ensure that the periorbital septa and adhesions are adequately released. If this is not performed, then the brow cannot be fully elevated, as the soft-tissue attachments to the bone at the supraorbital rim will limit its upward movement.

Common approaches to endoscopic brow lift involve three incisions placed behind the anterior hairline. A small central incision is combined with two lateral incisions placed in the temple region. Some surgeons prefer to use two additional paramedian incisions as well. These allow access for dissection and the camera port to be placed. Once the midline incision has been made down through galea, dissection can proceed centrally, either subperiosteally or subgaleally. Both of these approaches provide relatively avascular planes that are easily elevated, but choice of plane will differ according to surgeon's preference. There remains debate as to which of the two planes will provide a more durable result.[1,2] The subcutaneous plane should be avoided, as it is slow and tedious to dissect and is the wrong plane to achieve either adequate soft-tissue release or muscle resection. Where a subperiosteal dissection is used, initial dissection can be performed blindly using a periosteal elevator to within a few centimeters of the supraorbital rim. The temporal dissection is performed just above the deep temporal fascia (not below), as this safely preserves the frontal branch of the facial nerve. The central and temporal planes of dissection are then joined up, and the endoscope can be used to complete the dissection to the supraorbital rim with direct visualization of the supraorbital and supratrochlear sensory nerves. If required, the glabellar musculature can then be weakened by incising the periosteum and performing partial muscle resection/denervation. There is no proven benefit of fixation with screws over other products and the fixation method of choice is often surgeon's preference.[3]

REFERENCES

1. Flowers RS, Caputy GG, Flowers SS. The biomechanics of brow and frontalis function and its effect on blepharoplasty. Clin Plast Surg 1993;20(2):255–268
2. Troilius C. A comparison between subgaleal and subperiosteal brow lifts. Plast Reconstr Surg 1999;104(4):1079–1090, discussion 1091–1092
3. Nahai F, ed. The Art of Aesthetic Surgery: Principles and Techniques. 2nd ed. St Louis, MO: Quality Medical Publishing; 2011

TYPES OF BROW LIFTING SURGERY

12. Which one of the following procedures is best avoided in patients with a high hairline and high forehead?

  C. Endoscopic brow lift

An endoscopic brow lift is a very useful technique but should be avoided in patients with both a high hairline and a high forehead, particularly when the hairline is situated on the oblique part of the forehead in the lateral view. This is because it is technically difficult to advance the scope around the curvature of the forehead and achieve adequate reach to safely release the supraorbital attachments. The best candidates for endoscopic approaches to brow lift are patients with short, flat foreheads with nonreceding, thick hairlines and normal skin. Poor candidates are those with a high convex forehead, a high receding hairline with thin hair, thick skin, and deep rhytids with true excess skin on the forehead and brow.[1]

A direct brow lift may be favored in patients who want or need a local anesthetic procedure and are willing to accept a visible scar on the brow. The coronal brow lift has fallen out of favor but can be useful for elevating a low hairline with a concealed scar. The temporal brow lift can be used as an isolated procedure to elevate the lateral brow with hidden scars or combined with an endoscopic approach. A transpalpebral approach is useful where a hidden scar is desired, blepharoplasty is being performed and a less invasive overall procedure is preferred. In summary, there is no single best option for brow lift surgery, hence the number of different and varied approaches that are practiced. The surgeon should be able to offer a range of options for patients such that treatment can be individualized for each case.[1-3]

REFERENCES

1. Nahai F, ed. The Art of Aesthetic Surgery: Principles and Techniques. 2nd ed. St Louis, MO: Quality Medical Publishing; 2011
2. Ramirez OM. Endoscopically assisted biplanar forehead lift. Plast Reconstr Surg 1995;96(2):323–333
3. McCord CD Jr, Codner MA. Eyelid and Periorbital Surgery. St Louis, MO: Quality Medical Publishing; 2008

MECHANICS OF BROW ELEVATION SURGERY

13. What does the elastic band principle refer to with respect to brow lift?

D. That the lift is best when the suspension point is close to the brow.

The elastic band principle has clinical relevance to brow-lift procedures, as it states that the further away the suspension point is from the brow, the lift will be less effective.[1]

Therefore, placement of the fixation point should, in theory, be kept as close to the brow as possible. For this reason, a transpalpebral approach may be ideal, as the fixation will be close to the brow. When performing an open coronal or endoscopic approach, fixation is usually just behind the hairline and is therefore quite distant from the brow. However, there is no consensus on the best site of fixation or best device for fixation in brow-lift procedures. Furthermore, some surgeons debate whether fixation is even required, given the rebalancing of soft tissues that occurs following the procedure. In practice, maintaining fixation as close to the brow as possible is probably beneficial, given the underlining biomechanical principles.

Recurrence of brow ptosis can occur after brow lift and patients must be made aware of this preoperatively. The soft tissues of the brow do have elastic properties, but this is not described by the elastic band principle. Rigid fixation devices (not flexible) are used in brow lifts such as Endotine devices, screws, bone anchor devices, and sutures with or without cortical drill holes.

REFERENCE

1. Flowers RS, Caputy GG, Flowers SS. The biomechanics of brow and frontalis function and its effect on blepharoplasty. Clin Plast Surg 1993;20(2):255–268

POSTOPERATIVE COMPLICATIONS AFTER BROW LIFT

14. You assess a patient 6 months after performing an endoscopic brow-lift procedure. She has paresthesia at the scar within the hairline. Which nerve is most likely affected?

D. Deep branch of the supraorbital nerve

The forehead and scalp are supplied by the bilateral supraorbital nerves. These nerves divide into superficial and deep branches. The superficial branch enters the frontalis muscle 2 to 3 cm above the rim and then supplies the forehead. The deep branch supplies the scalp posterior to the hairline and runs laterally up to 0.5 to 1.5 cm medial to the temporal crest. Transection of the deep branch can result in postoperative scalp paresthesias. There is no specific division of the supratrochlear nerve into superficial or deep branches and this supplies sensation to the central forehead. The lesser occipital nerve supplies the lower part of the ear and is too distant from the brow to be involved.[1,2]

REFERENCES

1. Nahai F, ed. The Art of Aesthetic Surgery: Principles and Techniques. 2nd ed. St Louis, MO: Quality Medical Publishing; 2011
2. Moore KL, Dalley AF, eds. Clinically Oriented Anatomy. 4th ed. New York, NY: Lippincott, Williams, & Wilkins; 1999

110. Blepharoplasty

See *Essentials of Plastic Surgery*, third edition, pp. 1525–1545

MUSCLES OF THE EYELID AND GLOBE

1. *Correctly identify the anatomic components of the eyelid and extraocular region on the diagram below (Fig. 110.1). Five of the nine options will be used.*

   Options:
   A. Levator palpebrae superioris
   B. Superior rectus muscle
   C. Inferior rectus muscle
   D. Superior oblique muscle
   E. Müller's muscle
   F. Inferior oblique muscle
   G. Pretarsal orbicularis oculi
   H. Preseptal orbicularis oculi
   I. Preorbital orbicularis oculi

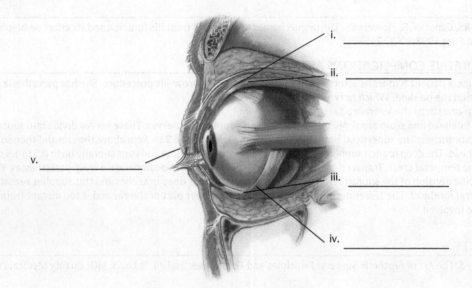

i. _____

ii. _____

iii. _____

iv. _____

v. _____

Fig. 110.1 Anatomy of the eyelid.

COMPONENTS OF THE EYELID

2. *Correctly identify the anatomic components of the eyelid and extraocular region on the diagram (Fig. 110-3). Six of the nine options will be used.*

   Options:
   A. Superior orbital rim
   B. Arcus marginalis
   C. Levator aponeurosis
   D. Retro-orbicularis oculi fat (ROOF)
   E. Suborbicularis oculi fat (SOOF)
   F. Conjunctiva
   G. Tarsal plate
   H. Capsulopalpebral fascia
   I. Postseptal fat pad

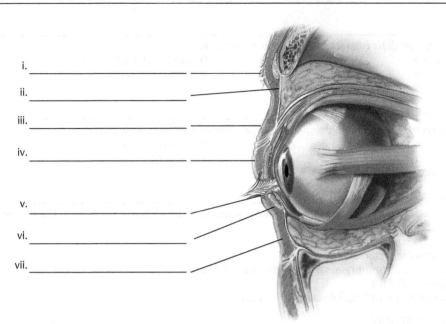

i. _____

ii. _____

iii. _____

iv. _____

v. _____

vi. _____

vii. _____

Fig. 110.3   Anatomy of the eyelid.

PERIORBITAL ANATOMY

3. *When asking a patient to keep their eyes tightly closed against resistance, which muscle is chiefly responsible?*
   A. Inferior rectus
   B. Superior rectus
   C. Pretarsal orbicularis
   D. Preseptal orbicularis
   E. Orbital orbicularis

SURGICAL ANATOMY OF THE EYELID

4. You are undertaking an upper lid blepharoplasty and have removed the skin and underlying orbicularis muscle as a single composite. *What is the most likely next layer of tissue?*
   A. Muscle
   B. Fascia
   C. Fat
   D. Fibrous tissue
   E. Mucosa

PERIOCULAR MUSCULATURE

5. *Which muscle of the eye has its vector of pull altered by Whitnall's ligament?*
   A. Superior oblique
   B. Inferior oblique
   C. Levator palpebrae superioris
   D. Orbicularis oculi
   E. Superior rectus

PERIOCULAR MUSCULATURE

6. *Which one of the following structures is responsible for causing subtle downward migration of the lower eyelid when asking a patient to look down at the floor?*
   A. Capsulopalpebral fascia
   B. Orbital septum
   C. Lockwood's ligament
   D. Orbicularis oculi
   E. Arcus marginalis

CLINICAL ASSESSMENT OF THE PERIORBITAL REGION

7. You see a patient in clinic before blepharoplasty surgery and note that there is a very subtle ptosis on the left side. On further examination, you also notice that the pupil is slightly smaller on this side. The patient is still able to elevate the eyelid. *Which muscle is primarily affected?*
   A. Superior oblique
   B. Superior rectus
   C. Levator palpebrae superioris
   D. Müller's muscle
   E. Pretarsal orbicularis

ORBITAL FAT

8. *How does orbital fat differ from fat in other anatomic locations?*
   A. Larger cell size
   B. Less saturated
   C. More lipoprotein lipase
   D. More metabolically active
   E. Less affected by diet

FAT COMPARTMENTS OF THE EYELIDS

9. *What separates the medial and middle postseptal fat compartments in the upper eyelid?*
   A. Lateral rectus muscle
   B. Inferior oblique muscle
   C. Superior rectus muscle
   D. Superior oblique muscle
   E. Lacrimal gland

AESTHETIC MEASUREMENTS OF THE EYELID

10. *When examining the normal eye during an aesthetic assessment, which one of the following measurements is most likely to be observed?*
    A. A palpebral fissure measuring 12×28 mm
    B. 12 mm of visible pretarsal skin
    C. A vertical lash line to supratarsal crease distance of 17 mm
    D. A negative canthal tilt
    E. A vertical brow-to-midpupil distance of 15 mm

ASIAN EYELID ANATOMY

11. Asians have different aesthetic eyelid features compared with white individuals. *Which one of the following is a common feature of the Asian eyelid?*
    A. A high supratarsal crease
    B. An increased tarsal height
    C. Descent of the preaponeurotic fat
    D. Absence of the eyelashes
    E. Dermal connection with the levator

DEFORMITIES OF THE EYELIDS

12. A 24-year-old woman presents with a history of recurrent bilateral swelling in the periorbital region. She has concerns regarding the appearance of her eyes, which have thin, puffy upper and lower eyelid skin. *Which one of the following is the most likely diagnosis?*
    A. Blepharoptosis
    B. Blepharochalasis
    C. Steatoblepharon
    D. Dermatochalasis
    E. Pseudoblepharoptosis

PREOPERATIVE PLANNING IN EYELID SURGERY

13. *Which one of the following preoperative test findings suggests a high risk of developing scleral show and ectropion following blepharoplasty?*
    A. A negative Bell's phenomenon
    B. A negative vector globe position
    C. A positive Schirmer's test
    D. A positive brow compensation test
    E. A positive vector globe position

TECHNIQUE SELECTION IN EYELID SURGERY

14. You are assessing a patient's upper eyelid during a cosmetic consultation and note a lateral fullness to the lid. *What is the most likely procedure to benefit this condition?*
    A. Fat transfer
    B. Excision of ROOF
    C. Excision of post septal fat
    D. Septal redraping
    E. Lacrimal glandulopexy

DECISION-MAKING IN BLEPHAROPLASTY

15. You see a 50-year-old woman who is eager to proceed with upper and lower eyelid rejuvenation surgery. She is otherwise healthy and states she has not undergone any recent surgery. You make a plan with her for upper and lower blepharoplasty surgery in 1 month. At the end of the consultation, you are finalizing the date, and she mentions that this will fit nicely with her planned corrective laser eye surgery and time off from work. *How would this statement alter your management plan?*
    A. Cancel the surgery
    B. Proceed with surgery as planned
    C. Postpone the surgery for 1 year after the laser correction
    D. Postpone the surgery for 6 weeks after the laser correction
    E. Assess her status in the office once her laser treatment is complete

SKIN MARKING FOR UPPER BLEPHAROPLASTY SURGERY

16. *When marking a patient for upper eyelid blepharoplasty, which one of the following is true?*
    A. The upper line should be performed first and placed 15 mm below the brow.
    B. The lower line should be marked with the eyelids open and placed 5 mm above the lash line.
    C. The skin resection pattern should be a symmetrical ellipse.
    D. The skin markings should not pass medially or laterally beyond the canthi.
    E. The markings should be made with the patient upright with eyes closed then open.

TECHNIQUES FOR EYELID CORRECTION

17. You see a 66-year-old man with prominent lower eyelid bags. He has an excess of skin, fat, and muscle with improvement of his festoon on forcible eye closure (positive squinch test). *Which one of the following procedures is most likely to address his eyelid concerns?*
    A. Lower eyelid pinch blepharoplasty
    B. Transconjunctival lower eyelid blepharoplasty with fat and muscle resection
    C. Subciliary lower eyelid blepharoplasty with skin-only resection
    D. Subciliary lower eyelid blepharoplasty with skin and muscle resection
    E. Subciliary lower eyelid blepharoplasty with skin, fat, and muscle resection and septal reset

TECHNIQUES FOR EYELID CORRECTION

18. You see a 50-year-old woman with marked unilateral ectropion, a positive snap test, mild scleral show, 5 mm of anterior lid distraction, but satisfactory skin volume following a previous lower eyelid blepharoplasty. *Which one of the following procedures is most likely to address her eyelid problems?*
    A. Kuhnt-Szymanowski procedure
    B. Lateral canthoplasty with tarsal strip
    C. Loeb procedure
    D. Lateral canthopexy
    E. Lateral canthoplasty

SURGERY FOR THE ASIAN EYELID

19. A 22-year-old Asian model attends clinic keen to have surgery on her eyelids to have a "more-white" appearance. *Which one of the following adjuncts to blepharoplasty would be most beneficial for her to help achieve this?*
    A. Tarsal fixation
    B. Tarsal shortening
    C. Lid tightening
    D. Fat grafting
    E. Septal reset

EARLY COMPLICATIONS AFTER BLEPHAROPLASTY

20. A 59-year-old patient undergoes upper and lower blepharoplasties with postseptal fat removal and is initially well on postoperative rounds. An hour later you are called to see the patient, who has described decreased clarity of vision on the left side with increasing eye pain. On examination, there is mild left-side proptosis and ecchymosis with reduced eye movement. The direct pupillary light response is diminished, but the consensual reflex is maintained. *Which one of the following actions should you perform first?*
    A. Lie the patient flat
    B. Give oral mannitol
    C. Apply topical acetazolamide
    D. Remove the sutures
    E. Perform medial cantholysis

Answers

MUSCLES OF THE EYELID AND GLOBE

1. *Correctly identify the anatomic components of the eyelid and extraocular region on the diagram below (Fig. 110.1). Five of the nine options will be used.*
   Options:
   Answer is given in Fig. 110.2.

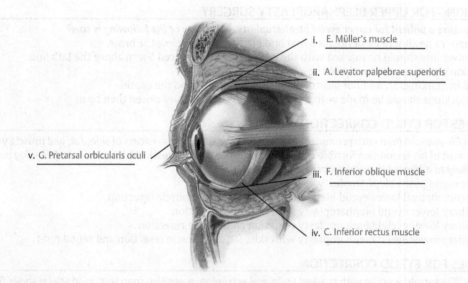

i. E. Müller's muscle

ii. A. Levator palpebrae superioris

v. G. Pretarsal orbicularis oculi

iii. F. Inferior oblique muscle

iv. C. Inferior rectus muscle

Fig. 110.2   Anatomy of the eyelid.

REFERENCES

1. Codner MA, Burke RM. Blepharoplasty. In: Chung KC, Gosain AK, Gurtner GC, Mehrara BJ, Rubin JP, Spear SL, eds. Grabb and Smith's Plastic Surgery. 7th ed. Philadelphia, PA: Wolters Kluwer; 2019
2. Carraway JH. Surgical anatomy of the eyelids. Clin Plast Surg 1987;14(4):693–701
3. Furnas DW. The orbicularis oculi muscle. Management in blepharoplasty. Clin Plast Surg 1981;8(4):687–715
4. Muzaffar AR, Mendelson BC, Adams WP Jr. Surgical anatomy of the ligamentous attachments of the lower lid and lateral canthus. Plast Reconstr Surg 2002;110(3):873–884, discussion 897–911
5. Nahai F, ed. The Art of Aesthetic Surgery: Principles and Techniques. 2nd ed. St Louis, MO: Quality Medical Publishing; 2011

COMPONENTS OF THE EYELID

2. *Correctly identify the anatomic components of the eyelid and extraocular region on the diagram (Fig. 110.3). Six of the nine options will be used.*
   Answer is in Fig. 110.4.

i. D. ROOF

ii. I. postseptal fat pad

iii. C. Levator aponeurosis

iv. G. Tarsal plate

v. G. Tarsal plate

vi. H. Capsulopalpebral fascia

vii. B. Arcus marginalis

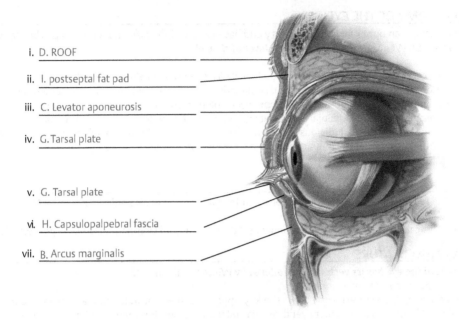

Fig. 110.4 Anatomy of the eyelid.

REFERENCES

1. Codner MA, Burke RM. Blepharoplasty. In: Chung KC, Gosain AK, Gurtner GC, Mehrara BJ, Rubin JP, Spear SL, eds. Grabb and Smith's Plastic Surgery. 7th ed. Philadelphia, PA: Wolters Kluwer; 2019
2. Carraway JH. Surgical anatomy of the eyelids. Clin Plast Surg 1987;14(4):693–701
3. Furnas DW. The orbicularis oculi muscle. Management in blepharoplasty. Clin Plast Surg 1981;8(4):687–715
4. Muzaffar AR, Mendelson BC, Adams WP Jr. Surgical anatomy of the ligamentous attachments of the lower lid and lateral canthus. Plast Reconstr Surg 2002;110(3):873–884, discussion 897–911
5. Nahai F, ed. The Art of Aesthetic Surgery: Principles and Techniques. 2nd ed. St Louis, MO: Quality Medical Publishing; 2011

PERIORBITAL ANATOMY

3. When asking a patient to keep their eyes tightly closed against resistance, which muscle is chiefly responsible?

E. Orbital orbicularis

The orbicularis oculi is a sphincter muscle surrounding the eye aperture. It has three portions: orbital, preseptal, and pretarsal which relate to the underlying structures, respectively. The functions of each are different. For example, the orbital part is under voluntary control and causes tight closure of the eye and medial brow depression. It is the outermost part and lies superficial to the corrugators and procerus. It is innervated by the frontal and zygomatic branches of the facial nerve (CN VII). The preseptal part is involved in both voluntary and involuntary actions including blinking. The pretarsal part is involuntary and also assists with blinking. Both parts are primarily innervated by the zygomatic branch of the facial nerve. The superior and inferior recti are both extraocular muscles involved in the movement of the globe, causing elevation and depression, respectively. They are innervated by the oculomotor nerve (CN III) and work in conjunction with the other extraocular muscles to coordinate eye movement.[1,2]

REFERENCES

1. Furnas DW. The orbicularis oculi muscle. Management in blepharoplasty. Clin Plast Surg 1981;8(4):687–715
2. Moore KL, Dalley AF, eds. Clinically Oriented Anatomy. 4th ed. New York, NY: Lippincott Williams & Wilkins; 1999

SURGICAL ANATOMY OF THE EYELID

4. You are undertaking an upper lid blepharoplasty and have removed the skin and underlying orbicularis muscle as a single composite. *What is the most likely next layer of tissue?*

   C. Fat

   The eyelid is composed of anterior and posterior lamella. The anterior lamella contains the skin and orbicularis oculi. The posterior lamella contains the tarsus and conjunctiva. The septum between them is sometimes referred to as the middle lamella. When undertaking an upper eyelid blepharoplasty, the next layer after orbicularis will be fat and this is termed the retro-orbicularis oculi fat layer or ROOF. It is clinically relevant, as it may be a cause of upper eyelid hooding and puffiness. Judicious reduction of this fat may be indicated to reduce fullness. This must not be confused with the preseptal fat compartments, which are accessed by incising the septum beneath the ROOF layer.[1,2]

REFERENCES

1. Nahai F, ed. The Art of Aesthetic Surgery: Principles and Techniques. 2nd ed. St Louis, MO: Quality Medical Publishing; 2011

2. Nowinski TS. Clinical surgical anatomy of the upper eyelid. Trans Pa Acad Ophthalmol Otolaryngol 1990;42:959–963

PERIOCULAR MUSCULATURE

5. *Which muscle of the eye has its vector of pull altered by Whitnall's ligament?*

   C. Levator palpebrae superioris

   The levator palpebrae superioris (LPS) is the key upper eyelid elevator. It originates from the lesser wing of sphenoid and inserts into the upper eyelid dermis and upper tarsus. It is innervated by the oculomotor nerve CN III. The natural vector of pull of this muscle would be posterior, given the attachments. Whitnall's ligament is a fascial condensation that translates this posterior vector into a superior vector. This allows LPS to provide 10 to 15 mm of upper eyelid excursion. The superior and inferior oblique muscles are extraocular muscles involved in movement of the globe assisting with abduction and adduction, respectively. The superior rectus is one of the other extraocular muscles that causes elevation of the globe. Orbicularis oculi is a sphincter muscle located beneath the skin of the periorbital area that serves to close the eye and assists with the lacrimal gland system function, thereby having a protective role for the globe.[1–3]

REFERENCES

1. Nahai F, ed. The Art of Aesthetic Surgery: Principles and Techniques. 2nd ed. St Louis, MO: Quality Medical Publishing; 2011

2. Collin JR, Beard C, Wood I. Experimental and clinical data on the insertion of the levator palpebrae superioris muscle. Am J Ophthalmol 1978;85(6):792–801

3. Kakizaki H, Takahashi Y, Nakano T, Ikeda H, Selva D, Leibovitch I. Whitnall ligament anatomy revisited. Clin Exp Ophthalmol 2011;39(2):152–155

PERIOCULAR MUSCULATURE

6. *Which one of the following structures is responsible for causing subtle downward migration of the lower eyelid when asking a patient to look down at the floor?*

   A. Capsulopalpebral fascia

   The capsulopalpebral fascia is the lower eyelid equivalent of the levator muscle. It originates from the inferior oblique muscle fascia and inserts on the septum below the tarsus. In contrast to the levator muscle, it has only a subtle action on the lower eyelid, resulting in a couple of millimeters of migration only (**Fig. 110.5**). Lockwood's ligament is a hammock-like structure that supports the globe; it is part of the tarsoligamentous complex shown in **Fig. 110.5**.

   The tarsoligamentous complex is a connective tissue framework supporting the eyelids and globe. It also includes the upper and lower tarsal plates and the medial and lateral canthal ligament complexes. The orbital septum is an extension of orbital periosteum that extends from the orbital rim to the eyelid retractors. The *arcus marginalis* is the fibrous attachment of the eyelid to the inferior orbital rim and represents the origin of the septum from the periosteum. It is released during some lower eyelid blepharoplasty techniques, but it does not cause downward migration of the eyelid.[1–3]

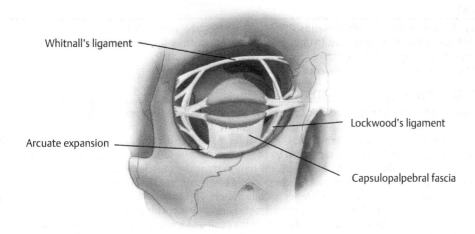

Whitnall's ligament

Lockwood's ligament

Arcuate expansion

Capsulopalpebral fascia

Fig. 110.5 The capsulopalpebral fascia is shown as it originates from the inferior fascia and inserts on the inferior portion of the tarsus and orbital septum.

REFERENCES

1. Codner MA, Burke RM. Blepharoplasty. In: Chung KC, Gosain AK, Gurtner GC, Mehrara BJ, Rubin JP, Spear SL, eds. Grabb and Smith's Plastic Surgery. 7th ed. Philadelphia, PA: Wolters Kluwer; 2019
2. Furnas DW. The orbicularis oculi muscle. Management in blepharoplasty. Clin Plast Surg 1981;8(4):687–715
3. Hamra ST. The role of the septal reset in creating a youthful eyelid-cheek complex in facial rejuvenation. Plast Reconstr Surg 2004;113(7):2124–2141, discussion 2142–2144

CLINICAL ASSESSMENT OF THE PERIORBITAL REGION

7. You see a patient in clinic before blepharoplasty surgery and note that there is a very subtle ptosis on the left side. On further examination, you also notice that the pupil is slightly smaller on this side. The patient is still able to elevate the eyelid. *Which muscle is primarily affected?*
   D. Müller's muscle
   Müller's muscle is a component of the upper eyelid. It is a small muscle responsible for 2 to 3 mm of eyelid elevation. It originates from the levator palpebrae superioris and is essentially the deep continuation of this muscle where it inserts on the superior edge of the tarsus. It has sympathetic innervation and, when denervated, results in a subtle ptosis on the affected side.[1] This clinical appearance is classically seen as a triad of features due to loss of sympathetic function known as Horner's syndrome. This includes upper eyelid ptosis, meiosis (pupillary constriction), and anhidrosis (loss of sweating on the affected side). Causes include tumor compression of the nerves, cerebrovascular injury, and spinal cord injury.[2]

REFERENCES

1. Esperidião-Antonio V, Conceição-Silva F, De-Ary-Pires B, Pires-Neto MA, de Ary-Pires R. The human superior tarsal muscle (Müller's muscle): a morphological classification with surgical correlations. Anat Sci Int 2010;85(1):1–7
2. Martin TJ. Horner syndrome: a clinical review. ACS Chem Neurosci 2018;9(2):177–186

ORBITAL FAT

8. *How does orbital fat differ from fat in other anatomic locations?*
   E. Less affected by diet
   Orbital fat is physiologically different from normal body fat and is minimally affected by diet. In addition, the fat cells are smaller, the fat is more saturated, and it is less metabolically active and has less lipoprotein lipase. There are also subtle differences in fat type within the orbit; for example, the medial compartment fat of the upper eyelid is more vascular than the others and has more pallor, smaller lobules, and more fibrous tissue. Fat content of the periocular region is important, as it affects the appearance of the eyes. The Eisler fat pad is a small pocket of fat above the lateral canthus, which is a good landmark for canthoplasty and canthopexy procedures.[1–3]

REFERENCES

1. Carraway JH. Surgical anatomy of the eyelids. Clin Plast Surg 1987;14(4):693–701
2. Codner MA, Burke RM. Blepharoplasty. In Chung KC, Gosain AK, Gurtner GC, Mehrara BJ, Rubin JP, Spear SL, eds. Grabb and Smith's Plastic Surgery. 7th ed. Philadelphia, PA: Wolters Kluwer; 2019
3. Chen WP. Oculoplastic Surgery. The Essentials. New York, NY: Thieme; 2001

FAT COMPARTMENTS OF THE EYELIDS

9. *What separates the medial and middle postseptal fat compartments in the upper eyelid?*

   D. Superior oblique muscle

   The upper eyelid has two postseptal fat compartments: middle and medial (the lacrimal gland occupies the lateral compartment. These are separated by the trochlea of the superior rectus muscle which acts to abduct, depress, and internally rotate the globe. It is the only extraocular muscle to be innervated by the fourth cranial nerve (trochlear nerve). In contrast, the lower eyelid has three fat compartments, and the lateral and central compartments are separated by the inferior oblique muscle. This abducts and elevates the globe and is innervated by the oculomotor nerve CN III. The fat compartments are relevant to blepharoplasty, as they can be manipulated during the procedure. In some cases, the fat within the compartments can cause excessive bulkiness to the eyelids and is therefore removed or cauterized during blepharoplasty. In the lower eyelid, redraping of the fat may also be undertaken to smooth off the eyelid cheek junction.[1-3]

REFERENCES

1. Carraway JH. Surgical anatomy of the eyelids. Clin Plast Surg 1987;14(4):693–701
2. Chen WP. Oculoplastic Surgery. The Essentials. New York, NY: Thieme; 2001
3. Sand JP, Zhu BZ, Desai SC. Surgical anatomy of the eyelids. Facial Plast Surg Clin North Am 2016;24(2):89–95

AESTHETIC MEASUREMENTS OF THE EYELID

10. *When examining the normal eye during an aesthetic assessment, which one of the following measurements is most likely to be observed?*

    A. A palpebral fissure measuring 12 × 28 mm

    There is individual variation in the measurements of the eyelids and brow. However, in most individuals, there are some standard measurements usually quoted during forward gaze[1]

    • Palpebral fissure: 12 to 14 mm vertically, 28 to 30 mm horizontally
    • Visible pretarsal skin: 3 to 6 mm
    • Lash line to supratarsal crease: 8 to 10 mm
    • Lateral canthus: 1 to 2 mm above medial canthus (i.e., positive canthal tilt)
    • In the midpupillary line:
    Anterior hairline to brow: 5 to 6 cm
    Brow to orbital rim: 1 cm
    Brow to supratarsal crease: 12 to 16 mm
    Brow to midpupil: 2.5 cm[1-5]

REFERENCES

1. Jelks GW, Jelks EB. Preoperative evaluation of the blepharoplasty patient. Bypassing the pitfalls. Clin Plast Surg 1993;20(2):213–223, discussion 224
2. Codner MA, Kikkawa DO, Korn BS, Pacella SJ. Blepharoplasty and brow lift. Plast Reconstr Surg 2010;126(1):1e–17e
3. Flowers RS, DuVal C. Blepharoplasty and periorbital aesthetic surgery. In: Aston SJ, Beasley RW, Thorne HM, et al, eds. Grabb and Smith's Plastic Surgery. 6th ed. Philadelphia, PA: Lippincott Williams & Wilkins; 2007
4. Guyuron B. Blepharoplasty and ancillary procedures. In: Achauer BH, Eriksson E, Guyuron B, et al, eds. Plastic Surgery: Indications, Operations, and Outcomes. St Louis, MO: Mosby-Year Book; 2000
5. Nahai F. The Art of Aesthetic Surgery: Principles and Techniques. 2nd ed. St Louis, MO: Quality Medical Publishing; 2011

ASIAN EYELID ANATOMY

11. Asians have different aesthetic eyelid features compared with white individuals. *Which one of the following is a common feature of the Asian eyelid?*

    C. Descent of the preaponeurotic fat

    The Asian eyelid is distinctly different from other races. The key differences are descent of the preaponeurotic fat and absence of the supratarsal fold (or short supratarsal crease). This gives the upper eyelid a fuller and less well-defined appearance. In addition, the tarsus is also shorter (**Fig. 110.6**).[1]

Absence of the eyelashes is termed *madarosis*. It is associated with multiple conditions ranging from skin conditions such as eczema, through autoimmune diseases such as lupus and scleroderma, to malignancies such as sebaceous gland and squamous cell carcinomas. It is not specifically related to a particular racial group.[2]

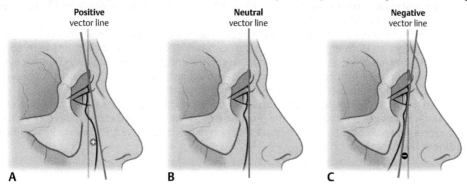

| Positive | Neutral | Negative |
| vector line | vector line | vector line |

A   **B**   **C**

Fig. 110.6 *A–C* On sagittal view, a line between the most anterior projection of the globe and the malar eminence. A positive vector exists when the most anterior projection of the malar eminence is anterior to the most anterior projection of the globe.

REFERENCES

1. Lee CK, Ahn ST, Kim N. Asian upper lid blepharoplasty surgery. Clin Plast Surg 2013;40(1):167–178
2. Khong JJ, Casson RJ, Huilgol SC, Selva D. Madarosis. Surv Ophthalmol 2006;51(6):550–560

DEFORMITIES OF THE EYELIDS

12. A 24-year-old woman presents with a history of recurrent bilateral swelling in the periorbital region. She has concerns regarding the appearance of her eyes, which have thin, puffy upper and lower eyelid skin. *Which one of the following is the most likely diagnosis?*

    B. Blepharochalasis

    Blepharochalasis is a condition with thin, excessive upper and lower eyelid skin caused by repeated bouts of painless edema. It most often occurs before the age of 20 years and is refractory to antihistamines and steroids.[1] Dermatochalasis refers to an excess of upper eyelid skin and is a common indication for upper eyelid blepharoplasty. Steatoblepharon is a condition where fat protrudes through a lax septum. Again, this can be an indication for blepharoplasty. Blepharoptosis is drooping of the upper eyelid that may be caused by muscle weakness, nerve injury, or traumatic disruption of the levator mechanism. This condition may be an indication for specialized lid repair, depending on cause and its degree of resulting dysfunction.[2] Pseudoblepharoptosis is an appearance of ptosis with a normal lid position, commonly due to a ptotic brow and excess brow skin. Brow lift may be indicated in such cases.

REFERENCES

1. Collin JR. Blepharochalasis. A review of 30 cases. Ophthal Plast Reconstr Surg 1991;7(3):153–157
2. Ahmad SM, Della Rocca RC. Blepharoptosis: evaluation, techniques, and complications. Facial Plast Surg 2007;23(3):203–215

PREOPERATIVE PLANNING IN EYELID SURGERY

13. *Which one of the following preoperative test findings suggests a high risk of developing scleral show and ectropion following blepharoplasty?*

    B. A negative vector globe position

    Understanding the concept of positive and negative vectors in blepharoplasty is critical in decision-making for surgery. This term refers to the relationship of the lower eyelid to the orbital rim, as seen on lateral view. It considers the anterior projection of the globe compared with the most anteriorly projecting portion of the lateral orbital rim.

    A **prominent** eye is described as having a *negative* vector, where the anterior portion of the globe is anterior to the orbital rim. In this case, a lower eyelid blepharoplasty risks development of downward "clothes lining" of the lower eyelid below the inferior limbus (i.e., the lower lid becomes too tight and slides under the globe, leading to a low eyelid with scleral show and ectropion).

    A **deep-set** eye has a *positive* vector, and in mild cases this does not represent a problem for a standard lower lid blepharoplasty, because tightening the lower lid will tend to act as a snug hammock for the globe. In more severe cases, patients will need lower and deeper lateral canthal anchoring, however, because a standard canthal position would cause upward "clothes lining" of the lower lid with narrowing of the eye fissure and a reduction in the size of the lateral scleral angle.[1]

Eye prominence and vector assessment can be formally measured using a Hertel exophthalmometer. With this tool, a normal globe prominence should be 16 to 18 mm. A prominent eye would be 19 mm or more, and a deep-set eye would be 15 mm or less.[1]

The Bell's phenomenon is a natural protective reflex and refers to upward movement of the globe during eye closure. Where this is absent the patient is at increased risk of dry-eye symptoms with postoperative lagophthalmos. Schirmer's test assesses the lacrimal function and, if positive, indicates that dry eye is present preoperatively. It can be performed with or without local anesthetic depending on whether reflex secretion is to be assessed or not. Blepharoplasty should be avoided in these patients.

It is vital to test for compensated brow ptosis before blepharoplasty, as this needs to be addressed before blepharoplasty, otherwise it is likely that the problem will not be corrected and may even be exacerbated. In addition, excess skin may be removed, and once brow correction is achieved, there may be insufficient eyelid skin leading to lagophthalmos.[1-3]

REFERENCES

1. Codner MA, Mejia JD. Lower eyelid blepharoplasty. In: Nahai F, ed. The Art of Aesthetic Surgery: Principles and Techniques. 2nd ed. St Louis, MO: Quality Medical Publishing; 2011
2. Lyon DB. Upper blepharoplasty and brow lift: state of the art. Mo Med 2010;107(6):383–390
3. Rajabi MT, Makateb A, Hassanpoor N, et al. Determinative factors in surgical planning of eyebrow cosmetic and reconstructive surgery. Clin Ophthalmol 2017;11:1333–1336

TECHNIQUE SELECTION IN EYELID SURGERY

14. You are assessing a patient's upper eyelid during a cosmetic consultation and note a lateral fullness to the lid. *What is the most likely procedure to benefit this condition?*

   E. Lacrimal glandulopexy

   Lateral upper-lid fullness is most likely caused by ptosis of the lacrimal gland. The upper eyelid has only two (central and medial) postseptal fat pads, and the lacrimal gland fills the lateral aspect. Awareness of the location of the lacrimal gland is vital when performing eyelid surgery, since damage to this structure can lead to a dry-eye condition. Although not commonly required, lacrimal glandulopexy is preferable to resection of some of the gland from a functional standpoint. Caution should always be taken when considering removing anything other than skin and orbicularis from the upper eyelid. For example, postseptal fat removal from the upper eyelid can lead to a sunken, aged appearance that can be difficult to later correct.[1,2]

   Conversely, if fullness is in the lower eyelids, then careful removal or cautery of some postseptal fat may be indicated to decrease fullness, although again this should be done with caution. Fat transfer is not commonly performed in the eyelids, though it may be used to improve a tear-trough deformity at the eyelid–cheek junction. Septal redraping is another lower lid technique that may be useful to improve the tear-trough deformity. This releases the tight band created by the septum as it joins the maxilla and allows the fat to be used to soften the interface between the two facial zones—eyelid and cheek.[3,4]

REFERENCES

1. Friedhofer H, Orel M, Saito FL, Alves HR, Ferreira MC. Lacrimal gland prolapse: management during aesthetic blepharoplasty: review of the literature and case reports. Aesthetic Plast Surg 2009;33(4):647–653
2. Yuksel D, Yakin M, Kosker M, Simsek S. The treatment of lacrimal gland prolapse in blepharoplasty by repositioning the glands. Semin Ophthalmol 2013;28(4):230–232
3. Hamra ST. The role of the septal reset in creating a youthful eyelid-cheek complex in facial rejuvenation. Plast Reconstr Surg 2004;113(7):2124–2141, discussion 2142–2144
4. Barton FE Jr, Ha R, Awada M. Fat extrusion and septal reset in patients with the tear trough triad: a critical appraisal. Plast Reconstr Surg 2004;113(7):2115–2121, discussion 2122–2123

DECISION-MAKING IN BLEPHAROPLASTY

15. You see a 50-year-old woman who is eager to proceed with upper and lower eyelid rejuvenation surgery. She is otherwise healthy and states she has not undergone any recent surgery. You make a plan with her for upper and lower blepharoplasty surgery in 1 month. At the end of the consultation, you are finalizing the date, and she mentions that this will fit nicely with her planned corrective laser eye surgery and time off from work. *How would this statement alter your management plan?*

   E. Assess her status in the office once her laser treatment is complete

This patient will be at increased risk of developing dry-eye syndrome following her laser eye surgery. Although there are no strict rules or guidelines, it would be most sensible to defer eyelid correction surgery until after the laser surgery is complete; 6 months is generally thought to be adequate. Given the situation, it would be most appropriate to assess this woman again a few months after her laser eye surgery to review and discuss her options. The timing of surgery can then be revisited.

It is not uncommon for patients to request their surgery at times to suit logistics of life in terms of their family, work, and other health commitments. It does make sense to be efficient with treatment timings, but this case does highlight the potential risks, when doing so, of moving toward performing procedures at a suboptimal time. Doing so can lead to increased complications and poor outcomes.[1,2]

REFERENCES

1. Drolet BC, Sullivan PK. Evidence-based medicine: blepharoplasty. Plast Reconstr Surg 2014;133(5):1195–1205
2. Jelks GW, Jelks EB. Preoperative evaluation of the blepharoplasty patient. Bypassing the pitfalls. Clin Plast Surg 1993;20(2):213–223, discussion 224

SKIN MARKING FOR UPPER BLEPHAROPLASTY SURGERY

16. *When marking a patient for upper eyelid blepharoplasty, which one of the following is true?*

E. The markings should be made with the patient upright with eyes closed then open.

Markings for upper eyelid blepharoplasty are key to get right in order to achieve the optimal outcome. These must be performed with the patient upright to take account of gravity on the brow position. The patient will need to close and open their eyes repeatedly during the marking procedure, as the markings need to be done with eyes closed, but the skin excess and scar placement is best guided with them open.

The lower line is marked first and is placed close to the supratarsal crease usually around 10 mm from the lash line. Following this, skin excess can be assessed using non-toothed forceps. The excess, which can be safely taken without causing lagophthalmos, is noted and the upper line can then be drawn. This mark cannot be set at a specific numerical value as it will differ according to skin excess and eye shape characteristics. The skin pattern created will not normally be a symmetrical ellipse but will involve extension laterally by canting upward from the lower line to the upper line, thereby removing more tissue laterally and keeping the scar within a rhytid in the crow's foot area (**Fig. 110.7**).

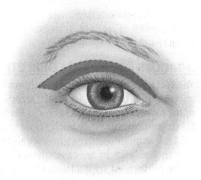

Fig. 110.7 Blepharoplasty markings.

The planned excision should not pass medially to the medial canthus but should pass laterally beyond the lateral canthus in order to remove adequate lateral tissue and blend the scar discretely.[1–3]

REFERENCES

1. Flowers RS, DuVal C. Blepharoplasty and periorbital aesthetic surgery. In: Aston SJ, Beasley RW, Thorne HM, et al, eds. Grabb and Smith's Plastic Surgery. 6th ed. Philadelphia, PA: Lippincott Williams & Wilkins; 2007
2. Hashem AM, Couto RA, Waltzman JT, Drake RL, Zins JE. Evidence-based medicine: a graded approach to lower lid blepharoplasty. Plast Reconstr Surg 2017;139(1):139e–150e
3. Nahai F, ed. The Art of Aesthetic Surgery: Principles and Techniques, 2nd ed. St Louis, MO: Quality Medical Publishing; 2011

TECHNIQUES FOR EYELID CORRECTION

17. You see a 66-year-old man with prominent lower eyelid bags. He has an excess of skin, fat, and muscle with improvement of his festoon on forcible eye closure (positive squinch test). *Which one of the following procedures is most likely to address his eyelid concerns?*

E. Subciliary lower eyelid blepharoplasty with skin, fat and muscle resection and septal reset

This man needs attention to multiple layers of the lower eyelid with reduction of skin, muscle, and fat. A lower lid blepharoplasty in his case would be best achieved through a subciliary skin approach allowing composite muscle and skin removal with fat redraping and or removal. This procedure should help tighten the lax muscle which will likely have a weak septum beneath it and allow redraping of the overlying soft tissues to smooth the lid–cheek junction. Most surgeons would also resuspend the lower eyelid following this with either a lateral suspension suture through the orbicularis oculi flap into periosteum at the lateral orbit or with a lateral canthopexy. No description of his lower eyelid laxity preoperatively was mentioned, and it is crucial that this is assessed. One would expect from the age of the patient and the description that there was lower lid laxity and so resuspension would be indicated.

A pinch blepharoplasty is a procedure indicated in patients with good lower eyelid support, either naturally or following facelift who just have a small volume of excess lower eyelid skin with or without muscle and but no other significant eyelid concerns. In the right patient, this can be a rewarding procedure as the downtime is low, the risk of ectropion and postoperative swelling is low, and the scar is very subtle. In this case, however, it would not address the key problems listed for this patient. Transconjunctival blepharoplasty can be a discrete way to reshape the lower eyelid without creating a skin scar. However, it does not allow adjustment of skin excess, which this patient has.[1-6]

REFERENCES

1. Hamra ST. The role of the septal reset in creating a youthful eyelid-cheek complex in facial rejuvenation. Plast Reconstr Surg 2004;113(7):2124–2141, discussion 2142–2144
2. Barton FE Jr, Ha R, Awada M. Fat extrusion and septal reset in patients with the tear trough triad: a critical appraisal. Plast Reconstr Surg 2004;113(7):2115–2121, discussion 2122–2123
3. Rohrich RJ, Ghavami A, Mojallal A. The five-step lower blepharoplasty: blending the eyelid-cheek junction. Plast Reconstr Surg 2011;128(3):775–783
4. Casson P, Siebert J. Lower lid blepharoplasty with skin flap and muscle split. Clin Plast Surg 1988;15(2):299–304
5. Aston SJ. Skin-muscle flap lower lid blepharoplasty. Clin Plast Surg 1988;15(2):305–308
6. Tomlinson FB, Hovey LM. Transconjunctival lower lid blepharoplasty for removal of fat. Plast Reconstr Surg 1975; 56(3):314–318

TECHNIQUES FOR EYELID CORRECTION

18. You see a 50-year-old woman with marked unilateral ectropion, a positive snap test, mild scleral show, 5 mm of anterior lid distraction, but satisfactory skin volume following a previous lower eyelid blepharoplasty. *Which one of the following procedures is most likely to address her eyelid problems?*

    B. Lateral canthoplasty with tarsal strip

    This woman requires lower eyelid tightening, which can be achieved with either a lateral canthopexy or a canthoplasty. In her case, given the degree of laxity, a canthoplasty is probably preferable. This would likely be performed with a lateral tarsal strip which involves denuding some of the lateral lower eyelid (overlying the canthal tendon) of skin and conjunctiva, dividing the lateral canthus, and re-securing the canthus deep in the lateral orbit with sutures passed through the inner layer of periosteum or drilled through bone. The skin and conjunctiva are removed because this part of the lid becomes buried as the lid is tightened and effectively shortened. A canthopexy is a useful and less invasive procedure where the lateral canthal tendon is not divided, but instead just resuspended deep and often higher in the lateral orbit. This can be performed using a double-ended polypropylene suture passing both needles from the lower canthal tendon through the lateral inner orbit periosteum and securing them via an upper blepharoplasty access incision. For less tightening, a Kuhnt-Szymanowski procedure would be appropriate. This involves a pentagonal excision of the lower eyelid including some tarsus and is therefore ideally indicated where there is a true tarsal excess as opposed to a lower lid laxity alone. The Loeb procedure is a technique used to improve the lower eyelid–cheek junction and involves sliding the medial postseptal fat out of its compartment into the tear trough before it is sutured to the angular muscles.[1-4]

REFERENCES

1. Loeb R. Fat pad sliding and fat grafting for leveling lid depressions. Clin Plast Surg 1981;8(4):757–776
2. Fagien S. Algorithm for canthoplasty: the lateral retinacular suspension: a simplified suture canthopexy. Plast Reconstr Surg 1999;103(7):2042–2053, discussion 2054–2058
3. Carraway JH, Mellow CG. The prevention and treatment of lower lid ectropion following blepharoplasty. Plast Reconstr Surg 1990;85(6):971–981
4. Tepper OM, Steinbrech D, Howell MH, Jelks EB, Jelks GW. A retrospective review of patients undergoing lateral cantho-plasty techniques to manage existing or potential lower eyelid malposition: identification of seven key preoperative findings. Plast Reconstr Surg 2015;136(1):40–49

SURGERY FOR THE ASIAN EYELID

19. A 22-year-old Asian model attends clinic keen to have surgery on her eyelids to have a "more-white" appearance. *Which one of the following adjuncts to blepharoplasty would be most beneficial for her to help achieve this?*

A. Tarsal fixation

Tarsal fixation techniques are used to help create a high supratarsal fold. These may be suture or no suture techniques. An example of a suture technique is the anchor blepharoplasty approach described by Flowers,[1,2] which uses a permanent suture passing from the skin to the tarsus and levator. Baker et al[3] described a different approach without sutures that involved resection of a section of the orbicularis oculi and allowing the skin to scar to the septum.

These techniques are particularly useful in the Asian eyelid, which has an absent or short supratarsal crease. They may also be useful in other scenarios including secondary blepharoplasty, men with brow ptosis, and patients with low preoperative eyelid folds.

The Asian eyelid tends to have a shorter tarsus and descent of the aponeurotic fat; so, tarsal shortening and fat transfer would not be indicated. Lid tightening is indicated in lax lower eyelids, but this is not a characteristic of the young Asian eyelid. Septal reset is used to improve a tear-trough deformity, which is not typically present in the Asian eyelid, either.

REFERENCES

1. Flowers RS. Upper blepharoplasty by eyelid invagination. Anchor blepharoplasty. Clin Plast Surg 1993;20(2):193–207
2. Flowers RS, DuVal C. Blepharoplasty and periorbital aesthetic surgery. In: Aston SJ, Beasley RW, Thorne CM, et al, eds. Grabb and Smith's Plastic Surgery. 6th ed. Philadelphia, PA: Lippincott Williams & Wilkins; 2006
3. Baker TJ, Gordon HL, Mosienko P. Upper lid blepharoplasty. Plast Reconstr Surg 1977;60(5):692–698

EARLY COMPLICATIONS AFTER BLEPHAROPLASTY

20. A 59-year-old patient undergoes upper and lower blepharoplasties with postseptal fat removal and is initially well on postoperative rounds. An hour later you are called to see the patient, who has described decreased clarity of vision on the left side with increasing eye pain. On examination, there is mild left-side proptosis and ecchymosis with reduced eye movement. The direct pupillary light response is diminished, but the consensual reflex is maintained. *Which one of the following actions should you perform first?*

D. Remove the sutures

Patients who undergo blepharoplasty with removal of postseptal fat have a very small but appreciable risk of developing retrobulbar hematoma.[1] This is a clinical emergency that without appropriate treatment within 1 to 2 hours can result in permanent blindness.

The patient above has key signs and symptoms of this condition: proptosis, altered vision and pain, and bruising around the eye. The pathophysiology is similar to that of compartment syndrome where there is an expanding volume (continued bleeding/swelling) held within a fixed space (the bony orbit).

Removal of the sutures should be performed immediately, as this will help decompress the area. The patient should be placed with the head up (approximately 30 degrees) to help venous drainage and reduce swelling. Other measures also directed at relieving intraorbital pressure can be medical (such as steroids, mannitol, and acetazolamide) or surgical (such as release of the lateral canthus to decompress the globe).

Mannitol and acetazolamide both act to shrink the vitreous humor, thereby reducing intraocular pressure. Mannitol is an osmotic agent that should be given intravenously in boluses of 12.5 g over 3 to 5 minutes. Acetazolamide is a carbonic anhydride inhibitor also administered intravenously (not topically) in 500 mg doses. Lateral cantholysis is required and the patient should be transferred to the operating room so that release can be performed and the hematoma fully evacuated. The risk of blindness after blepharoplasty remains exceedingly low, but given the significance of losing vision, it must still be discussed with patients preoperatively.[1,2]

REFERENCES

1. Winterton JV, Patel K, Mizen KD. Review of management options for a retrobulbar hemorrhage. J Oral Maxillofac Surg 2007;65(2):296–299
2. Christie B, Block L, Ma Y, Wick A, Afifi A. Retrobulbar hematoma: a systematic review of factors related to outcomes. J Plast Reconstr Aesthet Surg 2018;71(2):155–161

111. Blepharoptosis

See *Essentials of Plastic Surgery*, third edition, pp. 1546–1559

EYELID MUSCULATURE

1. *Which one of the following is true regarding Müller's muscle in the upper eyelid?*
   A. It is the primary upper eyelid elevator.
   B. It is formed from the posterior lamella of the levator muscle.
   C. It has both conscious and unconscious control.
   D. It develops directly from the superior oblique muscle.
   E. Its dysfunction is the main cause of acquired ptosis.

TRUE VERSUS PSEUDOPTOSIS OF THE EYELID

2. It is important to be able to differentiate between true ptosis and pseudoptosis of the upper eyelid. *Which one of the following clinical scenarios would be considered an example of true upper eyelid ptosis?*
   A. A patient with enophthalmos following facial trauma
   B. A patient with contralateral exophthalmos
   C. A patient with unilateral blepharospasm
   D. A patient with Grave's disease
   E. A patient with a CN III nerve palsy

CONGENITAL BLEPHAROPTOSIS

3. You see a 6-month-old infant in clinic. His parents are concerned about the appearance of his left eye, as the upper lid sits lower on this side, partially covering the iris. He is otherwise healthy and developing normally. *Which one of the following is true of his condition?*
   A. It is very likely to be present in other close family members.
   B. It probably reflects abnormal levator development.
   C. His upper eyelid excursion is still likely to be normal.
   D. A normal supratarsal crease would be expected on examination.
   E. The aesthetic appearance is likely to become worse over time.

DIAGNOSIS IN BLEPHAROPTOSIS

4. A young boy is referred to your pediatric clinic with congenital ptosis. His parents have noticed the child's left eyelid consistently elevates while he is eating. *What is the most likely diagnosis?*
   A. Neurofibromatosis
   B. Duane's syndrome
   C. A chronic squint
   D. Marcus Gunn syndrome
   E. Blepharophimosis syndrome

ACQUIRED PTOSIS

5. *What is the most common type of acquired blepharoptosis?*
   A. Physiologic
   B. Neurogenic
   C. Involutional
   D. Mechanical
   E. Traumatic

DIFFERENTIATION OF CONGENITAL AND ACQUIRED PTOSIS

6. *When examining a young patient with ptosis of the upper eyelids, which one of the following may be useful to differentiate between congenital and acquired causes?*
   A. Strabismus
   B. Amblyopia
   C. Telecanthus
   D. Lagophthalmos
   E. Hypoglobus

DIAGNOSING ABNORMAL UPPER EYELID ANATOMY

7. *In an adult patient with a unilateral elevated supratarsal fold, mild ptosis, and an accentuated supratarsal hollow, which one of the following is the most likely diagnosis?*
   A. Prior botulinum toxin injection
   B. Levator dehiscence
   C. Reduced sympathetic innervation
   D. Myasthenia gravis
   E. CN III compression

TECHNIQUE SELECTION FOR BLEPHAROPTOSIS SURGERY

8. *Which one of the following is considered the single most important factor when selecting a technique for correction of blepharoptosis?*
   A. Lid height position
   B. Duration of ptosis
   C. Degree of ptosis
   D. Amount of lid elevation
   E. Presence of lagophthalmos

SURGICAL MANAGEMENT OF BLEPHAROPTOSIS

9. A 60-year-old patient is seen with a chronic unilateral visual impairment resulting from obstruction from the right upper eyelid. Examination of the affected eye shows moderate blepharoptosis, with 8 mm of levator excursion. *Which one of the following is the best surgical approach to management?*
   A. Müller's muscle–conjunctival resection
   B. Levator advancement
   C. Frontalis suspension
   D. Levator reinsertion
   E. Aponeurosis repair

SURGICAL CORRECTION OF EYELID PTOSIS

10. *When undertaking surgical correction of upper eyelid ptosis in adult patients, which one of the following is correct?*
   A. Undercorrection should be performed when using epinephrine in the local anesthetic.
   B. Correction is best achieved with the use of general anesthetic because of patient compliance difficulties.
   C. When using local anesthetic agents, overcorrection may be required to achieve satisfactory results.
   D. In patients who wear contact lenses, a Schirmer's test must be performed before surgery.
   E. All patients must be counseled about and should receive appropriate management for lagophthalmos.

THE FASANELLA-SERVAT TECHNIQUE

11. You have a patient with blepharoptosis and have decided to perform the Fasanella-Servat technique. *Which one of the following is correct regarding this procedure?*
   A. It is ideal when levator function is poor.
   B. It involves a transverse skin incision.
   C. It may result in a floppy upper lid.
   D. It has highly predictable outcomes.
   E. It is a levator advancement technique.

LEVATOR APONEUROSIS SURGERY

12. A 58-year-old patient has moderate unilateral upper lid ptosis, and a plan is made for the advancement of the levator aponeurosis under general anesthesia. Preoperative lid height is 3 mm below the upper limbus and levator excursion is 9 mm. *When performing this surgery, which one of the following is true?*
   A. A transconjunctival approach should be made at the superior tarsal border.
   B. Correction of ptosis will require 6 mm of levator advancement.
   C. The upper lid should be set to lie above the upper limbus.
   D. Using the gapping method, a distance of 9 mm should be used to set advancement.
   E. A single central mattress suture should be used to repair the aponeurosis.

FRONTALIS SUSPENSION IN BLEPHAROPTOSIS

13. A young patient has unilateral blepharoptosis with poor levator function. They are seen by your assistant and scheduled to undergo frontalis suspension. *Which one of the following is true in this case?*
   A. This technique is not well suited to treat this patient's condition.
   B. Surgery would involve resection of the remaining viable Müller's muscle.
   C. Suspension is achieved by direct suturing of the upper tarsus to the frontalis.
   D. Simultaneous surgery to the contralateral eyelid would not normally be required.
   E. Long-term nighttime patching and ointment will be required after surgery.

POSTOPERATIVE PROBLEMS AFTER PTOSIS CORRECTION

14. You assess a patient in the clinic after a left unilateral levator aponeurosis advancement. She is satisfied with the improvement gained to the left eye but is concerned that the right eye now appears ptotic. **Which one of the following explains these clinical findings?**
    A. Putterman's test
    B. Schirmer's test
    C. Hering's law
    D. Fasanella's law
    E. Hering's test

Answers

EYELID MUSCULATURE

1. *Which one of the following is true regarding Müller's muscle in the upper eyelid?*

   B. It is formed from the posterior lamella of the levator muscle.

   Müller's muscle is an important component of the upper eyelid levator mechanism; however, the primary lid elevator is the levator palpebrae superioris (LPS), which originates from the lesser wing of sphenoid and inserts into the superior aspect of the tarsus and orbicularis oculi and its overlying dermis. The LPS has two lamellae and the anterior one forms the aponeurosis inserting into the tarsus and orbicularis, while the posterior one forms Muller's muscle. Muller's muscle is under involuntary control with sympathetic innervation. It adds a few millimeters of lift to the eyelids and its dysfunction is associated with acquired ptosis, although it is not the main cause of this.

   The LPS and Muller's muscle develop from the superior rectus (not superior oblique muscle) embryologically. The other muscle that is clinically relevant to eyelid ptosis is the frontalis muscle, as this is the primary brow elevator and thus also an elevator of the upper eyelid skin. Ptosis of the brow itself can result in drooping of the eyelids into the visual field, although frontalis dysfunction is not a cause of eyelid ptosis specifically. Overactivity of the frontalis can sometimes assist in compensating for genuine eyelid ptosis.[1-3]

REFERENCES

1. McCord CD Jr, Ford DT. Ptosis in the blepharoplasty patient. In: Nahai F, eds. The Art of Aesthetic Surgery Principles and Techniques. St Louis, MO: Quality Medical Publishing, Inc.; 2005:752–767
2. McCord CD Jr, Codner MA, eds. Eyelid and Periorbital Surgery. St Louis, MI: Quality Medical Publishing; 2008
3. Jubbal KT, Kania K, Braun TL, Katowitz WR, Marx DP. Pediatric Blepharoptosis. Semin Plast Surg 2017;31(1):58–64

TRUE VERSUS PSEUDOPTOSIS OF THE EYELID

2. It is important to be able to differentiate between true ptosis and pseudoptosis of the upper eyelid. *Which one of the following clinical scenarios would be considered an example of true upper eyelid ptosis?*

   E. A patient with a CN III nerve palsy

   Upper eyelid ptosis is known as blepharoptosis and is defined as a drooping of the upper eyelid margin to a position that is lower than normal. The normal position for the upper eyelid to rest when upright and in forward gaze is around the level of the upper limbus in the midpupillary line. Apparent drooping of the eyelid can be either true ptosis, as caused by dysfunction of the levator mechanism, or another cause, which is described as *pseudoptosis* as it is not a primary levator mechanism problem. CN III is the main nerve involved with innervation of the levator mechanism of the upper eyelid and therefore a palsy of this nerve would leave to significant ptosis.

   A patient with enophthalmos after facial trauma may have one eyelid sitting lower than the other because the globe is sitting in a larger space than on the other side (i.e., the orbital space is increased), so the soft tissues fall further over the eyelid. In a patient with contralateral exophthalmos, the eyelid will also appear lower on the index side, but this is due to abnormal elevation on the contralateral side, as the soft tissues have further to reach. Blepharospasm can give the appearance of a lowered upper lid due to unwanted contractions of orbicularis oculi. Patients with Grave's disease may have unilateral lid retraction, which also gives the appearance of a contralateral ptosis. They may also have lagophthalmos on downward gaze known as "Von Graef's sign."[1-4]

REFERENCES

1. McCord CD Jr, Ford DT. Ptosis in the blepharoplasty patient. In: Nahai F, eds. The Art of Aesthetic Surgery Principles and Techniques. St Louis, MI: Quality Medical Publishing, Inc.; 2005:752–767
2. McCord CD Jr, Codner MA, eds. Eyelid and Periorbital Surgery. St Louis, MI: Quality Medical Publishing; 2008
3. Jubbal KT, Kania K, Braun TL, Katowitz WR, Marx DP. Pediatric blepharoptosis. Semin Plast Surg 2017;31(1):58–64
4. McCord CD Jr. The evaluation and management of the patient with ptosis. Clin Plast Surg 1988;15(2):169–184

CONGENITAL BLEPHAROPTOSIS

3. You see a 6-month-old infant in clinic. His parents are concerned about the appearance of his left eye, as the upper lid sits lower on this side, partially covering the iris. He is otherwise healthy and developing normally. *Which one of the following is true of his condition?*

   B. It probably reflects abnormal levator development.

Congenital ptosis is due to developmental dysgenesis of the LPS muscle. It is usually noticed shortly after birth and can be unilateral or bilateral, with a slight predominance for occurrence on the left. It is most often a sporadic, isolated occurrence and does not have a clear inheritance pattern. It has been associated with dominant, recessive, and X-linked cases as well as rare syndromes. Because the levator is poorly formed and fibrosed, upper lid excursion is usually reduced and the supratarsal crease is absent or elevated. Other physical findings include a decreased palpebral aperture, a reduced margin to light reflex, and lagophthalmos on downward gaze. The condition is not usually progressive, so is unlikely to become worse over time.[1,2]

REFERENCES

1. Jubbal KT, Kania K, Braun TL, Katowitz WR, Marx DP. Pediatric Blepharoptosis. Semin Plast Surg 2017;31(1):58–64
2. SooHoo JR, Davies BW, Allard FD, Durairaj VD. Congenital ptosis. Surv Ophthalmol 2014;59(5):483–492

DIAGNOSIS IN BLEPHAROPTOSIS

4. **A young boy is referred to your pediatric clinic with congenital ptosis. His parents have noticed the child's left eyelid consistently elevates while he is eating. *What is the most likely diagnosis?***

   D. **Marcus Gunn syndrome**

   This child displays findings in keeping with trigeminal oculomotor nerve synkinesis, also known as Marcus Gunn syndrome. This involves unwanted upper eyelid elevation during activation of the muscles of mastication, such as when chewing or biting.[1] It occurs in 5% of children with congenital ptosis and is caused by aberrant CN V innervation to the levator muscle. There is also another condition called inverse Marcus Gunn syndrome that involves unwanted eyelid closure during biting and is an extremely rare, acquired condition. A similar condition is Marin-Amat syndrome, which is a rare synkinesis in which eye closure occurs on full opening of the jaw.[2]

   Neurofibromatosis (NF1) can be associated with ptosis of the upper eyelid, due to the increased physical bulk of the eyelid because of neurofibroma formation. Lesions may need debulking if they begin to compromise vision, but commonly recur over time following surgery. Other key features of NF1 include café au lait spots, pigmented lesions on the iris (Lisch nodules), optic nerve tumors, and skin nodules.

   Duane's syndrome is a congenital condition that results in pseudoptosis and strabismus. It is caused by abnormal development of the abducens nerve, and subsequently lateral rectus muscle function is impaired. A squint refers to a misalignment of the eyes and an uncontrolled squint can lead to a lazy eye (amblyopia). It can also give the appearance of a ptotic upper lid. Blepharophimosis syndrome is a rare inherited condition involving a complex eyelid malformation. It is characterized by ptosis, blepharophimosis (narrowing of the horizontal aperture), telecanthus, and epicanthus inversus (a skin fold arising from the lower eyelid).

REFERENCES

1. Gunn RM. Congenital ptosis with peculiar associated movements of the affected lid. Trans Ophthalmol Soc U K 1883;3:283–287
2. Jethani J. Marin-Amat syndrome: a rare facial synkinesis. Indian J Ophthalmol 2007;55(5):402–403

ACQUIRED PTOSIS

5. ***What is the most common type of acquired blepharoptosis?***

   C. **Involutional**

   Acquired ptosis may be classified as myogenic, neurogenic, traumatic, or mechanical. Involutional ptosis is the most common type of acquired ptosis. It represents a subtype of myogenic ptosis and is caused by stretching of the levator aponeurosis attachments to the tarsal plate. Dermal attachments remain in place. Traumatic causes are the next most common, where there is disruption of the levator aponeurosis. These can be secondary to cataract surgery, due to use of hard contact lenses, or due to blunt trauma to the eye leading to soft-tissue swelling. Neurogenic causes include CN III palsy and Horner's syndrome, as the latter will cause weakness to Muller's muscle. Mechanical causes tend to refer to external physical causes that counteract normal lid elevation, such as upper lid tumors and excess upper eyelid skin (dermatochalasis).[1–3]

REFERENCES

1. McCord CD Jr. The evaluation and management of the patient with ptosis. Clin Plast Surg 1988;15(2):169–184
2. McCord CD Jr, Ford DT. Ptosis in the Blepharoplasty patient. In: Nahai F, eds. The Art of Aesthetic Surgery Principles and Techniques. St Louis, MI: Quality Medical Publishing, Inc.; 2005:752–767
3. McCord CD Jr, Codner MA, eds. Eyelid and Periorbital Surgery. St Louis, MI: Quality Medical Publishing; 2008

DIFFERENTIATION OF CONGENITAL AND ACQUIRED PTOSIS

6. *When examining a young patient with ptosis of the upper eyelids, which one of the following may be useful to differentiate between congenital and acquired causes?*

    D. Lagophthalmos

    Differentiation between congenital and acquired causes of blepharoptosis is usually straightforward, given the timing of symptoms. In the event that the diagnosis is less obvious, it may be useful to differentiate between the two, based on the presence or absence of lagophthalmos on downward gaze. This occurs secondary to levator fibrosis which is more commonly seen in congenital cases.

    Strabismus refers to a misalignment of the eyes as a result of impaired extraocular muscle function. Amblyopia is a lazy eye where there is decreased vision secondary to abnormal visual development during infancy. Telecanthus is an increase in distance between the medial canthi. The interpupillary distance remains normal. Hypoglobus is downward displacement of the eye in the orbit and may give the appearance of ptosis. None of these features specifically help differentiate between congenital and acquired ptosis, although many of them can be associated with congenital ptosis.[1-5]

REFERENCES

1. Jubbal KT, Kania K, Braun TL, Katowitz WR, Marx DP. Pediatric Blepharoptosis. Semin Plast Surg 2017;31(1):58–64
2. McCord CD Jr. The evaluation and management of the patient with ptosis. Clin Plast Surg 1988;15(2):169–184
3. McCord CD. Evaluation of the ptosis patient. In: McCord CD Jr, Codner MA, Hester TR, eds. Eyelid Surgery: Principles and Techniques. 2nd ed. New York, NY: Lippincott Williams & Wilkins; 2006
4. SooHoo JR, Davies BW, Allard FD, Durairaj VD. Congenital ptosis. Surv Ophthalmol 2014;59(5):483–492
5. Tuli SY, Kelly M, Giordano B, Fillipps DJ, Tuli SS. Blepharoptosis: assessment and management. J Pediatr Health Care 2012;26(2):149–154

DIAGNOSING ABNORMAL UPPER EYELID ANATOMY

7. *In an adult patient with a unilateral elevated supratarsal fold, mild ptosis, and an accentuated supratarsal hollow, which one of the following is the most likely diagnosis?*

    B. Levator dehiscence

    This patient is likely to have dehiscence of the LPS. The other options may all lead to ptosis, but an elevated fold and supratarsal hollowing are classic signs of levator dehiscence. Botulinum toxin inadvertently placed into the levator during treatment of glabellar or forehead rhytids can lead to isolated temporary brow or eyelid ptosis. Keeping injections high in the brow and superficial can help minimize this. Reduced sympathetic innervation could reduce Müller's muscle function leading to a subtle ptosis in conjunction with meiosis and anhidrosis (Horner's syndrome). This can occur secondary to tumors at the lung apex, or within the neck or spine. Myasthenia gravis is a systemic autoimmune neuromuscular disorder which can cause diplopia with ptosis that is typically worse toward the end of the day. Patients can also have problems with facial movement, swallowing, and speaking. Compression of CN III can cause loss of levator function, also leading to an isolated ptosis.[1-3]

REFERENCES

1. McCord CD Jr. The evaluation and management of the patient with ptosis. Clin Plast Surg 1988;15(2):169–184
2. McCord CD. Evaluation of the ptosis patient. In: McCord CD Jr, Codner MA, Hester TR, eds. Eyelid Surgery: Principles and Techniques. 2nd ed. New York, NY: Lippincott Williams & Wilkins; 2006
3. Tuli SY, Kelly M, Giordano B, Fillipps DJ, Tuli SS. Blepharoptosis: assessment and management. J Pediatr Health Care 2012;26(2):149–154

TECHNIQUE SELECTION FOR BLEPHAROPTOSIS SURGERY

8. *Which one of the following is considered the single most important factor when selecting a technique for correction of blepharoptosis?*

    D. Amount of lid elevation

    When assessing patients for surgical correction of blepharoptosis, an assessment should be made of levator function (**Fig. 111.1**). The amount of lid elevation is graded as mild (>10 mm lift), moderate (5–10 mm lift), or severe (0–5 mm lift), and this is the most important factor in determining surgical management. Naturally, this will be linked to the cause of the ptosis. For example, if there is good elevation in the presence of ptosis, the levator mechanism is probably elongated or stretched.

    Other factors which are important in surgical planning include the degree of ptosis and lid height position, which are essentially the same thing. The duration of ptosis is not usually relevant, other than if sudden onset which may suggest a traumatic cause. Lagophthalmos is often present in congenital ptosis. Furthermore, it is highly likely to occur after ptosis surgery and can exacerbate dry-eye symptoms.[1,2]

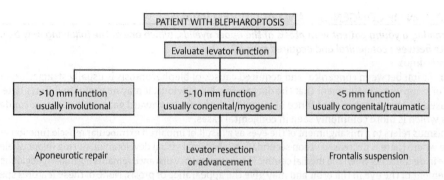

Fig. 111.1 Algorithm for ptosis repair.

REFERENCES

1. McCord CD Jr, Codner MA, Hester TR Jr. Eyelid Surgery: Principles and Techniques. Philadelphia, PA: Lippincott-Raven; 1995:148–153
2. Chang S, Lehrman C, Itani K, Rohrich RJ. A systematic review of comparison of upper eyelid involutional ptosis repair techniques: efficacy and complication rates. Plast Reconstr Surg 2012;129(1):149–157

SURGICAL MANAGEMENT OF BLEPHAROPTOSIS

9. A 60-year-old patient is seen with a chronic unilateral visual impairment resulting from obstruction from the right upper eyelid. Examination of the affected eye shows moderate blepharoptosis, with 8 mm of levator excursion. *Which one of the following is the best surgical approach to management?*

   B. Levator advancement

   There are a number of surgical procedures available for the correction of upper eyelid ptosis,[1] but at present there have been no randomized controlled studies comparing the effectiveness of these techniques. McCord et al[2] proposed a treatment algorithm for blepharoptosis based on levator function (see **Fig. 111.1**). According to this, the patient could have either resection or advancement procedures. Levator advancement is useful for mild to moderate ptosis and requires good levator function with an aponeurotic defect. It involves a blepharoplasty type skin incision and dissection to the aponeurosis which is sutured to the tarsus to elevate it.

   A patient with more than 10 mm of levator function would probably have a formal aponeurotic repair or Müllerectomy, and a patient with less than 5 mm of levator elevation would probably be a candidate for frontalis suspension.

   More recently, Chang et al[3] have undertaken a systematic review of blepharoptosis studies and proposed a treatment algorithm more specifically for involutional blepharoptosis, which would also advocate the use of an advancement procedure for this patient. According to this algorithm (**Fig. 111.2**), a patient with minimal to moderate ptosis and good levator function would be a candidate for Müller's muscle–conjunctival resection.

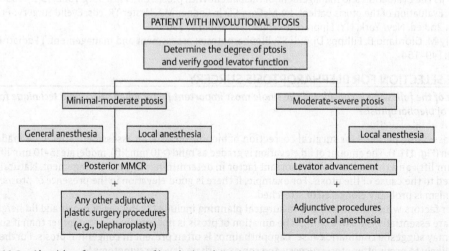

Fig. 111.2 Algorithm for treatment of involutional ptosis. (*MMCR*, Müller's muscle–conjunctival resection.)

REFERENCES

1. Beard C, Sullivan JH. Ptosis--current concepts. Int Ophthalmol Clin 1978;18(3):53–73
2. McCord CD Jr, Codner MA, Hester TR Jr. Eyelid Surgery: Principles and Techniques. Philadelphia, PA: Lippincott-Raven; 1995
3. Chang S, Lehrman C, Itani K, Rohrich RJ. A systematic review of comparison of upper eyelid involutional ptosis repair techniques: efficacy and complication rates. Plast Reconstr Surg 2012;129(1):149–157

SURGICAL CORRECTION OF EYELID PTOSIS

10. **When undertaking surgical correction of upper eyelid ptosis in adult patients, which one of the following is correct?**

    E. All patients must be counseled about and should receive appropriate management for lagophthalmos.
    Lagophthalmos is very likely to occur following correctional surgery for eyelid ptosis; so, patients must be advised about this risk and its potential postoperative management prior to undergoing surgery. The secondary problems of lagophthalmos include corneal exposure, keratitis, and dry-eye syndrome. Treatment includes daytime eye drops and night time ointments and patching.

    When undertaking ptosis correction surgery, care must be taken to avoid overcorrection or undercorrection. The use of epinephrine can increase the sympathetic tone to Müller's muscle; so, slight overcorrection may be required to take this into account. When using local anesthetic agents, the levator muscles may be paralyzed, so undercorrection may be required. Although a general anesthetic avoids difficulties with patient compliance, where possible, local anesthetic is preferable because it allows assessment of lid position during surgery. Undercorrection of ptosis will necessitate revision surgery to further elevate the eyelid, and overcorrection is usually managed nonoperatively in the first instance by early stretching and massage. If it does not settle with time, surgical revision may be indicated. Schirmer's test is performed to assess for the presence of dry eye. It involves placing a Schirmer paper strip into the eye for 5 minutes and wetting on the strip is then assessed at the end of the 5-minute period. Patients who regularly wear contact lenses are unlikely to suffer from dry eyes, so this test is not typically indicated for them.[1]

REFERENCE

1. McCord CD Jr. Complications of ptosis surgery and their management. In: McCord CD Jr, Codner MA, Hester TR, eds. Eyelid Surgery: Principles and Techniques. New York, NY: Lippincott-Raven; 1995

THE FASANELLA-SERVAT TECHNIQUE

11. You have a patient with blepharoptosis and have decided to perform the Fasanella-Servat technique. **Which one of the following is correct regarding this procedure?**

    C. It may result in a floppy upper lid.
    The Fasanella-Servat technique is used for mild cases of blepharoptosis in patients with excellent levator function. It involves a transconjunctival approach and thereby avoids a skin scar, but the outcomes can be unpredictable. It is a resection technique, not an advancement technique, and involves removal of Müller's muscle, part of the tarsus and levator, and the conjunctiva. It can result in a floppy upper lid as a result of the tarsal resection. Many modifications and variations of the technique have been described since its first description in 1961.[1-4]

REFERENCES

1. McCord CD Jr, Ford DT. Ptosis in the blepharoplasty patient. In: Nahai F, eds. The Art of Aesthetic Surgery Principles and Techniques. St Louis, MI: Quality Medical Publishing, Inc.; 2005:752–767
2. Samimi DB, Erb MH, Lane CJ, Dresner SC. The modified Fasanella-Servat procedure: description and quantified analysis. Ophthal Plast Reconstr Surg 2013;29(1):30–34
3. Jubbal KT, Kania K, Braun TL, Katowitz WR, Marx DP. Pediatric blepharoptosis. Semin Plast Surg 2017;31(1):58–64
4. Bentz ML, Bauer BS, Zuker RM. Principles and Practice of Pediatric Plastic Surgery. St Louis: Quality Medical Publishing; 2008

LEVATOR APONEUROSIS SURGERY

12. A 58-year-old patient has moderate unilateral upper lid ptosis, and a plan is made for the advancement of the levator aponeurosis under general anesthesia. Preoperative lid height is 3 mm below the upper limbus and levator excursion is 9 mm. **When performing this surgery, which one of the following is true?**

    D. Using the gapping method, a distance of 9 mm should be used to set advancement.
    The gapping method is useful for achieving correct advancement when patients undergoing levator aponeurosis advancement or external levator resection are under general anesthesia. The preoperative excursion measurement (9 mm in this case) is used as a guide to set advancement so that the distance between the upper and lower eyelids matches the excursion measurement.

Levator aponeurosis advancement is indicated for mild to moderate ptosis and is undertaken using a skin incision at the desired supratarsal fold rather than a transconjunctival approach. The upper lid is set according to excursion such that with good excursion, as in this case, the upper lid should be set just below (not just above) the upper limbus. Only if the excursion was poor, should the lid be set above the upper limbus.

In general, a 4:1 ratio of advancement to ptosis correction is required with this technique. Therefore 12 mm of levator advancement (not 6 mm) would probably be needed to achieve correction of the 3-mm ptosis. Although a central lifting suture is used initially to secure the levator to the superior tarsus, this is not sufficient by itself and therefore an additional two sutures are placed, one medial and one lateral to the central suture. In addition, supratarsal crease fixation may be performed (see Fig. 111.2).[1-3]

REFERENCES

1. Chang S, Lehrman C, Itani K, Rohrich RJ. A systematic review of comparison of upper eyelid involutional ptosis repair techniques: efficacy and complication rates. Plast Reconstr Surg 2012;129(1):149–157
2. Carraway JH, Vincent MP. Levator advancement technique for eyelid ptosis. Plast Reconstr Surg 1986;77(3):394–403
3. de la Torre JI, Martin SA, De Cordier BC, Al-Hakeem MS, Collawn SS, Vásconez LO. Aesthetic eyelid ptosis correction: a review of technique and cases. Plast Reconstr Surg 2003;112(2):655–660, discussion 661–662

FRONTALIS SUSPENSION IN BLEPHAROPTOSIS

13. A young patient has unilateral blepharoptosis with poor levator function. They are seen by your assistant and scheduled to undergo frontalis suspension. *Which one of the following is true in this case?*

E. Long-term nighttime patching and ointment will be required after surgery.

Frontalis suspension can provide 1 cm of excursion with a good result in a straightforward gaze but will likely produce lagophthalmos during sleep. Therefore, nighttime patching and ointment will be required to protect the globe. The main indication for this surgery is congenital blepharoptosis with poor excursion, so it is an appropriate technique in this scenario. This surgery does not involve resection of Müller's muscle. This is part of the Putterman conjunctival technique and the external levator resection techniques as described by Beard and Burke, respectively. Suspension is not achieved by direct suturing, instead it requires slips of fascia lata, other fascia, or similar tissue to suspend the upper eyelid to the frontalis (see Fig. 111.4). Bilateral suspension is often required, even where there is a unilateral ptosis, in order to achieve good symmetry.[1-3]

REFERENCES

1. Crawford JS. Repair of ptosis using frontalis muscle and fascia lata: a 20-year review. Ophthalmic Surg 1977;8(4):31–40
2. Beard C. Ptosis. 2nd ed. Saint Louis: The C V Mosby Company; 1976:173–175
3. Berke RN. A simplified Blaskovics operation for blepharoptosis; results in ninety-one operations. AMA Arch Opthalmol 1952;48(4):460–495

POSTOPERATIVE PROBLEMS AFTER PTOSIS CORRECTION

14. You assess a patient in the clinic after a left unilateral levator aponeurosis advancement. She is satisfied with the improvement gained to the left eye but is concerned that the right eye now appears ptotic. *Which one of the following explains these clinical findings?*

C. Hering's law

The levator muscles receive bilateral equal innervation. The presence of severe ptosis on one side will create an impulse for bilateral lid retraction. If, as in this case, a patient undergoes unilateral correction, the innervation for lid retraction decreases, leading to ptosis on the nonoperated side. This is described in Hering's law.

Hering's test should therefore be performed preoperatively to avoid this occurrence; this involves immobilizing the brow and having the patient maintain a straightforward gaze. The affected upper eyelid is then gently elevated using a cotton-tipped applicator to alleviate the ptosis. The presence of contralateral ptosis should then be assessed. [1,2] Putterman and Fasanella are both names associated with blepharoptosis surgical techniques, not tests. Schirmer's test is for the evaluation of tear production.[3,4]

REFERENCES

1. Chen AD, Lai YW, Lai HT, et al. The impact of Hering's law in blepharoptosis: literature review. Ann Plast Surg 2016;76(Suppl 1):S96–S100
2. Jubbal KT, Kania K, Braun TL, Katowitz WR, Marx DP. Pediatric Blepharoptosis. Semin Plast Surg 2017;31(1):58–64
3. Guyuron B, Davies B. Experience with the modified Putterman procedure. Plast Reconstr Surg 1988;82(5):775–780
4. Tuli SY, Kelly M, Giordano B, Fillipps DJ, Tuli SS. Blepharoptosis: assessment and management. J Pediatr Health Care 2012;26(2):149–154

112. Face Lift

See *Essentials of Plastic Surgery*, third edition, pp. 1560–1579

CHRONOLOGIC AGING

1. *Which one of the following is most likely to be increased in aging skin?*
   A. Epidermal thickness
   B. Cell turnover
   C. The number of fibroblasts
   D. The amount of collagen and elastin
   E. The ratio of collagen type III to I

CHANGES IN THE AGING FACE

2. *Which one of the following is typically observed in the aging face?*
   A. Deflation and volume loss in the lower face
   B. Fat accumulation in the upper and midface
   C. Retrusion of the anterior maxilla and inferior orbital rim
   D. Cessation of bony growth irrespective of dentition
   E. Soft-tissue ptosis at the inferior orbital rim

THE AGING PROCESS

3. *Where on the aging face are the effects of "radial expansion" most apparent?*
   A. Glabella
   B. Orbital rim
   C. Nasolabial fold
   D. Neck
   E. Lateral cheek

INCISION PLACEMENT IN FACE LIFTING

4. You are planning a primary face lift on a 52-year-old man who has long hair and long sideburns. He has descent of the facial soft tissues with only mild skin excess. *Which one of the following incisions should be used?*
   A. A preauricular incision passing behind the tragus
   B. A temporal incision placed behind the anterior hairline
   C. A postauricular incision running vertically 1 cm behind the sulcus
   D. An occipital incision running along the hairline
   E. A retroauricular transverse incision level with the tragus

VECTORS AND FIXATION FOR FACE LIFTING

5. *When considering face-lifting procedures, which one of the following is true with regard to the superficial musculoaponeurotic system (SMAS)?*
   A. It should ideally be elevated with a posterolateral vector.
   B. It should ideally be elevated with a predominantly vertical vector.
   C. It should ideally be elevated with the same vector as the skin.
   D. It should ideally be supported with a permanent internal mesh.
   E. It should be fixed after elevation with long-acting absorbable sutures.

SUBCUTANEOUS FACE LIFT PROCEDURES

6. *Which one of the following is true regarding skin-only face lifts?*
   A. They remain the most popular face-lifting approach.
   B. They are best suited to thin patients with skin excess.
   C. They are best suited to overweight patients with skin excess.
   D. They should no longer be used in clinical practice.
   E. The results are proven to be significantly worse than other techniques.

MINIMAL ACCESS CRANIAL SUSPENSION FACE LIFT (MACS-LIFT)

7. A patient comes to clinic for a second opinion to discuss face-lift procedures, having been offered MACS-lift by another clinician. *Which one of the following is true of this procedure?*
   A. It is reliant on the skin for providing soft-tissue elevation.
   B. It is usually performed using an endoscopic approach.
   C. It carries a theoretical risk of compression damage to facial nerve branches.
   D. It commonly uses a vector of elevation perpendicular to the nasolabial fold.
   E. It most often involves elevation and resection of the SMAS layer.

MINIMAL ACCESS CRANIAL SUSPENSION FACE LIFT (MACS-LIFT)

8. You are undertaking a MACS-lift on a 50-year-old patient who wishes to address the jowls, the neck/jawline, and the midface with a single procedure. *Intraoperatively which one of the following is true in this case?*
   A. The suspension will involve two separate continuous purse-string sutures per side.
   B. The suspension will be anchored to the deep temporal fascia just above the zygomatic arch.
   C. Two lengths of nonabsorbable monofilament suture will be optimal for this procedure.
   D. Each suture placed will be passed in a circular pattern encompassing SMAS tissue.
   E. The skin and SMAS will ultimately be elevated with differing vectors obliquely.

THE SKOOG FACE LIFT

9. *What was the main limitation of the face-lift technique originally described by Skoog?*
   A. It had a high risk of skin slough.
   B. It had a short-lasting result.
   C. It failed to improve the nasolabial folds.
   D. It required separate dissection of the skin and SMAS layers.
   E. Skin excess was difficult to treat.

THE DEEP PLANE FACE LIFT

10. *In which plane of dissection would a deep plane face lift be performed?*
    A. Subcutaneous
    B. Sub-SMAS
    C. Supraperiosteal
    D. Deep fascial
    E. Subperiosteal

SUBPERIOSTEAL FACE LIFTS

11. *What is the main perceived advantage of using a subperiosteal approach to face lifting?*
    A. Technically easier and quicker dissection
    B. Enhanced manipulation of skin tissue fat compartments
    C. Avoidance of the need for endoscopic skills
    D. A reduced risk of facial palsy
    E. It targets large skin excesses of the jawline and neck

THE AGING LIP

12. *Which one of the following changes would be expected when examining the upper lip of an elderly patient during an aesthetic consultation?*
    A. Increased dental show
    B. Increased lip volume
    C. Increased visible vermilion
    D. Decreased commissure width
    E. Decreased dental show

FAT INJECTION FOR FACIAL REJUVENATION

13. You are undertaking a face and neck lift with submental liposuction and the patient asks if it is possible to enhance the malar and nasolabial regions with fat taken from the chin at the same time. *Which one of the following is true in this case?*
    A. Injection of fat into these locations at the same time as a face lift is contraindicated.
    B. Long-term fat viability would be highly predictable following injection into these sites.
    C. Injection of fat in this scenario should be placed deeply with a slight overcorrection.
    D. These areas would be better treated with a transblepharoplasty midface procedure.
    E. Extension of the sub-SMAS dissection to the nasolabial fold would be the optimal approach for this patient.

PERIOPERATIVE MANAGEMENT FOR RHYTIDECTOMY

14. A female patient comes to the clinic to discuss a face-lift procedure. She is 40 years old and recently separated from her long-term partner. She smokes 10 cigarettes per day and takes a range of herbal medications. She takes regular analgesics for lower back pain, but no other prescription drugs. *When assessing this woman for a face lift, which one of the following is correct?*
    - A. She should consider a consult with your clinical psychologist after surgical treatment.
    - B. Neither her prescribed nor over-the-counter remedies will increase her risk of complications.
    - C. She would need to undertake smoking cessation before treatment.
    - D. Her risk of skin slough would be about 5% if she proceeded with a sub-SMAS face lift.
    - E. She is very likely to be satisfied with her surgical outcome postoperatively.
        lift patient. Plast Reconstr Surg 1984;73(6):911–915

POSTOPERATIVE MANAGEMENT FOLLOWING RHYTIDECTOMY

15. You are asked to see a patient in recovery after a face lift. On examination, he has visible unilateral swelling overlying the mandibular border and neck. The neck drain is empty. Blood pressure has been well maintained at 125 mm Hg systolic. *What is your next step in the management of this patient?*
    - A. Give an intravenous dose of chlorpromazine
    - B. Flush and re-vacuum the drain
    - C. Remove sutures and suction a hematoma in recovery
    - D. Return the patient to the operating room
    - E. Observe, document, and reassess in 30 minutes

COMPLICATIONS IN FACE-LIFT SURGERY

16. *When discussing informed consent with a patient for a face lift, which one of the following represents the most common early complication?*
    - A. Facial nerve weakness
    - B. Infection
    - C. Hematoma
    - D. Skin slough
    - E. Altered sensation to the lobule

PERIOPERATIVE MANAGEMENT OF RHYTIDECTOMY PATIENTS

17. *When planning perioperative care for a patient undergoing a face lift, which one of the following is most likely to lower the risk of hematoma formation?*
    - A. Insertion of vacuum drains beneath the skin flaps
    - B. Use of fibrin glue before closure
    - C. Preoperative injection with epinephrine
    - D. Tumescent infiltration with saline solution after induction
    - E. Administration of a prophylactic dose of low-molecular-weight heparin daily

STIGMATA OF FACE LIFTS

18. A patient is seen before a face lift and is noted to have marked submalar hollowing. *What are the deformities that are at increased risk of developing after rhytidectomy?*
    - A. Lateral sweep
    - B. Joker's lines
    - C. Smile blocks
    - D. Pixie deformity
    - E. Hairline distortion

SECONDARY FACE LIFTS

19. *Which one of the following is true when considering secondary face lifts?*
    - A. The average duration between primary face lift and the secondary face lift is around four years.
    - B. The operation note from the primary procedure must be obtained before proceeding.
    - C. The SMAS is generally thicker and more robust when undertaking a secondary face lift procedure.
    - D. The skin flap vascularity is likely to be reduced compared with a primary face lift procedure.
    - E. The risk of facial nerve damage is likely to be increased when performing sub-SMAS approaches.

Answers

CHRONOLOGIC AGING

1. Which one of the following is most likely to be increased in aging skin?

   E. The ratio of collagen type III to I

   A number of intrinsic changes occur in aging skin. The ratio of collagen subtypes alters with an increase in the ratio of type III to type I while the diameter of collagen fibers decreases. Other changes include dermal and epidermal thinning with a less well-organized stratum corneum. Cell turnover decreases; so, there are also fewer fibroblasts, mast cells, and blood vessels, as well as a reduction in the total number of collagen and elastin fibers.[1] Dermal thickness decreases approximately 6% per decade and is accelerated by sun exposure, fluctuations in weight, and smoking. Subdermal adipose tissue also decreases. These skin and soft-tissue changes are further compounded by gravitational forces that cause deep wrinkles as facial fat descends and the dynamic forces from mimetic muscles that cause rhytids in the overlying skin. Approaches to improve skin quality include actinic damage prevention by using sun block and daily skin care, while reducing sun exposure and smoking. Techniques to address changes once they have developed include laser resurfacing and chemical peels.

REFERENCE

1. Sauermann K, Clemann S, Jaspers S, et al. Age related changes of human skin investigated with histometric measurements by confocal laser scanning microscopy in vivo. Skin Res Technol 2002;8(1):52–56

CHANGES IN THE AGING FACE

2. Which one of the following is typically observed in the aging face?

   C. Retrusion of the anterior maxilla and inferior orbital rim

   There are a number of changes within the bone and facial soft tissues during aging. These include retrusion of the anterior maxilla and inferior orbital rim, downward rotation of the facial skeleton with respect to the cranial base, and expansion of the orbital socket volume which leads to a sunken eye appearance and contributes to the tear-trough deformity. The adult facial skeleton continues to grow in dentate patients. In edentulous patients, however, there is a reduction in facial height because of loss of alveolar bone in the mandible and maxilla.

   Soft-tissue changes with advancing age include deflation and volume loss in the upper two-thirds of the face, while there is accumulation of fat in the lower face and neck. The appearance of these volume changes is exacerbated by descent of the remaining upper soft tissues from gravity and a combination of attenuation and tethering of retaining ligaments. There may be an appearance of ptosis along the inferior orbital rim, but this is really a pseudoptosis due to the effects of soft-tissue volume loss.[1-4]

REFERENCES

1. Coleman SR. Facial recontouring with lipostructure. Clin Plast Surg 1997;24(2):347–367
2. Lambros V. Observations on periorbital and midface aging. Plast Reconstr Surg 2007;120(5):1367–1376
3. Lambros V. Models of facial aging and implications for treatment. Clin Plast Surg 2008;35(3):319–327, discussion 317
4. Warren RJ, Aston SJ, Mendelson BC. Face lift. Plast Reconstr Surg 2011;128(6):747e–764e

THE AGING PROCESS

3. Where on the aging face are the effects of "radial expansion" most apparent?

   C. Nasolabial fold

   The four main mechanisms of soft-tissue aging in the face are the effects of gravity, upper and midface volume loss, lower face and neck volume gain, and radial expansion. Radial expansion refers to a process where repeated animation stretches the retaining ligaments of the face and allows the soft tissues to expand away from the face. This is most apparent at the nasolabial fold during smiling, because the skin of the lip is forced under the subcutaneous fat of the cheek, allowing the soft tissues to prolapse outward from the skeleton.[1]

   The nasolabial folds represent one of the key areas patients request attention to as part of facial rejuvenation. Deep nasolabial folds have been treated by various techniques including surgical and nonsurgical options. Nonsurgical approaches generally involve facial fillers placed directly in the fold or in the midface to increase cheek fullness and secondarily elevated and reduce the fold appearance. Hyaluronic acid is the most popular filler choice as it is reliable and reversible with low rates of complication. Surgical approaches include face lift, midface lift, and, in some cases, direct excision or dermal graft/fat graft surgery.

REFERENCE

1. Stuzin JM. Restoring facial shape in face lifting: the role of skeletal support in facial analysis and midface soft-tissue repositioning. Plast Reconstr Surg 2007;119(1):362–376, discussion 377–378

INCISION PLACEMENT IN FACE LIFTING

4. You are planning a primary face lift on a 52-year-old man who has long hair and long sideburns. He has descent of the facial soft tissues with only mild skin excess. *Which one of the following incisions should be used?*

B. A temporal incision placed behind the anterior hairline

There are four areas of the face-lift scar to consider: temporal, preauricular, postauricular, and occipital. The location of incisions should be individualized for each patient with the aim of making them the most aesthetically discrete and as short and neat as possible, while allowing for adequate skin removal and redraping. In situations where more significant amounts of skin are to be resected, it is best to place incisions at the interface between skin and hair; otherwise, the hairline will be altered, producing an unnatural appearance. In the case described, the temporal incision can be placed within the hairline as a vertical extension of the preauricular incision or passing through the hair above the sideburn because only a small amount of skin is to be removed. The preauricular incision should normally be placed at the junction between the ear and cheek passing behind the tragus in women and in front in men. The pretragal approach is generally preferred for men otherwise transfer of facial hair onto the tragus occurs and the gap between the ear and sideburn is artificially reduced.

The vertical component of the postauricular incision should run in the sulcus (not behind it) because it will be well hidden in this site. An extension of the postauricular incision along the occipital hairline incision is generally reserved for patients with large amounts of skin redundancy in the face and neck as this allows it to be removed without excess bunching. A smaller extension can be made transversely from the postauricular incision directly into hair-bearing area at various levels. In this scenario, the transverse extension, if needed, could be placed high at a level above the helical root.[1,2]

REFERENCES

1. Nahai F, ed. The Art of Aesthetic Surgery: Principles and Techniques. St Louis: Quality Medical Publishing; 2005
2. Barton FE Jr. Aesthetic surgery of the face and neck. Aesthet Surg J 2009;29(6):449–463, quiz 464–466

VECTORS AND FIXATION FOR FACE LIFTING

5. *When considering face-lifting procedures, which one of the following is true with regard to the superficial musculoaponeurotic system (SMAS)?*

B. It should ideally be lifted with a predominantly vertical vector.

During face lifts with manipulation of the SMAS, the key elements are to elevate and resuspend the SMAS in a largely vertical direction. In some cases, a vertical oblique direction will also work well. In contrast, most techniques use a more posterior or lateral vector in combination with some vertical lift for the skin. The fact that the two vectors are often different highlights one of the benefits of having two separately dissected layers, i.e., SMAS and a skin flap for independent manipulation rather than a composite flap with skin and SMAS moving as a single unit. The vertical vector on the SMAS is critical and improves the jawline and perioral areas, and the high SMAS can help restore the midface. The vertical/diagonal vector on the platysma improves the neck and submental areas. Once elevated, it is normal to then resuspend and support the SMAS with a permanent suture depending on surgeon's preference and technique used. Use of a long-acting absorbable suture would not be first choice for most surgeons, as it may not provide sufficient long-term support. Some surgeons may prefer to incorporate an absorbable mesh (such as Vicryl) to suspend the SMAS.[1–3]

REFERENCES

1. Nahai F, ed. The Art of Aesthetic Surgery: Principles and Techniques. St Louis: Quality Medical Publishing; 2005
2. Barrett DM, Casanueva FJ, Wang TD. Evolution of the rhytidectomy. World J Otorhinolaryngol Head Neck Surg 2016;2(1):38–44
3. Jacono AA, Bryant LM, Alemi AS. Optimal facelift vector and its relation to zygomaticus major orientation. Aesthet Surg J 2020;40(4):351–356

SUBCUTANEOUS FACE LIFT PROCEDURES

6. *Which one of the following is true regarding skin-only face lifts?*

B. They are best suited to thin patients with skin excess

Skin-only face lifts have generally fallen out of favor to be superseded by techniques that manipulate the SMAS layer as well as the overlying skin. The thinking behind using the SMAS is to lift and suspend the deeper tissues of the face and then redrape the skin over the top without tension. This is thought to provide the most stable and natural long-term result. By avoiding tension on the skin, the scars are less likely to stretch or be of poor quality. There is less likely to be over-resection of skin in order to achieve an adequate lift and the classic overdone windswept look of early face lifts can be avoided.

Perhaps if there is an indication for a skin-only approach, it would be for thin patients without much deep tissue ptosis yet with significant skin excess. In an overweight patient with ptotic deep soft tissues, a skin-only approach would be unlikely to provide a satisfactory result.

Theoretical advantages of a skin-only lift are that it is safe (with low risk of motor nerve injury), relatively easy to perform, and the downtime is short. Potential disadvantages are that even where early results are pleasing, longevity of the effects may be reduced.

There is no strong evidence to direct surgeons in their specific choice of face-lift technique because there is no robust evidence to prove one technique is better than another. Most surgeons choose one that works well in their hands, based on their training and personal experiences. Some senior surgeons have described their results over a career of plastic surgery and have reflected on the fact that a skin-only approach can provide results comparable to other techniques and that the additional risks of more complex procedures are not justified. The skin is a powerful tool to manipulate in a number of ptotic structures and forms part of direct brow lift, neck lift, mastopexy, abdominoplasty, brachioplasty, and thigh lift, so it must not be underestimated. It just should be remembered that ideally deeper soft-tissue bony layers should be repositioned and the skin used as a secondary rather than a primary elevator of the aged face.[1-3]

REFERENCES

1. Gonyon DL Jr, Barton FE Jr. The aging face: rhytidectomy and adjunctive procedures. Sel Read Plast Surg 2012
2. Hoefflin SM. The extended supraplatysmal plane (ESP) face lift. Plast Reconstr Surg 1998;101(2):494–503
3. Barrett DM, Casanueva FJ, Wang TD. Evolution of the rhytidectomy. World J Otorhinolaryngol Head Neck Surg 2016;2(1):38–44

MINIMAL ACCESS CRANIAL SUSPENSION FACE LIFT (MACS-LIFT)

7. A patient comes to clinic for a second opinion to discuss face-lift procedures, having been offered MACS-lift by another clinician. *Which one of the following is true of this procedure?*

C. It carries a theoretical risk of compression damage to facial nerve branches.

The MACS-lift is a popular supra-SMAS plication technique that uses continuous purse-string sutures placed within the SMAS to elevate the face and neck in a vertical vector. Plication techniques in general are used to tighten the SMAS layer and avoid reliance on skin to hold the required lift. A perceived advantage of SMAS plication compared with other SMAS manipulation techniques is that sub-SMAS dissection is avoided and therefore the risk of facial nerve damage is decreased. However, risk of facial nerve damage is still present because the SMAS is not elevated, and therefore the sutures passed to tighten the SMAS are done so blindly in relation to facial nerve branches. Consequently, branches of the facial nerve may be inadvertently caught within the suture. Intraoperatively, it is therefore important to ensure sutures are placed superficially through the SMAS and recognize any mimetic muscle twitches during passing of this suture. If there is any doubt that the suture may have contacted or compressed a facial nerve branch, it should be removed and replaced.[1]

MACS stands for "minimal access cranial suspension" because it uses a short scar (not an endoscopic) approach and elevates soft tissues vertically/cranially. A lateral SMASectomy elevates facial tissues parallel to the nasolabial fold and involves excision of a small patch of SMAS over the parotid. Techniques that involve elevation and resection of the SMAS are termed deep plane techniques and include low and high SMAS approaches, where both subcutaneous and sub-SMAS planes are elevated and SMAS is secured in a posterior and vertical direction.[2,3]

REFERENCES

1. Tonnard PL, Verpaele AM. The MACS-Lift: Short-Scar Rhytidectomy. St Louis: Quality Medical Publishing; 2004
2. Verpaele A, Tonnard P, Gaia S, Guerao FP, Pirayesh A. The third suture in MACS-lifting: making midface-lifting simple and safe. J Plast Reconstr Aesthet Surg 2007;60(12):1287–1295
3. Tonnard PL, Verpaele A, Gaia S. Optimising results from minimal access cranial suspension lifting (MACS-lift). Aesthetic Plast Surg 2005;29(4):213–220, discussion 221

MINIMAL ACCESS CRANIAL SUSPENSION FACE LIFT (MACS-LIFT)

8. You are undertaking a MACS-lift on a 50-year-old patient who wishes to address the jowls, the neck/jawline, and the midface with a single procedure. *Intraoperatively which one of the following is true in this case?*

B. The suspension will be anchored to the deep temporal fascia just above the zygomatic arch.

The MACS-lift is a vertical vector face lift with short scars and SMAS suspension without SMAS elevation or resection. It involves raising subcutaneous skin flaps around a preauricular incision passing from the lobule to the temporal hairline. Dissection proceeds anteriorly and inferiorly in the subcutaneous plane to allow access to the underlying SMAS in the face and neck. The original technique described placement of two continuous purse-string sutures placed within the SMAS, both anchored to the deep temporal fascia (DTF) just above the zygomatic arch. The first of the two sutures is placed in a U-shaped loop commencing at the DTF passing in front of the ear vertically down into the neck ensuring bites of platysma are incorporated. A U-turn is then made and the continuous suture passed vertically upward approximately 1 cm in front of the descending line to be completed and tied at the level of DTF. A second suture is passed toward the nasolabial fold from the same DTF location, but this time with a more oval rather than U-shaped purse-string shape loop. For many patients, this combination of sutures will be sufficient to achieve a nice shape to the neck and jowls. If as in this case, the patient wishes to address the midface, a third optional suture may be indicated. This would be passed in a small loop just posterior to the orbital rim in order to lift the midface soft tissues and support them onto periosteum of the zygomatic arch.

Suture selection for this procedure is personal choice but most would advocate a permanent suture to maintain the lift. There is debate between monofilament and braided alternatives. The benefit of a monofilament is reduced risk of infection but increased risk of loosening. In contrast a braided suture (such as Ethibond) will be less likely to loosen but carries a greater risk of infection or extrusion. When performing this surgery, it is possible to vary the vectors of the SMAS and skin relative to one another. Overall modifications of this technique remain very popular with many surgeons, as the results are reliable and reproducible, the risks are relatively low, and the technique is straightforward to master. Many surgeons will use this SMAS suspension with varied skin incision lengths based on the skin extent required for removal.[1-3]

REFERENCES

1. Tonnard PL, Verpaele AM. The MACS-Lift: Short-Scar Rhytidectomy. St Louis: Quality Medical Publishing; 2004
2. Verpaele A, Tonnard P, Gaia S, Guerao FP, Pirayesh A. The third suture in MACS-lifting: making midface-lifting simple and safe. J Plast Reconstr Aesthet Surg 2007;60(12):1287–1295
3. Tonnard PL, Verpaele A, Gaia S. Optimising results from minimal access cranial suspension lifting (MACS-lift). Aesthetic Plast Surg 2005;29(4):213–220, discussion 221

THE SKOOG FACE LIFT

9. What was the main limitation of the face-lift technique originally described by Skoog?

C. It failed to improve the nasolabial folds.

Skoog described a technique for face lifting in 1974[1] that involved elevation of the skin and SMAS as a single unit, advancing the entire skin-SMAS unit posteriorly onto the cheek and neck. The main limitation of this technique was that it failed to address the nasolabial folds and anterior neck. Hamra[2] later modified this approach to better treat the nasolabial folds. His "composite" technique incorporates the lower lid orbicularis muscle into the single dissected soft-tissue unit. Each of these techniques has a robust blood supply to the skin because it is elevated in conjunction with the SMAS, rather than as a separate layer independent of it. Results are long lasting as the SMAS is able to support the elevated soft tissues. Skin excess can be managed as required with these techniques.[2]

REFERENCES

1. Skoog T, ed. Plastic Surgery: New Methods and Refinements. Philadelphia: WB Saunders; 1974
2. Hamra ST. Composite rhytidectomy. Plast Reconstr Surg 1992;90(1):1–13

THE DEEP PLANE FACE LIFT

10. In which plane of dissection would a deep plane face lift be performed?

B. Sub-SMAS

Face-lift procedures can be categorized by the plane of dissection. Common dissection planes for face lifts are subcutaneous and sub-SMAS. Less commonly, subperiosteal and supraperiosteal planes are used. The term "deep plane" refers to a sub-SMAS dissection and this is performed so that the SMAS can be elevated and resuspended to provide support for redraped soft tissues such as skin, fat, and muscle. The intended benefit is to obtain long-term support for the face lift without reliance on skin fixation alone. Many, but not all, deep plane techniques also involve separate subcutaneous dissection, so that skin and SMAS layers can be moved with different vectors. This means that SMAS can be elevated and fixed in a more vertical or diagonally vertical direction, while skin can be elevated and fixed in a more posterior and vertical direction. Deep plane face lifts can be either low SMAS or high SMAS. This relates to the craniocaudal dissection in relation to the zygomatic arch, respectively. A low

SMAS technique will, in theory, treat the lower face but not affect the midface, perioral, or infraorbital tissues. A high SMAS technique should be able to do both areas as the malar fat pad can be elevated.[1-4]

REFERENCES

1. Barton FE Jr. Rhytidectomy and the nasolabial fold. Plast Reconstr Surg 1992;90(4):601–607
2. Nahai F, ed. The Art of Aesthetic Surgery: Principles and Techniques. St Louis: Quality Medical Publishing; 2005
3. Jacono A, Bryant LM. Extended deep plane facelift: incorporating facial retaining ligament release and composite flap shifts to maximize midface, jawline and neck rejuvenation. Clin Plast Surg 2018;45(4):527–554
4. Jacono AA. A novel volumizing extended deep-plane facelift: using composite flap shifts to volumize the midface and jawline. Facial Plast Surg Clin North Am 2020;28(3):331–368

SUBPERIOSTEAL FACE LIFTS

11. What is the main perceived advantage of using a subperiosteal approach to face lifting?

D. A reduced risk of facial palsy

The subperiosteal approach to face lifting involves elevation of the midface periosteum as a single unit and then redraping of the composite face to achieve tissue repositioning. The main perceived advantage is that the facial nerve and its branches are protected because dissection is deep to them. A further advantage is that visible scarring can be minimized by using temporal and intraoral approaches. There are, however, a number of disadvantages to this technique. First, it is technically difficult and may need to be performed using endoscopic techniques. This can make for a steep learning curve, particularly for surgeons not used to working on the bony facial skeleton nor using the endoscope regularly. Second, it does not allow for skin and fat excesses to be treated; so, it is less effective at managing skin redundancy of the nasolabial folds, jawline, and neck compared with other techniques.[1,2]

REFERENCES

1. Tessier P. [Subperiosteal face-lift]. Ann Chir Plast Esthet 1989;34(3):193–197
2. Gonyon DL Jr, Barton FE Jr. The aging face: rhytidectomy and adjunctive procedures. Sel Read Plast Surg 2012

THE AGING LIP

12. Which one of the following changes would be expected when examining the upper lip of an elderly patient during an aesthetic consultation?

E. Decreased dental show

The upper lip becomes longer and less full with increasing age; so, there is decreased dental show. Because a long upper lip is characteristic of aging, techniques have been developed to address this. The appearance of a long upper lip can be improved using a vermillion advancement technique. However, this does leave a visible scar on the lip margin. Alternatively, the lip height can be shortened by using a skin incision at the base of the nose which effectively hides the scar at the lip–nose interface. Lip volume can be enhanced using fillers such as hyaluronic acid and autologous fat grafting. This also addresses the decreased (not increased) vermillion exposure characteristic of the aging lip. The oral commissure does not specificity alter with age.[1]

REFERENCE

1. Gonyon DL Jr, Barton FE Jr. The aging face: rhytidectomy and adjunctive procedures. Sel Read Plast Surg 2012

FAT INJECTION FOR FACIAL REJUVENATION

13. You are undertaking a face and neck lift with submental liposuction and the patient asks if it is possible to enhance the malar and nasolabial regions with fat taken from the chin at the same time. Which one of the following is true in this case?

B. Injection of fat in this scenario should be placed deeply with a slight overcorrection.

Fat injection is a popular technique used predominantly in the head, neck, and breast regions following reconstruction or as part of a rejuvenation procedure. It can help restore age-associated volume loss and improve skin appearance. Advantages of fat over other injectable materials are that it is autologous and relatively permanent. In this scenario, fat is being harvested from the neck anyway, so it would be reasonable to recycle and redistribute this soft-tissue volume by reinjection at the sites requested by the patient. Disadvantages are that fat does resorb over time so the injection process may need to be repeated. It is safe to combine this with a face lift, bearing in mind that fat requires a well-vascularized recipient site. Fat can be placed in the lips, nasolabial folds, chin, jawline, tear trough, malar region, and periorbicular areas. When injecting with fat, it is standard practice to overcorrect the defect on the understanding that once swelling has gone and some of the fat has resorbed, the result will still be satisfactory. The resorption following fat injection can be unpredictable, but most surgeons anticipate up to 50% loss.

Deep nasolabial folds and midface volume loss have been treated by various techniques and there is no single best technique for either of them. A sub-SMAS face lift that goes through the SMAS medially to the subcutaneous plane at the level of the belly of the zygomaticus major muscle can stretch the nasolabial fold if sufficient tension is placed on the anterior cheek skin. Alternatively, dermal attachments of the fold can be released and filled with fat or dermal fat grafts. Malar augmentation can be provided by implants, fillers (fat, hydroxyapatite, hyaluronic acid), or autologous tissues (e.g., SMAS). Improved malar fullness and nasolabial contour can be achieved with a midface lift via a transblepharoplasty approach and suspension of deep structures to the lateral orbital periosteum.[1-3]

REFERENCES

1. Nahai F, ed. The Art of Aesthetic Surgery: Principles and Techniques. St Louis: Quality Medical Publishing; 2005
2. Molina-Burbano F, Smith JM, Ingargiola MJ, et al. Fat grafting to improve results of facelift: systematic review of safety and effectiveness of current treatment paradigms. Aesthet Surg J 2021;41(1):1–12
3. Schreiber JE, Terner J, Stern CS, et al. The boomerang lift: a three-step compartment-based approach to the youthful cheek. Plast Reconstr Surg 2018;141(4):910–913

PERIOPERATIVE MANAGEMENT FOR RHYTIDECTOMY

14. A female patient comes to the clinic to discuss a face-lift procedure. She is 40 years old and recently separated from her long-term partner. She smokes 10 cigarettes per day and takes a range of herbal medications. She takes regular analgesics for lower back pain, but no other prescription drugs. *When assessing this woman for a face lift, which one of the following is correct?*

C. **She would need to undertake smoking cessation before treatment.**

Smoking is a contraindication to a face lift, and the incidence of skin slough is much higher than 5% among smokers with a sub-SMAS technique. Their risk is estimated to be 12 times greater than non-smokers.[1] Therefore, patients should be advised to stop smoking before face-lift surgery. Because this woman has recently separated from her partner, there is a risk that this is the trigger for her desire to have a face lift, and it may be a poor time for her to proceed with this surgery. Recent major life changes and social instability are red flags to proceeding with some plastic surgical procedures. Patients need to be fully supported in the preoperative meetings to ensure they are undergoing the right procedure for them at the right time in their life. In this case, she is also relatively young to need or want her first face lift. As with any cosmetic procedure, unrealistic expectations must be assessed, and if that is determined to be the case, surgery should be avoided. A consult with a clinical psychologist preoperatively is strongly advised given the above. The risk of bleeding during and immediately after a face lift should be minimized, and many herbal medications can increase bleeding or negatively affect wound healing. Her regular analgesics may include nonsteroidal anti-inflammatory drugs that can also increase bleeding risk.

REFERENCE

1. Rees TD, Liverett DM, Guy CL. The effect of cigarette smoking on skin-flap survival in the face lift patient. Plast Reconstr Surg 1984;73(6):911–915

POSTOPERATIVE MANAGEMENT FOLLOWING RHYTIDECTOMY

15. You are asked to see a patient in recovery after a face lift. On examination, he has visible unilateral swelling overlying the mandibular border and neck. The neck drain is empty. Blood pressure has been well maintained at 125 mm Hg systolic. *What is your next step in the management of this patient?*

D. **Return the patient to the operating room**

A hematoma is a common early complication following a face lift, occurring in 2 to 3% of female patients and 8% of male patients. Although it may be prudent to release the suture line if there is an area of vascularly compromised skin, it would be better to promptly return to the operating room to ensure formal evacuation of the hematoma and hemostasis. The patient in this scenario has maintained a stable and appropriate blood pressure, so no action for this needs to be taken. In rebound hypertension, intravenous chlorpromazine at 1 and 3 hours after surgery can be very effective. Other options include clonidine or labetalol. Discussion with the anesthesiologist is advised in such circumstances. In this case, they are not warranted, as blood pressure is satisfactory and the hematoma has already occurred. Small hematomas may be left to resolve spontaneously or drained a few days after surgery, once they have liquefied.[1-5]

REFERENCES

1. Baker DC, Stefani WA, Chiu ES. Reducing the incidence of hematoma requiring surgical evacuation following male rhytidectomy: a 30-year review of 985 cases. Plast Reconstr Surg 2005;116(7):1973–1985, discussion 1986–1987
2. Jones BM, Grover R. Avoiding hematoma in cervicofacial rhytidectomy: a personal 8-year quest. Reviewing 910 patients. Plast Reconstr Surg 2004;113(1):381–387, discussion 388–390
3. Por YC, Shi L, Samuel M, Song C, Yeow VK. Use of tissue sealants in face-lifts: a metaanalysis. Aesthetic Plast Surg 2009;33(3):336–339
4. Baker DC, Aston SJ, Guy CL, Rees TD. The male rhytidectomy. Plast Reconstr Surg 1977;60(4):514–522
5. Jones BM, Grover R, Hamilton S. The efficacy of surgical drainage in cervicofacial rhytidectomy: a prospective, randomized, controlled trial. Plast Reconstr Surg 2007;120(1):263–270

COMPLICATIONS IN FACE-LIFT SURGERY

16. When discussing informed consent with a patient for a face lift, which one of the following represents the most common early complication?

C. **Hematoma**

The most common complication during or after a face lift is hematoma. It is most likely to occur within the first 24 hours. The risk can be minimized by meticulous intraoperative hemostasis and careful perioperative blood pressure control. The reported rate is about 2 or 3% in women and 8% in men. Other avenues to reduce this risk are commonsense and include patient selection, systemic factors, and intraoperative techniques.

The first step to minimizing hematoma is patient selection. Patients with uncontrolled hypertension should not be booked for face lifting surgery. It is reasonable to discuss face lifts and a patient's suitability for this, but surgery should be deferred until blood pressure is well controlled. Patients who require anticoagulants such as Plavix, Rivaroxaban, or Coumadin are likely to have additional health risks anyway and stopping their medications may be unwise. These patients should generally be discouraged from undergoing face lifting surgery, as their risks of bleeding or other postoperative complications maybe high. Herbal supplements which can affect bleeding should also be stopped. Once you and your patient have committed to surgery, intraoperative steps to minimize bleeding include stable, normotensive blood pressure throughout and meticulous hemostasis. Avoiding rebound hypertension postoperatively needs to be achieved. Postoperative management is also important and the patient should be nursed with the head elevated and the patient must be advised to avoid stooping or straining for the first 48 to 72 hours.

Neck drains are used by many, but not by all surgeons and these can be helpful at removing fluid from the neck but won't themselves be a substitute for adequate hemostasis. Other surgeons use fibrin sealants at wound closure, but these again are unlikely to stop a hematoma while they may reduce bruising and overall drainage. Use of epinephrine should be with caution as rebound bleeding can occur. However, the benefits of a clear surgical field by using the outweigh the risk on most cases.

The other complications listed are common but less than that of hematomas. Altered sensation to the lobule represents injury to the greater auricular nerve and is the most common nerve injury in face lifting (approximately 7%). Facial nerve weakness is much less common (<1%) and tends to be transient. Infection and skin slough tend to be associated with patients who have other comorbidities such as smoking or diabetes and specific techniques.[1-3]

REFERENCES

1. Baker DC, Conley J. Avoiding facial nerve injuries in rhytidectomy. Anatomical variations and pitfalls. Plast Reconstr Surg 1979;64(6):781–795
2. Stuzin JM. MOC-PSSM CME article: face lifting. Plast Reconstr Surg 2008;121(1, Suppl):1–19
3. Jones BM, Grover R. Avoiding hematoma in cervicofacial rhytidectomy: a personal 8-year quest. Reviewing 910 patients. Plast Reconstr Surg 2004;113(1):381–387, discussion 388–390

PERIOPERATIVE MANAGEMENT OF RHYTIDECTOMY PATIENTS

17. When planning perioperative care for a patient undergoing a face lift, which one of the following is most likely to lower the risk of hematoma formation?

D. **Tumescent infiltration with saline solution after induction**

Jones and Grover[1] reported that tumescent infiltration of around 200 mL per side without epinephrine reduced the rate of postoperative hematomas without significantly increasing wound bleeding or facial edema.

The use of drains will not lower the risk of hematoma formation but can reduce postoperative bruising. Many surgeons use fibrin glue under the skin flaps, but there is no evidence to show that this action actually reduces hematoma occurrence either. Preoperative injection of epinephrine may limit early intraoperative bleeding but could lead to a rebound effect part way through the case. Prophylactic administration of low-molecular-weight heparin may increase postoperative bleeding without decreasing the risk of venous thrombosis.

REFERENCE

1. Jones BM, Grover R. Avoiding hematoma in cervicofacial rhytidectomy: a personal 8-year quest. Reviewing 910 patients. Plast Reconstr Surg 2004;113(1):381–387, discussion 388–390

STIGMATA OF FACE LIFTS

18. A patient is seen before a face lift and is noted to have marked submalar hollowing. *What are the deformities that are at increased risk of developing after rhytidectomy?*

   B. Joker's lines

   Face lifting can lead to unnatural appearances if the lift is performed with incorrect or inappropriate vectors and preexisting deformities may be amplified. For example, Joker's lines were described by Lambros and Stuzin[1] and refer to the appearance of the oral commissure extending onto the cheek following a face lift. This is a potential sequela of performing a face lift in a patient who has submalar hollowing preoperatively. Prevention of this deformity requires careful patient selection and for those with submalar hollowing, a more limited SMAS and skin release in combination with a more subtle vertical lift should be performed. Established Joker's lines are difficult to treat but may be improved by fat-transfer procedures.

   Hamra introduced the term "lateral sweep" caused by an excess of lateral pull in the lower face without treatment of the midface.[2] This allows natural descent from aging over time to sag over the lateral pleat in the lower face. It can be avoided by using vectors that provide a more vertical lift and avoid excessive lateral tightening, while ensuring that the midface is adequately supported. Smile blocks have been described as hypodynamic cheek mounds that do not move appropriately with animation and these may be improved with fat transfer. A pixie-ear deformity may arise from distortion of the lobule because of excessive tension on the skin flap. It can be minimized by securing SMAS to the postauricular region (mastoid) in order to minimize caudal pull on the lobule. Hairline distortion can generally be avoided by thoughtful incision placement and then ensuring that skin is not excessively removed and that tension during closure is minimized.

REFERENCES

1. Lambros V, Stuzin JM. The cross-cheek depression: surgical cause and effect in the development of the "joker line" and its treatment. Plast Reconstr Surg 2008;122(5):1543–1552
2. Hamra ST. Frequent face lift sequelae: hollow eyes and the lateral sweep: cause and repair. Plast Reconstr Surg 1998;102(5):1658–1666

SECONDARY FACE LIFTS

19. *Which one of the following is true when considering secondary face lifts?*

   E. The risk of facial nerve damage is likely to be increased when performing sub-SMAS approaches.

   It is not uncommon for patients to present requesting their second or third face lift procedure. The timing of this can vary and the average duration between the primary and secondary face lift in one large series was 9 years.[1] In most cases, it probably is around the 10-year mark and this is something to discuss with patients preoperatively when considering their first procedure. Patients may seek secondary face lifts not only to treat the natural aging process but also deal with an unfavorable result or a combination of the two. Preexisting deficits in sensation and facial animation must be identified and documented thoroughly. Though it is prudent to obtain the surgical report from the patient's previous operation, it often is not available, and this should not preclude surgery.

   From a technical perspective, some things need to be considered when undertaking secondary face lift. As with all secondary procedures, the natural tissue planes will have been disrupted and the presence of scarring can complicate the procedure. Because of this, sub-SMAS dissection may increase the risk of facial nerve damage and patients must be advised of this. The SMAS is generally thinner in secondary face lifts and some of this may have been excised or imbricated. The skin flaps are probably more robust, if anything, having been elevated before. Secondary face lift may be an ideal opportunity to correct some of the stigmata of face lifts if these are present, e.g., pixie ears, smile blocks, or poor scars.[1,2]

REFERENCES

1. Rasko YM, Beale E, Rohrich RJ. Secondary rhytidectomy: comprehensive review and current concepts. Plast Reconstr Surg 2012;130(6):1370–1378
2. Beale EW, Rasko Y, Rohrich RJ. A 20-year experience with secondary rhytidectomy: a review of technique, longevity, and outcomes. Plast Reconstr Surg 2013;131(3):625–634

113. Neck Lift

See *Essentials of Plastic Surgery*, third edition, pp. 1580–1601

ANATOMY OF THE NECK

1. **Which one of the following is true regarding the platysma?**
   A. The origin is the lower border of the mandible.
   B. It represents a continuation of the deep cervical fascia.
   C. The dominant blood supply arises from the suprasternal artery.
   D. Motor innervation is received from the cervical plexus.
   E. Most commonly, the right and left sides interdigitate.

THE MARGINAL MANDIBULAR BRANCH OF THE FACIAL NERVE

2. **When performing surgery in the neck, which one of the following statements is true regarding the marginal mandibular nerve?**
   A. It normally travels 1 cm below the lower mandibular border throughout its course.
   B. It can be identified in the supraplatysmal plane as it passes anteromedially across the neck.
   C. Iatrogenic damage is unlikely to occur during neck rejuvenation surgery, as the nerve is away from the operative field.
   D. Inadvertent nerve transection will cause denervation of the platysma, risorius, and lower lip depressors.
   E. The nerve is most at risk of damage within a circle with a 2-cm radius, 2-cm inferior and posterior to the oral commissure.

RELATIONS OF THE GREAT AURICULAR NERVE

3. **On which muscle does the great auricular nerve travel 6 cm inferior to the external auditory canal?**
   A. Platysma
   B. Sternocleidomastoid
   C. Trapezius
   D. Splenius capitis
   E. Posterior scalene

THE DIGASTRIC MUSCLES

4. **What do the two bellies of digastric have in common?**
   A. The same nerve supply
   B. A similar length
   C. A shared central tendon
   D. An origin on the mandible
   E. An insertion on the mastoid

RETAINING LIGAMENTS OF THE FACE AND NECK

5. **You are assessing a patient in clinic before neck rejuvenation surgery. They are concerned regarding soft-tissue overhang beyond the lower border of the mandible, just lateral to the chin. *Tethering of which ligament is responsible for this appearance?***
   A. Mandibulo-cutaneous
   B. Platysma-auricular
   C. Masseteric-cutaneous
   D. Zygomatico-cutaneous
   E. Mandibulo-auricular

FAT CONTENTS WITHIN THE NECK

6. **Which one of the following sites normally contains the greatest volume of fat within the neck and lower face and is the primary target for liposuction when recontouring this area?**
   A. Jowl fat
   B. Supraplatysmal fat
   C. Subplatysmal fat
   D. Periauricular fat
   E. Central chin fat

CLINICAL ASSESSMENT OF THE NECK

7. **When examining the neck of a young, healthy patient in clinic, the outline of which one of the following should normally be visible?**
   A. The submandibular gland
   B. The thyroid gland
   C. The digastric muscle
   D. The sternocleidomastoid muscle
   E. The hyoid bone

NONSURGICAL MANAGEMENT OF THE NECK

8. You see a patient in the office requesting improvement in chin/neck contour definition which is lacking due to fat excess. *Which one of the following treatments should be considered as an alternative to undergoing submental liposuction in this case?*
   A. Ulthera
   B. Kybella
   C. Vobella
   D. Botulinum toxin
   E. Triamcinolone

SELECTION OF SURGICAL PROCEDURES IN NECK REJUVENATION

9. You see a 63-year-old, mildly obese woman with loss of neck contour and jowling. She has a large excess of neck skin and fat with prominent platysmal banding at rest. *Which one of the following surgical procedures is most likely to be optimal for her?*
   A. Liposuction alone
   B. Submental neck lift
   C. Isolated neck lift
   D. Short scar neck lift with liposuction
   E. Full scar face and neck lift with liposuction

SELECTION OF SURGICAL PROCEDURES IN NECK REJUVENATION

10. You see a 39-year-old woman with excellent skin quality and moderate submental fat excess. She has no platysmal banding at rest, but banding becomes apparent on animation. A skin pinch test reveals no alteration in pinch size on animation. *Which one of the following surgical procedures is most likely to be optimal for her?*
   A. Liposuction only
   B. Submental neck lift
   C. Submental neck lift with liposuction
   D. Short-scar face and neck lift
   E. Full-scar face and neck lift

LIPOSUCTION OF THE NECK

11. **When performing suction-assisted liposuction to the neck in a patient with submental fat excess, which one of the following is correct?**
   A. A single-access point should be used.
   B. A 7-mm multihole cannula should be used.
   C. Subplatysmal fat volumes should be cautiously reduced.
   D. Small quantities of aspirate will normally provide satisfactory results.
   E. Drains and compression garments should be used.

SUBMENTAL NECK LIFT

12. **When considering the submental approach to neck lift, which one of the following is true?**
   A. It is primarily indicated to address skin excess.
   B. It avoids the need for liposuction.
   C. It facilitates access to allow platysmal plication.
   D. The incision should be placed within the submental crease.
   E. A lateral incision is most often also required.

DIFFERENT TYPES OF NECK LIFT

13. **Which one of the following is a key technical difference between performing an isolated neck lift and a combined face and neck lift?**
   A. The primary plane of dissection
   B. The risk of sensory nerve damage
   C. The need for adjunctive liposuction
   D. The length of periauricular scars
   E. The need for a submental incision

ADJUNCTIVE PROCEDURES DURING NECK REJUVENATION

14. *Which one of the following is most commonly performed during correction of the deep plane (deep to the platysma) in neck rejuvenation?*
    A. Full resection of the anterior belly of the digastric muscle
    B. Extracapsular excision of the deep lobe of submandibular gland
    C. Resection of subplatysmal and interplatysmal fat
    D. Excision of suprahyoid fascia to improve the cervical angle
    E. Resection of multiple central lymph nodes

PLATYSMAL PROCEDURES IN NECK REJUVENATION

15. You see a patient after previous aesthetic surgery to the neck. On examination she has a visible transverse step in the neck and a window shading effect. *Which one of the procedures has most likely been undertaken?*
    A. Platysma flap
    B. Suspension sutures
    C. Corset platysmaplasty
    D. Platysma muscle sling
    E. Percutaneous platysma myotomy

POSTOPERATIVE COMPLICATIONS FOLLOWING NECK REJUVENATION

16. A patient referred to you has undergone neck rejuvenation at another clinic and is dissatisfied with the appearance of her neck contour. On examination, she has an irregular contour with thin, visible bilateral bulges and adjacent hollowing in the anterior aspect of the neck just below the mandible. *What is the most likely explanation for this appearance?*
    A. Dehiscence of platysma plication
    B. Excessive submental liposuction
    C. Inadequate resection of the submandibular gland
    D. Excessive botulinum toxin use
    E. Excessive resection of the digastric muscles

NERVE INJURY IN NECK LIFTS

17. A patient undergoes a neck lift and subsequently develops symptoms of a marginal mandibular nerve injury. *Which one of the following is true in this case?*
    A. The patient should be taken back to the operating room to explore the nerve and decompress or repair it, if necessary.
    B. The patient will display lower lip paralysis due to the triad of mentalis, depressor anguli oris, and buccinator weakness.
    C. On clinical examination, the injury is indistinguishable from a complex cervical branch injury.
    D. While waiting for recovery to occur, neurotoxin may be injected into the contralateral depressor anguli inferioris.
    E. A full recovery would be expected within 72 hours, so no action needs to be taken.

Answers

ANATOMY OF THE NECK

1. *Which one of the following is true regarding the platysma?*

   E. Most commonly, the right and left sides interdigitate.

   The platysma is a broad, thin muscle situated in the subcutaneous plane of the neck that is a key instrument for controlling neck and lower face contour. It originates from the pectoralis and deltoid fascia caudally, with insertions to the mandibular symphysis and superficial musculoaponeurotic system (SMAS) cranially. It receives its main blood supply from the submental artery, which is a branch of the facial artery, and receives a secondary supply from the suprasternal artery. Innervation is from the facial nerve (cervical branch), not the cervical plexus. The platysma is not a continuation of the deep cervical fascia, which, instead, lies beneath it. Three different anatomic patterns related to its decussation were described by de Castro[1] in 50 patients (**Fig. 113.1**). Type I was most common (75%), in which limited decussation of the muscles for 1 to 2 cm below the mandibular symphysis was present. In type II, the decussation was more extensive and passed down to the thyroid cartilage. In type III, no decussation was present. A subsequent anatomic study was undertaken by Kim et al[2] in 70 Korean patients; this showed that subtypes I and II were equally common (43% each), and this may reflect racial differences. The benefit of a midline decussation is the provision of a supportive sling without which the free medial edges of the muscle can fall away laterally creating vertical platysmal bands.

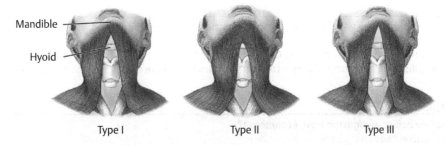

Mandible

Hyoid

Type I   Type II   Type III

Fig. 113.1 Three anatomic patterns of the neck. *A*, Type I is most common and occurs in 75% of individuals. This type demonstrates a limited decussation of the platysma muscles, extending 1 to 2 cm below the mandibular symphysis. *B*, Type II occurs in 15% and demonstrates decussation of the platysma from the mandibular symphysis to the thyroid cartilage. *C*, Type III occurs in 10% and demonstrates no decussation or interdigitations.

REFERENCES

1. de Castro CC. The anatomy of the platysma muscle. Plast Reconstr Surg 1980;66(5):680–683
2. Kim HJ, Hu KS, Kang MK, Hwang K, Chung IH. Decussation patterns of the platysma in Koreans. Br J Plast Surg 2001;54(5):400–402

THE MARGINAL MANDIBULAR BRANCH OF THE FACIAL NERVE

2. *When performing surgery in the neck, which one of the following statements is true regarding the marginal mandibular nerve?*

   E. The nerve is most at risk of damage within a circle with a 2-cm radius, 2-cm inferior and posterior to the oral commissure.

   The marginal mandibular nerve is at risk of damage during neck rejuvenation procedures and neck dissection surgery. The danger zone is usually within a circle of 2-cm radius, located 2-cm posterior and inferior to the oral commissure overlying the lower border of the mandible. This region corresponds to where the facial vessels cross the lower mandibular border and the nerve. The marginal mandibular nerve originates from the lower division of the facial nerve and passes close by the tail of the parotid, from lateral to anteromedial in the subplatysmal plane. It is important to remember this, as any subplatysmal dissection in the region of the lower mandibular border can risk iatrogenic damage. The nerve travels close to the lower border of the mandible and most commonly runs above the lower border throughout its course, although this can change with advancing age. Before the point at which it crosses the facial vessels, it runs above the inferior border in more than 80% of cases. Beyond the facial vessels, all of its branches are above the inferior border. The marginal mandibular nerve innervates the lower lip depressors, the risorius, and part of the orbicularis oris. It does not usually innervate the platysma, as this is innervated by the cervical branches. Injury to it leads to weakness of the lower lip with an inability to evert the lips.[1-3]

REFERENCES

1. Yang HM, Kim HJ, Park HW, et al. Revisiting the topographic anatomy of the marginal mandibular branch of facial nerve relating to the surgical approach. Aesthet Surg J 2016;36(9):977–982
2. Atlas of Human Anatomy. 5th ed. Summit, NJ: CIBA-GEIGY; 2010
3. Seckel BR. Facial Danger Zones: Avoiding Nerve Injury in Facial Plastic Surgery. 2nd ed. St. Louis, MO: Quality Medical Publishing; 2010: xi, 52p

RELATIONS OF THE GREAT AURICULAR NERVE

3. *On which muscle does the great auricular nerve travel 6 cm inferior to the external auditory canal?*

   B. Sternocleidomastoid

   The great auricular nerve is at risk of damage during neck-lift and face-lift surgery. The main danger zone is located within a circle with a 3-cm radius dropped approximately 6.5 cm inferior to the external auditory canal. This corresponds to the midpoint of the sternocleidomastoid (SCM) muscle and the nerve emerges beneath the SCM just below this site, which is also known as McKinney's point. This nerve supplies sensation to the lobule of the ear via its lobular branch as well as the lower anterior and posterior aspects of the ear. It is the most commonly injured nerve during a face lift because of its superficial location; so, it is important to discuss this possibility with patients preoperatively.[1-3]

REFERENCES

1. Seckel BR. Facial Danger Zones: Avoiding Nerve Injury in Facial Plastic Surgery. 2nd ed. St. Louis, MO: Quality Medical Publishing; 2010:xi, 52p
2. Atlas of Human Anatomy. 5th ed. Summit, NJ: CIBA-GEIGY; 2010
3. McKinney P, Katrana DJ. Prevention of injury to the great auricular nerve during rhytidectomy. Plast Reconstr Surg 1980;66(5):675–679

THE DIGASTRIC MUSCLES

4. *What do the two bellies of digastric have in common?*

   C. A shared central tendon

   The digastric muscle is so named because it has two heads. Each of these has a different bony origin (anterior belly originates from the mandibular symphysis; posterior belly originates from the mastoid process), but they share a central tendon. The posterior belly is longer than the anterior belly and together they form the lower border of the submandibular triangle. Embryologically they originate from different branchial arches and so have different motor innervation. The anterior digastric develops from the first arch and has trigeminal innervation. The posterior digastric develops from the second arch and has facial nerve innervation. The digastric muscles are sometimes addressed during neck surgery to debulk them if they are overly prominent.[1-4]

REFERENCES

1. Baker DC. Face lift with submandibular gland and digastric muscle resection: radical neck rhytidectomy. Aesthet Surg J 2006;26(1):85–92
2. Connell BF, Shamoun JM. The significance of digastric muscle contouring for rejuvenation of the submental area of the face. Plast Reconstr Surg 1997;99(6):1586–1590
3. Nahai F, ed. The Art of Aesthetic Surgery: Principles and Techniques. St Louis: Quality Medical Publishing; 2005
4. Feldman JJ. Neck lift my way: an update. Plast Reconstr Surg 2014;134(6):1173–1183

RETAINING LIGAMENTS OF THE FACE AND NECK

5. You are assessing a patient in clinic before neck rejuvenation surgery. They are concerned regarding soft-tissue overhang beyond the lower border of the mandible, just lateral to the chin. *Tethering of which ligament is responsible for this appearance?*

   A. Mandibulo-cutaneous

   Tethering of the mandibulo-cutaneous ligament produces the appearance of jowls. These can be assessed by inspection and palpation near the lower border of the mandible at the lateral edge of the chin. Assessment of jowl volume with the patient supine helps plan surgical intervention. An excess of soft tissue alone may be treated with liposuction, whereas laxity of the deeper soft tissues will require SMAS-platysma tightening. The masseteric-cutaneous ligament is also relevant to the formation of jowls, as this attenuates with age allowing ptosis of the midfacial tissues.

The platysma-auricular ligament is also relevant to neck-lift procedures because it marks the posterior extent of the platysma and also the site where the platysma is often anchored to provide elevation of the neck. Weakening of the zygomatico-cutaneous ligament causes downward migration of the malar soft tissues and creates redundant skin that hangs over the fixed nasolabial fold.[1-4]

REFERENCES

1. Furnas DW. The retaining ligaments of the cheek. Plast Reconstr Surg 1989;83(1):11–16
2. Lamb J, Surek C. Facial Volumization: An Anatomic Approach. 1st ed. New York, New York. Thieme Medical Publishers; 2017
3. Nahai F, ed. The Art of Aesthetic Surgery: Principles and Techniques. St Louis: Quality Medical Publishing; 2005
4. Alghoul M, Codner MA. Retaining ligaments of the face: review of anatomy and clinical applications. Aesthet Surg J 2013;33(6):769–782

FAT CONTENTS WITHIN THE NECK

6. *Which one of the following sites normally contains the greatest volume of fat within the neck and lower face and is the primary target for liposuction when recontouring this area?*

B. **Supraplatysmal fat**

Fat is located in a number of different subunit areas within the lower face and neck. The most inferior facial fat compartment is the jowl area and this is adherent to the depressor anguli oris, which forms the medial boundary of the compartment. The inferior border is formed by a membranous fusion of the platysma muscle.[1] Fat within the neck itself may be located above, below, or between the two platysma muscles. Supraplatysmal fat is bordered by the anterior border of mandible superiorly, the sternal notch inferiorly, and the anterior border of SCM laterally. It contains 45% of fat in the neck[1], approximately 14 to 15 g in many patients and is the primary target for liposuction.[2] The subplatysmal fat is bordered by the anterior border of mandible superiorly, thyroid cartilage inferiorly, and the anterior border of SCM laterally. It contains 31% of fat in the neck,[2] approximately 3.7 to 5.5 g and care must be taken if removing this fat, as over-resection here can lead to scarring between the platysma and mylohyoid muscle, causing a contour deformity which is difficult to correct. Furthermore, deeper liposuction between the two platysma muscles risks damage to the anterior jugular veins, which can cause significant bleeding and bruising (**Fig. 113.2**).[3]

There are five periauricular fat compartments relevant to the lower face and neck contour; these are the superior, middle, inferior, subauricular, and preauricular areas. The inferior and subauricular compartments are divided by the subauricular membrane, which can be an area of tethering in the lateral neck. The subauricular membrane is associated with the great auricular nerve.[4] There is no specific central chin compartment, and this would probably lie over mentalis between the jowl fat areas if it was described.

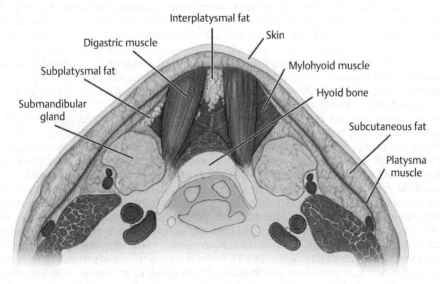

Fig. 113.2 Practical anatomy of the neck.

REFERENCES

1. Rohrich RJ, Pessa JE. The fat compartments of the face: anatomy and clinical implications for cosmetic surgery. Plast Reconstr Surg 2007;119(7):2219–2227, discussion 2228–2231
2. Larson JD, Tierney WS, Ozturk CN, Zins JE. Defining the fat compartments in the neck: a cadaver study. Aesthet Surg J 2014;34(4):499–506
3. Raveendran SS, Anthony DJ, Ion L. An anatomic basis for volumetric evaluation of the neck. Aesthet Surg J 2012;32(6):685–691
4. Narasimhan K, Stuzin JM, Rohrich RJ. Five-step neck lift: integrating anatomy with clinical practice to optimize results. Plast Reconstr Surg 2013;132(2):339–350

CLINICAL ASSESSMENT OF THE NECK

7. *When examining the neck of a young, healthy patient in clinic, the outline of which one of the following should normally be visible?*

   D. The sternocleidomastoid muscle

   When examining a normal neck, the SCM muscle should be visible at its anterior border. Ellenbogen and Karlin[1] classified features of the youthful neck that change with age. Features of a youthful neck involve a visible thyroid cartilage (not the thyroid gland), subhyoid depression (not the hyoid), and the inferior mandibular border. A normal cervicomental angle of between 105 and 120 degrees should also be observed. The submandibular gland and digastric muscle should not be visible. A bulge below the mandibular rim within the submandibular triangle may represent a ptotic or enlarged submandibular gland. Sometimes prominent digastric muscles may be observed bulging below the inferior mandibular border. This may only become apparent following neck rejuvenation.[1-3]

REFERENCES

1. Ellenbogen R, Karlin JV. Visual criteria for success in restoring the youthful neck. Plast Reconstr Surg 1980;66(6):826–837
2. Nahai F, ed. The Art of Aesthetic Surgery: Principles and Techniques. St Louis: Quality Medical Publishing; 2005
3. Matarasso A. Managing the components of the aging neck: from liposuction to submentalplasty, to neck lift. Clin Plast Surg 2014;41(1):85–98

NONSURGICAL MANAGEMENT OF THE NECK

8. You see a patient in the office requesting improvement in chin/neck contour definition which is lacking due to fat excess. *Which one of the following treatments should be considered as an alternative to undergoing submental liposuction in this case?*

   B. Kybella

   Patients commonly request treatments to the neck to improve its contour and this may be focusing on the skin, platysma, fat, or other deeper tissues. Traditionally, fat excesses have been treated with liposuction and this still remains a popular approach to the neck. However, there are nonsurgical alternatives that should be considered. Kybella is a preparation of deoxycholic acid that can be injected into the subcutaneous tissues in order to cause adipocytosis (fat dissolving). It should be injected in 0.2-mL aliquots spaced 1 to 1.5 cm apart in the preplatysmal, submental fat using a 30-gauge, 0.5-inch needle. It usually requires multiple treatment sessions (up to 6), spaced 1 month apart. Most patients experience a response within 2 to 4 treatments.[1] It should be avoided in patients with preplatysmal bands, skin laxity, prior submental surgery, dysphagia, or facial nerve paralysis. It can cause damage to the marginal branch of the facial nerve leading to lip and chin weakness and this must be discussed with the patient prior to treatment.

   Ulthera is a technique that uses microfocused ultrasound to tighten skin rather than deal with adipose tissue excess. It can cause thermally induced contracture of tissue in addition to stimulating collagen and elastin remodeling. It affects a very small area of dermis or SMAS but spares the epidermis. It is thought to work best in patients with a BMI < 30, although its use should not be kept exclusively for this patient group. Vobella is a type of hyaluronic acid that is used for superficial injections as a facial filler. It is commonly used for lip enhancement. This would add, not subtract, volume to the area. Botulinum toxin is used in the neck for management of platysmal bands, particularly where there is little or no skin excess. Up to 20 units of neurotoxin is typically injected per band. Potential complications include dysphagia at high doses, edema, ecchymosis, neck discomfort, and weakness. Use of neurotoxins in the neck should generally be reserved for patients with good skin elasticity and minimal submental fat. Otherwise, results may be indiscernible, and benefits outweighed by the risk of dysphagia. Triamcinolone is a glucocorticoid that is injected into the skin to soften scars (particularly hypertrophic or keloid types) or used to help musculoskeletal injuries such as tennis elbow, carpal tunnel, or De Quervain's. It is not used in the neck as part of a facial rejuvenation procedure unless there are firm areas of scar post–neck surgery, which are resistant to massage therapy.[1-4]

REFERENCES

1. Dayan SH, Schlessinger J, Beer K, et al. Efficacy and safety of ATX-101 by treatment session: pooled analysis of data from the Phase 3 REFINE trials. Aesthet Surg J 2018;38(9):998–1010
2. Humphrey S, Sykes J, Kantor J, et al. ATX-101 for reduction of submental fat: a phase III randomized controlled trial. J Am Acad Dermatol 2016;75(4):788–797.e7
3. Jones DH, Kenkel JM, Fagien S, et al; Proper Technique for Administration of ATX-101. Proper technique for administration of ATX-101 (deoxycholic acid injection): insights from an injection practicum and roundtable discussion. Dermatol Surg 2016;42(Suppl 1):S275–S281
4. Oni G, Hoxworth R, Teotia S, Brown S, Kenkel JM. Evaluation of a microfocused ultrasound system for improving skin laxity and tightening in the lower face. Aesthet Surg J 2014;34(7):1099–1110

SELECTION OF SURGICAL PROCEDURES IN NECK REJUVENATION

9. You see a 63-year-old, mildly obese woman with loss of neck contour and jowling. She has a large excess of neck skin and fat with prominent platysmal banding at rest. *Which one of the following surgical procedures is most likely to be optimal for her?*

   E. Full scar face and neck lift with liposuction

   Selection of an appropriate technique for neck rejuvenation is highly patient specific and needs to be chosen to address the key areas of concern to the individual patient. The patient in this scenario has multiple problems to be dealt with. She has excess submental fat and platysmal banding, so will require an open submental approach to her neck. This entails resection of fat with platysmal midline plication. She will also require a lateral face lift with scars placed around the ear in order to address her skin excess and jowls. The other techniques would be unlikely to provide her with a satisfactory improvement addressing all the issues present.[1-3]

REFERENCES

1. Rohrich RJ, Rios JL, Smith PD, Gutowski KA. Neck rejuvenation revisited. Plast Reconstr Surg 2006;118(5):1251–1263
2. Narasimhan K, Stuzin JM, Rohrich RJ. Five-step neck lift: integrating anatomy with clinical practice to optimize results. Plast Reconstr Surg 2013;132(2):339–350
3. Matarasso A. Managing the components of the aging neck: from liposuction to submentalplasty, to neck lift. Clin Plast Surg 2014;41(1):85–98

SELECTION OF SURGICAL PROCEDURES IN NECK REJUVENATION

10. You see a 39-year-old woman with excellent skin quality and moderate submental fat excess. She has no platysmal banding at rest, but banding becomes apparent on animation. A skin pinch test reveals no alteration in pinch size on animation. *Which one of the following surgical procedures is most likely to be optimal for her?*

    B. Submental neck lift with liposuction

    Selection of appropriate procedure in neck rejuvenation is based on the parameters which need to be addressed. The main approaches are liposuction only, a submental neck lift, an isolated neck lift, a short scar face and neck lift, or a full--scar face and neck lift. These may be performed with additional adjunctive procedures where required.

    The patient in this scenario has moderate subcutaneous fat without subplatysmal fat excess as evidenced by the skin pinch test. She could therefore be a good candidate for liposuction only but will also need to have her platysmal bands treated, because these are likely to become evident at rest following liposuction. For this reason, she should have liposuction combined with an open submental approach. If her skin pinch test had revealed a diminished pinch size during animation, then this would suggest she had evidence of subplatysmal fat, and an open submental approach to remove this would be indicated too. In patients in whom there is skin excess and facial tissue ptosis, a face and neck lift approach need to be combined, with acceptance of the increased scars this would create.[1-3]

REFERENCES

1. Rohrich RJ, Rios JL, Smith PD, Gutowski KA. Neck rejuvenation revisited. Plast Reconstr Surg 2006;118(5):1251–1263
2. Nahai F, ed. The Art of Aesthetic Surgery: Principles and Techniques. St Louis: Quality Medical Publishing; 2005
3. Matarasso A. Managing the components of the aging neck: from liposuction to submentalplasty, to neck lift. Clin Plast Surg 2014;41(1):85–98

LIPOSUCTION OF THE NECK

11. *When performing suction-assisted liposuction to the neck in a patient with submental fat excess, which one of the following is correct?*

    D. Small quantities of aspirate will normally provide satisfactory results.

    Neck liposuction carries a risk of over-resection of fat, which will lead to suboptimal results. This is difficult to correct, so it is better to slightly under-resect instead. Even small volumes of aspirate can make a significant difference to aesthetics (e.g., 5–10 cc). When undertaking liposuction of the neck, some key principles should be employed. Wetting solution containing epinephrine should be infiltrated before skin preparation and allowed to take effect for 10 minutes. Three incisions are usually required, especially if there is lateral fat to be harvested (a single submental incision is combined with two postauricular incisions). This approach facilitates feathering which can be useful to minimize irregularities. Small, flat cannulas (2–3 mm) should be used with a single hole facing toward deeper tissues, ensuring that no more than one or two passes are made within a given tunnel. (Multihole cannulas are normally used for infiltration, not harvest, and a 7-mm cannula would be too coarse for the detailed contouring required in the neck.)

Liposuction is intended to treat subcutaneous fat excess, not subplatysmal fat, which would risk damage to other subplatysmal structures such as blood vessels and nerves. If there is subplatysmal excess, an open approach is required. A drain is not required, but a compression garment should be worn.[1,2]

REFERENCES

1. Nahai F. Neck lift. In: Nahai F, ed. The Art of Aesthetic Surgery: Principles and Practices. 2nd ed. St Louis: Quality Medical Publishing; 2011
2. Koehler J. Complications of neck liposuction and submentoplasty. Oral Maxillofac Surg Clin North Am 2009;21(1): 43–52, vi

SUBMENTAL NECK LIFT

12. When considering the submental approach to neck lift, which one of the following is true?

   B. It facilitates access to allow platysmal plication.

   The submental approach to the neck is very useful as it allows manipulation of a number of key areas with minimal visible scarring. The main indications are for patients with platysmal banding that will benefit from plication or other maneuver, and where there is modest or no skin excess and deeper fat manipulation is required.

   It can address some skin excess if wide undermining is performed, but it may be better to use additional periauricular or lateral incisions to facilitate this instead. It is often used in conjunction with liposuction, as this can recontour the preplatysmal fat and then the inter- and subplatysmal fat layers can be further manipulated with direct excision, if needed. The submental incision should be placed just behind the natural submental crease to prevent scarring that may deepen the crease. It is usually made around 4 cm in length. Other adjunctive procedures can be incorporated with the submental approach such as refining the digastric muscles or releasing the mandibular septum and retaining ligament.[1–3]

REFERENCES

1. Knize DM. Limited incision submental lipectomy and platysmaplasty. Plast Reconstr Surg 2004;113(4):1275–1278
2. Matarasso A. Managing the components of the aging neck: from liposuction to submentalplasty, to neck lift. Clin Plast Surg 2014;41(1):85–98
3. Feldman JJ. Neck lift my way: an update. Plast Reconstr Surg 2014;134(6):1173–1183

DIFFERENT TYPES OF NECK LIFT

13. Which one of the following is a key technical difference between performing an isolated neck lift and a combined face and neck lift?

   B. The length of periauricular scars

   Surgery to the face and neck is on a continuum with an isolated neck lift being toward one end of the spectrum and a full-scar face and neck lift on the other.

   Each of the procedures will address the neck contour in terms of the jowls and neckline, but only the face lift will do this while also addressing the cheeks at the same time. From a technical perspective, a key difference is the length and placement of the lateral scar around the ear as well as the extent of associated subcutaneous undermining.

   In an isolated neck lift, the scar typically starts at the level of the tragus and extends posteriorly to the retroauricular sulcus. It can be continued onto the retroauricular hairline if there is a large skin excess to be removed. In contrast, a short scar face and neck lift will involve a hairline incision that starts at the sideburn or temple and extends to the lobule. A full-scar face and neck lift will normally have scar extension both in front of and behind the ear, often into the postauricular hairline.

   In general, within plastic surgery, required scar length will be related to skin excess and this is seen at other body sites such as breast (reduction/mastopexy), abdomen (abdominoplasty), and limbs (brachioplasty and thigh lift).

   The primary plane of dissection is subcutaneous for both an isolated neck or face and neck procedure is being performed. Only when a sub-SMAS technique is used in the facelift component, will an additional dissection plane be created. The risk of nerve damage, the need for a submental incision, and the need for adjunctive liposuction will apply to each technique.

The indications for an isolated neck lift are patients with skin excess and inelastic skin tone who do not want or need to have a facelift. Incorporating a submental incision is generally recommended with this approach to avoid future problems with platysmal banding. The indications for short-scar facelift in conjunction with neck lift include mild jowling, slight neck skin excess (good-quality skin), and patients who do not want scarring behind the ears. Indications for full-scar face and neck lift include patients with more significant skin laxity and jowling, who are accepting of the longer scars in front of, and behind the ears.[1-3]

REFERENCES

1. Rohrich RJ, Rios JL, Smith PD, Gutowski KA. Neck rejuvenation revisited. Plast Reconstr Surg 2006;118(5):1251–1263
2. Nahai F, ed. The Art of Aesthetic Surgery: Principles and Techniques. St Louis: Quality Medical Publishing; 2005
3. Matarasso A. Managing the components of the aging neck: from liposuction to submentalplasty, to neck lift. Clin Plast Surg 2014;41(1):85–98

ADJUNCTIVE PROCEDURES DURING NECK REJUVENATION

14. **Which one of the following is most commonly performed during correction of the deep plane (deep to the platysma) in neck rejuvenation?**

C. **Resection of subplatysmal and interplatysmal fat**

During the deep plane component of neck rejuvenation, a number of factors may be addressed. Interplatysmal and subplatysmal fat may be performed in addition to subcutaneous defatting. Care must be exercise when performing subplatysmal fat, as this can lead to tethering of the platysma to the underlying mylohyoid muscle. The anterior belly of digastric may also be resected, but this is most commonly performed tangentially to debulk it, rather than completely excise it. Intracapsular piecemeal resection of the superficial (not deep) lobe of submandibular gland may be performed if the gland is large or ptotic. It is unwise to perform an extracapsular dissection, because this risks damage to the facial artery and marginal mandibular nerve. The suprahyoid fascia is occasionally released to improve the cervical angle in patients with a high hyoid. During the resection of interplatysmal and subplatysmal fat, there are often one or two lymph nodes taken with the specimen, but no attempt is made to specifically resect nodes.[1-3]

REFERENCES

1. Vaca EE, Sinno S. Rejuvenation of the neck. Advances in Cosmetic Surgery. 2018;1(1):23–30
2. Feldman JJ. Neck Lift. St. Louis, MO: Quality Medical Publishing; 2006: xvi, 532p
3. Matarasso A. Managing the components of the aging neck: from liposuction to submentalplasty, to neck lift. Clin Plast Surg 2014;41(1):85–98

PLATYSMAL PROCEDURES IN NECK REJUVENATION

15. **You see a patient after previous aesthetic surgery to the neck. On examination she has a visible transverse step in the neck and a window shading effect. Which one of the procedures has most likely been undertaken?**

D. **Platysma muscle sling**

The platysma muscle sling technique involves dividing the platysma horizontally across the entire width. This creates a wide gap that is potentially visible. Retraction of the platysma superiorly results in a window shading effect which has diminished the popularity of this procedure.

Platysmal suspension involves placement of sutures along the inferior mandibular border over the superficial fascia on platysma.

Platysmal flap cervical rhytidectomy involves a sectional myotomy of the medial edge of platysma so that lateral rotation and advancement of flap edges can be achieved.

Corset platysmaplasty is used to eliminate static paramedian muscle bands and reshape the neck. No muscle resection is performed, but platysma is plicated in the midline (**Fig. 113.3**).[1-5]

REFERENCES

1. Marten T, Elyassnia D. Management of the platysma in neck lift. Clin Plast Surg 2018;45(4):555–570
2. Narasimhan K, Ramanadham S, O'Reilly E, Rohrich RJ. Secondary neck lift and the importance of midline platysmaplasty: review of 101 cases. Plast Reconstr Surg 2016;137(4):667e–675e
3. Knize DM. Limited incision submental lipectomy and platysmaplasty. Plast Reconstr Surg 2004;113(4):1275–1278

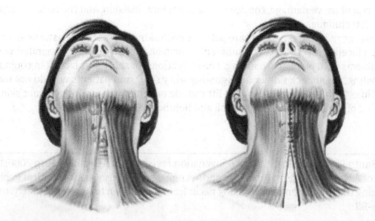

Fig. 113.3   Coaptation of decussated platysmal fibers in the midline creates a corset-type effect.

4. Fuente del Campo A. Midline platysma muscular overlap for neck restoration. Plast Reconstr Surg 1998;102(5): 1710–1714, discussion 1715
5. Feldman JJ. Corset platysmaplasty. Plast Reconstr Surg 1990;85(3):333–343

POSTOPERATIVE COMPLICATIONS FOLLOWING NECK REJUVENATION

16. A patient referred to you has undergone neck rejuvenation at another clinic and is dissatisfied with the appearance of her neck contour. On examination, she has an irregular contour with thin, visible bilateral bulges and adjacent hollowing in the anterior aspect of the neck just below the mandible. *What is the most likely explanation for this appearance?*

   B. Excessive submental liposuction

   The appearance described is in keeping with excessive submental liposuction that has left visible prominent digastric muscles (**Fig. 113.4**). Liposuction should be performed with caution in the neck, as this case illustrates. Only small quantities of aspirate should be harvested, and 3 to 5 mm of subcutaneous fat should be left to provide a natural, soft contour. This is a difficult problem to address and may require fat grafting. As with many other plastic surgical procedures, a "less-is-more" approach is often best. Patients want to look better, and feel and look younger and fresher than they started when undergoing aesthetic surgery. They do not (usually) want to look odd or unnatural. If in doubt when operating, it is preferable to under resect tissues giving an improvement that is too subtle rather than one that is overdone and subsequently difficult to correct.[1–3]

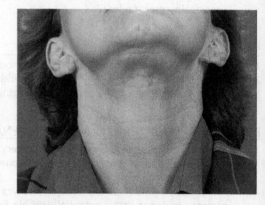

Fig. 113.4   Overaggressive fat removal from the neck and submental area has unmasked platysma bands and prominent digastric muscles.

REFERENCES

1. Batniji RK. Complications/sequelae of neck rejuvenation. Facial Plast Surg Clin North Am 2014;22(2):317–320
2. Koehler J. Complications of neck liposuction and submentoplasty. Oral Maxillofac Surg Clin North Am 2009;21(1):43–52, vi
3. Nahai F. The Art of Aesthetic Surgery: Principles and Techniques. 2nd ed. St. Louis, MO: Quality Medical Publishing; 2011

NERVE INJURY IN NECK LIFTS

17. A patient undergoes a neck lift and subsequently develops symptoms of a marginal mandibular nerve injury. *Which one of the following is true in this case?*

   D. While waiting for recovery to occur, neurotoxin may be injected into the contralateral depressor anguli inferioris.

The marginal mandibular branch of the facial nerve is at risk of injury during neck-lift procedures. It is most often a transient problem due to neuropraxia or use of local anesthetic agents. Where there is evidence of a neuropraxia and the patient is distressed by their appearance during a smile, it may be helpful to inject neurotoxin into the contralateral depressor anguli oris and depressor labii inferioris. These muscles are responsible for pulling the lower lip down in a full denture smile and injury to the marginal mandibular branch will cause weakness to them on the affected side leading to asymmetry. Weakening the working muscles on a temporary basis can therefore be helpful to improve symmetry. It is unlikely that exploration of the nerve is warranted unless the surgeon had suspected nerve division and if this were the case, primary repair would have been indicated.

Injury to the marginal mandibular branch can be differentiated from a cervical branch injury, although the two can have similarities. A cervical branch injury can be distinguished from the former, because the patient is able to evert the lower lip (mentalis muscle and the other depressors are still functioning). Platysma, which is innervated by the cervical branches of the facial nerve, is another lip depressor, hence the overlap in clinical appearances between these two nerve injures. Marginal mandibular nerve injuries are managed conservatively because the majority are due to neuropraxia from traction in the operating room and are expected to resolve spontaneously within 3 months.[1,2]

REFERENCES

1. Vaca EE, Sinno S. Rejuvenation of the neck. Advances in Cosmetic Surgery. 2018;1(1):23–30
2. Gonyon D, Barton F. the aging face: rhytidectomy and adjunctive procedures. Sel Read Plast Surg. 2005;10:21

114. Perioral Rejuvenation

See *Essentials of Plastic Surgery*, third edition, pp. 1602–1611

ANATOMY OF THE PERIORAL REGION

1. **When considering the anatomy of the perioral region, which one of the following is true?**
   A. It excludes the lower part of the nose and chin.
   B. It is bounded inferolaterally by the nasolabial folds.
   C. It includes the single midline mentalis muscle.
   D. It extends vertically from the subnasale to the menton.
   E. It is highly variable between different patients.

MUSCULAR ANATOMY OF THE PERIORAL REGION

2. **Which one of the following perioral muscles attaches to the midline of the upper lip and may be targeted during aesthetic injectable procedures?**
   A. Levator labii superioris
   B. Levator labii superioris alaeque nasi
   C. Zygomaticus major
   D. Zygomaticus minor
   E. Depressor septi nasi

SURFACE ANATOMY OF THE LIP

3. **How is the characteristic V-shape area of the central upper lip described?**
   A. Cupid's bow
   B. Tubercle
   C. Philtral column
   D. White roll
   E. Vermillion

CLINICAL HISTORY FOR PERIORAL REJUVENATION

4. **When conducting an interview with a patient considering perioral rejuvenation, which one of the following is true?**
   A. The interview will be most effective if closed questions are used to explore the patient's aims and objectives.
   B. Although diabetes is an issue to consider for surgical procedures, it has little relevance for nonoperative interventions.
   C. It is key to explore previous surgical and nonsurgical treatments received by the patient.
   D. For the most part, current skin care regimens need not form part of the detailed discussion.
   E. Unusually, undergoing injectable therapies while smoking does not result in increased complication risks

PHYSICAL EXAMINATION FOR PERIORAL REJUVENATION

5. **When examining a patient considering perioral rejuvenation, which one of the following is true?**
   A. The three key things that need to be considered for the skin are its thickness, texture, and pigmentation.
   B. The examination needs to be performed at rest and during animation including normal speech.
   C. Resting incisal display should be recorded and would normally be around 5 mm for both men and women.
   D. The upper and lower lips should have similar volumes and the surface area ratio between them should normally be 1:1.
   E. Complete photographic evaluation should consist of frontal and lateral views in repose.

CHRONOLOGICAL AGING OF THE LIP

6. **Which one of the following occurs in the lip with advancing age?**
   A. Upper lip lengthening with eversion
   B. Loss of lip volume/architecture
   C. Increased orbicularis oris tone to the lower lip
   D. Decreasing display of teeth at rest
   E. Loss of pigment from the vermillion

TRETINOIN USE IN FACIAL REJUVENATION

7. *What is the proposed benefit of using tretinoin prior to undergoing ablative perioral resurfacing?*
   A. It improves penetration of the treatment.
   B. It reduces pain during treatment.
   C. It reduces posttreatment erythema.
   D. It prevents development of milia.
   E. It protects against development of cold sores

NEUROTOXINS IN PERIORAL REJUVENATION

8. A patient is seen in the office with concerns about the vertical lines evident on her lips and is keen to trial botulinum toxin therapy to help with this having been satisfied with neurotoxin treatment to her brow and crow's feet areas previously. *When injecting in this case, which one of the following is true?*
   A. Treatment should involve a single injection to each lip.
   B. Dosage should mirror that used previously for her crow's feet.
   C. Neurotoxin should ideally be combined with hyaluronic acid.
   D. She will be at risk of experiencing speech and eating difficulties.
   E. She should be warned this treatment is likely to need repeating annually.

FILLER INJECTION TO THE LIPS

9. A patient is seen in clinic requesting improved definition of her lips. *When injecting nonpermanent filler into the lip for this patient, which one of the following is true?*
   A. A 21-gauge needle is generally preferred to deliver the filler
   B. Filler will need to be used "*off label*" as the FDA has not approved its use.
   C. Collagen is currently the only injectable recommended for the lips.
   D. Injection technique is the same whether adding volume or defining structural elements.
   E. Use of an infraorbital nerve block is highly recommended.

TREATMENT OF THE DEEP NASOLABIAL FOLD AND MARIONETTE LINE

10. *When injecting filler in a patient to improve the nasolabial folds and marionette lines, which one of the following is true?*
   A. Injection of filler along the nasolabial fold should be performed using an inverted cone shape.
   B. The marionette lines typically require larger volumes of filler than the nasolabial folds.
   C. Neither nasolabial nor marionette line injection is beneficial to the downturned oral commissure.
   D. Direct injection to the fold should be avoided and instead the malar region should be injected.
   E. The nasolabial folds are generally better treated with direct excision or dermal grafts.

TREATMENT OF THE DOWNTURNED ORAL COMMISSURE

11. A patient comes to see you requesting treatment for the oral commissure, which she feels appears downturned. She has decided upon undergoing a commissure-lift procedure. *What is the key benefit of this procedure?*
   A. It involves minimal scarring.
   B. It offers an immediate result.
   C. It avoids a smile deformity.
   D. It avoids a need for skin resurfacing.
   E. It is less invasive than alternative approaches.

MANAGEMENT OF THE LONG LIP

12. You see a 50-year-old patient in clinic who is unhappy with the appearance of her upper lip and feels that with age her dental show has reduced. She has normal occlusion and her own teeth which are in good condition. Cupid's bow lip anatomy is preserved. *Which one of the following interventions would be most suitable for this patient?*
   A. LeFort I osteotomy
   B. Dental crowns
   C. Injectable fillers
   D. Subnasal lip lift
   E. Vermillion border lip lift

Answers

ANATOMY OF THE PERIORAL REGION

1. When considering the anatomy of the perioral region, which one of the following is true?

D. It extends vertically from the subnasale to the menton

The perioral region extends vertically from the subnasale to the menton (the inferior-most point on the chin), thereby including both upper and lower lips, the labiomental fold, and the chin. It is bounded superolaterally by the paired nasolabial (NL) folds and inferolaterally by the marionette (M) lines, which represent extensions of the nasolabial folds onto the chin. Each of these is commonly treated during perioral rejuvenation and face lifting. The perioral region does not include the nose, the base of which instead marks the limit of its cranial extent. The perioral region consists of skin, subcutaneous fat, and a number of key muscles of facial expression including the orbicularis oris, depressor labii inferioris, depressor anguli oris, and mentalis. It also includes the insertions of the zygomaticus major, zygomaticus minor, levator labii superioris, levator labii superioris alaeque nasi, depressor septi nasi, and buccinators where they join with the orbicularis oris. The mentalis muscles are vertically and obliquely oriented paired muscles of the chin located on the mandible. These muscles originate from the incisive fossa of the mandible and insert into the skin of the chin creating the mentolabial sulcus or groove. They serve to elevate, evert, and protrude the lower lip and cause wrinkling during animation. While there are differences between patients in terms of soft tissue and bony anatomy, the fundamentals of the perioral region are consistent across patient groups.[1]

REFERENCE

1. Perenack J. Lip and perioral cosmetic surgery. In: Guttenberg SA, ed. Cosmesis of the Mouth, Face and Jaws. Wiley Online Books; 2012:59–81

MUSCULAR ANATOMY OF THE PERIORAL REGION

2. Which one of the following perioral muscles attaches to the midline of the upper lip and may be targeted during aesthetic injectable procedures?

E. Depressor septi nasi

The depressor septi nasi is one of the facial mimetic muscles of the upper lip. It is a paired muscle located on either side of the nasal septum with attachments to the medial crura of the lower lateral cartilages, the anterior nasal spine, and the orbicularis oris muscle. In some patients, it acts to either pull the nasal tip downward or shorten and elevate the upper lip during animation which some patients do not like. Accordingly, it may be chemically denervated with botulinum toxin injection or surgically severed, as an independent procedure or as part of a rhinoplasty procedure.[1,2]

The other muscles all serve to elevate the upper lip during a smile with the zygomaticus major being the primary smile muscle. They each insert onto the orbicularis oris, which acts as a concentric muscle to close the oral commissure. In relation to perioral rejuvenation, knowledge of the underlying muscles is important and learning to modify their action can be important in improving aesthetics.

REFERENCES

1. Moina DG, Moina GM. Depressor septi nasi muscle resection or nerve block. Miniinvasive Tech Rhino 2016;3:57
2. Rohrich RJ, Huynh B, Muzaffar AR, Adams WP Jr, Robinson JB Jr. Importance of the depressor septi nasi muscle in rhinoplasty: anatomic study and clinical application. Plast Reconstr Surg 2000;105(1):376–383, discussion 384–388

SURFACE ANATOMY OF THE LIP

3. How is the characteristic V-shape area of the central upper lip described?

A. Cupid's bow

The upper lip has defined anatomic components and knowledge of them is key to perioral rejuvenation, planning and executing its treatment, and ensuring clear, concise documentation. The key anatomic structures may each be targeted with filler in a structural manner or the lip more generally volumized with filler.

The lips comprise the orbicularis oris muscle which is lined internally with mucosa of the oral cavity. Externally, the lips have skin and subcutaneous tissue over the orbicularis. Linking the surfaces of the external skin and internal mucosa is the vermilion which is the red colored zone of the lip that has a specialized stratified squamous epithelial surface. The vermillion is subdivided into wet (internal) and dry (external) components. The join between the skin of the lip and the vermillion is called the white roll or white line.

Cupid's bow represents the central **V**-shaped section of the upper lip at the junction of vermilion and skin. The vertical ridges that link this to the nose are the philtral columns and these represent ridges formed by decussation of the orbicularis oris. The channel they create is called the "philtral column." The tubercle is the term normally used to describe the midline prominence at the lower part of the upper lip. Sometimes multiple tubercles are described: three to the upper lip and two to the lower lip in relation to aesthetics of the lips. These simply represent natural areas of fullness of prominence that may also be enhanced with injectable fillers (**Fig. 114.1**).[1,2]

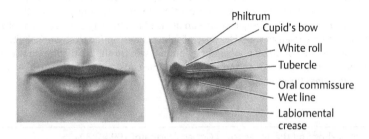

Fig. 114.1   Lip architecture. (From Coleman SR. Structural Fat Grafting. Thieme, 2004.)

REFERENCES

1. Thornton J, Carboy J, eds. Facial Reconstruction after Mohs Surgery. 1st ed. Thieme; 2018
2. Mckee D, Remington K, Swift A, Lambros V, Comstock J, Lalonde D. Effective rejuvenation with hyaluronic acid fillers: current advanced concepts. Plast Reconstr Surg 2019;143(6):1277e–1289e

CLINICAL HISTORY FOR PERIORAL REJUVENATION

4. *When conducting an interview with a patient considering perioral rejuvenation, which one of the following is true?*
   C. It is key to explore previous surgical and nonsurgical treatments received by the patient.
   When meeting a patient in the office to discuss perioral rejuvenation, the same approach should be considered when conducting a standard medical or surgical history. One of the key elements is to ensure that you are aware of what treatments the patient has tried previously, what has worked well, and what has not. This helps you filter the best treatments likely to benefit them.

Sometimes patients are vague about what they have had done and this may be simply because they are unsure what filler or neurotoxin was used, nor where exactly it was placed or the dose given. Conversely, some patients know exactly what was done and have fine detail about it to provide to you. The interview will be most effective if open-ended questions are used to explore the patient's aims and objective. This forms a basis to develop a plan that is likely to be effective and provide patient's satisfaction. A series of closed questions alone may be time-efficient but may miss key elements required. The usual risks for surgery such as diabetes, smoking, and hypertension all apply to nonsurgical and surgical interventions and so must be explored. Smoking and diabetes can lead to increased risks for infection, either following injections or after the procedures. Understanding what current skin care is being used (this can range from nothing to a complex recipe of products) is important, as certain treatments may affect options for further treatment under your care. Key things otherwise to pick up on include a history of hypertrophic or keloid scarring, of acne and treatment, and a history of herpes labialis.[1-3]

REFERENCES

1. Perenack J. Lip and perioral cosmetic surgery. In: Guttenberg SA, ed. Cosmesis of the Mouth, Face and Jaws. Wiley Online Books; 2012:59–81
2. Lamb JP, Surek CC. Facial Volumization: An Anatomic Approach. Thieme; 2017
3. Nahai F, ed. The Art of Aesthetic Surgery: Principles and Techniques. St Louis: Quality Medical Publishing; 2005

PHYSICAL EXAMINATION FOR PERIORAL REJUVENATION

5. *When examining a patient considering perioral rejuvenation, which one of the following is true?*

    B. The examination needs to be performed at rest and during animation including normal speech.

The key element to consider when performing an examination of the perioral area with a view to rejuvenation is that the exam must include assessment at rest and animated in order to assess static and dynamic rhytids, the smile dynamics, the nasolabial and marionette folds, the lip competence, facial symmetry, and hyperactivity of orbicularis oris. Assessment of the skin is also key, but there are more than three elements to consider. Skin characteristics that need to be assessed include its thickness, abnormal pigmentation, texture, scarring, wrinkling patterns (static vs. dynamic), acne activity and its sequelae, and evidence of pathological skin lesions and actinic damage (i.e., actinic keratosis, squamous cell carcinoma, basal cell carcinoma, melanoma). The Fitzpatrick skin type classification is useful to quantify when deciding upon treatment plans as skin resurfacing approaches differ according to skin type. The Glogau scale can be used to quantify and record photoaging.[1] Lip volume and architecture should be assessed as well. The ratio of subnasale–stomion to stomion–submentum should normally be 1:2, and the surface area of lip display of upper lip to lower lip should display a ratio of 2:3.[2] The relationship of the lips to dental structure at repose and smile should be considered. Incisal display in repose should be 3 to 4 mm for women but is less for men at 2 to 3 mm.

REFERENCES

1. Glogau RG. Chemical peeling and the aging skin. J Geriatr Dermatol 1994;2:30–35
2. Perenack J. Lip and perioral cosmetic surgery. In: Guttenberg SA, ed. Cosmesis of the Mouth, Face and Jaws. Wiley Online Books; 2012:59–81

CHRONOLOGICAL AGING OF THE LIP

6. *Which one of the following occurs in the lip with advancing age?*

    B. Loss of lip volume/architecture

There are a number of predictable changes in the lip that occur with advancing age. These include a loss of volume and subsequent loss of architecture, lengthening of the lip with inversion, loss of orbicularis oris tone, and an increased display of teeth at rest. In addition, there are often skin changes with skin thinning and development of both fine vertical lines and deeper static rhytids (**Fig. 114.2**).

These changes are addressed with perioral rejuvenation techniques. The loss of volume and definition can be improved with injection of temporary or permanent fillers. The fine rhytids can be improved with skin resurfacing techniques and the lip length can be addressed with surgery to reduce its overall height.[1–3]

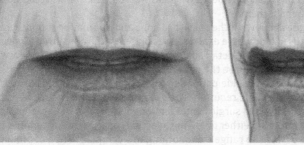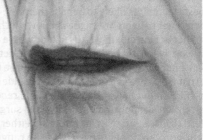

Fig. 114.2   Aging changes in the lips. (From Coleman SR. Structural Fat Grafting. Thieme, 2004.)

REFERENCES

1. Perenack JD, Biggerstaff T. Lip modification procedures as an adjunct to improving smile and dental esthetics. Atlas Oral Maxillofac Surg Clin North Am 2006;14(1):51–74
2. Perenack J. Treatment options to optimize display of anterior dental esthetics in the patient with the aged lip. J Oral Maxillofac Surg 2005;63(11):1634–1641
3. Rozner L, Isaacs GW. Lip lifting. Br J Plast Surg 1981;34(4):481–484

TRETINOIN USE IN FACIAL REJUVENATION

7. *What is the proposed benefit of using tretinoin prior to undergoing ablative perioral resurfacing?*

A. It improves penetration of the treatment

When planning for ablative facial resurfacing, patients should undergo topical home treatment of tretinoin (up to 0.1%) four times per day for at least 3 to 4 weeks. This provides a uniform thinning of the epidermis, which can improve penetration of chemical peels and decreased healing times after ablative skin treatments.

Pretreatment with topical hydroquinone 4% twice daily for 3 to 4 weeks prior to ablative skin resurfacing procedures, and 1 to 2 months postprocedure after re-epithelialization has begun, is intended to reduce unwanted pigmentary changes. It is generally indicated for darker skin tones. Antiviral prophylaxis when undergoing skin resurfacing of the perioral region is warranted even when there is no history of cold sores. An antiviral such as acyclovir rather than tretinoin is used for this. All patients undergoing resurfacing should start this 1 day prior to treatment and continue for 2 weeks after treatment. Following ablative skin resurfacing treatment, the treated area should be kept moist with ointment or an occlusive dressing. Sunscreen should be worn for 3 months posttreatment once healing is complete to minimize unwanted pigmentary changes. Milia, acne, and prolonged erythema are all potential complications of skin resurfacing, but tretinoin does not specifically target these problems.[1–6]

REFERENCES

1. De Boulle K, Heydenrych I. Patient factors influencing dermal filler complications: prevention, assessment, and treatment. Clin Cosmet Investig Dermatol 2015;8:205–214
2. Gazzola R, Pasini L, Cavallini M. Herpes virus outbreaks after dermal hyaluronic acid filler injections. Aesthet Surg J 2012;32(6):770–772
3. Lamb JP, Surek CC. Facial Volumization: An Anatomic Approach. Thieme; 2017
4. Hevia O, Nemeth AJ, Taylor JR. Tretinoin accelerates healing after trichloroacetic acid chemical peel. Arch Dermatol 1991;127(5):678–682
5. Nemeth AJ, Eaglstein WH, Falanga V, Hevia O, Taylor JR. Methods to speed healing after skin biopsy or trichloroacetic acid chemical peel. Prog Clin Biol Res 1991;365:267–277
6. Mandy SH. Tretinoin in the preoperative and postoperative management of dermabrasion. J Am Acad Dermatol 1986;15(4, Pt 2):878–879, 888–889

NEUROTOXINS IN PERIORAL REJUVENATION

8. A patient is seen in the office with concerns about the vertical lines evident on her lips and is keen to trial botulinum toxin therapy to help with this having been satisfied with neurotoxin treatment to her brow and crow's feet areas previously. *When injecting in this case, which one of the following is true?*

D. She will be at risk of experiencing speech and eating difficulties.

Vertical fine lines on the lips can be troublesome for patients and are often associated with prior smoking and high levels of sun exposure. They are difficult to eradicate, but methods to improve them include skin resurfacing, volume-enhancing fillers, and neurotoxin injections. When injecting botulinum toxin into the lips, it is normal to inject once in each lip quadrant (not once to each lip). The toxin is injected into the muscle (orbicularis oris). It is key to use small doses only, otherwise there will be a high risk of causing problems with speech and eating secondary to lip weakness and oral incompetence, which patients will find extremely distressing. The dosage will therefore be far less than that usually required for periorbital rejuvenation. The effects are temporary and repeat treatments will be needed well before 1 year. It is reasonable to combine filler and neurotoxin treatments as they target different problems but are complimentary to one another. However, the two do not need to be physically mixed together.[1,2]

REFERENCES

1. Perenack J. Lip and perioral cosmetic surgery. In: Guttenberg SA, ed. Cosmesis of the Mouth, Face and Jaws. Wiley Online Books; 2012:59–81
2. Levy LL, Emer JJ. Complications of minimally invasive cosmetic procedures: prevention and management. J Cutan Aesthet Surg 2012;5(2):121–132

FILLER INJECTION TO THE LIPS

9. A patient is seen in clinic requesting improved definition of her lips. *When injecting nonpermanent filler into the lip for this patient, which one of the following is true?*

   E. Use of an infraorbital nerve block is highly recommended.

   Injection of nonpermanent fillers into the lip is most commonly performed with hyaluronic acid, as this is safe, easy to use, has a low risk of adverse reactions, is reasonably cost-effective, and can be reversed if the effect is undesired. The main products available are FDA approved, although some are used *"off label."* For example, Restylane Silk and Juvederm Volbella do have specific FDA approval for lip augmentation, where many other products have approval for other areas including the nasolabial fold. Products such as Juvederm, Restylane, Prevelle Silk, and Belotero balance contain local anesthetic in the form of lidocaine but can still be painful to inject especially in the lip. It is therefore ideal to use an infraorbital nerve block prior to injecting the lips, as just a small volume of local anesthetic placed into the upper gums can provide patient comfort without distorting the lip appearance. Alternatively, topical anesthetic such as EMLA or LMX4 can be used but is less effective than a nerve block.

   When injecting nonpermanent filler into the lip, it can be for an overall volume increase, or to define certain anatomic elements of the lip such as the white roll, Cupid's bow, tubercle, or the philtral columns. There are similarities in the technique with either approach, but they are subtly different. For example, when placing filler to improve structural elements, a threading technique with a 30-gauge needle superficially into the dermal and subdermal plane would usually be preferred. Volumes should be very low and product placement needs to be very precise. When injecting primarily for overall lip volume increases, product placement can be less precise and delivered in greater volumes more deeply within tissue to minimize surface irregularity. A larger needle such as a 25-gauge may be used instead with a volumizing technique. Alternative products for injection include calcium hydroxylapatite (CaHA) such as Radiesse, poly-L-lactic acid such as Sculptra, polymethylmethacrylate (PMMA) such as Bellafill, and collagen based such as Zyderm. These tend to be used for deeper injections than hyaluronic acid which is well suited to the lips.[1-4]

REFERENCES

1. Eccleston D, Murphy DK. Juvéderm(®) Volbella™ in the perioral area: a 12-month prospective, multicenter, open-label study. Clin Cosmet Investig Dermatol 2012;5:167–172
2. Rohrich RJ, Bartlett EL, Dayan E. Practical approach and safety of hyaluronic acid fillers. Plast Reconstr Surg Glob Open 2019;7(6):e2172
3. Fitzgerald R, Vleggaar D. Facial volume restoration of the aging face with poly-l-lactic acid. Dermatol Ther (Heidelb) 2011;24(1):2–27
4. Mckee D, Remington K, Swift A, Lambros V, Comstock J, Lalonde D. Effective rejuvenation with hyaluronic acid fillers: current advanced concepts. Plast Reconstr Surg 2019;143(6):1277e–1289e

TREATMENT OF THE DEEP NASOLABIAL FOLD AND MARIONETTE LINE

10. *When injecting filler in a patient to improve the nasolabial folds and marionette lines, which one of the following is true?*

    A. Injection of filler along the nasolabial fold should be performed using an inverted cone shape.

    The nasolabial folds are a frequent primary focus for patients attending clinic. They tend to deepen with age due to a combination of factors including the effects of repeated animation, relaxation of facial ligamentous supporting structures, and prominence of the malar regions. Noninvasive treatments for minimizing the nasolabial folds include fillers. These may be temporary such as hyaluronic acid or permanent such as fat.

    When injecting the nasolabial fold directly, it is useful to do so with an inverted cone shape which leaves a greater volume of filler close to the alar grooves and less toward the commissure. Marionette lines are also treated similarly with the nasolabial folds, but with less product volume. Filling the marionette lines may give a secondary benefit to the downturned oral commissure, by providing a subtle lift to it. There has been debate regarding placement of filler to enhance the nasolabial fold and in techniques such as the "liquid" or "injectable" facelift, filler is placed in a number of specific locations throughout the face to volumize areas and provide a lift. These injections are often at the level of periosteum. Doing so in the malar region can help reduce the nasolabial fold depth and appearance. Often a combination of the malar and nasolabial injections is helpful. The nasolabial folds may be treated with surgery either by placing dermal grafts or by direct excision. The downside to the latter, in particular, is that permanent scars are placed in the folds, which may be unacceptable to many patients.[1,2]

REFERENCES

1. Mckee D, Remington K, Swift A, Lambros V, Comstock J, Lalonde D. Effective rejuvenation with hyaluronic acid fillers: current advanced concepts. Plast Reconstr Surg 2019;143(6):1277e–1289e
2. de Maio M. MD Codes™: a methodological approach to facial aesthetic treatment with injectable hyaluronic acid fillers. Aesthetic Plast Surg 2021;45(2):690–709

TREATMENT OF THE DOWNTURNED ORAL COMMISSURE

11. A patient comes to see you requesting treatment for the oral commissure, which she feels appears downturned. She has decided upon undergoing a commissure-lift procedure. *What is the key benefit of this procedure?*

B. It offers an immediate result.

Surgical treatment of the severely drooping oral commissure may be considered where more conservative approaches have been exhausted. The "commissure lift" involves resection of skin around the corner of the mouth. The markings for this procedure are as follows.

With the patient in the sitting position, mark the commissure and draw a line diagonally toward the superior tragus extending 1 to 1.5 cm (this should not pass beyond the NL fold). A second diagonal line of equal length should then be drawn medially from the commissure vermillion. A third line completing the triangle superiorly in a curvilinear fashion is then drawn. The height of the arched line is approximately 5 to 7 mm (**Fig. 114.3**).

This surgical approach has the advantage of effectively lifting the commissure and reducing the "miserable" appearance a downturned commissure can create, in a permanent fashion and with immediate changes evident. The downside is that it leaves a permanent visible scar lateral to the commissure that can be unacceptable to some patients. This can be described as a "Joker smile deformity" and may benefit from postsurgery resurfacing to help conceal it.[1–3]

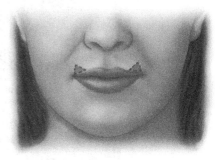

Fig. 114.3 M lines and downturned oral commissure.

REFERENCES

1. Vidal P, Berner JE, Castillo P, Rochefort G, Loubies R. Descended mouth corner: an ignored but needed feature of facial rejuvenation. Arch Plast Surg 2013;40(6):783–786
2. Goldman A, Wollina U. Elevation of the corner of the mouth using botulinum toxin type a. J Cutan Aesthet Surg 2010;3(3):145–150
3. Perkins SW. The corner of the mouth lift and management of the oral commissure grooves. Facial Plast Surg Clin North Am 2007;15(4):471–476, vii

MANAGEMENT OF THE LONG LIP

12. You see a 50-year-old patient in clinic who is unhappy with the appearance of her upper lip and feels that with age her dental show has reduced. She has normal occlusion and her own teeth which are in good condition. Cupid's bow lip anatomy is preserved. *Which one of the following interventions would be most suitable for this patient?*

D. Subnasal lip lift

The subnasal lip lift may be optimal for patients with a long upper lip and decreased incisal display where there is a normal cupid's bow. It involves removal of 4 to 5 mm of skin and soft tissue from the junction between the upper lip and nose. It should therefore be used only in patients with lips longer or taller than 15 mm. The scar is generally well hidden in cupid's bow, but this procedure can cause distortion of the nasal sill (**Fig. 114.4**).

An alternative to the subnasal technique for addressing the long upper lip is the vermillion border lip lift. This has the added advantage of correcting an inadequate cupid's bow which was not required in this scenario. The incision is made at the vermillion–skin junction. A disadvantage with this technique is that it leaves a less well concealed scar and can obliterate the white roll of the upper lip.

In the setting of a maxillary deficiency, an apparently long lip may be improved with maxillofacial intervention such as a LeFort osteotomy with bone grafts. It would not be required in this case. Manipulation of the dentition can be advantageous in order to change dental show; however, in the setting described, it would be addressing a different problem to the one that exists and making the dentition excessively long can affect function while eating and speaking. Injectable approaches to the lip can be helpful to fill out lip volume and thereby reduce length; they can also help increase length by adding volume in some cases. In this case, however, a surgical approach would be preferable and longer lasting.[1–3]

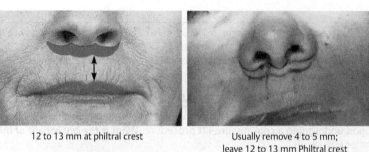

12 to 13 mm at philtral crest

Usually remove 4 to 5 mm;
leave 12 to 13 mm Philtral crest

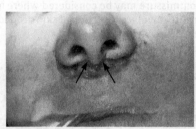

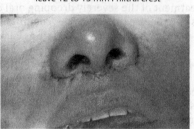

Crest points anchored to septal perichondrium
do not take excision lateral to alar base

Everted closure

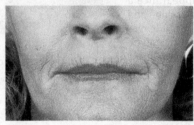

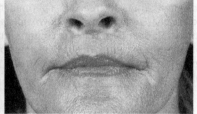

Preoperatively

1 year postoperatively

Fig. 114.4   Subnasal lip lift. (From Barton FE Jr. Facial Rejuvenation. Thieme, 2008.)

References

1. Yamin F, McAuliffe PB, Vasilakis V. Aesthetic surgical enhancement of the upper lip: a comprehensive literature review. Aesthetic Plast Surg 2021;45(1):173–180
2. Talei B. The modified upper lip lift: advanced approach with deep-plane release and secure suspension: 823-patient series. Facial Plast Surg Clin North Am 2019;27(3):385–398
3. Salibian AA, Bluebond-Langner R. Lip lift. Facial Plast Surg Clin North Am 2019;27(2):261–266

115. Rhinoplasty

See *Essentials of Plastic Surgery*, third edition, pp. 1612–1641

NASAL ANATOMY

1. *Correctly identify the anatomic components of the nose on the diagram below. Five of the nine options will be used (Fig. 115.1).*
   A. Nasal bone
   B. Upper lateral cartilage
   C. Medial crus of lower lateral cartilage
   D. Lateral crus of lower lateral cartilage
   E. Middle crus of lower lateral cartilage
   F. Nasal septum
   G. Inferior nasal spine
   H. Keystone area
   I. Scroll area

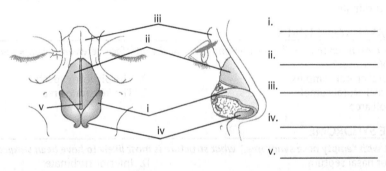

i. _____

ii. _____

iii. _____

iv. _____

v. _____

Fig. 115.1 Nasal anatomy.

NASAL OBSTRUCTION

2. A patient with unresolving unilateral Bell's palsy is seen in clinic, as they are experiencing problems with nasal obstruction. *Paralysis of which one of the following muscles is most likely to be responsible for their symptoms?*
   A. Nasalis
   B. Depressor septi nasi
   C. Buccinator
   D. Levator labii alaeque nasi
   E. Levator labii superioris

CLINICALLY ORIENTED NASAL ANATOMY

3. A 30-year-old woman is seen in clinic requesting rhinoplasty. She has two issues: the first is a mild dorsal hump and the second is nasal obstruction on the left side. On examination, you note that her nasal tip frequently drops during animation and on discussion with her and her partner, you find that they have noticed this and like the aesthetics this produces. *In this case, what muscle should be specifically preserved to maintain the aesthetics described?*
   A. Levator labii superioris
   B. Levator labii alaeque nasi
   C. Depressor septi nasi
   D. Depressor anguli oris
   E. Depressor labii inferioris

VASCULAR SUPPLY TO THE NOSE

4. *What provides the main arterial supply to the nasal tip after an open rhinoplasty?*
   A. Lateral nasal
   B. Columellar
   C. Angular
   D. Dorsal nasal
   E. Superior labial

SENSORY INNERVATION TO THE EXTERNAL NOSE

5. *What is the sensory nerve supply to the nasal tip?*
   A. Anterior ethmoid
   B. Posterior ethmoid
   C. Infraorbital
   D. Supratrochlear
   E. Supraorbital

KEY ANATOMIC STRUCTURES IN THE NOSE

6. *Which one of the following structures is formed predominantly by the caudal edge of the lateral crus of the lower lateral cartilage and the nasal septum.*
   A. External nasal valve
   B. Lower turbinate
   C. Middle turbinate
   D. Internal nasal valve
   E. Lateral crural complex

INTERNAL NASAL STRUCTURES

7. *What is the term given to describe the anatomic area at the interface between the upper and lower lateral cartilages of the nose?*
   A. The lateral crural complex
   B. The medial crural complex
   C. The scroll area
   D. The piriform aperture
   E. The keystone area

EMPTY NOSE SYNDROME

8. *In a patient with "empty nose syndrome," what structure is most likely to have been surgically resected?*
   A. Posterior nasal septum
   B. Anterior nasal septum
   C. Superior turbinate
   D. Inferior turbinate
   E. Lower lateral cartilages

NASAL AIRFLOW PHYSIOLOGY

9. *Which one of the following is correct regarding nasal airflow physiology?*
   A. During inhalation, the nostrils and internal nasal valve narrow due to negative pressure generation.
   B. The nasal airway normally contributes less than a quarter of the overall airway resistance.
   C. Constant nasal obstruction is due to a fixed structural abnormality, but rarely requires surgical intervention.
   D. Gradual worsening of nasal obstruction warrants further investigation, including endonasal scoping, and possibly biopsy.
   E. Rhinitis medicamentosus should be treated with oxymetazoline (Afrin) and oral antibiotics for 2 months.

TYPES OF GRAFTS USED IN RHINOPLASTY

10. *Which one of the following graft types is used to improve internal nasal valve patency or correct an open-roof deformity?*
    A. Radix graft
    B. Alar spreader graft
    C. Septal extension graft
    D. Spreader graft
    E. Alar rim graft

NASAL TIP GRAFTS

11. *Which one of the following involves placement of a cartilage graft vertically between the medial crura of the lower lateral cartilages to maintain or increase tip projection and help shape the columellar–lobular angle?*
    A. Cap graft
    B. Columellar strut graft
    C. Shield graft
    D. Soft triangle graft
    E. Onlay tip graft

SURGICAL APPROACHES TO RHINOPLASTY

12. *When discussing the merits of open versus closed rhinoplasty techniques, which one of the following represents an advantage to using an open approach?*
   A. A reduced operative duration
   B. A reduced postoperative recovery time
   C. A reduction in postoperative swelling
   D. A better intraoperative view for the surgeon
   E. The avoidance of external scars

SURGICAL APPROACHES TO RHINOPLASTY

13. A patient is undergoing an endonasal rhinoplasty. *Which one of the following septal approaches may result in a loss of tip support and projection?*
   A. Complete transfixion
   B. Limited partial transfixion
   C. Partial transfixion
   D. Hemitransfixion
   E. High septal transfixion

SURGICAL APPROACHES TO RHINOPLASTY

14. *When undertaking the alar access component of a rhinoplasty, which one of the following approaches is made between the upper and lower lateral cartilages?*
   A. Intercartilaginous
   B. Supracartilaginous
   C. Subcartilaginous
   D. Transcartilaginous
   E. Infracartilaginous

NASAL TIP PROCEDURES

15 You are performing an open rhinoplasty and want to increase tip rotation and projection. *Which one of the following techniques would be most helpful?*
   A. Shortening of the medial crura
   B. Lengthening of the lateral crura
   C. Placement of medial crural septal sutures
   D. Resection of both lateral and medial crura
   E. Placement of medial crural sutures

MANAGEMENT OF THE DORSAL HUMP IN RHINOPLASTY

16. *When managing the prominent dorsal hump during a rhinoplasty, which one of the following is true?*
   A. Hump reduction should be performed once the septal cartilage harvest and refinements to the tip have been made.
   B. Hump reduction should be performed incrementally after separation of the upper lateral cartilages from the septum.
   C. Hump reduction should routinely involve removal of septum, nasal bone, and upper lateral cartilages.
   D. Hump reduction occasionally requires additional measures to augment the area with cartilage or synthetic grafts.
   E. Hump reduction is sometimes associated with creation of an inverted-V deformity, but only when the nasal bones are long.

GRAFT MATERIALS IN RHINOPLASTY

17. You are undertaking an open rhinoplasty where you expect to need cartilage grafts. *Which one of the following is true in this case?*
   A. Septal cartilage is the preferred donor site as it is always plentiful.
   B. Auricular cartilage is ideal for nasal reconstruction due to its shape and rigidity.
   C. Costal cartilage works particularly well, as it does not warp when placed in the nasal framework.
   D. Irradiated costal cartilage is prone to warp but avoids a requirement for a donor site.
   E. Synthetic alternatives should be avoided for nasal reconstruction due to poor outcomes and high complication rates.

OSTEOTOMIES IN RHINOPLASTY

18. *Which one of the following is correct regarding osteotomies in rhinoplasty?*
    A. They are rarely required after dorsal hump correction.
    B. Lateral osteotomies should be performed before medial osteotomies.
    C. There are two main types of lateral osteotomy, each with similar indications.
    D. They may be contraindicated in elderly patients and in individuals of some ethnic groups.
    E. They are used to reduce rather than widen the nasal vault.

ALAR DEFORMITIES

19. A patient is seen in clinic with alar flaring. *Which one of the following techniques is most effective at correcting this deformity?*
    A. Full-thickness alar wedge excision
    B. Partial-thickness alar wedge excision
    C. Medial crural suture placement
    D. Lateral crural strut graft
    E. Alar contour graft

NASAL AIRWAY MANAGEMENT

20. You assess a 25-year-old woman who complains of long-term nasal obstruction that is relieved when she moves her cheek laterally. She has a mild septal deviation and a narrow midvault. *Which one of the following interventions is most likely to improve her symptoms?*
    A. Submucosal turbinate resection
    B. Infracture of the inferior turbinate
    C. Closed septoplasty
    D. Insertion of spreader grafts
    E. Placement of a lateral nasal wall graft

MANAGEMENT OF THE DEVIATED NOSE

21. You are performing an open rhinoplasty on a patient with a deviated nose. He has a caudal deformity and an apparent straight tilt to the septum. *Which one of the following should preferentially be performed?*
    A. A swinging door flap secured to the nasal spine
    B. Cartilage scoring with batten grafts
    C. Cartilage weakening and spreader grafts
    D. Horizontal mattress sutures to the upper lateral cartilages
    E. Osteotomy and infracture of the nasal bones

SEQUELA OF RHINOPLASTY SURGERY

22. You see a patient in clinic following closed rhinoplasty. They are concerned about the appearance of their nasal bridge, which is wide and flat just distal to the radix. *What procedure would you ideally use to correct this deformity?*
    A. Hump reduction
    B. Dorsal and sidewall augmentation
    C. Osteotomy and infracture
    D. An A-frame graft
    E. A U-frame graft

PRINCIPLES OF RHINOPLASTY SURGERY

23. You see a patient in clinic who desires a rhinoplasty because they are unhappy with the appearance and function of their nose. They have unilateral airway problems, with breathing difficulties at night. They also dislike the appearance of their nose because of a dorsal hump, bulbous tip, and wide alar bases. *What is the main benefit of performing a cephalic trim during rhinoplasty for this patient?*
    A. Improved airway patency
    B. Reduced dorsal hump
    C. Reduced tip rotation
    D. Refinement of the nasal tip
    E. Reduction of alar flaring

Answers

NASAL ANATOMY

1. *Correctly identify the anatomic components of the nose on the diagram below. Five of the nine options will be used (Fig. 115.1).*

For Fig. 115.1, the labels are as follows:

The nose comprises a bony cartilaginous framework with three components: upper, middle, and lower thirds. The upper third is formed by the paired nasal bones and nasal septum, the middle third is formed by the paired upper lateral cartilages and nasal septum, and the lower third is formed by the paired lower lateral cartilages and nasal septum. Having a good understanding of this anatomy is vital to both rhinoplasty and nasal reconstruction surgery. The nasal bones are around 2.5 cm long and are continuous with the frontal processes of the maxilla. They overlap the upper lateral cartilages for around 6 to 8 mm. At this point, the upper lateral cartilages and nasal septum join to form a T-shape construct. The upper lateral cartilages continue caudally to join with the paired lower lateral cartilages, which also overlap the upper lateral cartilages. The lower lateral cartilages have three different components: lateral, middle, and medial crura. They join with the nasal septum in the midline at the medial crus. The lower lateral cartilages are intimately related to tip projection, rotation, and definition and are usually modified during rhinoplasty. It is important to realize that the nasal alae do not contain cartilage, as the lower lateral cartilage finishes more cranially than the alae. Alar support is instead provided by the fibrous nature and shape of the alar construct.[1-3]

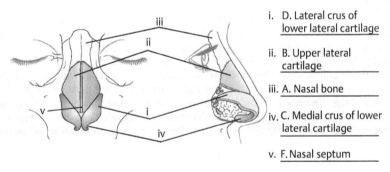

i. D. Lateral crus of lower lateral cartilage

ii. B. Upper lateral cartilage

iii. A. Nasal bone

iv. C. Medial crus of lower lateral cartilage

v. F. Nasal septum

Fig. 115.1 Algorithm for correction of a deviated nose. (ULCs, upper lateral cartilages.)

REFERENCES

1. Gunter JP, Rohrich RJ, Adams WP Jr. Dallas Rhinoplasty: Nasal Surgery by the Masters. 2nd ed. St Louis: Quality Medical Publishing; 2007
2. Sheen JH, Sheen AP. Aesthetic Rhinoplasty. 2nd ed. St Louis: Quality Medical Publishing; 1998
3. Constantian M. Rhinoplasty, Craft and Magic. New York: Thieme Publishers; 2009

NASAL OBSTRUCTION

2. A patient with unresolving unilateral Bell's palsy is seen in clinic, as they are experiencing problems with nasal obstruction. *Paralysis of which one of the following muscles is most likely to be responsible for their symptoms?*

D. Levator labii alaeque nasi

In patients with Bell's palsy, the muscles of facial expression are paralyzed, either temporarily or permanently. A number of muscles will affect nasal obstruction in a facial palsy patient, but the levator labii superioris alaeque nasi muscle is the most important in this regard. It originates from the upper frontal process of the maxilla and inserts into the skin of the lateral nostril and upper lip. It is innervated by the buccal branch of the facial nerve and elevates the medial nasolabial fold and nasal alae. The nasalis has two components that affect nasal airway patency. There are both compressor and dilator components which cause reduction or enlargement of the nasal alae, respectively. Paralysis of this muscle will therefore also contribute to nasal obstruction in this patient, but less so than the levator labii alaeque muscle. The buccinator muscle pulls the corner of the mouth laterally and compresses the cheek, the levator labii superioris muscle elevates the lip and midportion of the nasolabial fold, and the depressor septi nasi muscle pulls the septum inferiorly.[1–3]

There are a number of other potential causes of nasal obstruction with or without rhinoplasty. A recent systematic review found that common causes postrhinoplasty included collapse of the internal nasal valve, a deviated septum, and loss of mucosa to the inferior turbinate. Other causes included disruption of the external nasal valve, alar rim, and alterations to the nasal bones.[4]

REFERENCES

1. Freilinger G, Gruber H, Happak W, Pechmann U. Surgical anatomy of the mimic muscle system and the facial nerve: importance for reconstructive and aesthetic surgery. Plast Reconstr Surg 1987;80(5):686–690
2. Soler ZM, Rosenthal E, Wax MK. Immediate nasal valve reconstruction after facial nerve resection. Arch Facial Plast Surg 2008;10(5):312–315
3. Gunter JP, Rohrich RJ, Adams WP Jr. Dallas Rhinoplasty: Nasal Surgery by the Masters. 2nd ed. St Louis: Quality Medical Publishing; 2007
4. Wright L, Grunzweig KA, Totonchi A. Nasal obstruction and rhinoplasty: a focused literature review. Aesthetic Plast Surg 2020;44(5):1658–1669

CLINICALLY ORIENTED NASAL ANATOMY

3. A 30-year-old woman is seen in clinic requesting rhinoplasty. She has two issues: the first is a mild dorsal hump and the second is nasal obstruction on the left side. On examination, you note that her nasal tip frequently drops during animation and on discussion with her and her partner, you find that they have noticed this and like the aesthetics this produces. *In this case, what muscle should be specifically preserved to maintain the aesthetics described?*

C. Depressor septi nasi

The depressor septi nasi muscle is a small muscle that arises from the incisive fossa of the maxilla or orbicularis oris and inserts into the nasal septum, the medial crura of the lower lateral cartilages, and part of the nasalis muscle. It acts to depress the nasal septum and tip, acting as an antagonist to the other muscles of the nose. It is innervated by the buccal branch of the facial nerve and is relevant to rhinoplasty because it can accentuate a drooping nasal tip on animation of the upper lip. Many surgeons resect or divide this muscle in certain patients to prevent these effects. An anatomic study of this muscle found that it is most commonly in continuity with the orbicularis oris and they describe a procedure to dissect and transpose this muscle during rhinoplasty in order to improve tip and upper lip appearance in some patients.[1] In the scenario described, the patient has activity of the depressor that is clearly liked by her and her partner. For this reason, preservation of the depressor is indicated in this case.[1,2]

REFERENCES

1. Rohrich RJ, Huynh B, Muzaffar AR, Adams WP Jr, Robinson JB Jr. Importance of the depressor septi nasi muscle in rhinoplasty: anatomic study and clinical application. Plast Reconstr Surg 2000;105(1):376–383, discussion 384–388
2. Gunter JP, Rohrich RJ, Adams WP Jr. Dallas Rhinoplasty: Nasal Surgery by the Masters. 2nd ed. St Louis: Quality Medical Publishing; 2007

VASCULAR SUPPLY TO THE NOSE

4. *What provides the main arterial supply to the nasal tip after an open rhinoplasty?*

A. Lateral nasal

Understanding the blood supply to the nasal tip is crucial when undertaking an open rhinoplasty, because inadvertent damage of the lateral nasal artery (e.g., during alar base resection) may lead to soft-tissue necrosis of the tip.[1] The nose normally receives its blood supply from both the ophthalmic and facial arteries. The ophthalmic artery branches supply the cranial aspect, and the facial artery branches supply the caudal aspect. In most patients, the superior labial artery gives rise to the columellar artery, which supplies the nasal tip. After an open rhinoplasty, this vessel is divided, so the blood supply becomes dependent on a branch of the angular artery called the "lateral nasal artery," which passes from the nasojugal groove over the alar.[1,2]

REFERENCES

1. Rohrich RJ, Gunter JP, Friedman RM. Nasal tip blood supply: an anatomic study validating the safety of the transcolumellar incision in rhinoplasty. Plast Reconstr Surg 1995;95(5):795–799, discussion 800–801
2. Rohrich RJ, Muzaffar AR, Gunter JP. Nasal tip blood supply: confirming the safety of the transcolumellar incision in rhinoplasty. Plast Reconstr Surg 2000;106(7):1640–1641

SENSORY INNERVATION TO THE EXTERNAL NOSE

5. *What is the sensory nerve supply to the nasal tip?*
   A. Anterior ethmoid

   Sensory innervation of the external nose is from the trigeminal nerve (CN V) divisions I and II. The supraorbital and supratrochlear nerves from the ophthalmic division supply the cephalad portion, while the external nasal branch of anterior ethmoid supplies the middle vault and nasal tip. Following open rhinoplasty, patients typically experience reduced sensation to the nasal tip, but in most cases this fully recovers with time. Discussing this preoperatively is important so that they have some expectation of this.[1-3]

REFERENCES

1. Bafaqeeh SA, al-Qattan MM. Alterations in nasal sensibility following open rhinoplasty. Br J Plast Surg 1998;51(7):508–510
2. Moore KL, Dalley AF, eds. Clinically Oriented Anatomy. 4th ed. New York, NY: Lippincott Williams and Wilkins; 1999
3. Sheen JH, Sheen AP. Aesthetic Rhinoplasty. 2nd ed. St Louis: Quality Medical Publishing; 1998

KEY ANATOMIC STRUCTURES IN THE NOSE

6. *Which one of the following structures is formed predominantly by the caudal edge of the lateral crus of the lower lateral cartilage and the nasal septum.*
   A. External nasal valve

   The nose is considered to have two valves: internal and external. Both of these are important in relation to nasal airflow characteristics and problems with nasal obstruction. The external nasal valve is created primarily by the caudal edge of the lateral crus and nasal septum, with contributions from the ala and nasal sill soft tissues. External valve collapse may be seen with nostril collapse on inspiration. This can occur following surgery to the alar or refinement of the tip with alteration to the lower lateral cartilages. Cartilage grafts such as alar contour grafts, lateral crural strut grafts, or alar batten grafts can help address problems with the external nasal valve to reinforce the alar. Also correction of a deviated septum can be effective if this is the underlying cause.

   The internal nasal valve is the narrowest portion of the nasal airway and is therefore particularly important in regulating airflow resistance. It provides a significant amount of total airway resistance. It is formed by the junction of the caudal border of the upper lateral cartilages and the nasal septum where they form a T shape. A normal internal valve angle is 10 to 15 degrees and if this angle becomes more acute, obstruction is likely to occur. Where there is internal valve obstruction, cartilage spreader grafts may be placed between the upper lateral cartilages and the septum cranially to alleviate the problem. The turbinates are also relevant to airflow through the nose. They are paired bony structures that regulate and humidify inspired air. There are three turbinates each side: superior, middle, and inferior. The lateral crural complex is the term used to describe the lateral crus of the lower lateral cartilage and the accessory cartilage of the nose as a single entity.[1-3]

REFERENCES

1. Gunter JP, Rohrich RJ, Adams WP Jr. Dallas Rhinoplasty: Nasal Surgery by the Masters. 2nd ed. St Louis: Quality Medical Publishing; 2007
2. Wexler DB, Davidson TM. The nasal valve: a review of the anatomy, imaging, and physiology. Am J Rhinol 2004;18(3):143–150
3. Bloching MB. Disorders of the nasal valve area. GMS Curr Top Otorhinolaryngol Head Neck Surg 2007;6:Doc07

INTERNAL NASAL STRUCTURES

7. *What is the term given to describe the anatomic area at the interface between the upper and lower lateral cartilages of the nose?*
   C. The scroll area

   The scroll area is the region of abutment between the upper and lower lateral cartilages. The lateral crural complex is formed by the lateral crus and accessory cartilage (**see Fig. 115.1**). There is no named medial crural complex. The piriform aperture (derived from the Latin "piri," meaning pear) is a pear-shaped opening of the skull where the nose is situated. The keystone area of the nose refers to the point at which the upper and middle vaults meet (**see Fig. 115.1**). It usually represents the widest part of the nose. The keystone area is one of the most challenging areas to refine well during rhinoplasty. It is frequently manipulated when undertaking component reduction and refinement of the dorsal hump. Given the three-dimensional structure of the keystone area and the fact that it represents an interface between nasal bone, upper lateral cartilage, and septum likely accounts for this.[1,2]

REFERENCES

1. Gunter JP, Rohrich RJ, Adams WP Jr. Dallas Rhinoplasty: Nasal Surgery by the Masters. 2nd ed. St Louis: Quality Medical Publishing; 2007
2. Constantian M. Rhinoplasty, Craft and Magic. New York: Thieme Publishers; 2009

EMPTY NOSE SYNDROME

8. *In a patient with "empty nose syndrome," what structure is most likely to have been surgically resected?*

   D. Inferior turbinate

   Empty nose syndrome describes a situation in which a patient has nasal obstruction and a dry nose following nasal or sinus surgery.[1] Most commonly, it occurs after resection of the inferior turbinate. Symptoms may be delayed for months or years after surgery and are counterintuitive, as there is no physical obstruction present. The turbinates are paired bony structures that regulate and humidify inspired air. The inferior turbinate is the primary turbinate treated in rhinoplasty, and a severely deviated septum may induce contralateral turbinate hypertrophy to balance bilateral nasal cavities. A hypertrophied turbinate may be responsible for up to two-thirds of airway resistance. The two most common approaches to surgical correction of turbinate hypertrophy are outfracture (using a Boise elevator or a Vienna speculum), or submucosal resection and removal of underlying anterior bone.

REFERENCE

1. Coste A, Dessi P, Serrano E. Empty nose syndrome. Eur Ann Otorhinolaryngol Head Neck Dis 2012;129(2):93–97

NASAL AIRFLOW PHYSIOLOGY

9. *Which one of the following is correct regarding nasal airflow physiology?*

   D. Gradual worsening of nasal obstruction warrants further investigation, including endonasal scoping, and possibly biopsy.

   Gradual worsening of an airway obstruction, particularly in smokers or in association with epistaxis, may indicate a neoplasm and warrants further investigation. The nasal airway contributes around half of total nasal obstruction and can significantly reduce airflow when mucosal swelling is present, such as during a cold. During inspiration, the internal nasal valve narrows from negative pressure, but the nostrils usually open to facilitate airflow. Nasal obstruction can be either anatomic or physiologic; constant obstruction is more likely, but not exclusively, caused by a structural problem such as a deviated septum. These frequently require surgical intervention in the form of a septoplasty. Rhinitis medicamentosus is a condition arising secondary to excessive use of nasal congestants such as Afrin. Treatment involves stopping the offending agent (not continuing with it) and may include antihistamines and steroids.[1-3]

REFERENCES

1. Howard BK, Rohrich RJ. Understanding the nasal airway: principles and practice. Plast Reconstr Surg 2002;109(3):1128–1146, quiz 1145–1146
2. Lund VJ, Clarke PM, Swift AC, McGarry GW, Kerawala C, Carnell D. Nose and paranasal sinus tumours: United Kingdom National Multidisciplinary Guidelines. J Laryngol Otol 2016;130(S2):S111–S118
3. Ramey JT, Bailen E, Lockey RF. Rhinitis medicamentosa. J Investig Allergol Clin Immunol 2006;16(3):148–155

TYPES OF GRAFTS USED IN RHINOPLASTY

10. *Which one of the following graft types is used to improve internal nasal valve patency or correct an open-roof deformity?*

   D. Spreader graft

   The cartilage spreader graft is placed between the septum and upper lateral cartilages near to the nasal bone to increase the distance between them and open the angle of the internal nasal valve. It can additionally be used to help straighten a deviated dorsal septum or smooth the dorsal aesthetic lines, as well as correct an open roof deformity. The radix graft involves placing a small piece of cartilage within a soft-tissue pocket over the proximal nasal bone. This can help mask deformity or bony deficiency in this region by augmenting the nasofrontal angle or redefining the radix further cephalad. This can provide the appearance of a lengthened nose. The alar spreader graft is placed between the lateral crura and vestibular skin to improve external nasal valve function and correct a pinched nasal tip deformity. The septal extension graft controls projection, rotation, and support of the nasal tip and helps create a supratip break. The alar rim graft is placed within the intranasal rim to correct notching and retraction (see Fig. 115.14–115.16, *Essentials of Plastic Surgery*, third edition).[1-4]

REFERENCES

1. Gunter JP, Landecker A, Cochran CS. Frequently used grafts in rhinoplasty: nomenclature and analysis. Plast Reconstr Surg 2006;118(1):14e–29e
2. Gunter JP, Rohrich RJ, Adams WP Jr. Dallas Rhinoplasty: Nasal Surgery by the Masters. 2nd ed. St Louis: Quality Medical Publishing; 2007
3. Sheen JH, Sheen AP. Aesthetic Rhinoplasty. 2nd ed. St Louis: Quality Medical Publishing; 1998
4. Sinkler MA, Wehrle CJ, Elphingstone JW, Magidson E, Ritter EF, Brown JJ. Surgical management of the internal nasal valve: a review of surgical approaches. Aesthetic Plast Surg 2021;45(3):1127–1136

NASAL TIP GRAFTS

11. Which one of the following involves placement of a cartilage graft vertically between the medial crura of the lower lateral cartilages to maintain or increase tip projection and help shape the columellar–lobular angle?

B. Columellar strut graft

There are many different cartilage grafts used to improve the nasal tip appearance or projection.[1] A columellar strut graft is commonly used in rhinoplasty. It involves placement of a strip of cartilage, most commonly harvested from the dorsal septum, vertically between the medial crura of the lower lateral cartilages. During an open rhinoplasty, it is normally fixed directly to the nasal spine or premaxilla and inserted into a tight soft-tissue pocket. It may also be secured with transfixion sutures through the caudal septum and lower lateral cartilages. It helps maintain or increase tip projection and aids in shaping the columellar–lobular angle, while providing structural support to the caudal part of the nose.[2]

The cap graft is placed between the tip-defining points and the medial crura. It serves to increase projection or refine the infratip lobule. Shield grafts are placed on the anterior middle crura and extend to the nasal tip to improve tip projection and definition. Not all grafts use solid pieces of cartilage. Instead, some use morselized cartilage by itself or mixed with a product such as a fibrin glue or placed within a soft-tissue pocket of fascia like a small pillow. One example of this is a soft triangle graft which involves placement of morselized cartilage graft adjacent to the infratip lobule and deep to the soft tissues. It is useful for closing dead space and supporting the soft triangles. The onlay tip graft is a piece of cartilage placed horizontally over the alar domes. The objective is to increase tip projection and definition and improve the contour of the infratip lobule.[1-3]

REFERENCES

1. Gunter JP, Landecker A, Cochran CS. Frequently used grafts in rhinoplasty: nomenclature and analysis. Plast Reconstr Surg 2006;118(1):14e–29e
2. Bitik O, Uzun H, Kamburoğlu HO, Çaliş M, Zins JE. Revisiting the role of columellar strut graft in primary open approach rhinoplasty. Plast Reconstr Surg 2015;135(4):987–997
3. Constantian M. Rhinoplasty, Craft and Magic. New York: Thieme Publishers; 2009

SURGICAL APPROACHES TO RHINOPLASTY

12. When discussing the merits of open versus closed rhinoplasty techniques, which one of the following represents an advantage to using an open approach?

D. A better intraoperative view for the surgeon

Rhinoplasty can be performed via open or closed (endonasal) approaches. The choice between the two will depend on many factors including surgeon's and patient's preferences and the elements of the nose, which require alteration.

There continues to be debate at international conferences as to which is better and there will be some surgeons who only do open, some who only do closed, and others who will vary their approach according to patient factors. For example, some will do secondary or revision rhinoplasty open even when they do most primary rhinoplasties closed. Overall, there is no strong evidence to show one technique is better than another.

The main advantage of using an open approach is that the underlying framework of the nose is exposed and is therefore easier to directly visualize and make incremental changes to it. In contrast, endonasal approaches can be more challenging to view the anatomy clearly. Open rhinoplasty facilitates alterations to the nasal tip, alae, dorsum, septum, nasal bone, and radix. However, it does leave a small but permanent scar within the columella. Provided this is closed with care and attention to detail, it becomes very difficult to see further down the line. Intraoperatively, the open approach frees up one of the surgeon's hands, allows direct control of bleeding with electrocautery, and increases options for cartilage grafts. In contrast, closed approaches avoid the external scar, minimize postsurgical edema, allow visualization of the incremental changes to the underlying framework through an intact skin envelope, and may decrease surgical duration and recovery, although this is likely to be surgeon dependent.[1,2]

REFERENCES

1. Sheen JH. Closed versus open rhinoplasty--and the debate goes on. Plast Reconstr Surg 1997;99(3):859–862
2. Adams WP Jr, Rohrich RJ, Hollier LH, Minoli J, Thornton LK, Gyimesi I. Anatomic basis and clinical implications for nasal tip support in open versus closed rhinoplasty. Plast Reconstr Surg 1999;103(1):255–261, discussion 262–264

SURGICAL APPROACHES TO RHINOPLASTY

13. A patient is undergoing an endonasal rhinoplasty. *Which one of the following septal approaches may result in a loss of tip support and projection?*

A. **Complete transfixion**

Endonasal approaches to rhinoplasty require septal incisions in order to access the septum and lateral cartilages. They include complete and partial subtypes. During a complete (full) transfixion, the entire septum is incised at the membranous and caudal cartilaginous junction. This releases the tip completely and exposes the nasal spine and depressor septi muscle. It disrupts the attachments of the medial crural footplates to the caudal septum and can result in a loss of tip support and consequent loss of projection. In contrast, a partial transfixion begins caudal to the anterior septal angle and ends just short of the medial crural attachments to the caudal septum. A limited partial transfixion provides less tip access but allows preservation of attachments between the medial crural footplates and the caudal septum. A hemitransfixion approach is created unilaterally at the junction of the caudal septum and columella. A high septal transfixion does not violate the junction of the caudal septum and the medial crura or membranous septum.[1,2]

REFERENCES

1. Sheen JH. Closed versus open rhinoplasty--and the debate goes on. Plast Reconstr Surg 1997;99(3):859–862
2. Constantian M. Rhinoplasty, Craft and Magic. New York: Thieme Publishers; 2009

SURGICAL APPROACHES TO RHINOPLASTY

14. When undertaking the alar access component of a rhinoplasty, which one of the following approaches is made between the upper and lower lateral cartilages?

A. **Intercartilaginous**

Rhinoplasty can be performed as an open or closed procedure. Both open and closed rhinoplasty approaches require internal nasal incisions. These are classified as those made through the alar mucosa and those made to the septum. Open rhinoplasty will also require an additional columellar incision but avoid the septal incision. Alar incisions are made between the upper and lower lateral cartilages (intercartilaginous), through the lower lateral cartilage (transcartilaginous/intracartilaginous), or below the lower lateral cartilage (infracartilaginous). This is sometimes called a marginal approach. There are advantages and disadvantages to each. For example, an intercartilaginous approach avoids incising through the cartilage and causing damage to it. A transcartilaginous approach can be useful when removing some of the lower lateral cartilages, as the cephalic trim can be incorporated into the incision.

The infracartilaginous approach also avoids cartilage incision and consequent damage. There is a risk of causing notching, however, where the incision is placed too close to the nostril edge (see Fig. 115.5, *Essentials of Plastic Surgery*, third edition).[1–3]

REFERENCES

1. Constantian M. Rhinoplasty, Craft and Magic. New York: Thieme Publishers; 2009
2. Sheen JH. Closed versus open rhinoplasty--and the debate goes on. Plast Reconstr Surg 1997;99(3):859–862
3. Gunter JP, Rohrich RJ, Adams WP Jr. Dallas Rhinoplasty: Nasal Surgery by the Masters. 2nd ed. St Louis: Quality Medical Publishing; 2007

NASAL TIP PROCEDURES

15. You are performing an open rhinoplasty and want to increase tip rotation and projection. *Which one of the following techniques would be most helpful?*

C. **Placement of medial crural septal sutures**

Medial crural septal sutures are placed between the medial crura and the septum and are used for correction of a drooping tip or aging nose and help increase both tip projection and rotation.

The "tripod" model is useful for understanding the relationship between nasal tip projection and rotation. When the lateral crura are shortened, the tip will be rotated, while projection is decreased. Shortening of the medial crura will derotate and deproject the tip (both options A and B will therefore derotate the tip). If equivalent portions of both medial and lateral crura are resected, the projection is decreased, while the rotation should remain the same (option D).

Medial crural sutures differ from medial crural septal sutures. They involve horizontal mattress sutures placed between the medial crura that unify the lower lateral cartilages and stabilize the columellar strut to resist flaring of the medial crura.[1-3]

REFERENCES

1. Rohrich RJ, Griffin JR. Correction of intrinsic nasal tip asymmetries in primary rhinoplasty. Plast Reconstr Surg 2003;112(6):1699–1712, discussion 713–715
2. Ghavami A, Janis JE, Acikel C, Rohrich RJ. Tip shaping in primary rhinoplasty: an algorithmic approach. Plast Reconstr Surg 2008;122(4):1229–1241
3. Guyuron B, Behmand RA. Nasal tip sutures part II: the interplays. Plast Reconstr Surg 2003;112(4):1130–1145, discussion 1146–1149

MANAGEMENT OF THE DORSAL HUMP IN RHINOPLASTY

16. *When managing the prominent dorsal hump during a rhinoplasty, which one of the following is true?*

B. Hump reduction should be performed incrementally after separation of the upper lateral cartilages from the septum.

Dorsal hump reduction is probably the most common motivation for patients to undergo rhinoplasty. The dorsal hump usually comprises an excess of bone, soft tissue, and cartilage. It relates to the keystone area of the nose at the junction of the nasal bones, upper lateral cartilages, and septum. When performing a reduction, it is important to first separate out the anatomic structures so that each can be individually manipulated. This involves a subperichondrial dissection along the septum to separate the upper lateral cartilages from it all the way up to the nasal bones. Once free, assessment can be made of the excesses that need to be removed and incremental reduction can be performed primarily on the cartilaginous septum and the nasal bones. These are usually refined using blades, scissors, osteotomes, and rasps. Both palpation and visualization are undertaken throughout to ensure the desired reduction is achieved.

It is common practice to perform the dorsal hump reduction early in the procedure and then make refinements to the nasal tip once this has been completed. In most cases, the upper lateral cartilages should not be reduced, as this risks leaving them short when reconstructing the nasal framework. This would otherwise contribute to the creation of an open roof deformity. In order to smooth the refined dorsum well, it may be necessary to implement other techniques including suturing the upper lateral cartilages to the septum, performing osteotomies, and placing spreader grafts. Spreader grafts are often used, not only to provide a satisfactory dorsal shape but also to ensure the internal nasal valves remain patent and avoid an inverted-V–shape deformity. The inverted-V deformity as viewed from the front is where an upside-down V-shaped indentation exists between the end of the nasal bones and the start of the upper lateral cartilages. In this situation, the cartilaginous area caudal to the nasal bones is noticeably thinner and indented compared with the width of the nasal bones. It is more likely to occur in patients with short nasal bones, but can occur where the nasal bones are long too. In a situation where an inverted-V deformity already exists, spreader graft placement between the septum and upper lateral cartilages is one of the main corrective approaches. These grafts may be harvested from the septum itself. Where there is a true excess of the upper lateral cartilages, some surgeons will flip the excess upper lateral cartilage between the septum to achieve the spreader effect.[1-3]

REFERENCES

1. Rohrich RJ, Muzaffar AR, Janis JE. Component dorsal hump reduction: the importance of maintaining dorsal aesthetic lines in rhinoplasty. Plast Reconstr Surg 2004;114(5):1298–1308, discussion 1309–1312
2. Lee MR, Unger JG, Rohrich RJ. Management of the nasal dorsum in rhinoplasty: a systematic review of the literature regarding technique, outcomes, and complications. Plast Reconstr Surg 2011;128(5):538e–550e
3. Gunter JP, Rohrich RJ. Augmentation rhinoplasty: dorsal onlay grafting using shaped autogenous septal cartilage. Plast Reconstr Surg 1990;86(1):39–45

GRAFT MATERIALS IN RHINOPLASTY

17. You are undertaking an open rhinoplasty where you expect to need cartilage grafts. *Which one of the following is true in this case?*

D. Irradiated costal cartilage is prone to warp but avoids a requirement for a donor site.

There are a number of options available for cartilage grafts in rhinoplasty. The most popular choice would usually be the septum itself, as cartilage can be harvested from this site without creating any functional deficit or a separate donor site.[1] However, while septal cartilage may be plentiful in the primary rhinoplasty setting, where grafts are most often needed, i.e., in secondary rhinoplasty or nasal reconstruction, the nose may be cartilage deficient and grafts will need to be harvested from elsewhere. Other options therefore include auricular[2] and costal donor sites,[3] using irradiated cadaveric cartilage[4] or synthetic alternatives.

Auricular cartilage is useful where curved contour grafts are required such as alar grafts in nasal reconstruction but is less useful where larger flat pieces are required, for example when septal extension grafts are needed. Auricular cartilage also lacks rigidity for structural support of the nose. Costal cartilage provides a useful supply but will lead to additional donor-site scars. Furthermore, it does have a propensity for warping and techniques have been described to limit this, including cross-sectional carving, placement of the concave side downward, and using percutaneous wires. Irradiated costal cartilage is another useful graft source, which avoids the need for a rib donor site and hence the skill set required to harvest this. Unfortunately, it too risks warping in the medium to longer term.[4] Diced or morselized cartilage can be very useful for contouring the nose, particularly the dorsum when this has a deficiency perhaps following a poor primary rhinoplasty or in the setting of vasculitis and a saddle nose deformity.[5,6] Synthetic implants remain a popular option for many surgeons. These include silicone, Gore-Tex, polyethylene, Dacron, and dermal substitutes.

REFERENCES

1. Gunter JP, Rohrich RJ. Augmentation rhinoplasty: dorsal onlay grafting using shaped autogenous septal cartilage. Plast Reconstr Surg 1990;86(1):39–45
2. Lee M, Callahan S, Cochran CS. Auricular cartilage: harvest technique and versatility in rhinoplasty. Am J Otolaryngol 2011;32(6):547–552
3. Lopez MA, Shah AR, Westine JG, O'Grady K, Toriumi DM. Analysis of the physical properties of costal cartilage in a porcine model. Arch Facial Plast Surg 2007;9(1):35–39
4. Adams WP Jr, Rohrich RJ, Gunter JP, Clark CP, Robinson JB Jr. The rate of warping in irradiated and nonirradiated homograft rib cartilage: a controlled comparison and clinical implications. Plast Reconstr Surg 1999;103(1):265–270
5. Daniel RK. Diced cartilage grafts in rhinoplasty surgery: current techniques and applications. Plast Reconstr Surg 2008;122(6):1883–1891
6. Gibson T, Davis WB. The distortion of autogenous cartilage grafts: its cause and prevention. Br J Plast Surg 1958;10:257

OSTEOTOMIES IN RHINOPLASTY

18. *Which one of the following is correct regarding osteotomies in rhinoplasty?*

D. They may be contraindicated in elderly patients and in individuals of some ethnic groups.

Osteotomies are useful to allow repositioning of the nasal bones during rhinoplasty. Relative contraindications to their use include elderly patients with thin nasal bones, ethnic noses that are low and broad, and patients who wear heavy glasses.

Osteotomies in rhinoplasty are described as either medial or lateral. They can be used independent of one another or may be combined. Lateral osteotomies are classified by the level at which they are performed in relation to the face of the maxilla (low to low, low to high, or double level). They are commonly used after dorsal hump reduction to correct an open-roof deformity or narrow a wide bony dorsum. Medial osteotomies are used to narrow the bony vault but may be used to widen it when combined with lateral osteotomies. Medial osteotomies should be performed before lateral osteotomies; otherwise, the bones will have little support, making them a moving target during the medial osteotomies.[1-3]

REFERENCES

1. Gunter JP, Rohrich RJ, Adams WP Jr. Dallas Rhinoplasty: Nasal Surgery by the Masters. St Louis: Quality Medical Publishing; 2002
2. Rohrich RJ, Krueger JK, Adams WP Jr, Hollier LH Jr. Achieving consistency in the lateral nasal osteotomy during rhinoplasty: an external perforated technique. Plast Reconstr Surg 2001;108(7):2122–2130, discussion 2131–2132
3. Rohrich RJ, Gunter JP, Deuber MA, Adams WP Jr. The deviated nose: optimizing results using a simplified classification and algorithmic approach. Plast Reconstr Surg 2002;110(6):1509–1523, discussion 1524–1525

ALAR DEFORMITIES

19. A patient is seen in clinic with alar flaring. *Which one of the following techniques is most effective at correcting this deformity?*

B. Partial-thickness alar wedge excision

Flared alae are best corrected with partial-thickness wedge excisions that preserve the alar base and do not extend into the nasal vestibule. Alar base width reduction is also performed with wedge excisions, but in this case, full-thickness incisions are made. Alar base reduction will alter the alar–cheek junction and may alter the appearance of nasal projection. Medial crural suture placement is used to improve tip definition and provide tip support. Lateral crural strut grafts and alar contour grafts are used to treat alar rim deformities and provide internal alar support. Alar rim deformities are commonly due to excessive lateral crural resection during previous rhinoplasty.[1,2]

REFERENCES

1. Rohrich RJ, Malafa MM, Ahmad J, Basci DS. Managing alar flare in rhinoplasty. Plast Reconstr Surg 2017;140(5):910–919
2. Unger JG, Lee MR, Kwon RK, Rohrich RJ. A multivariate analysis of nasal tip deprojection. Plast Reconstr Surg 2012;129(5):1163–1167

NASAL AIRWAY MANAGEMENT

20. You assess a 25-year-old woman who complains of long-term nasal obstruction that is relieved when she moves her cheek laterally. She has a mild septal deviation and a narrow midvault. *Which one of the following interventions is most likely to improve her symptoms?*

   D. Insertion of spreader grafts

   There are a number of structural factors that may lead to nasal obstruction, and management is specific to the cause. This patient displays a positive Cottle's sign, in which lateral displacement of the cheek opens the internal nasal valve and improves airflow. The obstruction is usually caused by a decreased nasal valve angle (<15 degrees) or weak upper lateral cartilage where the septum and upper lateral cartilages meet. This is addressed by placing a cartilage graft between the upper lateral cartilages and the septum. Submucosal turbinate resection or outfracture (not infracture) may be helpful if the obstruction has resulted from turbinate hypertrophy. If the lateral nasal wall is weak, strengthening it with lateral grafts may be helpful. A septoplasty can also help correct nasal obstruction, depending on the cause.[1–4]

REFERENCES

1. Rohrich RJ, Hollier LH. Use of spreader grafts in the external approach to rhinoplasty. Clin Plast Surg 1996;23(2):255–262
2. Gunter JP, Rohrich RJ, Adams WP Jr. Dallas Rhinoplasty: Nasal Surgery by the Masters. 2nd ed. St Louis: Quality Medical Publishing; 2007
3. Lee M, Unger JG, Gryskiewicz J, Rohrich RJ. Current clinical practices of the Rhinoplasty Society members. Ann Plast Surg 2013;71(5):453–455
4. Sinkler MA, Wehrle CJ, Elphingstone JW, Magidson E, Ritter EF, Brown JJ. Surgical management of the internal nasal valve: a review of surgical approaches. Aesthetic Plast Surg 2021;45(3):1127–1136

MANAGEMENT OF THE DEVIATED NOSE

21. You are performing an open rhinoplasty on a patient with a deviated nose. He has a caudal deformity and an apparent straight tilt to the septum. *Which one of the following should preferentially be performed?*

   A. A swinging door flap secured to the nasal spine

   Rohrich et al[1] proposed a treatment algorithm for managing patients with deviated noses (**Fig. 115.2**). Correction is performed through an open rhinoplasty technique and differs, depending on whether deviation is caudal or dorsal and whether the septum is **C**-shaped, **S**-shaped, or has a straight tilt. In the case of a straight tilt with the septum incorrectly located, the approach is to reduce the caudal septum onto the nasal spine, and this may require vertical sectioning to create a "swinging door."

   If this is insufficient, small wedges of cartilage can also be excised from the convex side of the deviation, with cartilage scoring on the concave side to decrease the cartilage memory and straighten the septum. The caudal septum is sutured to the nasal spine and may be secured using a piece of septal cartilage.

   Cartilage scoring with batten grafts may be useful to treat **C**-shaped or **S**-shaped caudal deformity. Cartilage weakening and spreader grafts may be used to treat **C**-shaped or **S**-shaped dorsal deformity. Horizontal mattress sutures to the upper lateral cartilages may be used to control any residual deviation after correction with the other techniques. Osteotomies are generally used to correct a proximal (cranial) bony deviation.

REFERENCE

1. Rohrich RJ, Gunter JP, Deuber MA, Adams WP Jr. The deviated nose: optimizing results using a simplified classification and algorithmic approach. Plast Reconstr Surg 2002;110(6):1509–1523, discussion 1524–1525

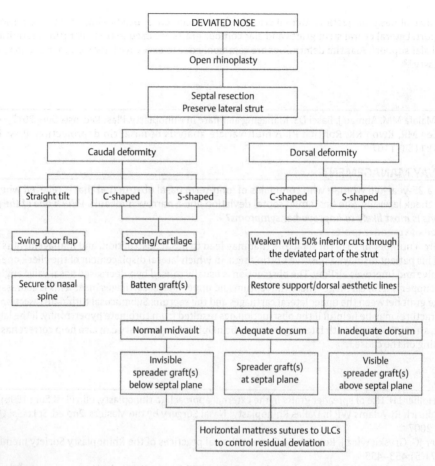

Fig. 115.2   Algorithm for correction of a deviated nose. (ULCs, Upper lateral cartilages.)

SEQUELA OF RHINOPLASTY SURGERY

22. You see a patient in clinic following closed rhinoplasty. They are concerned about the appearance of their nasal bridge, which is wide and flat just distal to the radix. *What procedure would you ideally use to correct this deformity?*

   C. Osteotomy and infracture

   This patient has an open-roof deformity of the nasal bridge following their previous rhinoplasty. The open-roof deformity occurs when a dorsal hump is reduced without bringing the nasal bones together in the midline. It may be conceptualized as shaving the top of a triangular prism structure and not folding the open edges back together again. The usual way to correct or prevent an open-roof deformity is to perform osteotomies and infracture of the nasal bones to bring them together and reconstruct the "roof." It is possible to augment an open-roof deformity with a graft, but osteotomies are generally preferred, as they correct rather than mask the deformity.

   There are a number of techniques used to augment the nasal dorsum and these include septal, auricular, and costal cartilage grafts. Graft shapes include inverted-V, inverted-U, and A-shaped examples.[1,2]

REFERENCES

1. Rohrich RJ, Krueger JK, Adams WP Jr, Hollier LH Jr. Achieving consistency in the lateral nasal osteotomy during rhinoplasty: an external perforated technique. Plast Reconstr Surg 2001;108(7):2122–2130, discussion 2131–2132
2. Gunter JP, Landecker A, Cochran CS. Frequently used grafts in rhinoplasty: nomenclature and analysis. Plast Reconstr Surg 2006;118(1):14e–29e

PRINCIPLES OF RHINOPLASTY SURGERY

23. You see a patient in clinic who desires a rhinoplasty because they are unhappy with the appearance and function of their nose. They have unilateral airway problems, with breathing difficulties at night. They also dislike the appearance of their nose because of a dorsal hump, bulbous tip, and wide alar bases. *What is the main benefit of performing a cephalic trim during rhinoplasty for this patient?*

D. Refinement of the nasal tip

A cephalic trim refers to removal of some of the lower lateral cartilages along their superior aspect. It may be beneficial in this patient in order to reduce the bulbous nasal tip and refine its appearance. It is also useful for increasing (not decreasing) tip rotation when this is required, but this was not a problem identified in this patient. Sometimes cephalic trims are further augmented with suture techniques in order to refine and support the nasal tip.

A cephalic trim is unlikely to affect airway patency. Depending on the cause, patency may be improved with manipulation of the septum or nasal valves. Reduction of a dorsal hump removes the prominent nasal septum and nasal bones, as well as the upper lateral cartilages. It does not affect the lower lateral cartilages. Alar flaring is not usually affected by tip work and reduction of alar bases in this case would require a wedge excision.[1-4]

REFERENCES

1. Ghavami A, Janis JE, Acikel C, Rohrich RJ. Tip shaping in primary rhinoplasty: an algorithmic approach. Plast Reconstr Surg 2008;122(4):1229–1241
2. Nagarkar P, Stark RY, Pezeshk RA, Amirlak B, Rohrich RJ. Role of the cephalic trim in modern rhinoplasty. Plast Reconstr Surg 2016;137(1):89–96
3. Tebbetts JB. Shaping and positioning the nasal tip without structural disruption: a new, systematic approach. Plast Reconstr Surg 1994;94(1):61–77
4. Guyuron B, Behmand RA. Nasal tip sutures part II: the interplays. Plast Reconstr Surg 2003;112(4):1130–1145, discussion 1146–1149

116. Secondary Rhinoplasty

See *Essentials of Plastic Surgery*, third edition, pp. 1642–1649

REVISION RHINOPLASTY

1. *Which one of the following is true regarding revision rhinoplasty?*
   A. The primary reason for requiring revision is a new-onset airway problem.
   B. The internationally quoted revision rates are normally between 1 and 3%.
   C. The overall revision rates are significantly different between open and closed approaches.
   D. The most commonly cited revision rates of 5 to 10% are most likely underestimated.
   E. The main reason for needing revision is poor technique in the primary setting.

PATIENT SELECTION FOR SECONDARY RHINOPLASTY

2. You are assessing a patient in the office to consider secondary rhinoplasty. *Which one of the following is most reassuring to move forward with surgery in their case?*
   A. That you know the original operating surgeon and know them to be competent.
   B. That you have personally operated on the patient previously for a different cosmetic procedure.
   C. That they decided not to take medicolegal proceedings against their previous rhinoplasty surgeon.
   D. That you share a similar aesthetic sense with the patient regarding nasal form.
   E. That the patient is able to produce images of the nose they would like you to create.

AIRWAY ISSUES FOLLOWING RHINOPLASTY

3. *Which one of the following causes of obstruction would not be addressed effectively with secondary rhinoplasty?*
   A. Septal deviation
   B. Internal valve collapse
   C. External valve dysfunction
   D. Turbinate hypertrophy
   E. Chronic rhinosinusitis

PREOPERATIVE DISCUSSIONS FOR SECONDARY RHINOPLASTY

4. *Which one of the following will carry greater emphasis when counseling someone specifically for a secondary rhinoplasty?*
   A. Emphasizing what things can be done
   B. Emphasizing what things should be done
   C. Emphasizing what things will be done
   D. Emphasizing what things cannot be done
   E. Emphasizing how things will be done

DEFORMITIES REQUIRING SECONDARY RHINOPLASTY

5. A 35-year-old male is seen in clinic following rhinoplasty elsewhere. He dislikes the shape of his nasal tip as well as the shape of the dorsum. He says he initially disliked the previous large dorsal hump, and acknowledges this was improved by his prior surgery, although perhaps excessively. On examination, he has thick skin to the nasal tip with excess fullness and drooping of the tip with under rotation. *Which one of the following best describes his deformity?*
   A. An inverted-V deformity
   B. A saddle-nose deformity
   C. A pinched tip deformity
   D. A hanging columella
   E. A pollybeak deformity

EXAMINATION IN SECONDARY RHINOPLASTY

6. *When examining a patient in preparation for secondary rhinoplasty, which one of the following body sites would be least likely to need to be examined with respect to graft donor sites?*
   A. Scalp
   B. Chest
   C. Ear
   D. Mouth
   E. Thigh

REOPERATIVE DIGITAL SIMULATION IN RHINOPLASTY

7. *What is the primary objective in using preoperative simulation with digital photography in patients considering secondary rhinoplasty?*
   A To marry the nose type they select from bank images with images of their face.
   B. To provide them with an accurate "airbrushed" image of their expected final outcome.
   C. To allow them to make requests for small refinements to the proposed nose shape prior to undergoing surgery.
   D. To facilitate the preoperative discussions on goals of surgery between the patient and their surgeon.
   E. To provide medicolegal evidence of the preoperative discussions which were undertaken prior to surgery.

PATIENT COMMUNICATION IN SECONDARY RHINOPLASTY

8. *Which one of the following is the key message to convey to patients prior to undergoing secondary rhinoplasty?*
   A. That the primary surgeon probably did nothing technically wrong.
   B. The opinions of their friends and family are likely to be positive following surgery.
   C. That the term "perfection" should be used cautiously in rhinoplasty.
   D. That the surgeon will have a clear understanding what to expect intraoperatively.
   E. That both patient and surgeon must be realistic about their goals of surgery.

DECISION-MAKING IN SECONDARY RHINOPLASTY

9. You meet a 29-year-old patient who wishes to discuss revision rhinoplasty. On further inquiry, you find out she has had three previous open rhinoplasties, the last of which was 1 year ago. She feels overall her nasal appearance has improved since she started; however, she now wishes to further refine her nose and asks you to consider making some additional small changes for her. *What would concern you most about this patient in relation to further rhinoplasty surgery?*
   A. That she has significant psychological issues
   B. That she did not come to you first for her surgery
   C. That she has not gone back to her last surgeon on this occasion
   D. That she has unrealistic expectations about further surgery
   E. That she needs to wait longer before undergoing rhinoplasty

THE APPROACH TO SECONDARY RHINOPLASTY

10. *When considering the surgical approach to revision rhinoplasty, which one of the following represents a disadvantage of using an open approach?*
   A. How well the deformity can be visualized
   B. How precisely the deformities may be corrected
   C. The lack of release of deforming soft-tissue forces
   D. The effect on long-term nasal tip edema
   E. The challenges of achieving intraoperative hemostasis

TRANSCOLUMELLAR SCAR MANAGEMENT IN SECONDARY RHINOPLASTY

11. A patient comes to the office requesting secondary rhinoplasty following a previous open approach. There are many areas of the nose to be corrected, including the dorsum, septum, and tip. On examination, you note that the previous scar is incorrectly placed too near to the columellar base. *In this situation, what should you do in terms of further nasal approaches?*
   A. Automatically opt for a closed approach to optimize safety
   B. Excise the scar and perform an open approach at the same level
   C. Incise the scar and perform an open approach at the same level
   D. Ignore the original scar and use an open approach at the correct level
   E. Avoid operating on this patient and decline surgery

PATIENT SELECTION IN SECONDARY RHINOPLASTY

12. *In which one of the following patients should fillers be avoided following rhinoplasty?*
   A. A patient who is not prepared to undergo further surgery to correct a deformity.
   B. A patient who has undergone a surgical rhinoplasty within the past year.
   C. A patient who wants to see the potential results of surgery before committing to surgery.
   D. A patient who has had undergone multiple rhinoplasties and has a heavily scarred nose with a thin soft-tissue envelope.
   E. A patient with only subtle irregularities to the nasal dorsum after one rhinoplasty.

Answers

REVISION RHINOPLASTY

1. *Which one of the following is true regarding revision rhinoplasty?*

   D The most commonly cited revision rates of 5 to 10% are most likely underestimated.

   The revision rates for rhinoplasty are estimated to be between 5 and 10%; however, these rates are very likely to be underestimated.[1-3] The main reason why these rates may be difficult to accurately assess is that these data are not well recorded. Surgeons may be cagey about discussing their actual revision rates or indeed have no idea of the true rates, especially when patients go elsewhere for their second or third procedure.

   There are a number of reasons why patients will seek revision rhinoplasty, and these may be functional, aesthetic, or a combination of both. A requirement for secondary rhinoplasty can be due to poor surgical technique, first time round, and can also be due to other factors such as incorrect technique selection, unpredictable scarring, or other complication such as hematoma, infection, or delayed healing. It may be that there are patient factors such as subsequent trauma to the nose or noncompliance with postoperative care such as continued smoking perioperatively. Of course, there are instances where patients request secondary rhinoplasty because they have unrealistic expectations about what can be achieved or has been achieved. These patients typically do not require secondary rhinoplasty and should not be offered this. There is no proven evidence that more revision surgery is required with a closed versus an open approach. Revision need will be affected by patient selection, surgeon experience, and the changes that are being implemented by any given approach.[1-3]

REFERENCES

1. Rohrich RJ, Ahmad J. Why primary rhinoplasty fails. In: Rohrich RJ, Ahmad J, eds. Secondary Rhinoplasty: By the Global Masters. 1st ed. Boca Raton, FL: CRC Press, Inc.; 2017:3–14
2. Neaman KC, Boettcher AK, Do VH, et al. Cosmetic rhinoplasty: revision rates revisited. Aesthet Surg J 2013;33(1):31–37
3. Bouaoud J, Loustau M, Belloc JB. Functional and aesthetic factors associated with revision of rhinoplasty. Plast Reconstr Surg Glob Open 2018;6(9):e1884

PATIENT SELECTION FOR SECONDARY RHINOPLASTY

2. You are assessing a patient in the office to consider secondary rhinoplasty. *Which one of the following is most reassuring to move forward with surgery in their case?*

   D. That you share a similar aesthetic sense with the patient regarding nasal shape.

   When considering secondary rhinoplasty for a patient, it is important to have a frank and open discussion preoperatively of what is possible and not possible to achieve for them. There are many factors to consider in general when deciding with a patient whether you should proceed with surgery for them. A key element of this is feeling that you and the patient are on the "same page" with what you would like to correct and have a similar aesthetic sense regarding what constitutes a balanced nose for them. Both the surgeon and the patient must understand that neither primary nor secondary rhinoplasty will ever create the "perfect nose."[1-3] **If either surgeon or patient has unrealistic goals or expectations of surgery, surgery should not proceed.**[1]

   It is easy to be flattered by a patient putting their trust into you to correct another surgeon's work, but one should always take a moment to pause and reflect, to be sure that you are likely to improve things and ask the question, "why is the original result suboptimal in the first place?"

   Knowing the competence of the original operating surgeon can be a useful piece of information here because if they are likely to have performed the surgery well, this should make you question whether you can really make it any better second time round especially when scarring is present, and the stakes are higher. Likewise, just because you have operated on the patient before, that does not mean you will necessarily have a great outcome for them in secondary rhinoplasty having been uninvolved before. That said, having insight into the patient's background can be useful and hopefully shows you have a proven track record with them and a good working relationship. That their decision of not to take medicolegal proceedings is not necessarily of great significance, unless of course you have made a conscious decision to avoid such a case mix where claims have been made before. When patients bring photos of noses they like, this can be helpful but can also be a concern. If the purpose is to help the surgeon understand what the patient likes, then this is helpful. However, if the patient is unrealistic and wishes to create someone else's nose, this is a red flag to avoid operating on them.

REFERENCES

1. Rohrich RJ, Ahmad J. Why primary rhinoplasty fails. In: Rohrich RJ, Ahmad J, eds. Secondary Rhinoplasty: By the Global Masters. 1st ed. Boca Raton, FL: CRC Press, Inc.; 2017:3–14
2. Fattahi T. Considerations in revision rhinoplasty: lessons learned. Oral Maxillofac Surg Clin North Am 2011;23(1):101–108, vi
3. Bagal AA, Adamson PA. Revision rhinoplasty. Facial Plast Surg 2002;18(4):233–244

AIRWAY ISSUES FOLLOWING RHINOPLASTY

3. *Which one of the following causes of obstruction would not be addressed effectively with secondary rhinoplasty?*

D. Chronic rhinosinusitis

Rhinoplasty can unfortunately cause problems with the airway, even where no issues were present preoperatively. This can be due to technical error or due to postoperative swelling and scarring. In some cases, only marginal alterations in the airflow mechanism can unmask a problem with the airway. Structural causes of nasal airway obstruction are common in patients presenting for rhinoplasty, but patients are often unaware that these problems exist. The most common anatomic areas for obstruction are the septum, the inferior turbinates, and internal nasal valve. Techniques to address airway issues will be directed to the underlying cause, for example, septoplasty for the septum, spreader grafts for the internal nasal valve, and turbinate fracture for the turbinates. Some conditions are not amenable to improvement by rhinoplasty including allergic rhinitis, acute or chronic rhinosinusitis, rhinitis medicamentosa, and atrophic rhinitis but instead may benefit from medical management. Evaluation of the patient's nasal airway for causes that are amenable to surgical correction is required prior to undertaking rhinoplasty surgery and the patient should be informed of those conditions which are not amenable to improvement.[1–4]

REFERENCES

1. Ahmad J, Rohrich RJ. Restoring the nasal airway during secondary rhinoplasty. In: Rohrich RJ, Ahmad J, eds. Secondary Rhinoplasty: By the Global Masters, 1st ed. Boca Raton, FL: CRC Press, Inc.; 2017:111–132
2. Rohrich RJ, Ahmad J. Preoperative evaluation and patient selection. In: Rohrich RJ, Ahmad J, eds. Secondary Rhinoplasty: By the Global Masters. 1st ed. Boca Raton, FL: CRC Press, Inc.; 2017:15–32
3. Ballert JA, Park SS. Functional considerations in revision rhinoplasty. Facial Plast Surg 2008;24(3):348–357
4. Sedaghat AR. Chronic rhinosinusitis. Am Fam Physician 2017;96(8):500–506

PREOPERATIVE DISCUSSIONS FOR SECONDARY RHINOPLASTY

4. *Which one of the following will carry greater emphasis when counseling someone specifically for a secondary rhinoplasty?*

D. Emphasizing what things cannot be done

Although the focus of consultation with primary rhinoplasty patients is centered around what the surgeon can do, the discussion with secondary rhinoplasty patients is about what the surgeon cannot do and cannot improve. It is critically important to make it clear from the outset what cannot be done and why you feel this is the case, so patients are not under any illusion that these things can be provided when they cannot. This ties in with patient expectations. Patients who desire perfection will be disappointed regardless of how successful the surgeon believes the operation has been and how ideal the outcome is. Because of this, such patients should not undergo revision rhinoplasty, as they stand to be further disappointed and yet will have been subject to additional risk and financial costs. The other things are also important to cover in both primary and secondary rhinoplasty; i.e., what can be done, then how it will be done intraoperatively. For example, if a patient has a pinched tip deformity, then to discuss the fact this can be improved and that the surgery might involve cartilage grafts and suture placement to support the lower lateral cartilages would be an appropriate discussion. One should avoid stating what "should" be done as, it is in most cases, there just needs to be a two-way discussion about options and plans, which the patient must drive forward. Telling patients, they "should" do something might be construed as encouraging them down a particular pathway.[1,2]

REFERENCES

1. Rohrich RJ, Ahmad J. Why primary rhinoplasty fails. In: Rohrich RJ, Ahmad J, eds. Secondary Rhinoplasty: By the Global Masters. 1st ed. Boca Raton, FL: CRC Press, Inc.; 2017 3–14
2. Rohrich RJ, Ahmad J. Preoperative evaluation and patient selection. In: Rohrich RJ, Ahmad J, eds. Secondary Rhinoplasty: By the Global Masters. 1st ed. Boca Raton, FL: CRC Press, Inc.; 2017:15–32

DEFORMITIES REQUIRING SECONDARY RHINOPLASTY

5. A 35-year-old male is seen in clinic following rhinoplasty elsewhere. He dislikes the shape of his nasal tip as well as the shape of the dorsum. He says he initially disliked the previous large dorsal hump, and acknowledges this was improved by his prior surgery, although perhaps excessively. On examination, he has thick skin to the nasal tip with excess fullness and drooping of the tip with under rotation. *Which one of the following best describes his deformity?*

    E. A pollybeak deformity

    The pollybeak deformity is one of the most common complications after rhinoplasty. It is characterized by fullness in the supratip area with derotation and caudal displacement of the nasal tip. This effect is said to resemble a parrot's beak. Common causes of the pollybeak deformity following primary rhinoplasty include a lack of tip support leading to underprojection of the tip, excess scarring in the supratip creating excess fullness, and over resection of the nasal dorsum more cranially.

    The principles of correction for a pollybeak deformity are to address the underlying causes on an individualized basis. Therefore, the tip support likely needs to be reinforced and the tip scar tissue may need to be reduced. The tip then typically needs elevation with or without upward rotation and the dorsum may also need correction with grafts to build it back up.[1,2]

    Other common deformities in secondary rhinoplasty include the inverted-V deformity, dorsal irregularity, saddle-nose deformity, a pinched tip, and a hanging columella.[3,4]

    A saddle nose deformity corresponds to a loss of projection of the cartilaginous and or bony structure of the nasal dorsum and may be caused by trauma, rhinoplasty, infection, or autoimmune disorders such as Wegener's granulomatosis. The inverted-V deformity is observed at the keystone area of the nose where there is separation of the upper laterals from the dorsal septum and the caudal margin of the nasal bones. A pinch-tip deformity is as it sounds, where the tip appears to be pinched. This deformity can present when there has been over-resection of the lower lateral cartilages. The hanging columellar can be a developmental or acquired issue where the soft tissues of the columellar area protrude and appear to hang beneath the columella.[5]

REFERENCES

1. Rohrich RJ, Shanmugakrishnan RR, Mohan R. Rhinoplasty refinements: addressing the pollybeak deformity. Plast Reconstr Surg 2020;145(3):696–699
2. Hoehne J, Brandstetter M, Gubisch W, Haack S. How to reduce the probability of a pollybeak deformity in primary rhinoplasty: a single-center experience. Plast Reconstr Surg 2019;143(6):1620–1624
3. Rohrich RJ, Ahmad J. Systematic nasal analysis and common deformities in secondary rhinoplasty. In: Rohrich RJ, Ahmad J, eds. Secondary Rhinoplasty: By the Global Masters. 1st ed. Boca Raton, FL: CRC Press, Inc.; 2017:33–50
4. Ahmad J, Rohrich RJ. Understanding the anatomy of nasal deformities in secondary rhinoplasty. In: Rohrich RJ, Ahmad J, eds. Secondary Rhinoplasty: By the Global Masters. 1st ed. Boca Raton, FL: CRC Press, Inc.; 2017:51
5. Rohrich RJ, Afrooz PN. Components of the hanging columella: strategies for refinement. Plast Reconstr Surg 2018;141(1):46e–54e

EXAMINATION IN SECONDARY RHINOPLASTY

6. *When examining a patient in preparation for secondary rhinoplasty, which one of the following body sites would be least likely to need to be examined with respect to graft donor sites?*

    D. Mouth

    Secondary rhinoplasty may require additional cartilage grafts in order to correct underlying nasal deformities such as an inverted-V, saddle nose, pollybeak, or pinch-tip deformity. Unfortunately, patients who have undergone previous rhinoplasty may be cartilage deficient if key sites have been overly resected and the septum has been used before. Therefore, it is vital to plan for needing additional cartilage and there are a number of potential donor sites for this.

    These include the ear and the ribs. In addition to cartilage, fascia may be required, for example, to create a "pillow of diced cartilage" to help build and recontour the nose. Facia may be obtained from the temporal scalp, mastoid area, or thigh (fascia lata). Cadaveric tissues can also be used such as irradiated rib and fascia.[1–3]

    The mouth tends to be a donor site where buccal mucosa is required, and this perhaps is more likely in some nasal and eyelid reconstructions rather than rhinoplasty. When autologous tissue is not sufficient, alloplastic material such as polyethylene and polydiaxone may be used.

REFERENCES

1. Romo T III, Kwak ES. Nasal grafts and implants in revision rhinoplasty. Facial Plast Surg Clin North Am 2006;14(4):373–387, vii

2. Bussi M, Palonta F, Toma S. Grafting in revision rhinoplasty. Acta Otorhinolaryngol Ital 2013;33(3):183–189
3. Ahmad J, Sajjadian A, Hofer SOP, Rohrich RJ. Grafting materials in secondary rhinoplasty. In: Rohrich RJ, Ahmad J, eds. Secondary Rhinoplasty: By the Global Masters. 1st ed. Boca Raton, FL: CRC Press, Inc.; 2017:133–152

PREOPERATIVE DIGITAL SIMULATION IN RHINOPLASTY

7. *What is the primary objective in using preoperative simulation with digital photography in patients considering secondary rhinoplasty?*

D. To facilitate the preoperative discussions on goals of surgery between the patient and their surgeon.

Standardized preoperative photographs are a vital component of any rhinoplasty consult whether for primary or revision surgery. They serve many purposes including supporting the discussions between patient and surgeon, providing objective evidence of the starting point before/after surgery, and medicolegal purposes.

The standard rhinoplasty views should include frontal, lateral, oblique, basal, bird's eye, and any additional views that may be required to better show specific deformities.

It is possible to take this to the next level and use simulation technology to show what the planned changes in surgery may look like postsurgery. Some surgeons and patients feel this is a helpful practice, but others do not as a computer-generated image may not be effectively replicated in life following surgery, no matter how well the surgery is performed. It is therefore best indicated to facilitate the preoperative discussions on goals of surgery between the patient and their surgeon.

Preoperative digital imaging can give the patient an idea of the possible surgical outcome, but its use should be limited to providing a dialogue between them and the surgeon. It should be used to represent the surgical goals, not the final result and so may be helpful to discuss expectations and to provide education regarding the proposed operation.[1]

Patients cannot select images of other individuals and expect a rhinoplasty to give them such a nose. Use of patient's preferred images can, however, still help the preoperative discussions to guide what they like and dislike.

Simulation technology does not provide patients with images of the exact final outcome, nor enable them to request and expect subtle changes they would like.

Indeed, one should be wary of a patient who requests multiple simulations and miniscule alterations to these images, as these patients likely have unrealistic expectations of what surgery can deliver. There may be little medicolegal benefit in showing a proposed image; in fact, it may be unhelpful if the result does not match it as the patient may claim they were promised such a result.[1-4]

REFERENCES

1. Rohrich RJ, Ahmad J. Why primary rhinoplasty fails. In: Rohrich RJ, Ahmad J, eds. Secondary Rhinoplasty: By the Global Masters. 1st ed. Boca Raton, FL: CRC Press, Inc.; 2017:3–14
2. Rohrich RJ, Ahmad J. Preoperative evaluation and patient selection. In: Rohrich RJ, Ahmad J, eds. Secondary Rhinoplasty: By the Global Masters. 1st ed. Boca Raton, FL: CRC Press, Inc.; 2017:15–32
3. Lekakis G, Claes P, Hamilton GS III, Hellings PW. Evolution of preoperative rhinoplasty consult by computer imaging. Facial Plast Surg 2016;32(1):80–87
4. Punthakee X, Rival R, Solomon P. Digital imaging in rhinoplasty. Aesthetic Plast Surg 2009;33(4):635–638

PATIENT COMMUNICATION IN SECONDARY RHINOPLASTY

8. *Which one of the following is the key message to convey to patients prior to undergoing secondary rhinoplasty?*

E. That both patient and surgeon must be realistic about their goals of surgery.

There has to be an emphasis on realistic expectations in all aesthetic surgery, perhaps none more so than in secondary rhinoplasty. Taking time to find out what specific elements of the nose patients are unhappy with is the first step. Then assessing which of the changes will not be possible and which may be possible to effect should come next. During this discussion, it is paramount to ensure patients have understood and have realistic expectations. Multiple consults are often required to do so with support from patient information leaflets. Without this, the surgeon and patient are at risk of postoperative disappointment and conflict.

It may be that the primary surgeon did nothing wrong and, in some cases, this warrants exploration. In other circumstances, this may not be known and may have no place for discussion. Some patients are disproportionately bothered about what friends and family say and need to have reassurance from them about results. This response from others is completely unpredictable and patients should be reminded of this. The term "perfection' should not be used in rhinoplasty and in fact expecting imperfection is the right approach even following high-quality surgery, especially in complex revision cases in the same way that this is highlighted to patients undergoing nasal reconstruction. Things will never return to an unscarred normal.

A real technical issue for surgeons undertaking revision surgery, particularly of the nose is that the underlying anatomy will be distorted, and the intraoperative findings may be unpredictable. They must therefore prepare for this and consider what tricks and techniques might be required so that they can be incorporated at the time. Patients must be made aware of this during the consenting process, as this will have an impact on likely outcomes and the potential need for grafts and specific techniques.[1-3]

REFERENCES

1. Rohrich RJ, Ahmad J. Preoperative evaluation and patient selection. In: Rohrich RJ, Ahmad J, eds. Secondary Rhinoplasty: By the Global Masters. 1st ed. Boca Raton, FL: CRC Press, Inc.; 2017:15–32
2. Bagal AA, Adamson PA. Revision rhinoplasty. Facial Plast Surg 2002;18(4):233–244
3. Rohrich RJ, Ahmad J. Systematic nasal analysis and common deformities in secondary rhinoplasty. In: Rohrich RJ, Ahmad J, eds. Secondary Rhinoplasty: By the Global Masters. 1st ed. Boca Raton, FL: CRC Press, Inc.; 2017:33–50

DECISION-MAKING IN SECONDARY RHINOPLASTY

9. You meet a 29-year-old patient who wishes to discuss revision rhinoplasty. On further inquiry, you find out she has had three previous open rhinoplasties, the last of which was 1 year ago. She feels overall her nasal appearance has improved since she started; however, she now wishes to further refine her nose and asks you to consider making some additional small changes for her. *What would concern you most about this patient in relation to further rhinoplasty surgery?*

   D. That she has unrealistic expectations about further surgery

   One of the main issues in rhinoplasty in general is ensuring patients have realistic expectations about the possible outcomes following this procedure. There is a large amount of media coverage and extensive online information ranging from reliable scientific clinical data to forums for open discussion by patients and surgeons. It is easy for people to review such data and develop unrealistic expectations for surgery. This can range from wanting to change subtle, barely noticeable irregularities and imperfections as they see them to wanting nasal shapes that are not achievable nor would suit their face shape.

   It seems this patient has had improvements in her nasal appearance and probably just needs a fresh pair of eyes to review things with her and provide honest feedback about the current status of things. She may also benefit from clinical psychology input to help her obtain a more balanced perspective on things.

   Revision rhinoplasty should be reserved for patients who have an identifiable problem that has the potential for improvement and that outweighs the risk of further surgery. It is key to remind patients considering undergoing revision surgery of any sort that the process may actually make things worse, rather than better, especially if the benefits are marginal or they experience a postoperative complication.

   While some patients will have psychological issues relating to their nasal appearance combined with deeper underlying personal issues, it would be wrong to conclude this patient has significant psychological issues based on the information provided.

   In general, it is preferable for patients to see their primary surgeon in the first instance to discuss and review outcomes and this patient may have already done so. One should be cautious with patients who focus on the previous surgeon's inadequate abilities or incompetence or who persist in blaming the previous surgeon for the result. In general, revision following rhinoplasty should be delayed until 1 year postsurgery, as this allows time for the soft tissues to settle fully. Therefore, in this case if a further revision was indicated, she has waited sufficient time already.[1-3]

REFERENCES

1. Bagal AA, Adamson PA. Revision rhinoplasty. Facial Plast Surg 2002;18(4):233–244
2. Rohrich RJ, Ahmad J. Preoperative evaluation and patient selection. In: Rohrich RJ, Ahmad J, eds. Secondary Rhinoplasty: By the Global Masters. 1st ed. Boca Raton, FL: CRC Press, Inc.; 2017:15–32
3. Naraghi M, Atari M. Development and validation of the expectations of aesthetic rhinoplasty scale. Arch Plast Surg 2016;43(4):365–370

THE APPROACH TO SECONDARY RHINOPLASTY

10. *When considering the surgical approach to revision rhinoplasty, which one of the following represents a disadvantage of using an open approach?*

    D. The effect on long-term nasal tip edema

    There will continue to be debate about the advantages of the open and closed approaches in rhinoplasty with proponents for either approach. However, for secondary rhinoplasty, there are potential benefits of using an open technique over a closed approach. These advantages include binocular vision, the ability to use both hands, a more effective evaluation of the deformity without distortion and subsequent precision in deformity correction. The deforming forces from soft-tissue scarring can be released and scar tissue can be removed. The options for both graft and suture techniques are increased over a closed approach and bleeding can be well controlled under direct vision.

The disadvantages of an open approach are minimal but include the transcolumellar scar which will not be present if the primary rhinoplasty was performed closed, problems with wound healing, continued tip edema, and a greater potential for devascularization of the soft-tissue envelope. For these reasons, an open approach is more popular for secondary rhinoplasty in most people's practice.[1-4]

REFERENCES

1. Ahmad J, Rohrich RJ. Choosing the approach in secondary rhinoplasty. In: Rohrich RJ, Ahmad J, eds. Secondary Rhinoplasty: By the Global Masters. 1st ed. Boca Raton, FL: CRC Press, Inc.; 2017:155–172
2. Schreiber JE, Marcus E, Tepper O, Layke J. Discovering the true resolution of postoperative swelling after rhinoplasty using 3-dimensional photographic assessment. Plast Reconstr Surg Glob Open 2019;7(8, Suppl):11–12
3. Rohrich RJ, Lee MR. External approach for secondary rhinoplasty: advances over the past 25 years. Plast Reconstr Surg 2013;131(2):404–416
4. Lee M, Unger JG, Gryskiewicz J, Rohrich RJ. Current clinical practices of the Rhinoplasty Society members. Ann Plast Surg 2013;71(5):453–455

TRANSCOLUMELLAR SCAR MANAGEMENT IN SECONDARY RHINOPLASTY

11. A patient comes to the office requesting secondary rhinoplasty following a previous open approach. There are many areas of the nose to be corrected, including the dorsum, septum, and tip. On examination, you note that the previous scar is incorrectly placed too near to the columellar base. *In this situation, what should you do in terms of further nasal approaches?*

  D. Ignore the original scar and use an open approach at the correct level
  One of the main caveats of an open approach to rhinoplasty is the presence of a transcolumellar scar, which can be a giveaway that rhinoplasty surgery has been undertaken. However, if done well, in most cases, the scar will be subtle and imperceptible in the longer term.

  When faced with patients requiring revision surgery, making decisions about scar placement can be complicated by where they were placed by their previous surgeon. This applies to any aspects of plastic surgery, not only the nose, and in some cases, it will be best to excise the original scars and thereby reuse the same approach, while in other cases it will be better to ignore them and use incisions at the ideal place.

  Deciding about the transcolumellar incision for a secondary rhinoplasty is a challenge because if the scar was too low or too high previously, then trying to correct this risks potential compromise of the skin and soft-tissue vascular supply and subsequent problems with necrosis and poor wound healing, which in a rhinoplasty can make a huge difference to outcome. It may also be that the shape of the scar is suboptimal.

  A recent retrospective study reviewed 100 cases of secondary open rhinoplasty from a single center over a 10-year period where the original transcolumellar scar had been ignored and a new preferred incision made. There were no problems with wound healing, tissue necrosis, or poor scars by taking this approach. The authors suggested that unless the patient has high-risk factors for wound healing problems such as diabetes and smoking, this is a safe and reliable approach to take even when the original incision was placed too high on the columella.

  They do suggest caution though in terms of patient selection and would not advocate this in patients undergoing surgery at less than 1-year post rhinoplasty or in active smokers. Most surgeons would not operate on active smokers for revision rhinoplasty or on any patients earlier than 1-year postsurgery.[1]

REFERENCE

1. Unger JG, Roostaeian J, Cheng DH, et al. The open approach in secondary rhinoplasty: choosing an incision regardless of prior placement. Plast Reconstr Surg 2013;132(4):780–786

PATIENT SELECTION IN SECONDARY RHINOPLASTY

12. *In which one of the following patients should fillers be avoided following rhinoplasty?*

  D. A patient who has had undergone multiple rhinoplasties and has a heavily scarred nose with a thin soft-tissue envelope.
  Soft-tissue fillers can be very useful for correcting subtle imperfections of the face due to ageing or following previous surgery. The "liquid rhinoplasty" has been marketed as an alternative to surgery for many patients and certainly does have a place for patients with contour deformities and volume deficiencies of the nose. Unfortunately, the vast majority of patients wishing to improve their nasal shape will need volume reduction and reshaping that only surgery can achieve. Many would also prefer a permanent result. The patient with residual dorsal excess would be better served with further surgical revision to reduce the cartilaginous excess rather than trying to mask it by building up other areas.

There is, however, a role for using injectables either before or after surgical rhinoplasty for certain cases. These include the following:

- Patients who do not want to undergo further surgery to correct a nasal deformity.
- Patients who are awaiting the appropriate time interval before undergoing further nasal surgery.
- Patients who want to "wear a secondary rhinoplasty" before committing to surgery.
- Patients who are not surgical candidates for rhinoplasty due to health reasons.
- Patients with subtle irregularities that may not be predictably treated with surgery.

Hyaluronic acid–based soft-tissue fillers are preferred because of their characteristics and safety profile. A variety of hyaluronic acid–based soft-tissue fillers are available and range in characteristics such as gel hardness, hydrophilicity, and dwell time.

Complications are generally low with hyaluronic acid filler; however, even in the best hands, complications can occur. Aside from the risks of blindness, tissue necrosis can occur where skin and soft-tissue vascularity is compromised, and the tissues are thin with altered blood supply such as a patient following multiple surgical rhinoplasties.

Tissue necrosis may occur following injection because of inadvertent direct intravascular injection of the product or, more likely, secondary to pressure ischemia by the product on adjacent tissues. If blanching is observed during injection of hyaluronic acid fillers, the injection must be stopped and Hyalase may need to be injected if it does not recover. Other components of the management plan when tissues are felt to be compromised by intravascular injection or severe soft-tissue compromise would include aspirin and nitro paste. Hyperbaric oxygen may also be considered for more extreme cases.[1-3]

REFERENCES

1. Ahmad J, Kurkjian TJ, Rohrich RJ. Soft tissue fillers in secondary rhinoplasty. In: Rohrich RJ, Ahmad J, eds. Secondary Rhinoplasty: By the Global Masters. 1st ed. Boca Raton, FL: CRC Press, Inc.; 2017:63–75
2. Johnson ON III, Kontis TC. Nonsurgical rhinoplasty. Facial Plast Surg 2016;32(5):500–506
3. Chen Q, Liu Y, Fan D. Serious vascular complications after nonsurgical rhinoplasty: a case report. Plast Reconstr Surg Glob Open 2016;4(4):e683

117. Genioplasty

See *Essentials of Plastic Surgery*, third edition, pp. 1650–1662

ANATOMY OF THE CHIN AND LOWER LIP

1. *Failure to repair which muscle during a genioplasty via an intraoral approach can lead to a "witch's chin" deformity?*
   A. Depressor anguli oris
   B. Depressor labii inferioris
   C. Mentalis
   D. Geniohyoid
   E. Genioglossus

IATROGENIC NERVE INJURY DURING GENIOPLASTY

2. *Which nerve is most at risk of inadvertent injury during a sliding genioplasty?*
   A. Marginal mandibular nerve
   B. Hypoglossal nerve
   C. Mandibular nerve
   D. Inferior alveolar nerve
   E. Mental nerve

OCCLUSION AND MALOCCLUSION

3. *What is the most common type of malocclusion in North American Caucasian individuals?*
   A. Angle class I
   B. Angle class II
   C. Angle class III
   D. Angle class IV
   E. Angle class V

EVALUATION OF SOFT TISSUES OF THE CHIN

4. *When evaluating chin prominence in clinic, which one of the following structures should normally lie on Riedel's plane?*
   A. Upper lip
   B. Nasal tip
   C. Alar base
   D. Labiomental crease
   E. Modiolus

OSSEOUS GENIOPLASTY

5. *Which one of the following statements is true regarding osseous genioplasty?*
   A. Malocclusion can be corrected with osseous genioplasty.
   B. A large vertical excess of the mandible is best corrected with a jumping genioplasty.
   C. Soft-tissue movement during advancement genioplasty predictably parallels skeletal changes.
   D. Complex deficiencies are better treated by prosthetic augmentation.
   E. Shallow labiomental folds are exacerbated by advancing genioplasty techniques.

IMPLANT GENIOPLASTY

6. *What is the main indication for performing an implant genioplasty?*
   A. An isolated mild horizontal chin excess
   B. An isolated mild vertical chin deficiency
   C. An isolated mandibular asymmetry
   D. An isolated mild horizontal chin deficiency
   E. An isolated large horizontal chin deficiency

APPROACHES TO IMPLANT GENIOPLASTY

7. Implant genioplasty can be undertaken through intraoral or submental approaches. *Which one of the following is a benefit of an intraoral approach?*
   A. A lower infection rate
   B. More precise placement of the implant
   C. Reduced visible scarring
   D. Less chance of mental nerve injury
   E. Reduced operative time

COMPLICATIONS OF GENIOPLASTY

8. *Which one of the following complications is most commonly observed following genioplasty?*
   A. Hematoma
   B. Infection
   C. Extrusion of implant or metalwork
   D. Lower lip weakness
   E. Lower lip paresthesia

Answers

ANATOMY OF THE CHIN AND LOWER LIP

1. *Failure to repair which muscle during a genioplasty via an intraoral approach can lead to a "witch's chin" deformity?*

   C. Mentalis

   A *witch's chin deformity* is present when there is soft-tissue ptosis of the chin caudal to the menton that results in an exaggerated submental crease. During an intraoral approach to genioplasty, the mentalis muscle is transected. To prevent subsequent ptosis, the mentalis should be reattached to the mandible and repaired during closure. The remaining muscles are relevant to local anatomy of the chin and lower lip but are neither specifically relevant to the witch's chin deformity nor genioplasty.[1,2] Alternative methods to avoid a witch's chin deformity following osseous genioplasty include minimizing soft-tissue dissection or degloving in the first instance.[3] The depressor anguli oris and depressor labii inferioris are paired muscles of facial animation that pull the lower lip downward due to their attachments from the mandible to the orbicularis oris and lower lip dermis. The geniohyoid muscles are paired narrow muscles that pass from the hyoid to the mandible. They have a role in swallowing by elevating the tongue and hyoid. The genioglossus muscles are paired extrinsic muscles of the tongue. They form most of the tongue mass and serve to protrude and deviate the tongue.

REFERENCES

1. Cohen SR. Genioplasty. In: Achauer BH, Eriksson E, Guyuron B, et al, eds. Plastic Surgery: Indications, Operations, and Outcomes, Vol. 5. St Louis, MO: Mosby-Year Book; 2000
2. Guyuron B, Michelow BJ, Willis L. Practical classification of chin deformities. Aesthetic Plast Surg 1995;19(3):257–264
3. Lambi AG, Byrd R, Bradley C, Volpicelli E, Bradley JP. Abstract QS05: Osseous genioplasty: prevention of witch's chin deformity with custom-milled plates. Plast Reconstr Surg Glob Open 2018;6(4 Suppl):116–117

IATROGENIC NERVE INJURY DURING GENIOPLASTY

2. *Which nerve is most at risk of inadvertent injury during a sliding genioplasty?*

   E. Mental nerve

   The mental nerve is at risk of damage during a sliding genioplasty if the osteotomy is placed too high or if the mental foramen is lower than anticipated. The mental nerve supplies sensation to the lower lip and dentition and is a continuation of the inferior alveolar nerve which passes through the mandible. There have been a number of anatomical and clinical studies undertaken to assess the location of the mental foramen and mental nerve, particularly relevant in the micrognathic mandible in order to reduce risk of this complication.[1–3] The inferior alveolar nerve is a branch of the mandibular division of the trigeminal nerve. These two nerves are too proximal to be at significant risk during genioplasty. The hypoglossal nerve supplies motor function to the tongue but is well protected during a genioplasty. The marginal mandibular nerve is also protected during a genioplasty, as it lies above the lower border of the mandible and lateral to the area of dissection.

REFERENCES

1. Lin HH, Denadai R, Sato N, Hung YT, Pai BCJ, Lo LJ. Avoiding inferior alveolar nerve injury during osseous genioplasty: a guide for the safe zone by three-dimensional virtual imaging. Plast Reconstr Surg 2020;146(4):847–858
2. Ousterhout DK. Sliding genioplasty, avoiding mental nerve injuries. J Craniofac Surg 1996;7(4):297–298
3. Hwang K, Lee WJ, Song YB, Chung IH. Vulnerability of the inferior alveolar nerve and mental nerve during genioplasty: an anatomic study. J Craniofac Surg 2005;16(1):10–14, discussion 14

OCCLUSION AND MALOCCLUSION

3. *What is the most common type of malocclusion in North American Caucasian individuals?*

   B. Angle class II

   There are three types of malocclusion as originally described by Edward Angle.[1,2] These are numbered I to III, and of these, the most common type in North American Caucasian individuals is type II. In simple terms, occlusion is a description of the relationship between the dentition of the upper and lower jaws when the mouth is gently closed. It is described by the upper to lower first molar relationships. The precise definition for type II malocclusion is that the mesiobuccal cusp of the maxillary first molar rests mesial to the buccal groove of the mandibular first molar. This means that the maxillary dentition sits more anterior to the mandibular dentition than normal in the lateral view. This is also called retrognathia or an overjet.

A normal occlusion involves the mesiobuccal cusp of the maxillary first molar resting in the buccal groove of the mandibular first molar without any teeth being malrotated or malpositioned. This means that the maxillary dentition is only slightly anterior to the mandibular dentition in the lateral view. A class I malocclusion is where the mesiobuccal cusp of the first molar sits in the buccal groove of the mandibular first molar, but teeth are malpositioned or malrotated. Class III malocclusion is where the mesiobuccal cusp of the first maxillary molar sits distal to the buccal groove of the mandibular first molar. This means that the mandibular dentition sits anterior to the maxillary dentition in the lateral view. Often, though not always, patients with micrognathia have a class II malocclusion, and those with prognathism have a class III malocclusion. However, this cannot be guaranteed, as occlusion and chin prominence may not always be linked. For this reason, the two must be assessed independently. There is actually much debate as to the finer detail of occlusion and what this means in terms of dentition and function of mastication, and also more widely in terms of both bone and soft-tissue anatomy and relations of the jaw (**Fig. 117.1**).[3]

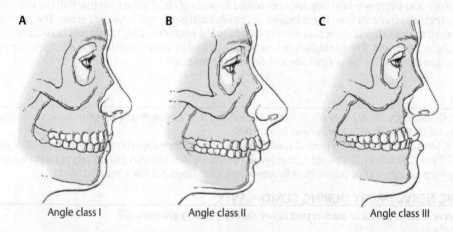

Fig. 117.1   Occlusion types. *A,* Angle class I. *B,* Angle class II. *C,* Angle class III.

REFERENCES

1. Angle EH. Classification of malocclusion. Dent Cosmos 1899;41:248–264, 350–357
2. Peck S. A biographical portrait of Edward Hartley Angle, the first specialist in orthodontics, part 1. Angle Orthod 2009;79(6):1021–1027
3. Türp JC, Greene CS, Strub JR. Dental occlusion: a critical reflection on past, present and future concepts. J Oral Rehabil 2008;35(6):446–453

EVALUATION OF SOFT TISSUES OF THE CHIN

4. *When evaluating chin prominence in clinic, which one of the following structures should normally lie on Riedel's plane?*
   A. Upper lip

   When assessing the profile of a patient before genioplasty, the relationship between the upper and lower lips and pogonion needs to be considered. Ideally, the upper lip should be just anterior to the lower lip, and the lower lip just anterior to the soft-tissue pogonion.[1] Riedel's plane is a straight line that connects the most prominent parts of the upper and lower lip in lateral view, which on a balanced face should also touch with the soft-tissue pogonion (the soft-tissue pogonion is the most projected soft-tissue point covering the mandible; **Fig. 117.2**).

   (Note there is slight variation between males and females in ideal chin prominence, with the male chin having greater prominence). Chin advancement beyond the lower lip will result in an artificial appearance with poor aesthetics; so, it must be avoided.[1]

REFERENCE

1. Guyuron B. Genioplasty. Boston, MA: Little, Brown; 1992

Riedel's plane

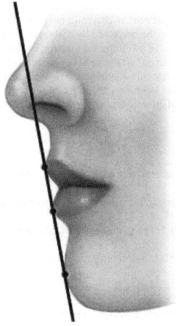

Fig. 117.2 Riedel's plane is a simple line that connects the most prominent portion of the upper and lower lip, which on a balanced face should touch the pogonion.

OSSEOUS GENIOPLASTY

5. *Which one of the following statements is true regarding osseous genioplasty?*

    C. Soft-tissue movement during advancement genioplasty predictably parallels skeletal changes.

    Soft-tissue movement during genioplasty follows bony advancement predictably, with a ratio close to 1:1 (the precise amount varies slightly between 0.8:1 and 1:1). However, this ratio does not hold true for posterior repositioning of the chin, which may be reduced. For this reason, outcomes are less predictable for prominent chin correction, and the potential soft-tissue effects must be taken into account during preoperative planning.

    Osseous genioplasty provides good flexibility for the correction of chin deformities in multiple planes, and this represents an advantage over prosthetic techniques.[1] Most commonly, it is used for horizontal (sagittal) advancement but can also be used to increase or decrease vertical deformities and amend symphyseal asymmetries. A jumping genioplasty is indicated for very minor vertical excess correction, where there is horizontal deficiency. Larger excesses are better treated by reduction genioplasty. A jumping genioplasty involves movement of the inferior-most part of the mandible anteriorly and superiorly as an onlay to augment a horizontal deficiency. The labiomental crease should normally be about 4 mm deep in women and 6 mm deep in men. Deep (not shallow) labiomental folds will be exacerbated by horizontal chin advancement or by shortening the vertical chin height. Therefore, when advancing the chin in patients with a normal or short lower face height, vertical advancement of the chin can be incorporated into the sliding genioplasty to compensate and thus maintain a normal labiomental fold depth. This approach must not be used in patients with long lower faces, and these patients are better served with orthognathic procedures.[1-3]

REFERENCES

1. Rosen HM. Osseous genioplasty. In: Thorne CH, ed. Grabb & Smith's Plastic Surgery. 6th ed. Philadelphia, PA: Lippincott Williams & Wilkins; 2006
2. Jones BM, Vesely MJ. Osseous genioplasty in facial aesthetic surgery--a personal perspective reviewing 54 patients. J Plast Reconstr Aesthet Surg 2006;59(11):1177–1187
3. Guyuron B. Genioplasty. Plast Reconstr Surg 2008;121(4, Suppl):S1–S7

IMPLANT GENIOPLASTY

6. *What is the main indication for performing an implant genioplasty?*

D. An isolated mild horizontal chin deficiency

In general, alloplastic augmentation of the chin should only be used for patients with a mild horizontal chin deficiency in the sagittal plane and with a shallow labiomental fold. It may be preferred by cosmetic surgery patients and can be incorporated into face and neck lift procedures where a submental incision is already planned. Implant types include silicone and porous polyethylene. These can be "off the shelf" or customized to each individual patient. The latter are typically custom 3D printed. Alloplastic chin augmentation cannot correct excess horizontal deficiency, vertical deficiency of any severity, mandibular asymmetry, significant microgenia, or malocclusion. Contraindications to implant use include the presence of infection, poor dentition with active dental disease, diabetes, immunocompromise, and smoking.[1-4]

REFERENCES

1. Guyuron B, Raszewski RL. A critical comparison of osteoplastic and alloplastic augmentation genioplasty. Aesthetic Plast Surg 1990;14(3):199–206
2. Zide BM, Pfeifer TM, Longaker MT. Chin surgery: I. Augmentation--the allures and the alerts. Plast Reconstr Surg 1999;104(6):1843–1853, discussion 1861–1862
3. Cohen SR. Genioplasty. In: Achauer BH, Eriksson E, Guyuron B, et al, eds. Plastic Surgery: Indications, Operations, and Outcomes, Vol. 5. St Louis, MO: Mosby-Year Book; 2000
4. Aston SJ, Smith DM. Taking it on the chin: recognizing and accounting for lower face asymmetry in chin augmentation and genioplasty. Plast Reconstr Surg 2015;135(6):1591–1595

APPROACHES TO IMPLANT GENIOPLASTY

7. Implant genioplasty can be undertaken through intraoral or submental approaches. *Which one of the following is a benefit of an intraoral approach?*

C. Reduced visible scarring

Implant genioplasty may be performed via intraoral or extraoral approaches. The advantage of an intraoral approach is that external scars are completely avoided. The alternative to the intraoral approach is a submental approach, which involves a short, transverse skin incision placed just behind the submental crease. This hides the scar discretely and provides access, which can also be useful when combined procedures such as a neck lift or corset platysmaplasty are required. Further potential benefits of using the submental approach are a more precise implant placement, reduced risk of mental nerve damage and avoidance of the creation of a witch's chin deformity. The two approaches have similar rates of infection, which may be counterintuitive as one may expect infection rates to be higher when inserting a prosthesis through the oral cavity, because of the high number of pathogens within the mouth. However, this element does not need to be a major factor to consider when selecting the preferred approach. Operative times are comparable with either approach and are more likely to be affected by surgeon and patient factors rather than the approach itself.[1-3]

REFERENCES

1. White JB, Dufresne CR. Management and avoidance of complications in chin augmentation. Aesthet Surg J 2011;31(6):634–642
2. Yaremchuk MJ. Improving aesthetic outcomes after alloplastic chin augmentation. Plast Reconstr Surg 2003;112(5):1422–1432, discussion 1433–1434
3. Cohen SR. Genioplasty. In: Achauer BH, Eriksson E, Guyuron B, et al, eds. Plastic Surgery: Indications, Operations, and Outcomes, Vol. 5. St Louis, MO: Mosby-Year Book; 2000

COMPLICATIONS OF GENIOPLASTY

8. *Which one of the following complications is most commonly observed following genioplasty?*

E. Lower lip paresthesia

The most common complication of those listed following genioplasty is a transient lower lip paresthesia which is seen almost universally. This resolves in almost all patients who have solely undergone genioplasty without other combined procedures such as orthognathic surgery, where rates of continued paresthesia are between 15 and 29%.[1,2]

Hematomas are rare and most often occur at the osteotomy site in association with an osseous genioplasty. Infection is less than 5% for implant genioplasty and 3% for osseous genioplasty. Extrusion of implant or metalwork is also rare. Lower lip weakness can occur leading to drooling, but again is usually temporary and not common.

The most common complication following genioplasty is a poor aesthetic outcome, but in spite of this, patient satisfaction rates are very high (>90%). Poor aesthetic outcomes include overcorrection, undercorrection, and asymmetry.[1,3]

REFERENCES

1. Hoenig JF. Sliding osteotomy genioplasty for facial aesthetic balance: 10 years of experience. Aesthetic Plast Surg 2007;31(4):384–391
2. Lindquist CC, Obeid G. Complications of genioplasty done alone or in combination with sagittal split-ramus osteotomy. Oral Surg Oral Med Oral Pathol 1988;66(1):13–16
3. Rosen HM. Aesthetic guidelines in genioplasty: the role of facial disproportion. Plast Reconstr Surg 1995;95(3):463–469, discussion 470–472

118. Liposuction

See *Essentials of Plastic Surgery*, third edition, pp. 1663–1676

HISTORICAL DEVELOPMENT IN LIPOSUCTION

1. *Which one of the following changes in practice has been key in the development of current liposuction techniques?*
   A. Introduction of taper-tipped cannulae as standard practice
   B. Evacuation using pressures greater than 1 atmosphere
   C. Phasing out of wetting solutions containing epinephrine
   D. A focus on preserving zones of adherence
   E. A trend toward fat aspiration from the superficial fat layer

ANATOMY RELEVANT TO LIPOSUCTION

2. *Which layer of fat is considered safest to target when performing liposuction on the buttock?*
   A. Superficial
   B. Intermediate
   C. Deep
   D. Cellulite
   E. All areas are equally safe

ZONES OF ADHERENCE IN LIPOSUCTION

3. *Which one of the following is a zone of adherence found only in male patients?*
   A. Distal iliotibial tract
   B. Gluteal crease
   C. Lateral gluteal depression
   D. Iliac crest
   E. Distal posterior thigh

PHYSICS OF LIPOSUCTION

4. *What is the main benefit of selecting a smaller-diameter cannula for traditional suction-assisted liposuction (SAL)?*
   A. To reduce the chances of damaging blood vessels
   B. To achieve a more even fat removal
   C. To allow better control of the instrument
   D. To accelerate the process of fat removal
   E. To make the process more comfortable for the operator

WETTING SOLUTIONS IN LIPOSUCTION

5. You are working as a fellow during your aesthetic fellowship preparing a patient for liposuction to the trunk and abdomen. Your attending asks you to begin the infiltration. She estimates the patient requires removal of 400 to 500 cc of fat and wishes to use a tumescent technique. *What approximate volume of infiltrate should you use?*
   A. 250 cc
   B. 500 cc
   C. 750 cc
   D. 1,500 cc
   E. 2,000 cc

EPINEPHRINE USE IN LIPOSUCTION

6. *When preparing a typical solution for infiltration in liposuction, what is the most common dilution used for epinephrine?*
   A. 1:200,000
   B. 1:1,000
   C. 1:10,000
   D. 1:100,000
   E. 1:1,000,000

LIDOCAINE USE IN TUMESCENT LIPOSUCTION

7. You are preparing a solution to infiltrate for tumescent liposuction in a patient requiring comprehensive body contouring under local anesthetic and sedation. You plan to target the trunk, thighs, and buttocks. The patient weighs 86 kg and has a body mass index (BMI) of 33. *What is the approximate maximum dose of lidocaine that can be used for this procedure according to work undertaken by Klein?*
   A. 600 mg
   B. 1,000 mg
   C. 1,600 mg
   D. 3,000 mg
   E. 3,600 mg

ULTRASOUND-ASSISTED LIPOSUCTION

8. You have been trained in the use of SAL and move to a new facility where ultrasound-assisted liposuction (UAL) is being used. *Which one of the following is correct about the UAL technique?*
   A. An oscillating reciprocating cannula is used at rates of 4,000 cycles per minute.
   B. It is a four-stage procedure involving subdermal skin stimulation.
   C. The sole mechanism of action is cavitation by collapse of intracellular microbubbles.
   D. It still requires the use of SAL.
   E. It carries a minimal risk of thermal injury compared with laser-assisted techniques.

POWER-ASSISTED LIPOSUCTION

9. *Which one of the following situations best suits the use of PAL?*
   A. When subtle fine contouring is required
   B. When patients are conscious and low noise is preferable
   C. When vibration transmission to the surgeon must be avoided
   D. When overlying skin perfusion is felt to be compromised
   E. When large volumes of fibrofatty tissue are to be removed

LASER-ASSISTED LIPOSUCTION

10. *What is the proposed benefit of using laser-assisted liposuction over PAL?*
    A. It is faster and less labor intensive.
    B. Fewer stages need to be undertaken.
    C. Conventional evacuation techniques are not required.
    D. The machinery is less expensive.
    E. There may be a potential skin-tightening effect.

FLUID RESUSCITATION FOLLOWING LIPOSUCTION

11 *When should a patient receive both maintenance and intravenous crystalloid fluid therapy after liposuction?*
    A. In all cases
    B. In all patients with a BMI greater than 30
    C. When the aspirate-to-infiltrate ratio is 1:1
    D. In ASA grade 3 patients
    E. When more than 5 L is aspirated

LIPOSUCTION STAGES

12. *Which one of the following is true when performing SAL?*
    A. The entire process has three stages.
    B. There should be a 4-minute gap between the first and second stages.
    C. The cannula should be progressively moved from superficial to deep.
    D. The primary clinical endpoint of the final stage is guided by a pinch test.
    E. The port sites must be protected with wet towels.

LIPOSUCTION BY ANATOMIC AREA

13 When performing body contouring procedures using liposuction, it is important to have a concept of the "ideal" or "normal" aesthetically pleasing form for both males and females. This may differ according to personal tastes and with racial variations. *Which one of the following is not a feature of the ideal female body contour?*
    A. A flat contour to the lower abdomen
    B. Convexity over the hips and thighs
    C. Concavity below the rib cage
    D. A rounded contour to the lateral buttock crease
    E. Shallow convexities to the upper thighs

CLINICAL DECISION-MAKING IN LIPOSUCTION

14. A 34-year-old woman is seeking lower abdominal recontouring following pregnancy and weight loss. Her weight is stable within 30% of her ideal and she is otherwise healthy. On examination, she has an excess of fat in the infraumbilical region and loose skin with striae. *She has a Pfannenstiel scar and significant cellulite. Which one of the following is correct?*
    A. Liposuction alone is likely to give her a good result.
    B. Further weight loss is required before liposuction.
    C. She may be better served by an abdominoplasty.
    D. Her skin changes will improve with SAL.
    E. Liposuction is the best modality to address her cellulite.

Answers

HISTORICAL DEVELOPMENT IN LIPOSUCTION

1. Which one of the following changes in practice has been key in the development of current liposuction techniques?

D. A focus on preserving zones of adherence

A better understanding of natural soft-tissue zones of adherence[1] has led to surgeons tending to preserve these zones during liposuction to avoid undesirable contour changes (**Fig. 118.1**).

Current liposuction techniques have been developed from work performed by doctors in France and Italy in the 1970s. They have been regularly practiced in the United States since the early 1980s, following presentation by a French team at the 1982 American Society of Plastic Surgeons (ASPS) conference.

The first description of liposuction can be traced back to the 1920s, and this tragically ended in eventual amputation of the involved lower limb. An Italian father and son team by the name of Fischer were the first to develop liposuction techniques using a blunt hollow cannula attached to a suction source. The Italians' ideas were further developed by surgeons in Paris including Illouz, Fournier, and Otteni, who were instrumental in popularizing the technique in France. Illouz developed the wet infiltration technique to decrease bleeding and ease suctioning. Fournier originally preferred a dry harvesting technique, although later converted to a wet technique. He made further contributions such as refinements to contoured harvesting and postoperative compression, and spent time widely teaching these techniques.

Liposuction techniques generate variable degrees of negative pressure less than 1 atmosphere pressure. Rodriguez and Condé-Green[2] quantified the degree of negative pressure generated using syringe techniques between 2,165 and 2,718 mm Hg (a maximum of 20.94 atmospheric pressure).

The introduction of epinephrine into solutions has been attributed to Hetter, who showed that large decreases in postoperative hematocrit level could be reduced when incorporating epinephrine into the liposuction infiltrate.[3,4] The tumescent approach currently used by many plastic surgeons was later introduced by Klein in the 1980s. Most surgeons recommend caution in using liposuction in the superficial fat plane, as there is a high risk of creating surface irregularities.

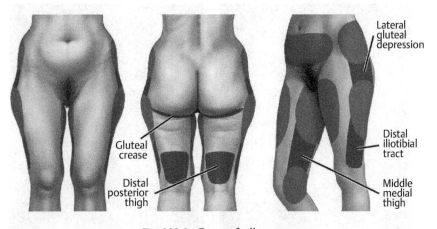

Fig. 118.1 Zones of adherence.

REFERENCES

1. Rohrich RJ, Smith PD, Marcantonio DR, Kenkel JM. The zones of adherence: role in minimizing and preventing contour deformities in liposuction. Plast Reconstr Surg 2001;107(6):1562–1569
2. Rodriguez RL, Condé-Green A. Quantification of negative pressures generated by syringes of different calibers used for liposuction. Plast Reconstr Surg 2012;130(2):383e–384e
3. Hetter GP. The effect of low-dose epinephrine on the hematocrit drop following lipolysis. Aesthetic Plast Surg 1984;8(1):19–21
4. Coleman WP III. The history of liposuction and fat transplantation in America. Dermatol Clin 1999;17(4):723–727, v

ANATOMY RELEVANT TO LIPOSUCTION

2. *Which layer of fat is considered safest to target when performing liposuction on the buttock?*

    B. Intermediate

In general, it is safest to perform liposuction in the intermediate fat layer, as it is least likely to result in surface irregularities or deep tissue damage. Depth of liposuction is also affected by anatomic area. For example, in most anatomic regions, it is safe to liposuction the deep layers of fat; however, in the buttock region, this should be avoided. Liposuction in the superficial fat layer must always be done with caution, as there is a risk of creating visible surface irregularities that can subsequently be difficult to correct.[1,2] Cellulite is caused by hypertrophy of the superficial fat within septa that connects the superficial fascial system and the epidermis. It is more appropriately treated with skin-tightening procedures than liposuction.[2,3]

REFERENCES

1. Markman B, Barton FE Jr. Anatomy of the subcutaneous tissue of the trunk and lower extremity. Plast Reconstr Surg 1987;80(2):248–254
2. Illouz YG. Study of subcutaneous fat. Aesthetic Plast Surg 1990;14(3):165–177
3. Lockwood TE. Superficial fascial system (SFS) of the trunk and extremities: a new concept. Plast Reconstr Surg 1991;87(6):1009–1018

ZONES OF ADHERENCE IN LIPOSUCTION

3. *Which one of the following is a zone of adherence found only in male patients?*

    D. Iliac crest

Zones of adherence are areas where the superficial fascial system has dense connections with the deep/investing layer of muscle fascia, meaning that the superficial subcutaneous plane is adherent to the muscle fascia.[1] There are gender differences in the zones of adherence that result in different effects with weight gain. In men, there is a zone of adherence along the iliac crest, and this defines the inferior margin of the flank. In contrast, women carry fat from this area over the iliac crest due to an absence of adherence (**Fig. 118.2**). The fat is held by the next zone of adherence, which lies with the gluteal depression overlying the greater trochanter.

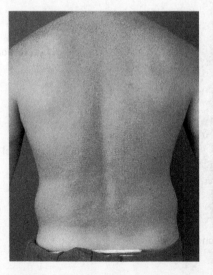
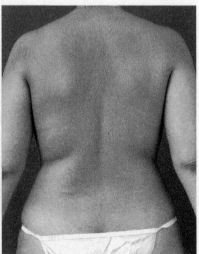

Fig. 118.2　Sex differences in the zones of adherence result in different weight gain effects. Males have a zone of adherence along the iliac crest that women lack.

REFERENCE

1. Rohrich RJ, Smith PD, Marcantonio DR, Kenkel JM. The zones of adherence: role in minimizing and preventing contour deformities in liposuction. Plast Reconstr Surg 2001;107(6):1562–1569

PHYSICS OF LIPOSUCTION

4. *What is the main benefit of selecting a smaller-diameter cannula for traditional suction-assisted liposuction (SAL)?*

   B. To achieve a more even fat removal

   The main benefit of using a smaller-diameter cannula for SAL is that it helps ensure even removal of fat. This is at the expense of making the process more work and more time consuming for the operator, as the resistance increases dramatically with a decrease in the cannula diameter. Cannulas are designed with blunt tips to minimize damage to vessels, nerves, and fascia. A larger, blunt cannula is less likely to damage these anatomic structures, but both should tend to move them out of the way. Control is improved when using a shorter cannula, especially for fine work, but this does not directly affect the evenness of fat removal.[1,2]

REFERENCES

1. Hetter GP. Lipoplasty: The Theory and Practice of Blunt Suction Lipectomy. Boston. MA: Little Brown; 1984
2. Fodor PB, Cimino WW, Watson JP, Tahernia A. Suction-assisted lipoplasty: physics, optimization, and clinical verification. Aesthet Surg J 2005;25(3):234–246

WETTING SOLUTIONS IN LIPOSUCTION

5. You are working as a fellow during your aesthetic fellowship preparing a patient for liposuction to the trunk and abdomen. Your attending asks you to begin the infiltration. She estimates the patient requires removal of 400 to 500 cc of fat and wishes to use a tumescent technique. *What approximate volume of infiltrate should you use?*

   D. 1,500 cc

   There are three types of infiltration ratio used for liposuction: wet, superwet, and tumescent. They differ in their volume-to-aspiration ratios. A wet technique involves infiltration of 200 to 300 mL per treated area. A superwet technique involves a 1:1 ratio between infiltrate and planned aspirate. A tumescent technique involves infiltration-to-aspiration ratios of 3:1; so in this case, 1.2 to 1.5 L should be administered.[1,2]

REFERENCES

1. Rohrich RJ, Beran SJ, Fodor PB. The role of subcutaneous infiltration in suction-assisted lipoplasty: a review. Plast Reconstr Surg 1997;99(2):514–519, discussion 520–526
2. Iverson RE, Pao VS. MOC-PS(SM) CME article: liposuction. Plast Reconstr Surg 2008; 121(4, Suppl):1–11

EPINEPHRINE USE IN LIPOSUCTION

6. *When preparing a typical solution for infiltration in liposuction, what is the most common dilution used for epinephrine?*

   E. 1:1,000,000

   Epinephrine is used to induce vasoconstriction in liposuction techniques. It forms an important component of the infiltrate. A typical dilution involves 1 mg of epinephrine diluted in 1 L of normal saline or Hartman's solution. Each 1 mg vial of epinephrine normally has a concentration of 1:1,000. Following dilution in the liter bag of saline/Hartman's solution, the epinephrine will be diluted to a final concentration of 1:1,000,000. This still represents a relatively low concentration in comparison to local anesthetics such as lidocaine which are often packaged with 1:200,000 epinephrine or 1:100,000 for dental syringes. Therefore, it represents a safe dosage to adopt. It is important to allow 7 minutes following infiltration before commencing liposuction, to allow time for the effects of epinephrine to be observed.[1-3]

REFERENCES

1. Farkas JP, Stephan PJ, Kenkel JM. Liposuction: basic techniques and safety considerations. In: Nahai F, ed. The Art of Aesthetic Surgery: Principles and Techniques. 2nd ed. St Louis, MO: Quality Medical Publishing; 2011
2. Rohrich RJ, Beran SJ, Fodor PB. The role of subcutaneous infiltration in suction-assisted lipoplasty: a review. Plast Reconstr Surg 1997;99(2):514–519, discussion 520–526
3. Rohrich RJ, Kenkel JM, Janis JE, Beran SJ, Fodor PB. An update on the role of subcutaneous infiltration in suction-assisted lipoplasty. Plast Reconstr Surg 2003;111(2):926–927, discussion 928

LIDOCAINE USE IN TUMESCENT LIPOSUCTION

7. You are preparing a solution to infiltrate for tumescent liposuction in a patient requiring comprehensive body contouring under local anesthetic and sedation. You plan to target the trunk, thighs, and buttocks. The patient weighs 86 kg and has a body mass index (BMI) of 33. *What is the approximate maximum dose of lidocaine that can be used for this procedure according to work undertaken by Klein?*

   D. 3,000 mg

   The maximum dose of subcutaneous lidocaine when using epinephrine is often quoted as 7 mg/kg. In this case, the maximum dose would be just 602 mg for this patient. However, Klein[1] published an article on the use of far greater doses of lidocaine for tumescent liposuction with no adverse effects. In 1990, he published a study in which plasma concentrations of lidocaine were measured after injection of dilute lidocaine and epinephrine in patients undergoing liposuction. He found that peak doses of lidocaine were reached 12 to 14 hours after injection. He concluded that a combination of lidocaine dilution, epinephrine, and liposuction limits the systemic absorption and potential toxicity of lidocaine in this setting. He estimated a maximum safe dose of 35 mg/kg for tumescent infiltration, and this has been widely accepted in clinical practice. For the patient described in this scenario, this would equate to an absolute maximum of 3,010 mg. However, it is recommended that attention be paid to the concentration of lidocaine administered, as well as the overall dose. Concentrations over 0.05% are not recommended in large-volume liposuction infiltration fluid.[2]

REFERENCES

1. Klein JA. Tumescent technique for regional anesthesia permits lidocaine doses of 35 mg/kg for liposuction. J Dermatol Surg Oncol 1990;16(3):248–263
2. Pace MM, Chatterjee A, Merrill DG, Stotland MA, Ridgway EB. Local anesthetics in liposuction: considerations for new practice advisory guidelines to improve patient safety. Plast Reconstr Surg 2013;131(5):820e–826e

ULTRASOUND-ASSISTED LIPOSUCTION

8. You have been trained in the use of SAL and move to a new facility where ultrasound-assisted liposuction (UAL) is being used. *Which one of the following is correct about the UAL technique?*

   D. It still requires the use of SAL.

   UAL was first described by Zocchi in Italy in the 1990s. It works by creating alternating currents with piezoelectric crystals that expand and contract, releasing ultrasonic waves. It is a three-stage process involving infiltration, ultrasound treatment to emulsify fats, and then evacuation of fat and final contouring with SAL. Emulsification is achieved by three mechanisms: micromechanical, thermal, and cavitation. It is a very effective treatment but carries a risk of thermal injury; for this reason, many surgeons prefer not to use it.

   Power-assisted liposuction (PAL) uses an oscillating reciprocating cannula and may reduce risks of thermal injury while providing a more efficient method compared with standard liposuction. Laser-assisted liposuction involves four phases, one of which is direct dermal stimulation for skin tightening. It has shown promising results, but no prospective trials have shown a benefit over conventional techniques.[1-3]

REFERENCES

1. Kenkel JM, Janis JE, Rohrich RJ, Beran SJ. Aesthetic body contouring: ultrasound-assisted liposuction. In: Matarasso A, ed. Operative Techniques in Plastic and Reconstructive Surgery. Philadelphia, PA: Saunders-Elsevier; 2003
2. Zocchi ML. Ultrasonic assisted lipoplasty. Technical refinements and clinical evaluations. Clin Plast Surg 1996;23(4):575–598
3. Rohrich RJ, Kenkel JM, Beran SJ. Ultrasound-assisted liposuction. St Louis, MO: Quality Medical Publishing; 1998

POWER-ASSISTED LIPOSUCTION

9. *Which one of the following situations best suits the use of PAL?*

   E. When large volumes of fibrofatty tissue are to be removed

   PAL uses an externally powered cannula that oscillates in a 2-mm reciprocating motion at rates of 4,000 to 6,000 cycles per minute. The main advantage of this technique is that liposuction is faster and less labor intensive. It is therefore ideal for performing liposuction in larger areas, particularly in fibrofatty tissues and those that have had prior liposuction. The disadvantages are significant noise generation, mechanical vibration transmission to the operator, and the system tends to be more bulky and cumbersome than traditional equipment. It is therefore not well suited to fine-contouring changes. Radiographic dye studies show that UAL, not PAL, reduces the vascular disruption to skin and soft tissues following liposuction. However, no form of liposuction is advisable in areas where skin vascularity is compromised.[1,2]

REFERENCES

1. Farkas JP, Stephan PJ, Kenkel JM. Liposuction: basic techniques and safety considerations. In: Nahai F, ed. The Art of Aesthetic Surgery: Principles and Techniques. 2nd ed. St Louis, MO: Quality Medical Publishing; 2011
2. Wall SH Jr, Lee MR. Separation, aspiration, and fat equalization: SAFE liposuction concepts for comprehensive body contouring. Plast Reconstr Surg 2016;138(6):1192–1201

LASER-ASSISTED LIPOSUCTION

10. *What is the proposed benefit of using laser-assisted liposuction over PAL?*

    E. There may be a potential skin-tightening effect.

Laser-assisted liposuction involves insertion of a laser fiber through a small skin incision. This may either be housed within the cannula or a standalone device. The main proposed advantage of laser-assisted liposuction is that it may produce a skin-tightening effect secondary to heating of the subdermal tissues. However, this is anecdotal, and no large prospective studies have proven a difference between laser-assisted and conventional techniques. The process involves four stages with infiltration, application of energy, evacuation, and then subdermal skin stimulation. It therefore is more time and labor intensive than other techniques and the equipment is expensive.[1-3]

REFERENCES

1. Farkas JP, Stephan PJ, Kenkel JM. Liposuction: basic techniques and safety considerations. In: Nahai F, ed. The Art of Aesthetic Surgery: Principles and Techniques. 2nd ed. St Louis, MO: Quality Medical Publishing; 2011
2. Prado A, Andrades P, Danilla S, Leniz P, Castillo P, Gaete F. A prospective, randomized, double-blind, controlled clinical trial comparing laser-assisted lipoplasty with suction-assisted lipoplasty. Plast Reconstr Surg 2006;118(4):1032–1045
3. DiBernardo BE, Reyes J. Evaluation of skin tightening after laser-assisted liposuction. Aesthet Surg J 2009;29(5):400–407

FLUID RESUSCITATION FOLLOWING LIPOSUCTION

11. *When should a patient receive both maintenance and intravenous crystalloid fluid therapy after liposuction?*

    E. When more than 5 L is aspirated

Fluid balance must be carefully assessed and managed during the perioperative period for liposuction, as infiltration of large volumes can lead to significant fluid shifts. Only a quarter of the infiltration fluid is removed during suctioning. The remainder is therefore reabsorbed over a 6- to 12-hour period. Most patients can be managed with maintenance fluids alone. The requirement for additional intravenous crystalloid is only for patients who have more than 5 L of aspirate removed. In such patients, the recommended fluid is 0.25 mL of intravenous crystalloid per mL of aspirate over 5 L. As with all guidelines, the actual fluid given must be tailored to the patient's parameters such as blood pressure, urine output, and tissue characteristics.[1-3]

REFERENCES

1. Grazer FM, de Jong RH. Fatal outcomes from liposuction: census survey of cosmetic surgeons. Plast Reconstr Surg 2000;105:436–446, discussion 447–448
2. Trott SA, Beran SJ, Rohrich RJ, Kenkel JM, Adams WP Jr, Klein KW. Safety considerations and fluid resuscitation in liposuction: an analysis of 53 consecutive patients. Plast Reconstr Surg 1998;102(6):2220–2229
3. Wang G, Cao WG, Zhao TL. Fluid management in extensive liposuction: a retrospective review of 83 consecutive patients [published correction appears in Medicine (Baltimore). 2018;97(44):e13212

LIPOSUCTION STAGES

12. *Which one of the following is true when performing SAL?*

    D. The primary clinical endpoint of the final stage is guided by a pinch test.

The process of SAL has two main stages: infiltration and evacuation/contouring. There should be a 10-minute gap between the two stages to allow for the epinephrine effects on vasoconstriction to occur. The endpoint to stage 1 is uniform blanching and skin turgor. In stage 2, the cannula should be moved from deep to superficial. When using UAL, this is reversed. The primary clinical endpoint of the final stage is guided by the final contour appearance and the symmetry of pinch test results. When using UAL, port sites must be protected and wet towels are used to cool the area. However, this is not applicable to standard SAL.[1-3]

REFERENCES

1. Farkas JP, Stephan PJ, Kenkel JM. Liposuction: basic techniques and safety considerations. In: Nahai F, ed. The Art of Aesthetic Surgery: Principles and Techniques. 2nd ed. St Louis, MO: Quality Medical Publishing; 2011

2. Klein JA. The tumescent technique. Anesthesia and modified liposuction technique. Dermatol Clin 1990;8(3):425–437
3. Shridharani SM, Broyles JM, Matarasso A. Liposuction devices: technology update. Med Devices (Auckl) 2014;7:241–251

LIPOSUCTION BY ANATOMIC AREA

13. When performing body contouring procedures using liposuction, it is important to have a concept of the "ideal" or "normal" aesthetically pleasing form for both males and females. This may differ according to personal tastes and with racial variations. *Which one of the following is not a feature of the ideal female body contour?*

A. A flat contour to the lower abdomen

The "ideal" female body form has a curvy silhouette, often described as an hourglass shape. It is wider at the shoulder and hip and narrower at the waist when viewed from the front (**Fig. 118.3,** A). This involves concavity below the ribcage and convexity over the hips and thighs. The convexity should continue over the proximal thighs and buttocks. In the lateral view, the abdomen should be concave in the epigastric area but slightly convex lower down in the periumbilical region. Since individual preferences vary, these must be discussed in detail with patients before surgery. Males have a more linear silhouette, with only limited convexity and concavity (**Fig. 118.3,** B). The flanks should taper from the lower ribs to the iliac crest. The abdomen should be flat in the periumbilical region.[1,2]

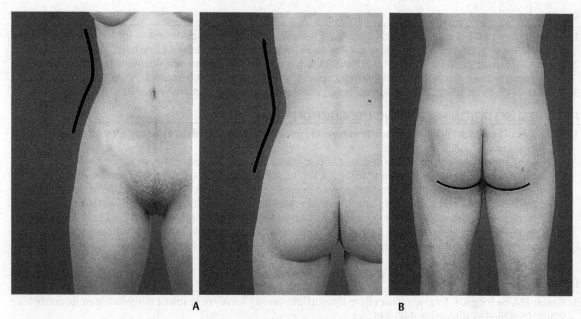

Fig. 118.3 A, An aesthetic female contour begins as a concavity at the flare of the lower ribcage that changes to a convexity over the hips and thighs. **B,** The male form has relative concavities above the pelvic area and convexities in the buttock area. The buttock crease is more angular and square than in females.

REFERENCES

1. Rohrich RJ, Smith PD, Marcantonio DR, Kenkel JM. The zones of adherence: role in minimizing and preventing contour deformities in liposuction. Plast Reconstr Surg 2001;107(6):1562–1569
2. Nahai F, ed. The Art of Aesthetic Surgery: Principles and Techniques. 2nd ed. St Louis, MO: Quality Medical Publishing; 2011

CLINICAL DECISION-MAKING IN LIPOSUCTION

14. A 34-year-old woman is seeking lower abdominal recontouring following pregnancy and weight loss. Her weight is stable within 30% of her ideal and she is otherwise healthy. On examination, she has an excess of fat in the infraumbilical region and loose skin with striae. She has a Pfannenstiel scar and significant cellulite. *Which one of the following is correct?*

C. She may be better served with an abdominoplasty.

Understanding the limitations of liposuction is vital for practitioners and patients. Given the clinical features described, this woman may be best managed with an abdominoplasty rather than liposuction, as this will address both the skin and fat excesses. From a technical perspective, she is unlikely to obtain a good outcome following liposuction as her skin is thin and stretched, as evidenced by the striae. Removing the residual volume in this case will lead to an exaggerated residual skin excess. Liposuction is generally indicated in patients with fat excess but minimal skin excess. Patients should also be close to their ideal weight (within 30%). Therefore, further weight loss is not required in this case. Cellulite probably represents a combination of fat hypertrophy within fibrous septae and skin laxity. It is not well treated with liposuction and it is important to inform patients of this preoperatively. It may be more effectively treated using skin-tightening procedures. Where mild skin-tightening effects are desired, then laser liposuction may be helpful, but SAL is not beneficial.[1,2]

REFERENCES

1. Illouz YG. Study of subcutaneous fat. Aesthetic Plast Surg 1990;14(3):165–177
2. Lockwood TE. Superficial fascial system (SFS) of the trunk and extremities: a new concept. Plast Reconstr Surg 1991;87(6):1009–1018

119. Brachioplasty

See *Essentials of Plastic Surgery*, third edition, pp. 1677–1690

ANATOMY IN RELATION TO BRACHIOPLASTY

1. Six months following brachioplasty, a patient complains of continued pain around the elbow and paresthesia in the forearm. *What nerve is most likely to have been injured during the procedure?*
   A. Anterior brachial cutaneous nerve
   B. Ulnar nerve
   C. Musculocutaneous nerve
   D. Lateral antebrachial cutaneous nerve
   E. Medial antebrachial cutaneous nerve

SURGICAL ANATOMY IN BRACHIOPLASTY

2. *Where in the arm is most subcutaneous fat generally found?*
   A. Anterior
   B. Posterior
   C. Medial
   D. Lateral
   E. Distal

CONTRAINDICATIONS TO BRACHIOPLASTY

3. *Which one of the following represents an absolute contraindication to brachioplasty?*
   A. Connective tissue disorders
   B. Diabetes mellitus
   C. Lymphedema
   D. Rheumatoid arthritis
   E. Raynaud's disease

PATIENT EDUCATION IN BRACHIOPLASTY

4. *What is the main limitation of a standard brachioplasty procedure in terms of patient satisfaction when compared to many other commonly performed aesthetic procedures?*
   A. The pain incurred following the procedure
   B. The downtime following the procedure
   C. The visibility of the scars
   D. The residual contour deformity
   E. The functional outcome after surgery

CLINICAL DECISION-MAKING IN BRACHIOPLASTY

5. A 35-year-old woman has lost 14 pounds and currently has a body mass index (BMI) of 29. She is unhappy with the appearance of her arms which she feels still look fat. Examination shows she has good quality skin and soft tissues with moderate fat excess. *How best would her arms be treated?*
   A. Liposuction only
   B. Radiofrequency-assisted liposuction
   C. Mini brachioplasty only
   D. Brachioplasty with liposuction
   E. Mini brachioplasty with liposuction

PATIENT EVALUATION IN BRACHIOPLASTY

6. A 28-year-old woman has achieved a sustained weight loss after gastric banding. Her BMI has reduced from 39 to 28, but this has left her with significant skin redundancy in a number of areas. Examination shows scars from a belt lipectomy and medial thigh lift. She has minimal fat excess in the upper arms but has significant skin laxity passing onto the chest wall, with empty ptotic breasts. *Which one of the following procedures would best manage her upper arm condition?*
   A. Brachioplasty with horizontal skin excision only
   B. Brachioplasty with vertical skin excision only
   C. Liposuction and brachioplasty with vertical skin excision
   D. Brachioplasty with combined vertical and horizontal skin excision
   E. Extended brachioplasty with vertical and horizontal skin excision

TECHNIQUE SELECTION IN BRACHIOPLASTY

7. A 50-year-old man has lost 40 pounds over the past 3 years by diet and exercise modification. Examination shows his BMI to be 34, with moderate fat excess and vertical skin excess along the length of the upper arm. *Which one of the following surgical approaches would be best indicated in his case?*
   A. Liposuction and brachioplasty with vertical skin excision
   B. Liposuction and brachioplasty with horizontal skin excision
   C. Brachioplasty with horizontal skin excision only
   D. Brachioplasty with vertical skin excision only
   E. Avulsion brachioplasty without liposuction

COMMUNICATION IN BRACHIOPLASTY

8. A patient is seen in clinic having decided to undergo brachioplasty under your care. Since the last meeting she has heard about a mini brachioplasty technique and wishes to know how this differs from a standard brachioplasty. *What should you tell her?*
   A. Skin excision is usually avoided.
   B. Liposuction is usually avoided.
   C. The incision is usually limited to the axilla.
   D. The incision is usually limited to the posterior arm.
   E. It relies solely on fascial suspension.

STANDARD BRACHIOPLASTY APPROACHES

9. *When marking a patient for a standard brachioplasty, which one of the following is correct?*
   A. The patient should face you with arms extended at the elbows and abducted 90 degrees at the shoulder.
   B. A dotted line should be placed in the bicipital groove from the axilla to the elbow to mark the lower incision.
   C. The amount of planned skin excision can be estimated using a pinch test so that the upper incision can be marked.
   D. With experience, it may be beneficial to place the scar inferior/posterior to the bicipital groove.
   E. Placement of the scar more posteriorly will usually provide a less favorable scar quality.

CLINICAL DECISION-MAKING IN BRACHIOPLASTY

10. You are performing simultaneous bilateral brachioplasties with your resident. You have decided that no liposuction is required and have jointly marked the patient preoperatively with a 3 cm × 20 cm ellipse. *Which one of the following is the most useful advice for you to give to your resident?*
    A. Infiltration of a wetting solution will offer little benefit in this case.
    B. He or she should begin with excision of the marked area as an ellipse.
    C. Some undermining may be required to facilitate wound closure.
    D. Two-layer closure should be performed with a short-acting monofilament suture.
    E. Wound closure should be staggered by partial closure as tissue is excised.

NERVE INJURY IN BRACHIOPLASTY

11. You are performing a brachioplasty and note you have cut through a medium-size sensory nerve at the distal arm. There is segmental loss as a portion of the nerve has been excised with the redundant skin, which has already been discarded. *What should you do before continuing with the procedure?*
    A. Do nothing with the nerve
    B. Remove a larger segment of nerve
    C. Repair the nerve with a nerve graft
    D. Cauterize the nerve end
    E. Cauterize the nerve end and bury it in muscle

Answers

ANATOMY IN RELATION TO BRACHIOPLASTY

1. Six months following brachioplasty, a patient complains of continued pain around the elbow and paresthesia in the forearm. *What nerve is most likely to have been injured during the procedure?*

   E. Medial antebrachial cutaneous nerve

   Most nerves in the arm such as the median, radial, ulnar, and musculocutaneous nerve lie deep to the deep fascia and are not at risk of injury during brachioplasty. However, the cutaneous nerves of the arm and forearm lie superficial to the deep fascia and are therefore at risk of damage. The median antebrachial cutaneous nerve (MABC; also known as the medial cutaneous nerve of the forearm) travels with the basilic vein and is most at risk of injury just proximal to the elbow, resulting in a painful neuroma, as in this scenario. The initial treatment of a neuroma is nonsurgical with massage, desensitization, physiotherapy, and analgesics. If the problem persists for more than 6 months as in this case, surgical intervention with resection of the neuroma and insertion of the ends into the triceps muscle may be beneficial.[1]

   The anterior brachial and lateral antebrachial cutaneous nerves are both superficial but should remain outside of the zone of dissection during brachioplasty. The lateral antebrachial cutaneous nerve is the continuation of the musculocutaneous nerve that supplies sensation to the lateral (radial) aspect of the forearm. The other nerve that is at risk during brachioplasty when close to the axilla is the intercostobrachial nerve. Injury to this would result in altered sensation to the axilla and upper arm.

REFERENCE

1. Stahl S, Rosenberg N. Surgical treatment of painful neuroma in medial antebrachial cutaneous nerve. Ann Plast Surg 2002;48(2):154–158, discussion 158–160

SURGICAL ANATOMY IN BRACHIOPLASTY

2. *Where in the arm is most subcutaneous fat generally found?*

   B. Posterior

   Subcutaneous fat in the arms tends to collect posteriorly and inferiorly with very little medially. It also tends to be found more proximally than distally. Therefore, when performing liposuction, the main target zone is the posterior arm with more subtle suctioning performed on the medial aspect, taking care not to overly thin the soft tissues such that 0.5 cm of subcutaneous fat is left in the skin and contour irregularities are avoided. The fat of the arm is supported by two fascial systems relevant to brachioplasty: the superficial system and the longitudinal system. The superficial system encases the fat circumferentially from the axilla to the elbow. The longitudinal fascial system begins at the clavicle and extends to the axillary fascia and superficial system. This is used in some techniques to support the arm tissues using permanent sutures to anchor the superficial system to the longitudinal fascia.[1] The skin is also thinner medially than it is posteriorly or laterally; so, there is less dermal support for scars, particularly when closed under tension.[1,2]

REFERENCES

1. Lockwood T. Brachioplasty with superficial fascial system suspension. Plast Reconstr Surg 1995;96(4):912–920
2. Knoetgen J III, Moran SL. Long-term outcomes and complications associated with brachioplasty: a retrospective review and cadaveric study. Plast Reconstr Surg 2006;117(7):2219–2223

CONTRAINDICATIONS TO BRACHIOPLASTY

3. *Which one of the following represents an absolute contraindication to brachioplasty?*

   C. Lymphedema

   Brachioplasty risks compromise to lymphatic flow from the upper limb and therefore should be avoided in patients who have chronic lymphedema, even if this is mild, as further interruption of lymphatic flow can be detrimental. Liposuction only in these patients may be beneficial as a treatment for their lymphedema, but compression garments will need to be worn long term.

   Other absolute contraindications to brachioplasty include reflex sympathetic dystrophy, smoking, and unrealistic patient expectations. Relative contraindications include symptomatic Raynaud's disease, connective tissue disorders, advanced rheumatoid arthritis, residual obesity, and diabetes mellitus. Minimizing complication risk is paramount in brachioplasty and as always in aesthetic surgery, careful patient selection for the procedure must be performed.[1,2]

REFERENCES

1. Nahai F, ed. The Art of Aesthetic Surgery: Principles and Techniques. 2nd ed. St Louis, MO: Quality Medical Publishing; 2011
2. Sisti A, Cuomo R, Milonia L, et al. Complications associated with brachioplasty: a literature review. Acta Biomed 2018;88(4):393–402

PATIENT EDUCATION IN BRACHIOPLASTY

4. *What is the main limitation of a standard brachioplasty procedure in terms of patient satisfaction when compared to many other commonly performed aesthetic procedures?*

    C. The visibility of the scars

    Brachioplasty is a good operation for recontouring the upper arms after weight loss in patients with excess skin with or without fat, but the main limitation is that the scarring is extensive and visible. Furthermore, the scars can become stretched, as there will be some tension across the wound during closure and the medial arm skin is relatively thin. For this reason, it is vital that patients have a clear understanding of the scars preoperatively. Markings should be made on the patient to show them the site, orientation, and extent of the scars during their preoperative consultation. This should be documented in the medical record. Postoperative photos of other patients can also be useful to illustrate the scar pattern.[1]

    This procedure is not particularly painful for patients and the downtime is short. Early ambulation is advised postoperatively, and most cases are performed as day cases.[1] The postoperative contour is usually good and patients tend to be satisfied with this. There is no functional loss following this surgery. In fact, it often helps function where larger skin volumes are resected.[1,2]

REFERENCES

1. Aly AS, Capella JF. Staging, reoperation, and treatment of complications after body contouring in the massive-weight-loss patient. In: Grotting J, ed. Reoperative Aesthetic and Reconstructive Surgery. 2nd ed. St Louis, MO: Quality Medical Publishing; 2007
2. Nahai F, ed. The Art of Aesthetic Surgery: Principles and Techniques. 2nd ed. St Louis, MO: Quality Medical Publishing; 2011

CLINICAL DECISION-MAKING IN BRACHIOPLASTY

5. A 35-year-old woman has lost 14 pounds and currently has a body mass index (BMI) of 29. She is unhappy with the appearance of her arms which she feels still look fat. Examination shows she has good quality skin and soft tissues with moderate fat excess. *How best would her arms be treated?*

    A. Liposuction only

    This patient requires liposuction only because there is fat excess in the absence of skin excess. As she is young and her skin quality is good, she should respond well to the liposuction with subsequent progressive natural skin tightening over time. In patients with mild to moderate skin laxity and small to medium adipose tissue excess, radiofrequency-assisted liposuction may be considered instead. This is thought to cause soft-tissue contraction and collagen formation secondary to thermal effects on the fibroseptal network in the subcutaneous space as well as a nonablative, inflammatory heating of the dermis. The combination of radiofrequency and liposuction can potentially result in a lower complication profile and greater skin tightening than liposuction alone.[1,2] However, in this scenario, skin quality is good without excess, so liposuction alone would be sufficient. A mini brachioplasty is indicated where there is mild skin laxity and mild to moderate fat in the upper arm. It combines fat removal with liposuction and skin removal from the axilla with or without upper arm. Brachioplasty with liposuction is indicated in patients with moderate to severe skin and fat excess rather than fat only as in this scenario.

REFERENCES

1. Chia CT, Theodorou SJ, Hoyos AE, Pitman GH. Radiofrequency-assisted liposuction compared with aggressive superficial, subdermal liposuction of the arms: a bilateral quantitative comparison. Plast Reconstr Surg Glob Open 2015;3(7):e459
2. Duncan DI. Improving outcomes in upper arm liposuction: adding radiofrequency-assisted liposuction to induce skin contraction. Aesthet Surg J 2012;32(1):84–95

PATIENT EVALUATION IN BRACHIOPLASTY

6. A 28-year-old woman has achieved a sustained weight loss after gastric banding. Her BMI has reduced from 39 to 28, but this has left her with significant skin redundancy in a number of areas. Examination shows scars from a belt lipectomy and medial thigh lift. She has minimal fat excess in the upper arms but has significant skin laxity passing onto the chest wall, with empty ptotic breasts. *Which one of the following procedures would best manage her upper arm condition?*

    E. **Extended brachioplasty with vertical and horizontal skin excision**

    When deciding on a surgical plan for patients requesting brachioplasty, a stepwise approach is helpful. The first step is to decide whether there is any fat excess. If there is, then liposuction may be useful, otherwise further weight loss may be advised. The next step is to see whether there is any skin excess and to note the anatomic location of this. When considering treatment for skin excess, it should be remembered that the resection is performed in the "opposite" vector from the direction of excess (i.e., vertical excess is removed through a horizontal [longitudinal] excision and horizontal excess is removed through a vertical [axillary] excision). These descriptors, vertical and horizontal, assume the patient is standing for the assessment with the shoulder abducted and elbow flexed to 90 degrees.

    Therefore, if the skin excess is horizontal, then a vertical scar in the axilla is used. If there is a vertical excess, then a longitudinal scar is used. If there are both horizontal and vertical excesses, then a combination of horizontal and vertical scars is used. If the skin excess is restricted to the proximal arm only, then a short T-scar can be used. The patient in this scenario requires an extended brachioplasty as shown in **Fig. 119.1**, because they have a large volume of skin excess that extends beyond the arm and axilla to the lateral chest wall. As can be seen in the figure, the excision pattern passes the full length of the arm to the axilla and onto the chest wall. It has both horizontal and vertical components. If there was additional fat excess, then liposuction could also be incorporated into this procedure.[1]

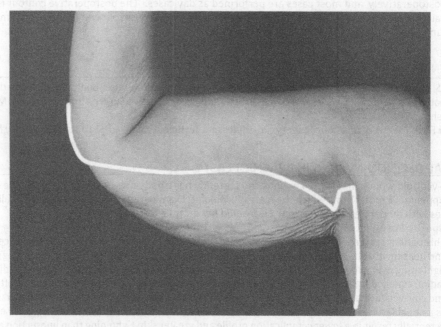

Fig. 119.1   Laxity in this patient extends onto the lateral chest wall and requires extended brachioplasty technique.

REFERENCE

1. Appelt EA, Janis JE, Rohrich RJ. An algorithmic approach to upper arm contouring. Plast Reconstr Surg 2006;118(1):237–246

TECHNIQUE SELECTION IN BRACHIOPLASTY

7. A 50-year-old man has lost 40 pounds over the past 3 years by diet and exercise modification. Examination shows his BMI to be 34, with moderate fat excess and vertical skin excess along the length of the upper arm. *Which one of the following surgical approaches would be best indicated in his case?*
   B. Liposuction and brachioplasty with horizontal skin excision
      This patient requires a standard brachioplasty with a horizontal incision placed in the brachial groove as shown in **Fig. 119.2**. As can be seen in the figure, the excision pattern passes the full length of the arm to the axilla, but without extension onto the chest wall or a vertical component into the axillary crease. This is to accommodate the vertical skin excess he has when the arm is positioned flexed at the elbow to 90 degrees and abducted at the shoulder to 90 degrees. He will also benefit from liposuction given the excess fat present, and this will allow slightly more skin to be resected. Scar placement would traditionally be on the medial aspect of the arm as shown in **Fig. 119.2**, but it can be more aesthetically placed by moving it slightly more posteriorly; so, ideally it is barely visible with the arm placed relaxed by the side and the scar is located in thicker dermis, less likely to stretch.[1]

      The avulsion brachioplasty is a technique that relies on liposuction as part of the process and cannot be performed in isolation without it. It is an alternative to standard brachioplasty, and can be used for patients such as this man with moderate-to-severe excess skin with excess fat. The procedure begins by planning the resection margin then aggressively liposuctioning this area until all the subcutaneous fat is removed. After completion of liposuction, there should be a very distinct, "dished-out" deformity. Incisions are then made through the skin and superficial fascial system to allow complete release around the area of planned resection. The tissue is grasped proximally with a Kocher clamp, and avulsed proximally to distally. The procedure is completed with hemostasis and two-layer wound closure.[2]

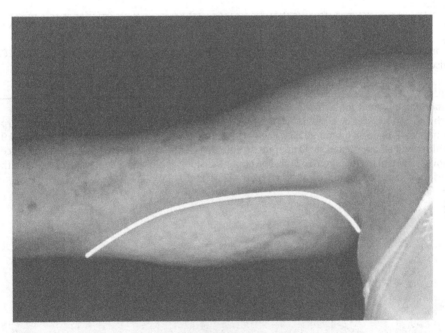

Fig. 119.2 This patient has isolated vertical skin redundancy that is treated with a horizontal excision along the brachial/bicipital groove.

REFERENCES

1. Appelt EA, Janis JE, Rohrich RJ. An algorithmic approach to upper arm contouring. Plast Reconstr Surg 2006;118(1):237–246
2. Knotts CD, Kortesis BG, Hunstad JP. Avulsion brachioplasty: technique overview and 5-year experience. Plast Reconstr Surg 2014;133(2):283–288

COMMUNICATION IN BRACHIOPLASTY

8. A patient is seen in clinic having decided to undergo brachioplasty under your care. Since the last meeting she has heard about a mini brachioplasty technique and wishes to know how this differs from a standard brachioplasty. *What should you tell her?*

    C. The incision is usually limited to the axilla.

    The main difference between a mini brachioplasty and a standard brachioplasty is the site and size of the skin excision and subsequent scars. In a mini brachioplasty, the incision is hidden in the axilla (**Fig. 119.3**). It still includes liposuction in the posteromedial upper arm where necessary. In some cases, a short dart extension onto the medial arm (not posterior) may be required, creating a **T**-shaped scar. Lockwood described a technique for anchoring the superficial fascia to the longitudinal fascial system (dense axillary and clavipectoral fascia) in order to correct the laxity of the upper arm. However, this is not always performed and is not exclusive to a mini brachioplasty approach. The mini brachioplasty is indicated in select patients only. They should have mild skin excess and mild to moderate fat excess. The most important step in successful mini brachioplasty is patient selection, and in the right patient it can be highly effective. However, patients who have more significant excess skin will benefit from a standard or full brachioplasty approach.[1,2]

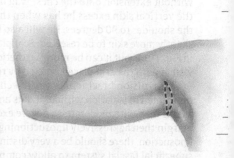

Fig. 119.3   Placement of the axillary incision for a mini brachioplasty.

REFERENCES

1. Nahai F, ed. The Art of Aesthetic Surgery: Principles and Techniques. 2nd ed. St Louis, MO: Quality Medical Publishing; 2011
2. Abramson DL. Minibrachioplasty: minimizing scars while maximizing results. Plast Reconstr Surg 2004;114(6):1631–1634, discussion 1635–1637

STANDARD BRACHIOPLASTY APPROACHES

9. *When marking a patient for a standard brachioplasty, which one of the following is correct?*

    D. With experience, it may be beneficial to place the scar inferior/posterior to the bicipital groove.

    During marking for a brachioplasty, the patient should face you with their arms abducted 90 degrees at the shoulder and elbows flexed to 90 degrees as if flexing the biceps. A dotted line should be placed in the bicipital groove to help mark the planned scar. The upper incision should then be marked 1 cm above this, and the lower incision can then be estimated by pinching the skin (**Fig. 119.4**).

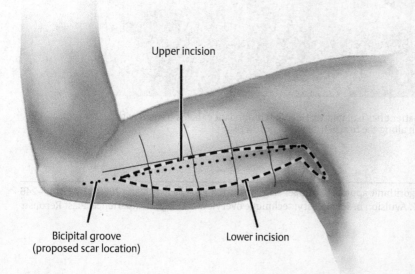

Upper incision

Fig. 119.4   Preoperative markings for a standard brachioplasty.

Bicipital groove
(proposed scar location)

Lower incision

Placement of the scar posteriorly may provide a more favorable quality of scar but one that is more visible from behind. A compromise between the two may be chosen, as this can help make the scar placement more discrete and located in better quality skin than in the medial arm. This is worth considering with experience of the procedure, although should be done with caution to avoid skin over resection and the incision falling too far posteriorly. Vertical crosshatch markings are made to divide the incision into fifths and facilitate correct wound edge approximation, once the skin resection has been performed.[1,2]

REFERENCES

1. Nahai F, ed. The Art of Aesthetic Surgery: Principles and Techniques. 2nd ed. St Louis, MO: Quality Medical Publishing; 2011
2. Aly AS. Body Contouring After Massive Weight Loss. St Louis, MO: Quality Medical Publishing; 2006

CLINICAL DECISION-MAKING IN BRACHIOPLASTY

10. You are performing simultaneous bilateral brachioplasties with your resident. You have decided that no liposuction is required and have jointly marked the patient preoperatively with a 3 cm × 20 cm ellipse. *Which one of the following is the most useful advice for you to give to your resident?*

    E. Wound closure should be staggered by partial closure as tissue is excised.

When undertaking a brachioplasty, the order of excision and closure must be modified from standard excisional and closure techniques. It is easy to over-resect skin during this procedure; so, a single upper incision is made first and a posteriorly based skin flap is carefully elevated. Closure is tested before committing to the lower incision. The excision and closure are staged to close each part of the wound segmentally to minimize arm swelling that might otherwise prevent closure. A three-layer closure should be used without undermining. The superficial fascial system is closed with a long-lasting absorbable suture, and the skin closed in two layers (deep dermal and subcuticular) with shorter-acting ones. Infiltration is useful to limit bleeding, regardless of whether liposuction is to be performed.[1,2]

REFERENCES

1. Nahai F, ed. The Art of Aesthetic Surgery: Principles and Techniques. 2nd ed. St Louis, MO: Quality Medical Publishing; 2011
2. Aly AS. Body Contouring After Massive Weight Loss. St Louis, MO: Quality Medical Publishing; 2006

NERVE INJURY IN BRACHIOPLASTY

11. You are performing a brachioplasty and note you have cut through a medium-size sensory nerve at the distal arm. There is segmental loss as a portion of the nerve has been excised with the redundant skin, which has already been discarded. *What should you do before continuing with the procedure?*

    E. Cauterize the nerve end and bury it in muscle

The main problem with transection of a sensory nerve, such as the MABC during brachioplasty, is the risk of subsequent neuroma formation, leaving the patient with chronic pain in the upper limb. The loss of sensation tends to be much better tolerated than the neuroma symptoms. For this reason, when a sensory nerve is divided, it should either be repaired or managed such that a neuroma is unlikely to occur. By cauterizing the nerve and burying it in muscle, the risk of neuroma formation will be reduced. Smaller nerve branches can just be cauterized. Use of a graft is not indicated, as the harvest will create a similar defect elsewhere anyway.[1-3]

REFERENCES

1. Nahai F, ed. The Art of Aesthetic Surgery: Principles and Techniques. 2nd ed. St Louis, MO: Quality Medical Publishing; 2011
2. Sisti A, Cuomo R, Milonia L, et al. Complications associated with brachioplasty: a literature review. Acta Biomed 2018;88(4):393–402
3. Stahl S, Rosenberg N. Surgical treatment of painful neuroma in medial antebrachial cutaneous nerve. Ann Plast Surg 2002;48(2):154–158, discussion 158–160

120. Abdominoplasty

See *Essentials of Plastic Surgery*, third edition, pp. 1691–1710

CLINICAL ANATOMY OF THE ABDOMEN

1. *When elevating an abdominal skin flap during a traditional abdominoplasty, which one of the following statements is correct?*
   A. The flap receives its blood supply from vessels in Huger's zone I.
   B. Striae present on the flap will normally be improved by this procedure.
   C. Sensory innervation from the lateral branches of intercostal nerves T10–T12 is divided.
   D. If flap thinning is required, it should be performed in the subscarpal fat layer.
   E. Umbilical blood supply becomes dependent on the ligamentum teres and median umbilical ligament.

CLINICAL ANATOMY OF THE ANTERIOR ABDOMINAL WALL

2. *What is the clinical relevance of the arcuate line with respect to performing surgery on the anterior abdominal wall?*
   A. It represents the ideal vertical anatomic position for the umbilicus.
   B. It marks the superior extent of the abdominoplasty flap dissection.
   C. It represents the point at which rectus diastasis repair must be started.
   D. It marks the distinction between superficial and deep fat layers.
   E. It marks the point below which the posterior rectus sheath is absent.

PREOPERATIVE EVALUATION FOR ABDOMINOPLASTY

3. You are consenting a patient for abdominoplasty and find out that she has been smoking approximately five cigarettes per day since you met her in clinic to plan surgery 1 month ago. She previously denied smoking. *How should you now proceed knowing this information?*
   A. Proceed with surgery as planned without further discussion.
   B. Start her on nicotine replacement therapy and proceed as planned.
   C. Check her blood and urine nicotine levels then proceed as planned.
   D. Proceed with surgery, explaining the increased risk of complications.
   E. Postpone surgery until smoking cessation is complete.

CLINICAL ASSESSMENT OF THE ABDOMINOPLASTY PATIENT

4. *When assessing a patient for an abdominoplasty, what is the key clinical relevance of a positive diver's test?*
   A. That there is an excess of lower abdominal fat
   B. That there is an excess of lower abdominal skin
   C. That there is rectus diastasis present
   D. That there is myofascial laxity present
   E. That there is a hernia present

CONTRAINDICATIONS TO ABDOMINOPLASTY SURGERY

5. *Which one of the following scars represents the most significant contraindication to standard abdominoplasty surgery?*
   A. McBurney (appendectomy)   D. Lower midline
   B. Kocher's (subcostal)   E. Periumbilical laparoscopic
   C. Pfannenstiel (cesarian)

INFORMED CONSENT FOR ABDOMINOPLASTY

6. You are consenting a patient preoperatively to undergo a full abdominoplasty with rectus sheath plication. She has a moderate amount of skin and soft-tissue excess and wants to know about the likely outcomes. *Which one of the following is least likely in her case?*
   A. A long transverse scar will curve from hip to hip but should be hidden in her underwear.
   B. Her umbilicus will need to be relocated, leaving a visible scar around it.
   C. She will need a short vertical scar given her current tissue laxity.
   D. Minor scar revision may be necessary after her original procedure.
   E. The rectus plication is likely to increase her recovery time.

PATIENT COMMUNICATION IN ABDOMINOPLASTY

7. A patient returns to the clinic after an initial consultation for an abdominoplasty where she was seen by your resident. She has since read through the information sheet describing the risks of surgery and wants to know why she was advised that she may have "dog-ears" after her surgery. She asks you to clarify exactly what this means. **Which one of the following would be correct to tell her about "dog-ears"?**
   A. They are the result of abnormal scarring at the wound edge.
   B. They can occur at any point along the transverse scar.
   C. They usually resolve spontaneously with massage and scar maturation.
   D. They normally occur secondary to surgical error.
   E. They are treated with liposuction or surgical excision.

EXPECTATIONS FOR PATIENTS UNDERGOING ABDOMINOPLASTY

8. A 46-year-old nurse is scheduled to undergo standard abdominoplasty surgery and wants to clarify some aspects of the surgical procedure and downtime. **Regarding the perioperative and postoperative periods surrounding her surgery, which one of the following statements is true?**
   A. It is standard practice to include concomitant liposuction to the central and upper abdomen.
   B. Her surgery would normally be performed under local anesthetic with sedation.
   C. She may be unable to stand up straight for several days following surgery.
   D. Two weeks off work will provide her with sufficient time to fully recover.
   E. She will be unable to use the gym for 9 months following surgery.

PROCEDURE SELECTION IN LOWER ABDOMINAL WALL CONTOURING

9. A 44-year-old woman has a mild soft-tissue and moderate skin excess involving the lower abdomen and back after major weight loss. She is otherwise healthy, has a stable weight for the past year, and is a nonsmoker. **How best should this be managed surgically?**
   A. Mini abdominoplasty
   B. Traditional abdominoplasty
   C. Circumferential abdominoplasty
   D. Reverse abdominoplasty
   E. Fleur-de-lis abdominoplasty

PROCEDURE SELECTION IN ABDOMINOPLASTY

10. An otherwise healthy 24-year-old woman has a moderate infraumbilical skin and soft-tissue excess following pregnancy. Her skin quality is average, and she has multiple striae in the lower abdomen. She is generally slim, but this area seems unresponsive to diet and physical exercise. **Which one of the following surgical procedures would be indicated in this case?**
   A. Mini abdominoplasty
   B. Traditional abdominoplasty
   C. Circumferential abdominoplasty
   D. Reverse abdominoplasty
   E. Targeted liposuction only

PERIOPERATIVE MANAGEMENT

11. **Which one of the following is true of the perioperative management of patients undergoing abdominoplasty?**
   A. The pubic area should be shaved the day before surgery.
   B. Intravenous antibiotics should be given 30 to 60 minutes before starting surgery.
   C. Intraoperative TED hose (stockings) are usually reserved for high-risk individuals.
   D. A single dose of low-molecular-weight heparin should be given on induction.
   E. Postoperative antibiotics should continue for 7 days after surgery.

INTRAOPERATIVE TIPS IN ABDOMINOPLASTY

12. **What is the main benefit of leaving a layer of fat over the anterior superior iliac spine (ASIS) during abdominoplasty?**
   A. A reduction in seroma rate
   B. A reduction in hematoma rate
   C. A better abdominal wall contour
   D. A reduced risk of nerve damage
   E. A reduced rate of fat necrosis

RECTUS PLICATION IN ABDOMINOPLASTY

13. *Which one of the following is correct when incorporating rectus plication into a standard abdominoplasty technique?*
    A. The upper skin flap should be elevated widely to allow access for plication.
    B. Plication is best achieved using a long-acting resorbable or permanent suture.
    C. Plication should begin 2 inches below the xiphisternum.
    D. Plication should be performed with a single layer of interrupted sutures.
    E. Plication negates the need for progressive tension sutures.

MINI ABDOMINOPLASTY

14. You are discussing the relative merits of using a mini abdominoplasty with a patient. She is of slim build and has modest lower abdominal soft-tissue excess. She has had a previous cesarean section and wants to minimize further scarring. Examination shows mild rectus diastasis. *Which one of the following is true of this procedure?*
    A. It involves a standard abdominoplasty transverse scar.
    B. It is mainly indicated for infraumbilical skin and fat excess.
    C. It is contraindicated in the presence of rectus diastasis.
    D. It should be avoided after cesarean section.
    E. The umbilicus is normally at relocated level with the iliac crest.

PROGRESSIVE TENSION SUTURES

15. *Which one of the following is not a recognized benefit of using progressive tension sutures during closure of an abdominoplasty?*
    A. Reduced seroma formation
    B. Reduced hematoma formation
    C. Reduced operative time
    D. Improved scar appearance
    E. Reduced wound-edge necrosis

FLEUR-DE-LIS ABDOMINOPLASTY

16. *Which one of the following is the main advantage of using the fleur-de-lis abdominoplasty technique?*
    A. Postoperative scars are easier to conceal in underwear.
    B. Postoperative complications are less likely to occur.
    C. Rectus plication is avoided.
    D. Horizontal and vertical abdominal tissue excess is addressed.
    E. Anterior and lateral thigh soft-tissue excess is addressed.

POSTOPERATIVE MANAGEMENT FOLLOWING ABDOMINOPLASTY

17. You see a 44-year-old otherwise healthy woman the morning after an abdominoplasty. She previously had two pregnancies by cesarean section and has undergone previous breast surgery in the past, coping well with postoperative pain management. On this occasion she is really quite sore, despite having access to a morphine pump (patient controlled analgesia [PCA]) and acetaminophen. She is wearing an external abdominal binder and lying with knees on a pillow. Her abdomen remains soft but tender and is otherwise unremarkable. Her CRP is elevated to 20 (normal range is <5) and her observations are normal. *What is the most likely explanation for her continued discomfort?*
    A. Abdominoplasty is generally a very painful procedure.
    B. She is not regularly using her morphine PCA.
    C. She is developing a postoperative infection.
    D. She has an intraperitoneal injury and developing peritonitis.
    E. She has undergone correction surgery for rectus diastasis.

COMPLICATIONS OF ABDOMINOPLASTY

18. A patient who underwent traditional abdominoplasty surgery 6 months ago has called your office concerned about residual fullness to the epigastric region. She had a standard abdominoplasty approach with rectus plication, but no liposuction. *What is the most likely cause of the bulge in this area?*
    A. Inadequate flap dissection
    B. Inadequate fat excision
    C. Chronic seroma
    D. Solidified hematoma
    E. Postoperative weight gain

Answers

CLINICAL ANATOMY OF THE ABDOMEN

1. *When elevating an abdominal skin flap during a traditional abdominoplasty, which one of the following statements is correct?*[2]

   D. If flap thinning is required, it should be performed in the subscarpal fat layer.

   Abdominal fat has two layers separated by a layer of superficial fascia. These layers have different vascular supplies. The overlying skin is reliant on blood supply through the superficial fat layer, whereas the deep fat vascularity is distinct from the skin. For this reason, superficial fat should be preserved when flap thinning is required.

   After raising a skin flap during an abdominoplasty, the blood supply arises from superolateral, which will correspond to Huger's zone III. Huger's zone I normally supplies the central area of the flap through the rectus abdominis muscles, but these perforating vessels are divided during flap elevation (**Fig. 120.1**).[1] Vascularity of the soft tissue of the elevated abdominoplasty flap is reduced compared with normal levels of perfusion in the surrounding tissues.[2]

   The normal sensory innervation to this part of the abdomen arises from T7–T12 (ventral) intercostal nerves, which have anterior and lateral branches. The lateral branches are preserved during an abdominoplasty and travel within the superficial tissues anterior to the anterior axillary line. The anterior branches remain deep to the internal intercostal until they reach the rectus sheath. At this point they pass anteriorly through the sheath to supply overlying skin and will be divided during flap elevation. Patients probably will not have long-term sensory loss at this level because of sensory nerve arborization and reinnervation.[3]

   The umbilicus normally receives its vascular supply through perforators from the deep inferior epigastric arteries (DIEAs), the subdermal plexus, the medial umbilical ligament, and the ligamentum teres.[4] During an abdominoplasty, the subdermal supply is divided, but the main perforators from the DIEA are still preserved. The blood supply would normally rely only on the medial umbilical ligament and ligamentum teres, if, for example, a bilateral DIEP flap had been performed. Striae are caused by thinning or absence of the dermis. Those present below the umbilicus will be excised during a standard abdominoplasty procedure. However, those above this line will remain and are likely to appear worse, as the flap will be stretched during wound closure. This is a key concept to convey to patients preoperatively.[1-5]

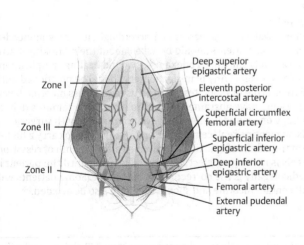
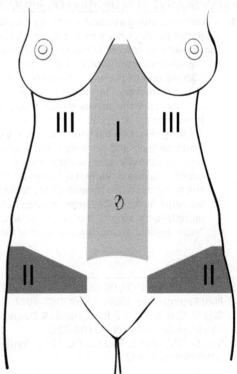

Fig. 120.1 Huger's vascular zones of the abdominal wall.

REFERENCES

1. Huger WE Jr. The anatomic rationale for abdominal lipectomy. Am Surg 1979;45(9):612–617
2. Mayr M, Holm C, Höfter E, Becker A, Pfeiffer U, Mühlbauer W. Effects of aesthetic abdominoplasty on abdominal wall perfusion: a quantitative evaluation. Plast Reconstr Surg 2004;114(6):1586–1594
3. Moore KL, Dalley AF, eds. Clinically Oriented Anatomy. 4th ed. New York, NY: Lippincott, Williams, and Wilkins; 1999
4. Stokes RB, Whetzel TP, Sommerhaug E, Saunders CJ. Arterial vascular anatomy of the umbilicus. Plast Reconstr Surg 1998;102(3):761–764
5. Hunstad JP, Repta R. Atlas of Abdominoplasty. Philadelphia, PA: Elsevier Health Sciences; 2008

CLINICAL ANATOMY OF THE ANTERIOR ABDOMINAL WALL

2. *What is the clinical relevance of the arcuate line with respect to performing surgery on the anterior abdominal wall?*
   E. **It marks the point below which the posterior rectus sheath is absent.**

   The arcuate line is located halfway between the umbilicus and symphysis pubis. Above this line there are both anterior and posterior rectus sheaths. Below this line there is only an anterior rectus sheath present, therefore making this area of the abdomen more prone to weakness and herniation. It is particularly relevant when performing abdominal wall reconstruction and raising rectus abdominis flaps, as this area will need reinforcement if the anterior sheath is deficient. There may be deficiency in this area in patients undergoing abdominoplasty particularly if they have previously had significant weight loss or multiple pregnancies.

   The ideal anatomic position for the umbilicus is the midline at the level of the iliac crest, although in less than 2% of patients is the umbilicus truly sited in the midline. Diastasis should be repaired from the xiphisternum down to the top of the symphysis in most cases. For this reason, the superior limit of skin flap dissection in an abdominoplasty is also the xiphisternum. Scarpa's fascia marks the junction between superficial and deep fat layers of the abdominal wall.[1–3]

REFERENCES

1. Nahai F. The Art of Aesthetic Surgery: Principles and Techniques. New York, NY: Thieme Publishers; 2005
2. Landfair AS, Rubin JP. Applied anatomy in body contouring. In: Nahai F, ed. The Art of Aesthetic Surgery: Principles and Techniques. New York, NY: Thieme Publishers; 2005
3. Hunstad JP, Repta R. Atlas of Abdominoplasty. Philadelphia, PA: Elsevier Health Sciences; 2008

PREOPERATIVE EVALUATION FOR ABDOMINOPLASTY

3. **You are consenting a patient for abdominoplasty and find out that she has been smoking approximately five cigarettes per day since you met her in clinic to plan surgery 1 month ago. She previously denied smoking. *How should you now proceed knowing this information?***
   E. **Postpone surgery until smoking cessation is complete.**

   Abdominoplasty places a large stress on the abdominal wall flap vasculature and, accordingly, is not recommended in active smokers. During the preoperative consultation, patients should be asked about their smoking status and advised of the increased risks of surgery while actively smoking. For example, wound healing complications in smokers are nearly 50% as compared to 15% in nonsmokers.[1] Any plans for surgery should be postponed until smoking cessation has been successfully completed. Urine or blood tests can be used to assess nicotine levels (cotinine test)[2] and can help confirm whether patients have abstained from smoking. There remains debate regarding the effects of nicotine replacement therapy on wound healing; however, continuing with surgery in a patient who has recently stopped smoking and is on nicotine replacement therapy is still likely to carry a higher risk of postoperative complications. While some of the effects of smoking are reversed after a month of cessation, but other factors take longer to reverse. Given this is nonurgent elective surgery, waiting until the patient is optimized for surgery is common sense and medicolegally is the correct approach to take. Some patients will "vape" instead of smoking, but some of these still contain nicotine and should therefore also be avoided.[1–3]

REFERENCES

1. Manassa EH, Hertl CH, Olbrisch RR. Wound healing problems in smokers and nonsmokers after 132 abdominoplasties. Plast Reconstr Surg 2003;111(6):2082–2087, discussion 2088–2089
2. Raja M, Garg A, Yadav P, Jha K, Handa S. Diagnostic methods for detection of cotinine level in tobacco users: a review. J Clin Diagn Res 2016;10(3):ZE04–ZE06
3. Shestak KC, Rios L, Pollock TA, Aly A. Evidenced-based approach to abdominoplasty update. Aesthet Surg J 2019;39(6):628–642

CLINICAL ASSESSMENT OF THE ABDOMINOPLASTY PATIENT

4. *When assessing a patient for an abdominoplasty, what is the key clinical relevance of a positive diver's test?*
   D. That there is myofascial laxity present

   Myofascial laxity of the anterior abdominal wall must be assessed before undertaking an abdominoplasty so that a plan to treat it can be made in advance of surgery. Laxity can be measured by the diver test, a pinch test, and by assessment of rectus diastasis. The diver test is performed with the patient standing and then flexing at the waist. Worsening of lower abdominal wall fullness indicates myofascial laxity is present (**Figs. 120.2,** A and B).

   The pinch test assesses abdominal fullness with the patient both relaxed and actively tensing the abdominal wall (**Fig. 120.2,** C). If the amount of fullness that can be pinched is significantly decreased by tensing the abdominal wall, then significant myofascial laxity is present. Midline rectus diastasis is assessed by asking the patient to raise their legs off the examination table while lying supine. This allows palpation of the rectus muscles in most patients. Examination of a hernia can also be undertaken at this time. Myofascial laxity can be reduced intraoperatively in most patients with a selection of suture-tightening techniques either laterally or medially depending on the anatomic location of the relative myofascial weakness.[1-3]

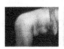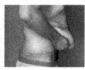

Fig. 120.2 *A* and *B*, Diver's test. *C*, Pinch test.

REFERENCES

1. Nahai F, ed. The Art of Aesthetic Surgery: Principles and Techniques. 2nd ed. St Louis, MO: Quality Medical Publishing; 2011
2. Hunstad JP, Repta R. Atlas of Abdominoplasty. Philadelphia, PA: Elsevier Health Sciences; 2008
3. Friedland JA, Maffi TR. MOC-PS(SM) CME article: abdominoplasty. Plast Reconstr Surg 2008; 121(4, Suppl):1–11

CONTRAINDICATIONS TO ABDOMINOPLASTY SURGERY

5. *Which one of the following scars represents the most significant contraindication to standard abdominoplasty surgery?*
   B. Kocher's (subcostal)

   Scars represent an alteration of the blood supply to the abdominal wall. Those in the subcostal area, such as a Kocher for cholecystectomy, are of particular concern, as they interrupt the superolateral blood supply on which the abdominoplasty flap will be reliant. For this reason, a traditional abdominoplasty is contraindicated in these patients. It would be more appropriate to perform a procedure that avoids undermining such as a fleur-de-lis procedure for patients with subcostal scars. The other scars would not usually present a problem for a traditional abdominoplasty. The McBurney, the Pfannenstiel, and lower midline scars could all be excised during the procedure and so do not affect the decision-making in procedure selection in regard to vascularity of the tissues. Periumbilical laparoscopic surgery can affect blood supply to the umbilicus and patients must be made aware of this; however, it does not represent a contraindication to surgery. Any of these scars may be associated with abdominal wall weakness and hernia formation. They can also distort the planes of dissection and make surgery more challenging. An awareness and respect for them is warranted prior to undergoing surgery.[1-4]

REFERENCES

1. Hunstad JP, Repta R. Atlas of Abdominoplasty. Philadelphia, PA: Elsevier Health Sciences; 2008
2. Landfair AS, Rubin JP. Applied anatomy in body contouring. In: Nahai F, ed. The Art of Aesthetic Surgery: Principles and Techniques. New York, NY: Thieme Publishers; 2005
3. Roostaeian J, Harris R, Farkas JP, Barton FE, Kenkel JM. Comparison of limited-undermining lipoabdominoplasty and traditional abdominoplasty using laser fluorescence. Aesthet Surg J 2014;34(5):741–747
4. Abdominal incisions in general surgery: a review. Ann Ib Postgrad Med 2007;5(2):59–63

INFORMED CONSENT FOR ABDOMINOPLASTY

6. You are consenting a patient preoperatively to undergo a full abdominoplasty with rectus sheath plication. She has a moderate amount of skin and soft-tissue excess and wants to know about the likely outcomes. *Which one of the following is least likely in her case?*
   C. She will need a short vertical scar given her current tissue laxity.

   This woman must be made aware of the extent of potential scarring that an abdominoplasty carries with it. She is unlikely to need a vertical component to the scar, but consent for this should be obtained in case she does not have sufficient laxity to fully remove the original periumbilical site, which subsequently closes with a vertical scar. She must also be informed of the risk of umbilical necrosis and be made aware that the periumbilical scar will still be visible in a bikini or underwear. In most cases, the transverse scar can be well hidden in underwear or swimwear, but a short vertical scar may not be. Minor revision surgery may be required following an abdominoplasty and this is usually done 3 to 6 months after the original surgery. Rectus plication can increase recovery time, due to discomfort and decreased mobility.[1-3]

REFERENCES

1. Jeffrey E. Janis. Essentials of Plastic Surgery 3rd ed. New York, NY: Thieme Publishers; 2021
2. Nahai F, ed. The Art of Aesthetic Surgery: Principles and Techniques, 2nd ed. St Louis, MO: Quality Medical Publishing; 2011
3. Hunstad JP, Repta R. Atlas of Abdominoplasty. Philadelphia, PA: Elsevier Health Sciences; 2008

PATIENT COMMUNICATION IN ABDOMINOPLASTY

7. A patient returns to the clinic after an initial consultation for an abdominoplasty where she was seen by your resident. She has since read through the information sheet describing the risks of surgery and wants to know why she was advised that she may have "dog-ears" after her surgery. She asks you to clarify exactly what this means. *Which one of the following would be correct to tell her about "dog-ears"?*

  E. They are treated with liposuction or surgical excision.

Dog-ears (also known as "standing cones") represent an excess of skin and subcutaneous fat at the end of a closed wound. Their formation is affected by wound geometry, and traditional thinking is that elliptical wounds with a length:width ratio of 3:1 or 4:1 (or maintaining closing angles of <30 degrees) can avoid dog-ear formation.[1] However, other factors may also be responsible such as tissue dynamics, surface contour, and surgical technique.

Dog-ears may be present after abdominoplasty where there is lateral skin and fat excess not incorporated into the original excision pattern. The decision to exclude this area from the abdominoplasty is normally made to limit lateral scar length, so it is not a surgical error. In cases where there is lateral and posterior soft-tissue excess, patients must be made aware that lateral fullness or dog-ears are likely to occur. Such patients may require belt lipectomy or liposuction to fully address these areas. Minimizing dog-ears during surgery is achieved by careful closure of the wound apex and serial halving or feeding in the shorter side of asymmetric wounds. In abdominoplasty, this usually means advancing the upper skin flap medially relative to the lower skin flap. Temporary tacking closure with staples can help ensure minimal dog ears and overall symmetry especially where two different operators are closing a side of the abdomen each simultaneously. Surgical removal of dog-ears will lengthen the original scar and a compromise must be reached between scar length and residual contour. Dog-ears do not usually resolve spontaneously unless they are very small. Massage to the scar will still be useful to help it soften. They should ideally be left to settle for at least a few months before revision.[1-3]

REFERENCES

1. Weisberg NK, Nehal KS, Zide BM. Dog-ears: a review. Dermatol Surg 2000;26(4):363–370
2. Nahai F, ed. The Art of Aesthetic Surgery: Principles and Techniques. 2nd ed. St Louis, MO: Quality Medical Publishing; 2011
3. Hunstad JP, Repta R. Atlas of Abdominoplasty. Philadelphia, PA: Elsevier Health Sciences; 2008

EXPECTATIONS FOR PATIENTS UNDERGOING ABDOMINOPLASTY

8. A 46-year-old nurse is scheduled to undergo standard abdominoplasty surgery and wants to clarify some aspects of the surgical procedure and downtime. *Regarding the perioperative and postoperative periods surrounding her surgery, which one of the following statements is true?*

  C. She may be unable to stand up straight for several days following surgery.

Following abdominoplasty, patients will have to initially mobilize slightly flexed at the hip due to the relatively tight wound closure, which is most often performed with the patient flexed. Postoperatively, they should be nursed with knees flexed on pillows and the hips also flexed. This takes tension off the wound repair during the early phase of healing. A standard abdominoplasty does not necessarily include liposuction, although it may do so. It is used to target lateral fullness that is not addressed by the abdominoplasty technique. Therefore, it is commonly directed at the flanks, rather than the central and upper abdomen which may risk flap viability, particularly if the suprascarpal fat is aspirated. The procedure is performed under general anesthetic and can typically be performed as an outpatient or overnight stay. This patient has an active job with heavy manual lifting of patients. She will require more than a week off work, even if light duties are possible. She will need to avoid heavy abdominal exercise such as sit-ups or heavy weights in the immediate postoperative period, but she can resume lighter cardiovascular work after a few weeks. She will certainly be recovered enough to resume going to the gym after 9 months.[1,2]

REFERENCES

1. Nahai F, ed. The Art of Aesthetic Surgery: Principles and Techniques. 2nd ed. St Louis, MO: Quality Medical Publishing; 2011
2. Hunstad JP, Repta R. Atlas of Abdominoplasty. Philadelphia, PA: Elsevier Health Sciences; 2008

PROCEDURE SELECTION IN LOWER ABDOMINAL WALL CONTOURING

9. A 44-year-old woman has a mild soft-tissue and moderate skin excess involving the lower abdomen and back after major weight loss. She is otherwise healthy, has a stable weight for the past year, and is a nonsmoker. *How best should this be managed surgically?*

C. Circumferential abdominoplasty

This woman has an excess of skin and fat to both the anterior and posterior abdominal walls and therefore will not be served well with a traditional abdominoplasty procedure. This would only address the anterior and some of the lateral excess for her. The best surgical procedure for this patient is a circumferential abdominoplasty, also termed a belt lipectomy or lower body lift, as this will address the circumferential tissue excess. It allows elevation of the buttocks and lateral thighs for a comprehensive lower body lift. The downside for the patient is that the scar will pass circumferentially and therefore be visible from behind. From a surgical perspective, there will be multiple patient turns required intraoperatively which will impact on timing and efficiency.[1,2] The umbilical stalk may need to be shortened to accommodate the refined abdominal contour.

A mini abdominoplasty would be unable to address the anterior excess, let alone the posterior excess. A reverse abdominoplasty would be used to address upper anterior abdominal excesses perhaps in the context of previous lower abdominoplasty with residual upper abdominal tissues, or where breast procedures are being performed concurrently. A fleur-de-lis procedure will address vertical and horizontal excesses anteriorly and laterally but not posteriorly.[3]

REFERENCES

1. Aly A, Mueller M. Circumferential truncal contouring: the belt lipectomy. Clin Plast Surg 2014;41(4):765–774
2. Landfair AS, Rubin JP. Applied anatomy in body contouring. In: Nahai F, ed. The Art of Aesthetic Surgery: Principles and Techniques. New York, NY: Thieme Publishers; 2005
3. Dellon AL. Fleur-de-lis abdominoplasty. Aesthetic Plast Surg 1985;9(1):27–32

PROCEDURE SELECTION IN ABDOMINOPLASTY

10. An otherwise healthy 24-year-old woman has a moderate infraumbilical skin and soft-tissue excess following pregnancy. Her skin quality is average, and she has multiple striae in the lower abdomen. She is generally slim, but this area seems unresponsive to diet and physical exercise. *Which one of the following surgical procedures would be indicated in this case?*

A. Mini abdominoplasty

This patient could benefit from a mini abdominoplasty procedure. It will target both the excess skin and fat, as well as remove some of the striae. It will, however, have a tendency to lower the umbilicus, and she must be counseled about this. Furthermore, it will fail to address many of the striae if located near to or above the umbilicus. She would not be a good candidate for liposuction, given her skin quality. A full abdominoplasty would be excessive in her case. A reverse abdominoplasty would be ineffective at removing her tissue excess given its location and leave her with scars high in the abdomen which would be poorly hidden given her overall shape.

The mini abdominoplasty is a great procedure for the right patient as in this scenario. It involves little or no soft-tissue flap undermining (unless rectus plication is to be incorporated), a relatively short intraoperative duration and overall recovery time. Often the transverse scar can be kept short and well hidden low on the abdominal wall. It effectively addresses the excess that slim patients can generate postpregnancy.

PERIOPERATIVE MANAGEMENT

11. *Which one of the following is true of the perioperative management of patients undergoing abdominoplasty?*

B. Intravenous antibiotics should be given 30 to 60 minutes before starting surgery.

Current guidelines from the Surgical Care Improvement Project (SCIP)[1] suggest that intravenous antibiotics are given 30 to 60 minutes before surgery begins. Cefazolin (Ancef) 1 g or clindamycin 900 mg are recommended, but institutions usually have their own individual guidelines based on local microbiological data. A full week's course is not required. The pubic area should not be shaved in advance, as skin damage can increase the risk of infection, but clipping is acceptable shortly before skin prep is applied. Thrombo-embolic deterrent (TED) hose (stockings) are recommended in all patients undergoing abdominoplasty, as it carries a high risk of thromboembolic events. Patients must be educated about this risk and the potential effects of either a deep vein thrombosis (DVT) or pulmonary embolism. In addition to TED hose, calf compression devices should also be used intraoperatively.

Most patients should be considered for prophylactic low-molecular-weight heparin (e.g., Lovenox 40 mg) on the evening of surgery and for 7 days after.[2]

Early ambulation and good hydration are also advocated to minimize problems with thrombus formation and chest complications. DVTs occur or at least are clinically recognized in less than 1% of patients undergoing abdominoplasty. Where there is doubt about risk stratification for each patient, use of the Caprini score may be helpful to guide their prophylactic management.[3]

REFERENCES

1. Bratzler DW, Houck PM, Richards C, et al. Use of antimicrobial prophylaxis for major surgery: baseline results from the National Surgical Infection Prevention Project. Arch Surg 2005;140(2):174–182
2. Buck DW II, Mustoe TA. An evidence-based approach to abdominoplasty. Plast Reconstr Surg 2010;126(6):2189–2195
3. Shestak KC, Rios L, Pollock TA, Aly A. Evidenced-based approach to abdominoplasty update. Aesthet Surg J 2019;39(6):628–642

INTRAOPERATIVE TIPS IN ABDOMINOPLASTY

12. What is the main benefit of leaving a layer of fat over the anterior superior iliac spine (ASIS) during abdominoplasty?

D. A reduced risk of nerve damage

It is very important to leave a small amount of fat on the fascia overlying the ASIS, as this helps prevent injury to the lateral femoral cutaneous nerve. Damage to this nerve can lead to significant postoperative pain, numbness, and dysesthesia in the hip and lateral thigh region. This condition is known as *meralgia paresthetica*.[1,2]

There is no proven benefit on seroma development of leaving this small area of fascia covered with fat, although in general leaving a thin layer of tissue overlying the rectus and external oblique fascia may help reduce seroma formation by preserving lymphatic channels. Quilting sutures may also reduce seroma formation following abdominoplasty.[3] There is no reduction in hematoma rate secondary to leaving a layer of tissue over the fascia and there is no discernible difference on abdominal wall contour, as the layer preserved is very thin.

REFERENCES

1. Chowdhry S, Davis J, Boyd T, et al. Safe tummy tuck: anatomy and strategy to avoid injury to the lateral femoral cutaneous nerve during abdominoplasty. Eplasty 2015;15:e22
2. Tomaszewski KA, Popieluszko P, Henry BM, et al. The surgical anatomy of the lateral femoral cutaneous nerve in the inguinal region: a meta-analysis. Hernia 2016;20(5):649–657
3. Pollock TA, Pollock H. Progressive tension sutures in abdominoplasty: a review of 597 consecutive cases. Aesthet Surg J 2012;32(6):729–742

RECTUS PLICATION IN ABDOMINOPLASTY

13. Which one of the following is correct when incorporating rectus plication into a standard abdominoplasty technique?

B. Plication is best achieved using a long-acting resorbable or permanent suture.

Rectus diastasis is where the distance between the two vertical rectus abdominis muscles is increased. It is common after pregnancy and weight loss. Closing this gap can be helpful during abdominoplasty to optimize the overall abdominal contour. The repair is termed rectus plication. Choice of suture for repair of rectus diastasis is very important with regard to longevity of the repair and should be performed using a long-acting resorbable or permanent suture. Recurrence of diastasis following rectus plication is much higher when a short-acting resorbable suture is used.[1-5] When using an absorbable suture, there was a 40% recurrence rate by 5 years as confirmed by ultrasound imaging.[1] In contrast, a study conducted when a permanent suture material was used found no diastasis recurrence observed at 5 to 7 years after surgery. The findings were confirmed by CT imaging in this case.[2] The upper skin flap needs to be elevated up to the xiphisternum during the abdominoplasty to allow access for rectus plication and a central area of undermining is adequate. Lateral undermining is unnecessary and reduces blood supply to the flap. Rectus plication must start just below the xiphisternum, otherwise a postoperative bulge may form and is apparent to the patient. It must also stop around the umbilicus to avoid strangulation and subsequent necrosis. There are different techniques of plication, but a typical example would be to use a two-layer approach combining interrupted and then continuous sutures to reinforce the repair. The use of plication does not negate the use of progressive tension sutures, as these are used to advance and distribute tension of wound closure away from the suture line. They may also reduce hematoma and seroma formation.[1-5]

REFERENCES

1. van Uchelen JH, Kon M, Werker PM. The long-term durability of plication of the anterior rectus sheath assessed by ultrasonography. Plast Reconstr Surg 2001;107(6):1578–1584
2. Nahas FX, Augusto SM, Ghelfond C. Should diastasis recti be corrected? Aesthetic Plast Surg 1997;21(4):285–289
3. Nahas FX, Ferreira LM, Mendes JdeA. An efficient way to correct recurrent rectus diastasis. Aesthetic Plast Surg 2004;28(4):189–196
4. Nahas FX, Ferreira LM, Augusto SM, Ghelfond C. Long-term follow-up of correction of rectus diastasis. Plast Reconstr Surg 2005;115(6):1736–1741, discussion 1742–1743
5. ElHawary H, Abdelhamid K, Meng F, Janis JE. A comprehensive, evidence-based literature review of the surgical treatment of rectus diastasis. Plast Reconstr Surg 2020;146(5):1151–1164

MINI ABDOMINOPLASTY

14. You are discussing the relative merits of using a mini abdominoplasty with a patient. She is of slim build and has modest lower abdominal soft-tissue excess. She has had a previous cesarean section and wants to minimize further scarring. Examination shows mild rectus diastasis. *Which one of the following is true of this procedure?*

   B. It is mainly indicated for infraumbilical skin and fat excess.

   The mini abdominoplasty is a useful technique for correcting small to moderate fat and skin excesses in the infraumbilical region. The benefits over a full abdominoplasty are that it creates a shorter transverse scar and avoids the periumbilical scar completely. Rectus plication is still possible but access will require transection of the umbilicus at the level of deep fascia, and the small fascial weak point this leaves must be closed over to prevent a hernia. Any upper or lateral abdominal wall skin and fat excess is not addressed. Because the umbilicus is not dissected and relocated, the umbilicus may be artificially lowered on the abdominal wall and will not sit level with the iliac crest. Transection of the umbilical stalk at the deep fascia will remove the dominant blood supply to it, but there will be sufficient blood supply from the surrounding subdermal plexus. In this case, the previous section scar can be excised and extended as required. Where the undermining is limited to below the umbilicus, i.e., where no rectus plication is required, the downtime will likely also be reduced compared to a full abdominoplasty. Overall this is a very useful procedure for a select number of patients, although the limitations must be fully explained preoperatively to the patient in order to minimize unrealistic expectations and dissatisfaction risk.[1,2]

REFERENCES

1. Landfair AS, Rubin JP. Applied anatomy in body contouring. In: Nahai F, ed. The Art of Aesthetic Surgery: Principles and Techniques. New York: Thieme Publishers; 2005
2. Nahai F. The Art of Aesthetic Surgery: Principles and Techniques. New York: Thieme Publishers; 2005

PROGRESSIVE TENSION SUTURES

15. *Which one of the following is not a recognized benefit of using progressive tension sutures during closure of an abdominoplasty?*

   C. Reduced operative time

   Progressive tension sutures have many benefits but tend to increase, not decrease, surgical time. Progressive tension sutures involve placement of interrupted resorbable sutures between the musculofascia and the underside of the abdominal flap. As the flap is advanced, progressive tension is exerted on each suture and thereby directed away from the incision. Decreased tension on the incision helps prevent wound-edge necrosis and hypertrophic scars. The dead space underneath the flap is closed, thereby reducing hematoma and seroma formation. Pollock and Pollock[1,2] have shown extremely low rates of seroma formation when using this technique.

REFERENCES

1. Pollock H, Pollock T. Progressive tension sutures: a technique to reduce local complications in abdominoplasty. Plast Reconstr Surg 2000;105(7):2583–2586, discussion 2587–2588
2. Pollock TA, Pollock H. Progressive tension sutures in abdominoplasty: a review of 597 consecutive cases. Aesthet Surg J 2012;32(6):729–742

FLEUR-DE-LIS ABDOMINOPLASTY

16. *Which one of the following is the main advantage of using the fleur-de-lis abdominoplasty technique?*

   D. Horizontal and vertical abdominal tissue-excess is addressed.

   The main advantage of the fleur-de-lis abdominoplasty is that it facilitates correction of combined horizontal and vertical soft-tissue and skin excesses of the anterior abdominal wall. It is possible to achieve a good contour of the waistline with this technique at the expense of a long, vertical midline scar on the anterior abdomen. It is often a good choice in patients who may otherwise need a circumferential approach, such as a belt lipectomy, to address these areas. It can therefore avoid a posterior or very lateral scar for such patients. It is also particularly well suited to patients who have previous scarring to the upper abdominal wall that may compromise the vascularity of a standard abdominoplasty skin flap and those who already have a paramedian scar following laparotomy. It is important that no flap undermining is performed during this procedure.

When performing a fleur-de-lis abdominoplasty, a standard lower abdominoplasty incision is made and the lower tissue ellipse is excised at the level of the umbilicus with no undermining of the flap above this point. The horizontal excess can be estimated at this stage by pinching the supraumbilical tissues together. A vertical elliptical excision can then be made from the umbilicus to the xiphisternum. It is important when performing this technique not to overestimate the amount of tissue that needs to be removed. It can also be difficult to avoid leaving epigastric fullness with this technique, particularly in massive-weight-loss patients. Careful feathering and thinning of the subcutaneous tissues at the apex can help minimize this. Following massive weight loss, this can be a particularly rewarding technique to use. The benefits and risks should be fully discussed with the patient before surgery.

Postoperative complications are similar to a standard abdominoplasty.

Rectus plication is generally required in patients undergoing fleur-de-lis abdominoplasty, because they tend to have been through significant fluctuations in body shape, such as multiple pregnancies or massive weight loss. This technique facilitates easy access to perform plication.[1-3] The Lockwood high-lateral-tension technique addresses tissue excess on the thigh, but the fleur-de-lis does not.

REFERENCES

1. Dellon AL. Fleur-de-lis abdominoplasty. Aesthetic Plast Surg 1985;9(1):27–32
2. Mitchell RT, Rubin JP. The fleur-de-lis abdominoplasty. Clin Plast Surg 2014;41(4):673–680
3. Friedman T, O'Brien Coon D, Michaels V J, et al. Fleur-de-lis abdominoplasty: a safe alternative to traditional abdominoplasty for the massive weight loss patient. Plast Reconstr Surg 2010;125(5):1525–1535

POSTOPERATIVE MANAGEMENT FOLLOWING ABDOMINOPLASTY

17. You see a 44-year-old otherwise healthy woman the morning after an abdominoplasty. She previously had two pregnancies by cesarean section and has undergone previous breast surgery in the past, coping well with postoperative pain management. On this occasion she is really quite sore, despite having access to a morphine pump (patient controlled analgesia [PCA]) and acetaminophen. She is wearing an external abdominal binder and lying with knees on a pillow. Her abdomen remains soft but tender and is otherwise unremarkable. Her CRP is elevated to 20 (normal range is <5) and her observations are normal. *What is the most likely explanation for her continued discomfort?*

E. She has undergone correction surgery for rectus diastasis.

Abdominoplasty is generally well tolerated by patients providing no adjunctive procedures have been performed. However, correction of rectus diastasis can be very painful in the early postoperative period. This is the most likely explanation in this case. It is often well controlled by using continuous local anesthetic infusion catheters placed near to the rectus or within the sheath. Alternatively, local anesthetic blocks placed intraoperatively into either the rectus sheath or the transversus abdominus plane can be highly effective.[1-3] It is too early for a postoperative soft-tissue infection to be likely in a healthy patient and there would usually be evidence of swelling, cellulitis, or warmth to the abdomen if this were the case. CRP will be elevated as a result of surgery and does not by itself suggest infection. If peritonitis was present the patient would be acutely unwell and have guarding or a rigid abdomen. The possibility of a rectus sheath hematoma should also be considered.

REFERENCES

1. Fiala T. Tranversus abdominis plane block during abdominoplasty to improve postoperative patient comfort. Aesthet Surg J 2015;35(1):72–80
2. Morales R Jr, Mentz H III, Newall G, Patronella C, Masters O III. Use of abdominal field block injections with liposomal bupivicaine to control postoperative pain after abdominoplasty. Aesthet Surg J 2013;33(8):1148–1153
3. Abo-Zeid MA, Al-Refaey AK, Zeina AM. Surgically-assisted abdominal wall blocks for analgesia after abdominoplasty: a prospective randomized trial. Saudi J Anaesth 2018;12(4):593–598

COMPLICATIONS OF ABDOMINOPLASTY

18. A patient who underwent traditional abdominoplasty surgery 6 months ago has called your office concerned about residual fullness to the epigastric region. She had a standard abdominoplasty approach with rectus plication, but no liposuction. *What is the most likely cause of the bulge in this area?*
    A. Inadequate flap dissection

    The patient in this scenario most likely has epigastric fullness because the rectus plication was not started high enough. Failure to elevate the flap up to the xiphisternum is the most likely cause in this case. A dog-ear can occur here following a fleur-de-lis abdominoplasty if there has been inadequate fat removal or if the skin flaps are particularly thick. Seromas can present late but are unlikely at this stage, and usually occur around the waist rather than superiorly as in this case. Postoperative weight gain can often be a reason for late changes in appearance and patient dissatisfaction following surgery, but fat gain affecting this area alone is not likely.[1-3]

REFERENCES

1. Winocour J, Gupta V, Ramirez JR, Shack RB, Grotting JC, Higdon KK. Abdominoplasty: risk factors, complication rates, and safety of combined procedures. Plast Reconstr Surg 2015;136(5):597e–606e
2. Neaman KC, Armstrong SD, Baca ME, Albert M, Vander Woude DL, Renucci JD. Outcomes of traditional cosmetic abdominoplasty in a community setting: a retrospective analysis of 1008 patients. Plast Reconstr Surg 2013;131(3):403e–410e
3. Gutowski KA. Evidence-based medicine: abdominoplasty. Plast Reconstr Surg 2018;141(2):286e–299e

121. Medial Thigh Lift

See *Essentials of Plastic Surgery*, third edition pp. 1711–1716

ANATOMY OF THE THIGH

1. *Which one of the following statements is correct regarding the anatomy of the thigh?*
   A. Thigh skin is of uniform thickness throughout.
   B. There are three distinct fat layers within the thigh.
   C. Colles' fascia lies within the superficial fat of the thigh.
   D. The femoral nerve runs adjacent to the femoral triangle to supply all thigh sensation.
   E. Colles' fascia anatomy is particularly relevant to thigh-lift techniques.

ANATOMY OF THE FEMORAL TRIANGLE

2. *What marks the medial border of the femoral triangle?*
   A. The medial border of the sartorius
   B. The medial border of the adductor longus
   C. The medial border of the adductor magnus
   D. The lateral border of the biceps femoris
   E. The lateral border of the gracilis

CLINICAL ANATOMY IN RELATION TO MEDIAL THIGH LIFTS

3. *When performing a medial thigh lift, what superficial muscle is particularly useful to guide location of the anatomic shelf of Colles' fascia used to suspend the thigh soft tissues?*
   A. Sartorius
   B. Gluteus maximus
   C. Adductor longus
   D. Vastus medialis
   E. Semitendinosus

TECHNIQUE SELECTION IN MEDIAL THIGH LIFTS

4. A 28-year-old woman has moderate skin laxity and subcutaneous fat extending from the distal third of her thigh up to the medial thigh crease. *Which one of the following operative procedures would be optimal in her case?*
   A. Liposuction only
   B. Liposuction and horizontal skin excision
   C. Liposuction with horizontal and vertical skin excision
   D. Horizontal skin excision only
   E. Vertical skin excision only

TECHNIQUE SELECTION IN MEDIAL THIGH LIFTS

5. A 45-year-old woman has an excess of fat to both medial and lateral aspects of the thigh. Her skin quality is good and there is minimal skin excess. *Which one of the following procedures would be best indicated in this case?*
   A Nonsurgical cryolipolysis procedure
   B. Liposuction only
   C. Single stage liposuction with horizontal skin excision
   D. Staged liposuction and horizontal skin excision
   E. Single stage liposuction and vertical skin excision

APPROACHES TO MEDIAL THIGH LIFT

6. A 30-year-old woman has lost more than 40 pounds and has recently undergone a lower body lift. She has a moderate excess of subcutaneous fat in the medial thigh and skin laxity in the upper to middle thirds, which represents a predominantly horizontal excess. *Which one of the following represents a key advantage for considering a skin avulsion technique during her planned medial thigh lift procedure?*
   A. A reduced surgical procedure time
   B. A reduced downtime following surgery
   C. A reduced risk of subsequent lymphedema
   D. A reduced risk of venous thromboembolism
   E. A reduced risk of contour irregularity

MARKING A PATIENT FOR A MEDIAL THIGH LIFT

7. *How should a patient be positioned when performing preoperative marking for a medial thigh lift?*
   A. Standing straight with feet placed together
   B. Standing straight with knees placed slightly apart
   C. Lying supine with legs straight and externally rotated
   D. Lying supine in the frog-leg position
   E. Lying prone with legs slightly apart

MARKING A PATIENT FOR A MEDIAL THIGH LIFT

8. *When marking a patient for a classic medial thigh lift to address a proximal one-third skin excess, which one of the following is correct?*
   A. A transverse incision should be marked 2 cm distal and parallel to the medial thigh crease.
   B. A vertical incision should be marked along the anterior border of adductor longus.
   C. A transverse incision should be marked parallel to the inguinal ligament on the anterior thigh.
   D. A transverse incision should pass from the pubic tubercle to the buttock crease in the medial thigh crease.
   E. The transverse skin resection is usually around 5 cm but should be estimated using a pinch test.

PATIENT POSITIONING DURING A MEDIAL THIGH LIFT

9. *How should the patient be positioned on the operating table during a classic medial thigh lift?*
   A. Lateral with pillows between the legs
   B. Supine with knees on pillows
   C. Supine with legs elevated in stirrups
   D. Supine in frog-leg position
   E. Prone with hips flexed

INTRAOPERATIVE TECHNIQUE DURING MEDIAL THIGH LIFT

10. *During a medial thigh lift, why is it particularly important to preserve the soft tissue that lies between the mons pubis and femoral triangle?*
   A. To avoid nerve damage
   B. To minimize vulval distortion
   C. To reduce infection risk
   D. To minimize risk of hypertrophic scarring
   E. To minimize risk of lymphedema

MEDIAL THIGH LIFT IN MASSIVE-WEIGHT-LOSS PATIENTS

11. You are planning a medial thigh lift on a patient following a belt lipectomy after massive weight loss. On examination, the patient has type V lipodystrophy, with moderate residual fat excess in the medial thigh. The skin excess is very large and extends from the groin crease to the knee. *Which one of the following is correct regarding the excisional component of the procedure?*
   A. It requires a full-length longitudinal incision in the medial thigh without a transverse component.
   B. Anchoring the superficial fascia to Colles' fascia is not required in this case.
   C. The patient should be placed supine on the operating table with stirrups to hold the ankles.
   D. The long saphenous vein should be identified and carefully tied off to avoid bleeding risk.
   E. Segmental excision and closure, as used for a brachioplasty, is not required in this case.

FASCIO-FASCIAL SUSPENSION TECHNIQUE FOR MEDIAL THIGH LIFT

12. The fascio-fascial suspension technique for medial thigh lift uses a different fixation than a standard medial thigh lift. *What structures are used to suspend the thigh in this technique?*
   A. Superficial fascia and inguinal ligament
   B. Superficial fascia and Colles' fascia
   C. Adductor fascia and inguinal ligament
   D. Gracilis fascia and adductor fascia
   E. Gracilis fascia and inguinal ligament

Answers

ANATOMY OF THE THIGH

1. **Which one of the following statements is correct regarding the anatomy of the thigh?**

   E. **Colles' fascia anatomy is particularly relevant to thigh-lift techniques.**

   The superficial anatomy of the thigh is highly relevant to thigh-lift procedures, and knowledge and understanding of Colles' fascia is particularly important. Colles' fascia is a thick, strong fascial layer found deep to the subcutaneous fat of the thigh. It attaches to the ischiopubic rami of the bony pelvis, Scarpa's fascia of the abdominal wall, and the posterior border of the urogenital diaphragm. It has a particularly strong area at the junction of the perineum and medial thigh, where it defines the perineal thigh crease. The Colles' fascia is relevant to medial thigh lift, as it is used to resuspend the elevated soft tissues.[1-3]

   Thigh skin thickness differs according to anatomic location and is thinner medially than laterally. The medial skin also contains fewer hairs. The thigh has two distinct fat layers and between the two is a weak superficial fascial system also relevant to thigh-lift procedures. The femoral nerve travels in the femoral triangle (not adjacent to it) and provides some sensation to the thigh through its branches. The medial femoral cutaneous nerve supplies most of the medial thigh (L1–L2). The proximal aspect of the medial thigh close to the groin crease is supplied by the ilioinguinal nerve (L1). The genitofemoral nerve (L1 component) supplies the skin over the femoral triangle. The lateral aspect of the thigh is supplied by the lateral cutaneous nerve of the thigh (L2–L3) and this may be damaged during an abdominoplasty over the anterior superior iliac spine (ASIS; **Fig. 121.1**).

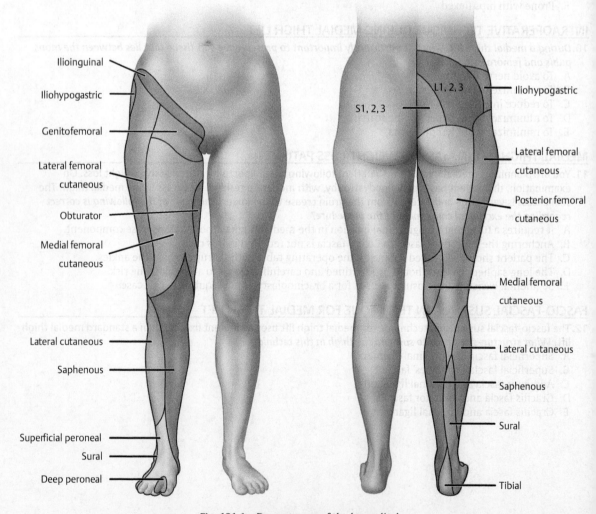

Fig. 121.1 Dermatomes of the lower limb.

REFERENCES

1. Mathes DW, Kenkel JM. Current concepts in medial thighplasty. Clin Plast Surg 2008;35(1):151–163
2. Lockwood TE. Fascial anchoring technique in medial thigh lifts. Plast Reconstr Surg 1988;82(2):299–304
3. Armijo BS, Campbell CF, Rohrich RJ. Four-step medial thighplasty: refined and reproducible. Plast Reconstr Surg 2014;134(5):717e–725e

ANATOMY OF THE FEMORAL TRIANGLE

2. *What marks the medial border of the femoral triangle?*
   B. **The medial border of the adductor longus**
      The femoral triangle is bounded by three structures: the medial border of the sartorius (laterally), the medial border of the adductor longus (medially), and the inguinal ligament superiorly (**Fig. 121.2**). The triangle contains the femoral vessels and nerve and lymphatic channels. It is relevant to a medial thigh lift, in that it should not be violated to avoid damage to these structures. Its anatomy is also relevant to other areas of plastic surgery including groin dissection and management of necrotizing fasciitis of the groin and medial thigh.[1]

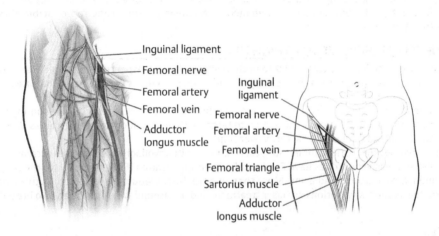

Fig. 121.2 Boundaries of the femoral triangle.

REFERENCE

1. Moore KL, Dalley AF, eds. Clinically Oriented Anatomy. 4th ed. New York, NY: Lippincott, Williams, and Wilkins; 1999

CLINICAL ANATOMY IN RELATION TO MEDIAL THIGH LIFTS

3. *When performing a medial thigh lift, what superficial muscle is particularly useful to guide location of the anatomic shelf of Colles' fascia used to suspend the thigh soft tissues?*
   C. **Adductor longus**
      The junction of the perineum and medial thigh represents a particularly strong area of Colles' fascia that is the site of fixation when performing a traditional medial thigh lift. This site is found by following the origin of the adductor muscles at the ischiopubic ramus and retracting the skin and superficial fat of the pubis medially. The adductor longus is the best guide to locating this area, as it lies superficially and can be palpated easily in most patients when their hips are externally rotated and knees flexed. The adductor magnus and gracilis origins are close to this area but deep to the longus muscle. The sartorius origin is the anterior superior iliac spine (ASIS) and therefore lies lateral to the medial thigh crease. The gluteus maximus lies posterior to the adductor insertion, as does the semitendinosus, which originates from the ischial tuberosity. The vastus medialis is one of the quadriceps muscles that originates from the femur.[1]

REFERENCE

1. Moore KL, Dalley AF, eds. Clinically Oriented Anatomy. 4th ed. New York, NY: Lippincott, Williams, and Wilkins; 1999

TECHNIQUE SELECTION IN MEDIAL THIGH LIFTS

4. A 28-year-old woman has moderate skin laxity and subcutaneous fat extending from the distal third of her thigh up to the medial thigh crease. *Which one of the following operative procedures would be optimal in her case?*

   C. Liposuction with horizontal and vertical skin excision

   The approach to medial thigh lift is both straightforward and logical. If there is excess fat, then liposuction or further weight loss is required. If there is excess skin, then resection is required. If both fat and skin excess are present, a combination of the two is required. If skin excess is confined to the upper third of the thigh, then a horizontal excision is performed in the groin crease, if skin excess affects the majority of the thigh, then a vertical excision is performed on the medial thigh itself. In some cases, such as in this scenario, both horizontal and vertical excisions are combined to create a **T** or **L**-shaped excision. If there are other areas that need to be addressed, such as the abdomen, back, and lateral thighs, then these are generally performed first. If there is severe fat excess, then the procedure may be staged with liposuction first and then skin resection is performed secondarily.[1–3]

REFERENCES

1. Mathes DW, Kenkel JM. Current concepts in medial thighplasty. Clin Plast Surg 2008;35(1):151–163
2. Capella JF, Matarasso A. Management of the postbariatric medial thigh deformity. Plast Reconstr Surg 2016;137(5):1434–1446
3. Armijo BS, Campbell CF, Rohrich RJ. Four-step medial thighplasty: refined and reproducible. Plast Reconstr Surg 2014;134(5):717e–725e

TECHNIQUE SELECTION IN MEDIAL THIGH LIFTS

5. A 45-year-old woman has an excess of fat to both medial and lateral aspects of the thigh. Her skin quality is good and there is minimal skin excess. *Which one of the following procedures would be best indicated in this case?*

   B. Liposuction only

   The patient in this scenario has only fat excess without a need for skin resection. Assuming that her weight is stable, she is best managed with liposuction to target both medial and lateral thigh areas. As her skin is in good condition, it should tighten satisfactorily over time.

   There may be other options for nonsurgical treatment with cryolipolysis which uses extreme cold to breakdown fat cells noninvasively. It does have Food and Drug Administration (FDA) approval for the thighs as well as the abdomen, hips, buttock, and arms. More than one treatment would be expected to give a noticeable result. Alternative noninvasive options are laser treatment and ultrasound which each can also breakdown fat.[1–3]

REFERENCES

1. Nahai F, ed. The Art of Aesthetic Surgery: Principles and Techniques. 2nd ed. St Louis, MO: Quality Medical Publishing; 2011
2. Capella JF, Matarasso A. Management of the postbariatric medial thigh deformity. Plast Reconstr Surg 2016;137(5):1434–1446
3. Kenkel JM, Janis JE, Rohrich RJ, Beran SJ. Aesthetic body contouring: ultrasound-assisted liposuction. In: Matarasso A, ed. Operative Techniques in Plastic and Reconstructive Surgery. Philadelphia, PA: Saunders-Elsevier; 2003

APPROACHES TO MEDIAL THIGH LIFT

6. A 30-year-old woman has lost more than 40 pounds and has recently undergone a lower body lift. She has a moderate excess of subcutaneous fat in the medial thigh and skin laxity in the upper to middle thirds, which represents a predominantly horizontal excess. *Which one of the following represents a key advantage for considering a skin avulsion technique during her planned medial thigh lift procedure?*

   C. A reduced risk of subsequent lymphedema

   This is a massive weight loss patient who is likely to benefit from medial thigh surgery to reduce the residual excess skin and fat present in the thigh. As she has both skin and fat excesses, the approach should include skin resection with liposuction. A more traditional approach is to perform liposuction followed by blade or monopolar skin and subcutaneous fat excision. More recently, combining aggressive liposuction with avulsion of excess skin has become a recognized alternative approach.[1] In this technique, the liposuction is performed to leave very little subcutaneous tissue on the underside of the dermis, which is then excised around the periphery and avulsed using a pair of Kocher forceps or similar in a proximal to distal direction. The key proposed advantage of this technique is that the underlying lymphatics are preserved resulting in reduced problems with subsequent lymphedema and lymphocele formation. In addition, because sensory nerves and connective tissue are preserved, wound healing issues and sensory nerve problems should also be reduced.

   Supplementary liposuction may be performed to other areas of the thigh to further improve overall contour, and this would be performed in a far less aggressive manner to more gently recontour the areas where no skin resection is planned.

This approach to medial thigh lift is unproven to significantly affect surgical duration or downtime. This is more likely to be affected by surgeon experience and patient factors. This approach can still lead to contour deformities and these again will most likely be dependent on surgeon experience and characteristics of the patient thighs. There is no reason why this approach should affect venous thromboembolism risk and patients should still be risk assessed to guide chemoprophylaxis.

REFERENCE

1. Hunstad JP, Kortesis BG, Knotts CD. Avulsion thighplasty: technique overview and 6-year experience. Plast Reconstr Surg 2016;137(1):84–87

MARKING A PATIENT FOR A MEDIAL THIGH LIFT

7. *How should a patient be positioned when performing preoperative marking for a medial thigh lift?*
   B. Standing straight with knees placed slightly apart

   When marking a patient for a medial thigh lift, it is important to perform this with them standing upright with knees apart. This should be performed in the presence of a chaperone of the same sex as the patient, given the intimate nature of the markings. It is important to do these markings with the patient standing, as it more reliably allows assessment of the location and extent of excess soft tissue. Where necessary, subtle refinements may be made on table to these markings.[1–3]

REFERENCES

1. Nahai F, ed. The Art of Aesthetic Surgery: Principles and Techniques. 2nd ed. St Louis, MO: Quality Medical Publishing; 2011
2. Armijo BS, Campbell CF, Rohrich RJ. Four-step medial thighplasty: refined and reproducible. Plast Reconstr Surg 2014;134(5):717e–725e
3. Capella JF, Matarasso A. Management of the postbariatric medial thigh deformity. Plast Reconstr Surg 2016;137(5):1434–1446

MARKING A PATIENT FOR A MEDIAL THIGH LIFT

8. *When marking a patient for a classic medial thigh lift to address a proximal one-third skin excess, which one of the following is correct?*
   E. The transverse skin resection is usually around 5 cm but should be estimated using a pinch test.

   When marking a patient for a medial thigh lift, it is best to assess the amount of excess skin that can safely be removed by performing a pinch test. This is done by gently grasping the soft tissues and lifting them toward the thigh crease. The exact amount that can be taken is patient dependent, but on average 5 to 7 cm is excised. A further 3 to 5 cm of lift is achieved secondary to anchoring of the skin flap to the Colles' fascia.

   The approach to a medial thigh lift will be guided by skin and soft-tissue excess. A standard approach for the patient described involves a transverse incision placed in the medial thigh crease, passing from the pubic tubercle to the perineal thigh crease. It is not necessary to extend the incision all the way posterior to the buttock crease. A vertical extension is required only where skin laxity extends beyond the upper third of the thigh, and is therefore not required in this case. When performing a fascio-fascial suspension technique, the transverse incision may be placed parallel to and 6 to 7 cm below the inguinal crease, but not in a classic thigh lift.[1]

REFERENCE

1. Armijo BS, Campbell CF, Rohrich RJ. Four-step medial thighplasty: refined and reproducible. Plast Reconstr Surg 2014;134(5):717e–725e

PATIENT POSITIONING DURING A MEDIAL THIGH LIFT

9. *How should the patient be positioned on the operating table during a classic medial thigh lift?*
   D. Supine in frog-leg position

   Patients undergoing classic medial thigh lift should normally be positioned supine in a frog-leg position.[1] Stirrups were previously used but are no longer needed because the incision ends at the perineal crease without extension to the buttocks. A prone position is unnecessary for the same reason and is less favorable from an anesthetic perspective. Lateral positioning would entail changing position and redraping intraoperatively when moving from one side to the next. This would have implications on surgical timings which would naturally be increased. Some authors describe performing this procedure with the patient supine on leg boards so that the legs are flat but abducted. This can offer some advantages with regard to surgeon comfort and minimizing repositioning of the patient intraoperatively.[2]

REFERENCES

1. Armijo BS, Campbell CF, Rohrich RJ. Four-step medial thighplasty: refined and reproducible. Plast Reconstr Surg 2014;134(5):717e–725e
2. Kenkel JM, Eaves FF III. Medial thigh lift. Plast Reconstr Surg 2008;122(2):621–622

INTRAOPERATIVE TECHNIQUE DURING MEDIAL THIGH LIFT

10. *During a medial thigh lift, why is it particularly important to preserve the soft tissue that lies between the mons pubis and femoral triangle?*

   E. To minimize risk of lymphedema

     It is important to carefully preserve the soft tissue that lies between the mons pubis and femoral triangle to prevent damage to the lymphatics and subsequent lymphedema.[1] Lymphedema is difficult to manage, and medial thigh lift carries a small risk of this and must be discussed during the preoperative consent process. The risk of nerve damage is low and the risk of infection is not affected. Hypertrophic scarring is not common at this site and a small volume resection of this soft tissue is unlikely to significantly distort the vulva.

REFERENCE

1. Armijo BS, Campbell CF, Rohrich RJ. Four-step medial thighplasty: refined and reproducible. Plast Reconstr Surg 2014;134(5):717e–725e

MEDIAL THIGH LIFT IN MASSIVE-WEIGHT-LOSS PATIENTS

11. You are planning a medial thigh lift on a patient following a belt lipectomy after massive weight loss. On examination, the patient has type V lipodystrophy, with moderate residual fat excess in the medial thigh. The skin excess is very large and extends from the groin crease to the knee. *Which one of the following is correct regarding the excisional component of the procedure?*

   B. Anchoring the superficial fascia to Colles' fascia is not required in this case.

     This patient has a significant horizontal excess of skin, and this requires a longitudinal (vertical), elliptical excision pattern. The addition of a short transverse upper incision will likely be required to avoid formation of a dog-ear. Because the vector of lift is horizontal instead of vertical, it is not necessary to anchor the skin flap to Colles' fascia. Stirrups are not required in this case.

     A similar approach to a brachioplasty should be adopted, where excision and closure are staged to minimize the effects of soft-tissue swelling and the risk of over-resection. This may not hold true if an avulsion technique is being used. The long saphenous vein should be identified and preserved. Injury to it can result in prolonged swelling of the lower extremity. A compression garment should be used after surgery for 2 to 4 weeks.[1-3]

REFERENCES

1. Gusenoff JA, Coon D, Nayar H, Kling RE, Rubin JP. Medial thigh lift in the massive weight loss population: outcomes and complications. Plast Reconstr Surg 2015;135(1):98–106
2. Capella JF, Matarasso A. Management of the postbariatric medial thigh deformity. Plast Reconstr Surg 2016;137(5):1434–1446
3. Schmidt M, Pollhammer MS, Januszyk M, Duscher D, Huemer GM. Concomitant liposuction reduces complications of vertical medial thigh lift in massive weight loss patients. Plast Reconstr Surg 2016;137(6):1748–1757

FASCIO-FASCIAL SUSPENSION TECHNIQUE FOR MEDIAL THIGH LIFT

12. The fascio-fascial suspension technique for medial thigh lift uses a different fixation than a standard medial thigh lift. *What structures are used to suspend the thigh in this technique?*

   D. Gracilis fascia and adductor fascia

     The fascio-fascial suspension technique was described by Candiani et al[1] as an alternative to a classic medial thigh lift. It employs a transverse skin excision with a vertical vector of pull. Instead of relying on anchoring of the Colles' fascia, the technique relies on the strength of overlap between the gracilis and the adductor longus muscles. Instead of making an incision in the medial thigh crease, it is made 6 to 7 cm below the inguinal crease. The skin and fat are undermined down to the fascia of the adductor longus and gracilis muscles. The fascia between the two muscles is then overlapped and closed to support the lift and allow skin closure under minimal tension.[1]

REFERENCE

1. Candiani P, Campiglio GL, Signorini M. Fascio-fascial suspension technique in medial thigh lifts. Aesthetic Plast Surg 1995;19(2):137–140

122. Body Contouring in the Massive-Weight-Loss Patient

See *Essentials of Plastic Surgery*, third edition, pp. 1717–1734

BODY MASS INDEX

1. *How is body mass index (BMI) calculated?*
   A. Height (m) divided by weight (kg)^2
   B. Weight (kg) divided by height (m)^2
   C. Height (m) multiplied by weight (kg)^2
   D. Weight (kg) multiplied by height (m)^2
   E. Height (m)^2 divided by weight (kg)

BODY MASS INDEX AND HEALTH STATUS

2. A patient is seen in clinic before surgery. The patient is 1.72 meters tall and weighs 86 kg. *How would you describe their current health status according to their calculated BMI?*
   A. Underweight
   B. Normal weight
   C. Overweight
   D. Morbidly obese
   E. Super obese

BARIATRIC SURGERY TECHNIQUES

3. A patient is seen in clinic having undergone gastric bypass surgery and subsequent major weight loss. *Why is gastric bypass considered to be a better procedure than gastric banding?*
   A. The surgery is less invasive.
   B. Nutritional supplements are not required.
   C. It is more easily reversed.
   D. It reduces small bowel food absorption.
   E. The effects can be adjusted postoperatively.

BARIATRIC SURGERY TECHNIQUES

4. *Which one of the following procedures has become the most common bariatric procedure to promote massive weight loss?*
   A. Adjustable gastric band
   B. Roux-en-Y gastric bypass
   C. Biliopancreatic diversion (BPD)
   D. Gastric sleeve
   E. Vertical band gastroplasty

PRIORITIES IN WEIGHT LOSS CONTOURING

5. *When planning body contouring after massive weight loss, which one of the following areas is commonly targeted first?*
   A. Breasts
   B. Trunk
   C. Face and neck
   D. Arms
   E. Medial thighs

TIMING OF BODY CONTOURING AFTER BARIATRIC SURGERY

6. A 30-year-old patient is seeking breast and trunk recontouring 9 months after undergoing gastric bypass. She has lost 22 kg (44 pounds), to move from a BMI of 40.5 to a BMI of 32. Her breasts and abdomen have significant skin excess. Her weight has been stable for 3 months. *Which one of the following is correct?*
   A. She is ready to proceed with an initial panniculectomy.
   B. She is ready to proceed with a breast reduction.
   C. Body contouring surgery should be postponed until her BMI is less than 25.
   D. Body contouring surgery should be postponed for an additional 3 months.
   E. Body contouring surgery should be postponed for an additional year.

FUNCTIONS OF A BELT LIPECTOMY

7. *Which one of the following areas is ineffectively addressed with a belt lipectomy procedure?*
   A. Lower abdominal pannus
   B. Central buttock region
   C. Lateral and medial thighs
   D. Lower and mid-back rolls
   E. Waistline and mons pubis

BELT LIPECTOMY PROCEDURE

8. *When marking a massive-weight-loss patient for a belt lipectomy, which one of the following is correct?*
   A. Preoperative markings are best done on the day of surgery with the patient standing.
   B. Upper and lower anterior transverse markings are placed at the same level as for an abdominoplasty.
   C. Strict adherence to preoperative markings during surgery is essential for good outcomes.
   D. The patient must bend forward while the posterior vertical excess is marked to avoid over excision.
   E. Posterior and lateral areas are most important to the final outcome, so warrant generous resection.

PERFORMING A BELT LIPECTOMY

9. *Which of the following is correct when performing a belt lipectomy in a massive-weight-loss patient?*
   A. The combination of supine and prone positioning provides optimal access.
   B. Umbilical lengthening is usually required during a standard belt lipectomy.
   C. Liposuction to the lateral thigh should preserve the zones of adherence.
   D. Posterior skin flap elevation should be performed at the level of the lumbar fascia.
   E. Incisions should be sited to place postoperative scars below the pelvic brim.

BREAST SURGERY AFTER MASSIVE WEIGHT LOSS

10. A patient has lost 98 pounds after gastric banding. Her breasts are flat and underfilled. She has sternal notch-to-nipple distances of 30 cm on both sides and has a BMI of 26. *How best should this be managed surgically?*
    A. Augmentation only
    B. Mastopexy only
    C. Reduction only
    D. Augmentation–mastopexy
    E. Autoaugmentation

BREAST SURGERY AFTER MASSIVE WEIGHT LOSS

11. A patient has lost 42 pounds with diet and exercise. Her BMI is now 23. Her breasts measure an A cup, and she has sternal notch-to-nipple distances of 22 cm. *Which one of the following procedures would be most beneficial in her case?*
    A. Augmentation only
    B. Mastopexy only
    C. Fat transfer only
    D. Augmentation–mastopexy
    E. Autoaugmentation

BREAST SURGERY AFTER MASSIVE WEIGHT LOSS

12. A patient has had body contouring surgery to the trunk after massive weight loss, but still has concerns regarding her breasts which are ptotic and empty. On examination, she has sternal notch-to-nipple distances of 28 cm with grade III ptosis and a significant lateral soft-tissue excess passing from the breasts toward the axillae. Her BMI is 33. *How might her breasts be best managed from a surgical perspective?*
    A. Augmentation only
    B. Mastopexy only
    C. Reduction only
    D. Augmentation–mastopexy
    E. Autoaugmentation

THIGH CONTOURING SURGERY AFTER MASSIVE WEIGHT LOSS

13. When considering the thighs in a massive weight loss patient, which one of the following is true?
    A. The lateral thighs should be treated before the medial thighs.
    B. A horizontal skin excision pattern should preferentially be used.
    C. Liposuction should generally be avoided in this patient group.
    D. Superficial tissues should be anchored to Colles' fascia with a permanent suture.
    E. A medial thigh lift will help reduce any existing problems with lymphedema.

COMPLICATIONS AFTER MASSIVE-WEIGHT-LOSS SURGERY

14. You are discussing the risks of surgery with a patient who has reduced their BMI from 40 to 30 after bariatric surgery. *Which one of the following complications is most common after major body contouring surgery?*
    A. Venous thromboembolism
    B. Skin necrosis
    C. Wound infection
    D. Hematoma
    E. Wound dehiscence

Answers

BODY MASS INDEX

1. ***How is body mass index (BMI) calculated?***
    B. **Weight (kg) divided by height (m)²**
    Body mass index is a measurement of body fat based on weight and height. It is calculated using the following equation:
    Weight in kg/Height (m)²
      It is useful when assessing patients before and after massive-weight-loss surgery and can be used to subclassify the degree of obesity. It was described by Keys et al in 1972 where they compared a number of different measures used to assess a patient's build.[1] It has since become a uniformly accepted measurement as a marker of obesity.
      Body mass index should be recorded for all plastic surgery patients, not only those who have undergone massive weight loss. It will help guide treatments and patient's suitability for them as well as their risks of certain complications including venous thromboembolism, chest infection, cardiac events, and risks of viral complications.[2,3]

REFERENCES

1. Keys A, Fidanza F, Karvonen MJ, Kimura N, Taylor HL. Indices of relative weight and obesity. J Chronic Dis 1972;25(6):329–343
2. Aly AS. Body Contouring After Massive Weight Loss. St Louis, MO: Quality Medical Publishing; 2006
3. Hamad GG. The state of the art in bariatric surgery for weight loss in the morbidly obese patient. Clin Plast Surg 2004;31(4):591–600, vi

BODY MASS INDEX AND HEALTH STATUS

2. **A patient is seen in clinic before surgery. The patient is 1.72 meters tall and weighs 86 kg. *How would you describe their current health status according to their calculated BMI?***
    C. **Overweight**
    This patient has a BMI of 29 kg/m² based on their height and weight, using the calculation: Weight in kg/Height (m)². The National Institute of Health (NIH) classification for BMI is as follows:
    - BMI <18.5: Underweight
    - BMI 18.5–24.9: Normal/healthy weight
    - BMI 25–29.9: Overweight
    - BMI 30–34.9: Obese
    - BMI 35–39.9: Severely obese
    - BMI > or = 40: Morbidly obese
    - BMI > or = 50: Super obese

    Most patients following massive weight loss will reach a plateau to remain with a BMI around 30. Some will be able to go further and achieve a BMI less than this, but most patients tend to remain slightly overweight. The relevance of BMI to body contouring surgery is that operative risks are markedly reduced once patients reduce their BMI to less than 30 or are close to their ideal body weight. They are also more likely to achieve good cosmetic outcomes after surgery. The patient described remains overweight at present but remains in a weight category where plastic surgery would be appropriate. Patients with a BMI above 35 should be encouraged to lose more weight prior to surgery.[1,2]

REFERENCES

1. Nuttall FQ. Body mass index: obesity, BMI, and health: a critical review. Nutr Today 2015;50(3):117–128
2. Available at: https://www.nhlbi.nih.gov/health/educational/lose_wt/BMI/bmi_dis.htm. Accessed June 10, 2021

BARIATRIC SURGERY TECHNIQUES

3. **A patient is seen in clinic having undergone gastric bypass surgery and subsequent major weight loss. *Why is gastric bypass considered to be a better procedure than gastric banding?***
    D. **It reduces small bowel food absorption.**
    Techniques commonly used to achieve massive weight loss are either restrictive (such as gastric banding or sleeve) or both restrictive and malabsorptive, such as gastric bypass and biliopancreatic diversion (**Fig. 122.1**). Restrictive procedures simply reduce the size of the stomach such that patients feel full sooner and reduce their food intake accordingly. In contrast, malabsorptive procedures bypass food through parts of the small intestine to reduce its

absorption. In general, procedures that are both restrictive and malabsorptive achieve more rapid and sustained weight loss at the expense of potentially causing nutritional deficiencies. The main benefit of the gastric bypass procedure over gastric banding, therefore, is the fact that it reduces both food intake and absorption.

Both procedures are performed laparoscopically and surgery is similarly invasive for both procedures, but is simpler and lower risk, due to the absence of bowel anastomoses in gastric banding. Nutritional supplements are required for patients following absorptive procedures. The gastric band procedure is reversible and more adjustable than gastric bypass, as the port can be inflated or deflated in clinic. In contrast, the gastric bypass requires surgical intervention to reverse or adjust.[1-4]

REFERENCES

1. Hamad GG. The state of the art in bariatric surgery for weight loss in the morbidly obese patient. Clin Plast Surg 2004; 31(4):591–600, vi
2. A review of bariatric surgery procedures. Plast Reconstr Surg 2006;117(1, Suppl):8S–13S
3. Gilbert EW, Wolfe BM. Bariatric surgery for the management of obesity: state of the field. Plast Reconstr Surg 2012; 130(4):948–954
4. Arterburn D, Gupta A. Comparing the outcomes of sleeve gastrectomy and Roux-en-Y gastric bypass for severe obesity. JAMA 2018;319(3):235–237

BARIATRIC SURGERY TECHNIQUES

4. *Which one of the following procedures has become the most common bariatric procedure to promote massive weight loss?*

D. Gastric sleeve

The gastric sleeve procedure (see **Fig. 122.1, B**) has become the most commonly performed procedure to assist in weight loss, although the gastric bypass remains the "gold standard," as it is more effective at achieving weight loss and putting diabetes into remission. The sleeve gastrectomy is a permanent restrictive procedure that involves creation of a gastric tube by resecting the greater curvature of the stomach, effectively turning it into a sleeve rather than a pouch. It has become more popular than the bypass, as it is more straightforward, less invasive, and incurs a lower complication risk of leakage of bowel contents. Following this procedure, the mean excess weight loss is around 50% at 6 years and there is an associated 70% remission in type 2 diabetes. This is, however, less than with gastric bypass where it is over 90% remission.

Gastric banding is usually performed laparoscopically and involves placement of an adjustable band around the top of the stomach. A separate port is connected to the band with silicone tubing and is sited in the subcutaneous tissues. This allows for adjustment of the band when required (see **Fig. 122.1, A**).

The Roux-en-Y gastric bypass is the current benchmark procedure for weight loss. It involves reducing the size of the stomach to create a pouch that is in continuity with the esophagus and intestine. Food consequently passes directly into the small intestine, while the stomach still releases gastric juices that also enter the small intestine and assist with digestion. This procedure means that food intake is restricted, as patients feel full rapidly. The absorption is also affected, but less so than with other malabsorptive techniques (see **Fig. 122.1, C**).

The biliopancreatic diversion (BPD) involves removal of part of the stomach to reduce its size by approximately 75%. The remaining stomach is then directly anastomosed to the lower portion of the small intestine. It is an effective procedure for achieving weight loss of 75 to 80% with good long-term maintenance. However, it may lead to significant nutritional deficiencies, such that patients require lifelong vitamin supplementation and experience foul smelling flatulence and loose stools (see **Fig. 122.1, D**).

The vertical band gastroplasty is a restrictive procedure (also referred to as "stomach stapling") that typically involves a reduction in stomach size by a combination of staples and a band with mesh wrapped around the stomach opening to help maintain the restriction. It is not very effective and around half of patients are unable to maintain their weight loss with this procedure.[1-4]

REFERENCES

1. Arterburn D, Gupta A. Comparing the outcomes of sleeve gastrectomy and Roux-en-Y gastric bypass for severe obesity. JAMA 2018;319(3):235–237
2. Metabolic and Bariatric Surgery Accreditation and Quality Improvement Program (MBSAQIP) Semiannual Report (SAR), July 2019: Data from January 1, 2018 to December 31, 2018, American College of Surgeons
3. Hamad GG. The state of the art in bariatric surgery for weight loss in the morbidly obese patient. Clin Plast Surg 2004;31(4):591–600, vi
4. Gilbert EW, Wolfe BM. Bariatric surgery for the management of obesity: state of the field. Plast Reconstr Surg 2012;130(4):948–954

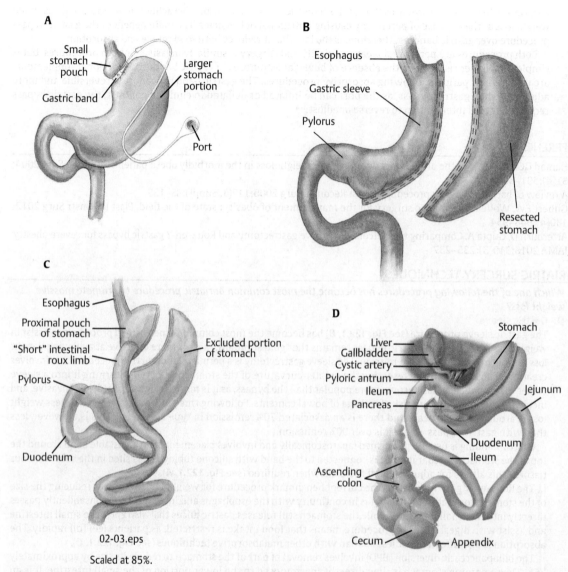

A

Small stomach pouch

Gastric band

Larger stomach portion

Port

B

Esophagus

Gastric sleeve

Pylorus

Resected stomach

C

Esophagus

Proximal pouch of stomach

"Short" intestinal roux limb

Pylorus

Duodenum

Excluded portion of stomach

D

Stomach

Liver

Gallbladder

Cystic artery

Pyloric antrum

Ileum

Pancreas

Jejunum

Duodenum

Ileum

Ascending colon

Cecum

Appendix

02-03.eps

Scaled at 85%.

Fig. 122.1 Restrictive procedures for bariatric surgery. *A*, Laparoscopic adjustable gastric band. *B*, Sleeve gastrectomy. *C*, Roux-en-Y gastric bypass. *D*, Biliopancreatic diversion with duodenal switch.

PRIORITIES IN WEIGHT LOSS CONTOURING

5. When planning body contouring after massive weight loss, which one of the following areas is commonly targeted first?

B. Trunk

The goals of plastic surgery following massive weight loss are to alleviate functional, aesthetic, and psychological impairments associated with skin redundancy and poor contour. Often the functional component is most important, since this can limit the patient's ability to exercise fully and find clothing to fit well. The order of treatment should always be patient specific, but, in general, the trunk is treated first with a lower body lift, abdominoplasty, or panniculectomy, because an overhanging abdominal pannus and trunk rolls can be quite restrictive in terms of exercising and achieving further weight loss. The breasts and arms would normally be targeted next, followed by the medial thighs, face, and neck.[1,2]

Most patients will require multiple procedures to correct the skin and soft-tissue excesses following massive weight loss. Some of these can be combined in one operation such as abdomen and breast, or breast and arms as they can be complimentary to one another and help reduce both hospital attendances and overall downtime. They can also help make the process more cost-effective for the patient, although this has to be a secondary aim behind optimal clinical decision-making. Patients need to understand the limitations of such surgical intervention and see the process as a work in progress. Many younger patients will not need any intervention to the face or neck at all.

REFERENCES

1. Aly AS. Body Contouring After Massive Weight Loss. St Louis, MO: Quality Medical Publishing; 2006
2. Nahai F, ed. The Art of Aesthetic Surgery: Principles and Techniques. 2nd ed. St Louis, MO: Quality Medical Publishing; 2011

TIMING OF BODY CONTOURING AFTER BARIATRIC SURGERY

6. A 30-year-old patient is seeking breast and trunk recontouring 9 months after undergoing gastric bypass. She has lost 22 kg (44 pounds), to move from a BMI of 40.5 to a BMI of 32. Her breasts and abdomen have significant skin excess. Her weight has been stable for 3 months. *Which one of the following is correct?*

    D. Body contouring surgery should be postponed for an additional 3 months.

    Although this patient has made excellent steps in her weight reduction, it is too early to proceed with body contouring surgery at this stage because she has not maintained a steady weight for sufficient time. Stability for at least 6 months is recommended before proceeding with body contouring surgery. This usually corresponds to at least 12 to 18 months after gastric bypass. The benefits of delaying surgery include a reduction in the risk of perioperative complications, improved aesthetic outcomes, and better wound healing. This delay helps achieve metabolic and nutritional homeostasis. In addition, it provides the patient and surgeon time for discussion and reflection on the best operative plan. Most patients following massive weight loss stabilize at a BMI of 30 to 35 and may benefit from an initial panniculectomy or breast reduction to assist further lifestyle changes such as diet or exercise. Although it may be optimal to wait until patients have a BMI less than 25, it is neither necessary nor realistic to wait until this time, given most patients' weight stabilizes around BMI 30, and they are unlikely to ever reach the BMI 25 target.[1-3]

REFERENCES

1. Aly AS. Body Contouring After Massive Weight Loss. St Louis, MO: Quality Medical Publishing; 2006
2. Rubin JP, Nguyen V, Schwentker A. Perioperative management of the post-gastric-bypass patient presenting for body contour surgery. Clin Plast Surg 2004;31(4):601–610, vi
3. Taylor J, Shermak M. Body contouring following massive weight loss. Obes Surg 2004;14(8):1080–1085

FUNCTIONS OF A BELT LIPECTOMY

7. *Which one of the following areas is ineffectively addressed with a belt lipectomy procedure?*

    C. Lateral and medial thighs

    A belt lipectomy has the benefit of addressing multiple areas of trunk skin and soft-tissue excess and accompanying ptosis that are characteristic of the inverted cone physique following massive weight loss. The circumferential excision pattern will address the anterior abdominal panniculus, the lateral abdominal excess, and the lower and mid-back folds. It cannot safely address the upper back fold, which is separately addressed during breast procedures or as an isolated procedure. It also lifts the ptotic tissues from the buttocks, mons pubis, and lateral thighs. This improves the contour of these areas while improving the waistline. The medial thigh will need to be addressed separately with a combination of skin resection and liposuction.[1-4]

REFERENCES

1. Aly AS. Body Contouring After Massive Weight Loss. St Louis, MO: Quality Medical Publishing; 2006
2. Zomerlei T, Janis JE. Liposuction, abdominoplasty and belt lipectomy. In: Chung KC, ed. Grabb and Smith's Plastic Surgery 8th ed. Philadelphia, PA: Wolters Kluwer; 2019:632–642
3. Losco L, Roxo AC, Roxo CW, et al. Lower body lift after bariatric surgery: 323 consecutive cases over 10-year experience. Aesthetic Plast Surg 2020;44(2):421–432
4. Aly A, Mueller M. Circumferential truncal contouring: the belt lipectomy. Clin Plast Surg 2014;41(4):765–774

BELT LIPECTOMY PROCEDURE

8. *When marking a massive-weight-loss patient for a belt lipectomy, which one of the following is correct?*

    D. The patient must bend forward while the posterior vertical excess is marked to avoid over excision.

    The preoperative markings can be done on the day of surgery, but it is preferable to do them the day before. This enables the surgeon to review photographs of the markings and make any necessary changes. It also increases time efficiency on the day of surgery. The markings will be made with the patient standing for some parts and supine with hips slightly flexed for others (**Fig. 122.2**).

The key aspect when marking is to ensure that sufficient excess will be removed anteriorly and laterally, where the patient can most easily see the result. It is important to ensure the posterior excision is not overdone, because this will lead to tension at the point of closure.

In massive-weight-loss patients, the anterior horizontal markings will differ from those for a standard abdominoplasty. The lower incision should be lower to correct mons pubis ptosis. The upper incision may be higher than the abdominoplasty level because of the presence of excess tissue. It will continue away from the midline, oriented horizontally, and will not taper back toward the lower incision. Preoperative markings must be used as a guide and may require adjustment in the operating room to optimally refine the procedure.[1-4]

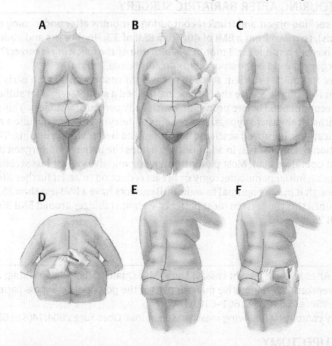

Fig. 122.2 Markings for belt lipectomy. **A,** The midline is marked initially. The horizontal pubic incision is marked below the natural hairline to allow elevation of the mons. The inferior midline of the closure should be level with the pubic symphysis. The pannus is elevated superiorly and medially to allow marking of the lateral extension of the inferior incision to just below the anterior superior iliac spine. **B,** The superior markings are made anteriorly using the pinch technique to determine the extent of resection. **C,** The midline of the back is marked with the inferior point at the coccyx. **D,** The patient is slightly bent at the waist, and the pinch test is used to estimate the superior extent of resection. **E** and **F,** The superior and inferior back marks are made to meet the abdominal marks laterally.

REFERENCES

1. Aly AS, Cram AE, Heddens C. Truncal body contouring surgery in the massive weight loss patient. Clin Plast Surg 2004;31(4):611–624, vii
2. Zomerlei T, Janis JE. Liposuction, abdominoplasty and belt lipectomy. In: Chung KC, ed. Grabb and Smith's Plastic Surgery 8th ed. Philadelphia, PA: Wolters Kluwer; 2019:632–642
3. Losco L, Roxo AC, Roxo CW, et al. Lower body lift after bariatric surgery: 323 consecutive cases over 10-year experience. Aesthetic Plast Surg 2020;44(2):421–432
4. Aly A, Mueller M. Circumferential truncal contouring: the belt lipectomy. Clin Plast Surg 2014;41(4):765–774

PERFORMING A BELT LIPECTOMY

9. *Which of the following is correct when performing a belt lipectomy in a massive-weight-loss patient?*

   E. Incisions should be sited to place postoperative scars below the pelvic brim.

   When performing a belt lipectomy procedure, scars should be placed to minimize their appearance in most undergarments and swimwear, and this can be achieved by designing them to lie below the pelvic brim. Patients undergoing belt lipectomy will need to be placed in supine, prone, and lateral decubitus positions during the procedure to achieve adequate access. Umbilical lengthening is not required; however, an umbilicoplasty (shortening) is required regardless of the contouring technique used, because the umbilical stalk will have become stretched and elongated during the period of excess weight gain and will not shrink with weight loss. This can help create an aesthetically pleasing umbilicus with some superior hooding and inferior retraction. Liposuction to the lateral thighs should be performed with release of the zones of adherence, in this case to facilitate lateral thigh elevation. The anterior resection is made at the level of the deep fascia or just above it, as per a standard abdominoplasty, but posteriorly the resection is limited to the level of superficial fascia, as this minimizes seroma formation. In addition, the level at which the posterior inferior flap is raised can affect buttock projection. In massive-weight-loss patients, the buttocks are usually under-projected, so it is wise to elevate the posterior flap at the level of the superficial fascia to maximize the soft-tissue volume maintained in this region.[1-5]

REFERENCES

1. Aly A, Mueller M. Circumferential truncal contouring: the belt lipectomy. Clin Plast Surg 2014;41(4):765–774
2. Aly AS. Body Contouring After Massive Weight Loss. St Louis, MO: Quality Medical Publishing; 2006
3. Aly AS, Cram AE, Heddens C. Truncal body contouring surgery in the massive weight loss patient. Clin Plast Surg 2004;31(4):611–624, vii
4. Zomerlei T, Janis JE. Liposuction, abdominoplasty and belt lipectomy. In: Chung KC, ed. Grabb and Smith's Plastic Surgery, 8th ed. Philadelphia, PA. Wolters Kluwer; 2019:632–642
5. Losco L, Roxo AC, Roxo CW, et al. Lower body lift after bariatric surgery: 323 consecutive cases over 10-year experience. Aesthetic Plast Surg 2020;44(2):421–432

BREAST SURGERY AFTER MASSIVE WEIGHT LOSS

10. A patient has lost 98 pounds after gastric banding. Her breasts are flat and underfilled. She has sternal notch-to-nipple distances of 30 cm on both sides and has a BMI of 26. *How best should this be managed surgically?*

   D. Augmentation–mastopexy

   The patient in this scenario most probably needs additional volume for her breasts but is likely to be fairly slim following her weight loss based on her BMI of 26. She is unlikely to have sufficient autologous tissue to augment her breasts and will therefore need prosthetic augmentation to restore adequate volume. Her sternal notch-to-nipple distances are large and should ideally be reduced. This requires skin excision in the form of a mastopexy. The best procedure for this patient is therefore a combined augmentation–mastopexy. This may be as a single- or two-stage procedure. The starting point for discussions will be to see what the patient wishes to achieve in terms of breast shape and volume and whether she would consider a two-stage procedure or only a single stage. She needs to understand that mastopexy or augment alone will not provide her with the optimal result. If performing a two-stage procedure, the breasts can be reshaped in the first instance with a Wise pattern skin excision and coning of the native breast. After 6 to 12 months, implants may be placed in the submuscular/dual plane via an inframammary approach. In contrast, if a single stage is to be performed, then placement of the implant or a temporary sizer should be performed first and the skin reduced accordingly to suit.[1-4]

REFERENCES

1. Losken A. Breast reshaping following massive weight loss: principles and techniques. Plast Reconstr Surg 2010;126(3):1075–1085
2. Nahai F, ed. The Art of Aesthetic Surgery: Principles and Techniques. 2nd ed. St Louis, MO: Quality Medical Publishing; 2011
3. Hurwitz DJ, Golla D. Breast reshaping after massive weight loss. Semin Plast Surg 2004;18(3):179–187
4. Beidas OE, Rubin JP. Breast reshaping after massive weight loss. Clin Plast Surg 2019;46(1):71–76

BREAST SURGERY AFTER MASSIVE WEIGHT LOSS

11. A patient has lost 42 pounds with diet and exercise. Her BMI is now 23. Her breasts measure an A cup, and she has sternal notch-to-nipple distances of 22 cm. *Which one of the following procedures would be most beneficial in her case?*

   A. Augmentation only

   The patient in this scenario has a relatively modest weight loss and is now slim. Her breasts are not ptotic but are just underfilled. She should have an augmentation procedure only. When consulting patients like this patient, it is really important to consider whether mastopexy will be required as well as augmentation as otherwise the wrong procedure may be selected, leading to patient dissatisfaction. In cases where there is mild ptosis and good quality soft tissues, augmentation can provide a degree of uplift to the breasts. Conversely if the breasts are more significantly ptotic, the addition of implants may exacerbate the appearance of ptosis.[1-3]

REFERENCES

1. Losken A. Breast reshaping following massive weight loss: principles and techniques. Plast Reconstr Surg 2010;126(3):1075–1085
2. Nahai F, ed. The Art of Aesthetic Surgery: Principles and Techniques. 2nd ed. St Louis:, MO Quality Medical Publishing; 2011
3. Hurwitz DJ, Golla D. Breast reshaping after massive weight loss. Semin Plast Surg 2004;18(3):179–187

BREAST SURGERY AFTER MASSIVE WEIGHT LOSS

12. A patient has had body contouring surgery to the trunk after massive weight loss, but still has concerns regarding her breasts which are ptotic and empty. On examination, she has sternal notch-to-nipple distances of 28 cm with grade III ptosis and a significant lateral soft-tissue excess passing from the breasts toward the axillae. Her BMI is 33. *How might her breasts be best managed from a surgical perspective?*

    E. Autoaugmentation

        The patient in this scenario requires additional breast volume and an uplift procedure with skin resection. She remains obese and has excess lateral tissue in the upper trunk which can be used to autoaugment her breasts. Autoaugmentation typically utilizes residual soft-tissue excess from the lateral and inferior breasts as local flaps. A Wise pattern skin approach is used, and this may have additional extension laterally compared with a standard breast reduction pattern depending on tissue excess and volume requirements. Both medial and lateral inferiorly based flaps are de-epithelialized with a central dermal extension including the nipple areola complex. The medial and lateral flaps are then transposed superiorly and fixed to rib periosteum along with the central pedicle to the midline of the breast. Plication of the flaps is then performed to provide maximal internal support. Wounds are closed in a similar way to a standard Wise pattern breast reduction (**Fig. 122.3**).[1-6]

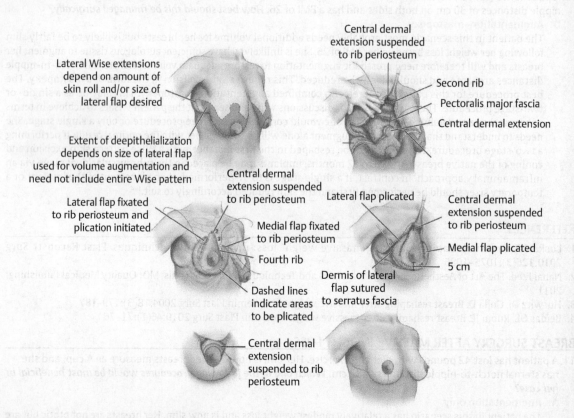

Fig. 122.3 Breast reconstruction in massive-weight-loss patients. (From Nahai F, ed. The Art of Aesthetic Surgery: Principles and Techniques, 2nd ed. St Louis, MO: Quality Medical Publishing, 2011.)

REFERENCES

1. Losken A. Breast reshaping following massive weight loss: principles and techniques. Plast Reconstr Surg 2010; 126(3):1075–1085
2. Nahai F, ed. The Art of Aesthetic Surgery: Principles and Techniques. 2nd ed. St Louis, MO: Quality Medical Publishing; 2011
3. Hurwitz DJ, Golla D. Breast reshaping after massive weight loss. Semin Plast Surg 2004;18(3):179–187
4. Söderman M, Ikander P, Boljanovic S, Gunnarsson GL, Sørensen JA, Thomsen JB. Utilizing the lateral excess for autologous augmentation in massive weight loss patients. Gland Surg 2019;8(Suppl 4):S271–S275
5. Song AY, Jean RD, Hurwitz DJ, Fernstrom MH, Scott JA, Rubin JP. A classification of contour deformities after bariatric weight loss: the Pittsburgh Rating Scale. Plast Reconstr Surg 2005;116(5):1535–1544, discussion 1545–1546
6. Swanson E. A critical appraisal of breast autoaugmentation in post-bariatric surgery patients. Aesthet Surg J 2020; 40(7):NP429–NP432

THIGH CONTOURING SURGERY AFTER MASSIVE WEIGHT LOSS

13. When considering the thighs in a massive weight loss patient, which one of the following is true?

A. The lateral thighs should be treated before the medial thighs.

There are some key principles to consider when addressing the massive-weight-loss patient, particularly with regard to the order of procedures. Before treating the medial thigh, the lateral thigh, waist, and hips should be treated first and this would normally involve a lower body lift. This procedure can target multiple areas including the lower abdomen, flanks, lower back, pubic area, lateral thighs, hips, and buttocks. It may be that treating these areas initially will avoid the need for any subsequent surgical treatment to the medial thigh area.

Where treatment is required, the most likely skin excess will be in the horizontal plane (not the vertical); so, a vertical skin pattern resection would be indicated. Liposuction is safe to incorporate into the procedure and actually has become a preferred integral component when using a skin avulsion technique. This involves aggressive liposuction to the area of skin on the medial thigh which is to be excised. Once left with only dermis, the area is incised peripherally and avulsed from the underlying soft tissues. The rationale for this is a reduction in damage to the underlying nerves, blood vessels, and lymphatic channels. Because the skin resection is performed vertically, there is no requirement to lift and support the superficial tissues to Colles' fascia as part of this procedure.

A medial thigh lift is contraindicated in patients with preexisting lymphedema and may actually exacerbate this. Although liposuction is a recognized treatment modality for lymphedema, long-term compression garments would be required following this. The avulsion technique is intended to minimize risk for patients of developing lymphedema.[1-5]

REFERENCES

1. Aly AS, Cram AE, Heddens C. Truncal body contouring surgery in the massive weight loss patient. Clin Plast Surg 2004;31(4):611–624, vii
2. Aly AS. Body Contouring After Massive Weight Loss. St Louis, MO: Quality Medical Publishing; 2006
3. Mathes DW, Kenkel JM. Current concepts in medial thighplasty. Clin Plast Surg 2008;35(1):151–163
4. Capella JF, Matarasso A. Management of the postbariatric medial thigh deformity. Plast Reconstr Surg 2016;137(5): 1434–1446
5. Hunstad JP, Kortesis BG, Knotts CD. Avulsion thighplasty: technique overview and 6-year experience. Plast Reconstr Surg 2016;137(1):84–87

COMPLICATIONS AFTER MASSIVE-WEIGHT-LOSS SURGERY

14. You are discussing the risks of surgery with a patient who has reduced their BMI from 40 to 30 after bariatric surgery. Which one of the following complications is most common after major body contouring surgery?

E. Wound dehiscence

There are a number of common complications that can occur in patients undergoing body contouring following massive-weight-loss surgery and many of these relate to the wounds themselves. The most common complication of those listed is wound dehiscence (22–30%), and this may be due to excess tension across the wounds, the extent of the wounds, or an underlying nutritional deficiency. Most of the time, this is self-limiting and wounds will heal with prolonged wound care. Other complications include wound infection (1–7%) and skin necrosis (6–10%). These will obviously contribute to wound dehiscence. Patients are also at risk of venous thromboembolism (1%) and this is affected by BMI and procedure type. Prophylaxis is generally recommended with low-molecular-weight heparin shortly after surgery and continued for 7 days, although a more precise individualized risk can be calculated using the Caprini score to guide chemoprophylaxis requirements. Calf-compression garments should be used intraoperatively and thrombo-embolic deterrent hose postoperatively. Hematomas occur in 1 to 5% of cases following body contouring surgery and are most often seen in the early phase. The other common complication is seroma and the range for these varies from 13 to 37% according to procedure and series reviewed. The risk tends to be higher with increased BMI. Drains are used intraoperatively to help minimize seroma development and where they do develop, early aspiration is advocated before capsule formation occurs.[1-6]

REFERENCES

1. Aly AS. Body Contouring After Massive Weight Loss. St Louis, MO: Quality Medical Publishing; 2006
2. Rubin JP, Nguyen V, Schwentker A. Perioperative management of the post-gastric-bypass patient presenting for body contour surgery. Clin Plast Surg 2004;31(4):601–610, vi Med
3. Taylor J, Shermak M. Body contouring following massive weight loss. Obes Surg 2004;14(8):1080–1085
4. Michaels J V, Coon D, Rubin JP. Complications in postbariatric body contouring: postoperative management and treatment. Plast Reconstr Surg 2011;127(4):1693–1700
5. Zomerlei T, Janis JE. Liposuction, abdominoplasty and belt lipectomy. In: Chung KC, ed. Grabb and Smith's Plastic Surgery 8th ed. Philadelphia, PA: Wolters Kluwer; 2019:632–642
6. Janis JE, Khansa L, Khansa I. Strategies for postoperative seroma prevention: a systematic review. Plast Reconstr Surg 2016;138(1):240–252

123. Buttock Augmentation

See *Essentials of Plastic Surgery*, third edition, pp. 1735–1746

ANATOMY OF THE BUTTOCKS

1. *When considering the anatomy of the buttocks, which one of the following is true?*
   A The buttocks extend from the sacrum superiorly to the infragluteal fold inferiorly.
   B. The piriformis muscle divides the gluteal muscles into deep, intermediate, and superficial subdivisions.
   C. The posterior-superior ischial spine, greater trochanter, and coccyx help delineate piriformis surface anatomy.
   D. The buttock skin and underlying musculature are primarily supplied by the superior gluteal artery and vein.
   E. The buttock skin and underlying musculature are primarily supplied by the sciatic nerve and its subdivisions.

NERVE ANATOMY OF THE BUTTOCK

2. *Which one of the following structures passes through the greater sciatic foramen above the piriformis muscle?*
   A. Sciatic nerve
   B. Pudendal nerve
   C. Obturator nerve
   D. Superior gluteal nerve
   E. Inferior gluteal nerve

AESTHETICS OF THE FEMALE BUTTOCK

3. *When considering aesthetics of the female buttock, which one of the following is true?*
   A. The buttock is traditionally subdivided into three key anatomic subunits for analysis.
   B. A **V**-shaped buttock is generally thought to represent the "ideal" buttock shape.
   C. The top of the natal cleft normally represents the superior boundary of the buttock.
   D. A waist-to-hip ratio of 0.7 in both posterior and lateral views is generally preferred.
   E. Visible supragluteal fossettes represent a good indication for buttock surgery.

IMPLANT-BASED BUTTOCK AUGMENTATION

4. You see a slim patient in clinic who is considering buttock enhancement with an implant-based approach. She has a neat round buttock which is mildly flattened and underfilled especially more laterally. She wishes to enhance the natural shape of her buttock by adding additional volume medially and laterally. *Which one of the following is true in this case?*
   A. An oval silicone buttock implant should ideally be used.
   B. A silicone gel–filled implant should be used to comply with Food and Drug Administration (FDA) guidance.
   C. The patient may be disappointed with the effect on her lateral buttock area.
   D. A single midline incision should be used to minimize wound-healing complications.
   E. The implant should ideally be placed in the subcutaneous tissue plane.

GLUTEAL FAT GRAFT AUGMENTATION

5. *Which one of the following is true of fat augmentation for buttock enhancement?*
   A. It is ideally combined with liposuction exceeding that required for harvest.
   B. It should ideally be reserved for patients with a BMI between 30 and 40.
   C. It fails to address lateral buttock emptiness consistently well.
   D. Overfilling during grafting is associated with an increased graft take.
   E. Expansion vibration lipofilling should be reserved for low-volume fat transfers.

INTRAMUSCULAR MIGRATION THEORY

6. You are attending a conference session on aesthetic buttock surgery and hear colleagues talking about intramuscular migration theory. *How does this relate to buttock augmentation?*
   A. It explains how fat is able to generate a new blood supply after reinjection.
   B. It explains why fat resorbs unpredictably following fat injection.
   C. It explains why fat embolism occurs even when intramuscular injection is avoided.
   D. It explains why muscles hypertrophy after fat injection creating additional volume.
   E. It explains why a single injection site can consistently fill the entire buttock.

PRACTICALITIES OF PERFORMING BUTTOCK AUGMENTATION WITH FAT

7. *What is the most important technical point on performing gluteal fat injections?*
   A. To ensure that no more than 300 mL of fat is injected per side.
   B. To ensure that fat is only injected in a retrograde fashion.
   C. To ensure that fat is placed only within the subcutaneous tissues.
   D. To ensure that a standardized protocol for fat processing is used.
   E. To ensure the patient does not sit or lay supine for 72 hours afterward.

CONSENTING PATIENTS FOR FAT GRAFTING TO THE BUTTOCKS

8. *When discussing fat grafting to the buttocks with a patient preoperatively, what is the most commonly occurring complication to discuss with them?*
   A. Fat necrosis
   B. Venous thromboembolism
   C. Seroma development
   D. Lower limb paralysis
   E. Death

FLAP-BASED BUTTOCK AUTOAUGMENTATION

9. *In which patient group would flap-based buttock reconstruction usually be best indicated?*
   A. Following pregnancy
   B. Following massive weight loss
   C. In patients with BMI less than 30
   D. In diabetic patients who cannot have fat injections
   E. In male patients

NONSURGICAL BUTTOCK AUGMENTATION

10. A patient presents to your clinic to discuss their options for gluteal enhancement with a synthetic filler. *What would be the main caveat of selecting this technique?*
    A. That the initial procedure is poorly tolerated by patients.
    B. That the volume and cost of the product required would be prohibitive.
    C. That good short- to medium-term outcomes have not been clearly demonstrated.
    D. That the associated complication risk is unacceptably high.
    E. That the results are maintained only for 3 to 6 months.

Answers

ANATOMY OF THE BUTTOCKS

1. *When considering the anatomy of the buttocks, which one of the following is true?*

   C. The posterior-superior ischial spine, greater trochanter, and coccyx help delineate piriformis surface anatomy.

   The piriformis muscle is landmarked by drawing a line connecting the posterior-superior ischial spine (PSIS) and the coccyx. Piriformis courses from the midpoint of this line to the greater trochanter in a transverse/oblique direction. The clinical relevance of piriformis is that it passes through and divides the greater sciatic foramen transversely and provides a useful clinical landmark for key neurovascular structures within the buttock region such as the superior and inferior gluteal vessels. These lie superior and inferior to the muscle, respectively.

   The buttock extends from the posterior iliac crest superiorly to the infragluteal fold inferiorly. It comprises of a number of layers from superficial to deep. These are the skin, subcutaneous fat, Scarpa's fascia, deep muscle fascia, superficial and deep muscles, periosteum, and bone. The subcutaneous fat, as in other places has multiple layers with superficial, intermediate, and deep components. The muscles of the buttock may be divided into superficial and deep; those within the superficial layer are the gluteus maximus, medius and minimus, as well as the tensor fascia lata. Those in the deep layer are the piriformis, obturator externus, gemelli, and quadratus femoris. The gluteal muscles form the bulk of the buttock volume and shape. The underlying bony structures provide supporting framework for this and are formed by the ilium, ischium, sacrum, and coccyx. The buttocks receive blood supply primarily from the superior and inferior gluteal vessels. Innervation of the buttock musculature mainly arises from the superior and inferior gluteal nerves as well as the nerve to piriformis, obturator nerve and nerve to obturator internus. Skin sensation to the buttocks is provided by perforating cutaneous cluneal nerves from the posterior branches of T12–TS3.[1-3]

REFERENCES

1. Moore KL, Dalley AF, eds. Clinically Oriented Anatomy. 4th ed. New York, NY: Lippincott, Williams, and Wilkins; 1999
2. Nahai F, ed. The Art of Aesthetic Surgery: Principles and Techniques. 2nd ed. St Louis, MO: Quality Medical Publishing; 2011
3. Da Rocha RP. Surgical anatomy of the gluteal region's subcutaneous screen and its use in plastic surgery. Aesthetic Plast Surg 2001;25(2):140–144

NERVE ANATOMY OF THE BUTTOCK

2. *Which one of the following structures passes through the greater sciatic foramen above the piriformis muscle?*

   D. Superior gluteal nerve

   The greater sciatic foramen is an opening in the pelvis through which pass a number of key neurovascular structures. The greater sciatic foramen is formed by the sacroiliac, sacrotuberous, and sacrospinous ligaments along with the greater sciatic notch and ischial spine. The nerves which exit the pelvis through this foramen include the inferior gluteal, pudendal, sciatic, posterior femoral cutaneous, nerve to obturator internus, and nerve to quadratus femoris. However, these all pass below the level of piriformis and the only nerve passing above this muscle is the superior gluteal nerve. The superior gluteal nerve (L4–S1) is a motor-only nerve that innervates gluteus medius, gluteus minimus, and tensor fascia lata, but does not supply gluteus maximus. It travels with the superior gluteal vessels. The inferior gluteal nerve (L5–S2) supplies the gluteus maximus and the hip capsule. It travels with the inferior gluteal vessels. The sciatic nerve (L4–S3) supplies the hamstring muscles in the thigh. It then divides at the knee to form the common peroneal and tibial nerves which supply both motor and sensory innervation to the leg. The pudendal nerve (S2–S4) is the main nerve of the perineum. It innervates the external

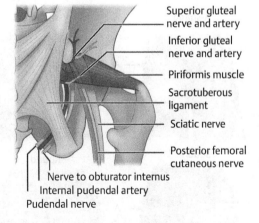

Superior gluteal nerve and artery

Inferior gluteal nerve and artery

Piriformis muscle

Sacrotuberous ligament

Sciatic nerve

Posterior femoral cutaneous nerve

Nerve to obturator internus
Internal pudendal artery
Pudendal nerve

Fig. 123.1 Nerve anatomy in relation to piriformis muscle.

genitalia and skin around the anus and perineum. It also innervates some of the pelvic muscles and urethral and anal sphincters. It runs with the internal pudendal artery and vein. The obturator nerve (L2–L4) innervates the adductor muscles of the medial thigh including obturator externus, adductor longus, brevis and magnus, as well as gracilis. It also provides sensory innervation to the skin of the medial thigh. It does not pass through the greater sciatic foramen. In contrast, the nerve to obturator internus (L5–S2) does and this supplies the obturator internus and superior gemelli (**Fig. 123.1**).[1–3]

REFERENCES

1. Moore KL, Dalley AF, eds. Clinically Oriented Anatomy. 4th ed. New York, NY: Lippincott, Williams, and Wilkins; 1999
2. Nahai F, ed. The Art of Aesthetic Surgery. Principles and Techniques. 2nd ed. Thieme; 2010
3. Cohen M, Thaller S, eds. The Unfavorable Result in Plastic Surgery: Avoidance and Treatment. 4th ed. Thieme; 2018

AESTHETICS OF THE FEMALE BUTTOCK

3. *When considering aesthetics of the female buttock, which one of the following is true?*
   D. **A waist-to-hip ratio of 0.7 in both posterior and lateral views is generally preferred.**
   A waist-to-hip ratio of 0.7 in both lateral and posterior views is regarded as the ideal in female gluteal aesthetics. Other elements in the ideal gluteal shape include a short infragluteal fold, a lumbar curvature of 45 degrees, visible supragluteal dimples, hollowing of the presacral "V," and a smooth skin envelope. Buttock shape is defined by the underlying framework, including the bony skeleton, the gluteal muscles, subcutaneous tissue distribution, and the overlying skin characteristics. Buttock shape should be assessed in both the posterior and lateral views. In the posterior view, buttock shape can be classified based on the dimensions of upper lateral hip ("point A"), the lateral thigh ("point B"), and the lateral mid-buttock ("point C"). There are four common buttock shapes when considering this assessment method (**Fig. 123.2**).
   * **A-shape ("pear-shaped," 30%):** Outward slope from point A to point B
   * **V-shape ("apple-shaped," 15%):** Inward slope from point A to point B
   * **Square** (40%): Equal volumes at point A and point B
   * **Round (15%):** Excess fullness at point C creates a gentle curve between points A and B

An **A**-shape buttock would be most in keeping with the ideal contour, especially in females. In males, a square variant may be preferred. The buttock extends from the iliac crest superiorly to the infragluteal fold inferiorly and extends laterally to the trochanteric depression of the lateral thighs. The superior border also coincides with the top of the gluteal muscles but not the natal cleft which normally lies lower than this. The posterior buttock region can be further divided into seven (not three) aesthetic subunits. These are the presacral, flank, lower back, gluteal, upper lateral buttock, midlateral buttock, and lower lateral buttock. As visible supragluteal fossettes represent a feature of the ideal buttock, their presence would not represent a good indication for buttock surgery (**Fig. 123.3**).[1–6]

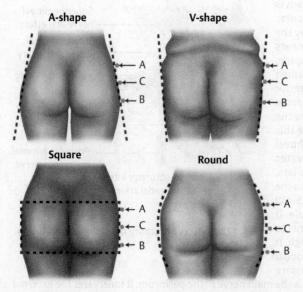

Fig. 123.2   The four different buttock shapes. **A-shape ("pear-shaped," 30%):** Outward slope from point A to point B. **V-shape ("apple-shaped," 15%):** Inward slope from point A to point B. **Square** (40%): Equal volumes at point A and point B. **Round (15%):** Excess fullness at point C creates a gentle curve between points A and B.

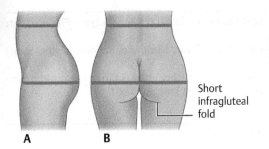

Fig. 123.3 (A, B) Characteristics of ideal female buttock shape. Note the waist-to-hip ratio of 0.7 in both the posterior and lateral views.

Short infragluteal fold

A   B

REFERENCES

1. Mendieta CG, Sood A. Classification system for gluteal evaluation: revisited. Clin Plast Surg 2018;45(2):159–177
2. Mendieta CG. Gluteal reshaping. Aesthet Surg J 2007;27(6):641–655
3. Heidekrueger PI, Sinno S, Tanna N, et al. The ideal buttock size: a sociodemographic morphometric evaluation. Plast Reconstr Surg 2017;140(1):20e–32e
4. Wong WW, Motakef S, Lin Y, Gupta SC. Redefining the ideal buttocks: a population analysis. Plast Reconstr Surg 2016;137(6):1739–1747
5. Singh D. Body shape and women's attractiveness: the critical role of waist-to-hip ratio. Hum Nat 1993;4(3):297–321
6. Cuenca-Guerra R, Quezada J. What makes buttocks beautiful? A review and classification of the determinants of gluteal beauty and the surgical techniques to achieve them. Aesthetic Plast Surg 2004;28(5):340–347

IMPLANT-BASED BUTTOCK AUGMENTATION

4. You see a slim patient in clinic who is considering buttock enhancement with an implant-based approach. She has a neat round buttock which is mildly flattened and underfilled especially more laterally. She wishes to enhance the natural shape of her buttock by adding additional volume medially and laterally. *Which one of the following is true in this case?*
   C. The patient may be disappointed with the effect on her lateral buttock area.
   Gluteal implants can be used to restore volume and projection to the medial two-thirds of the buttock with a similar concept to breast augmentation. It is a useful technique to adopt in patients with insufficient fat for autologous fat graft augmentation who are prepared to accept the long-term implications of implants and the access scars created. However, this patient is likely to be disappointed as the implants will not improve her lateral buttock emptiness.
   To address the lateral deficiency, buttock implants can be combined with gluteal fat grafting as a hybrid augmentation in some patients. This can provide predictable volume augmentation of the medial two-thirds of the buttock (implant) with correction of the lateral one-third and the waist-to-hip ratio (liposuction and fat grafting).[1] However given this woman is slim, this may not be a feasible option. The limitations of using implants alone must be explained preoperatively to set realistic expectations, otherwise with this patient's remit there will be disappointment. Patient selection is important when considering implant-based buttock augmentation and patients must have a stable weight, sufficient soft tissue to accommodate a gluteal implant, and realistic expectations.
   Buttock implants are either round or oval. A round implant would probably suit this patient best as she has a short, rounded buttock. Oval implants are better suited to patients with taller buttocks, but as with anatomic breast implants, malrotation can be a problem. Buttock implants can be gel filled with silicone shells as per current breast implants, or solid silicone devices. At present, only soft-solid silicone implants are FDA-approved for buttock augmentation in the United States. Silicone gel implants are widely used elsewhere, for example, in Central and South America. Implants are available with smooth or textured external surfaces. Buttock implants may be placed through a single midline incision, or two separate parasacral incisions placed within the gluteal cleft. Separate incisions reduce tension across the wound and so may reduce the risk of wound dehiscence. Buttock implants can be placed subcutaneously, subfascially, intramuscularly, or submuscularly (between gluteus maximus and medius). However, subcutaneous or submuscular placement is no longer recommended due to high complications rates. Intramuscular placement gives low implant visibility and palpability, so may be well suited to this patient. However, it is a more challenging pocket dissection and risks sciatic nerve injury. In contrast, subfascial placement provides an easier plane of dissection and can help projection, especially in the lower pole. However, it may be more palpable and visible; so, it would be less preferable in this slim patient.[1–3]

REFERENCES

1. Aslani A, Del Vecchio DA. Composite buttock augmentation: the next frontier in gluteal aesthetic surgery. Plast Reconstr Surg 2019;144(6):1312–1321
2. Senderoff DM. Aesthetic surgery of the buttocks using implants: practice-based recommendations. Aesthet Surg J 2016;36(5):559–576
3. Mofid MM, Gonzalez R, de la Peña JA, Mendieta CG, Senderoff DM, Jorjani S. Buttock augmentation with silicone implants: a multicenter survey review of 2226 patients. Plast Reconstr Surg 2013;131(4):897–901

GLUTEAL FAT GRAFT AUGMENTATION

5. *Which one of the following is true of fat augmentation for buttock enhancement?*
   A. It is ideally combined with liposuction exceeding that required for harvest.

   Gluteal fat grafting (a.k.a. Brazilian buttock lift) allows for volume augmentation and reshaping of the buttock. It is obviously combined with liposuction for fat harvest, but enhancement of shape can be more dramatic when additional targeted liposuction to the waist, lower back, and flanks is performed. This can help narrow down the waist and improve the waist-to-hip ratio. Fat grafting provides superior precision for buttock reshaping than implant-based augmentation alone and is particularly useful for the lateral one-third that cannot be addressed with implant-based augmentation. It is an ideal technique for patients with mild to moderate lipodystrophy. Patients with minimal excess body fat (body mass index [BMI] < 20) and obese patients (BMI > 30) are not ideal candidates for gluteal fat graft augmentation. Graft volume maintenance in gluteal fat grafting depends on the ability of the fat to revascularize within the recipient bed. The amount of fat that the recipient site can tolerate depends on soft-tissue compliance and characteristics including vascularity. Significant overfilling of the recipient site increases pressure and reduces oxygen diffusion capabilities, which can decrease percentage volume maintenance. Therefore, is should be avoided.[1] Expansion vibration lipofilling is a technique that allows for large volume fat grafting by expanding the recipient bed while simultaneously back-filling the recipient site.[2]

REFERENCES

1. Del Vecchio DA, Del Vecchio SJ. The graft-to-capacity ratio: volumetric planning in large-volume fat transplantation. Plast Reconstr Surg 2014;133(3):561–569
2. Del Vecchio D, Wall S Jr. Expansion vibration lipofilling: a new technique in large-volume fat transplantation. Plast Reconstr Surg 2018;141(5):639e–649e

INTRAMUSCULAR MIGRATION THEORY

6. You are attending a conference session on aesthetic buttock surgery and hear colleagues talking about intramuscular migration theory. *How does this relate to buttock augmentation?*
   C. It explains why fat embolism occurs even when intramuscular injection is avoided.

   In recent years, there has been a major focus on the risks of developing a life-threatening pulmonary fat embolism (PFE) during or following fat augmentation to the buttocks. This is a situation where macroembolism of fat into the venous circulation occurs, such that fat globules are transported to the heart and lungs, causing obstructive cardiopulmonary dysfunction.[1] PFE in gluteal fat grafting (macroembolism) is a different clinical entity to fat embolism syndrome (microembolism) and the signs and symptoms differ greatly.

   Traditionally, PFE was attributed to direct cannulation of gluteal vessels during fat injection. However, PFE has been observed in cases where deep intramuscular injection was not reported. Given this fact, the "Deep intramuscular migration" theory of PFE has been described.[2,3] In this theory, gluteus maximus muscle fascia acts as a barrier to prevent deep intramuscular migration of fat. However, when fat is injected deep to superficial gluteal fascia, it migrates along a path of least resistance, through gluteus maximus muscle fibers. A lack of deep fascia of the gluteus maximus muscle allows fat to collect in the submuscular space. Increased pressure in the submuscular space places traction on the gluteal veins. Traction-induced tears of the gluteal veins create a siphon effect, drawing fat into the venous circulation. Deep intramuscular migration theory explains how PFE might occur even in cases where no injections were performed in the deep intramuscular plane. The estimated risk of death in buttock fat transfer due to PFE is between 1 in 2,351 and 1 in 6,241.[4] Death is rapid in onset, typically occurring intraoperatively or < 24 hours postoperatively.

   There does not seem to be an association with PFE and the volume of fat injected. However, gluteal fat grafting is associated with the highest risk of mortality in aesthetic surgery; so, care must be taken when considering whether to perform this surgery and make steps to minimize risk of PFE occurring.[4–7]

REFERENCES

1. Cárdenas-Camarena L, Bayter JE, Aguirre-Serrano H, Cuenca-Pardo J. Deaths caused by gluteal lipoinjection: what are we doing wrong? Plast Reconstr Surg 2015;136(1):58–66
2. Del Vecchio DA, Villanueva NL, Mohan R, et al. Clinical implications of gluteal fat graft migration - a dynamic anatomic study. Plast Reconstr Surg 2018;142(5):1180–1192
3. Wall S Jr, Delvecchio D, Teitelbaum S, et al. Subcutaneous migration: a dynamic anatomical study of gluteal fat grafting. Plast Reconstr Surg 2019;143(5):1343–1351
4. Mofid MM, Teitelbaum S, Suissa D, et al. Report on mortality from gluteal fat grafting: recommendations from the ASERF Task Force. Aesthet Surg J 2017;37(7):796–806
5. Mills DC II, Rubin JP, Saltz R. Urgent warning to surgeons performing fat grafting to the buttocks (Brazilian butt lift or "BBL"). Aesthetic Society News 2018;22(4):1, 7
6. Thorne C, Matarasso A, Richter D, Coleman S, Magalon G. (June 11, 2019). Gluteal fat grafting safety advisory. Available at: https://www.surgery.org/sites/default/files/Gluteal-Fat-Grafting-Safety-Advisory_0.pdf. Accessed June 10, 2021
7. Alvarez-Alvarez FA, González-Gutiérrez HO, Ploneda-Valencia CF. Safe gluteal fat graft avoiding a vascular or nervous injury: an anatomical study in cadavers. Aesthet Surg J 2019;39(2):174–184

PRACTICALITIES OF PERFORMING BUTTOCK AUGMENTATION WITH FAT

7. *What is the most important technical point on performing gluteal fat injections?*

C. **To ensure that fat is placed only within the subcutaneous tissues.**

When injecting fat into the buttock, placement must always be superficial to the gluteal muscles and muscle fascia. This is because deeper injections have been associated with fatal fat embolic events. Intraoperative measures to reduce the risk of this occurring commence with the surgeon having awareness of this eventuality and ensuring they have maintained an up-to-date knowledge of the buttock soft tissue and vascular anatomy. At all times, the operator should know exactly where the cannula tip is located in terms of depth and advancement and this can be achieved by palpation, proprioceptive feedback, visualization, and maintaining a three-dimensional awareness. Further measures to reduce risk include using a single-hole injection cannula at least 4 mm diameter, avoiding downward angulation of the cannula and positioning the patient in such a way to limit deep injection. Fat may be injected antegrade or retrograde, but the key point is to only inject while in motion so that large deliveries of fat to a single spot are avoided. There is no specific limit to the amount of fat that can be safely injected per side during buttock augmentation. However, common sense should prevail and volumes adjusted on a case-by-case basis. A good indicator of reaching the maximum fill is where there is a loss of resistance during injection and fat begins to drain from the injection-site incision. There is no standardized protocol for fat preparation and there are a number of accepted ways of doing this such as centrifugation, washing, sieving, and custom-made devices which filter the fat automatically. Postoperatively patients must be advised to refrain from sitting or lying supine for at least 2 weeks to avoid causing compression and ischemia to the transferred fat.[1-5]

REFERENCES

1. Wall S Jr, Delvecchio D, Teitelbaum S, et al. Subcutaneous migration: a dynamic anatomical study of gluteal fat grafting. Plast Reconstr Surg 2019;143(5):1343–1351
2. Mills DC II, Rubin JP, Saltz R. Urgent warning to surgeons performing fat grafting to the buttocks (Brazilian butt lift or "BBL"). Aesthetic Society News 2018;22(4):1, 7
3. Thorne C, Matarasso A, Richter D, Coleman S, Magalon G. (June 11, 2019). Gluteal fat grafting safety advisory. Available at: https://www.surgery.org/sites/default/files/Gluteal-Fat-Grafting-Safety-Advisory_0.pdf. Accessed June 10, 2021
4. Alvarez-Alvarez FA, González-Gutiérrez HO, Ploneda-Valencia CF. Safe gluteal fat graft avoiding a vascular or nervous injury: an anatomical study in cadavers. Aesthet Surg J 2019;39(2):174–184
5. Ordenana C, Dallapozza E, Said S, Zins JE. Objectifying the risk of vascular complications in gluteal augmentation with fat grafting: a latex casted cadaveric study. Aesthet Surg J 2020;40(4):402–409

CONSENTING PATIENTS FOR FAT GRAFTING TO THE BUTTOCKS

8. *When discussing fat grafting to the buttocks with a patient preoperatively, what is the most commonly occurring complication to discuss with them?*

C. Seroma development

There are a number of potential complications that must be discussed with patients prior to undergoing fat grafting to the buttock area. The most commonly recorded complication is seroma formation and this occurs in around 2.5 to 3.5% of cases. It is usually self-limiting unless it becomes complicated by infection. Fat necrosis is a complication that one may expect to be common after this procedure, yet this seems to occur in less than 1% of cases. It may be that fat necrosis occurs much more commonly, but at a subclinical level, and so goes unnoticed. Venous thromboembolism occurs in less than 1% of cases. This can be minimized with chemoprophylaxis and calf compression devices/TED hose. As with all aesthetic procedures, realistic expectations must be in place and an acceptance that there will be only modest improvements as well as asymmetry and imperfections. Under-correction and infection each occur in around 2% of cases; pain and or sciatic nerve problems occur in less than 2% of cases. It would be extremely unlikely (though not impossible) that a significant neuropraxia affecting lower limb function could occur. Contour irregularities and asymmetry occur in less than 1% of cases, which again seems lower than might be expected. Death can occur following fat augmentation to the buttocks. The estimated risk of this is 1 in 2,351 to 6,241, which is, of course, extremely high for an elective cosmetic procedure. The cause of this high risk is fatal fat embolism. Patients must be counseled on this risk and the evidence, which supports it.[1-7]

REFERENCES

1. Condé-Green A, Kotamarti V, Nini KT, et al. Fat grafting for gluteal augmentation: a systematic review of the literature and meta-analysis. Plast Reconstr Surg 2016;138(3):437e–446e
2. Sinno S, Chang JB, Brownstone ND, Saadeh PB, Wall S Jr. Determining the safety and efficacy of gluteal augmentation: a systematic review of outcomes and complications. Plast Reconstr Surg 2016;137(4):1151–1156
3. Oranges CM, Tremp M, di Summa PG, et al. Gluteal augmentation techniques: a comprehensive literature review. Aesthet Surg J 2017;37(5):560–569
4. Vasilakis V, Hamade M, Stavrides SA, Davenport TA. Bilateral sciatic neuropathy following gluteal augmentation with autologous fat grafting. Plast Reconstr Surg Glob Open 2018;6(3):e1696
5. Mofid MM, Teitelbaum S, Suissa D, et al. Report on mortality from gluteal fat grafting: recommendations from the ASERF task force. Aesthet Surg J 2017;37(7):796–806
6. Cárdenas-Camarena L, Bayter JE, Aguirre-Serrano H, Cuenca-Pardo J. Deaths caused by gluteal lipoinjection: what are we doing wrong? Plast Reconstr Surg 2015;136(1):58–66
7. Mofid MM, Teitelbaum S, Suissa D, et al. Report on mortality from gluteal fat grafting: recommendations from the ASERF task force. Aesthet Surg J 2017;37(7):796–806

FLAP-BASED BUTTOCK AUTOAUGMENTATION

9. *In which patient group would flap-based buttock reconstruction usually be best indicated?*

B. Following massive weight loss

Following massive weight loss, patients are often left with significant buttock ptosis, deflation, and a lack of buttock projection. To a degree, traditional techniques such as a circumferential body lift will improve the buttock area, but may still leave flattening and further loss of projection.[1] Therefore, in this patient cohort, local autoaugmentation flaps may be useful to restore gluteal volume and projection. These would normally be performed at the same time as the body lift itself and are based on similar principles to those used to revolumize the breast in this same patient group, where medial and lateral flaps are transposed more centrally to revolumize the middle part of the breast. Examples of local flaps described for gluteal autoaugmentation include dermal fat flaps, superior gluteal artery perforator flaps, split gluteal muscle flaps, and purse string gluteoplasty.[2-5] Gluteal autoaugmentation does not significantly influence complication rates in circumferential lower body contouring, although wound dehiscence is the most common complication associated with these procedures. Following pregnancy, most patients with residual soft-tissue excess would tend to have this located in the central lower abdomen rather than the buttock. Patients with a BMI of less than 30 tend to be deficient in soft tissue to augment with more generally. Diabetic patients are best discouraged from having aesthetic buttock surgery unless their glucose control is especially good. Female patients who have undergone massive weight loss may be good candidates for autoaugmentation, but not male patients, per se.

REFERENCES

1. Srivastava U, Rubin JP, Gusenoff JA. Lower body lift after massive weight loss: autoaugmentation versus no augmentation. Plast Reconstr Surg 2015;135(3):762–772
2. Colwell AS, Borud LJ. Autologous gluteal augmentation after massive weight loss: aesthetic analysis and role of the superior gluteal artery perforator flap. Plast Reconstr Surg 2007;119(1):345–356
3. Sozer SO, Agullo FJ, Palladino H. Split gluteal muscle flap for autoprosthesis buttock augmentation. Plast Reconstr Surg 2012;129(3):766–776
4. de Runz A, Brix M, Gisquet H, et al. Satisfaction and complications after lower body lift with autologous gluteal augmentation by island fat flap: 55 case series over 3 years. J Plast Reconstr Aesthet Surg 2015;68(3):410–418
5. Hunstad JP, Daniels MA, Crantford JC. Autologous flap gluteal augmentation: purse-string technique. Clin Plast Surg 2018;45(2):261–267

NONSURGICAL BUTTOCK AUGMENTATION

10. A patient presents to your clinic to discuss their options for gluteal enhancement with a synthetic filler. *What would be the main caveat of selecting this technique?*

  B. That the volume and cost of the product required would be prohibitive.

   Injection of soft-tissue fillers into the subcutaneous tissues of the buttock can be used to achieve temporary nonsurgical buttock augmentation. The two most likely products that would be used are stabilized hyaluronic acid (HA) gel such as Macrolane and poly-L-lactic acid such as Sculptra.[1]

   The main issue with this treatment is the volume that needs to be injected and the financial implications of doing this. Typically, in facial rejuvenation, products for injection such as HA are marketed in syringes of 2 mL. In order to achieve a meaningful volume enhancement in a buttock, 200 to 300 mL would normally be required, and the cost implication of doing so with current prices would be prohibitive. In addition, this is something that would need to be repeated on an annual basis thereby compounding the financial limitations of this technique. The other issue is that while it is accepted that small volumes can safely be injected into the face, which is well vascularized, should the product to native tissue ratio be changed dramatically, the risk of complications including infection, allergic reaction, or soft-tissue swelling could be markedly elevated. There has been one study which looked at the results of injecting large volumes of stabilized HA into the buttock. This prospective multicenter study involved 61 patients with a mean age of 41. Each patient had injection of HA to the subcutaneous area of the buttock with an average of 340 mL in total. They were then followed up for 2 years at regular intervals. The authors reported a low complication rate and high levels of patient satisfaction. Moreover, the results were maintained for more than 1 year in many cases.[1]

   Based on this study, it would seem that the concept may be reasonable as an alternative to other invasive procedures such as fat grafting or implants. However, this is not approved for such use by the FDA; so, it would be off label in the United States. The use of a permanent filler should be avoided, as this risks irreversible changes which may be unwanted. Permanent fillers are associated with a high risk of complications including infection, ulceration, granuloma formation, asymmetry, and permanent deformity of the buttocks.[2-6]

REFERENCES

1. Camenisch CC, Tengvar M, Hedén P. Macrolane for volume restoration and contouring of the buttocks: magnetic resonance imaging study on localization and degradation. Plast Reconstr Surg 2013;132(4):522e–529e
2. De Meyere B, Mir-Mir S, Peñas J, Camenisch CC, Hedén P. Stabilized hyaluronic acid gel for volume restoration and contouring of the buttocks: 24-month efficacy and safety. Aesthetic Plast Surg 2014;38(2):404–412
3. Singh M, Solomon IH, Calderwood MS, Talbot SG. Silicone-induced granuloma after buttock augmentation. Plast Reconstr Surg Glob Open 2016;4(2):e624
4. Nasseri E. Gluteal augmentation with liquid silicone of unknown purity causes granulomas in an adult female: case report and review of the literature. J Cutan Med Surg 2016;20(1):72–79
5. Blanco J, Gaines S, Arshad J, Sheele JM. Silicone pneumonitis, diffuse alveolar hemorrhage and acute respiratory distress syndrome from gluteal silicone injections. Am J Emerg Med 2018;36(12):2340.e3–2340.e4
6. Clark RF, Cantrell FL, Pacal A, Chen W, Betten DP. Subcutaneous silicone injection leading to multi-system organ failure. Clin Toxicol (Phila) 2008;46(9):834–837

124. Male Aesthetic Plastic Surgery

See *Essentials of Plastic Surgery*, third edition, pp. 1747–1761

AESTHETIC PROCEDURES IN MALE PATIENTS

1. There are gender differences in the uptake of aesthetic surgical and nonsurgical services. *According to ASPS and ASAPS, what proportion of all nonsurgical and surgical aesthetic procedures are undertaken on men?*
   A. Less than 10%
   B. 15 to 20%
   C. 25 to 30%
   D. 35 to 40%
   E. 45 to 50%

AESTHETIC PRINCIPLES IN THE MALE FACE

2. *When performing facial rejuvenation on a male patient, why should augmentation of the malar area be performed with caution?*
   A. To avoid wound healing problems
   B. To avoid motor nerve injury
   C. To avoid sensory nerve injury
   D. To avoid feminization of the central face
   E. To avoid problems with subsequent hair growth

COMPLICATIONS IN MALE FACELIFTING SURGERY

3. *Which one of the following complications tends to be higher in males undergoing facelift than in females undergoing the same procedure?*
   A. Venous thromboembolism (VTE)
   B. Fat necrosis
   C. Facial nerve injury
   D. Hematoma
   E. Seroma

"SIMON" IN RELATION TO AESTHETIC SURGERY

4. In relation to aesthetic surgery in the male patient, the term "SIMON" is sometimes used. *What is the main concern regarding a patient with such a label?*
   A. They will not comply with treatment.
   B. They do not require any surgery.
   C. They are likely to be dissatisfied with treatment.
   D. They are likely to develop complications.
   E. They are unlikely to accept revision surgery.

ANATOMICAL FEATURES OF THE MALE NOSE

5. *How does the male nose differ from that of the female nose?*
   A. The supratip break is more pronounced.
   B. The tip tends to be more rotated.
   C. The dorsal aesthetic lines are wider.
   D. The nasal tip tends to be more defined.
   E. The skin is thinner and more sebaceous.

AESTHETIC TREATMENTS IN THE MALE PATIENT

6. *Which one of the following is the most popular aesthetic nonsurgical procedure for male patients?*
   A. Neurotoxin injection
   B. Injectable fillers
   C. Laser hair removal
   D. Microdermabrasions
   E. Chemical peels

LOWER EYELID BLEPHAROPLASTY

7. *When performing a lower eyelid blepharoplasty in a 58-year-old male, which one of the following is normally the final step prior to closure when performing this procedure.*
   A. Skin excision
   B. Muscle excision
   C. Fat excision
   D. Canthoplasty
   E. Septal modification

HAIR TRANSPLANT IN MALE PATIENTS

8. *Which one of the following can cause a long-term problem when performing hair transplant in a young male patient?*
   A. Using follicular units
   B. Pretreating with platelet-rich plasma (PRP)
   C. Setting the anterior hairline low
   D. Post treating with minoxidil
   E. Omitting the posterior strip excision

HAIR TRANSPLANT COMPLICATIONS

9. About 2 weeks following hair transplant, a patient calls the office, worried as the hairs have been shedding. *Which one of the following is most likely to explain this?*
   A. Incorrect placement of the grafts
   B. Triangulation of the grafts
   C. Premature hair washing
   D. Omission of minoxidil treatment
   E. This is a normal and expected finding

NORMAL CHARACTERISTICS OF THE MALE CHEST WALL

10. *When considering the male chest wall, which one of the following characteristics would feminize its appearance?*
    A. A well-defined IMF
    B. A NAC 2 cm above the IMF
    C. An absent IMF
    D. A well-defined pectoralis major
    E. A NAC less than 2 cm diameter

Answers

AESTHETIC PROCEDURES IN MALE PATIENTS

1. There are gender differences in the uptake of aesthetic surgical and nonsurgical services. *According to ASPS and ASAPS, what proportion of all nonsurgical and surgical aesthetic procedures are undertaken on men?*

A. Less than 10%

Only around 9% of all aesthetic procedures are performed on males in the United States according to ASPS and ASAPS 2018 data.[1,2] However, the requirement for male aesthetic procedures is growing in numbers from year to year. Men seek nonsurgical procedures more commonly than they do surgical procedures and this is a particular area of market growth. The approach to the male patient is somewhat different to the female patient and must take into account general differences in structural anatomy of the face and body as well as the objectives set by males, which can differ greatly from those set by females. In general, men tend to want quick, simple procedures which have reliable, but subtle results and minimal downtime. They have a growing understanding of the availability of aesthetic procedures due to their promotion online and in the media. It is important to consider the requirements for male patients carefully. For surgeons interested in developing a practice in male aesthetics, there are many opportunities available depending on patient subgroup and procedure type they wish to offer, e.g., facial rejuvenation, breast surgery, and body contouring. Marketing style and web content should differ from clinics more focused on the female patient to ensure patients feel comfortable to seek treatments they require.[3]

REFERENCES

1. Available at: https://surgery.org/sites/default/files/ASAPS-Stats2018.pdf. Accessed June 10, 2021
2. Available at: https://www.plasticsurgery.org/documents/News/Statistics/2018/plastic-surgery-statistics-full-report-2018.pdf. Accessed June 10, 2021
3. Boxall M. Changing Faces: marketing to the male customer. Available at: https://aestheticsjournal.com/feature/changing-faces-marketing-to-the-male-customer. Accessed June 10, 2021

AESTHETIC PRINCIPLES IN THE MALE FACE

2. *When performing facial rejuvenation on a male patient, why should augmentation of the malar area be performed with caution?*

D. To avoid feminization of the central face

When performing aesthetic rejuvenation procedures on the male face, it is really important to avoid any intervention that will feminize facial appearance. In order to avoid this, it is vital that the practitioner has an understanding of the differences between male and female facial structure. The male face has less fullness in the malar region and the fullness in that area tends to sit lower (caudally) in the cheek. Overzealous augmentation in this area, with fillers such as fat or hyaluronic acid, or during facelift can lead to a more feminine appearance (**Fig. 124.1**).

Other areas that must be treated carefully to avoid causing feminization are the brow, which sits lower and more flat in males without the high arch seen in females, and the periorbital region which tends to have a longer upper lip which is thinner, deeper, and heavier nasolabial folds and a stronger, squarer chin.[1–4]

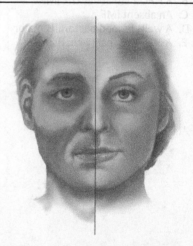

Fig. 124.1   Differences in the anatomy and characteristics of the male and female face.

REFERENCES

1. Steinbrech DS. Male Aesthetic Plastic Surgery. New York, NY: Thieme USA; 2020
2. de Maio M. Ethnic and gender considerations in the use of facial injectables: male patients. Plast Reconstr Surg 2015;136(5, Suppl):40S–43S
3. Keaney TC. Aging in the male face: Intrinsic and extrinsic factors. Dermatol Surg 2016;42(7):797–803
4. Jagdeo J, Keaney T, Narurkar V, Kolodziejczyk J, Gallagher CJ. Facial treatment preferences among aesthetically oriented men. Dermatol Surg 2016;42(10):1155–1163

COMPLICATIONS IN MALE FACELIFTING SURGERY

3. *Which one of the following complications tends to be higher in males undergoing facelift than in females undergoing the same procedure?*
   D. Hematoma

   Facelifting procedures can be very effective in male patients; however, their risk profile is different from that of females. Hematoma rates are higher for men and these range between 7 and 14%.[1,2] Reasons for this may include uncontrolled hypertension and increased vascularity of the tissues (due to hair-bearing skin) and may also reflect differences in postoperative behavior. In order to manage this, great care must be taken intraoperatively to ensure hemostasis is achieved. Normotensive anesthesia is recommended with smooth transition during wake up and recovery. Medications which are likely to increase bleeding must be avoided. Anticoagulant medication should be stopped 1 week prior to surgery, but antihypertensives should be continued perioperatively. Clonidine patches may be helpful to reduce fluctuations in blood pressure. Tranexamic acid may be used intraoperatively to help hemostasis. Vasoactive medications such as Viagra should be avoided for 4 weeks postsurgery, and patients must be advised to rest and avoid stooping, straining, and coughing in the early postoperative phase.

   In contrast to hematoma rate, there should be no significant difference in risk profile for venous thromboembolism (VTE), fat necrosis, facial nerve injury, or seroma development. To minimize VTE risk, thrombo-embolic deterrent hose should be prescribed as well as calf compression devices intraoperatively. Patients should normally receive low-molecular-weight heparin until fully mobile and remain well hydrated. A useful assessment tool to guide this is the Caprini score.[3]

REFERENCES

1. Rohrich RJ, Stuzin JM, Ramanadham S, Costa C, Dauwe PB. The modern male rhytidectomy: lessons learned. Plast Reconstr Surg 2017;139(2):295–307
2. Steinbrech DS. The male facelift. In: Aesthetic Plastic Surgery. Elsevier Health Sciences; 2009:155–167
3. Cronin M, Dengler N, Krauss ES, et al. Completion of the updated Caprini Risk Assessment Model (2013 version). Clin Appl Thromb Hemost 2019;25:1076029619838052

"SIMON" IN RELATION TO AESTHETIC SURGERY

4. In relation to aesthetic surgery in the male patient, the term "SIMON" is sometimes used. *What is the main concern regarding a patient with such a label?*
   C. They are likely to be dissatisfied with treatment.

   The term **"SIMON"** refers to a notional patient who has some specific traits and characteristics. These are as follows:
   • Single
   • Immature
   • Male
   • Obsessive
   • Narcissistic

   Clearly any individual may possess some or all of these characteristics, but when seen collectively in a patient they are a red flag for undergoing aesthetic procedures because they are likely to have unrealistic expectations, have more difficulty describing their objectives, and have selective hearing in terms of advice offered by the clinician. This can collectively lead to patient dissatisfaction with treatment. Undergoing aesthetic surgery in any individual can heighten focus on the body part or area treated, leading to obsessive behavior where individuals repeatedly analyze the results with a mirror and photographs multiple times each day. Photographs are often taken at a range of different unusual angles and with differing lighting settings, which do not represent the appearance of the area in everyday life. Patients will then have a tendency to compare images with those found online which may not be genuine, realistic, or comparable to their own images anyway.

   A patient with SIMON characteristics is highly likely to experience this type of behavior postsurgery and the situation should therefore be dodged by avoiding surgery in the first place. This is not to say that all male patients who are young and single should not undergo aesthetic surgery, but rather than the operator must take the responsibility to assess and evaluate the likelihood of such events occurring before they do so, based on their intuition in the office visit. For this reason, at least two consults prior to surgery is normally recommended to build appropriate rapport and make safe, sensible, and appropriate plans for patients.[1–3]

REFERENCES

1. Nahai F, ed. The Art of Aesthetic Surgery: Principles and Techniques. 2nd ed. St Louis, MO: Quality Medical Publishing; 2011

2. Bulstrode NW, Waterhouse N, Forrester P. Male aesthetic patients to avoid, SLAP-SIMON. Plast Reconstr Surg 2007;119(1):452
3. Adamson PA, Chen T. The dangerous dozen--avoiding potential problem patients in cosmetic surgery. Facial Plast Surg Clin North Am 2008;16(2):195–202, vii

ANATOMICAL FEATURES OF THE MALE NOSE

5. *How does the male nose differ from that of the female nose?*
   C. The dorsal aesthetic lines are wider.
   Understanding the differences between the male and female nose is important in rhinoplasty to ensure that male patients are not feminized and female patients are not masculinized. The key features of the male nose are that it is larger and longer, the dorsum is wider and straighter, there is no supratip break, and there is less tip rotation (with a reduced nasolabial angle of 90–95 degrees instead of 95–105 degrees). In addition, the nasal tip is broader and more bulbous and because the male skin is thicker, there are limitations in the ability to change its shape. The chin is also stronger and more prominent; so, the balance between the nose and chin is altered. The upper lip is usually taller and the lips are thinner in the male patient. The key aims of the male rhinoplasty should, in general terms, be to create a natural appearance and avoid feminization; preserve facial balance; avoid an excessively small, tweaked, upturned, or rounded nose; and avoid a nose that is too narrow, which will also lead to airway problems. In the lateral view, a straight dorsal line is generally preferred for the male patient (**Fig. 124.2**).[1-3]

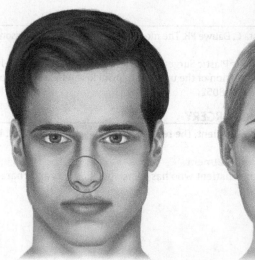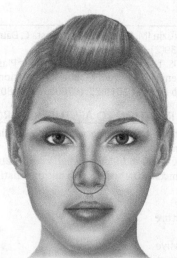

Fig. 124.2   Differences in the male and female nose.

REFERENCES

1. Rohrich RJ, Janis JE, Gunter JP. The male nose. In: Rohrich RJ, Adams WPA Jr., Ahmad J, Gunter JP, eds. Dallas Rhinoplasty: Nasal Surgery by the Masters. 3rd ed. St. Louis, MO: Quality Medical Publishing; 2014
2. Daniel RK. Rhinoplasty and the male patient. Clin Plast Surg 1991;18(4):751–761
3. Steinbrech DS. Male Aesthetic Plastic Surgery. New York, NY: Thieme; 2020

AESTHETIC TREATMENTS IN THE MALE PATIENT

6. *Which one of the following is the most popular aesthetic nonsurgical procedure for male patients?*
   A. Neurotoxin injection
   The most popular aesthetic nonsurgical procedure for males is neurotoxin therapy. This is frequently requested to improve the crow's feet area and the brow. Care must be taken to avoid over-treatment in males, as the glabellar region and brow can be feminized if excessive neurotoxin doses are used. The brow should remain flat in males rather than the high arch appearance seen in females. A subtle weakening of the mimetic muscles involved is preferable. Remembering to under-correct is always better than over-correcting as further injection top ups can be given, and considering reversal is not possible (unlike with hyaluronic acid injections). Males tend to have more powerful muscles especially in the brow and generally require larger doses to achieve the equivalent result

than females. For example, in the glabellar region, a starting dose for women is 20 to 30 units of Botox, where in men it is 30 to 40 units.

Other popular procedures for males include fillers, which may be commonly used to fill specific lines or furrows including the nasolabial folds, which tend to be deeper in males. Hair removal is another popular choice, although less so in the face. Sites such as the back and chest are more commonly targeted. Chemical peels and microdermabrasion are also popular for more general facial rejuvenation.[1-3]

REFERENCES

1. Sinno S, Lam G, Brownstone ND, Steinbrech DS. An assessment of gender differences in plastic surgery patient education and information in the United States: Are we neglecting our male patients? Aesthet Surg J 2016;36(1):107–110
2. Carruthers A, Carruthers J. Prospective, double-blind, randomized, parallel-group, dose-ranging study of botulinum toxin type A in men with glabellar rhytids. Dermatol Surg 2005;31(10):1297–1303
3. Scherer MA. Specific aspects of a combined approach to male face correction: botulinum toxin A and volumetric fillers. J Cosmet Dermatol 2016;15(4):566–574

LOWER EYELID BLEPHAROPLASTY

7. *When performing a lower eyelid blepharoplasty in a 58-year-old male, which one of the following is normally the final step prior to closure when performing this procedure.*

A. **Skin excision**

There are a number of key points to consider specific to the male blepharoplasty. The key goals of lower eyelid surgery are to remove any excess skin, fat, or muscle and improve the lid–cheek junction and tear trough areas, while ensuring that the lower eyelid remains well supported such that a natural shape is maintained and ectropion is avoided. Pitfalls that surgeons can run into include overly aggressive skin and or muscle resection without sufficient internal canthal support leading to poor results, and ongoing challenges in their subsequent correction. In order to avoid removing excess skin, this must be done conservatively in the lower eyelid, and AFTER the other components have been completed, including canthal suspension in the form of a canthoplasty or canthopexy where necessary. The difference between the two is that in a "pexy," the canthal tendon remains in continuity, where in a "plasty," it is divided and repaired during the tightening procedure. In general, skin removal in the lower eyelid should be no more than a few mm, in contrast to the upper lid where 10 to 15 mm may often be taken.

The approach to lower eyelid blepharoplasty may be with skin/orbicularis flap elevation to access the orbital septum and pre- and postseptal fat compartments. In this more invasive approach, many elements of the eyelid can be manipulated under direct vision. Alternatively, a pinch blepharoplasty approach may be preferred in younger patients who require only subtle changes and have good lower eyelid support. This is something that tends to be paired with procedures like a facelift where the malar tissues have been supported in a different manner.[1-3]

REFERENCES

1. Barrera JE, Most SP. Management of the lower lid in male blepharoplasty. Facial Plast Surg Clin North Am 2008;16(3):313–316, vi
2. Codner MA, Kikkawa DO, Korn BS, Pacella SJ. Blepharoplasty and brow lift. Plast Reconstr Surg 2010;126(1):1e–17e
3. Drolet BC, Sullivan PK. Evidence-based medicine: blepharoplasty. Plast Reconstr Surg 2014;133(5):1195–1205

HAIR TRANSPLANT IN MALE PATIENTS

8. *Which one of the following can cause a long-term problem when performing hair transplant in a young male patient?*

C. **Setting the anterior hairline low**

Hair transplant has advanced in recent years and the gold standard now is to use a follicular unit extraction technique with single follicles containing between one and four hairs each. As with all aesthetic procedures, it is vital to discuss things in detail with the patient beforehand, to ensure patients are well informed and have realistic expectations. Hair loss will continue to progress with time and patients must be aware of this. Of course, it is particularly true in younger patients undergoing hair transplant. Setting a hairline too low in these individuals must be avoided, as it will create problems in the future with an unnatural appearance. The hairline needs to look natural as the patient ages. Pretreatment with PRP or finasteride can be helpful in hair loss patients, as can posttreatment with minoxidil. The posterior strip excision is virtually obsolete and leaves a transverse scar in the posterior hair-bearing scalp.[1,2]

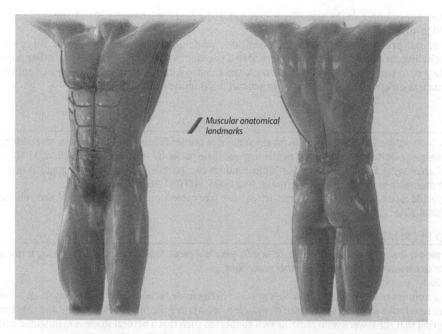

Fig. 124.3   Etching details for males undergoing abdominal liposuction.

REFERENCES

1. Unger W, Unger R, Shapiro R, et al, eds. Hair Transplantation. 5th ed. New York, NY: Thieme Medical Publishers; 2011
2. Rousso DE, Kim SW. A review of medical and surgical treatment options for androgenetic alopecia. JAMA Facial Plast Surg 2014;16(6):444–450

HAIR TRANSPLANT COMPLICATIONS

9. **About 2 weeks following hair transplant, a patient calls the office, worried as the hairs have been shedding. Which one of the following is most likely to explain this?**

   E. This is a normal and expected finding.

   Following hair transplant, it is normal for the transplanted hair to fall out at around 2 weeks. New hair growth begins around 12 weeks. It is vital to explain this to patients preoperatively and remind them postoperatively to avoid unnecessary anxiety as has occurred in this case. The usual posttreatment regimen includes oral antibiotics for a few days, and liposomal adenosine triphosphate (ATP) spray should be used every few hours throughout the day and a light covering used on the head for a few days. The ATP is thought to help graft growth by returning ATP levels to normal (ATP is presumed to be depleted because the hairs are deprived of blood and oxygen for a period of time), yet is important in hair growth. Normal washing may begin at day 5 and minoxidil or laser light therapy can begin around 3 weeks as adjunctive therapy. Usually 90% of follicles will grow. Intraoperatively, grafts should be placed snuggly and oriented with angulation flat in forward and lateral directions. Density of graft placement should increase moving posteriorly to help create a natural appearance. Triangulation involves random distribution of smaller and larger units.[1,2]

REFERENCES

1. Unger W, Unger R, Shapiro R, et al, eds. Hair Transplantation. 5th ed. New York, NY: Thieme Medical Publishers; 2011
2. Rousso DE, Kim SW. A review of medical and surgical treatment options for androgenetic alopecia. JAMA Facial Plast Surg 2014;16(6):444–450

NORMAL CHARACTERISTICS OF THE MALE CHEST WALL

10. **When considering the male chest wall, which one of the following characteristics would feminize its appearance?**

   A. A well-defined IMF

   Surgery for correction of gynecomastia (development of a female-shape breast in a male) is one of the most commonly performed aesthetic surgical procedures for males. Gynecomastia affects a large proportion of men at some point in their life, although most will not require surgery for it. Causes include certain medications, tumors, weight gain, and hormone imbalances. Gynecomastia can be glandular or fatty with or without excess skin and accompanying ptosis.

The male chest should ideally have the nipple areola complex (NAC) at least 1 to 2 cm above the inframammary fold (IMF) and it should normally be less than 2 cm in diameter. The IMF should be fairly indistinct with no breast ptosis. When it is well defined, this gives the breast a more feminine appearance. A larger IMF-to-NAC distance and a larger diameter NAC are both feminizing features of the breast. Upper and medial pectoralis major fullness is desirable in the male chest and any outer chest and axillary fullness should be corrected if surgery is performed, as this is less desirable.

Surgery should be aimed at resetting the chest to a male appearance with minimal tell-tale signs. If the consistency of the excess soft tissue is fatty, then liposuction is helpful, whereas if it is glandular, then formal surgical resection will be required. Skin excision will incur visible scars and the length of these is usually determined by the amount of skin excess. Trying to place these inconspicuously is a key factor in achieving a natural result and avoiding highlighting that breast surgery has been performed.[1-4]

REFERENCES

1. Rohrich RJ, Ha RY, Kenkel JM, Adams WP Jr. Classification and management of gynecomastia: defining the role of ultrasound-assisted liposuction. Plast Reconstr Surg 2003;111(2):909–923, discussion 924–925
2. Blau M, Hazani R. Correction of gynecomastia in body builders and patients with good physique. Plast Reconstr Surg 2015;135(2):425–432
3. Lista F, Ahmad J. Power-assisted liposuction and the pull-through technique for the treatment of gynecomastia. Plast Reconstr Surg 2008;121(3):740–747
4. Blugerman G, Schalvezon D, Mulholland RS, Soto JA, Siguen M. Gynecomastia treatment using radiofrequency-assisted liposuction (RFAL). Eur J Plast Surg 2013;36(4):231–236

125. Female Aesthetic Genital Plastic Surgery

See *Essentials of Plastic Surgery*, third edition, pp. 1762–1774

ANATOMY OF THE FEMALE EXTERNAL GENITALIA

1. *Which one of the following structures converges anteriorly on the ventral surface of the clitoris?*
   A. Labia majora
   B. Labia minora
   C. Vaginal vestibule
   D. Hymen
   E. Vestibular glands

ANATOMY OF THE FEMALE EXTERNAL GENITALIA

2. *Which one of the following is true regarding the anatomy of the female external genitalia?*
   A. All structures are supplied entirely by the internal pudendal artery.
   B. All structures are innervated entirely by the pudendal nerve.
   C. The clitoris is located within the vaginal vestibule.
   D. The labia majora lie medial to the labia minora.
   E. The urethral meatus lies dorsal to the clitoris.

PREOPERATIVE ASSESSMENT IN FEMALE GENITAL COSMETIC SURGERY

3. *Which one of the following must always form part of the examination for a patient considering genital aesthetic surgery?*
   A. Bimanual pelvic examination
   B. The presence of a female chaperone
   C. Assessment while the patient is standing and prone
   D. The use of a mirror to guide the examination
   E. Examination of the perineum and anus

INDICATIONS FOR FEMALE GENITAL COSMETIC SURGERY

4. The indications for female genital cosmetic surgery are categorized into four domains. *Which one of the following is NOT one of these domains?*
   A. Aesthetic
   B. Functional
   C. Psychosocial
   D. Sexual
   E. Reproductive

LABIAPLASTY

5. You review a 22-year-old woman in clinic with oversized labia minora. Examination shows significant bilateral soft-tissue excess and marked asymmetry. She experiences discomfort and chaffing and has researched the procedure thoroughly. She is interested in avoiding visible scarring and preserving the shape and color of the labia, including the border. *Which one of the following would best suit her requirements, while keeping the surgery minimally complex?*
   A. Edge excision labiaplasty
   B. Wedge resection labiaplasty
   C. W-plasty labiaplasty
   D. Z-plasty labiaplasty
   E. Central de-epithelialization labiaplasty

CLITORAL HOOD SURGERY

6. **When managing a patient with an excessively large clitoral hood, which one of the following is true?**
   A. The main indication for treating this is purely aesthetic.
   B. It would be adequately treated with a standard labiaplasty approach.
   C. It would be less evident following a standard labiaplasty
   D. Horizontal tissue excess is best managed with an inverted-V skin excision.
   E. Incisions are best kept superficial during surgical treatment.

LABIA MAJORA

7. A patient attends the office to discuss problems she is experiencing following surgery to the external genitalia at another hospital. She describes having had treatment to the labia majora and now her vaginal vestibule opens when she abducts her thighs. **What is the most likely explanation for this?**
   A. That skin excess has been removed without a Z-plasty being included.
   B. That lipomodeling has been performed with too much fat injected.
   C. That over-resection has been performed during labial reduction.
   D. That the scars for labial surgery have been placed incorrectly in the interlabial sulcus.
   E. That there has been abnormal scarring following this surgery.

VAGINOPLASTY

8. **What is the primary indication for performing a vaginoplasty procedure?**
   A. To tighten a lax vagina postpartum.
   B. To extend the length of the vagina following tumor extirpation.
   C. To recreate the vaginal vault following abdominoperineal (AP) resection.
   D. To increase the vaginal opening to facilitate sexual intercourse.
   E. To recreate a neovagina in a gender reassignment.

INDICATIONS FOR FEMALE GENITAL COSMETIC SURGERY

9. **Which one of the following procedures tends to be requested by patients based on their religious or ethical beliefs?**
   A. Labiaplasty
   B. Hymenoplasty
   C. Vaginoplasty
   D. Perineoplasty
   E. Monsplasty

SURGERY TO THE MONS PUBIS

10. A patient is seen in clinic with concerns about the appearance of her mons pubis. She has had an abdominoplasty at a nearby center and feels the mons has appeared droopy and full since this surgery. She also accepts she has put on weight since this was performed. **How best can this situation be managed?**
    A. Liposuction to the mons pubis
    B. Minimal access internal suspension sutures
    C. Revision abdominoplasty
    D. Formal monsplasty
    E. Skin excision to the mons via the abdominoplasty scar

VAGINISMUS

11. A patient is seen in clinic with a diagnosis of vaginismus. **Which one of the following is true regarding this condition?**
    A. It involves involuntary spasms and may be improved with neurotoxins.
    B. It is difficult to treat well even in a multidisciplinary setting.
    C. Surgery is generally indicated in more severe cases.
    D. Vaginal dilators have been shown to exacerbate this condition.
    E. The Lamont classification is based on the responses to treatment.

Answers

ANATOMY OF THE FEMALE EXTERNAL GENITALIA

1. *Which one of the following structures converges anteriorly on the ventral surface of the clitoris?*
   B. Labia minora

   The female external genitalia are also collectively termed the "vulva," which comprises the paired labia (two majora and two minora), the clitoris, the vaginal introitus, and urethral opening. It is in continuity with the mons pubis anteriorly, the perineum and anus posteriorly, and the medial thigh laterally **Fig. 125.1**.

   The paired labia minora are separated from the labia majora by the interlabial sulcus. They converge anteriorly on the ventral surface of the clitoral glans as the frenulum of the clitoris. The labia majora converge with the labia minora posterior to the vaginal vestibule to form the posterior fourchette. The clitoris comprises the glans (covered by the clitoral hood), the body, and the paired crura and vestibular bulbs. The suspensory ligament of the clitoris anchors the clitoral body to the pubic symphysis. The vaginal vestibule contains the urethral meatus (~2.5 cm ventral to the clitoral glans), the vaginal introitus (marked by the hymen), and the vestibular glands which provide lubrication of the vaginal vestibule.[1,2]

REFERENCES

1. Hamori CA. Aesthetic surgery of the female genitalia: labiaplasty and beyond. Plast Reconstr Surg 2014;134(4):661–673
2. Triana L, Robledo AM. Aesthetic surgery of female external genitalia. Aesthet Surg J 2015;35(2):165–177

ANATOMY OF THE FEMALE EXTERNAL GENITALIA

2. *Which one of the following is true regarding the anatomy of the female external genitalia?*
   E. The urethral meatus lies dorsal to the clitoris.

   Thorough knowledge of the anatomy of the female external genitalia is key to performing safe and effective surgery to this area. This is illustrated in **Fig. 125.1**. The urethral meatus is located in the vaginal vestibule along with the vaginal introitus and the vestibular glands which provide secretions to the vaginal vault. The clitoris and the clitoral hood lie ventral to the vaginal vestibule in the midline. The labia majora are located laterally next to the medial thigh and the minora are located medial to the majora at the edge of the vaginal opening, a part of which they form. The main arterial supply to the external female genitals is received from the internal

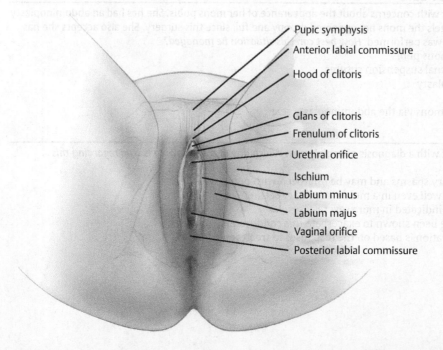

Pupic symphysis
Anterior labial commissure
Hood of clitoris
Glans of clitoris
Frenulum of clitoris
Urethral orifice
Ischium
Labium minus
Labium majus
Vaginal orifice
Posterior labial commissure

Fig. 125.1 Anatomy of the female external genitalia. (From Hamori C, Banwell C, Alinsod R. Female Cosmetic Genital Surgery. Thieme, 2017.)

pudendal artery and its branches, which is a branch of the internal iliac artery, but more laterally, the areas are supplied by the external pudendal artery, which is a branch of the femoral artery. The vulva is innervated by the anterior labial branches of the ilioinguinal and genitofemoral nerves as well as branches of the pudendal nerve. The pudendal nerve divides into three divisions near the ischial tuberosity to give the dorsal nerve of clitoris, perineal nerve (supplies the labia majora and perineum), and inferior rectal nerve (supplies the perianal area).[1-4]

REFERENCES

1. Hamori CA. Aesthetic surgery of the female genitalia: labiaplasty and beyond. Plast Reconstr Surg 2014;134(4):661–673
2. Triana L, Robledo AM. Aesthetic surgery of female external genitalia. Aesthet Surg J 2015;35(2):165–177
3. Georgiou CA, Benatar M, Dumas P, et al. A cadaveric study of the arterial blood supply of the labia minora. Plast Reconstr Surg 2015;136(1):167–178
4. Pauls RN. Anatomy of the clitoris and the female sexual response. Clin Anat 2015;28(3):376–384

PREOPERATIVE ASSESSMENT IN FEMALE GENITAL COSMETIC SURGERY

3. *Which one of the following must always form part of the examination for a patient considering genital aesthetic surgery?*
   B. The presence of a female chaperone
   Female genital cosmetic surgery is a highly sensitive and personal issue for many women and there needs to be a real emphasis on ensuring patients feel supported and safe during the consultation and examination process. It is vital for both the patient and clinician that a female chaperone is *always* present to ensure high standards of care are met. This approach protects both the patient and clinician and is a key component from a medicolegal perspective. The requirement for bimanual pelvic examination and examination of the perineum and anus will be dependent on the precise focus of the consultation and are not required in every case. The patient must be assessed supine in the frog-leg position, and, in some cases, also standing because this can highlight soft-tissue excesses and their appearance when gravity is acting upon them, for example, when labial or mons excess is a concern.
   The use of a mirror can be very helpful in a number of aesthetic surgery consultations, not just female genital surgery. However, it will not be required in every case, only those where it will help the dialogue and understanding between patient and physician.[1-4]

REFERENCES

1. Hamori CA. Aesthetic surgery of the female genitalia: labiaplasty and beyond. Plast Reconstr Surg 2014;134(4):661–673
2. Triana L, Robledo AM. Aesthetic surgery of female external genitalia. Aesthet Surg J 2015;35(2):165–177
3. Rogstad KE. Chaperones: protecting the patient or protecting the doctor? Sex Health 2007;4(2):85–87
4. Choudry U, Barta RJ, Kim N. Current trends in chaperone use by plastic and reconstructive surgeons. Ann Plast Surg 2013;70(6):709–713

INDICATIONS FOR FEMALE GENITAL COSMETIC SURGERY

4. The indications for female genital cosmetic surgery are categorized into four domains. *Which one of the following is NOT one of these domains?*
   E. Reproductive
   Motivation for women seeking female genital aesthetic surgery (FGCS) can be classified into four major domains. These **are aesthetic, functional** (e.g., pain, irritation), **psychosocial** (e.g., embarrassment, self-esteem issues, difficulty with relationships), and **sexual** (e.g., dyspareunia, laxity, lack of sensation). The primary indication for any FGCS procedure is any woman presenting with aesthetic or functional concerns regarding the vulva. Patients presenting with sexual or psychosocial concerns as a primary complaint may be FGCS candidates; however, caution should be taken preoperatively to clarify motivations and ensure these are appropriately addressed by a suitably qualified team.
   Negative genital self-image has been associated with lower sexual satisfaction; so, improvements in genital self-image can improve female sexual function.[1-4] That said, FGCS procedures should not be used in an attempt to solve patients' underlying relationship issues (e.g., save a relationship/marriage)[5] Furthermore, patients must never be coerced into any FGCS procedure; the decision must be a personal choice made of their own volition. Contraindications to FGCS include active or untreated pelvic infection or inflammatory process, pregnancy, pelvic malignancy, bleeding disorders, chronic pelvic pain, and unrealistic expectations. Reproductive problems are not generally associated with FGCS. These are associated with internal pathology.[6]

REFERENCES

1. Sharp G, Tiggemann M, Mattiske J. Factors that influence the decision to undergo labiaplasty: media, relationships, and psychological well-being. Aesthet Surg J 2016;36(4):469–478
2. Woertman L, van den Brink F. Body image and female sexual functioning and behavior: a review. J Sex Res 2012;49(2-3):184–211
3. Sharp G, Tiggemann M, Mattiske J. A retrospective study of the psychological outcomes of labiaplasty. Aesthet Surg J 2017;37(3):324–331
4. Goodman MP, Placik OJ, Matlock DL, et al. Evaluation of body image and sexual satisfaction in women undergoing female genital plastic/cosmetic surgery. Aesthet Surg J 2016;36(9):1048–1057
5. Schick VR, Calabrese SK, Rima BN, Zucker AN. Genital appearance dissatisfaction: implications for women's genital image self-consciousness, sexual esteem, sexual satisfaction, and sexual risk. Psychol Women Q 2010;34(3):394–404
6. Sharp G, Tiggemann M, Mattiske J. Psychological outcomes of labiaplasty. Plast Reconstr Surg 2016;138(6):1202–1209

LABIAPLASTY

5. **You review a 22-year-old woman in clinic with oversized labia minora. Examination shows significant bilateral soft-tissue excess and marked asymmetry. She experiences discomfort and chaffing and has researched the procedure thoroughly. She is interested in avoiding visible scarring and preserving the shape and color of the labia, including the border. *Which one of the following would best suit her requirements, while keeping the surgery minimally complex?***

   B. **Wedge resection labiaplasty**

   Labiaplasty involves reduction of the labia minora size and/or projection. This is usually performed for both functional and aesthetic reasons. For example, patients experience issues with discomfort, chafing, chronic irritation, and problems during sexual activity. They may also have issues with their appearance in and out of clothing.

   There are essentially four main techniques that can be utilized: wedge excision, free edge excision, central de-epithelialization, and W-plasty. There are no specific techniques based on Z-plasty. In this case, a wedge excision would suit her requirements best. This involves taking offset wedges from the inner and outer aspects of the minora. Usually, the skin/mucosal surface can be removed plus/minus some of the deeper tissues. Following resection, the wedge is closed so that scarring is well hidden medially in the introitus and laterally within the interlabial sulcus. The other advantage is that the wound edge scar between the upper and lower flaps is very small and the leading edge of the minora is preserved. This technique allows for symmetrization and large reductions as would be required in this case.

   With a free edge excision, the procedure is quicker to perform, but there will be scarring along the full leading edge of the minora. This technique does allow for fairly large reductions but may be less well suited to do so as a wedge and does risk over-resection, resulting in abnormal looking labia. The W-plasty is a variant of a wedge excision but is more complex and time consuming without a significant advantage. It may also be less well suited to large excisions and more challenging to achieve good symmetry. The central de-epithelialization approach is a technique that is useful to deproject the labia by de-epithelializing skin/mucosa from the medial and lateral labial surfaces with primary reapproximation of the edges. It is typically performed using a triangular or elliptical incision design. It also preserves the free border of the labia and preserves vascularity well but can be a little bulky due to the telescoping effect of deprojection.[1-5]

REFERENCES

1. Janis J, ed. Essentials of Aesthetic Surgery. 1st ed. Thieme; 2018
2. Oranges CM, Sisti A, Sisti G. Labia minora reduction techniques: a comprehensive literature review. Aesthet Surg J 2015;35(4):419–431
3. Lista F, Mistry BD, Singh Y, Ahmad J. The safety of aesthetic labiaplasty: a plastic surgery experience. Aesthet Surg J 2015;35(6):689–695
4. Ouar N, Guillier D, Moris V, Revol M, Francois C, Cristofari S. Postoperative complications of labia minora reduction. Comparative study between wedge and edge resection [in French]. Ann Chir Plast Esthet 2017;62(3):219–223
5. Alter GJ. A new technique for aesthetic labia minora reduction. Ann Plast Surg 1998;40(3):287–290

CLITORAL HOOD SURGERY

6. ***When managing a patient with an excessively large clitoral hood, which one of the following is true?***

   E. **Incisions are best kept superficial during surgical treatment.**

   Excess tissue of the clitoral hood can be quite bothersome, and women may complain of decreased sensitivity during sexual intercourse, and an inability to reach orgasm. They may also dislike the appearance, especially if it is perceived to look like a "small penis."

Incisions for clitoral hood reduction must be performed in a superficial plane to avoid injury to the clitoral glans and body. Furthermore, scars should not be placed on the clitoral hood itself to minimize the risk of scar hypersensitivity. Clitoral hood reduction is often performed at the same time as labiaplasty, as reduction of the labia minora can make the clitoral hood appear more prominent. However, it is not part of a standard labiaplasty approach. Clitoral hood excess may be present in the horizontal (more common) and/or vertical planes.

Horizontal excess is typically managed with a superficial skin excision placed in the sulcus between the labia majora and the clitoral hood. Vertical excess is typically managed with a superficial inverted-"V"–shape excision placed superior to the free-border of the clitoral hood. Clitoral hood reduction should be performed conservatively, and care must be taken to avoid permanent exposure of the clitoris, which can cause significant pain and hypersensitivity.[1-4]

REFERENCES

1. Triana L, Robledo AM. Aesthetic surgery of female external genitalia. Aesthet Surg J 2015;35(2):165–177
2. Hunter JG. Labia minora, labia majora, and clitoral hood alteration: experience-based recommendations. Aesthet Surg J 2016;36(1):71–79
3. Hamori CA. Postoperative clitoral hood deformity after labiaplasty. Aesthet Surg J 2013;33(7):1030–1036
4. Hamori C, Banwell P, Alinsod R, eds. Female Cosmetic Genital Surgery. 1st ed. Thieme; 2017

LABIA MAJORA

7. **A patient attends the office to discuss problems she is experiencing following surgery to the external genitalia at another hospital. She describes having had treatment to the labia majora and now her vaginal vestibule opens when she abducts her thighs. *What is the most likely explanation for this?***
   C. That over-resection has been performed during labial reduction.

Youthful appearing labia majora have a full, smooth contour and nearly approximate in the midline. Aesthetic concerns of the labia majora are typically related to either excessive fullness or deflation and ptosis. Excessive fullness can cause the labia majora to touch in the midline, creating a "closed clamshell" appearance in the standing position. Deflation/ptosis can cause the labia majora to appear or have redundant folds. When assessing the labia majora, it is important to examine the degree of skin excess and the amount of subcutaneous tissue present. Labia majora augmentation is appropriate for patients with mild skin excess and mild to moderate subcutaneous tissue atrophy. This would be achieved with either subcutaneous hyaluronic acid filler injection or autologous fat grafting, though soft-tissue flaps and dermal grafts have also been described.[1]

Labia majora reduction is appropriate for patients with either subcutaneous tissue excess alone, or moderate to severe skin excess. Mild subcutaneous tissue excess without skin excess can be treated with *liposuction* of the labia majora.[2] Moderate to severe skin or subcutaneous tissue excess can be treated with wedge resection of the labia majora. The incision for excisional labia majora reduction can be placed in the vulva-thigh crease, within the labia majora itself, or hidden in the interlabial sulcus (most common). Care must be taken to avoid over-resection of the labia majora, as this may result in opening of the vaginal vestibule with abduction of the thighs as has occurred in this case.

REFERENCES

1. Jabbour S, Kechichian E, Hersant B, et al. Labia majora augmentation: a systematic review of the literature. Aesthet Surg J 2017;37(10):1157–1164
2. Hunter JG. Labia minora, labia majora, and clitoral hood alteration: experience-based recommendations. Aesthet Surg J 2016;36(1):71–79

VAGINOPLASTY

8. *What is the primary indication for performing a vaginoplasty procedure?*
   A. To tighten a lax vagina postpartum.

Following pregnancy and vaginal childbirth, patients may experience vaginal laxity and pelvic floor weakness due to stretching of the tissues of the vagina and perineum with separation of the pelvic floor muscles. Patients subsequently experience problems with postpartum laxity leading to gaping of the perineum, difficulty maintaining tampon placement, decreased sexual satisfaction, and the potential for excessive vaginal secretions.

Vaginoplasty is a term that most commonly refers to a vaginal-tightening procedure. However, it is alternatively used more broadly to describe procedures on the vagina and could therefore be used less correctly to describe reconstruction or refinement of the vagina for a number of reasons. In the setting of vaginal tightening, the operation attempts to restore the damaged postpartum tissues of the vagina and perineum to their nulliparous state. While nonsurgical modalities have demonstrated some success in vaginal tightening, they tend to have more conservative improvements than a surgical procedure. At present, the long-term results of nonsurgical treatments such as radiofrequency stimulation or ablative laser are lacking. Vaginoplasty and perineoplasty share some common concepts but are distinctly different. Vaginoplasty refers to tightening of the vaginal canal above the level of the hymenal ring, where perineoplasty refers to tightening of the vaginal vestibule and perineum **below** the level of the hymenal ring. A perineoplasty is intended to restore perineal body length, correct gaping of the vaginal vestibule, and strengthen the pelvic floor by reapproximation of the superficial transverse perineal muscles. There are a number of different techniques used for vaginoplasty and the anterior, lateral, or posterior walls may be tightened. Particular care should be taken when performing posterior wall surgery, as this risks injury to the rectum where the levator ani muscles are repaired. Likewise, when performing anterior wall surgery, the bladder is at risk. If there are any concerns, this should ideally be performed with involvement of the gynecologist. Overall, vaginal tightening procedures have been associated with high patient and partner satisfaction outcome measures.[1,2]

REFERENCES

1. Furnas HJ, Canales FL. Vaginoplasty and perineoplasty. Plast Reconstr Surg Glob Open 2017;5(11):e1558
2. Qureshi AA, Tenenbaum MM, Myckatyn TM. Nonsurgical vulvovaginal rejuvenation with radiofrequency and laser devices: a literature review and comprehensive update for aesthetic surgeons. Aesthet Surg J 2018;38(3):302–311

INDICATIONS FOR FEMALE GENITAL COSMETIC SURGERY

9. *Which one of the following procedures tends to be requested by patients based on their religious or ethical beliefs?*
   A. Hymenoplasty
   The hymen is a thin, avascular membrane at the level of the vaginal introitus that separates the vaginal vestibule from the vaginal canal. There is significant variation in the native configuration of the hymen, with most common variants being "*annular*" and "*crescentic*" shapes. The hymen may be disrupted ("broken") for a number of reasons. These include trauma, vaginal tampon use, penetrative sexual intercourse, sexual assault, and medical interventions. Some cultures feel that an intact hymen confirms a girl's virginity. A hymenoplasty is a surgical procedure to restore the hymen back to its undisrupted form and is most commonly requested for ethnic/religious reasons in cultures where premarital virginity is highly valued. Bleeding during consummation of marriage is viewed as a sign of premarital chastity. Furthermore, premarital gynecological examination is required in some cultures to certify virginity. Because disruption of the hymen typically leaves remnants, known as carunculae myrtiformes ("caruncles"), these edges can be excised and repaired back together using absorbable sutures to restore integrity of the hymenal ring. Patients undergoing hymenoplasty should be warned that surgical restoration of the hymen cannot guarantee bleeding during first coitus. An adequate vaginal opening must be preserved (~1 cm) to allow for passage of vaginal secretions and menstrual fluids. The other procedures are requested based on functional and aesthetic grounds rather than religious beliefs.[1-3]

REFERENCES

1. Hamori C, Banwell P, Alinsod R, eds. Female Cosmetic Genital Surgery. 1st ed. Thieme; 2017
2. Vojvodic M, Lista F, Vastis P-G, Ahmad J. Luminal reduction hymenoplasty: a Canadian experience with hymen restoration. Aesthet Surg J 2018;38(7):802–806
3. Dobbeleir JM, Landuyt KV, Monstrey SJ. Aesthetic surgery of the female genitalia. Semin Plast Surg 2011;25(2):130–141

SURGERY TO THE MONS PUBIS

10. A patient is seen in clinic with concerns about the appearance of her mons pubis. She has had an abdominoplasty at a nearby center and feels the mons has appeared droopy and full since this surgery. She also accepts she has put on weight since this was performed. *How best can this situation be managed?*
    D. Formal monsplasty
    Deformities of the mons pubis are typically related to massive weight gain and/or loss. They can also become apparent following abdominoplasty where the mons has not been adequately treated. In this situation, the patient has put on weight since her original surgery which will compound the situation. In general terms, weight gain results in fat deposition in the mons and can lead to ptosis. Where significant weight loss occurs, the mons volume decreases leaving skin excess and further ptosis. Add into this an abdominoplasty, which treats the soft-tissue excess above the mons and creates a transverse scar that may tether to the underlying fascia. The result of this can, at the very least, make mons soft-tissue excess appear worse. A full monsplasty targets the three components which are problematic: fat excess, skin excess, and lack of internal support/ptosis. It involves removal of excess

skin, liposuction or direct excision of excess fat, and resuspension of the mons to the rectus fascia with long-acting or permanent sutures. Mild to moderate lipodystrophy without skin ptosis may be treated with liposuction alone. Skin excess alone may be treated with skin resection via the abdominoplasty scar. Internal suspension alone would be unsuccessful given the soft-tissue excesses. A revision abdominoplasty would only be indicated if there was residual soft-tissue excess above the scar or if there was a problem with contour or symmetry.[1,2]

REFERENCES

1. Alter GJ. Management of the mons pubis and labia majora in the massive weight loss patient. Aesthet Surg J 2009;29(5):432–442
2. Bykowski MR, Rubin JP, Gusenoff JA. The impact of abdominal contouring with monsplasty on sexual function and urogenital distress in women following massive weight loss. Aesthet Surg J 2017;37(1):63–70

VAGINISMUS

11. A patient is seen in clinic with a diagnosis of vaginismus. *Which one of the following is true regarding this condition?*

A. It involves involuntary spasms and may be improved with neurotoxins.

Vaginismus is a genitopelvic pain/penetration disorder characterized by involuntary spasm of the perineal muscles in addition to anxiety/fear with attempted vaginal penetration (e.g., sexual intercourse, tampon insertion, gynecologic examination, and childbirth). It has an incidence of 1 to 7% among women worldwide and unlike other pelvic pain disorders (e.g., vulvodynia, vestibulodynia), treatment for vaginismus is associated with a high success rate. One of the main treatment options is injection of neurotoxin into the muscles responsible for spasm. Other modalities include vaginal dilators, physical therapy with biofeedback, and psychological input with counseling. There is no surgical solution for vaginismus. Vaginismus is classified by the Lamont classification, which is based on the patient history and response to gynecologic examination:

Grade I: Tight vaginal muscles, can relax with coaxing to tolerate pelvic examination.
Grade II: Tight vaginal muscles, unable to relax but pelvic examination still possible.
Grade III: Patient elevates her buttocks to avoid examination.
Grade IV: Patient elevates buttocks, retracts, and adducts thighs to avoid examination.[1]

REFERENCE

1. Pacik PT, Geletta S. Vaginismus treatment: clinical trials follow up 241 patients. Sex Med 2017;5(2):e114–e123

126. Gender Affirmation Surgery

See *Essentials of Plastic Surgery*, third edition, pp. 1775–1796

DETERMINANTS OF FACIAL GENDER

1. *Which one of the following areas of the face and neck is said to represent the greatest determinant of facial gender?*
   A. Scalp
   B. Brow
   C. Ears
   D. Chin
   E. Cheeks

FACIAL FEMINIZATION SURGERY

2. *Which one of the following is true when considering facial feminization surgery for transfemale patients?*
   A. It is primarily aimed at reducing soft-tissue volume.
   B. The key surgical approaches all incur visible scarring.
   C. Prosthetic implant use may be indicated in the cheeks.
   D. Fat grafting is the mainstay of treatment in most cases.
   E. Standard rhinoplasty approaches are not generally useful.

MANAGEMENT OF THE NECK IN TRANSFEMALE PATIENTS

3. *A patient undergoing gender reassignment from male to female is unhappy with the appearance of the neck. When treating this area, which one of the following cartilage structures may be reduced to help this patient?*
   A. Cricoid cartilage
   B. Thyroid cartilage
   C. Arytenoid cartilage
   D. Tracheal cartilage
   E. Corniculate cartilages

PLANNING FACIAL FEMINIZATION SURGERY

4. *Which one of the following imaging modalities is preferred when considering feminizing facial surgery in a gender reassignment patient?*
   A. Computed tomography (CT)
   B. Magnetic resonance imaging (MRI)
   C. Plain radiograph
   D. Panorex radiograph
   E. Lateral cephalogram

FACIAL FEMINIZATION SURGERY

5. *You review a patient undergoing gender reassignment who wishes to feminize their forehead and brow. Which one of the following is true is this situation?*
   A. A minimally invasive (endoscopic) approach is most commonly utilized.
   B. Reduction of the bony excess is most often achieved with burring.
   C. Correction of a high hairline may be incorporated as part of the procedure.
   D. Frontal sinus repositioning is routinely required in almost every case.
   E. Forehead surgery should be performed separately from hair transplantation.

THE NORMAL MALE HAIRLINE

6. *How is the typical male hairline best described?*
   A. **A** shaped
   B. **C** shaped
   C. **Z** shaped
   D. **M** shaped
   E. **N** shaped

FACIAL MASCULINIZATION SURGERY

7. *Which one of the following is true regarding facial masculinization procedures?*
   A. Methyl methacrylate may be indicated to recontour the brow.
   B. Specialized rhinoplasty techniques are required to reshape the nose.
   C. Prosthetic implants are the preferred modality to recontour the chin.
   D. The pinna is the preferred cartilage source for reconstructing the Adam's apple.
   E. Fibula is the most commonly used donor site to augment the mandible.

INDICATIONS FOR BREAST SURGERY IN GENDER REASSIGNMENT

8. *When considering breast surgery in gender reassignment patients, which one is true according to the world professional association of transgender health?*
   A. The patient must have letters of support from at least three medical health professionals.
   B. The patient must be in a stable long-term relationship and ideally working.
   C. The patient must be over the age of 25 years at the time of surgery.
   D. The patient must have a persistent, well-documented history of gender dysphoria.
   E. The patient should have no documented history of mental health illness.

MALE-TO-FEMALE BREAST (TOP) SURGERY

9. *What is the first stage in reconstructing breasts for a transwoman patient?*
   A. Hormone therapy
   B. Staged fat grafting
   C. Placement of a tissue expander
   D. Placement of a permanent breast implant
   E. Performing a mastopexy procedure

BREAST SURGERY IN THE MALE-TO-FEMALE TRANSGENDER PATIENT

10. *When performing breast augmentation for a transgender patient, which one of the following is consistently true?*
   A. The implant should be placed centrally beneath the NAC.
   B. The implant should be placed as far medially as possible.
   C. The implant show be placed with its lower border at the inframammary fold.
   D. The implant should be placed in the submuscular plane.
   E. The implant should be placed through a periareolar incision.

BREAST SURGERY IN THE FEMALE-TO-MALE TRANSGENDER PATIENT

11. A patient is going through the transgender process from female to male and wishes to proceed with a mastectomy. They have large ptotic breasts with notch to nipple distances of **32 cm** and areola diameters of **6 cm**. *Which one of the following would be the most appropriate surgical approach for this patient?*
   A. Semicircular mastectomy preserving the NAC
   B. Transareolar mastectomy preserving the NAC
   C. Concentric circular mastectomy preserving the NAC
   D. Extended concentric mastectomy with free nipple grafts
   E. Double-incision mastectomy with free nipple grafts

TIMING OF TRANSGENDER SURGERY

12. *When patients are undergoing surgical procedures as part of their gender reaffirmation process, which area is normally targeted last?*
   A. Face
   B. Neck
   C. Chest
   D. Abdomen
   E. Genitals

GENITAL SURGERY FOR TRANSMALE PATIENTS

13. A 32-year-old patient is seen in clinic to discuss gender reaffirmation surgery. The patient has been living as a male for the past 5 years and wish to complete the process with genital surgery. The patient's main objective is to undergo single-stage surgery to create a neophallus and scrotum, and be able to micturate while standing. *Which one of the following procedures would best suit this patient?*
   A. Simple metoidioplasty
   B. Ring metoidioplasty
   C. Belgrade metoidioplasty
   D. Radial forearm phalloplasty
   E. Fibula flap phalloplasty

PHALLOPLASTY TECHNIQUES

14. A patient is interested in discussing phalloplasty as part of their transmale process. *Which one of the following techniques is most commonly used for this procedure?*
   A. Free radial forearm flap
   B. Free anterolateral thigh flap
   C. Pedicled anterolateral thigh flap
   D. Free fibula flap
   E. Free latissimus dorsi flap

PHALLOPLASTY

15. *What is the main advantage of performing a phalloplasty over a metoidioplasty in a transmale patient?*
   A. The number of procedures is reduced.
   B. Standing micturition may be possible.
   C. Penetrative sex may be possible.
   D. The ability to reach orgasm is more likely.
   E. A need for penile implants is avoided.

GENITAL (BOTTOM) SURGERY IN TRANSFEMALES

16. *Which one of the following approaches is most commonly used for transwomen to construct the neovagina?*
   A. Free radial forearm flap
   B. Penile and scrotal skin flap
   C. Pudendal artery flap
   D. Transverse colon
   E. Sigmoid colon

Answers

DETERMINANTS OF FACIAL GENDER

1. *Which one of the following areas of the face and neck is said to represent the greatest determinant of facial gender?*

    B. Brow

    The frontonasal–orbital complex includes the forehead, supraorbital ridge, orbit, frontomalar region, temporal ridges, and frontonasal transition. These areas collectively represent the greatest determinant of facial gender. The positions of the eyebrows and periorbital soft tissues including the eyelids are dictated by these areas. In males, they are typically more pronounced with greater bone volume and prominence. The brow tends to sit lower and flatter, the eyes are typically more deeply set, and the bony prominences are more marked.

    The scalp and hairline are also different in males and this can be most evident because of the hairline itself, which differs in shape and position. The ears tend to be larger in males than in females, but this is not consistently the case. The chin is more prominent in males due to greater volume in the mandible. Other differences include a longer upper lip in males, larger noses, squarer jaws, and facial hair growth.[1]

REFERENCE

1. Capitán L, Simon D, Kaye K, Tenorio T. Facial feminization surgery: the forehead. Surgical techniques and analysis of results. Plast Reconstr Surg 2014;134(4):609–619

FACIAL FEMINIZATION SURGERY

2. *Which one of the following is true when considering facial feminization surgery for transfemale patients?*

    C. Prosthetic implant use may be indicated in the cheeks.

    In general terms, the main focus of facial feminization surgery is to modify, reshape, and reduce bony structures such as the brow, periorbital area, nose, and jawline to soften masculine facial features. However, management of the cheeks is different. Fixed porous polyethylene implants may be used for augmentation of the cheeks as part of facial feminization surgery. This is because of gender differences in cheek fullness between males and females. Although males have greater malar bone volume, resulting in well-defined cheeks, females have a greater amount of fat in their cheeks and midface which gives them a more rounded appearance. Fixed porous polyethylene implants can be inserted using an intraoral approach which avoids any external scars. The results are generally stable over time. Alternatively, fat grafting may be performed and this should be deposited in a supraperiosteal plane. Injected fat does tend to partially resorb after injection so results may be less well maintained and repeat procedures are often required. While useful for some aspects, fat grafting does not represent the mainstay of treatment for facial feminization. There are differences between the male and female nose, with the male nose being larger and broader due to an increased volume of bone and cartilage. Therefore, standard rhinoplasty reduction techniques may successfully be applied.[1–3]

REFERENCES

1. Capitán L, Simon D, Kaye K, Tenorio T. Facial feminization surgery: the forehead. Surgical techniques and analysis of results. Plast Reconstr Surg 2014;134(4):609–619
2. Morrison SD, Vyas KS, Motakef S, et al. Facial feminization: systematic review of the literature. Plast Reconstr Surg 2016;137(6):1759–1770
3. Deschamps-Braly JC. Approach to feminization surgery and facial masculinization surgery: aesthetic goals and principles of management. J Craniofac Surg 2019;30(5):1352–1358

MANAGEMENT OF THE NECK IN TRANSFEMALE PATIENTS

3. A patient undergoing gender reassignment from male to female is unhappy with the appearance of the neck. *When treating this area, which one of the following cartilage structures may be reduced to help this patient?*

    B. Thyroid cartilage

    The thyroid cartilage is among the most prominent landmarks of male gender and is therefore something that is addressed during surgery when patients are transferring from male to female gender and vice versa. The primary function of the larynx is to protect the lower respiratory tract from aspirating food into the trachea while breathing. It also contains the vocal cords and functions as a voice box for phonation.

The thyroid cartilage is part of the laryngeal skeleton, which includes nine cartilages. These are the single thyroid, cricoid, and epiglottal cartilages, as well as the paired arytenoid, corniculate, and cuneiform cartilages.

The thyroid cartilage serves to protect the anterior part of the larynx and spans it vertically from top to bottom. It is the largest of all laryngeal cartilages and has the form of a half open book, with the back facing the front. Where the two halves meet in the middle, they form the protrusion which is best known as the "Adam's apple."

This most prominent portion of the thyroid cartilage can be modified during female feminization surgery. When such surgery is performed, the incision should be placed in the cervicomental fold in order to conceal the scar and prevent adhesions between the thyroid cartilage and the overlying soft tissues. This incision should be restricted to no more than 2 cm in length. The cartilage may be reduced with a combination of burring, rongeuring, or blade resection, depending on surgeon preference. Needless to say, sculpting close to the vocal cords must be avoided. When the reverse procedure is being performed, i.e., from female to male, the Adam's apple can be recreated with cartilage grafts.[1]

The cricoid cartilage is also known as the cricoid ring or signet ring, as it is the only cartilage to encircle the trachea completely. It sits in the inferior part of the larynx, at the level of C6 vertebra. The epiglottis is an elastic cartilaginous leaf-shaped flap covering the opening of the larynx. It is attached to the internal surface of the thyroid cartilage and projects over the pharynx, allowing the passage of air into the larynx, trachea, and lungs. As the hyoid bone rises, it draws the larynx upward during swallowing to allow food or drink into the esophagus, and to prevent food from entering the trachea. Arytenoid cartilages are a pair of small, hard but flexible pyramid-shaped cartilages that sit over the posterior portion of the cricoid cartilage. The vocal cords attach to them. The corniculate cartilages are small elastic cone-shaped cartilages that articulate with the apices of the arytenoid cartilages. The cuneiform cartilages are two elongated fibrous pieces of yellow cartilage that support the vocal folds and the lateral aspects of the epiglottis. None of these cartilages should be modified during facial feminization procedures, as this risks unacceptable and unnecessary risk for vocal cord damage and respiratory compromise.

REFERENCE

1. Deschamps-Braly JC, Sacher CL, Fick J, Ousterhout DK. First female-to-male facial confirmation surgery with description of a new procedure for masculinization of the thyroid cartilage (Adam's apple). Plast Reconstr Surg 2017;139(4):883e–887e

PLANNING FACIAL FEMINIZATION SURGERY

4. *Which one of the following imaging modalities is preferred when considering feminizing facial surgery in a gender reassignment patient?*
   A. Computed tomography
   Prior to undergoing facial feminization surgery, CT imaging including 3D reconstructions should ideally be obtained to assess anatomic features that can be addressed. In cases of financial restrictions, a panorex and lateral cephalogram will often provide adequate information, but remains a second choice. MRI scans are helpful to visualize the soft tissues of the head and neck region, but are more useful in oncologic and reconstructive cases rather than in the gender reaffirmation setting. Plain radiographic films generally add little to help planning treatment for facial feminization procedures.[1,2]

REFERENCES

1. Janis J. Essentials of Aesthetic Surgery. Thieme; 2018
2. Janis J. Essentials of Plastic Surgery. 3rd ed. Thieme; 2021

FACIAL FEMINIZATION SURGERY

5. *You review a patient undergoing gender reassignment who wishes to feminize their forehead and brow. Which one of the following is true is this situation?*
   C. Correction of a high hairline may be incorporated as part of the procedure.
   Forehead revision for transfemale patients modifies the frontonasal–orbital region to soften and feminize the patient's expression. The main goal is to reposition and remodel the forehead complex to soften frontal bossing, and to reduce the supraorbital rims, frontomalar buttresses, and temporal ridges. Forehead reshaping is usually performed with an open coronal approach rather than an endoscopic approach and takes two forms: anterior frontal wall sinus repositioning or frontal bone burring. The key factor which dictates which one of these will be used is the thickness of the outer table of the frontal bone. If the thickness of the anterior table is £3 mm, a frontal bone setback will be required rather than burring. In contrast, where there is more bone stock than this, burring alone may be acceptable.

In patients with a high hairline, simultaneous correction can be performed by placing the incision at the hairline and removing some excess skin anterior to this instead of using a coronal incision within the hairline. Brow reshaping may also be combined with hair transplantation in order to achieve upper third feminization in a single stage.[1,2]

REFERENCES

1. Capitán L, Simon D, Kaye K, Tenorio T. Facial feminization surgery: the forehead. Surgical techniques and analysis of results. Plast Reconstr Surg 2014;134(4):609–619
2. Capitán L, Simon D, Meyer T, et al. Facial feminization surgery: simultaneous hair transplant during forehead reconstruction. Plast Reconstr Surg 2017;139(3):573–584

THE NORMAL MALE HAIRLINE

6. How is the typical male hairline best described?

    D. M shaped

There are gender differences in the shape of the anterior hairline. Male patients tend to have an "**M**"-shaped hairline with this placed more anteriorly toward the midline and with more recession laterally in the temples (i.e., male pattern baldness). This may be exaggerated by androgenic alopecia. In contrast, females tend to have more rounded hairlines with implantation higher in the midline. Attention to the hairline can make a significant difference to a transmale or transfemale patient and this can be achieved with carefully placed hair transplantation. The primary goal for transfemale is to address the recessed corners of the hairline; the central section can also be addressed if hair density is also an issue. Two approaches include follicular unit strip and follicular unit extraction. In the former, follicles are obtained from a strip of scalp removed surgically, whereas in the latter, individual follicles are obtained nonsurgically. Any hair transplantation should ideally be performed after androgenic alopecia stabilizes.[1,2]

REFERENCES

1. Norwood OT. Male pattern baldness: classification and incidence. South Med J 1975;68(11):1359–1365
2. Nusbaum BP, Fuentefria S. Naturally occurring female hairline patterns. Dermatol Surg 2009;35(6):907–913

FACIAL MASCULINIZATION SURGERY

7. Which one of the following is true regarding facial masculinization procedures?

    A. Methyl methacrylate may be indicated to recontour the brow.

Facial masculinization surgery remains less common than facial feminization surgery and the procedures typically work in reverse to those used to feminize a face. To create a more masculine appearance to the brow, augmentation of the bony architecture is required. A coronal approach is undertaken to gain access to the brow area and methyl methacrylate can be applied directly to the forehead to build up the shape and contour. It is held in place temporarily with locking screws on each side and then contoured during the polymerization process. Management of the nose uses standard rhinoplasty and reconstructive techniques to alter the shape and size of the nose. Cartilage grafts are typically required to achieve this, and they may be harvested from the septum, pinna, or ribs.

The male chin is more prominent than the female chin in three dimensions: vertical height, width, and projection. Therefore, the most common way of addressing these three components is to perform segmental chin osteotomies using a sliding genioplasty. This is preferable to using implants or bone grafts where possible. In some cases, it is necessary to fill dead space created with hydroxyapatite granules to provide stability until subperiosteal calcification occurs. One of the key elements of a masculine neck is the presence of a visible and mobile "Adam's apple." To create this, a neck access incision is placed behind the submental crease and dissection is continued inferiorly beyond the thyroid cartilage. At this point, a deeper vertical incision is made between the strap muscles. A small piece of rib cartilage is used for the reconstruction and is placed over the thyroid cartilage and secured with permanent sutures. The cartilage is shaped into a narrow oblique pyramid with the base roughly three quarters of the width of the native thyroid cartilage. Fibula is commonly used to reconstruct the mandible following tumor resection, but not for gender reassignment.[1,2]

REFERENCES

1. Ousterhout DK. Dr. Paul Tessier and facial skeletal masculinization. Ann Plast Surg 2011;67(6):S10–S15
2. Deschamps-Braly JC, Sacher CL, Fick J, Ousterhout DK. First female-to-male facial confirmation surgery with description of a new procedure for masculinization of the thyroid cartilage (Adam's apple). Plast Reconstr Surg 2017;139(4):883e–887e

INDICATIONS FOR BREAST SURGERY IN GENDER REASSIGNMENT

8. *When considering breast surgery in gender reassignment patients, which one is true according to the world professional association of transgender health?*

    D. **The patient must have a persistent, well-documented history of gender dysphoria.**

    The World Professional Association for Transgender Health (WPATH) promotes a multidisciplinary approach for the care of transgender patients.[1] According to the WPATH, transgender patients should be under the care of primary care physicians, mental health services, endocrinologists, and surgical specialists. The WPATH have set guidelines for both top (breast) and bottom (genital) surgery and these differ slightly. These are as follows for top surgery:

    - A persistent, well-documented history of gender dysphoria
    - The capacity to make a fully informed decision and to give consent
    - Age of majority in a given country (not a specific age of 25)
    - If a prospective candidate for top surgery has a significant medical or mental health concern, it must be well controlled.
    - At least one letter from a qualified mental health professional recommending the patient to undergo the procedure is required.

    There is no requirement for the patient to be in a stable relationship or working.

    The guidelines for bottom (genital) surgery are as follows:

    - Two letters from the patient's mental health therapists recommending the patient for surgery.
    - The letters must include the duration of the patient–provider relationship, documentation of any associated diagnosis in addition to gender dysphoria, duration of time the patient has been living in their identified gender, a statement that the patient is mentally stable to undergo surgery, and a statement that the therapist is familiar with the WPATH Standards of Care (SOC) guidelines and that they recommend the patient to undergo surgery for transition.

REFERENCE

1. Coleman E, Bockting W, Botzer M, et al. Standards of care for the health of transsexual, transgender, and gender-non-conforming people, version 7. Int J Transgenderism 2012;13(4):165–232

MALE-TO-FEMALE BREAST (TOP) SURGERY

9. *What is the first stage in reconstructing breasts for a transwoman patient?*

    A. **Hormone therapy**

    The first step in reconstructing the breasts in a patient undergoing gender reassignment from male to female is to begin hormone therapy. There are obviously a number of more general systemic benefits for patients undergoing this treatment, but specifically for the breasts, it promotes mammogenesis, resulting in a softly pointed breast as seen in young girls or the small conical form found in young adolescents.

    Hormonal therapy can commonly provide an additional breast volume between half and one bra cup size of breast growth. Transwomen should undergo feminizing hormone therapy for a minimum of 1 year prior to breast augmentation surgery to maximize breast growth and obtain an optimal aesthetic result. Once they have reached this stage, their options will include prosthetic augmentation or fat transfer to add additional volume. They may require an adjunctive mastopexy to help reshape the breasts and address the nipple–areola complex (NAC) position, which may be too inferiorly or laterally placed. Breast expanders may be considered, to progressively expand tissues, although most patients tend to go straight to permanent implants.

    Fat grafting can be a good alternative to implants in patients with some breast volume from hormone treatment. It can provide a small to moderate augmentation of the breast, but patients need to be aware that variable amounts of the injected fat will be resorbed; so, they may require multiple grafting sessions to achieve the desired volume. Of course, fat grafting can also be used as an adjunct to augmentation to decrease implant visibility and help narrow a wide cleavage. Mastopexy can help correct the males NAC positioning and may help increase NAC diameter to some degree. It may be combined with fat grafting or implants, or may be performed as an isolated procedure in patients with higher body mass index.[1]

REFERENCE

1. Kanhai RC, Hage JJ, Karim RB, Mulder JW. Exceptional presenting conditions and outcome of augmentation mammaplasty in male-to-female transsexuals. Ann Plast Surg 1999;43(5):476–483

BREAST SURGERY IN THE MALE-TO-FEMALE TRANSGENDER PATIENT

10. *When performing breast augmentation for a transgender patient, which one of the following is consistently true?*

A. **The implant should be placed centrally beneath the NAC.**

Of all the surgical procedures performed in patients changing gender, breast surgery can be high on the priority list. As such, it can significantly facilitate their ability to live in a gender role congruent with their preferred gender identity. Prosthetic breast implants are therefore commonly desired by patients going from male to female gender to provide additional volume and feminize the chest.

Males tend to have wider chests with stronger pectoral fascia, more developed pectoralis muscles, and smaller NACs. It is key to ensure the NAC should always overlie the implant centrally, as an overly medial implant position can result in divergent nipple position. Unfortunately, even with large-volume wide implants, placed above pectoralis major, it is often not possible to avoid a wide cleavage between breasts, and the temptation to move them more medially to address this must be tempered.

Approaches to implant placement in this setting include the usual axillary, periareolar, and inframammary fold locations. The latter is usually preferred because it allows good access, with discrete scars, while the axillary approach limits the user to saline implants and the periareolar approach is limited by the small incision permitted. The implant should be placed lower than the preoperative inframammary fold because the inferior areolar margin and inframammary fold will expand after augmentation, much the same as when a large implant is placed in a slim female patient who has little breast tissue. This results in skin and subcutaneous tissue being recruited from the chest below the breasts. As with standard breast augmentation approaches, implants may be placed subglandular or submuscularly and decisions about placement will need to be made on an individualized patient basis. A subglandular placement is typically easier to perform, less painful, and has good aesthetic results in patients with more subcutaneous and glandular tissue. In contrast, subpectoral placement (or dual plane) provides more soft-tissue cover for implants and is necessary in thin patients.[1-3]

REFERENCES

1. Kanhai RC, Hage JJ, Karim RB, Mulder JW. Exceptional presenting conditions and outcome of augmentation mammaplasty in male-to-female transsexuals. Ann Plast Surg 1999;43(5):476–483
2. Coon D, Lee E, Fischer B, Darrach H, Landford WN. Breast augmentation in the transfemale patient: comprehensive principles for planning and obtaining ideal results. Plast Reconstr Surg 2020;145(6):1343–1353
3. Miller TJ, Wilson SC, Massie JP, Morrison SD, Satterwhite T. Breast augmentation in male-to-female transgender patients: technical considerations and outcomes. JPRAS Open 2019;21:63–74

BREAST SURGERY IN THE FEMALE-TO-MALE TRANSGENDER PATIENT

11. A patient is going through the transgender process from female to male and wishes to proceed with a mastectomy. They have large ptotic breasts with notch to nipple distances of 32 cm and areola diameters of 6 cm. *Which one of the following would be the most appropriate surgical approach for this patient?*

E. **Double-incision mastectomy with free nipple grafts**

Management of the breasts in female-to-male gender reassignment involves techniques similar to those used for gynecomastia in males and breast cancer treatment in females. The technique should be determined primarily by the amount of excess skin and skin elasticity rather than breast volume. The size and location of the NAC should also be considered. The most commonly performed procedure for transmale breast surgery is the double-incision mastectomy with free nipple grafts, and this would be indicated in this patient due to the characteristics of their breasts. The surface markings for this procedure are shown in **Fig. 126.1**.

The double-incision mastectomy with free nipple grafts is a versatile technique, as it allows skin reduction, volume reduction, and resizing and repositioning of the NAC. It also carries the lowest complication rate of all procedures. However, it does leave a long horizontal scar that passes close to the midline medially along the lower border of pectoralis major laterally. It also affects the appearance and sensitivity to the NAC and patients must understand this. It is optimal for cases such as this one where the breasts are large and ptotic with much skin excess.

The semicircular incision mastectomy is more like a gynecomastia technique and is ideal for patients with small breasts, but care must be taken to ensure sufficient glandular tissue is left under the NAC to prevent nipple depression. The scar is well-concealed, being confined to the edge of the lower half of the areola. However, this operation is technically challenging due to the small operative window. The transareolar approach is good for patients with small breasts and large prominent nipples, as it allows for immediate subtotal resection of the upper aspect of the nipple. It is the least commonly used technique, and carries the highest risk for complications. The scar traverses the areola horizontally and passes around the upper aspect of the nipple with optional extension medially and laterally. This technique is also technically challenging due to the small operative window. The concentric circular approach is recommended in patients with medium-size breasts with a good skin envelope or smaller breasts with poor skin elasticity. The concentric incision can be designed as a circle or an ellipse allowing for a precise amount of de-epithelialization to be performed (**Fig. 126.2**).

Access is made to the glandular tissue through the inferior aspect of the lateral incision. Because there is a dermal pedicle for the NAC, there is no need to leave excess glandular tissue beneath it. A permanent purse-string suture is used to set the desired areolar diameter.

The extended concentric approach involves triangular excision of skin and subcutaneous tissue medially and laterally. It can be undertaken with free nipple grafts to facilitate the resizing and repositioning of the NAC. It is a technique indicated for patients with larger breasts, e.g., C cup or above and with more significant ptosis.[1-3]

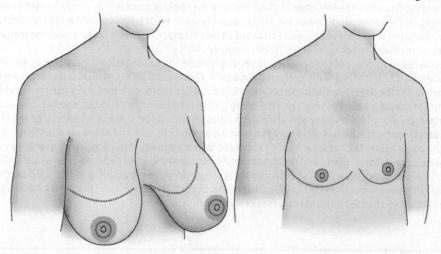

Fig. 126.1 Double-incision mastectomy with free nipple grafts showing surgical markings/incisions and final scar placement. Preoperative (left) and postoperative (right).

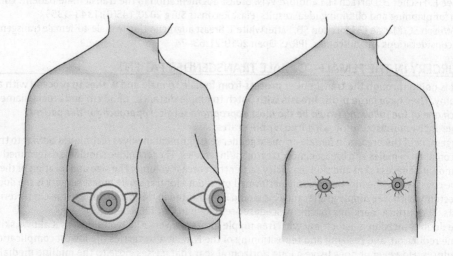

Fig. 126.2 Concentric circular technique for mastectomy in gender reassignment. Preoperative (left) and postoperative (right), incision/markings and scars shown.

REFERENCES

1. Monstrey S, Selvaggi G, Ceulemans P, et al. Chest-wall contouring surgery in female-to-male transsexuals: a new algorithm. Plast Reconstr Surg 2008;121(3):849–859
2. Hage JJ, Bloem JJ. Chest wall contouring for female-to-male transsexuals: Amsterdam experience. Ann Plast Surg 1995;34(1):59–66
3. Salgado CJ, Monstrey SJ, Djordjevic ML, eds. Gender Affirmation Medical and Surgical Perspectives. Stuttgart, Germany: Thieme Publishers; 2017

TIMING OF TRANSGENDER SURGERY

12. *When patients are undergoing surgical procedures as part of their gender reaffirmation process, which area is normally targeted last?*

E. Genitals

Gender reassignment surgery is normally the final surgical procedure in the surgical pathway for transgender patients. Prior to gender reassignment surgery, patients must complete WPATH SOC documentation which includes two letters from the patient's mental health therapists recommending the patient for surgery.

The letters must include the duration of the patient–provider relationship, documentation of any associated diagnosis in addition to gender dysphoria, duration of time the patient has been living in their identified gender, a statement that the patient is mentally stable to undergo surgery, and a statement that the therapist is familiar with the WPATH SOC guidelines and that they recommend the patient to undergo surgery for transition.

To reach the stage described earlier, patients need to have demonstrated their commitment and ability to live in their identified gender. Part of being able to do this effectively involves surgery to target the other areas which would otherwise give away their previous gender. This includes changes to the face and neck as well as the breasts and chest wall.[1]

REFERENCE

1. Coleman E, Bockting W, Botzer M, et al. Standards of care for the health of transsexual, transgender, and gender-non-conforming people, version 7. Int J Transgenderism 2012;13(4):165–232

GENITAL SURGERY FOR TRANSMALE PATIENTS

13. *A 32-year-old patient is seen in clinic to discuss gender reaffirmation surgery. The patient has been living as a male for the past 5 years and wish to complete the process with genital surgery. The patient's main objective is to undergo single-stage surgery to create a neophallus and scrotum, and be able to micturate while standing. Which one of the following procedures would best suit this patient?*

C. Belgrade metoidioplasty

Traditionally, genital or bottom surgery for transmen was relatively uncommon, as compared to genital or bottom surgery for transwomen and top or breast surgery for transmen, but this is probably becoming more common for a number of reasons including insurance coverage and patient awareness of the options available. Furthermore, the benefits of a metoidioplasty approach are now well documented and recognized.

In general terms, the main goals of female-to-male bottom surgery are threefold:

1. To make male appearing external genitalia
2. To facilitate standing micturition
3. To enable sexual activity ideally allowing both penetrative sexual intercourse and orgasm

A metoidioplasty is a surgical procedure that uses the hormonally enlarged clitoris to reconstruct a neophallus. The main advantages are the creation of an acceptable size and shape neophallus, while preserving erogenous sensation. This can also allow for standing micturition and the incorporation of other procedures such as vaginectomy, scrotoplasty, testicular implant placement, and hysterectomy with oophorectomy all within a single stage.

There are essentially three types of metoidioplasty performed: a simple variant, a ring variant, and the Belgrade variant. The Belgrade variant is based on the repair of the most severe forms of hypospadias and incorporates an advanced urethroplasty to achieve standing micturition for all patients. It also allows refashioning of the labia to create a scrotum which can receive implants at the same time. Belgrade metoidioplasty begins with removal of vaginal tissue except a small part around the urethral opening, which is used for urethral lengthening. The clitoris is degloved and lengthened by release of the suspensory ligaments and the urethral plate. Buccal grafts are used to line the lengthened urethra which are covered with labial flaps. The labia are also used to resurface the neophallus and create the new scrotum.

The other metoidioplasty techniques are more limited in what they achieve. A simple metoidioplasty also involves degloving and releasing the clitoris. However, the native urethral opening is left in place without urethral lengthening. Therefore, patients are unable to micturate while standing. One benefit of this technique is that the vagina may be left in situ if desired for penetrative intercourse and reproductive function can be maintained. A ring metoidioplasty involves additional dissection of the clitoris and elevation of a dorsal urethral ring flap from the vaginal introitus, which is used to extend the urethral plate. Some, but not all, patients will be able to micturate while standing following this procedure. The complication rate is higher than for the Belgrade approach. In contrast to metoidioplasty, phalloplasty is far more involved and has multiple stages to it. The main benefit is that penetrative intercourse may be possible once all stages are complete because the phallus size is more in keeping with a genetic male and rigidity may be achieved.[1,2]

REFERENCES

1. Djordjevic ML, Stojanovic B, Bizic M. Metoidioplasty: techniques and outcomes. Transl Androl Urol 2019;8(3):248–253
2. Djordjevic ML, Bizic M, Stanojevic D, et al. Urethral lengthening in metoidioplasty (female-to-male sex reassignment surgery) by combined buccal mucosa graft and labia minora flap. Urology 2009;74(2):349–353

PHALLOPLASTY TECHNIQUES

14. A patient is interested in discussing phalloplasty as part of their transmale process. *Which one of the following techniques is most commonly used for this procedure?*

   A. **Free radial forearm flap**

     Phalloplasty is a technique used to create a functional phallus while achieving the ability to micturate while standing and perform penetrative sex. It is usually the preferred approach for patients wishing to live fully as a male, although it is more involved and multifaceted than metoidioplasty. A range of different donor sites have been used for phalloplasty, including the anterolateral thigh, the latissimus dorsi, and the fibula. However, the radial forearm free flap (RFFF) remains the most frequently used surgical technique. It may be performed with a prelaminated urethra or using a tube within a tube technique.[1,2] The advantages of the radial forearm are that it provides thin, malleable, and sensate tissue with a long vascular pedicle. It can also subsequently accept a penile prosthesis to provide erection potential. The downside is the visible donor site even where scarring is optimal and of course microsurgical skills are required. Anterolateral thigh flaps can be useful alternatives in thin patients as can latissimus dorsi flap variants and both donor sites have the advantage over the RFFF of direct closure being possible and scars better hidden in clothing. Unfortunately, many patients' tissues at these donor sites will be too thick for these to work satisfactorily. The use of bone from either the radius or fibula has been used to provide rigidity to the neophallus; however, this is not popular due to high rates of bone resorption and donor-site morbidity. Instead, penile prostheses are normally used to provide stiffness.[2,3]

REFERENCES

1. Gottlieb LJ. Radial forearm. Clin Plast Surg 2018;45(3):391–398
2. Esmonde N, Bluebond-Langner R, Berli JU. Phalloplasty flap-related complication. Clin Plast Surg 2018;45(3):415–424
3. Garaffa G, Christopher NA, Ralph DJ. Total phallic reconstruction in female-to-male transsexuals. Eur Urol 2010;57(4):715–722

PHALLOPLASTY

15. *What is the main advantage of performing a phalloplasty over a metoidioplasty in a transmale patient?*

   C. **Penetrative sex may be possible.**

     The main advantage of performing a phalloplasty over a metoidioplasty is that greater penile size and stiffness are achieved, so the patient is more likely to be able to perform penetrative sexual intercourse. They should also more closely represent the appearance of a genetic male when unclothed. The main downsides to a phalloplasty are that multiple procedures are required and that patients are at high risk of urinary complications including urethrocutaneous fistulas and urinary strictures. Phalloplasty involves multiple components including creation of the shaft, the urethra, scrotoplasty, glansplasty, vaginectomy, and testicular and erectile implants. It also incurs a distant donor site. Standing micturition should be possible, but this is also possible with some metoidioplasty techniques. The ability to reach orgasm will be highly dependent on the patient's preoperative ability to do so. Furthermore, patients are commonly able to achieve this following metoidioplasty too. Erectile implants are not used for metoidioplasty but are normally required in phalloplasty patients to provide rigidity to the neophallus. Bone has been used as an alternative stiffener; however, integrating fibular and radial bone during phalloplasty has fallen out of favor due to high rates of bone resorption/erosion and donor-site morbidity.[1-4]

REFERENCES

1. Esmonde N, Bluebond-Langner R, Berli JU. Phalloplasty flap-related complication. Clin Plast Surg 2018;45(3):415–424
2. Garaffa G, Christopher NA, Ralph DJ. Total phallic reconstruction in female-to-male transsexuals. Eur Urol 2010; 57(4):715–722
3. Gottlieb LJ. Radial forearm. Clin Plast Surg 2018;45(3):391–398
4. Hu ZQ, Hyakusoku H, Gao JH, Aoki R, Ogawa R, Yan X. Penis reconstruction using three different operative methods. Br J Plast Surg 2005;58(4):487–492

GENITAL (BOTTOM) SURGERY IN TRANSFEMALES

16. *Which one of the following approaches is most commonly used for transwomen to construct the neovagina?*

   B. **Penile and scrotal skin flap**

   The use of penile and scrotal skin for creation of a neovagina remains the most commonly performed technique for transwomen undergoing genital (bottom) surgery. The advantages are that penile skin is robust, has a low tendency to contract, provides some sensibility inside the neovagina and where the penile shaft is hair free, and the neovagina will also be hairless. There is usually sufficient skin from the penis and scrotum to recreate the neofemale external genitalia including the internal vaginal vault and the external labia. The disadvantages include the risk of poor scarring, eventual shrinkage and contracture, a risk of insufficient vaginal cavity length, intravaginal hair growth in patients with penile hair growth, and the need for lubrication during intercourse. There will also be an ongoing need for regular dilation. The procedure begins with bilateral orchiectomy, and penile disassembly with dissection of the penile skin and glans, the urethra, corpus cavernosa, and the neurovascular bundle for the neoclitoris. The penile skin flap is used to create a tube, which is subsequently inverted and inset between the urethra, bladder, and rectum. Preservation of the subcutaneous tissue underlying the penile skin is essential for the formation of a long vascularized pedicle. A hole is made at the base of the pedicle, where the urethra and neoclitoris are passed through once the neovagina is inset. On the dorsal side of the skin tube flap, a superficial incision is made, leaving the subcutaneous layer intact; the urethral flap in then embedded along the tube and sutured in place. The distal end of the tube is closed prior to placement of the neovagina in the perineal space. The urethra is separated from the remaining dorsal tissue, and blood supply is maintained through preservation of the corpus spongiosum. Lining of the anterior neovagina is achieved with spatulation of the urethral flap. The clitoris is created from the remaining glans tissue. The remaining penile and scrotal skin is used to recreate the labia and clitoral hood. A tunnel is created in the perineal cavity between the urethra, bladder, and rectum and the neovagina is secured to the sacrospinous ligament to avoid prolapse of the urethral part of the vagina.[1]

   Colon vaginoplasty is an alternative to penile and scrotal skin use. The advantages are that vaginal depth may be better and the neovagina is self-lubricating. It is therefore indicated in patients in whom there is insufficient penile skin for penile inversion vaginoplasty and patients who have failed primary vaginoplasty and have insufficient vault depth or width due to stenosis or scar contracture. The sigmoid colon, not the transverse colon, is most commonly used. The main disadvantage is that it requires dual-specialty operating and risks potential problems with the bowel such as anastomotic leak, prolonged ileus, and adhesions. The radial forearm flap has many uses including phalloplasty, but is not normally used for the creation of a neovagina in this setting. The pudendal artery flap is a useful flap for vaginal reconstruction after tumor extirpation and can either be performed with unilateral or bilateral flaps. These are termed "Singapore flaps." They are not typically used for transgender neovagina reconstruction, as there are other tissues more readily available, although they could be used in principle if complications were present, and the vagina needed expansion.

REFERENCE

1. Salgado CJ, Monstrey SJ, Djordjevic ML, eds. Gender Affirmation Medical and Surgical Perspectives. Stuttgart, Germany: Thieme Publishers; 2017

127. Noninvasive Body Contouring

See *Essentials of Plastic Surgery*, third edition, pp. 1797–1803

NONINVASIVE BODY CONTOURING

1. *In general, what is the greatest challenge of using noninvasive body contouring treatments?*
   A. The high treatment cost
   B. The extended downtime
   C. The subtle effects of treatment
   D. The level of technical skills required
   E. The need for multiple treatments

NONINVASIVE TREATMENTS FOR FAT REDUCTION

2. *Which one of the following is true regarding noninvasive treatments for fat reduction and body contouring?*
   A. There are two main therapy types currently licensed for use.
   B. Their clinical effectiveness is somewhat inconsistent.
   C. Each treatment modality works by causing thermal changes to fat cells.
   D. Patient satisfaction following such treatments tends to be very high.
   E. Treatments represent an ideal alternative to traditional weight loss.

CRYOTHERMOLIPOLYSIS

3. *When undergoing cryolipolysis, which one of the following are patients most likely to experience?*
   A. Significant discomfort during treatment
   B. Significant discomfort after treatment
   C. Temporary erythema to the treated areas
   D. Decreased light touch sensitivity to the treated areas
   E. Temperature sensitivity to the treated areas

CRYOTHERMOLIPOLYSIS

4. *When considering the evidence base underpinning cryolipolysis, which one of the following is true?*
   A. The precise mechanism of action is well understood.
   B. Initial animal studies were ineffective at reducing fat volume.
   C. Initial clinical studies were ineffective at reducing fat volume.
   D. A systematic review has shown fat reduction as high as 28%.
   E. Evidence has shown that multiple treatments are required.

HIGH-INTENSITY FOCUSED ULTRASOUND FOR FAT REDUCTION

5. A patient is planning to undergo HIFU treatment to reduce excess abdominal fat. *Which one of the following represents the proposed mechanism of action for this treatment modality?*
   A. Coagulative necrosis
   B. Apoptosis
   C. Cold-induced thermogenesis
   D. Nonthermal cellular injury
   E. Mechanical emptying of fat cells

HIGH-INTENSITY FOCUSED ULTRASOUND FOR FAT REDUCTION

6. A female patient makes contact with your office to find out more about HIFU to address trunk fat excess. *Which one of the following should you tell her?*
   A. There is currently no strong evidence to support its use.
   B. The ideal candidate has a body mass index (BMI) of 30 to 35.
   C. It is not indicated for use on the trunk.
   D. Treatment usually takes around 90 minutes to perform.
   E. Results are not usually observed until 2 to 3 months.

LOW-LEVEL LASER THERAPY FOR FAT REDUCTION

7. *Which one of the following should you advise a female patient who is considering LLLT for targeted fat treatment?*
   A. She should expect a localized mild warming sensation during treatment.
   B. She should expect erythema that persists for up to a month after treatment.
   C. That following treatment, dressings will be applied for 2 weeks.
   D. Pain control will require opiate medication for 48 hours after treatment.
   E. That six consecutive monthly treatments will most likely be required.

LOW-LEVEL LASER THERAPY FOR FAT REDUCTION

8. You see a patient in the office who has recently undergone fat treatment to the abdomen with LLLT at a local aesthetic center. The patient is usually in good health, but now has areas of skin ulceration at the treatment sites. *Which one of the following would be most likely to explain this?*
   A. Poor patient selection
   B. Treatment at a setting too high
   C. Treatment continued for longer than advised
   D. Incorrect positioning of the laser diode panel
   E. Failure to adequately dress the wound posttreatment

PARADOXICAL ADIPOSE HYPERPLASIA

9. *Which one of the following is optimal to treat a patient with paradoxical adipose tissue hyperplasia to the abdomen?*
   A. Cryolipolysis
   B. HIFU
   C. LLLT
   D. Liposuction
   E. No treatment is usually required

CONTRAINDICATIONS TO NONINVASIVE BODY CONTOURING

10. *Which one of the following is a contraindication to all of the main noninvasive fat therapies?*
    A. Patients with cold urticaria
    B. Patients with mild skin laxity
    C. Patients older than 55 years
    D. Patients who are pregnant
    E. Patients who are fit for liposuction

Answers

NONINVASIVE BODY CONTOURING

1. *In general, what is the greatest challenge of using noninvasive body contouring treatments?*
   E. **The need for multiple treatments**
   Interest in noninvasive body contouring is growing due to the fact that it is effective, affordable, has a short downtime, and is easy to perform. In the United states, in almost three quarters of a million such treatments were delivered during 2018.[1] The main caveat is that multiple treatments are often required. The requirement for timing and number of treatments differs according to the specific treatment modality and the desired effects. It is important to ensure patients understand the limitations of these treatments and that they may well need repeating.

REFERENCE

1. American Society of Plastic Surgeons. National Clearinghouse of Plastic Surgery Statistics: 2019 Report of the 2018 Statistics. Arlington Heights, IL: American Society of Plastic Surgeons; 2019

NONINVASIVE TREATMENTS FOR FAT REDUCTION

2. *Which one of the following is true regarding noninvasive treatments for fat reduction and body contouring?*
   D. **Patient satisfaction following such treatments tends to be very high.**
   Noninvasive treatments for fat reduction have been shown to be effective and are associated with high rates of patient satisfaction. There are three (not two) main types of noninvasive treatment for fat reduction: cryolipolysis, high-intensity focused ultrasound (HIFU), and low-level laser therapy (LLLT). Each has a different mechanism of action and their own individual nuances. Only high-intensity ultrasound works by heating the fat cells to cause damage to them. Noninvasive treatments may be a reasonable alternative to surgical interventions such as liposuction, but they do not represent alternatives to weight loss, which should be encouraged in overweight patients.[1,2]

REFERENCES

1. Krueger N, Mai SV, Luebbberding S, Sadick NS. Cryolipolysis for noninvasive body contouring: clinical efficacy and patient satisfaction. Clin Cosmet Investig Dermatol 2014;7(7):201–205
2. Dierickx CC, Mazer JM, Sand M, Koenig S, Arigon V. Safety, tolerance, and patient satisfaction with noninvasive cryolipolysis. Dermatol Surg 2013;39(8):1209–1216

CRYOTHERMOLIPOLYSIS

3. *When undergoing cryolipolysis, which one of the following are patients most likely to experience?*
   C. **Temporary erythema to the treated areas**
   Cryolipolysis is a treatment used to reduce fat cells in localized areas of adipose tissue such as the flanks, thighs, abdomen, and neck. The technique involves first marking the areas for treatment and then applying conduction gel to these areas. A cooling applicator is then attached to the skin with a mild vacuum device that has either one or two panels. Tissue is drawn into the cooling panel and treatment is delivered for 30 to 60 minutes. Patients need to understand the process in advance of the treatment and the symptoms they will experience. Erythema posttreatment with cryolipolysis is a very consistent finding and patients must be aware of this. It resolves spontaneously over 7 days. Many patients are likely to also experience minor discomfort during treatment and then go on to experience 2 to 3 days of edema to the treated areas. The pain they experience is usually well controlled with simple topical and oral analgesics. In addition, patients often experience decreased light touch sensitivity and temperature sensitivity to the treated areas after treatment. This completely resolves spontaneously within 8 weeks of treatment. Patients should also understand the potential for undercorrection or overcorrection of fat areas, possible contour irregularities, and undesirable overlying skin changes. As with many interventions, there is no guarantee of a specific aesthetic outcome.[1-3]

REFERENCES

1. Manstein D, Laubach H, Watanabe K, Farinelli W, Zurakowski D, Anderson RR. Selective cryolysis: a novel method of non-invasive fat removal. Lasers Surg Med 2008;40(9):595–604

2. Coleman SR, Sachdeva K, Egbert BM, Preciado J, Allison J. Clinical efficacy of noninvasive cryolipolysis and its effects on peripheral nerves. Aesthetic Plast Surg 2009;33(4):482–488
3. Karcher C, Katz B, Sadick N. Paradoxical hyperplasia post-cryolipolysis and management. Dermatol Surg 2017;43(3):467–470

CRYOTHERMOLIPOLYSIS

4. When considering the evidence base underpinning cryolipolysis, which one of the following is true?

    D. **A systematic review has shown fat reduction as high as 28%.**

Cryolipolysis is a noninvasive treatment used to reduce fat volumes in specific body areas such as the arms, bra line, back, abdomen, flank, banana roll, and thighs. There is a large volume of evidence to support its use. For example, a systematic review of cryolipolysis treatment in 2015 showed average reductions in caliper measurement of subcutaneous tissues as high as 28.5% (range: 14.7–28.5%).[1] This evidence supports the clinical effectiveness of this treatment. Another study reviewed results in 53 patients in whom a single cryolipolysis treatment was delivered to the saddlebags. At 6 months posttreatment, mean thigh circumference had decreased 5.6 cm and the mean decrease in fat layer thickness measured by ultrasound was 1.3 cm. Patient satisfaction was also high (94% satisfaction rate).[2] The precise mechanism of action by which cryolipolysis works is not well understood; however, it is theorized to be related to apoptosis-mediated cell death and subsequent inflammatory response or through cold-induced thermogenesis.[3,4] Preclinical animal studies showed a 33% reduction in thickness of the superficial fat layer with maximal relative loss of nearly 80% with a single treatment.[3] Although it is generally accepted that multiple treatments are required with noninvasive body contouring techniques, these data show that with cryolipolysis, single-treatment delivery can achieve beneficial effects.

REFERENCES

1. Ingargiola MJ, Motakef S, Chung MT, Vasconez HC, Sasaki GH. Cryolipolysis for fat reduction and body contouring: safety and efficacy of current treatment paradigms. Plast Reconstr Surg 2015;135(6):1581–1590
2. Adjadj L, SidAhmed-Mezi M, Mondoloni M, Meningaud JP, Hersant B. Assessment of the efficacy of cryolipolysis on saddlebags: a prospective study of 53 patients. Plast Reconstr Surg 2017;140(1):50–57
3. Zelickson B, Egbert BM, Preciado J, et al. Cryolipolysis for noninvasive fat cell destruction: initial results from a pig model. Dermatol Surg 2009;35(10):1462–1470
4. Loap S, Lathe R. Mechanism underlying tissue cryotherapy to combat obesity/overweight: triggering thermogenesis. J Obes 2018 (epub ahead of print) doi: 10.1155/2018/5789647

HIGH-INTENSITY FOCUSED ULTRASOUND FOR FAT REDUCTION

5. A patient is planning to undergo HIFU treatment to reduce excess abdominal fat. Which one of the following represents the proposed mechanism of action for this treatment modality?

    A. **Coagulative necrosis**

HIFU is a noninvasive treatment used to reduce fat in specific body areas. It uses focused energy to thermally ablate subcutaneous adipose tissue and to induce neocollagenesis. HIFU increases the local temperature within the mid-lamellar fat layer leading to coagulative necrosis of adipocytes and subsequent reduction of fat layer.[1]

Apoptosis is programmed cell death and is believed to be one potential mechanism of action for cryolipolysis, a treatment that cools the subcutaneous tissues. The other proposed mechanism for cryolipolysis is cold-induced thermogenesis. Low-level laser energy (LLLT) is a nonthermal approach to fat reduction and the proposed mechanism of action is the induction of a transitory pore into an adipocyte resulting in release of lipids and adipocyte deflation.

REFERENCE

1. Fatemi A. High-intensity focused ultrasound effectively reduces adipose tissue. Semin Cutan Med Surg 2009;28(4):257–262

HIGH-INTENSITY FOCUSED ULTRASOUND FOR FAT REDUCTION

6. A female patient makes contact with your office to find out more about HIFU to address trunk fat excess. Which one of the following should you tell her?

    E. **Results are not usually observed until 2 to 3 months.**

HIFU is a noninvasive treatment used to reduce fat in specific body areas. It is indicated for waist circumference reduction and the ideal candidate is someone with a body mass index less than 30 and more than 2.5 cm of tissue on caliper pinch. There is a reasonable body of evidence to support its use. Two case series have been reported of 282 and 85 patients treated with HIFU to the abdomen and flank resulting in an average waist circumference decrease of 4.4 and 4.7 cm, respectively.[1,2] A multicenter, randomized, sham-controlled, single-blinded trial of 180 patients studying HIFU in trunk aesthetics showed a decrease of 2.5 cm in the treatment group (single treatment) compared with 1.2 cm in the sham group.[3] A multicenter, randomized, nonblinded study of 118 patients treated with a single HIFU treatment to the abdomen resulted in a decrease of 2.3 cm in waist circumference.[4]

The results are typically seen between 8 and 12 weeks posttreatment, so it is important to convey this information to patients prior to treatment to help set realistic expectations.

The actual treatment involves marking the areas with the patient standing, followed by treatment delivery with the patient supine. Topical anesthetic is applied to the treatment areas. Multiple passes are made with the HIFU transducer to deliver the appropriate amount of energy, with the treatment usually being completed in less than an hour.

REFERENCES

1. Fatemi A. High-intensity focused ultrasound effectively reduces adipose tissue. Semin Cutan Med Surg 2009;28(4): 257–262
2. Fatemi A, Kane MA. High-intensity focused ultrasound effectively reduces waist circumference by ablating adipose tissue from the abdomen and flanks: a retrospective case series. Aesthetic Plast Surg 2010;34(5):577–582
3. Jewell ML, Baxter RA, Cox SE, et al. Randomized sham-controlled trial to evaluate the safety and effectiveness of a high-intensity focused ultrasound device for noninvasive body sculpting. Plast Reconstr Surg 2011;128(1):253–262
4. Robinson DM, Kaminer MS, Baumann L, et al. High-intensity focused ultrasound for the reduction of subcutaneous adipose tissue using multiple treatment techniques. Dermatol Surg 2014;40(6):641–651

LOW-LEVEL LASER THERAPY FOR FAT REDUCTION

7. *Which one of the following should you advise a female patient who is considering LLLT for targeted fat treatment?*
   A. She should expect a localized mild warming sensation during treatment.

   LLLT is a noninvasive, nonthermal approach to fat reduction performed with a laser wavelength of 635 nm. The proposed mechanism is mechanical disruption of the adipocyte leading to adipocyte deflation. Treatment involves transdermal delivery of the 635-nm laser which can cause a warming sensation during the procedure. Posttreatment erythema does occur but resolves within 24 hours. No dressings are required following this treatment. Multiple treatments will be required, but these are more frequent than monthly. Studies have reported outcomes after six treatments over 2 weeks or six consecutive weekly treatments. with good results.[1-3] LLLT is not a particularly painful procedure, so opiate medications are not required. More simple oral and topical analgesia should suffice. Moreover, opiate analgesics should be avoided where possible due to their addictive nature.

REFERENCES

1. Jackson RF, Stern FA, Neira R, Ortiz-Neira CL, Maloney J. Application of low-level laser therapy for noninvasive body contouring. Lasers Surg Med 2012;44(3):211–217
2. Nestor MS, Zarraga MB, Park H. Effect of 635 nm low-level laser therapy on upper arm circumference reduction. J Clin Aesthet Dermatol 2012;5(2):42–48
3. Thornfeldt CR, Thaxton PM, Hornfeldt CS. A six-week low-level laser therapy protocol is effective for reducing waist, hip, thigh, and upper abdomen circumference. J Clin Aesthet Dermatol 2016;9(6):31–35

LOW-LEVEL LASER THERAPY FOR FAT REDUCTION

8. You see a patient in the office who has recently undergone fat treatment to the abdomen with LLLT at a local aesthetic center. The patient is usually in good health, but now has areas of skin ulceration at the treatment sites. *Which one of the following would be most likely to explain this?*
   D. Incorrect positioning of the laser diode panel

   LLLT is indicated for circumference reduction of the upper arms, waist, hips, and thighs secondary to localized fat deposits. It involves the application of a laser device at 635 nm to target the subcutaneous tissues. The patient is marked standing then placed supine on the treatment table, exposing the area or areas to be treated. Laser diode modules are suspended ~15 cm above the anterior and then the posterior aspect of the treatment area and transdermal delivery of the 635 nm laser can commence. Specific distances, wattage, wavelength, and delivery duration vary depending on the device used. Complications are rare when the laser diode panel is appropriately placed; however, when it is applied directly to the skin, persistent erythema and skin ulceration may occur.[1] This technical error is most likely to have occurred in this case and should be managed according to the principles of good wound care combined with an open and honest discussion with the patient.

   Patient selection is unlikely to be a cause of this problem unless they have a specific skin disorder. Contraindications otherwise are pregnancy, cancer, and large volume weight loss in obese patients. Too lengthy a treatment is also unlikely to cause this if the diode is correctly placed. No dressings are normally required after treatment, although they may be applied for patient comfort if desired.

REFERENCE

1. Jankowski M, Gawrych M, Adamska U, Ciescinski J, Serafin Z, Czajkowski R. Low-level laser therapy (LLLT) does not reduce subcutaneous adipose tissue by local adipocyte injury but rather by modulation of systemic lipid metabolism. Lasers Med Sci 2017;32(2):475–479

PARADOXICAL ADIPOSE HYPERPLASIA

9. *Which one of the following is optimal to treat a patient with paradoxical adipose tissue hyperplasia to the abdomen?*

   D. Liposuction

   Paradoxical adipose hyperplasia (PAH) is a condition where instead of reducing fat by performing noninvasive fat reduction, a process of hyperplasia ensures, leading to an increase in tissue firmness and fullness. PAH is specifically associated with cryolipolysis and has an incidence of just less than 1%.[1,2] When it does occur, it is unlikely to resolve spontaneously, and patients require an additional procedure to correct this. The primary treatment modality would be liposuction, although excisional surgery such as an abdominoplasty may also be considered. The main challenges of managing patients with PAH therefore are not only that they are in a worse position than when they started and will need some further surgical intervention, but they must also wait a number of months for the tissues to soften before any revision treatment can be undertaken. This would normally be at 6 to 9 months. The risk factors for developing PAH include male gender, Hispanic ethnicity, use of a large hand piece, and genetic predisposition.[1–3]

REFERENCES

1. Karcher C, Katz B, Sadick N. Paradoxical hyperplasia post-cryolipolysis and management. Dermatol Surg 2017;43(3):467–470
2. Kelly E, Rodriguez-Feliz J, Kelly ME. Paradoxical adipose hyperplasia after cryolipolysis: a report on incidence and common factors identified in 510 patients. Plast Reconstr Surg 2016;137(3):639e–640e
3. Stroumza N, Gauthier N, Senet P, Moguelet P, Nail Barthelemy R, Atlan M. Paradoxical adipose hypertrophy (PAH) after cryolipolysis. Aesthet Surg J 2018;38(4):411–417

CONTRAINDICATIONS TO NONINVASIVE BODY CONTOURING

10. *Which one of the following is a contraindication to all of the main noninvasive fat therapies?*

    D. Patients who are pregnant

    There are a number of contraindications to using noninvasive body contouring techniques. Pregnancy is a contraindication across the board for all treatments. Cold urticarial is a contraindication specific to cryolipolysis. Mild skin laxity is not a contraindication to treatment, as a mild skin tightening effect can often be seen as a secondary benefit of these procedures. However, greater amounts of skin laxity are a contraindication to noninvasive treatments because the skin will not retract well following the procedure, leading to a compromised aesthetic result. Age is not a contraindication to any of the treatment modalities for noninvasive fat reduction. Liposuction is a useful surgical intervention for managing specific fat deposits, but it should not always be the first-line choice for every patient. Even if a patient is healthy enough and agreeable to undergo liposuction, if they may benefit from a noninvasive approach this should be considered first.[1–3]

REFERENCES

1. Ingargiola MJ, Motakef S, Chung MT, Vasconez HC, Sasaki GH. Cryolipolysis for fat reduction and body contouring: safety and efficacy of current treatment paradigms. Plast Reconstr Surg 2015;135(6):1581–1590
2. Manstein D, Laubach H, Watanabe K, Farinelli W, Zurakowski D, Anderson RR. Selective cryolysis: a novel method of non-invasive fat removal. Lasers Surg Med 2008;40(9):595–604
3. Alizadeh Z, Halabchi F, Mazaheri R, Abolhasani M, Tabesh M. Review of the mechanisms and effects of noninvasive body contouring devices on cellulite and subcutaneous fat. Int J Endocrinol Metab 2016;14(4):e36727

Index